Computed Body Tomography with MRI Correlation

FOURTH EDITION

VOLUME 2

Computed Body Tomography with MRI Correlation

FOURTH EDITION

VOLUME 2

EDITORS

■ JOSEPH K. T. LEE, MD

E. H. Wood Distinguished Professor and Chair
Department of Radiology
University of North Carolina School of Medicine
Chapel Hill, North Carolina

■ STUART S. SAGEL, MD

Professor of Radiology
Director, Chest Radiology Section
Mallinckrodt Institute of Radiology
Washington University School of Medicine
St. Louis, Missouri

■ ROBERT J. STANLEY, MD, MSHA

Editor-in-Chief
American Journal of Roentgenology
Professor and Chair Emeritus, Department of Radiology
University of Alabama at Birmingham
Birmingham, Alabama

■ JAY P. HEIKEN, MD

Professor of Radiology
Director, Abdominal Imaging Section
Mallinckrodt Institute of Radiology
Washington University School of Medicine
St. Louis, Missouri

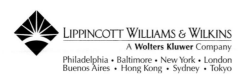
LIPPINCOTT WILLIAMS & WILKINS
A **Wolters Kluwer** Company
Philadelphia • Baltimore • New York • London
Buenos Aires • Hong Kong • Sydney • Tokyo

Acquisitions Editor: Lisa McAllister
Managing Editor: Kerry Barrett
Project Manager: Fran Gunning
Manufacturing Manager: Ben Rivera
Marketing Manager: Angela Panetta
Design Coordinator: Teresa Mallon
Production Services: Nesbitt Graphics, Inc.
Printer: Maple Press

© 2006 by LIPPINCOTT WILLIAMS & WILKINS

530 Walnut Street
Philadelphia, PA 19106 USA
LWW.com

Printed in the USA

Library of Congress Cataloging-in-Publication Data

Computed body tomography with MRI correlation / editors, Joseph K.T. Lee, Stuart S. Sagel.— 4th ed.
   p. ; cm.
 Includes bibliographical references and index.
 ISBN 0-7817-4526-8
 1. Tomography. 2. Magnetic resonance imaging. I. Lee, Joseph K. T. II. Sagel, Stuart S., 1940- . III. Title.
 [DNLM: 1. Tomography, X-Ray Computed. 2. Magnetic Resonance Imaging. WN 206 C7378 2005]
RC78.7.T6C6416 2005
616.07'57—dc22
                        2005029421

9 8 7 6 5 4 3 2 1

To our wives,
Christina, Beverlee, Sally, and Fran

To our children,
Alexander, Betsy, and Catherine; Scott, Darryl, and Brett;
Ann, Robert, Catherine, and Sara; and Lauren

And to our grandchildren

Contents

Contributing Authors

Kyongtae T. Bae, MD, PhD   Associate Professor of Radiology, Mallinckrodt Institute of Radiology, Washington University School of Medicine, St. Louis, Missouri

Dennis M. Balfe, MD   Professor of Radiology, Department of Diagnostic Radiology, Washington University School of Medicine, St. Louis, Missouri

Sanjeev Bhalla, MD   Assistant Professor of Radiology, Co-Chief, CT and Emergency Radiology, Mallinckrodt Institute of Radiology, Washington University School of Medicine, St. Louis, Missouri

Edward W. Bouchard, MD   Radiology Resident, University of North Carolina School of Medicine, Chapel Hill, North Carolina

Mark A. Brown, PhD   Senior Technical Instructor, Siemens Training and Development Center, Cary, North Carolina

Charles T. Burke, MD   Assistant Professor of Radiology, University of North Carolina School of Medicine, Chapel Hill, North Carolina

Cheri L. Canon, MD   Associate Professor, Vice Chair for Education, Department of Radiology, University of Alabama at Birmingham; Chief, Gastrointestinal Radiology, Department of Radiology, UAB Health System, Birmingham, Alabama

Mauricio Castillo, MD   Professor and Director of Neuroradiology, Department of Radiology, University of North Carolina School of Medicine, Chapel Hill, North Carolina

Khaled M. Elsayes, MD   Staff Radiologist, Theodore Bilhars Institute, Giza, Egypt

Julia R. Fielding, MD   Associate Professor and Director of Abdominal Imaging, Department of Radiology, University of North Carolina School of Medicine, Chapel Hill, North Carolina

David S. Gierada, MD   Associate Professor of Radiology, Mallinckrodt Institute of Radiology, Washington University School of Medicine, St. Louis, Missouri

Suzan Menasce Goldman, MD, PhD   Affiliated Professor, Imaging Diagnosis Department, UNIFESP/EPM, São Paulo, Brazil

Brett Gratz, MD   Instructor in Radiology, Mallinckrodt Institute of Radiology, Washington University School of Medicine, St. Louis, Missouri

Fernando R. Gutierrez, MD   Professor of Radiology, Cardiothoracic Imaging Section, Mallinckrodt Institute of Radiology, Washington University School of Medicine, St. Louis, Missouri

Jay P. Heiken, MD   Professor of Radiology, Department of Radiology, Mallinckrodt Institute of Radiology, Washington University School of Medicine, St. Louis, Missouri

Alvaro L. Huete-Garin, MD   Assistant Professor of Radiology, Catholic University, Santiago, Chile

Cylen Javidan-Nejad, MD   Assistant Professor of Cardiothoracic Imaging, Mallinckrodt Institute of Radiology, Washington University School of Medicine, St. Louis, Missouri

Philip J. Kenney, MD   Director of Outpatient Radiology and Chief, GU Section, Professor, Abdominal Imaging Section, Department of Radiology, University of Alabama at Birmingham, Birmingham, Alabama

Joseph K. T. Lee, MD   E. H. Wood Distinguished Professor and Chairman, Department of Radiology, University of North Carolina School of Medicine, Chapel Hill, North Carolina

Mark E. Lockhart, MD, MPH   Director, Abdominal Imaging Fellowship, Assistant Professor, Abdominal Imaging Section, Department of Radiology, University of Alabama at Birmingham, Birmingham, Alabama

Robert Lopez-Ben, MD   Associate Professor of Radiology, University of Alabama Medical School, Birmingham, Alabama

Matthew A. Mauro, MD   Professor and Vice Chair of Clinical Affairs, Department of Radiology, University of North Carolina School of Medicine, Chapel Hill, North Carolina

Christine O. Menias, MD   Assistant Professor, Department of Radiology, Mallinckrodt Institute of Radiology, Washington University School of Medicine, St. Louis, Missouri

Paul Lee Molina, MD   Professor of Radiology and Vice Chairman of Education, Department of Radiology, University of North Carolina School of Medicine, Chapel Hill, North Carolina

Daniel S. Moore, MD   Assistant Professor, Department of Radiology, University of Texas Southwestern Medical School, Dallas, Texas

Desiree E. Morgan, MD   Associate Professor and Medical Director—MRI, Department of Radiology, University of Alabama at Birmingham, Birmingham, Alabama

Harish Patel, MD   Clinical Instructor, Department of Radiology, University of North Carolina School of Medicine, Chapel Hill, North Carolina

Christine M. Peterson, MD   Clinical Fellow, Department of Radiology, Mallinckrodt Institute of Radiology, Washington University School of Medicine, St. Louis, Missouri

Michele T. Quinn, MD   Radiology Resident, University of North Carolina School of Medicine, Chapel Hill, North Carolina

Santiago Enrique Rossi, MD   Centro de Diagnostico, Hospital de Clínicas José de San Martín, Buenos Aires, Argentina

Zoran Rumboldt, MD   Associate Professor of Radiology, Medical University of South Carolina, Charleston, South Carolina

Stuart S. Sagel, MD   Professor of Radiology and Director, Chest Radiology Section, Mallinckrodt Institute of Radiology, Washington University School of Medicine, St. Louis, Missouri

Richard C. Semelka, MD   Professor and Vice Chair of Research, Department of Radiology, University of North Carolina School of Medicine, Chapel Hill, North Carolina

Marilyn Joy Siegel, MD   Professor of Radiology and Pediatrics, Mallinckrodt Institute of Radiology, Washington University School of Medicine, St. Louis, Missouri

Richard M. Slone, MD, FCCP   Virtual Radiologic Professionals, PLLC, Virtual Radiologic Consultants, Minneapolis, Minnesota

J. Kevin Smith, MD, PhD   Vice Chair for Veterans Affairs, Associate Professor, Abdominal Imaging Section, Department of Radiology, University of Alabama at Birmingham, Birmingham, Alabama

J. Keith Smith, MD, PhD   Associate Professor of Radiology, University of North Carolina School of Medicine, Chapel Hill, North Carolina

Robert J. Stanley, MD, MSHA   Professor and Chair Emeritus, Department of Radiology, University of Alabama at Birmingham, Birmingham, Alabama

Paul D. Stein, MD   St. Joseph Mercy Hospital, Pontiac, Michigan

Franklin N. Tessler, MD, CM   Professor of Radiology, Department of Radiology, University of Alabama at Birmingham, Birmingham, Alabama

D. Dean Thornton, MD   Clinical Assistant Professor, Department of Radiology, University of Alabama Medical School, Birmingham, Alabama

David M. Warshauer, MD   Professor of Radiology, University of North Carolina School of Medicine, Chapel Hill, North Carolina

Bruce R. Whiting, PhD   Research Assistant, Professor of Radiology, Mallinckrodt Institute of Radiology, Washington University School of Medicine, St. Louis, Missouri

Franz J. Wippold II, MD, FACR   Professor of Radiology, Chief of Neuroradiology, Mallinckrodt Institute of Radiology, Washington University Medical Center, St. Louis, Missouri; Adjunct Professor of Radiology and Nuclear Medicine, F. Edward Hébert School of Medicine, Uniformed Services University of the Health Sciences, Bethesda, Maryland

Pamela K. Woodard, MD   Associate Professor, Mallinckrodt Institute of Radiology, Washington University School of Medicine, St. Louis, Missouri

Preface

Since the publication of the third edition of our textbook *Computed Body Tomography with MRI Correlation* in 1998, major technologic advances have been made in both computed tomography (CT) and magnetic resonance imaging (MRI). The evolution from a single-detector-row helical (spiral) CT to multidetector-row CT (MDCT) has provided the unique opportunity to perform isotropic volumetric imaging and allowed new clinical indications. CT angiography now is routinely used for the detection of pulmonary emboli, for assessment of the aorta and its branches, for preoperative planning for resection of selected thoracic and abdominal tumors, and prior to donor nephrectomy. The 64 MDCT scanner now has replaced the electron beam scanner for assessing the coronary arteries as well as the cardiac anatomy and function. CT has become the procedure of choice for evaluating patients with acute abdominal pain and multiorgan trauma. Although controversial, largely because of cost–benefit and radiation-dose issues, CT also has been used to screen asymptomatic individuals in some centers. The development of PET-CT combines the metabolic information provided by PET with superb anatomic resolution provided by CT. PET-CT has now become an integral part of oncologic imaging.

During the same period of time, innovations and refinement in MR hardware and software technology have continued. Faster pulse sequences, improved coil design, and the development of parallel imaging all have contributed to the increased utilization of MR as a diagnostic tool. MRI is clearly the procedure of choice for evaluating many diseases of the central nervous system and the musculoskeletal system. Although MRI is well suited for assessing the cardiovascular system and has the advantage of not using ionizing radiation, the clear superiority of MRI over CT for imaging the cardiovascular system that was so evident several years ago is less apparent now because of the development of 64 MDCT scanners. However, MRI has been well established as a complementary imaging study in the abdomen and pelvis. The role of MRI in thoracic imaging is still limited.

This edition has been prepared to present a comprehensive text on the application of CT to the extracranial organs of the body. The role of MRI in these areas is also fully discussed, wherever applicable. The book is intended primarily for the radiologist to use in either clinical practice or training. Other physicians, such as the internist, pediatrician, and surgeon, also can derive state-of-the-art information about the relative value and indications for CT and MRI of the body. As in the first three editions, both normal and abnormal CT and MRI findings are described and illustrated. Instruction is provided to optimize the performance, analysis, and interpretation of CT and MR images. Information is provided on how to avoid technical and interpretative errors commonly encountered in CT and MRI examinations based on our collective experience.

The task of deciding which diagnostic test is most appropriate for a given clinical problem has remained a challenge in our practice. A thorough understanding of clinical issues, as well as the advantages and limitations of each imaging technique, is essential for determining the best imaging approach for establishing a specific diagnosis in a given situation. Our recommended uses of CT and MRI have been developed through the efforts of radiology colleagues at our three medical centers. We are fully aware that equally valid alternative imaging approaches to certain clinical problems exist. Furthermore, increasing knowledge, continued technologic improvement, and differences in available equipment and expertise will influence the selection of a particular imaging method at a given institution.

J.K.T.L.
S.S.S.
R.J.S.
J.P.H.

Acknowledgments

Providing recognition to everyone involved in the production of this edition is extremely difficult because of the large number of individuals from our three institutions who aided immeasurably in forming the final product. We graciously thank the various contributors who kindly provided chapters in their areas of expertise to bring depth and completeness to the book.

A special note of gratitude goes to our secretaries, Sue Day, Angela Lyght, Jama Rendell, Pam Schaub, and Trish Thurman, who spent endless hours typing manuscripts, checking references, and labeling images. Maurice Noble at the University of North Carolina Department of Radiology Photography Laboratory was extremely helpful in preparing the illustrative material. Our thanks go to our residents, fellows, and the many radiologic technologists who performed and monitored the CT and MRI studies. Their dedication is reflected in the high quality of the images used throughout this book.

We also would like to express our appreciation to Lippincott Williams and Wilkins for their professionalism in handling this project. Most particularly, we would like to thank Kerry Barrett and Lisa McAllister for their tireless dedication and advice during each stage in the production of this book.

The Biliary Tract

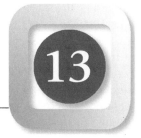

13

Franklin N. Tessler   Mark E. Lockhart

Dedicated computed tomography (CT) of the gallbladder and bile ducts is most often performed in the clinical setting of known or suspected biliary obstruction. CT has also come to play an increasingly important role in a variety of other conditions, such as congenital anomalies, inflammatory processes, and neoplasms. In addition, CT is often used to evaluate the secondary effects of nonbiliary pathology, notably pancreatic neoplasms, on the biliary system.

Historically, CT has competed with established contrast-based imaging procedures, including oral cholecystography, intravenous cholangiography, percutaneous transhepatic cholangiography (PTC), and endoscopic retrograde cholangiopancreatography (ERCP), all of which provide excellent detail within the confines of the biliary tract but are limited by their inability to directly visualize structures beyond the opacified lumen. Radionuclide biliary scintigraphy, which provides functional information at the expense of poorer spatial resolution, and sonography, which has gained acceptance because of its relatively low cost and ready availability, also continue to be widely used.

Most traditional imaging studies are still offered today, and indeed some have expanded their roles as newer variants, such as endoscopic ultrasound (EUS), have appeared. In recent years, magnetic resonance imaging (MRI) and magnetic resonance cholangiopancreatography (MRCP) have been added to the diagnostic armamentarium used to evaluate patients with biliary disease. MRCP, in particular, has seen growing application as a replacement for invasive traditional techniques such as ERCP and PTC.

Faced with an ever-expanding choice of imaging tests, the challenge for the clinician and the imaging specialist alike is to determine which imaging modality to use for a given patient and, in cases for which multiple studies must be performed, to know what sequence to use. This chapter reviews the basic anatomy and the normal and abnormal physiology of the biliary tract. Next, the role of CT and MRI in evaluating patients with biliary disease is discussed. Although a detailed discussion of other imaging modalities is beyond the scope of this chapter, the complementary role of tests such as sonography and EUS is described when appropriate.

NORMAL ANATOMY AND VARIATIONS

In most individuals, the right anterior and posterior segmental intrahepatic bile ducts converge to form the right hepatic duct, which joins the left hepatic duct to form the common hepatic duct (CHD). The gallbladder, drained by the cystic duct, is usually located at the inferior margin of the liver in a plane defined by the interlobar fissure. The cystic duct inserts into the CHD, which continues on as the common bile duct (CBD). At the ampulla of Vater, the CBD typically joins the main pancreatic duct. Anatomic variations of biliary drainage are common, however, and have particular significance in patients who are prospective living liver donors. In a recent study of 300 donors who underwent intraoperative cholangiography, seven different types of intrahepatic branching patterns were described, with the previously noted configuration found in only 63% of cases (38). In the second most common pattern, which was found in 11% of cases, the right posterior segmental duct emptied directly into either the CHD or the left hepatic duct. Almost as common was a third pattern, in which the right anterior and posterior ducts joined the left hepatic duct at a single point. Other variations, which included drainage of the right hepatic duct or accessory ducts into the cystic duct, were seen less often.

Multiple variations of gallbladder anatomy have also been described. The most frequent anomaly is the so-called "Phrygian cap," in which the gallbladder fundus has a folded configuration (as discussed later in this chapter) (132).

Complete agenesis of the gallbladder is exceedingly rare, with a reported incidence of less than one in 6,000 live births (172). Septation, duplication, and triplication of the gallbladder are slightly more common (132). Various sites of ectopic gallbladder development, including intrahepatic and suprahepatic locations, have also been reported (261,267), as has herniation of the gallbladder through the foramen of Winslow into the lesser sac (16). Likewise, variations of cystic duct anatomy are common. The cystic duct may empty into the CHD anywhere along its course, from the confluence to the ampulla. Direct communication between the intrahepatic bile ducts and the cystic duct also may occur. Finally, malrotation of the cystic duct can cause it to form a loop anterior or posterior to the CHD (217).

PATHOPHYSIOLOGY OF BILIARY OBSTRUCTION

Bile formation is a complex process that begins with the secretion of primary bile by the hepatocytes (233). Bile then passes along the intrahepatic ducts, which modify it extensively. The gallbladder further modifies the bile by concentrating and acidifying it before excreting it into the CBD and hence into the duodenum. Any process that results in excessive accumulation of bilirubin within the blood serum (hyperbilirubinemia) results in a spectrum of clinical manifestations, which include jaundice (a yellowish discoloration of the skin), scleral icterus, dark urine, and light stools (154). Jaundice appears when the serum bilirubin level is greater than 2 to 4 mg/dL.

The primary role of biliary imaging is to distinguish obstructive from nonobstructive hyperbilirubinemia, which is a diagnosis largely based on the detection of anatomic changes in the biliary tract in response to obstruction. The earliest such change is an increase in the diameter of the CBD (154), which usually measures no greater than 6 or 7 mm in normal adults (56). The time course for the development of biliary dilatation is variable, and the degree of dilatation also depends on whether the obstruction is continuous or intermittent. Importantly, biliary dilatation may be minimal early in the course of obstruction. Conversely, patients who have had a cholecystectomy may have a dilated CBD in the absence of functional obstruction (108).

If biliary obstruction is not relieved, intrahepatic biliary dilatation and enlargement of the gallbladder usually follow. Again, however, the time course for these anatomic changes to occur is quite variable. As well, the intrinsic ability of these structures to dilate in response to increased biliary pressure varies depending on their intrinsic compliance and on the compliance of adjacent tissues and structures. For example, intrahepatic bile ducts in cirrhotic livers with extensive fibrosis may be less able to expand in the setting of biliary obstruction.

GENERAL PRINCIPLES OF BILIARY IMAGING

The choice and sequence of imaging tests in patients with biliary disease is based on the clinical symptoms and signs, as well as findings on initial laboratory testing. A positive screening study is often further evaluated with a more specific invasive test, such as ERCP or PTC. However, a false positive result may necessitate additional studies to yield a diagnosis, with associated additional cost and risks. Therefore, the potential risks must be balanced against the need for a diagnosis in the individual patient.

Noninvasive imaging techniques include ultrasound, CT, MRI, and nuclear medicine studies. Sonography is often the initial imaging study to evaluate abnormal biliary laboratory tests because of its low cost, portability, and lack of ionizing radiation, which facilitate its use at the bedside. Ultrasound is highly sensitive for detecting biliary obstruction, and it is also very useful for detecting cholelithiasis, choledocolithiasis, or acute cholecystitis (25,162,163,200). However, ultrasound often has limited specificity in patients with biliary obstruction, and its sensitivity is limited in obese patients (184). Moreover, the clinical information gained from sonography depends greatly upon the skill of the operator who performs the study and the physician who interprets the images.

Nuclear cholescintigraphy is a noninvasive technique that lacks the spatial resolution of the other imaging modalities, but it can be very accurate in the diagnosis of cystic duct obstruction (146). Cholescintigraphy can accurately diagnose acute cholecystitis, and it also may characterize acalculous cholecystitis (50). However, cholescintigraphy is limited in patients who are receiving total parental nutrition or who are chronically hospitalized.

MRI provides excellent anatomic detail and contrast resolution, also without the use of ionizing radiation. MRI may detect most biliary abnormalities, and it is often preferred in place of ERCP if there is low suspicion that intervention will be needed. MRCP is able to demonstrate noncalcified gallstones as filling defects, but it may be less sensitive than CT for calcifications (101). Unfortunately, MRCP may be more susceptible to artifacts associated with breathing or motion, which may be limiting in ill patients who are unable to suspend respiration or lie still on the MRI couch. As well, neither MRI nor MRCP allow for direct evaluation of tenderness, which can be a valuable adjunctive finding on ultrasound in patients with acute cholecystitis (221).

CT is not a first-line choice in the evaluation of biliary colic because of its cost, lack of portability, and use of ionizing radiation. However, CT may detect biliary dilatation, biliary wall thickening, ductal stones, pancreatic mass, or adenopathy. CT is very sensitive and specific for calcified biliary duct stones, and it has excellent spatial resolution (193). When the etiology of symptoms is not confidently localized to the biliary system, CT is a robust technique that not only may localize a biliary abnormality, but may also detect a nonbiliary etiology for the patient's symptoms and signs. CT is also less susceptible to motion artifacts than MRI.

If direct active evaluation of the bile ducts or pathologic diagnosis is necessary, imaging with ERCP, PTC, or EUS may be performed. ERCP and PTC are invasive, but they provide the greatest anatomic and mucosal detail of the biliary ducts. These techniques suffer from higher rates of complication, but they allow potential sampling for malignant cells. In ERCP, the ampullary region is accessed endoscopically to cannulate the bile ducts and distend them with contrast for imaging. PTC similarly distends the bile ducts, but uses needle cannulation of an intrahepatic duct by placing a needle through the liver parenchyma transcutaneously. PTC is occasionally used for diagnosis, but it is more commonly performed to drain biliary obstruction when the biliary system cannot be accessed by ERCP.

ERCP and MRCP have significant different technical considerations that affect the appearance of the biliary system. ERCP distends the biliary system from the CBD using contrast injection, whereas MRCP relies on detection of signal from bile within the ducts without distension with contrast. Therefore, the ducts will be smaller and yield less signal intensity in the normal state on MRCP than is present on ERCP. In contrast, ERCP may not be able to cross a biliary stricture to allow evaluation of dilated intrahepatic bile ducts.

In summary, when considering a patient with potential biliary disease, a thorough history, physical examination, and laboratory evaluation should be performed. For detection of gallstones or acute cholecystitis, sonography is usually performed, but CT or nuclear medicine studies may yield the diagnosis. If the clinical suspicion is biliary obstruction or jaundice, sonography should be performed initially. If gallstones are present on ultrasound, ERCP is performed to detect ductal stones and provide therapy. If the duct cannot be cannulated, PTC may be performed. If there is no evidence of gallstone disease on ultrasound, CT or MRI may be used to evaluate for cholangiocarcinoma or other neoplasm and search for any evidence of metastatic disease. MRCP may be performed initially rather than sonography if there is high clinical suspicion of sclerosing cholangitis.

COMPUTED TOMOGRAPHY: TECHNIQUE AND NORMAL APPEARANCES

Even prior to the development of helical CT in the 1990s, the ability of axial CT to image the normal and abnormal gallbladder and bile ducts was well established. Nevertheless, CT was rarely considered as the primary imaging modality in patients with suspected biliary obstruction, particularly given the ready availability of ultrasound and the subsequent ability of MRCP to depict the biliary system in exquisite detail. During recent years, however, the rapid deployment of helical CT scanners and increasing

availability of multidetector row CT has led to an enhanced role for CT imaging of biliary pathology. Concurrently, there has been renewed interest in the use of oral and intravenous contrast agents to opacify the gallbladder and bile ducts prior to CT assessment. However, because the latter technique has not been widely accepted in clinical practice, this review will begin by describing the principles of CT imaging of the unopacified biliary tree.

Even in patients with suspected primary biliary pathology, CT is usually performed as much to detect and characterize abnormalities of the nonbiliary organs and structures (notably the liver, the pancreas, and adjacent lymph node chains and vessels) as to depict the bile ducts themselves. Consequently, it is vital that any "biliary" CT technique take this requirement into account. The examination begins with frontal and lateral projection scout images, which provide general anatomic landmarks for imaging, and which may occasionally demonstrate malpositioned stents or other instruments. Subsequently, unenhanced helical CT images of the upper abdomen are obtained using 5-mm collimation during a single breath-hold with a 1:1 pitch. This image set allows the operator to localize the bile ducts and pancreas and also facilitates identification of calcifications within the pancreas, gallbladder, and bile ducts. The type of oral contrast agent to opacify the gastrointestinal tract is open to debate and depends, to an extent, on ancillary indications for the study. If the CT examination is somewhat generalized in scope, it is best to administer water-soluble iodinated contrast orally prior to scanning. However, if the scan is primarily directed at the bile ducts or pancreas, the use of water as a negative oral "contrast agent" helps minimize artifacts and also increases the sensitivity for the detection of abnormalities in the duodenum and ampulla.

Next, arterial and portal venous phase imaging of the upper abdomen is performed during rapid intravenous administration of 125 to 150 mL of water-soluble contrast medium into an antecubital or other suitable vein at a flow rate of 4 or 5 mL per second. Imaging from the hepatic dome down to the porta hepatis uses 5 mm collimation, whereas 2.5-mm or thinner collimation is used from this level down through the uncinate process of the pancreas. In selected cases, thin-section imaging can be initiated higher in the liver to facilitate subsequent multiplanar reformatting or volume rendering. Arterial phase imaging is performed with a scan delay of approximately 25 to 30 seconds after the start of injection, whereas portal venous phase imaging begins at approximately 70 seconds. The delay times should be adjusted upward in patients with cardiac disease or other conditions that prolong the circulation time and lower in younger athletic patients. Although not required in all cases, multiplanar reformatting, maximum or minimum-intensity projection images, or volume-rendered images are often helpful to confirm impressions based on review of the axial images or to produce displays that mimic MRCP or ERCP for referring clinicians (107,183) (Fig. 13-1).

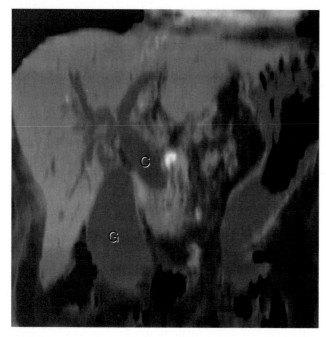

Figure 13-1 Computed tomography image reformatted in the coronal plane demonstrates intra- and extrahepatic biliary dilatation in a patient with a periampullary tumor. C, common bile duct; G, gallbladder.

In patients with known or suspected intrahepatic neoplasm, delayed imaging may be helpful to distinguish cholangiocarcinoma from other tumors, particularly hepatocellular carcinoma, because of the propensity of the former to show increased attenuation on delayed images (115,152). Loyer et al. (152) found that a delay time of 2 to 6 minutes after injection was adequate for this purpose, whereas Keogan et al. (115) suggested a longer scan delay of 10 to 20 minutes. Because patients may find it difficult to remain on the CT table for longer periods of time, 10 minutes seems to be a good compromise for so-called quadruple phase imaging.

As an alternative to the "negative contrast" images of the biliary system afforded by the previously noted technique, some investigators have evaluated oral or intravenous contrast agents to opacify the gallbladder and bile ducts prior to CT. In a pilot study of 5 healthy volunteers and 14 patients who ingested 6 g of iopanoic acid orally prior to CT, the examination was nondiagnostic in 5 of the patients, limiting its utility (33). In another study, Takahashi et al. performed CT cholangiography using iotroxic acid, a newer intravenous biliary contrast agent, in 133 patients with suspected pancreatic or biliary disease (235). Patients were scanned 45 to 75 minutes after the agent was completely infused. These authors diagnosed choledocholithiasis with a sensitivity of 89% and a specificity of 98% in a subset of 80 patients with confirmed diagnoses and concluded that CT cholangiography is a reliable technique. However, despite the low incidence of contrast reactions in this series (minor reactions were encountered in only three

patients), the historically high rate of life-threatening reactions with intravenous cholangiographic contrast agents may limit their acceptance in the near term.

The intrahepatic bile ducts bear a variable anatomic relationship to the hepatic vessels and are typically visualized as low attenuation structures adjacent to the portal venous branches (Fig. 13-2). Differentiation of normal-caliber from borderline dilated ducts can be difficult on noninvasive imaging; however, the normal bile ducts measure 1.8 mm peripherally (range, 1 to 3 mm), and 1.9 mm centrally (range, 1 to 2.8 mm) (142). Normal-caliber intrahepatic ducts are visualized on CT in 40% of normal patients. The CHD and CBD, in contrast, are visible in almost 100% of patients with or without biliary obstruction (Fig. 13-3). The maximal diameter of the normal CBD measures between 6 and 7 mm (56). Some investigators have found only a minimal increase in duct caliber with advancing age (191), whereas others have found an age-related increase in patients older than age 75 years (108). The cystic duct is usually not seen on CT unless it is dilated. The duct walls in the biliary system are typically paper-thin and enhance slightly.

The effect of cholecystectomy on the diameter of the extrahepatic bile ducts has also been open to debate. One study of 234 patients who were examined with ultrasound showed only a small increase in duct size postoperatively (mean diameter 5.9 mm before surgery versus 6.1 mm after cholecystectomy) (56). Puri et al. reported no significant change in common duct diameter in 34 patients who were followed up to 4 to 6 months after cholecystectomy (197). However, another study found significant dilation

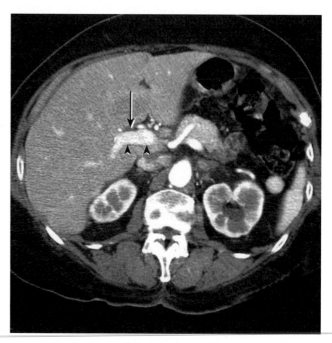

Figure 13-2 Normal intrahepatic ducts. Contrast-enhanced computed tomography CT shows non-dilated central right intrahepatic bile ducts (*arrow*) anterior to the right portal vein (*arrowheads*).

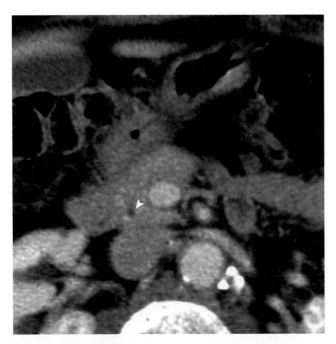

Figure 13-3 Normal common bile duct. Contrast-enhanced computed tomography shows normal caliber common duct (*arrowhead*) within the head of the pancreas.

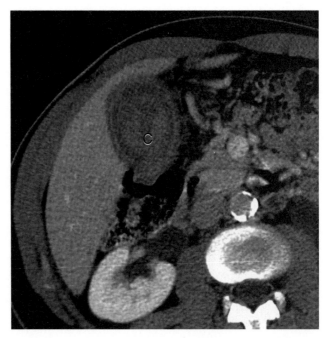

Figure 13-5 Hematobilia. Contrast-enhanced computed tomography image shows high-attenuation clot (C) in the gallbladder.

of the CBD (mean 8.7 mm, range 4.1 to 14.0 mm) in elderly patients after cholecystectomy (108).

The normal gallbladder is seen as a fluid-density structure (Fig. 13-4) in a fossa that occupies the same plane as the interlobar hepatic fissure, and the middle hepatic vein, which is usually easily identified on unenhanced and enhanced scans. Gallbladder attenuation typically is similar to that of water, but may be increased in patients with sludge, calculi, milk-of-calcium, or hematobilia (Fig. 13-5). The normal gallbladder wall measures between 1 and 3 mm in thickness, and typically enhances. Anatomic variations such as the Phrygian cap (Fig. 13-6), mentioned previously, are readily visualized when present, as are variations in gallbladder position.

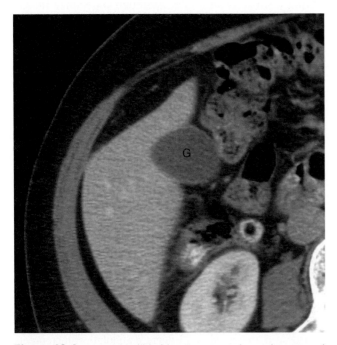

Figure 13-4 Normal gallbladder. Contrast-enhanced computed tomography demonstrates a fluid-attenuation gallbladder (G) with a thin wall.

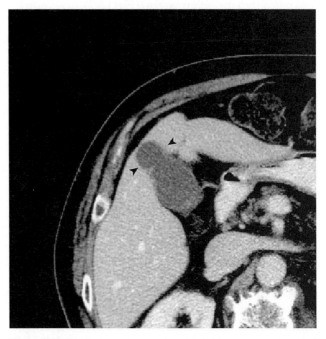

Figure 13-6 Phrygian cap. Axial computed tomography image of gallbladder fundus shows normal variant Phrygian cap (*arrowheads*).

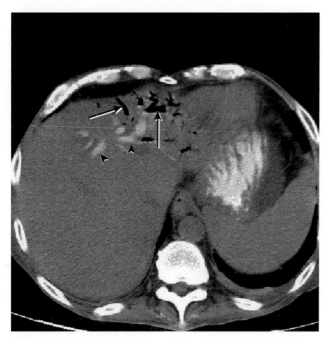

Figure 13-7 Pneumobilia and refluxed oral contrast into the biliary ducts. Contrast-enhanced computed tomography shows peripheral linear tracts of gas (*arrows*) in the expected location of the bile ducts. The peripheral location of the gas is related to dense oral contrast (*arrowheads*) that has also refluxed into the biliary tree.

Air in the bile ducts, or pneumobilia, is commonly seen following sphincterotomy, creation of biliary-enteric anastomoses, and placement of biliary stents. Demonstration of pneumobilia in this group of patients indicates a patent communication between the biliary tree and the gastrointestinal tract. Conversely, its absence suggests a lack of communication (as discussed later). Oral contrast may also reflux into the biliary system (Fig. 13-7).

MAGNETIC RESONANCE IMAGING: TECHNIQUE AND NORMAL APPEARANCES

MRCP uses signal produced by fluid within the ducts that can create images of the biliary and pancreatic ductal systems. Unlike ERCP and PTC studies, however, no extrinsic contrast injection is necessary. The MRCP techniques take advantage of the long spin-spin (T2) relaxation times of the static bile and pancreatic duct fluid. The long echo time allows the signal of most tissues, such as fat and solid organ signal, to decay, and only certain materials such as fluids with long T2 relaxation times produce significant signal. Earlier magnetic resonance sequences such as gradient-recalled echo and fast spin echo provided MRCP images, but these long sequences often suffered from motion artifact and poor spatial resolution. Images are now created with one of several magnetic resonance sequences that use heavy T2 weighting: single shot fast-spin echo (SSFSE), half Fourier single-shot turbo spin-echo (HASTE), and rapid-acquisition relaxation-enhanced (RARE) im-

aging have been commonly described. These ultrafast techniques obtain images rapidly and therefore reduce artifacts caused by patient motion and respiratory movement, thereby mitigating one of the previously described disadvantages of MRI compared with CT.

Proper patient preparation is crucial to optimize imaging of the biliary system with MRCP. For safety purposes, a checklist of exclusion criteria such as aneurysm clips or pacemakers should be discussed with the patient before the procedure. We recommend that the patient fast on the day of the procedure whenever possible to reduce bowel gas and peristalsis, but some centers do not require fasting before MRCP (251). A negative oral contrast agent may be given prior to the examination to reduce signal from the duodenum adjacent to the bile ducts. The patient removes all external metal items prior to entering the magnet, and is given earplugs. Once in the scanning room, the patient is instructed to lie supine and a phased-array torso coil is placed against the chest wall and upper abdomen. The coil acts as an antenna to improve the signal-to-noise ratio of the images. The patient is coached to remain very still and to pay special attention to the breathing instructions that are given during the study.

Most of our MRCP studies are performed using a 1.5 Tesla magnet. Multiplanar thin-slice images show excellent spatial resolution of the ducts. Stronger magnetic fields may provide better spatial resolution, but biliary MRI studies may be severely limited on magnets with field strengths of less than 1.0 Tesla. A combination of thin-slice and thick-slab sequences is performed. Unlike CT, MRI images may be prospectively acquired in any plane.

Generally, we use 1.6- to 4-mm-thick contiguous slices during a single breath-hold. Although the source images are sensitive for subtle details of the bile ducts, the entire duct cannot usually be displayed on a single slice. However, a series of slices may be "stacked" to form a maximum intensity projection (MIP) image that simulates the images produced with ERCP. The parameters for MRCP are usually echo time 900 to –1,000, repetition time infinite, 256 × 256 matrix, and a field-of-view that is small but does not have signal wrap over the biliary structures. MRCP images may be obtained without intravenous contrast, but it may be given for T1-axial imaging during the examination to evaluate for any pancreatic lesion that may cause biliary obstruction.

Thick-slab MRCP images may have less spatial resolution than thin slices, but they can also demonstrate most of the biliary system in a single view (Fig. 13-8), simulating the images obtained by ERCP. The slab thickness varies between 20 and 50 mm and may be limited by poor signal-to-noise ratio if the slab is thin. Each slab requires only a couple of seconds to obtain and is not often affected by motion artifact. Often, multiple planes of thick-slab imaging are obtained, and are varied at 15 degrees angulation increments centered on the common duct. An additional thick slab is chosen to specifically image most of the pancreatic duct.

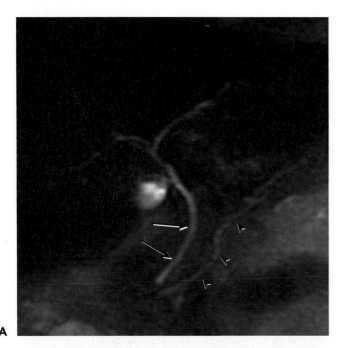

A

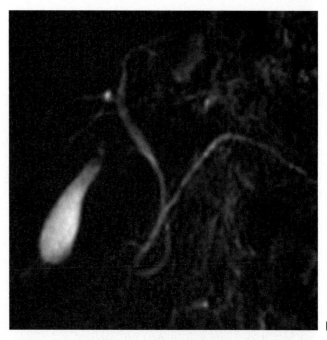

B

Figure 13-8 Normal magnetic resonance cholangiopancreatography. **A:** Thick-slab T2-weighted images of the biliary system shows normal-caliber smooth common duct (*arrows*) and smoothly tapering intrahepatic ducts. The pancreatic duct is well visualized (*arrowheads*). **B:** Magnetic resonance cholangiopancreatography of another patient with normal gallbladder, common duct, and pancreatic duct on oblique thick-slab image.

The slab may be repositioned or thinned to exclude signal from overlying structures, such as the renal collecting system. The bowel may contain fluid that will also show as high signal overlying and likely obscuring the extrahepatic bile ducts. Therefore, as previously noted, we usually give a negative oral contrast agent to reduce the amount of overlying signal from the bowel (91), although some authors do not use bowel contrast agents routinely (251).

There have been several publications regarding the use of MRCP in conjunction with intravenous injection of secretin to evaluate biliary function (159,160,165,166). Although the supply of secretin has been limited at times, it is currently available for functional evaluation of the biliary system. Secretin (1 mL/kg) stimulates secretion by the pancreas, which allows better distension of the pancreatic duct (159,165,166). The effect is rapid and resolves quickly. Repeated imaging with thick-slab MRCP every 15 to 30 seconds for 10 to 15 minutes is performed. This allows dynamic evaluation of the pancreatic duct and ampullary regions. Secretin stimulation allows improved visualization of the pancreatic duct as compared with standard MRCP (159). This technique also has been reported to improve the detection of pancreas divisum (165).

Limitations of Magnetic Resonance Cholangiopancreatography

Small or impacted biliary ductal calculi may be missed on MRCP (196). Air or metal artifacts may limit visualization of the entire duct. Another limitation of MRCP occurs when reconstructed images miss small ductal stones as a result of volume averaging of signal (12). Volume averaging can especially mask small stones in the thick-slab HASTE images, and the thin-slice MRCP source images should always be reviewed for filling defects (101).

Artifacts are commonly encountered in MRCP examinations. These are often from gas, clot, metallic clips, motion artifact, or pulsation artifact (123,203,228,258). Respiratory motion may artifactually simulate ductal stones or strictures (101). This occurs because of misregistration of data during breathing motion in a patient who is unable to adequately breath-hold (101). Pulsatility artifact from the hepatic artery may simulate stricture in the common duct. The CHD and left hepatic duct are most commonly involved (101). The left hepatic duct may be compressed by the right hepatic artery (101). The mid CBD may be narrowed extrinsically by the gastroduodenal artery (101). In the absence of other artifacts, MRCP may still overestimate the severity of a biliary stenosis on maximum intensity projection images. This can be overcome using thick-slab HASTE images to document the absence of a stricture in a region of question (101). In the absence of secretin stimulation, a normal collapsed pancreatic duct can simulate a pancreatic duct stricture.

In some patients, the examination cannot be performed because the patient has a pacemaker or cerebral aneurysm clips or suffers from claustrophobia. Furthermore, false-negative results of MRCP may occur if the level of obstruction is at the ampulla (247). RARE images may not visualize ducts that contain blood products. However, this weakness may occasionally be of benefit by showing that a signal from a vascular structure is not an abnormal biliary radical, because blood vessels are not visible on RARE imaging (90).

An inadequate MRCP may result from inappropriate selection of the region of imaging for thin- or thick-slab MRCP. Coronal oblique images are localized on axial images through the liver. It is possible that the CBD may be posterior to the levels selected at the level of the intrahepatic ducts. If the slices are not selected to include the entire duct, interpretative errors may occur (63). This interpretive error can be avoided by review of the thin-slice source images.

If a negative oral contrast agent is not used, fluid in the duodenum may obscure the common duct. Other structures such as the stomach or ureter may simulate an abnormality on MRCP. Proper selection of the slice location may be used to exclude overlying bowel signal, but it may be difficult to completely remove high signal bowel fluid that is adjacent to biliary structures.

Standard MRCP has limitations involving visualization and interpretation of the ampullary region (75,79,167). Because ERCP can directly visualize the ampulla, it should be performed if there is clinical concern for an ampullary lesion, even if no lesion is seen in this region on MRCP. Furthermore, MRCP cannot provide therapy and may not be as useful in patients with a very high likelihood of ductal stones that would require removal.

CONGENITAL ABNORMALITIES AND DISEASES OF THE GALLBLADDER

Congenital Abnormalities of the Gallbladder

As noted previously, congenital variations of gallbladder anatomy, including intrahepatic gallbladder and gallbladder duplication, are usually easily recognized on CT, MRI, or ultrasonography. Gallbladder folds and septations are also readily apparent, particularly on ultrasonography, because of its ability to image them in oblique planes. It is especially important to definitively identify the gallbladder when it is located in an atypical position. Occasionally, a long mesentery may permit the gallbladder to herniate through the foramen of Winslow into the lesser sac and undergo torsion and strangulation (16). If there is doubt whether a fluid-filled structure in the upper abdomen represents the gallbladder, radionuclide biliary imaging is usually definitive, unless the cystic duct is obstructed.

Diseases of the Gallbladder

Cholelithiasis and Sludge

Stones that develop in the gallbladder, in distinction to those that form within the biliary tree, are exceedingly common. It is estimated that 20 to 25 million adults in the United States have cholelithiasis, although the actual prevalence is unknown, because most are asymptomatic (26,109). Women are affected more frequently than men, and gallstones are more common with advancing age.

Approximately 70% to 80% of gallbladder stones are of the cholesterol variety, with pigment, mixed, and calcium carbonate calculi comprising the remainder. Of these, calcium carbonate stones are the least common. The pathogenesis of cholelithiasis is thought to be related to hypersaturation of bile with various constituents, and is associated with diminished gallbladder emptying and an increased intestinal transit time. The risk of cholesterol stones is increased by various clinical factors, including elevated estrogen levels (due to pregnancy, oral contraceptives, or postmenopausal hormone replacement therapy), obesity, rapid weight loss, hyperlipidemia, intestinal hypomotility, genetics, longstanding parenteral nutrition, certain drugs (e.g., octreotide, ceftriaxone), spinal cord injuries, and diseases of the terminal ileum (109).

Biliary sludge is a sediment consisting of various substances, including cholesterol crystals, which have precipitated from bile, and is associated with many of the same clinical factors as cholelithiasis (216). Although sludge is usually asymptomatic and often resolves spontaneously, it may cause biliary obstruction in the absence of cholelithiasis or it may be a precursor of biliary stones.

As noted previously, most patients with cholelithiasis are asymptomatic (109). Although patients with gallstones frequently report indigestion, intolerance to fatty foods, and belching, these symptoms are nonspecific. However, when gallstones migrate into and obstruct the gallbladder neck or the cystic duct, symptoms may ensue. Patients with transient ductal obstruction experience biliary colic, which is classically localized to the right upper quadrant, waxes and wanes over the course of 1 to 3 hours, and may be associated with nausea and vomiting (26,109). However, if obstruction persists, inflammation of the gallbladder wall (acute cholecystitis) may develop (as discussed later in this chapter).

Imaging of Cholelithiasis and Sludge

Approximately 80% to 85% of gallstones are invisible on conventional radiographs because they do not contain sufficient calcium (243). For many years, oral cholecystography was the procedure of choice to diagnose cholelithiasis, but has been largely replaced by cross sectional imaging in recent decades. In most patients, sonography is the best initial imaging test in a patient with suspected gallbladder calculi, because of its high accuracy, relatively low cost, its lack of ionizing radiation, its ability to evaluate the liver and bile ducts, and its availability at the bedside (26). Gallbladder calculi appear on ultrasound as echogenic intraluminal structures which are associated with posterior acoustic shadows (Fig. 13-9); mobility is another distinguishing feature in a patient who can be examined in the left lateral decubitus, prone, or upright position. The presence of acoustic

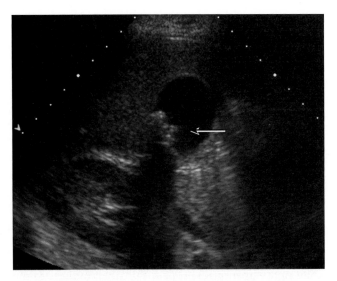

Figure 13-9 Cholelithiasis. Grayscale ultrasound shows round mobile echogenic structures (*arrow*) with shadowing (*arrow*) in the gallbladder lumen. There is no wall thickening or pericholecystic fluid.

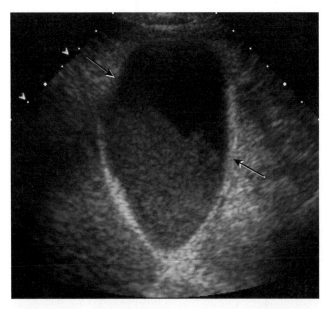

Figure 13-11 Layering sludge. Grayscale ultrasound of the gall-bladder shows smoothly layering echogenic material (*arrows*) within an otherwise normal gallbladder.

shadowing and mobility serves to distinguish stones from gallbladder polyps and focal aggregates of sludge, so-called tumefactive sludge (Fig. 13-10). Nontumefactive sludge is usually readily identified as layering, dependent material that is more echogenic than bile (Fig. 13-11).

Computed Tomography and Magnetic Resonance Imaging of Cholelithiasis.   Although the sonographic diagnosis of cholelithiasis is usually straightforward, patients who are large or uncooperative may prove challenging, and CT may be helpful. The density of gallstones on CT varies from heavily calcified to hypodense, with the latter appearance

characteristic of pure cholesterol stones (Fig. 13-12) (18). Large or medium-size calculi are usually easily recognized (Fig. 13-13), but minute stones may be easily overlooked.

As with ultrasonography, the diagnosis of cholelithiasis on CT can be challenging when the gallbladder is markedly contracted and therefore difficult to distinguish from adjacent opacified duodenum or other bowel. Sludge and minute calculi (so-called biliary sand) typically appear as a

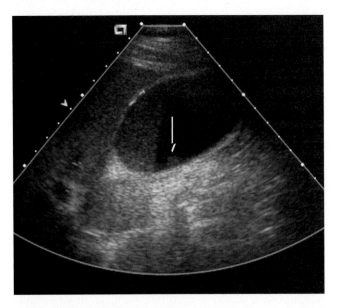

Figure 13-10 Tumefactive sludge. Grayscale ultrasound of the gallbladder shows a round echogenic structure (*arrow*) without shadowing. On further imaging, the debris changed configuration and layered dependently.

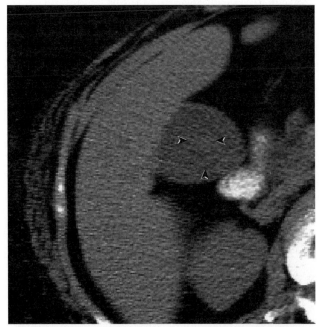

Figure 13-12 Subtle gallstones on computed tomography. Noncontrast computed tomography CT at the level of the gall-bladder shows mild heterogeneity (arrowheads) without well-de-fined gallstones. Gallstones were clearly visible on subsequent grayscale ultrasound of the gallbladder (not shown).

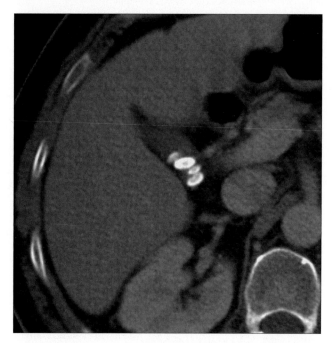

Figure 13-13 Cholelithiasis. Contrast-enhanced computed tomography shows multiple, calcified gallstones.

layer of dependent high attenuation within the gallbladder lumen, and cannot be reliably distinguished by CT. As well, dependent density mimicking sludge may be seen in patients with so-called vicarious excretion of water-soluble contrast media by the gallbladder (Fig. 13-14). Gallbladder excretion of intravenously-administered contrast is often not clinically significant, and is seen in patients with and without ureteral obstruction (51,95).

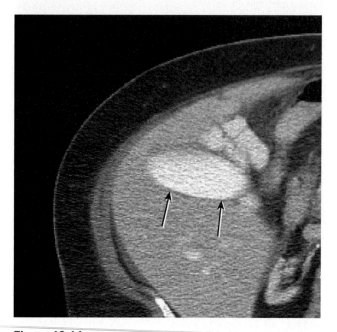

Figure 13-14 Contrast excretion by gallbladder. Dense contrast opacifies the gallbladder (*arrows*) with a small amount of layering of density in a patient who had another study using intravenous contrast prior to this computed tomography.

The sensitivity of MRCP for detecting gallstones is as high as 98% (31,202). Cholelithiasis usually appears as multiple dependent round structures within the high T2 signal bile of the gallbladder (Fig. 13-15). The stones usually have low T1 and low T2 signal characteristics. If there is water matrix within the stone, the signal may be variable (113).

Cholecystitis

Obstruction of the gallbladder by a stone in the gallbladder neck or cystic duct causes distension, increased intracholecystic pressure, mural ischemia, bacterial invasion, and acute inflammation. A minority of patients with acute cholecystitis have no evidence of stones. The pathogenesis of acalculous cholecystitis is not well understood, but is thought to be related to ischemia, biliary stasis, and inflammation. Clinically, patients typically present with acute right upper quadrant pain that often radiates to the right shoulder or back. Pronounced tenderness over the gallbladder (Murphy's sign) may also be seen. If left untreated, empyema of the gallbladder may ensue, or the gallbladder wall may become necrotic and perforate, leading to a localized abscess or peritonitis. In some patients, repeated episodes of acute inflammation lead to chronic cholecystitis, which is characterized by thickening, infiltration, and fibrosis of the gallbladder wall.

Imaging of Cholecystitis

As in patients with suspected cholelithiasis, ultrasound is the procedure of choice, with a reported sensitivity and specificity of greater than 95% (200). Sonographic signs include thickening of the gallbladder wall greater than 3 mm, pericholecystic fluid, and tenderness over the gallbladder, the so-called sonographic Murphy's sign (Fig. 13-16). Radionuclide cholescintigraphy is also highly sensitive for the diagnosis of acute calculous cholecystitis by demonstrating nonvisualization of the obstructed gallbladder, but is most useful as an adjunctive test in patients with indeterminate sonograms.

Although not the first-line imaging modality in patients with suspected uncomplicated acute cholecystitis, CT is nonetheless helpful in equivocal cases or in patients who are scanned for nonspecific abdominal pain. Some of the CT findings in acute cholecystitis, namely gallstones, mural thickening (Fig. 13-17), and pericholecystic fluid, parallel the features seen sonographically. However, CT is much better than ultrasound at demonstrating associated inflammatory changes, which appear as stranding or infiltration of pericholecystic tissues (Fig. 13-18). CT may also show hyperemia of the adjacent inflamed liver following administration of intravenous contrast medium, making it possible to distinguish inflammatory from noninflammatory gallbladder wall thickening (262). In the setting of acute trauma, gallbladder injury may mimic the findings of acute cholecystitis at CT (Fig. 13-19). In patients with emphysematous cholecystitis, which is most frequent in diabetic patients, CT can demonstrate intramural gas (Fig. 13-20).

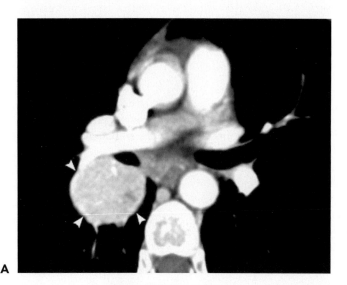

A

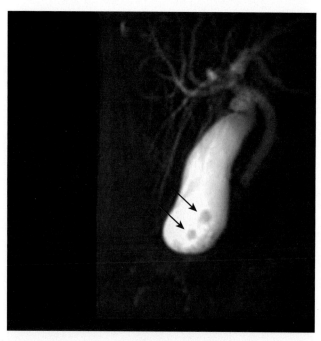

B

Figure 13-15 Magnetic resonance imaging. MRI of cholelithiasis. **A:** T2-weighted magnetic resonance imaging of the gallbladder shows multiple round signal voids within the normal high T2-weighted signal bile in the gallbladder. **B:** Thick-slab magnetic resonance cholangiopancreatography MRCP shows the stones (*arrows*) in the gallbladder fundus.

CT has also been reported to be helpful in patients with xanthogranulomatous cholecystitis, an unusual condition that is most common in older women (189). Although some of the CT findings are similar to those in the more common forms of acute cholecystitis, a hypodense band was seen in the gallbladder wall in 33% of the 26 patients studied. In this series, it was suggested that patients with xanthogranulomatous cholecystitis may experience an increased incidence of problems at laparoscopic cholecystectomy. More important, however, is the potential for xanthogranulomatous cholecystitis to mimic or be associated with gallbladder carcinoma (125,134).

CT is also valuable to assess adjacent organs and to diagnose complications of acute cholecystitis. In patients with

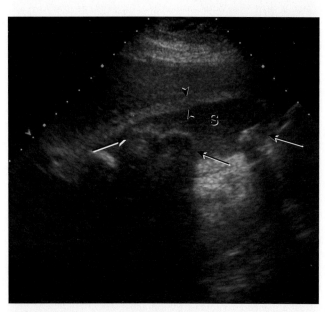

Figure 13-16 Cholecystitis. Sonogram of right upper quadrant shows gallbladder wall thickening (*arrowheads*), sludge (S), and stones (*arrows*).

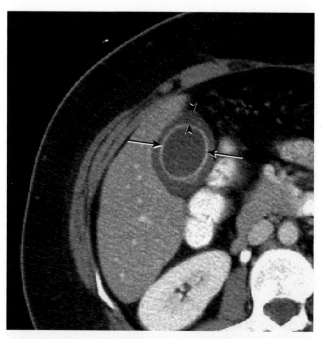

Figure 13-17 Acute cholecystitis. Contrast-enhanced computed tomography CT shows gallbladder wall thickening with bright mucosal enhancement (*arrows*) and wall thickening (*arrowheads*). Acute cholecystitis was confirmed at surgery.

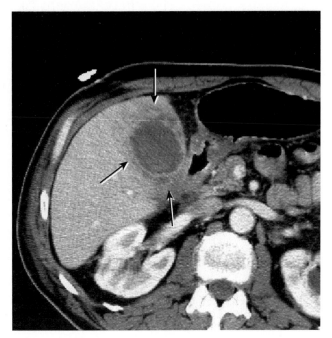

Figure 13-18 Severe acute cholecystitis. Contrast-enhanced computed tomography demonstrates diffuse gallbladder irregular wall thickening and pericholecystic infiltration (*arrows*).

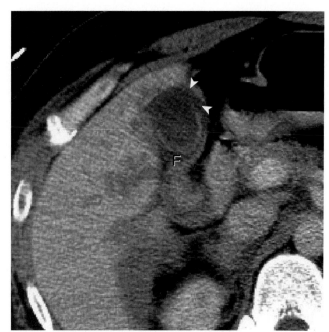

Figure 13-19 Gallbladder avulsion. Contrast-enhanced computed tomography in a patient being evaluated for trauma shows disrupted, non-enhancing anterior wall of the gallbladder (*arrowheads*) with pericholecystic fluid (F).

acute onset of right-sided abdominal pain, for example, CT may demonstrate acute pancreatitis or pyelonephritis, with can cause similar signs and symptoms. As well, complications such as gallbladder perforation with formation of a localized, pericholecystic abscess or peritonitis are depicted far better with CT than sonography. CT is also excellent for diagnosing small bowel obstruction in patients in whom a gallstone has gained access to the gastrointestinal tract via gallbladder perforation, termed *gallstone ileus*. Obstruction at the level of the duodenum is known as *Bouveret's syndrome* (Fig. 13-21) (192).

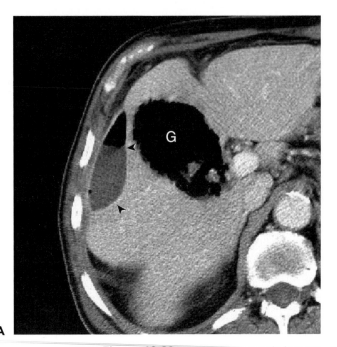

A

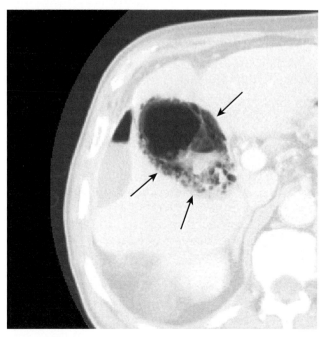

B

Figure 13-20 Emphysematous cholecystitis. Contrast-enhanced computed tomography with **A:** soft tissue windows shows gas-density filling the gallbladder (G). Perihepatic abscess with fluid and gas is also present (*arrowheads*). **B:** Image of the same level using lung windows better delineates the gas bubbles in the gallbladder and gallbladder wall (*arrows*).

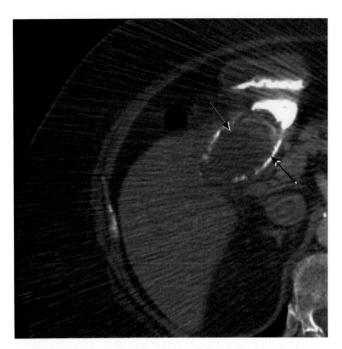

Figure 13-21 Bouveret's syndrome. Noncontrast computed tomography at the level of the gallbladder and duodenum shows a large filling defect within the second portion of the duodenum. The low-density oval stone (*arrows*) is outlined by dense contrast within the bowel. Gas was present within the gallbladder (not shown).

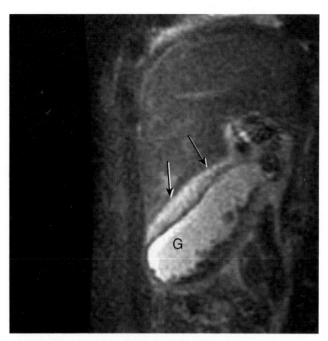

Figure 13-22 Acute cholecystitis. Non-enhanced T2-weighted MRI of the gallbladder shows gallbladder wall thickening and hyperintense T2 signal fluid (*arrows*) surrounding the gallbladder (G).

Magnetic Resonance Imaging of Acute Cholecystitis.

MRCP is very sensitive (91%) and shows good specificity (79%) and accuracy (89%) for acute cholecystitis (202). The MRI findings include gallbladder wall thickening and increased wall enhancement on T1-weighted images (151). There may be high T2 signal fluid around the gallbladder (Fig. 13-22). Gallbladder dilatation and gallstones are also associated findings. MRCP may detect the obstructing stone in the gallbladder neck or common duct to provide the etiology of the inflammation (188). On contrast-enhanced MRI, there may be abnormal enhancement of the liver parenchyma adjacent to the inflamed gallbladder due to hyperemia, a finding that has also been described on CT (151,262).

Gallbladder Polyps

Adenomatous and hyperplastic polyps are common incidental findings at gallbladder sonography, and also may be seen at thin-section CT (Fig. 13-23). Most gallbladder polyps are of no clinical significance, although it is difficult to absolutely exclude the rare possibility of very early gallbladder malignancy in a given patient. At present, the only imaging feature that can be used to distinguish innocuous lesions from those that should be followed or surgically removed is size (176). Polyps larger than 10 mm should be viewed with suspicion, whereas lesions that are 5 mm or smaller can be safely ignored. Polyps of intermediate size can be followed sonographically for signs of growth, although their clinical significance is doubtful in the majority of patients. Notably, however, it appears that

patients with primary sclerosing cholangitis (PSC) and polyps have an increased risk of gallbladder malignancy, suggesting that either cholecystectomy or close imaging surveillance is warranted (28).

Porcelain Gallbladder

The descriptive term *porcelain gallbladder* refers to calcification in the gallbladder wall, which usually is associated with chronic inflammation. Calcification may be partial or complete, and is easily recognized on CT (Fig. 13-24). At sonography, porcelain gallbladder must be distinguished from a contracted gallbladder containing a single, large calculus, in which the gallbladder wall is usually seen to be separate from the subadjacent stone (Fig. 13-25). If calcification is sufficiently dense, acoustic shadowing may preclude visualization of the gallbladder lumen on sonography, and CT may be helpful to exclude cholelithiasis. On MRI, calcification in the wall may appear as low T1 and low T2 signal.

Adenomyomatosis

Adenomyomatosis is a condition that is characterized by thickening of the muscularis of the gallbladder wall along with proliferation of the mucosa. Eventually, the overgrown mucosa protrudes through the thickened muscular layer to form so-called Rokitansky-Aschoff sinuses; if sufficiently large, they may be visible on sonography. Three variants of adenomyomatosis have been described: fundal, segmental, and diffuse (99). The fundal type, which is the most common, manifests as a discrete mass in the

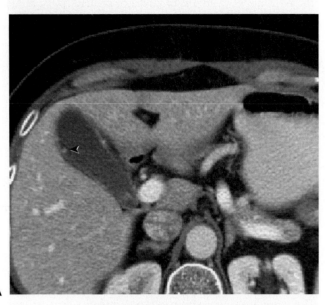

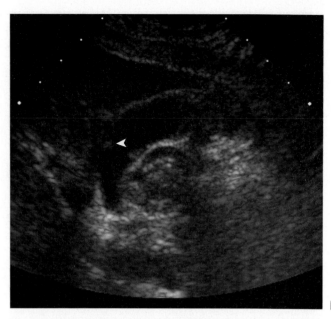

Figure 13-23 Small gallbladder polyp. **A:** Contrast-enhanced computed tomography of the gallbladder shows a small, nondependent structure (*arrowhead*) arising from the gallbladder wall, projecting into lumen. **B:** Grayscale ultrasound of the gallbladder in the same patient confirms a small, nondependent, nonshadowing polyp (*arrowhead*).

gallbladder fundus; the other two types of adenomyomatosis are characterized by a segmental stricture and by generalized thickening of the gallbladder wall, respectively.

Not surprisingly, the CT appearance of adenomyomatosis is nonspecific, unless the individual Rokitansky-Aschoff sinuses can be identified (99). Differentiating the fundal variant from gallbladder carcinoma or the diffuse form from chronic cholecystitis may be problematic. Sonography may be of benefit by demonstrating echogenic foci with so-called comet-tail artifacts within the mural sinuses (Fig. 13-26). The clinical significance of adenomyomatosis has been the subject of some debate; most authorities consider it to be an asymptomatic condition that is not associated with either cholelithiasis or gallbladder malignancy,

although there have been scattered reports of symptomatic cases (215).

Gallbladder Carcinoma

Carcinoma of the gallbladder is the sixth most common gastrointestinal malignancy in the United States (140). It is primarily a disease of the elderly, with a mean age at presentation of 72 years, and has a 3:1 female predominance. Certain ethnic groups, including Native and Hispanic Americans, are at increased risk, possibly because of their higher prevalence of gallbladder calculi. Cholelithiasis is a well-documented risk factor for gallbladder carcinoma, presumably because calculi lead to chronic inflammation and dysplasia. Porcelain gallbladder is also associated with

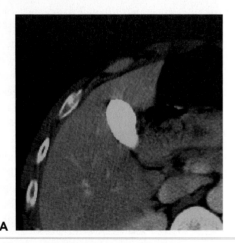

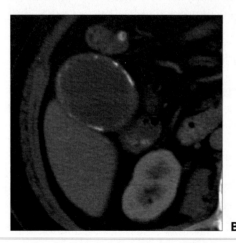

Figure 13-24 Porcelain gallbladder. **A:** Contrast-enhanced computed tomography (CT) shows extensive calcification in the wall of a contracted gallbladder. When it is this diffuse, the wall calcification may be difficult to differentiate from cholelithiasis. **B:** CT image of another patient demonstrates discontinuous mural calcification.

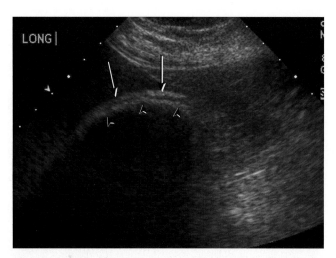

Figure 13-25 Wall-echo-complex sign. Grayscale ultrasound of the gallbladder shows a thin echogenic gallbladder wall (*arrows*) with a thin hypoechoic crescent of bile anterior to an echogenic, shadowing gallstone (*arrowheads*).

gallbladder carcinoma, although the association may not be as strong as previously thought (231). Interestingly, the diffuse form of mural calcification may not be associated with an increased risk of gallbladder malignancy (231).

Other conditions that are associated with an increased incidence of gallbladder carcinoma include congenital anomalies of the bile ducts (choledochal cyst, congenital cystic dilatation of the biliary tree, anomalous pancreaticobiliary junction, and low cystic duct insertion), and PSC. Early gallbladder carcinoma is usually clinically occult; therefore, patients most often have locally advanced or metastatic disease at presentation. The 5-year survival rate is poor (47,237). Symptoms include weight loss and abdominal pain, and patients may have a palpable mass in

the right upper quadrant or jaundice if there is associated biliary obstruction.

Pathologically, most gallbladder malignancies are adenocarcinomas, which arise from the mucosal layer, and range from poorly to well differentiated. Other primary malignancies of the gallbladder, such as sarcomas, lymphomas, and carcinoid tumors, are much less common, as are metastases to the gallbladder (most commonly from melanoma) (230). The majority (68%) of gallbladder carcinomas are infiltrating, whereas the remaining 32% are polypoid (223). Most arise in the gallbladder fundus, in which case they may be confused with the fundal variant of adenomyomatosis.

Computed Tomography of Gallbladder Carcinoma

The CT appearance reflects the gross presentation of the disease, which takes the form of a mass that completely replaces the gallbladder, focal or diffuse mural thickening, or an intraluminal mass, which is least common (Fig. 13-27). The mass-forming variants typically enhance to a varying degree, depending on the extent of tumor necrosis. Direct invasion into the contiguous hepatic parenchyma may be evident. CT also may be helpful to show involvement of the hepatic flexure of the colon or regional adenopathy. In patients in whom the primary tumor has grown along the bile ducts, biliary obstruction may be present. Hematogenous metastases are also well depicted by CT (Fig. 13-28).

Historically, the form of gallbladder carcinoma that produces focal or generalized wall thickening has been the most difficult to diagnose, as it has a similar appearance to chronic cholecystitis. It is therefore particularly important to look for signs of local or metastatic involvement in such

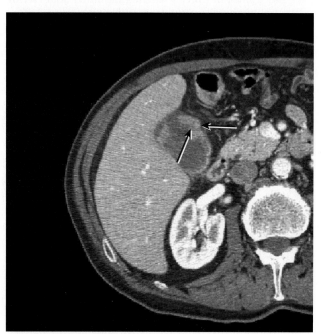

Figure 13-27 Localized gallbladder carcinoma. Contrast-enhanced computed tomography shows a heterogeneous, lobulated mass (*arrows*) projecting into the lumen of the gallbladder fundus.

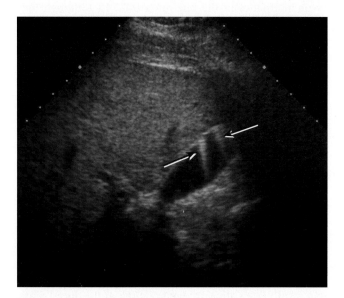

Figure 13-26 Adenomyomatosis. Grayscale ultrasound of the gallbladder demonstrates echogenic "comet tail" artifacts (*arrows*) arising from the wall and projecting into the gallbladder lumen.

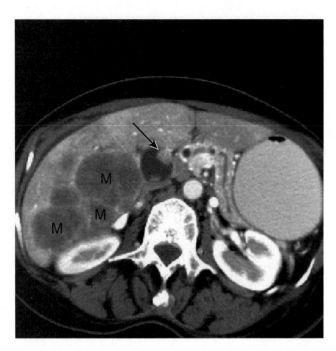

Figure 13-28 Gallbladder carcinoma. Axial computed tomography image shows multiple hepatic metastases (M). A discrete gallbladder mass also is seen (*arrow*).

cases. However, a recent report suggests that mural enhancement patterns may help to distinguish these two conditions. In a study of 82 patients, Yun et al. found that gallbladder carcinoma was characterized by arterial phase enhancement of a thickened inner wall, which remained hyperattenuating or became isodense to the liver parenchyma during the venous phase (268). Chronic cholecystitis, in contrast, showed a thin, isoattenuating inner wall during both phases. Metastases to the gallbladder may also present as mural masses, and cannot be reliably distinguished from the focal form of gallbladder carcinoma based on their CT appearance alone (Fig. 13-29).

Magnetic Resonance Imaging of Gallbladder Carcinoma

The MR appearance mirrors the appearance at CT. Findings include focal or diffuse thickening of the gallbladder wall. The mass usually will enhance rapidly and retain contrast. The appearance must be differentiated from benign gallbladder wall thickening due to inflammation or benign polyps, which are more uniform and do not retain contrast (266).

CONGENITAL ABNORMALITIES AND DISEASES OF THE BILE DUCTS

Choledochal Cysts and Choledochoceles

Choledochal cysts are characterized by cystic dilatation of the intrahepatic or extrahepatic bile ducts. A classification scheme was initially proposed by Alonso-Lej et al. (10), and was subsequently modified by Todani et al. (241) to include five types. Type I cysts consist of cystic (IA), focal

segmental (IB), and fusiform (IC) dilatation of the common duct. Type II cysts are true diverticula of the CBD. Type III choledochal cysts, also known as *choledochoceles*, represent cystic herniation of the distal CBD into the duodenum. Type IV cysts include multiple intra- and extrahepatic cysts (IVA) and multiple extrahepatic cysts (IVB). Finally, Type V choledochal cysts comprise multiple cystic dilatations of the intrahepatic bile ducts, also known as *Caroli disease* (discussed later in this chapter).

The true incidence of choledochal cysts is not known; however, they occur in approximately 1 in 15,000 live births in Western countries (213). As this suggests, choledochal cysts are thought to be congenital anomalies, although some may be acquired (81). Moreover, Babbitt has proposed a causative association with anomalies of the junction between the common bile and pancreatic ducts, which permits reflux of pancreatic enzymes into the common duct, leading to weakening and progressive dilatation (15).

Choledochal cysts are typically diagnosed in childhood, and may present with jaundice, abdominal pain, or vomiting. They are also associated with a range of complications, including biliary lithiasis, and, most importantly, malignancy of the biliary tract or pancreas (57). Depending on the type of choledochal cyst, treatment by surgical excision of the cyst or endoscopic sphincterotomy has been advocated to prevent complications (57,130).

At CT or MRI, choledochal cysts appear as fluid-filled structures, which are in continuity with the bile ducts (204) (Fig. 13-30). The presence of luminal nodularity or enhancement is suggestive of cholangiocarcinoma, and should prompt further investigation with ERCP. CT has also been shown to be capable of demonstrating an anomalous pancreaticobiliary junction in a patient with a choledochal cyst, and may be helpful for preoperative assessment (234).

Choledochoceles are rare, comprising less than 2% of cystic anomalies of the bile ducts (46,74). Although they are included in the Todani classification described previously, the association has been called into question by some researchers (199). Clinical manifestations include abdominal pain pancreatitis, nausea or vomiting, and jaundice (164). Cross-sectional imaging demonstrates a fluid-filled sac which protrudes into the duodenal lumen, but does not opacify with oral contrast (74). Management options range from endoscopic treatment to surgical resection.

Caroli Disease

Caroli disease, also known as *communicating cavernous ectasia of the intrahepatic bile ducts*, is a disorder that is primarily characterized by saccular or fusiform dilatation of the intrahepatic biliary tree (141). Although originally encompassed in the Todani classification as a type V choledochal cyst, this disorder is now thought to be a distinct entity that results from abnormal remodeling of the ductal plate, the embryologic precursor of the intrahepatic bile ducts (66,141,173). Nevertheless, the literature suggests an

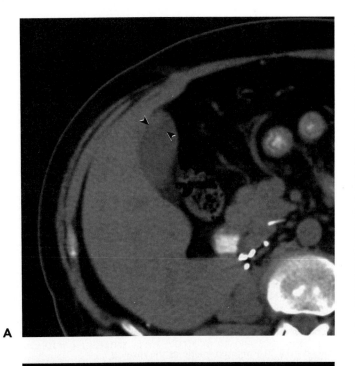

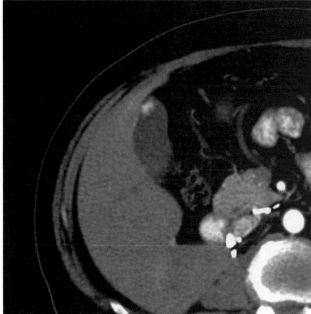

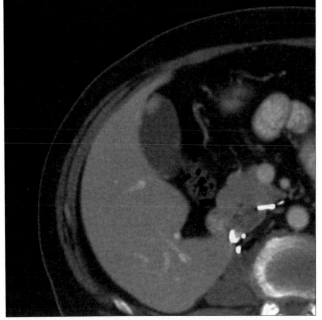

Figure 13-29 Metastasis to the gallbladder. **A:** Noncontrast computed tomography (CT) at the level of the gallbladder shows a subtle, peripheral, medium-density lesion (*arrowheads*), slightly higher in attenuation than adjacent bile. **B:** Contrast-enhanced CT at the same level demonstrates bright arterial enhancement of the gallbladder mass in the arterial phase. **C:** Portal phase image shows retention of contrast within the lesion. Metastatic renal cell carcinoma to the gallbladder was diagnosed.

association between Caroli disease and extrahepatic bile duct dilatation (141).

Two forms of Caroli disease have been described. The so-called simple or pure form of the disease, which most closely approximates the original description, is quite rare, and is characterized by ductal dilatation without fibrosis (66,170). Patients present with symptoms of cholangitis or hepatic abscess, including recurrent attacks of right upper quadrant pain and fever, but do not develop cirrhosis. The more common form of Caroli disease is hereditary, and is associated with periportal fibrosis, which leads to the development of cirrhosis and portal hypertension (77).

At cholangiography, alternating areas of ductal dilatation and stricture are seen. In one series, intraductal calculi were found in almost one half of cases and were visible cholangiographically in seven of eight patients with pathologically confirmed stones (141). CT typically demonstrates cystic structures, which represent the dilated bile ducts imaged in cross section. The extent of involvement may vary from focal to generalized. The finding of a central enhancing focus, termed the *central dot sign*, is helpful in distinguishing the dilated biliary segments of Caroli disease from other hepatic cysts (37) (Fig. 13-31). Pathologically, these dots have been shown

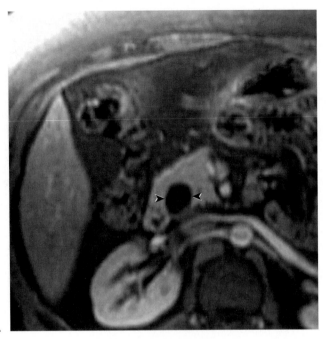

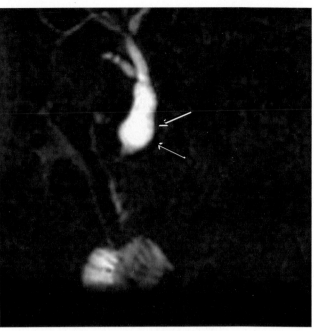

Figure 13-30 Choledochal cyst. **A:** Contrast-enhanced axial T1-weighted image at the level of the pancreatic head shows homogenous, well-marginated ductal dilatation (*arrowheads*) without enhancement. No mass or filling defect is detected. **B:** Thick-slab T2-weighted magnetic resonance cholangiopancreatography of the biliary ducts shows fusiform dilatation of the extrahepatic bile duct (*arrows*) without intrahepatic dilatation.

to correspond to portal vein radicals, which have been engulfed by the dilated ducts.

Guy et al. described three patterns of Caroli disease at MRI (77). In the first pattern, fusiform and cystic dilatation of the intrahepatic bile ducts was seen, and a central dot was demonstrated on gadolinium-enhanced scans. The second pattern was characterized by isolated, fusiform intrahepatic ductal dilatation, while the third pattern showed dilatation of left intrahepatic ducts, in addition to hepatic cysts.

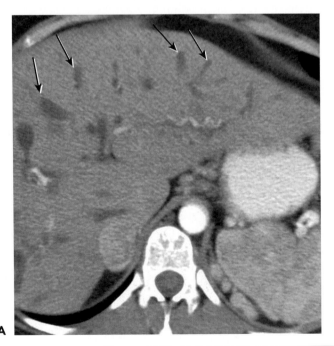

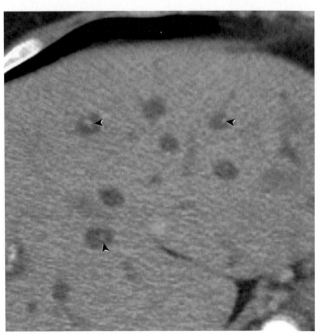

Figure 13-31 Caroli disease. **A:** Contrast-enhanced computed tomography of the liver shows numerous non-enhancing cystic structures (*arrows*) in the hepatic parenchyma. These represent focally dilated biliary ducts. **B:** Magnified image of the liver shows central foci of high density (*arrowheads*), which represent vessels surrounded by the dilated ducts, the "central dot" sign.

Choledocholithiasis

In most cases, stones within the bile duct migrate from the gallbladder. Calculi that primarily form within the bile ducts are relatively uncommon, and may be seen in patients with biliary strictures, cholangitis, choledochal cysts, or Caroli disease (4). A minority of patients with common duct stones are asymptomatic. More commonly, patients present with pain and jaundice, or possibly fever, if there is associated cholangitis.

Multiple noninvasive methods have been used for the diagnosis of calculi in the bile ducts, including sonography, unenhanced CT, enhanced CT, CT with oral or intravenous biliary contrast agents, and MRCP. As previously noted, sonography is often used as the first-line imaging modality in patients with suspected choledocholithiasis. However, sonography of the common duct is particularly limited by operator dependence. Although the reported sensitivity of ultrasound in the detection of choledocholithiasis is as high as 77% (97), the distal CBD may be obscured by overlying bowel gas, and a small stone in a nondilated duct can be missed (249). Cronan found that the sensitivity of sonography was higher in the proximal common duct than in its distal segment (40). Despite the availability of newer techniques, such as harmonic imaging, a normal sonogram still does not reliably exclude the diagnosis of choledocholithiasis (185,249).

Although CT is usually not performed specifically to diagnose choledocholithiasis, CT has demonstrated sufficient sensitivity and specificity to warrant its use as a screening test, particularly in patients in whom ERCP is contraindicated. In a study comparing unenhanced helical CT with sonography and ERCP, Pickuth and Spielmann found that unenhanced CT had a sensitivity of 86% and a specificity of 98% for the detection of common duct calculi (193). In another study by Neitlich et al. (179), unenhanced CT achieved a sensitivity and specificity of 88% and 97%, respectively, whereas Cuenca et al. (43) found a CT sensitivity of 80% and a specificity of 100%. In their series, the most common CT appearance of choledocolithiasis was a high-density calcification within the duct (Fig. 13-32) (43). A focal soft tissue density surrounded by bile or a high-attenuation ring surrounded by bile was seen less commonly.

When unenhanced CT is performed specifically to assess for choledocholithiasis, initial localizer scans are obtained to determine the level for subsequent imaging. Next, 5-mm images are obtained from above the gallbladder fossa through the bottom of the uncinate process of the pancreas in a single breath-hold. The data set is then reconstructed at 1-mm intervals. Reformatted multiplanar, maximum intensity projection, and shaded surface display images also may be generated in selected cases. Oral contrast should be withheld, as it may reduce the conspicuity of distal common duct calculi. As noted previously, the potential role of CT in conjunction with biliary contrast agents, so-called CT cholangiography, remains unclear, although some

investigators have achieved promising results. In a study of 101 patients who received the cholangiographic agent iotroxic acid intravenously, Giadas et al. achieved a 95.5% sensitivity for detection of ductal calculi (29).

MRCP has shown good sensitivity (86% to 100%) and specificity (85% to 100%) for ductal stones, relative to ERCP (48,147,149,150,158,227,246,247). The stones are detected as focal round or linear low signal voids partially or completely surrounded by high T2 signal bile within the ducts (62) (Fig. 13-33). An impacted stone may not be completely surrounded by bile, and it may simulate a stricture (21). Occasionally, intrahepatic biliary calculi may be detected on MRCP (127,224), and MRCP is significantly more sensitive than ERCP for intrahepatic calculi (97% versus 59%) (119).

The bile ducts are normally visible on MRCP in nonobstructed patients, but ductal stones are easily seen in the setting of biliary dilatation with a sensitivity and specificity of 94% and 93%, respectively (94). The thin-slice sequences are best for stone detection because the thick-slab images may obscure the stone due to volume averaging (34). However, some studies have shown similar ability of thick-slab HASTE and RARE compared with thin-slice imaging in the detection of ductal stones (226).

A limitation of MRCP for ductal stones relates to false positive findings due to artifacts. Air bubbles, clot, polyps, metal, and flow related artifacts may simulate duct calculi (85). In some cases, questionable findings on T2-weighted MRCP images may be answered with T1-weighted images. For instance, metal may have "bloom" artifact on T1 due to metal susceptibility artifact. The similar appearance of these other findings to ductal calculi may limit the usefulness of positive findings, but a negative study may preclude the need for invasive ERCP (63,257).

Cholangitis

Acute cholangitis usually results from bacterial infection of an obstructed biliary tree. Left untreated, acute cholangitis may be life-threatening by itself or lead to the formation of hepatic abscesses. Bacteria reach the obstructed bile ducts in retrograde fashion from the gastrointestinal tract or via the portal venous system (82). Imaging is usually directed toward identifying the source of obstruction or infection rather than making the diagnosis. Thickening of the bile duct may be seen with sonography, CT, or MRI, and contrast-enhanced CT or MRI may demonstrate mural enhancement (Fig. 13-34). In addition, Arai et al. found nodular, patchy, wedge-shaped, or geographic areas of heterogeneous arterial phase enhancement in 11 of 13 patients with acute cholangitis (13). Notably, these changes either decreased or resolved after treatment. MRCP may demonstrate irregularity and beading of the intrahepatic bile ducts (Fig. 13-35).

The term *Mirizzi syndrome* refers to obstruction of the CBD or CHD, usually in the setting of gallbladder neck

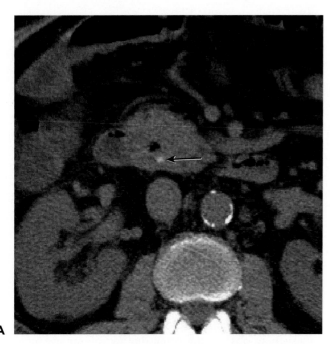

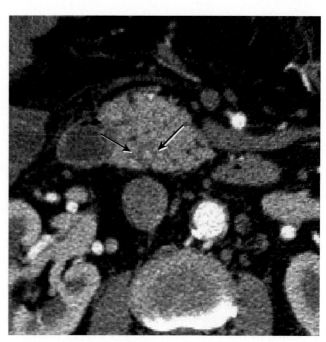

A

B

Figure 13-32 Choledocolithiasis. **A:** Noncontrast computed tomography through the level of the pancreatic head demonstrates a focal calcification within the distal CBD common bile duct (*arrow*). **B:** Contrast-enhanced computed tomography of the same region shows the calcification with an adjacent rim of lower-density bile (*arrows*), consistent with a bile duct stone (the crescent sign).

or cystic duct obstruction by one or more impacted stones (2). The propensity for the syndrome is enhanced in patients in whom the cystic duct parallels the CHD (153). Since the syndrome's original description, the definition has been expanded to include variants in which stones pass into the CHD via a cholecystocholedochal fistula (42). Patients typically present with obstructive jaundice, often with abdominal pain and fever. Both sonography and CT can demonstrate the impacted stone or stones as well as intrahepatic biliary dilatation and a normal caliber common duct below the site of obstruction (Fig. 13-36) (2).

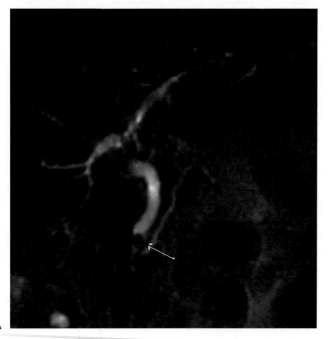

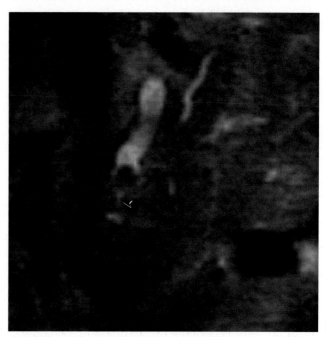

A

B

Figure 13-33 Choledocolithiasis. **A:** Thick-slab T2-weighted magnetic resonance cholangiopancreatography of the biliary system depicts a round signal void (*arrow*) in the distal duct within the hyperintense bile. **B:** Thin-slice T2-weighted magnetic resonance imaging MRI shows the normal caliber of the duct (*arrowhead*) distal to the stone.

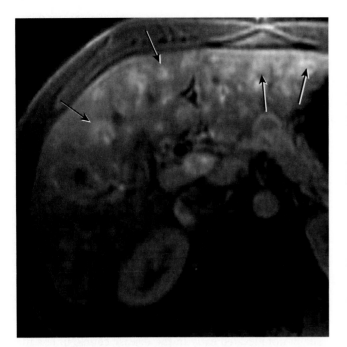

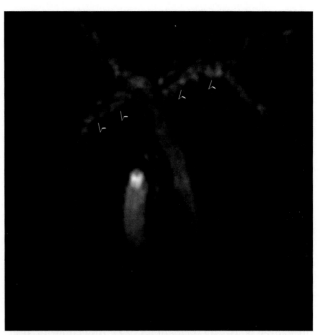

Figure 13-34 Cholangitis. Contrast-enhanced T1-weighted magnetic resonance image of the liver shows bright enhancement of the intrahepatic biliary radicals (*arrows*), consistent with biliary inflammation.

Figure 13-35 Cholangitis. Thick-slab magnetic resonance cholangiopancreatography shows irregularity of the intrahepatic bile ducts (*arrowheads*).

Recurrent Pyogenic Hepatitis

Formerly known as *oriental cholangiohepatitis*, recurrent pyogenic hepatitis is characterized by intra- and extrahepatic pigment stones, with resultant episodes of pyogenic

cholangitis (83). The disease is endemic to Southeast Asia, but is being seen with increasing frequency in the United States and other countries with large numbers of Southeast Asian immigrants. Patients present with recurrent attacks of abdominal pain accompanied by jaundice and fever.

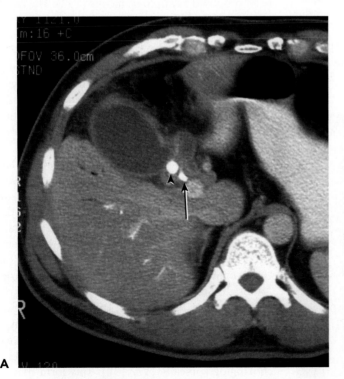

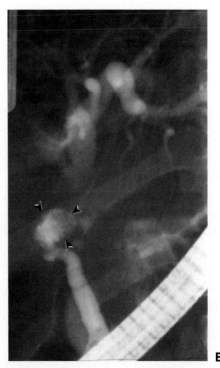

Figure 13-36 Mirizzi syndrome. **A:** Contrast-enhanced computed tomography of the gallbladder fossa shows a calculus in the cystic duct (*arrowhead*) adjacent to a common duct stent (*arrow*). **B:** Endoscopic retrograde cholangiopancreatography demonstrates a round filling defect in the cystic duct (*arrowheads*) and mild proximal biliary dilatation.

Pathologically, the affected bile ducts are dilated and contain multiple, soft, pigmented calculi and pus (144). CT or sonography may demonstrate multiple intra- or extrahepatic calculi and varying degrees of intrahepatic bile duct dilatation, which may be mild or segmental (145).

AIDS Cholangiopathy

AIDS cholangiopathy is a complication of AIDS. The symptoms are nonspecific, and patients present with abdominal pain, nausea, fever and jaundice. Most commonly, the causative organism is cryptosporidium, a parasite that causes only mild symptoms in hosts with intact immune systems. However, in immunocompromised patients, cryptosporidium may cause wasting and diarrhea (169). In some patients, CMV can be a secondary cause of AIDS cholangiopathy (71). Sonography may demonstrate biliary dilatation, mural thickening involving the gallbladder or bile ducts (Fig. 13-37), and increased echogenicity adjacent to the ducts (206,222). However, the gallbladder thickening is usually incidental (222). An echogenic nodule at the distal CBD, thought to represent an edematous papilla, has also been described (45). The CT appearance mirrors the appearance on ultrasound, with mural wall thickening and thickening of the gallbladder wall (71). Unfortunately, however, treatment options are limited.

Primary Sclerosing Cholangitis

PSC is a chronic cholestatic liver disease, which is characterized by inflammation, destruction, and fibrosis of the bile ducts (84,110,177). The smaller intrahepatic biliary radicals are obliterated, and the larger ducts develop irregular strictures. Eventually, these changes lead to the development of cirrhosis, portal hypertension, and liver failure.

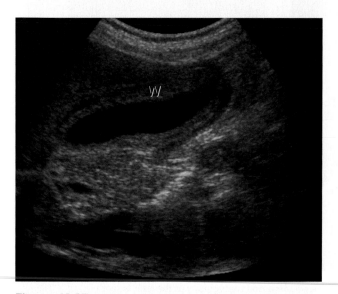

Figure 13-37 AIDS cholangiopathy. Grayscale ultrasound of the gallbladder shows diffuse symmetric gallbladder wall thickening (W) without gallstones.

Most PSC patients are male, and most have associated inflammatory bowel disease, typically ulcerative colitis or Crohn disease (5,84,110). There is also an association with other forms of fibrosis, including retroperitoneal and mediastinal fibrosis (19). Because symptoms usually develop insidiously, it is difficult to determine the precise age of onset, however the diagnosis is usually made late in the third or in the fourth decade (5,84). Patients usually present with pruritus, which may be more symptomatic at night and during warm weather (137). Steatorrhea, malabsorption of fat-soluble vitamins, osteoporosis, and cholangitis may also develop. As noted, cirrhosis and its manifestations may eventually ensue (as discussed later). Patients with PSC also have an increased incidence of cholangiocarcinoma, which is discussed in the section on malignant biliary neoplasm.

Although biochemical abnormalities are commonly found in patients with PSC, these findings are never diagnostic (138). The serum alkaline phosphatase and aminotransferase levels are usually elevated. Serum albumin is usually not elevated early in the disease course unless the patient also has active inflammatory bowel disease. Bilirubin levels are usually normal early on, but rise subsequently. Increased serum and hepatic copper levels are other features of PSC and are thought to reflect cholestasis (84,138). The majority of patients with PSC also exhibit antineutrophic cytoplasmic antibodies.

The cause of PSC remains speculative, although various factors that cause recurring injury to the bile ducts have been proposed as etiologic factors (138). The close association of PSC with ulcerative colitis has led some investigators to suggest that portal bacteremia or exposure to other toxins may play a role; however, little supportive evidence has been found for this theory (178). More recently, various genetic and immunological causes have been suggested. In particular, human leukocyte antigen profiles that have been associated with various autoimmune conditions, such as insulin-dependent diabetes mellitus and myasthenia gravis, have also been associated with PSC (245).

Liver biopsy is generally recommended for staging of PSC (177). Pathologically, the affected bile ducts show areas of mural fibrous thickening which alternate with segments of saccular or tubular dilatation (177). Varying degrees of inflammatory infiltration are seen within the ductal wall. As the disease progresses, there is more involvement of the adjacent hepatocytes, which leads to the final, cirrhotic stage. Unfortunately, treatment options are few and ineffective. Although orthotopic liver transplantation has been attempted, clinically significant PSC is likely to recur (128).

Several variants of PSC have been described. In so-called small bile duct PSC, also sometimes referred to a *pericholangitis*, the affected ducts are too small to be imaged cholangiographically (177,138). This form may occur in isolation in patients with ulcerative colitis or in association with large-duct PSC. As well, secondary forms of sclerosing cholangitis are being diagnosed with increasing frequency in a wide range of conditions, including immunodeficiency (severe combined form immunodeficiency or HIV), ischemia, drug toxicity, and recurrent cholangitis. There is another group of PSC patients in whom autoantibodies are found in the serum and who have histopathologic features of autoimmune hepatitis, termed the *autoimmune hepatitis and PSC overlap syndrome* (84,177). This variant is more common in children.

Chemotherapy-induced cholangitis is a specific form of secondary sclerosing cholangitis that is seen in patients who receive intra-arterial infusion of chemotherapeutic agents for metastatic colorectal cancer, particularly floxuridine. Effects on the bile ducts represent either direct toxicity or ischemia, and manifest radiologically as intra- or extrahepatic bile duct stenoses, which may worsen the prognosis of the underlying metastatic disease (8,254).

Imaging of Primary Sclerosing Cholangitis

Cholangiography remains the gold standard for the diagnosis of PSC. ERCP is generally preferred over direct, percutaneous cholangiography because the attenuated bile ducts may be difficult to cannulate percutaneously (138). Early in the disease process, the affected extrahepatic bile ducts may show only mild mural irregularity or nodularity (84,138,194). Subsequently, the characteristic findings include multifocal intra- and extrahepatic bile duct strictures with intervening normal or dilated segments, resulting in a so-called pruned and beaded appearance (Fig. 13-38). Multiple diverticulumlike outpouchings are another late finding (194).

For the most part, the CT appearance of PSC mirrors the cholangiographic findings. In a study of 20 patients with PSC by Teefey et al., CT demonstrated nodularity of the extrahepatic duct, pruning of the intrahepatic ducts, and stenosis and dilatation in both regions (238). However, neither pruning nor beading are specific for PSC because these findings are also present in patients with other types of benign and malignant biliary obstruction (239).

Interestingly, the hepatic morphologic abnormalities in PSC, which have generally been described as similar to those found in other forms of cirrhosis, do appear to be different, and may facilitate the diagnosis in patients with advanced cirrhosis (49). These findings include marked lobulation of the liver contour, atrophy of the posterior and lateral segments (30), and hypertrophy of the caudate. As well, the hypertrophied caudate lobe may be higher in attenuation than the rest of the liver on unenhanced scans, creating the appearance of a pseudotumor (Fig. 13-39).

Magnetic Resonance Imaging of Primary Sclerosing Cholangitis

The typical MRI findings of PSC include biliary strictures involving the intrahepatic or extrahepatic bile ducts, diverticula with beaded appearance of the ducts, webs, ductal stones, and duct irregularity (Fig. 13-40) (253). Ernst et al. noted peripheral ductal dilatation that did not communicate with central ducts due to strictures (53). There may be wall thickening or abnormal wall enhancement on contrast-enhanced T1-weighted images (102). The sensitivity and specificity of MRCP for PSC are 85% to 100%, and 92% to 100%, respectively (53,64).

Dilatation and good visualization of the peripheral ducts on MRCP are considered abnormal and are due to

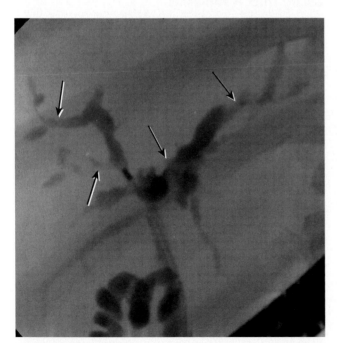

Figure 13-38 Primary sclerosing cholangitis. Endoscopic retrograde cholangiopancreatography shows multifocal strictures (*arrows*) involving the intrahepatic and extrahepatic biliary ducts.

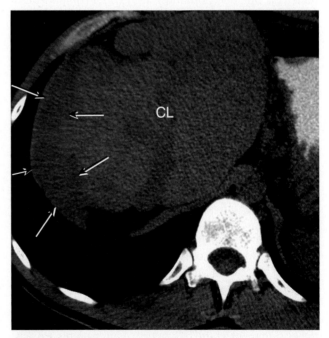

Figure 13-39 Primary sclerosing cholangitis with pseudotumor of caudate lobe. On a noncontrast computed tomography image, the massively enlarged caudate lobe (CL) appears slightly denser than the adjacent liver parenchyma (*arrows*).

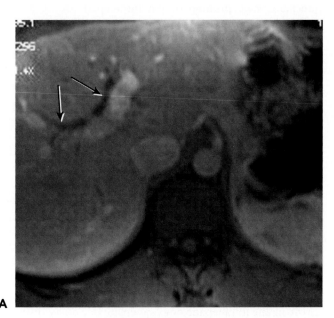

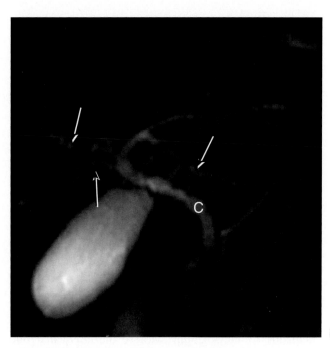

Figure 13-40 Primary sclerosing cholangitis. **A:** Contrast-enhanced T1-weighted images of the liver show intrahepatic biliary dilatation (*arrows*). **B:** Thick-slab magnetic resonance cholangiopancreatography shows multifocal strictures with a "beaded" appearance of the intrahepatic ducts (*arrows*). The common duct (C) is irregular, but has a normal caliber.

multiple strictures. In one study, the intrasegmental and peripheral ducts were more often visible in PSC patients than in a control group (86% versus 9%, and 67% versus 0%, respectively) (252). Furthermore, a proximal stricture in the setting of PSC may limit the visualization of the extrahepatic bile ducts on MRCP (251). In a comparison of MRCP and ERCP, the most common reason for disagreement between the modalities is a stricture suspected on MRCP that is not identified on ERCP (251).

Parasitic Infection of the Bile Ducts

Parasitic infection of the biliary tree is uncommonly encountered in North America, but is seen in endemic areas such as Southeast Asia. Intestinal ascariasis is caused by *Ascaris lumbricoides*, which is the most common cause of human helminthic infestation (98). The infection generally has a benign course, but worms may enter the biliary tree via the ampulla of Vater (6) and cause cholangitis and, rarely, liver abscesses. The CT appearance is nonspecific, but sonography may demonstrate tubular structures within the bile ducts or gallbladder. A similar appearance has been reported at MRCP (58,98). Dead worms may also act as a nidus for stone formation, usually in the gallbladder, the CBD, or the left intrahepatic ducts.

The liver flukes *Clinorchis sinensis* and *Opisthorchis viverrini* also may infect the biliary tree. As in patients with ascariasis, mild infections may go unnoticed. However, heavy infestations can lead to worms within the gallbladder, the extrahepatic bile ducts, and the pancreas (120). At CT, the diagnosis may be suspected in the presence of mild, extrahepatic biliary dilatation, enlargement of the body and/or tail of the pancreas, and small, peripherally enhancing cysts within the pancreas.

Biliary Duct Neoplasms

The bile ducts give rise to a variety of benign and malignant tumors, of which cholangiocarcinoma is the most common. Other bile duct neoplasms, including cystadenoma, adenoma, and papilloma, are encountered far less frequently, and will be discussed subsequently.

Cholangiocarcinoma

Cholangiocarcinoma is a malignant neoplasm that arises from cholangiocytes, which form the epithelial lining of the bile ducts (72). The vast majority are adenocarcinomas, although several other histologic subtypes have been described (263). The tumor is most commonly found in older patients, with 65% older than age 65 years (117). Although still relatively uncommon, there has been a recent increase in the incidence of cholangiocarcinoma (72). Between 1973 and 1997, the incidence and mortality rates increased markedly, with an estimated annual change of 9.11% and 9.44%, respectively (190).

Although the etiology of cholangiocarcinoma remains uncertain, a number of conditions have been identified as predisposing factors (35). Of these, PSC has the strongest association. Occult cholangiocarcinoma is found in up to 40% of autopsy specimens in PSC patients (1,27,36,207).

The incidence of cholangiocarcinoma is also increased in patients with biliary cystic disease, including choledochal cysts and Caroli disease, presumably because of chronic biliary inflammation (47). Patients with parasitic infections of the bile ducts, particularly *C. sinensis*, are also at higher risk for cholangiocarcinoma, as are patients with recurrent pyogenic hepatitis, chronic typhoid carriers, and patients with a history of Thorotrast exposure (35,117).

The common thread linking these risk factors to cholangiocarcinoma appears to be chronic inflammation, which is also associated with tumors in other parts of the gastrointestinal tract (72). Cytokines released by cholangiocytes and inflammatory cells cause the cholangiocytes to express inducible nitric oxide synthase, which generates nitric oxide, leading to DNA damage (104). Interleukin-6, another cytokine, also appears to play an important role as a mitogenic agent (187).

Clinical Aspects and Classification of Cholangiocarcinoma

Cholangiocarcinoma can arise from any point in the biliary epithelium, from the intrahepatic biliary radicals to the ampulla of Vater (35,80,136). Because the behavior of cholangiocarcinoma is in part related to its site of origin within the biliary tree, the most commonly employed classification scheme divides tumors into intra- and extrahepatic types.

Intrahepatic cholangiocarcinoma is further classified into peripheral and perihilar subtypes, with the former arising peripheral to the second bifurcation of the right or left hepatic duct (80,136). Perihilar cholangiocarcinomas, which arise at the confluence of the hepatic ducts, commonly known as *Klatskin tumors*, are the most common type of these tumors, comprising up to 60% of the total (35,117). Together, intrahepatic and perihilar tumors comprise approximately 75% to 80% of the total. Extrahepatic lesions, which arise along the CHD or CBD, make up the remainder, and are subdivided by their level along the common duct (upper, middle, or lower third). Some authors consider perihilar and extrahepatic cholangiocarcinomas as a single entity, since they tend to have similar growth patterns (72,80,136).

To a large extent, the clinical presentation of cholangiocarcinoma depends on its level of origin. Tumors with resultant biliary obstruction will cause painless jaundice, which is seen in up to 90% of cases, and weight loss is seen in 50% (263). Right upper quadrant pain, fever, and chills suggest superimposed cholangitis (117). Peripheral, intrahepatic cholangiocarcinomas, on the other hand, present with signs and symptoms of a liver mass, including pain, weight loss, night sweats, and malaise (72). The serum alkaline phosphatase level is often elevated, but the bilirubin level is usually normal. While there are no specific tumor markers for cholangiocarcinoma, levels of cancer antigen 19-9, carcinoembryonic antigen, and cancer antigen 125 may be abnormal (72,117,242).

Growth Patterns and Approach to Diagnosis and Staging of Cholangiocarcinoma

In addition to location within the biliary tract, growth pattern plays an important role in determining the imaging appearance of cholangiocarcinoma in a given patient. Four types of growth pattern have been described (136). The exophytic form, in which the tumor grows outside of the bile ducts and forms a mass, is the most common pattern encountered in peripheral cholangiocarcinomas (80,136). An infiltrative pattern, which is characterized by desmoplastic tumor that grows along and engulfs bile ducts and blood vessels, is more typical of perihilar and extrahepatic tumors (72,136). This pattern of direct spread occurs in more than 70% of perihilar lesions (80). A polypoid growth pattern, with predominantly intraluminal growth, is seen in a minority of intra- and extrahepatic cholangiocarcinomas. Finally, a combined growth pattern has also been described (136).

In patients who present with a peripheral hepatic mass, a pathologic diagnosis of cholangiocarcinoma can usually be obtained by percutaneous biopsy under CT or ultrasound guidance. Infiltrative tumors present more of a diagnostic challenge because the tumor often extends along the submucosal space (72). Bile sampling for cytology can be performed in conduction with ERCP or PTC, but is positive in only 30% of cases; combining brush cytology with biopsy increases the yield to 40% to 70% (117). Despite diligent effort, however, a pathologic diagnosis may not be feasible in some patients, and the diagnosis must be based on a composite of clinical criteria (72).

The goal of initial imaging in patients with suspected or known cholangiocarcinoma is to determine suitability for surgical resection, which currently offers the only possibility of cure. Although there is a tumor, node, metastasis (TNM) staging system for cholangiocarcinoma, it is not reliable for clinical assessment or prediction of survival (72,263). Another staging scheme devised by Bismuth classifies perihilar tumors by the degree of involvement of the right and left hepatic ducts, which is useful for surgical planning (24,210). Assessment of the extent of vascular involvement is also critical, as is the exclusion of metastatic disease to the liver, lymph nodes, or peritoneum. Because primary malignancies arising in other organs, notably the pancreas, stomach, breast, lung, and colon, may mimic cholangiocarcinoma, imaging may be required to exclude these possibilities if the diagnosis is in doubt (117).

Computed Tomography of Cholangiocarcinoma

The CT appearance of cholangiocarcinoma largely depends on its site of origin. Peripheral, mass-forming tumors appear as low attenuation lesions on unenhanced CT, with incomplete rim enhancement on arterial and portal venous phase images (Fig. 13-41) (60,80,118). A low-attenuation appearance of the mass without arterial phase enhancement is seen less frequently (244). Rarely, cholangiocarcinoma shows marked enhancement in the arterial

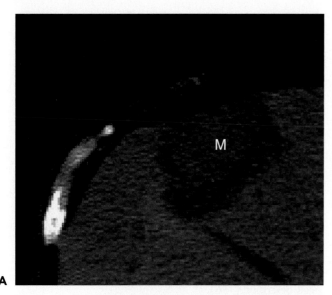
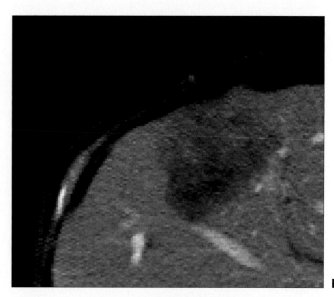

A
B

Figure 13-41 Intrahepatic cholangiocarcinoma. **A:** Noncontrast computed tomography (CT) image shows a heterogeneous, hypodense mass (M) without calcifications. **B:** Portal venous phase CT image shows mild enhancement.

phase (265). As noted previously, cholangiocarcinoma may exhibit delayed enhancement, which has been attributed to contrast diffusion into the interstitial space within the fibrous stroma (115,244) (Fig. 13-42). This pattern is variable, with a reported frequency ranging from 36% to 70% (115,152,244). However, when delayed enhancement occurs, it may permit a presumptive diagnosis of cholangiocarcinoma. Other ancillary CT findings of peripheral intrahepatic cholangiocarcinoma include regional lymphadenopathy, biliary dilatation, satellite nodules, and retraction of the liver capsule (80,244).

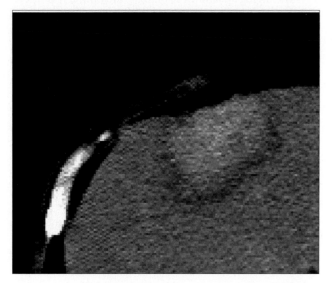

Figure 13-42 Intrahepatic cholangiocarcinoma. Computed tomography image of the same patient as in Figure 13-41 after a 10-minute delay shows retention of contrast in the mass, which is clearly denser than the adjacent liver.

In contrast to the mass-forming type of intrahepatic cholangiocarcinoma, intraductal tumors are characterized by segmentally-dilated bile ducts which are higher in attenuation than normal bile (80,133) (Fig. 13-43). These tumors are usually papillary adenocarcinomas and have a better prognosis than other types of cholangiocarcinoma (133,264). Notably, lesions that secrete large amounts of mucin are associated with ductal dilatation both proximal and distal to the tumor. Detection of the obstructing mass itself depends on its size, with masses larger than 1 cm being visible on CT.

Perihilar and extrahepatic cholangiocarcinomas typically exhibit an infiltrating growth pattern (80,136,240). These neoplasms are characterized by focal, circumferential thickening of the bile duct with proximal dilatation, which may be seen sonographically or at thin-section CT (Fig. 13-44). Conspicuity of perihilar cholangiocarcinoma is highest on arterial phase images (240). Occasionally, perihilar lesions may be similar in appearance to the intrahepatic, mass-forming type of cholangiocarcinoma, or may manifest as an intraluminal polypoid mass (80,136).

The diagnosis of cholangiocarcinoma in patients with PSC can be particularly challenging. At cholangiography, dominant benign strictures are often difficult to distinguish from malignant strictures, although progressive biliary dilatation on serial studies suggests complicating cholangiocarcinoma (32). Because of its ability to depict tumor masses, particularly those that invade the liver parenchyma, CT is helpful to monitor patients with PSC.

The role of positron emission tomography (PET) imaging in screening for cholangiocarcinoma or staging patients with known or suspected cholangiocarcinoma has yet to be determined, however, the technique shows promise.

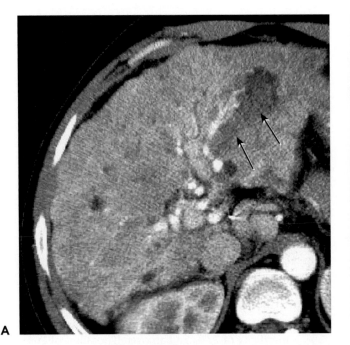

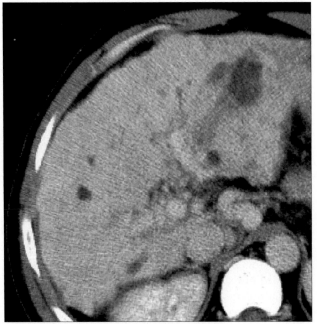

A   B

Figure 13-43 Intrahepatic cholangiocarcinoma. **A:** Contrast-enhanced computed tomography of the liver shows biliary dilatation with dense material (*arrows*) filling the bile ducts in the left hepatic lobe. **B:** Delayed image demonstrates persistent high density in this region.

In one study, visual analysis of ^{18}F-flurodeoxyglucose-PET images showed a sensitivity of 92% and a specificity of 93% in the diagnosis of 26 patients with cholangiocarcinoma, including 4 with underlying PSC (121). In this study, PET was also helpful to diagnose distant metastases, but it was not useful for the detection of regional lymph node involvement.

A variant malignancy which combines elements of cholangiocarcinoma and hepatocellular carcinoma (HCC) also deserves mention (70). This unusual neoplasm, which

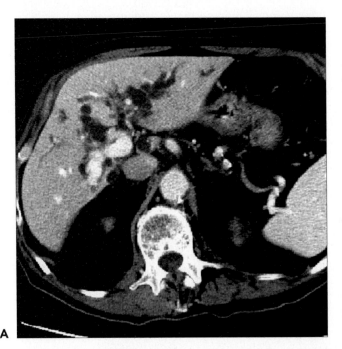

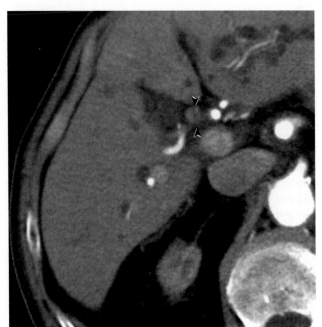

A   B

Figure 13-44 Extrahepatic cholangiocarcinoma. **A:** Contrast-enhanced computed tomography (CT) scan through the liver shows extensive intrahepatic ductal dilatation. **B:** Contrast-enhanced CT at the level of the liver hilum shows a short segment of a concentrically thickened common bile duct with mural enhancement (*arrowheads*).

comprises less than 5% of primary hepatic malignancies, behaves more like HCC clinically (52). Most patients with this type of tumor have cirrhosis or chronic hepatitis B or C, and the serum alpha-fetoprotein is elevated in most cases. At CT, combined cholangiocarcinoma-HCC exhibits imaging features of both types of tumor. These features include areas of arterial phase enhancement that appear hypodense on portal venous phase or delayed images, as well as areas that exhibit the commonly seen delayed hyperattenation and capsular retraction associated with cholangiocarcinoma.

Magnetic Resonance Imaging of Cholangiocarcinoma

MRI may show a low T1 signal lesion, and there may be increased enhancement on delayed images, as seen on CT. The lesion should be hyperintense on T2-weighted sequences (3,55,76,229,250) (Fig. 13-45). Occasionally, a thickened bile duct wall is visualized, and the wall of the duct may demonstrate abnormal enhancement. A wall thickness greater than 5 mm has been suggested to correlate with a malignant rather than a benign cause of obstructive jaundice (214). However, cholangitis may also cause thickening of the bile duct wall. For surgical planning, MRCP may depict the cranial extent of the mass (135) and determine whether both lobes of the liver are involved.

Unusual Bile Duct Tumors

Benign tumors of the bile ducts, mostly biliary adenomas or papillomas, are uncommon. Multifocal biliary papillomas, also known as biliary papillomatosis, are characterized by multiple polypoid filling defects within the bile ducts. CT, MRCP, and sonography may demonstrate a dilated biliary tree with endoluminal masses or poorly defined filling defects (156). Although they are benign, these neoplasms have a malignant potential (88).

Biliary cystadenomas are uncommon cystic lesions of the biliary tree. The typical CT appearance is a multilocular cystic mass with a well-defined capsule and mural nodules (173) (Fig. 13-46). Polypoid excrescences are suggestive of malignant transformation (23).

Biliary hamartomas, also known as *Von Meyenburg complex of the liver*, are benign malformations of the bile ducts which present as small, cyst-like deformed bile ducts embedded within dense connective tissue (259). CT shows multiple, nonenhancing foci throughout both lobes of the liver (173). At MRI, the lesions are hypointense on T1-weighted images and hyperintense on T2-weighted sequences. As with CT, enhancement is usually not seen after the intravenous administration of gadolinium.

Nonbiliary Tumors That Affect the Biliary Tree

A wide variety of primary and secondary nonbiliary neoplasms affect the bile ducts. Among these, the most important are periampullary tumors that arise from the ampulla of Vater or the adjacent duodenum. Traditionally, these tumors have been grouped with distal CBD cholangiocarcinomas and adenocarcinomas arising in the pancreatic head because they typically present with biliary and pancreatic duct obstruction (Fig. 13-47). At present, surgical resection offers the only possibility of cure (96,205,219). Apart from establishing a definitive diagnosis, the goal of preoperative imaging in these patients is to determine if resectability is feasible.

Criteria that exclude the possibility of curative surgical resection include (a) hepatic or distant metastases, (b) invasion of the contiguous organs or mesentery (apart from the duodenum), and (c) obstruction, encasement, or invasion of the portal vein, the superior mesenteric–portal vein confluence, the celiac axis, or the superior mesenteric artery (96,205).

In a study of 21 patients with periampullary malignancy, Howard et al. found that helical CT had a sensitivity of 63%, a specificity of 100%, and an overall accuracy of 86% in determining respectability (96). EUS was more sensitive but less specific than CT, with a sensitivity of 75%, a specificity of 77%, and an overall accuracy of 76%. A later study by Shoup et al. found that EUS was superior to CT in detecting tumor and in predicting vascular invasion (219). They recommended helical CT as the initial imaging modality for staging periampullary tumors, with EUS reserved for patients with high clinical suspicion but no identifiable mass at CT or for patients with equivocal CT evidence for vascular invasion.

Metastatic disease from any source can also obstruct the intra- or extrahepatic bile ducts if they are located fortuitously (Fig. 13-48). Not surprisingly, the CT appearance of these lesions is nonspecific. In addition, there have been case reports of patients with benign, fibrotic masses at the hepatic hilum mimicking perihilar cholangiocarcinoma (86,248). However, the CT appearance of these lesions is also nonspecific, and a preoperative diagnosis of benign fibrosis is usually not possible.

Biliary Tract Surgery

Liver Transplant Evaluation

The preoperative evaluation of the biliary system for cadaveric liver transplantation is typically based upon laboratory values, and imaging is not routinely performed. In living donor liver transplantation (LDLT), however, an understanding of the hepatic anatomy is critical, and extensive imaging is often obtained to evaluate arterial, venous, and biliary anatomy and look for variants. Of these, anomalous biliary anatomy is more common than variants of the portal venous or hepatic arterial systems (236). Most of the variations can be identified during surgery and will not affect the procedure if properly considered (100). However, cholangiography is commonly performed during surgery to precisely determine the anatomy for division of the left duct. The hepatic artery branches that supply the

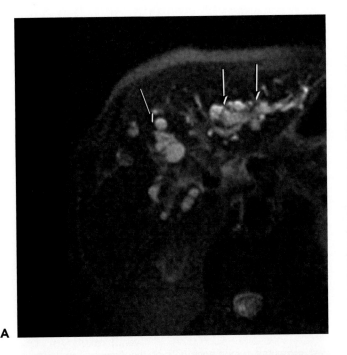

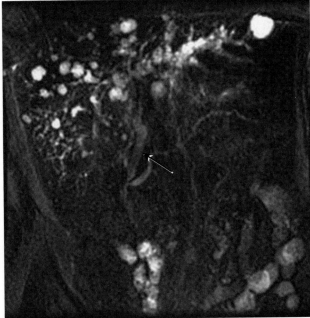

A

B

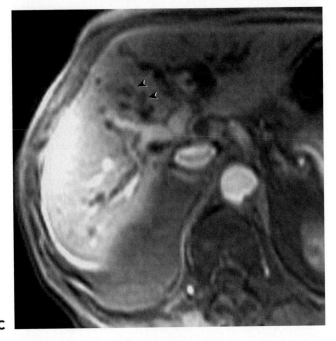

C

Figure 13-45 Magnetic resonance cholangiopancreatography (MRCP) of cholangiocarcinoma. **A:** Axial T2-weighted magnetic resonance image shows dilated intrahepatic ducts with homogenous high T2 signal (*arrows*). **B:** Coronal oblique thick-slab MRCP demonstrates extensive intrahepatic hyperintense T2 signal duct dilatation to the level of the hepatic hilum, with a normal caliber of the extrahepatic bile duct (*arrow*). **C:** Contrast-enhanced T1-weighted image of the liver shows low T1 signal in the dilated intrahepatic ducts (*arrowheads*).

ducts are also important because injury to the feeding artery may result in severe biliary necrosis. Although CT is useful for vascular delineation, preoperative CT is not sensitive for the biliary anatomy in the absence of biliary dilatation. Although uncommonly used, positive biliary contrast techniques allow CT imaging of the biliary system with intravenous biliary contrast (212).

After a patient has been approved to receive a liver transplant, significant time may pass before they receive a new liver. There is a significant wait-list for liver transplantation, and patients with liver disease may have extensive liver damage that can include biliary obstruction. If a liver allograft is not available, ERCP may be used to treat acute biliary problems, such as using balloon angioplasty for a stricture, until an organ is available. Drainage past strictures or removal of obstructing biliary stones are usually considered temporizing treatments in these patients.

Living Donor Liver Transplantation/Segmental Hepatectomy

LDLT has been used in the pediatric population with good success. In pediatric recipients, the lateral segment of the

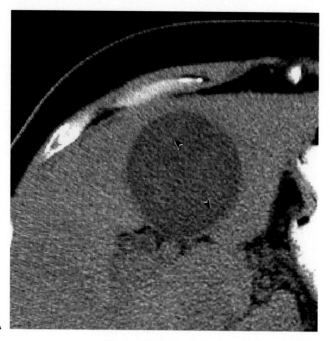

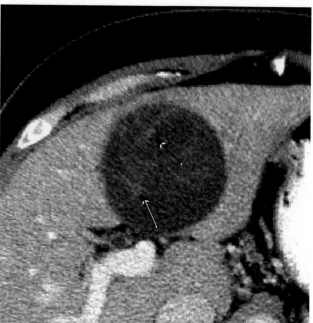

Figure 13-46 Biliary cystadenoma. **A:** Noncontrast computed tomography (CT) of the liver demonstrates a focal low-density mass with subtle septations (*arrowheads*). **B:** Contrast-enhanced CT shows enhancement of the septations (*arrows*), but no enhancement in the cystic components of the mass.

left hepatic lobe is removed from the donor and grafted to the hepatic vessels of the recipient. This procedure is more common in liver donation to a child, but the demands upon the liver in an adult are more substantial and will usually require right hepatic lobe transplantation (161). It is important to remember that an adequate amount of

liver must also remain to sustain the donor, so evaluation of the donor is critical.

The evaluation of the donor liver may involve a combination of multiple imaging modalities such as ultrasound, CT, MRI, MRCP, and angiography to evaluate different aspects of the liver. Of these, MRCP is best suited for

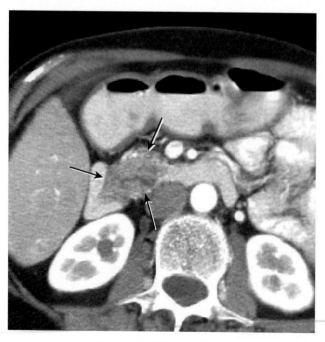

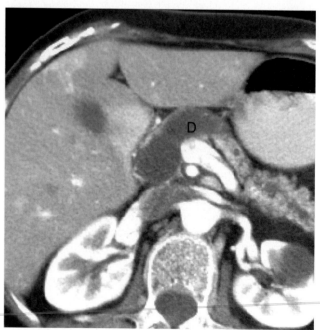

Figure 13-47 Ampullary mass. **A:** Hypodense irregular mass (*arrows*) in the region of the ampulla of Vater on contrast-enhanced computed tomography. **B:** Image through the level of the pancreas shows pancreatic ductal dilatation (D).

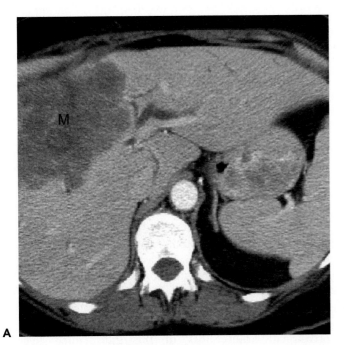

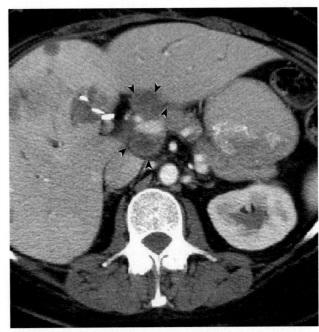

A   **B**

Figure 13-48 Colon carcinoma metastases causing biliary obstruction. **A:** Contrast- enhanced computed tomography (CT) shows intrahepatic biliary dilatation and a large, hypodense hepatic metastasis (M). **B:** CT image at the level of the common duct depicts multiple hypodense oval masses in the liver hilum and peripancreatic region (*arrowheads*).

evaluation of the biliary tree configuration. MRCP is helpful to detect variants in the biliary anatomy prior to surgery (61). MRI and MRCP may also detect any unsuspected biliary pathology within the donor that may preclude liver donation. The volume of the liver segments is evaluated by CT or MRI to ensure that adequate donated liver volume is available to the recipient (20,148). At the time of surgery, ultrasound may be helpful to identify the vascular anatomy and direct the location of the surgical resection plane.

Preoperative detection of a cholangiocarcinoma is an ominous finding in a patient waiting for liver transplant, even if a new liver is quickly found. It is considered a contraindication to transplantation because of a high recurrence rate in transplant recipients (201,208).

Postoperative Biliary Complications

Several possible complications of cholecystectomy involve the biliary system, and major bile duct injury is more common with laparoscopic cholecystectomy than open surgery (256). However, other studies have cited much lower rates of complications when intraoperative cholangiography is performed (59). Complications in these patients are due to mistaken identification of biliary structures (22,225). These complications include biliary injury, biliary stricture, and retained stones. Ultrasound is usually the initial imaging modality when a complication of surgery is a concern, but CT may also detect free fluid or a contained biloma (Fig. 13-49). However, biloma is rare after laparoscopic

cholecystectomy, occurring in less than 3% of patients (7,124,255).

Recently, there has been increasing usage of MRI to visualize the biliary ducts in patients with suspected biliary

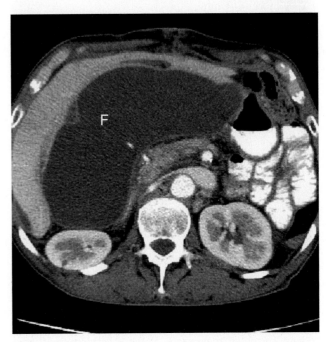

Figure 13-49 Complication of laparoscopic cholecystectomy. Contrast-enhanced computed tomography of the hepatic hilar region shows a large fluid collection (F), consistent with a biloma.

complications. The most common findings are biliary leak, retained biliary stones, and anastomotic stricture (116). Bile duct injury with biliary leak appears as hyperintense T2-weighted signal collections of bile within the liver or adjacent to the hepatic hilum on MRI, and occasionally the site of leakage can be identified (78). However, one study (39) showed that MRCP had difficulty differentiating complete bile duct transection from ductal occlusion. If MRCP is not available, intraoperative cholangiography is one alternative that may reduce the occurrence of or rapidly identify biliary complications associated with laparoscopic cholecystectomy (256).

Stricture is a common complication of biliary surgery. As many as 95% of benign biliary strictures occur as a sequela of surgery (131,143). MRCP is a noninvasive method to evaluate the extent of a stricture and to detect additional biliary abnormalities. Retained stones in the bile duct are another possible complication of cholecystectomy (Fig. 13-50). The stones are usually located in the CBD, but they may be found within intrahepatic bile ducts, as well.

Many biliary surgeries involve the creation of a biliary-enteric anastomosis, which may limit evaluation by ERCP. If there is suspicion of a biliary surgical complication, the bile ducts usually cannot be accessed endoscopically in these patients. MRCP allows noninvasive method of evaluation of the biliary system in these patients.

Liver Transplant Complications

In liver transplantation, the donor bile duct is anastomosed to the recipient common duct or to a loop of small

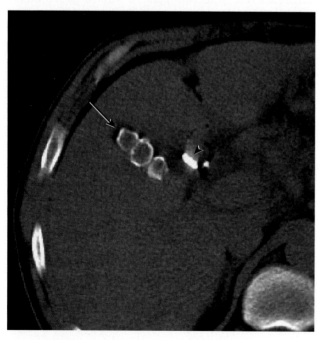

Figure 13-50 Retained gallstones after cholecystectomy. Noncontrast computed tomography of the gallbladder fossa after cholecystectomy shows multiple retained calcified gallstones (*arrow*). Note the adjacent cholecystectomy clip (*arrowhead*).

bowel. In most cases, a direct anastomosis is created between the donor and recipient bile ducts. Choledocojejunostomy is chosen if the recipient duct is too small or diseased (106,180). At the institution of these authors, a biliary T-tube is placed to allow easy evaluation of the ducts for early postoperative bile leak or stricture. The biliary tube is subsequently capped to allow internal drainage, and it is later removed.

Biliary complications are common within the recipient after cadaveric liver transplantation (181). As many as 15% to 19% of liver transplantation recipients experience a biliary complication (44,73,139,209,232). Typical complications include biliary leak, stricture, stone formation, or occasionally diffuse biliary necrosis. Early complications of liver transplantation are often related to surgical technique or local ischemia. They may be due to scarring, multifactorial causes, rejection, or cytomegalovirus infection (174). Bile leaks often occur early, but strictures may occur months after surgery (67). Although death is rare, biliary complications result in morbidity and may occasionally cause loss of the transplanted liver (14,17,73). In severe cases, diffuse biliary ischemia associated with arterial insufficiency may be catastrophic (Fig. 13-51) (269).

Doppler ultrasound should be the first imaging study if a transplant biliary abnormality is suspected. Biliary dilatation can be confidently detected by ultrasound, and the hepatic vessels may be evaluated for hepatic artery occlusion. Ultrasound may also detect perihepatic or hilar fluid collections. A biloma will appear as a hypoechoic or anechoic collection adjacent to the liver. Likewise, MRCP and CT may be useful to detect biliary dilatation or bile leaks, but these modalities are not commonly performed as the initial imaging study. Hepatic 2,6-dimethyl-iminodiacetic acid scan can detect leaks, but it is not sensitive for stricture. If there is suspicion of a stricture or stone, ERCP may allow therapeutic intervention. If sepsis develops, percutaneous decompression of the biliary system is often necessary by ERCP. PTC with drain or stent placement may also be used to relieve the obstruction. The procedure is invasive, but may be used in combination with antibiotics to improve the patient's condition until a liver allograft becomes available. Ultrasound is often requested to provide marking or direct guidance for liver biopsy, which may be used to diagnose ischemia or rejection.

Bile leak after transplantation may appear as a focal collection in the liver hilum that is low-density on CT or low T1 signal and high T2 signal on MRI. The fluid can track away from the liver if it is large (Fig. 13-52). The point of early leakage, usually at the T-tube site (198), can be demonstrated on MRCP images. Leaks may also occur from the cystic duct closure in the donor or recipient duct. Delayed leaks most commonly occur at the anastomotic site (186), and biliary stenosis at the anastomosis may be a

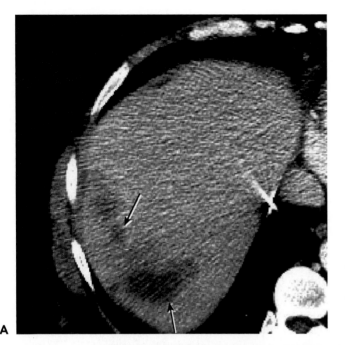
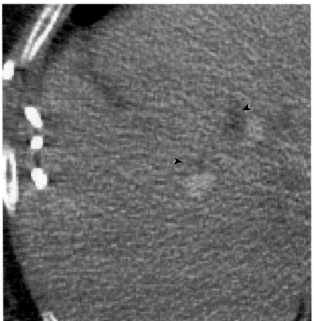

Figure 13-51 Biliary necrosis. **A:** Contrast-enhanced computed tomography of the liver after liver transplantation shows poor enhancement of the parenchyma with multiple areas of low-density necrosis in the liver periphery (*arrows*). **B:** Small areas of low-density necrosis (*arrowheads*) involve the biliary regions adjacent to the portal venous branches. Hepatic artery thrombosis was confirmed by Doppler ultrasound.

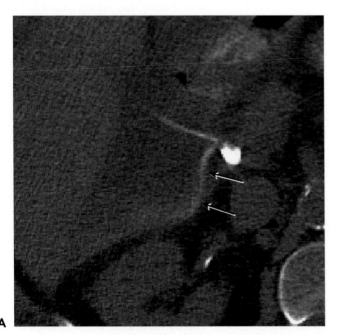
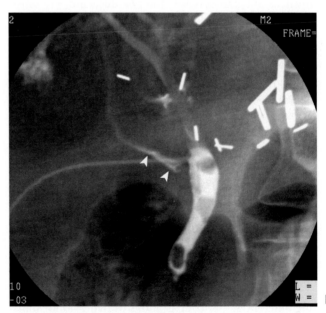

Figure 13-52 Biliary leak after liver transplantation. **A:** Noncontrast computed tomography shows a low-density perihepatic collection with a dense "waterfall" of opacified contrast (*arrows*) from the bile duct. **B:** T-tube cholangiogram depicts a similar tract of dense contrast (*arrowheads*) extending from the bile duct at the site of the T-tube insertion. Note the filling defects of retained bile duct stones in the recipient portion of the bile duct.

sequela of previous bile leak (11). If leakage is present, ERCP can be performed to place a stent across the point of extravasation. Removable plastic internal stents are left across the point of leakage for approximately 2 weeks (186). Occasionally, biliary collections require drainage catheter decompression, and ultrasound or CT may be employed to guide the procedure (218).

Dilatation of the bile ducts after liver transplantation should suggest biliary stenosis or occlusion. However, biliary stenosis may not create ductal dilatation in the transplanted liver, even if there is biliary obstruction caused by a significant stenosis (198). Active distention of the biliary ducts by PTC or ERCP may detect a stenosis that is not apparent on CT or MRI (198). Biliary stenosis may result from ductal injury during surgery or prolonged cold storage prior to transplantation (211).

In contrast, biliary dilatation is not always caused by stenosis. Dilatation of the duct also may result from Sphincter of Oddi dysfunction, possibly due to denervation of the duct (195). Other causes of biliary dilatation include biliary stone and sludge formation (114). Stones may form in the ducts as a result of stasis or infection or possibly the effects of cyclosporin A on the bile (168). Rarely, a mucocele may extrinsically compress and obstruct the common duct (54). In patients transplanted for PSC, recurrence of the original disease process may have an imaging appearance similar to the original disease with strictures and areas of biliary dilatation on CT or MRCP.

Bile duct ischemia and necrosis is often severe and threatens allograft survival. The bile ducts are very sensitive to ischemia and depend solely on hepatic arterial blood supply (103,269). Acute arterial occlusion can be life threatening and requires retransplantation. Partial thrombosis may result in strictures or biliary necrosis (89). Biliary necrosis may result in bile leak or abscess formation (93,111). Ultrasound is generally the first screening study to suggest hepatic arterial thrombosis by demonstrating decreased arterial flow or poststenotic waveforms on color and spectral Doppler imaging. There may be irregular biliary dilatation with communication to small bilomas on grayscale images. CT may show focal perfusional defects if the arterial thrombosis is segmental (89). However, the diagnosis is usually confirmed with angiography or at surgical exploration.

Living Donor Transplant Complications

LDLT is a subset of liver transplantation that has similar complications to cadaveric transplantation with some specific differences. The complications of living donor transplantation may simultaneously affect two individuals. In some cases, the donor can develop complications of the procedure and require additional surgery. Bile leak from the resected surface of the liver in the donor may cause biloma formation or peritonitis (186).

The complications in the recipient are similar to recipients of cadaveric livers, but occur more frequently (65).

In the recipient, biliary leak is the most common immediate complication and may occur at the liver edge or anastomosis (65).

Unlike cadaveric transplants, the biliary drainage for LDLT is most commonly created as Roux-en-Y hepaticojejunostomy, rather than a duct-duct anastomosis, because there is a higher rate of stenosis in adult LDLT recipients using duct-duct biliary drainage (112). However, when a biliary-enteric anastomosis is performed, biliary stenosis at the anastomosis is the most common complication and may be detected as biliary dilatation by MRCP or ultrasound (65). One benefit of LDLT is there is decreased "cold ischemic time" of the liver because the procedure is elective, and this type of cold injury should be minimized (67).

Biliary Complications of Radiofrequency Ablation

CT is a commonly used for surveillance after radiofrequency ablation (RFA) of primary or secondary liver malignancy. RFA may result in biliary injury, although this only occurs in approximately 1% of cases (175). The most common complication is biliary stricture. In central tumor treatment, the central biliary structures may require a stent placement after the procedure because of the risk of stricture formation (87,157,260). Other reported complications of RFA are biliary leakage and biloma, fistula, and hematobilia (175).

Assessment of Biliary Stents and Drains

Migration of a biliary stent occurs in up to 6% of patients, and the stent will often pass into the bowel (9). The location of a biliary stent or drain can be well depicted in an atypical location, such as within the small bowel (Fig. 13-53). A malpositioned stent may remain in the bile duct, but it may no longer cross a level of stenosis. Pancreatic stent migration further into the pancreas duct may require endoscopic or open surgical removal (Fig. 13-54). A large-caliber stent or a short stent has a higher risk of migration (9).

Although MRI may adequately show a drainage catheter, the spatial resolution is generally better for CT. Catheters are often dense on CT but only appear as a low signal linear structure on MRI. Also, motion artifact is more likely to limit visualization of the catheter by MRI. Bile duct drainage may help in cases of bile leak, but drainage alone is often not enough if the leakage is caused by biliary necrosis from arterial insufficiency (269).

Catheters can become blocked with biliary stones or sludge. Stasis of bile flow is a major cause of catheter obstruction. If the catheter is percutaneous, it may be exchanged for a new tube to improve tube function. Internal biliary stents require ERCP or PTC for stent exchange (220).

Hematobilia is a potential complication of liver instrumentation and is most common after liver biopsy or

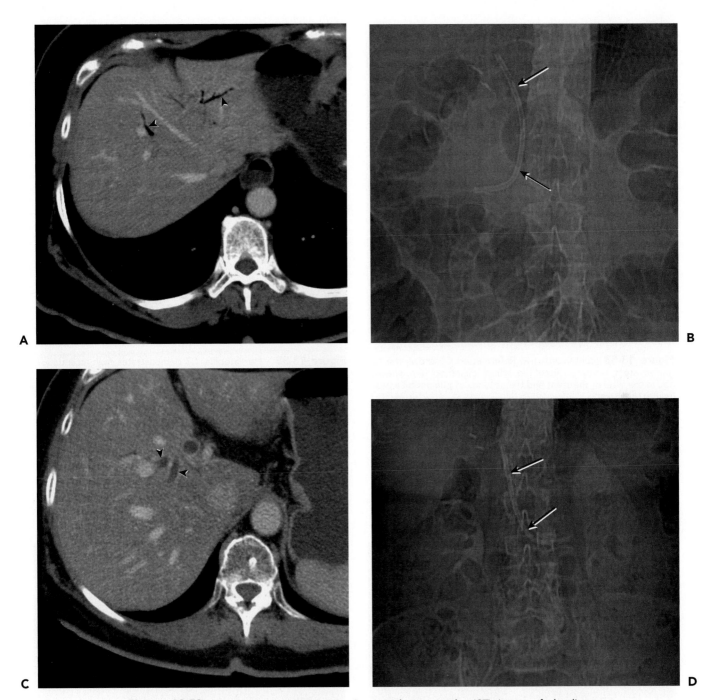

Figure 13-53 Biliary stent migration. **A:** Computed tomography (CT) image of the liver post–stent placement shows pneumobilia (*arrowheads*), indicating stent patency. **B:** Scout CT image demonstrates the biliary stent (*arrows*) in proper position. **C:** Image 3 months later shows intrahepatic bile duct dilatation (*arrowheads*) and absent pneumobilia, suggesting stent dysfunction. **D:** Scout CT image shows that the stent (*arrows*) has migrated distally. (*continued*)

percutaneous biliary drain placement. This complication occurs in 2% to 10% of cases (68,105,129,182). There is higher risk of hematobilia if drain placement is near the liver hilum (41). However, ultrasound guidance may help to avoid the central hepatic vessels and reduce the incidence of vascular injury (122). CT can show biliary dilatation with clot or a contrast collection in the ducts or gallbladder (Fig. 13-55) (126,155). Angiography is the definitive imaging study, but it is invasive and may detect injuries that are clinically self-limited. By angiographic assessment, there is arterial injury in up to 32% of biliary drainage procedures (92,171).

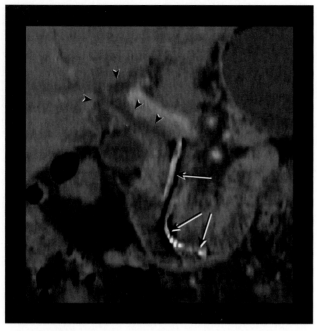

E

Figure 13-53 (continued)   **E:** Reformatted CT shows the migrated stent (*arrows*). Note the biliary dilatation (*arrowheads*) above the level of the stent and the absence of pneumobilia proximal to the stent.

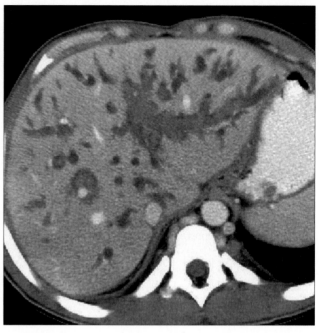

Figure 13-55   Hematobilia. CT demonstrates high attenuation clot throughout the biliary system after a liver biopsy.

Post–Whipple Procedure Assessment

Resection of pancreatic carcinoma often requires partial pancreatectomy, partial duodenectomy, and biliary-enteric anastomosis. Abnormal laboratory values may indicate biliary dysfunction, and should be evaluated by ultrasound or MRCP. Benign biliary strictures or leaks may be present as a result of the procedure. CT or ultrasound may detect a biloma as a focal fluid collection near the anastomotic regions. Imaging can also be used to guide percutaneous drainage catheter placement because ERCP is often no longer possible in these

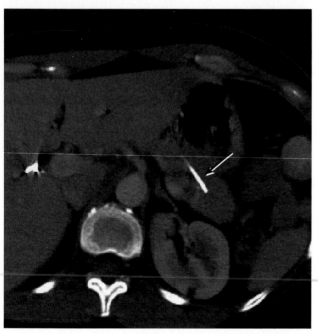

A

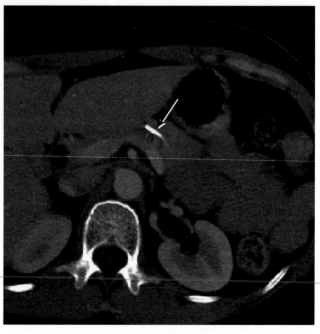

B

Figure 13-54   Pancreatic stent migration. **A, B:** Axial computed tomography images of the pancreatic tail show that a stent (*arrows*), which was previously placed across the ampulla, has migrated into the pancreatic tail. Surgery was required to remove the stent.

patients. If there is also a biliary stenosis, the biliary system must also be persistently drained to allow healing. Follow-up cholangiography must confirm healing of the point of leakage before the biloma drainage is discontinued (69). In a case of delayed new-onset biliary obstruction after Whipple procedure, recurrent malignancy obstructing the ducts should be a consideration.

REFERENCES

1. Aadland E, Schrumpf E, Fausa O, et al. Primary sclerosing cholangitis: a long-term follow-up study. *Scand J Gastroenterol.* 1987;22:655–664.
2. Abou-Saif A, Al-Kawas FH. Complications of gallstone disease: Mirizzi syndrome, cholecystocholedochal fistula, and gallstone ileus. *Am J Gastroenterol.* 2002;97:249–254.
3. Adjei ON, Tamura S, Sugimura H, et al. Contrast-enhanced MR imaging of intrahepatic cholangiocarcinoma. *Clin Radiol.* 1995; 50:6–10.
4. Ahmed A, Cheung RC, Keeffe EB. Management of gallstones and their complications. *Am Fam Physician.* 2000;61:1673–1680, 1687–1678.
5. Ahrendt SA, Pitt HA. Surgical treatment for primary sclerosing cholangitis. *J Hepatobiliary Pancreat Surg.* 1999;6:366–372.
6. Akata D, Ozmen MM, Kaya A, et al. Radiological findings of intraparenchymal liver Ascaris (hepatobiliary ascariasis). *Eur Radiol.* 1999;9:93–95.
7. Albasini JL, Aledo VS, Dexter SP, et al. Bile leakage following laparoscopic cholecystectomy. *Surg Endosc.* 1995;9:1274–1278.
8. Aldrighetti L, Arru M, Ronzoni M, et al. Extrahepatic biliary stenoses after hepatic arterial infusion (HAI) of floxuridine (FUdR) for liver metastases from colorectal cancer. *Hepatogastroenterology* 2001;48:1302–1307.
9. Aliperti G. Complications related to diagnostic and therapeutic endoscopic retrograde cholangiopancreatography. *Gastrointest Endosc Clin N Am.* 1996;6:379–407.
10. Alonso-Lej F, Rever WBJ, Pessagno DJ. Congenital choledochal cyst, with a report of 2, and an analysis of 94 cases. *Int Abstr Surg.* 1959;108:1–30.
11. Ametani F, Itoh K, Shibata T, et al. Spectrum of CT findings in pediatric patients after partial liver transplantation. *Radiographics* 2001;21:53–63.
12. Anderson CM, Saloner D, Tsuruda JS, et al. Artifacts in maximum-intensity-projection display of MR angiograms. *AJR Am J Roentgenol.* 1990;154:623–629.
13. Arai K, Kawai K, Kohda W, et al. Dynamic CT of acute cholangitis: early inhomogeneous enhancement of the liver. *AJR Am J Roentgenol.* 2003;181:115–118.
14. Asfar S, Metrakos P, Fryer J, et al. An analysis of late deaths after liver transplantation. *Transplantation* 1996;61:1377–1381.
15. Babbitt DP. Congenital choledochal cysts: new etiological concept based on anomalous relationships of the common bile duct and pancreatic bulb. *Ann Radiol* (Paris). 1969;12:231–240.
16. Bach DB, Satin R, Palayew M, et al. Herniation and strangulation of the gallbladder through the foramen of winslow. *AJR Am J Roentgenol.* 1984;142:541–542.
17. Backman L, Gibbs J, Levy M, et al. Causes of late graft loss after liver transplantation. *Transplantation* 1993;55:1078–1082.
18. Barakos JA, Ralls PW, Lapin SA, et al. Cholelithiasis: evaluation with CT. *Radiology* 1987;162:415–418.
19. Bartholomew LG, Cain JC, Woolner LB, et al. Sclerosing cholangitis: its possible association with Riedel's struma and fibrous retroperitonitis. Report of two cases. *N Engl J Med.* 1963;269: 8–12.
20. Bassignani MJ, Fulcher AS, Szucs RA, et al. Use of imaging for living donor liver transplantation. *Radiographics* 2001;21:39–52.
21. Becker CD, Grossholz M, Becker M, et al. Choledocholithiasis and bile duct stenosis: diagnostic accuracy of MR cholangiopancreatography. *Radiology* 1997;205:523–530.
22. Bernard HR, Hartman TW. Complications after laparoscopic cholecystectomy. *Am J Surg.* 1993;165:533–535.
23. Beutow PC, Midkiff RB. MR imaging of the liver. Primary malignant neoplasms in the adult. *Magn Reson Imaging Clin N Am.* 1997;5:289–318.
24. Bismuth H, Nakache R, Diamond T. Management strategies in resection of hilar cholangiocarcinoma. *Ann Surg.* 1992;215:31–38.
25. Blackbourne L, Earnhardt R, Sistrom C, et al. The sensitivity and role of ultrasound in the evaluation of biliary obstruction. *Am Surg.* 1994;60:683–690.
26. Bortoff GA, Chen MY, Ott DJ, et al. Gallbladder stones: imaging and intervention. *Radiographics* 2000;20:751–766.
27. Broome U, Lofberg R, Veress B, et al. Primary sclerosing cholangitis and ulcerative colitis: evidence for increased neoplastic potential. *Hepatology* 1995;22:1404–1408.
28. Buckles DC, Lindor KD, Larusso NF, et al. In primary sclerosing cholangitis, gallbladder polyps are frequently malignant. *Am J Gastroenterol.* 2002;97:1138–1142.
29. Cabada Giadas T, Sarria Octavio de Toledo L, Martinez-Berganza Asensio MT, et al. Helical CT cholangiography in the elevation of the biliary tract: application to the diagnosis of choledocholithiasis. *Abdom Imaging.* 2002;27:61–70.
30. Caldwell SH, Hespenheide EE, Harris D, et al. Imaging and clinical characteristics of focal atrophy of segments 2 and 3 in primary sclerosing cholangitis. *J Gastroenterol Hepatol.* 2001;16:220–224.
31. Calvo MM, Bujanda L, Heras I, et al. Magnetic resonance cholangiography versus ultrasound in the evaluation of the gallbladder. *J Clin Gastroenterol.* 2002;34:233–236.
32. Campbell WL, Peterson MS, Federle MP, et al. Using CT and cholangiography to diagnose biliary tract carcinoma complicating primary sclerosing cholangitis. *AJR Am J Roentgenol.* 2001; 177:1095–1100.
33. Caoili EM, Paulson EK, Heyneman LE, et al. Helical CT cholangiography with three-dimensional volume rendering using an oral biliary contrast agent: feasibility of a novel technique. *AJR Am J Roentgenol.* 2000;174:487–492.
34. Cesari S, Liessi G, Balestreri L, et al. Raysum reconstruction algorithm in MR cholangiopancreatography. *Magn Reson Imaging.* 2000;18:217–219.
35. Chamberlain RS, Blumgart LH. Hilar cholangiocarcinoma: a review and commentary. *Ann Surg Oncol.* 2000;7:55–66.
36. Chapman RW, Arborgh BA, Rhodes JM, et al. Primary sclerosing cholangitis: a review of its clinical features, cholangiography, and hepatic histology. *Gut* 1980;21:870–877.
37. Choi BI, Yeon KM, Kim SH, et al. Caroli disease: central dot sign in CT. *Radiology* 1990;174:161–163.
38. Choi JW, Kim TK, Kim KW, et al. Anatomic variation in intrahepatic bile ducts: an analysis of intraoperative cholangiograms in 300 consecutive donors for living donor liver transplantation. *Korean J Radiol.* 2003;4:85–90.
39. Coakley FV, Schwartz LH, Blumgart LH, et al. Complex postcholecystectomy biliary disorders: preliminary experience with evaluation by means of breath-hold MR cholangiography. *Radiology* 1998;209:141–146.
40. Cronan JJ. US diagnosis of choledocholithiasis: a reappraisal. *Radiology* 1986;161:133–134.
41. Croutch KL, Gordon RL, Ring EJ, et al. Superelective arterial embolization in the liver transplant recipient: a safe treatment for hemobilia caused by percutaneous transhepatic biliary drainage. *Liver Transpl Surg.* 1996;2:118–123.
42. Csendes A, Diaz JC, Burdiles P, et al. Mirizzi syndrome and cholecystobiliary fistula: a unifying classification. *Br J Surg.* 1989;76:1139–1143.
43. Cuenca IJ, Martinez del Olmo L, Perez Homs M. Helical CT without contrast in choledocholithiasis diagnosis. *Eur Radiol.* 2001;11:197–201.
44. D'Alessandro A M, Kalayoglu M, Pirsch JD, et al. Biliary tract complications after orthotopic liver transplantation. *Transplant Proc.* 1991;23:1563.
45. Da Silva F, Boudghene F, Lecomte I, et al. Sonography in AIDS-related cholangitis: prevalence and cause of echogenic nodule in the distal end of the common bile duct. *AJR Am J Roentgenol.* 1993;160:1205–1207.
46. De Backer AI, Van den Abbeele K, De Schepper AM, et al. Choledochocele: diagnosis by magnetic resonance imaging. *Abdom Imaging.* 2000;25:508–510.

47. de Groen PC, Gores GJ, LaRusso NF, et al. Biliary tract cancers. *N Engl J Med*. 1999;341:1368–1378.

48. Demartines N, Eisner L, Schnabel K, et al. Evaluation of magnetic resonance cholangiography in the management of bile duct stones. *Arch Surg*. 2000;135:148–152.

49. Dodd GD, 3rd, Baron RL, Oliver JH, 3rd, et al. End-stage primary sclerosing cholangitis: CT findings of hepatic morphology in 36 patients. *Radiology* 1999;211:357–362.

50. Drane WE. Nuclear medicine techniques for the liver and biliary system. Update for the 1990s. *Radiol Clin North Am*. 1991;29:1129–1150.

51. Dyer RB, Gilpin JW, Zagoria RJ, et al. Vicarious contrast material excretion in patients with acute unilateral ureteral obstruction. *Radiology* 1990;177:739–742.

52. Ebied O, Federle MP, Blachar A, et al. Hepatocellular-cholangiocarcinoma: helical computed tomography findings in 30 patients. *J Comput Assist Tomogr*. 2003;27:117–124.

53. Ernst O, Asselah T, Sergent G, et al. MR cholangiography in primary sclerosing cholangitis. *AJR Am J Roentgenol*. 1998;171:1027–1030.

54. Evans RA, Raby ND, O'Grady JG, et al. Biliary complications following orthotopic liver transplantation. *Clin Radiol*. 1990;41:190–194.

55. Fan ZM, Yamashita Y, Harada M, et al. Intrahepatic cholangio-carcinoma: spin-echo and contrast-enhanced dynamic MR imaging. *AJR Am J Roentgenol*. 1993;161:313–317.

56. Feng B, Song Q. Does the common bile duct dilate after cholecystectomy? Sonographic evaluation in 234 patients. *AJR Am J Roentgenol*. 1995;165:859–861.

57. Fieber SS, Nance FC. Choledochal cyst and neoplasm: a comprehensive review of 106 cases and presentation of two original cases. *Am Surg*. 1997;63:982–987.

58. Fitoz S, Atasoy C. MR cholangiography in massive hepatobiliary ascariasis. *Acta Radiol*. 2000;41:273–274.

59. Flum DR, Koepsell T, Heagerty P, et al. Common bile duct injury during laparoscopic cholecystectomy and the use of intraoperative cholangiography: adverse outcome or preventable error? *Arch Surg*. 2001;136:1287–1292.

60. Fukukura Y, Hamanoue M, Fujiyoshi F, et al. Cholangiolocellular carcinoma of the liver: CT and MR findings. *J Comput Assist Tomogr*. 2000;24:809–812.

61. Fulcher AS, Szucs RA, Bassignani MJ, et al. Right lobe living donor liver transplantation: preoperative evaluation of the donor with MR imaging. *AJR Am J Roentgenol*. 2001;176:1483–1491.

62. Fulcher AS, Turner MA. Benign diseases of the biliary tract: evaluation with MR cholangiography. *Semin Ultrasound CT MR*. 1999;20:294–303.

63. Fulcher AS, Turner MA. Pitfalls of MR cholangiopancreatography (MRCP). *J Comput Assist Tomogr*. 1998;22:845–850.

64. Fulcher AS, Turner MA, Franklin KJ, et al. Primary sclerosing cholangitis: evaluation with MR cholangiography-a case-control study. *Radiology* 2000;215:71–80.

65. Fulcher AS, Turner MA, Ham JM. Late biliary complications in right lobe living donor transplantation recipients: imaging findings and therapeutic interventions. *J Comput Assist Tomogr*. 2002;26:422–427.

66. Fulcher AS, Turner MA, Sanyal AJ. Case 38: Caroli disease and renal tubular ectasia. *Radiology* 2001;220:720–723.

67. Garcia-Criado A, Gilabert R, Bargallo X, et al. Radiology in liver transplantation. *Semin Ultrasound CT MR*. 2002;23:114–129.

68. Gazzaniga GM, Faggioni A, Bondanza G, et al. Percutaneous transhepatic biliary drainage - twelve years' experience. *Hepatogastroenterology* 1990;37:517–523.

69. Gervais DA, Fernandez-del Castillo C, O'Neill MJ, et al. Complications after pancreatoduodenectomy: imaging and imaging-guided interventional procedures. *Radiographics* 2001;21:673–690.

70. Goodman ZD, Ishak KG, Langloss JM, et al. Combined hepato-cellular-cholangiocarcinoma. A histiligic and immunohisto-chemical study. *Cancer* 1985;55:124–135.

71. Gore RM, Miller FH, Yaghmai V. Acquired immunodeficiency syndrome (AIDS) of the abdominal organs: imaging features. *Semin Ultrasound CT MR*. 1998;19:175–189.

72. Gores GJ. Cholangiocarcinoma: current concepts and insights. *Hepatology* 2003;37:961–969.

73. Greif F, Bronsther OL, Van Thiel DH, et al. The incidence, timing, and management of biliary tract complications after orthotopic liver transplantation. *Ann Surg*. 1994;219:40–45.

74. Groebli Y, Meyer JL, Tschantz P. Choledochocele demonstrated by computed tomographic cholangiography: report of a case. *Surg Today*. 2000;30:272–276.

75. Guibaud L, Bret PM, Reinhold C, et al. Bile duct obstruction and choledocholithiasis: diagnosis with MR cholangiography. *Radiology* 1995;197:109–115.

76. Guthrie JA, Ward J, Robinson PJ. Hilar cholangiocarcinomas: T2-weighted spin-echo and gadolinium-enhanced FLASH MR imaging. *Radiology* 1996;201:347–351.

77. Guy F, Cognet F, Dranssart M, et al. Caroli's disease: magnetic resonance imaging features. *Eur Radiol*. 2002;12:2730–2736.

78. Hakansson K, Leander P, Ekberg O, et al. MR imaging of upper abdomen following cholecystectomy. Normal and abnormal findings. *Acta Radiol*. 2001;42:181–186.

79. Hall-Craggs MA, Allen CE, Owens CM, et al. MR cholangiography: clinical evaluation in 40 cases. *Radiology* 1993;189:423–427.

80. Han JK, Choi BI, Kim AY, et al. Cholangiocarcinoma: pictorial essay of CT and cholangiographic findings. *Radiographics* 2002;22:173–187.

81. Han SJ, Hwang EH, Chung KS, et al. Acquired choledochal cyst from anomalous pancreatobiliary duct union. *J Pediatr Surg*. 1997;32:1735–1738.

82. Hanau LH, Steigbigel NH. Acute (ascending) cholangitis. *Infect Dis Clin North Am*. 2000;14:521–546.

83. Harris HW, Kumwenda ZL, Sheen-Chen SM, et al. Recurrent pyogenic cholangitis. *Am J Surg*. 1998;176:34–37.

84. Harrison PM. Diagnosis of primary sclerosing cholangitis. *J Hepatobiliary Pancreat Surg*. 1999;6:356–360.

85. Hartman EM, Barish MA. MR cholangiography. *Magn Reson Imaging Clin N Am*. 2001;9:841–855.

86. Hasegawa K, Kubota K, Komatsu Y, et al. Mass-forming inflammatory periductal fibrosis mimicking hilar bile duct carcinoma. *Hepatogastroenterology* 2000;47:1230–1233.

87. Havlik R. Radiofrequency thermal ablation in liver tumours. In: *Annual Course in Hepatobiliary and Pancreatic Surgery*, Hammersmith Hospital. London, 1999.

88. Helling TS, Strobach RS. The surgical challenge of papillary neoplasia of the biliary tract. *Liver Transpl Surg*. 1996;2:290–298.

89. Heneghan MA, Sylvestre PB. Cholestatic diseases of liver transplantation. *Semin Gastrointest Dis*. 2001;12:133–147.

90. Hennig J, Nauerth A, Friedburg H. RARE imaging: a fast imaging method for clinical MR. *Magn Reson Med*. 1986;3:823–833.

91. Hirohashi S, Hirohashi R, Uchida H, et al. MR cholangiopancreatography and MR urography: improved enhancement with a negative oral contrast agent. *Radiology* 1997;203:281–285.

92. Hoevels J, Nilsson U. Intrahepatic vascular lesions following nonsurgical percutaneous transhepatic bile duct intubation. *Gastrointest Radiol*. 1980;5:127–135.

93. Hoffer FA, Teele RL, Lillehei CW, et al. Infected bilomas and hepatic artery thrombosis in infant recipients of liver transplants. Interventional radiology and medical therapy as an alternative to retransplantation. *Radiology* 1988;169:435–438.

94. Holzknecht N, Gauger J, Sackmann M, et al. Breath-hold MR cholangiography with snapshot techniques: prospective comparison with endoscopic retrograde cholangiography. *Radiology* 1998;206:657–664.

95. Hopper KD, Weingast G, Rudikoff J, et al. Vicarious excretion of water-soluble contrast media into the gallbladder in patients with normal serum creatinine. *Invest Radiol*. 1988;23:604–608.

96. Howard TJ, Chin AC, Streib EW, et al. Value of helical computed tomography, angiography, and endoscopic ultrasound in determining resectability of periampullary carcinoma. *Am J Surg*. 1997;174:237–241.

97. Hunt DR. Common bile duct stones in non-dilated bile ducts? An ultrasound study. *Australas Radiol*. 1996;40:221–222.

98. Hwang CM, Kim TK, Ha HK, et al. Biliary ascariasis: MR cholangiography findings in two cases. *Korean J Radiol*. 2001;2:175–178.

99. Hwang JI, Chou YH, Tsay SH, et al. Radiologic and pathologic correlation of adenomyomatosis of the gallbladder. *Abdom Imaging*. 1998;23:73–77.

100. Imamura H, Makuuchi M, Sakamoto Y, et al. Anatomical keys and pitfalls in living donor liver transplantation. *J Hepatobiliary Pancreat Surg*. 2000;7:380–394.

101. Irie H, Honda H, Kuroiwa T, et al. Pitfalls in MR cholangiopancreatographic interpretation. *Radiographics* 2001;21:23–37.

102. Ito K, Mitchell DG, Outwater EK, et al. Primary sclerosing cholangitis: MR imaging features. *AJR Am J Roentgenol.* 1999;172:1527–1533.

103. Ito K, Siegelman ES, Stolpen AH, et al. MR imaging of complications after liver transplantation. *AJR Am J Roentgenol.* 2000;175:1145–1149.

104. Jaiswal M, LaRusso NF, Burgart LJ, et al. Inflammatory cytokines induce DNA damage and inhibit DNA repair in cholangiocarcinoma cells by a nitric oxide-dependent mechanism. *Cancer Res.* 2000;60:184–190.

105. Jeng KS, Ohta I, Yang FS. Reappraisal of the systematic management of complicated hepatolithiasis with bilateral intrahepatic biliary strictures. *Arch Surg.* 1996;131:141–147.

106. Johnson GK, Geenen JE, Venu RP, et al. Endoscopic treatment of biliary tract strictures in sclerosing cholangitis: a larger series and recommendations for treatment. *Gastrointest Endosc.* 1991;37:38–43.

107. Johnson PT, Heath DG, Hofmann LV, et al. Multidetector-row computed tomography with three-dimensional volume rendering of pancreatic cancer: a complete preoperative staging tool using computed tomography angiography and volume-rendered cholangiopancreatography. *J Comput Assist Tomogr.* 2003;27:347–353.

108. Kaim A, Steinke K, Frank M, et al. Diameter of the common bile duct in the elderly patient: measurement by ultrasound. *Eur Radiol.* 1998;8:1413–1415.

109. Kalloo AN, Kantsevoy SV. Gallstones and biliary disease. *Prim Care.* 2001;28:591–606.

110. Kaplan AA, Pagonini EP, Bosch JP. Effect of the dialysis membrane in acute renal failure. *N Engl J Med.* 1995;332:961–962.

111. Kaplan SB, Zajko AB, Koneru B. Hepatic bilomas due to hepatic artery thrombosis in liver transplant recipients: percutaneous drainage and clinical outcome. *Radiology* 1990;174(3 Pt 2):1031–1035.

112. Kawachi S, Shimazu M, Wakabayashi G, et al. Biliary complications in adult living donor liver transplantation with duct-to-duct hepaticocholedochostomy or Roux-en-Y hepaticojejunostomy biliary reconstruction. *Surgery* 2002;132:48–56.

113. Kelekis NL, Semelka RC. MR imaging of the gallbladder. *Top Magn Reson Imaging.* 1996;8:312–320.

114. Keogan MT, McDermott VG, Price SK, et al. The role of imaging in the diagnosis and management of biliary complications after liver transplantation. *AJR Am J Roentgenol.* 1999;173:215–219.

115. Keogan MT, Seabourn JT, Paulson EK, et al. Contrast-enhanced CT of intrahepatic and hilar cholangiocarcinoma: delay time for optimal imaging. *AJR Am J Roentgenol.* 1997;169:1493–1499.

116. Khalid TR, Casillas VJ, Montalvo BM, et al. Using MR cholangiopancreatography to evaluate iatrogenic bile duct injury. *AJR Am J Roentgenol.* 2001;177:1347–1352.

117. Khan SA, Davidson BR, Goldin R, et al. Guidelines for the diagnosis and treatment of cholangiocarcinoma: consensus document. *Gut* 2002;51 (Suppl VI):vi1–vi9.

118. Kim TK, Choi BI, Han JK, et al. Peripheral cholangiocarcinoma of the liver: two-phase spiral CT findings. *Radiology* 1997;204:539–543.

119. Kim TK, Kim BS, Kim JH, et al. Diagnosis of intrahepatic stones: superiority of MR cholangiopancreatography over endoscopic retrograde cholangiopancreatography. *AJR Am J Roentgenol.* 2002;179:429–434.

120. Kim YH. Pancreatitis in association with Clonorchis sinensis infestation: CT evaluation. *AJR Am J Roentgenol.* 1999;172:1293–1296.

121. Kluge R, Schmidt F, Caca K, et al. Positron emission tomography with [(18)F]fluoro-2-deoxy-D-glucose for diagnosis and staging of bile duct cancer. *Hepatology* 2001;33:1029–1035.

122. Koito K, Namieno T, Nagakawa T, et al. Percutaneous transhepatic biliary drainage using color Doppler ultrasonography. *J Ultrasound Med.* 1996;15:203–206.

123. Kondo H, Kanematsu M, Shiratori Y, et al. Potential pitfall of MR cholangiopancreatography: right hepatic arterial impression of the common hepatic duct. *J Comput Assist Tomogr.* 1999;23:60–62.

124. Kozarek R, Gannan R, Baerg R, et al. Bile leak after laparoscopic cholecystectomy. Diagnostic and therapeutic application of endoscopic retrograde cholangiopancreatography. *Arch Intern Med.* 1992;152:1040–1043.

125. Krishnani N, Shukla S, Jain M, et al. Fine needle aspiration cytology in xanthogranulomatous cholecystitis, gallbladder adenocarcinoma and coexistent lesions. *Acta Cytol.* 2000;44:508–514.

126. Krudy AG, Doppman JL, Bissonette MB, et al. Hemobilia: computed tomographic diagnosis. *Radiology* 1983;148:785–789.

127. Kubo S, Hamba H, Hirohashi K, et al. Magnetic Resonance cholangiography in hepatolithiasis. *Am J Gastroenterol.* 1997;92:629–632.

128. Kubota T, Thomson A, Clouston AD, et al. Clinicopathologic findings of recurrent primary sclerosing cholangitis after orthotopic liver transplantation. *J Hepatobiliary Pancreat Surg.* 1999;6:377–381.

129. L'Hermine C, Ernst O, Delemazure O, et al. Arterial complications of percutaneous transhepatic biliary drainage. *Cardiovasc Intervent Radiol.* 1996;19:160–164.

130. Ladas SD, Katsogridakis I, Tassios P, et al. Choledochocele, and overlooked diagnosis: report of 15 cases and review of 56 published reports from 1984 to 1992. *Endoscopy* 1995;27:233–239.

131. Laghi A, Pavone P, Catalano C, et al. MR cholangiography of late biliary complications after liver transplantation. *AJR Am J Roentgenol.* 1999;172:1541–1546.

132. Lamah M, Karanjia ND, Dickson GH. Anatomical variations of the extrahepatic biliary tree: review of the world literature. *Clin Anat.* 2001;14:167–172.

133. Lee JW, Han JK, Kim TK, et al. CT features of intraductal intrahepatic cholangiocarcinoma. *AJR Am J Roentgenol.* 2000;175:721–725.

134. Lee SB, Ryu KH, Ryu JK, et al. Acute acalculous cholecystitis associated with cholecystoduodenal fistula and duodenal bleeding. A case report. *Korean J Intern Med.* 2003;18:109–114.

135. Lee SS, Kim MH, Lee SK, et al. MR cholangiography versus cholangioscopy for evaluation of longitudinal extension of bilar cholangiocarcinoma. *Gastrointest Endosc.* 2002;56:25–32.

136. Lee WJ, Lim HK, Jang KM, et al. Radiologic spectrum of cholangiocarcinoma: emphasis on unusual manifestations and differential diagnoses. *Radiographics* 2001;21:S97–S116.

137. Lee YM, Kaplan MM. Medical treatment of primary sclerosing cholangitis. *J Hepatobiliary Pancreat Surg.* 1999;6:361–365.

138. Lee YM, Kaplan MM. Primary sclerosing cholangitis. *N Engl J Med.* 1995;332:924–933.

139. Lerut J, Gordon RD, Iwatsuki S, et al. Biliary tract complications in human orthotopic liver transplantation. *Transplantation* 1987;43:47–51.

140. Levy AD, Murakata LA, Rohrmann CA, Jr. Gallbladder carcinoma: radiologic-pathologic correlation. *Radiographics* 2001;21:295–314; questionnaire, 549–255.

141. Levy AD, Rohrmann CAJ, Murakata LA, et al. Caroli's disease: radiologic spectrum with pathologic correlation. *AJR Am J Roentgenol.* 2002;179:1053–1057.

142. Liddell RM, Baron RL, Ekstrom JE, et al. Normal intrahepatic bile ducts: CT depiction. *Radiology* 1990;176:633–635.

143. Lillemoe KD, Pitt HA, Cameron JL. Current management of benign bile duct strictures. *Adv Surg.* 1992;25:119–174.

144. Lim JH. Oriental cholangiohepatitis: pathologic, clinical, and radiologic features. *AJR Am J Roentgenol.* 1991;157:1–8.

145. Lim JH, Ko YT, Lee DH, et al. Oriental cholangiohepatitis: sonographic findings in 48 cases. *AJR Am J Roentgenol.* 1990;155:511–514.

146. Lin EC, Kuni CC. Radionuclide imaging of hepatic and biliary disease. *Semin Liver Dis.* 2001;21:179–194.

147. Liu TH, Consorti ET, Kawashima A, et al. The efficacy of magnetic resonance cholangiography for the evaluation of patients with suspected choledocholithiasis before laparoscopic cholecystectomy. *Am J Surg.* 1999;178:480–484.

148. Lo CM, Fan ST, Liu CL, et al. Adult-to-adult living donor liver transplantation using extended right lobe grafts. *Ann Surg.* 1997;226:261–270.

149. Lomas DJ, Bearcroft PW, Gimson AE. MR cholangiopancreatography: prospective comparison of a breath-hold 2D projection technique with diagnostic ERCP. *Eur Radiol.* 1999;9:1411–1417.

150. Lomas DJ, Gimson A. Magnetic resonance cholangiopancreatography. *Hosp Med.* 2000;61:395–399.

151. Loud PA, Semelka RC, Kettritz U, et al. MRI of acute cholecystitis: comparison with the normal gallbladder and other entities. *Magn Reson Imaging.* 1996;14:349–355.

152. Loyer EM, Chin H, DuBrow RA, et al. Hepatocellular carcinoma and intrahepatic peripheral cholangiocarcinoma: enhancement patterns with quadruple phase helical CT—a comparative study. *Radiology* 1999;212:866–875.

153. Lubbers EJ. Mirizzi syndrome. *World J Surg.* 1983;7:780–785.

154. Lucas WB, Chuttani R. Pathophysiology and current concepts in the diagnosis of obstructive jaundice. *Gastroenterologist* 1995;3:105–118.

155. Lutter DR, Berger ML. Diagnosis of nontraumatic hematobilia by computerized tomography of the abdomen. *Am J Gastroenterol.* 1988;83:329–330.

156. Ma KF, Iu PP, Chau LF, et al. Clinical and radiological features of biliary papillomatosis. *Australas Radiol.* 2000;44:169–173.

157. Machi J, Oishi AJ, Morioka WK, et al. Radiofrequency thermal ablation of synchronous metastic liver tumors can be performed safely in conjunction with colorectal cancer resection. *Cancer J.* 2000;6:S344–350.

158. Magnuson TH, Bender JS, Duncan MD, et al. Utility of magnetic resonance cholangiography in the evaluation of biliary obstruction. *J Am Coll Surg.* 1999;189:63–71; discussion 71–62.

159. Manfredi R, Costamagna G, Brizi MG, et al. Severe chronic pancreatitis versus suspected pancreatic disease: dynamic MR cholangiopancreatography after secretin stimulation. *Radiology* 2000;214:849–855.

160. Manfredi R, Costamagna G, Brizi MG, et al. Pancreas divisum and "santorinicele": diagnosis with dynamic MR cholangiopancreatography with secretin stimulation. *Radiology* 2000;217:403–408.

161. Marcos A, Fisher RA, Ham JM, et al. Right lope living donor liver transplantation. *Transplantation* 1999;68:798–803.

162. Martinez A, Bona X, Velasco M, et al. Diagnostic accuracy of ultrasound in acute cholecystitis. *Gastrointest Radiol.* 1986;11:334–338.

163. Marzio L, Innocenti P, Genovesi N, et al. Role of oral cholecystography, real-time ultrasound, and CT in evaluation of gallstones and gallbladder function. *Gastrointest Radiol.* 1992;17:257–261.

164. Masetti R, Antinori A, Coppola R, et al. Choledochocele: changing trends in diagnosis and management. *Surg Today.* 1996;26:281–285.

165. Matos C, Metens T, Deviere J, et al. Pancreas divisum: Evaluation with secretin-enhanced magnetic resonance cholangiopancreatography. *Gastrointest Endosc.* 2001;53:728–733.

166. Matos C, Metens T, Deviere J, et al. Pancreatic Duct: Morphologic and Functional evaluation with dynamic MR pancreatography after secretin stimulation. *Radiology* 1997;203:435–441.

167. Mehta SN, Reinhold C, Barkun AN. Magnetic resonance cholangiopancreatography. *Gastrointest Endosc Clin N Am.* 1997;7:247–270.

168. Milas M, Ricketts RR, Amerson JR, et al. Management of biliary tract stones in heart transplant patients. *Ann Surg.* 1996;223:747–756.

169. Miller FH, Gore RM, Nemcek AAJ, et al. Pancreaticobiliary manifestations of AIDS. *AJR Am J Roentgenol.* 1996;166:1269–1274.

170. Miller WJ, Sechtin AG, Campbell WL, et al. Imaging findings in Caroli's disease. *AJR Am J Roentgenol.* 1995;165:333–337.

171. Monden M, Okamura J, Kobayashi N, et al. Hemobilia after percutaneous transhepatic biliary drainage. *Arch Surg.* 1980;115:161–164.

172. Monroe SE. Congenital absence of the gallblader: a statistical study. *J Int Coll Surg.* 1959;32:369–373.

173. Mortele KJ, Ros PR. Cystic focal liver lesions in the adult: differential CT and MR imaging features. *Radiographics* 2001;21:895–910.

174. Moser MA, Wall WJ. Management of biliary problems after liver transplantation. *Liver Transpl.* 2001;7:S46–S52.

175. Mulier S, Mulier P, Ni Y, et al. Complications of radiofrequency coagulation of liver tumours. *Br J Surg.* 2002;89:1206–1222.

176. Myers RP, Shaffer EA, Beck PL. Gallbladder polyps: epidemiology, natural history and management. *Can J Gastroenterol.* 2002;16:187–194.

177. Nakanuma Y, Harada K, Katayanagi K, et al. Definition and pathology of primary sclerosing cholangitis. *J Hepatobiliary Pancreat Surg.* 1999;6:333–342.

178. Narayanan Menon KV, Wiesner R. Etiology and natural history of primary sclerosing cholangitis. *J Hepatobiliary Pancreat Surg.* 1999;6:343–351.

179. Neitlich JD, Topazian M, Smith RC, et al. Detection of choledocholithiasis: comparison of unenhanced helical CT and endoscopic retrograde cholangiopancreatography. *Radiology* 1997;203:753–757.

180. Nghiem HV. Imaging of hepatic transplantation. *Radiol Clin North Am.* 1998;36:429–443.

181. Nghiem HV, Tran K, Winter TC III, et al. Imaging of complications in liver transplantation. *Radiographics* 1996;16:825–840.

182. Nilsson U, Evander A, Ihse I, et al. Percutaneous transhepatic cholangiography and drainage. Risks and complications. *Acta Radiol Diagn* (Stockh). 1983;24:433–439.

183. Nino-Murcia M, Jeffrey RB, Jr., Beaulieu CF, et al. Multidetector CT of the pancreas and bile duct system: value of curved planar reformations. *AJR Am J Roentgenol.* 2001;176:689–693.

184. Oria HE. Pitfalls in the diagnosis of gallbladder disease in clinically severe obesity. *Obes Surg.* 1998;8:444–451.

185. Ortega D, Burns PN, Hope Simpson D, et al. Tissue harmonic imaging: is it a benefit for bile duct sonography? *AJR Am J Roentgenol.* 2001;176:653–659.

186. Ostroff JW. Post-transplant biliary problems. *Gastrointest Endosc Clin N Am.* 2001;11:163–183.

187. Park J, Tadlock L, Gores GJ, et al. Inhibition of interleukin 6-mediated mitogen-activated protein kinase activation attenuates growth of a cholangiocarcinoma cell line. *Hepatology* 1999;30:1128–1133.

188. Park MS, Yu JS, Kim YH, et al. Acute cholecystitis: comparison of MR cholangiography and US. *Radiology* 1998;209:781–785.

189. Parra JA, Acinas O, Bueno J, et al. Xanthogranulomatous cholecystitis: clinical, sonographic, and CT findings in 26 patients. *AJR Am J Roentgenol.* 2000;174:979–983.

190. Patel T. Increasing incidence and mortality of primary intrahepatic cholangiocarcinoma in the United States. *Hepatology* 2001;33:1353–1357.

191. Perret RS, Sloop GD, Borne JA. Common bile duct measurements in an elderly population. *J Ultrasound Med.* 2000;19:727–730.

192. Pickhardt PJ, Friedland JA, Hruza DS, et al. CT, MR cholangiopancreatography, and endoscopy findings in Bouveret's Syndrome. *AJR Am J Roentgenol.* 2003;180:1033–1035.

193. Pickuth D, Spielmann RP. Detection of choledocholithiasis: comparison of unenhanced spiral CT, US, and ERCP. *Hepatogastroenterology* 2000;47:1514–1517.

194. Ponsioen CY, Vrouenraets SME, Prawirodirdjo W, et al. Natural history of primary sclerosing cholangitis and prognostic value of cholangiography in a Dutch population. *Gut* 2002;51:562–566.

195. Porayko MK, Kondo M, Steers JL. Liver transplantation: late complications of the biliary tract and their management. *Semin Liver Dis.* 1995;15:139–155.

196. Prasad SR, Sahani D, Saini S. Clinical applications of magnetic resonance cholangiopancreatography. *J Clin Gastroenterol.* 2001;33:362–366.

197. Puri SK, Gupta P, Panigrahi P, et al. Ultrasonographic evaluation of common duct diameter in pre and post cholecystectomy patients. *Trop Gastroenterol.* 2001;22:23–24.

198. Quiroga S, Sebastia MC, Margarit C, et al. Complications of orthotopic liver transplantation: spectrum of findings with helical CT. *Radiographics* 2001;21:1085–1102.

199. Rabie ME, Al-Humayed SM, Hosni MH, et al. Choledochocele: the disputed origin. *Int Surg.* 2002;87:221–225.

200. Ralls PW, Colletti PM, Lapin SA, et al. Real-time sonography in suspected acute cholecystitis. Prospective evaluation of primary and secondary signs. *Radiology* 1985;155:767–771.

201. Redvanly RD, Nelson RC, Stieber AC, et al. Imaging in the preoperative evaluation of adult liver transplant candidates: goals, merits of various procedures, and recommendations. *AJR Am J Roentgenol.* 1995;164:611–617.

202. Regan F, Schaefer DC, Smith DP, et al. The diagnostic utility of HASTE MRI in the evaluation of acute cholecystitis. Half-Fourier acquisition single-shot turbo SE. *J Comput Assist Tomogr.* 1998;22:638–642.

203. Reinhold C, Bret PM. Current Status of MR Cholangiopancreatography. *AJR Am J Roentgenol.* 1996;166:1285–1295.

204. Rizzo RJ, Szucs RA, Turner MA. Congenital abnormalities of the pancreas and biliary tree in adults. *Radiographics.* 1995;15:49–68.

205. Robinson EK, Lee JE, Lowy AM, et al. Reoperative pancreaticoduodenectomy for periampullary carcinoma. *Am J Surg.* 1996;172:432–438.

206. Romano AJ, van Sonnenberg E, Casola G, et al. Gallbladder and bile duct abnormalities in AIDS: sonographic findings in eight patients. *AJR Am J Roentgenol.* 1988;150:123–127.

207. Rosen CB, Nagorney DM, Wiesner RH, et al. Cholangiocarcinoma complicating primary sclerosing cholangitis. *Ann Surg.* 1991;213:21–25.

208. Rosen HR, Shackleton CR, Martin P. Indications for and timing of liver transplantation. *Med Clin North Am.* 1996;80:1069–1102.

209. Rossi G, Lucianetti A, Gridelli B, et al. Biliary tract complications in 224 orthotopic liver transplantations. *Transplant Proc.* 1994; 26:3626–3628.

210. Rumalla A, Petersen BT. Diagnosis and therapy of biliary tract malignancy. *Semin Gastrointest Dis.* 2000;11:168–173.

211. Sanchez-Urdazpal L, Sterioff S, Janes C, et al. Increased bile duct complications in ABO incompatible liver transplant recipients. *Transplant Proc.* 1991;23(1 Pt 2):1440–1441.

212. Schroeder T, Malago M, Debatin JF, et al. Multidetector computed tomographic cholangiography in the evaluation of potential living liver donors. *Transplantation* 2002;73:1972–1973.

213. Sela-Herman S, Scharschmidt BF. Choledochal cyst, a disease for all ages. *Lancet* 1996;347:779.

214. Semelka RC, Shoenut JP, Koroeker MA, et al. Bile duct disease: prospective comparison of ERCP, CT, and fat suppression MRI. *Gastrointest Endosc.* 1992;17:347–352.

215. Sermon A, Himpens J, Leman G. Symptomatic adenomyomatosis of the gallbladder-report of a case. *Acta Chir Belg.* 2003; 103:225–229.

216. Shaffer EA. Gallbladder sludge: what is its clinical significance? *Curr Gastroenterol Rep.* 2001;3:166–173.

217. Shaw MJ, Dorsher PJ, Vennes JA. Cystic duct anatomy: an endoscopic perspective. *Am J Gastroenterol.* 1993;88:2102–2106.

218. Sherman S, Jamidar P, Shaked A, et al. Biliary tract complications after orthotopic liver transplantation. Endoscopic approach to diagnosis and therapy. *Transplantation* 1995;60:467–470.

219. Shoup M, Hodul P, Aranha GV, et al. Defining a role for endoscopic ultrasound in staging periampullary tumors. *Am J Surg.* 2000;179:453–456.

220. Shrestha R, Lasch H. Endoscopic therapy for biliary tract disease before orthotopic liver transplantation. *Gastrointest Endosc Clin N Am.* 2001;11:45–64.

221. Simeone JF, Brink JA, Mueller PR, et al. The sonographic diagnosis of acute gangrenous cholecystitis: importance of the Murphy sign. *AJR Am J Roentgenol.* 1989;152:289–290.

222. Smith FJ, Mathieson JR, Cooperberg PL. Abdominal Abnormalities in AIDS: detection at US in a large population. *Radiology* 1994;192:691–695.

223. Sons HU, Borchard F, Joel BS. Carcinoma of the gallbladder: autopsy findings in 287 cases and review of the literature. *J Surg Oncol.* 1985;28:199–206.

224. Soong TC, Lee RC, Cheng HC, et al. Dynamic MR imaging of hepatolithiasis. *Abdom Imaging.* 1998;23:515–519.

225. Soper NJ, Flye MW, Brunt LM, et al. Diagnosis and management of biliary complications of laparoscopic cholecystectomy. *Am J Surg.* 1993;165:663–669.

226. Soto JA, Barish MA, Alvarez O, et al. Detection of choledocholithiasis with MR cholangiography: comparison of three-dimensional fast spin-echo and single- and multisection half-Fourier rapid acquisition with relaxation enhancement sequences. *Radiology* 2000;215:737–745.

227. Soto JA, Barish MA, Alvarez O, et al. Detection of choledocholithiasis with MR cholangiography: comparison of three-dimensional fast spin-echo and single- and multisection half-fourier rapid acquisition with relaxation enhancement sequences. *Radiology* 2000;215:737–745.

228. Soto JA, Barish MA, Yucel EK, et al. MR Cholangiopancreatography: findings on 3D fast spin-echo imaging. *AJR Am J Roentgenol.* 1995;165:1397–1401.

229. Soyer P, Bluemke A, Sibert A, et al. MR imaging of intrahepatic cholangiocarcinoma. *Abdom Imaging.* 1995;20:126–130.

230. Sparwasser C, Krupienski M, Radomsky J, et al. Gallbladder metastasis of renal cell carcinoma. A case report and review of the literature. *Urol Int.* 1997;58:257–258.

231. Stephen AE, Berger DL. Carcinoma in the porcelain gallbladder: a relationship revisited. *Surgery* 2001;129:699–703.

232. Stratta RJ, Wood RP, Langnas AN, et al. Diagnosis and treatment of biliary tract complications after orthotopic liver transplantation. *Surgery* 1989;106:675–683.

233. Strazzabosco M, Spirli C, Okolicsanyi L. Pathophysiology of the intrahepatic biliary epithelium. *J Gastroenterol Hepatol.* 2000;15:244–253.

234. Sugiyama M, Haradome H, Takahara T, et al. Anomalous pancreaticobiliary junction shown on multidetector CT. *AJR Am J Roentgenol.* 2003;180:173–175.

235. Takahashi M, Saida Y, Itai Y, et al. Reevaluation of spiral CT cholangiography: basic considerations and reliability for detecting choledocholithiasis in 80 patients. *J Comput Assist Tomogr.* 2000;24:859–865.

236. Takayama T, Makuuchi M, Kawasaki S, et al. Outflow Y-Reconstruction for Living Related Partial Hepatic Transplantation. *J Am Coll Surg.* 1994;179:227–229.

237. Taner CB, Nagorney DM, Donohue JH. Surgical treatment of gallbladder cancer. *J Gastrointest Surg.* 2004;8:83–89.

238. Teefey SA, Baron RL, Rohrmann CA, et al. Sclerosing cholangitis: CT findings. *Radiology* 1988;169:635–639.

239. Teefey SA, Baron RL, Schulte SJ, et al. Patterns of intrahepatic bile duct dilatation at CT: correlation with obstructive disease processes. *Radiology* 1992;182:139–142.

240. Tillich M, Mischinger HJ, Preisegger KH, et al. Multiphasic helical CT in diagnosis and staging of hilar cholangiocarcinoma. *AJR Am J Roentgenol.* 1998;171:651–658.

241. Todani T, Watanabe Y, Narusue M, et al. Congenital bile duct cysts: Classification, operative procedures, and review of thirty-seven cases including cancer arising from choledochal cyst. *Am J Surg.* 1977;134:263–269.

242. Torok N, Gores GJ. Cholangiocarcinoma. *Semin Gastrointest Dis.* 2001;12:125–132.

243. Trotman BW, Petrella EJ, Soloway RD, et al. Evaluation of radiographic lucency or opaqueness of gallstones as a means of identifying cholesterol or pigment stones. *Gastroenterology* 1975; 68:1563–1566.

244. Valls C, Guma A, Puig I, et al. Intrahepatic peripheral cholangiocarcinoma: CT evaluation. *Abdom Imaging.* 2000;25:490–496.

245. van Milligen de Wit AW, Van Deventer SJ, Tytgat GN. Immunogenetic aspects of primary sclerosing cholangitis: implications for therapeutic strategies. *Am J Gastroenterol.* 1995;90:893–900.

246. Varghese JC, Farrell MA, Courtney G, et al. A prospective comparison of magnetic resonance cholangiopancreatography with endoscopic retrograde cholangiopancreatography in the evaluation of patients with suspected biliary tract disease. *Clin Radiol.* 1999;54:513–520.

247. Varghese JC, Liddell RP, Farrell MA, et al. The diagnostic accuracy of magnetic resonance cholangiopancreatography and ultrasound compared with direct cholangiography in the detection of choledocholithiasis. *Clin Radiol.* 1999;54:604–614.

248. Verbeek PC, van Leeuwen DJ, de Wit LT, et al. Benign fibrosing disease of the hepatic confluence mimicking Klatskin tumors. *Surgery* 1992;112:866–871.

249. Vilgrain V, Palazzo L. Choledocholithiasis: role of US and endoscopic ultrasound. *Abdom Imaging.* 2001;26:7–14.

250. Vilgrain V, Van Beers B, Flejou JF, et al. Intrahepatic cholangiocarcinoma: MRI and pathologic correlation in 14 patients. *J Comput Assist Tomogr.* 1997;21:59–65.

251. Vitellas KM, El-Dieb A, Vaswani KK, et al. MR cholangiopancreatography in patients with primary sclerosing cholangitis: interobserver variability and comparison with endoscopic retrograde cholangiopancreatography. *AJR Am J Roentgenol.* 2002;179: 399–407.

252. Vitellas KM, Enns RA, Keogan MT, et al. Comparison of MR cholangiopancreatographic techniques with contrast-enhanced cholangiography in the evaluation of sclerosing cholangitis. *AJR Am J Roentgenol.* 2002;178:327–334.

253. Vitellas KM, Keogan MT, Freed KS, et al. Radiologic manifestations of sclerosing cholangitis with emphasis on MR cholangiopancreatography. *Radiographics* 2000;20:959–975.

254. Vitellas KM, Keogan MT, Spritzer CE, et al. MR cholangiopancreatography of bile and pancreatic duct abnormalities with emphasis on the single-shot fast spin-echo technique. *Radiographics* 2000;20:939–957.

255. Walker AT, Shapiro AW, Brooks DC, et al. Bile duct disruption and biloma after laparoscopic cholecystectomy: imaging evaluation. *AJR Am J Roentgenol.* 1992;158:785–789.

256. Walsh RM, Henderson JM, Vogt DP, et al. Trends in bile duct injuries from laparoscopic cholecystectomy. *J Gastrointest Surg.* 1998;2:458–462.

257. Watanabe Y, Dohke M, Ishimori T, et al. Pseudo-obstruction of the extrahepatic bile duct due to artifact from arterial pulsatile compression: a diagnostic pitfall of MR cholangiopancreatography. *Radiology* 2000;214:856–860.

258. Watanabe Y, Dohke M, Ishimori T, et al. Diagnostic pitfalls of MR cholangiopancreatography in the evaluation of the biliary tract and gallbladder. *Radiographics* 1999;19:415–429.

259. Wohlgemuth WA, Bottger J, Bohndorf K. MRI, CT, US and ERCP in the evaluation of bile duct hamartomas (von Meyenburg complex): a case report. *Eur Radiol.* 1998;8:1623–1626.

260. Wood TF, Rose DM, Chung M, et al. Radiofrequency ablation of 231 unresectable hepatic tumors: indications, limitations, and complications. *Ann Surg Oncol.* 2000;7:593–600.

261. Wysong CB, Gorten RJ. Intrahepatic gallbladder. *South Med J* 1980;73:825–826.

262. Yamashita K, Jin MJ, Hirose Y, et al. CT finding of transient focal increased attenuation of the liver adjacent to the gallbladder in acute cholecystitis. *AJR Am J Roentgenol.* 1995;164:343–346.

263. Yee K, Sheppard BC, Domreis J, et al. Cancers of the gallbladder and biliary ducts. *Oncology* (Huntingt). 2002;16:939–946.

264. Yoon KH, Ha HK, Kim CG, et al. Malignant papillary neoplasms of the intrahepatic bile ducts: CT and histopathologic features. *AJR Am J Roentgenol.* 2000;175:1135–1139.

265. Yoshida Y, Imai Y, Murakami T, et al. Intrahepatic cholangiocarcinoma with marked hypervascularity. *Abdom Imaging.* 1999;24:66–68.

266. Yoshimitsu K, Honda H, Jimi M, et al. MR diagnosis of adenomyomatosis of the gallbladder and differentiation from gallbladder carcinoma: importance of showing Rokitansky-Aschoff sinuses. *AJR Am J Roentgenol.* 1999;172:1535–1540.

267. Youngwirth LD, Peters JC, Perry MD. The suprahepatic gallbladder. An unusual anatomical variant. *Radiology* 1983;149:57–58.

268. Yun EJ, Cho SG, Park S, et al. Gallbladder carcinoma and chronic cholecystitis: differentiation with two-phase spiral CT. *Abdom Imaging.* 2004;29:102–108.

269. Zajko AB, Campbell WL, Logsdon GA, et al. Cholangiographic findings in hepatic artery occlusion after liver transplantation. *AJR Am J Roentgenol.* 1987;149:485–489.

Spleen

David M. Warshauer

14

The spleen is well seen on computed tomography (CT) and magnetic resonance (MR) images of the abdomen in virtually every patient. Normally, it appears as an oblong or ovoid organ in the left upper abdomen. The contour of the superior lateral border of the spleen is convex, conforming to the shape of the adjacent abdominal wall and left hemidiaphragm. The margins of the spleen are smooth, and the parenchyma is sharply demarcated from the adjacent fat. The hilum usually is directed anteromedially, and the splenic artery and vein and their branches can be seen entering the spleen in this region (Fig. 14-1). The posteromedial surface of the spleen behind the hilum often is concave where it conforms to the shape of the adjacent left kidney. The medial surface anterior to the hilum is in contact with the stomach and also assumes a shallow concave shape in some patients (Fig. 14-2). On images performed without intravenous (IV) injection of contrast material, the normal spleen appears homogeneous in density, with CT attenuation values in the range of 55 to 65 Hounsfield units (HU), equal to or slightly less than those for the normal liver (210).

Like the liver, the spleen ordinarily has a small area that is not covered by peritoneum, a so-called bare area (341). Smaller than the bare area of the liver, this corresponds to an approximately 2 × 3 cm portion of the spleen's surface contained between the anterior and posterior leaves of the splenorenal ligament. This area overlies the renal fascia covering the anterior aspect of the upper pole of the left kidney. Ascites and other intraperitoneal left upper abdominal fluid collections tend to surround all surfaces of the spleen except this small area. Recognition of this feature is occasionally helpful in determining whether fluid lies in the peritoneal space or left pleural space.

The splenic vessels are seen even on non–contrast-enhanced CT images in most individuals. The splenic vein follows a fairly straight course toward the splenic hilum, running transversely along the posterior aspect of the body and tail of the pancreas. Unlike the splenic vein, the splenic artery often is tortuous, especially in older patients. On any given section, it may appear as a single curvilinear structure or it may wander in and out of the plane of the section and appear as a series of round densities, each of which represents a cross-sectional image of a portion of the artery. In older individuals, it is common to see calcified atheromas within the wall of the splenic artery.

USE OF CONTRAST MATERIAL

It is useful to administer iodinated contrast material intravenously (IV) when examining the spleen by CT. Dynamic scans performed during a bolus injection are optimal for clarifying the nature of soft-tissue structures in the splenic hilar and retropancreatic regions that can mimic abnormalities of the pancreas or left adrenal gland, but that may, in fact, be the result of normal splenic vasculature. The splenic artery and vein and their branches undergo dense contrast enhancement during bolus injection and are easily identified. Splenic parenchymal opacification also occurs and may be used to improve the detectability of mass lesions within the spleen. When contrast material is given by rapid IV injection and scans are obtained early in the injection, the splenic parenchyma initially appears heterogeneous (Fig. 14-3). Arciform and wave-like patterns can be seen during this phase. This heterogeneous enhancement is thought to be to the result of the dual circulatory routes through the splenic red pulp. Early enhancing areas reflect the fast circulation with its direct arteriole to venule connection, whereas the late enhancing areas reflect the slow circulation of arteriole to cords of Bilroth to venular flow (117,191,335). Only after a minute or more passes does the splenic parenchyma achieve uniform, homogeneous

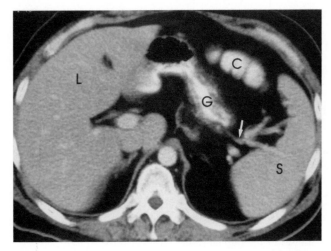

Figure 14-1 Computed tomography image of normal spleen (*S*). The outer border is convex and conforms to the shape of the adjacent body wall. The medial surface is concave. The splenic artery (*arrow*) enters the hilum. C, colon; G, stomach; L, liver.

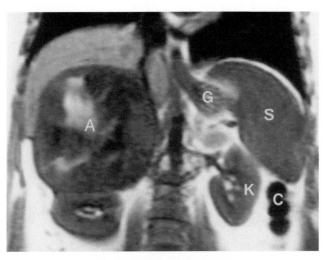

Figure 14-2 Coronal T1-weighted fast low-angle shot magnetic resonance image (repetition time, 140 ms; echo time, 4 ms; flip angle, 80 degrees) of normal spleen (S). Note the intimate relation of the spleen to the left hemidiaphragm, gastric fundus (G), left kidney (K), and colon (C). Also note a large right adrenal carcinoma (A).

enhancement. In work done with a pediatric population, this early heterogeneity has been shown to be related to injection rate, age, and splenomegaly, with heterogeneity occurring more frequently at higher injection rates, in patients older than 1 year of age, and in patients without splenomegaly (81). Care must be taken not to misinterpret this early postinjection heterogeneity as an indication of focal abnormality.

No significant difference in splenic parenchymal enhancement has been shown between ionic and nonionic contrast material (129,210). After administration of 180 mL of iothalamate-60%, iopamidol-300, or iohexol-300 at 2 mL per second, mean enhancement of splenic parenchyma ranges from 75 to 97 HU (210).

MAGNETIC RESONANCE IMAGING

The adult spleen has relatively long T1 and T2 relaxation times. Its signal intensity on T1-weighted images is less (i.e., darker) than that of liver and is similar to that of renal cortex. On T2-weighted images, the spleen appears brighter than liver, reflecting its greater free water content (Fig. 14-4). Unlike in the adult, the neonatal spleen is initially isointense or hypointense to liver on T2-weighted images during the first weeks of life, only assuming an adult appearance after 8 months. This increase in T2-weighted signal is thought

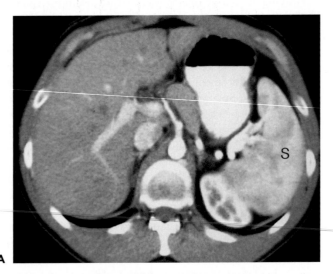

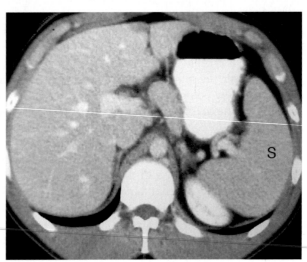

A   B

Figure 14-3 Computed tomography appearance of the normal spleen (S) during bolus intravenous injection of contrast material. **A:** Patchy pattern of early splenic parenchymal enhancement 30 seconds after the start of contrast injection. The aorta and splenic vessels are densely opacified. **B:** Uniform appearance of splenic parenchyma 70 seconds after the start of contrast injection.

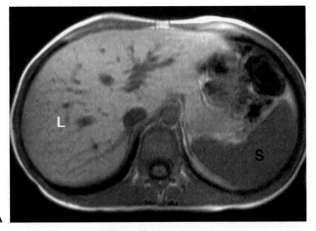
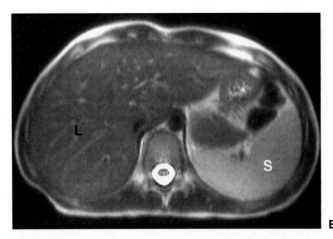

A   B

Figure 14-4 Magnetic resonance imaging appearance of the normal spleen (S). **A:** On this T1-weighted fast low-angle shot image (repetition time, 142 ms; echo time 4.4 ms; flip angle, 80 degrees), the signal intensity of the spleen (S) is less than that of the liver (L) and much less than that of the surrounding fat. **B:** On a T2-weighted half-Fourier acquisition single-shot turbo spin-echo magnetic resonance image (1,500/92), there is reversal of the relative signal intensities of the spleen (S) and liver (L).

to correlate with maturation of the lymphoproliferative system, with resulting increase in the white pulp to red pulp ratio (80). Breath-hold spoiled gradient echo techniques [e.g., fast low-angle shot (FLASH)] have proved to be useful in splenic evaluation by decreasing time of acquisition and hence respiratory-motion artifact. The flow void produced by moving blood allows the major splenic vessels to be seen well, without the use of IV contrast material. Because the tissue relaxation times of splenic parenchyma and many tumors of the spleen are similar (126), the use of IV contrast material for evaluating the spleen has become important (193,282). Gadolinium–diethylene-triamine penta-acetic acid (Gd-DTPA) is the agent used most commonly. Multisection T1-weighted spoiled gradient echo sequences can be employed at various times after contrast material injection to image the spleen in the early, mid-, and late perfusion phases (Fig. 14-5).

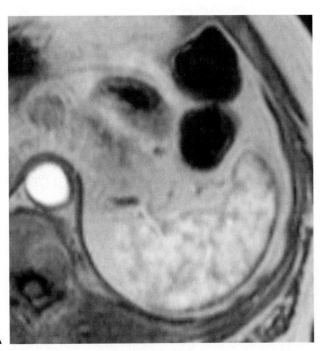
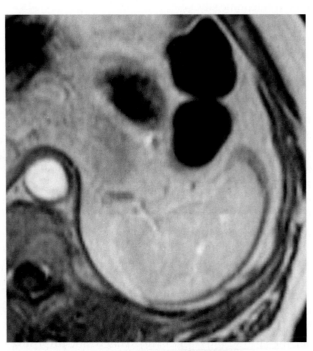

A   B

Figure 14-5 Magnetic resonance imaging appearance of the normal spleen (S). **A:** On this T1-weighted fast low-angle shot image (repetition time, 140 ms; echo time, 4 ms; flip angle, 80 degrees) performed during the perfusion phase of intravenous administration of gadolinium-diethylene-triamine penta-acetic acid, the splenic parenchyma shows heterogeneous enhancement. **B:** The spleen has assumed a more homogeneous appearance 45 seconds later.

Using this technique, approximately 80% of patients demonstrate normal heterogeneous or arciform enhancement on early perfusion images; 15% show uniform high signal (282). The significance of the early uniform enhancement is uncertain, although it has been speculated that it may represent a response to a coexisting inflammatory or neoplastic process (282).

At present, IV contrast–enhanced MRI appears to be as sensitive as or slightly more sensitive than CT for evaluation of the splenic parenchyma. The ability of MRI to directly image in the coronal and sagittal planes is advantageous in showing the relation of the spleen to the adjacent left kidney, adrenal, and hemidiaphragm, although this advantage has diminished with the availability of isotropic imaging with multislice CT. Respiratory motion artifact and the increased cost and time involved in an MRI study, however, limit its routine use.

SPLENIC SIZE

The spleen measures from 12 to 15 cm in length, 4 cm to 8 cm in width, and 3 to 4 cm in thickness (10). Because of the spleen's irregular shape and oblique orientation within the left upper quadrant, these measurements are of limited use as a guide to normal splenic size on CT. Many observers judge splenic volume by subjective evaluation of the CT image based on experience. Rounding of the normally crescentic spleen and extension of the spleen anterior to the aorta or below the right hepatic lobe or rib cage are further clues to splenomegaly.

A more accurate approach to the assessment of splenic volume is the splenic index (172,310), which is the product of the length, width, and thickness of the spleen as seen on CT (Fig. 14-6). Splenic length is determined by summing the number of contiguous CT slices on which the spleen is visible. The width is the longest splenic diameter that can be drawn on any transverse image. The thickness is measured at the level of the splenic hilum and is the distance between the inner and outer (peripheral) borders of the spleen. When the thicknesses of the anterior and posterior portions of the spleen differ significantly, two or three measurements of thickness are averaged. When determined in this way, the normal splenic size corresponds to an index of 120 to 480 cm (172). The correlation between splenic index (and other simplified linear measures) and actual splenic volume calculated on a per-slice basis is good (245,270,276), although the correlation with the weight of the surgically excised spleen is an imperfect one. It has been demonstrated that the weight of the excised spleen in grams averages from one third to one half the splenic index (113,310). This is not surprising, because the size and weight of the excised spleen are affected by the amount of blood that drains from the specimen before it is weighed. The splenic index as determined by CT is probably a better indicator of splenomegaly than is the

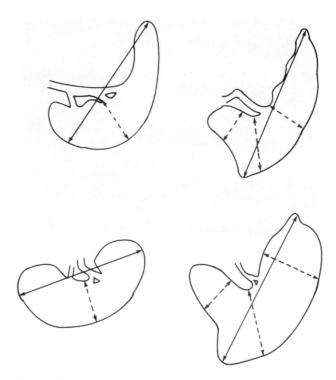

Figure 14-6 Diagrammatic representation of the measurements used in calculating the splenic index from transverse computed tomography or magnetic resonance images of spleens of various shapes. The width (solid lines) and thickness (dashed lines) are shown. (See text for details.)

weight of the spleen as determined in the operating room or pathology laboratory.

Most accurate of all are computer programs for calculating actual splenic volume from a series of CT or MR images. Calculated adult splenic volume has ranged in various studies of normal volunteers from a mean of 112 cm^3 (range 32 to 209 cm^3) to 214 cm^3 (range 107 to 315 cm^3) (149,246). Splenic volume did not correlate with gender, body mass index, or body weight (149,246). Although an inverse correlation was noted with age in one study, this was not seen in any other report (149,246).

NORMAL VARIANTS AND CONGENITAL ANOMALIES

The spleen forms from multiple mesenchymal cell aggregates in the dorsal mesogastrium. As the dorsal mesentery bows to the left with the developing stomach, these aggregates coalesce. The left side of the dorsal mesentery fuses with the parietal peritoneum covering the left adrenal and kidney to form Gerota's fascia. This fusion brings the developing dorsal pancreas and splenic vasculature into the retroperitoneum. The spleen, however, remains intraperitoneal, with its vasculature running in the splenorenal ligament. The gastrosplenic ligament represents the remaining anterior portion of the dorsal mesogastrium and connects the spleen to the greater curvature of the stomach. The

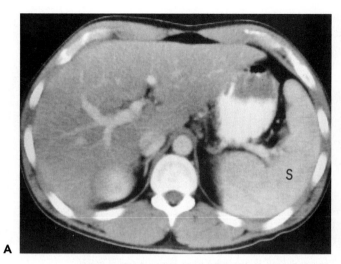
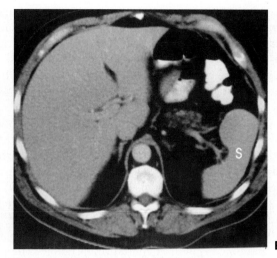

A

B

Figure 14-7 Normal variations in splenic shape. **A:** A prominent lobule of splenic tissue is seen extending medially from the posterior margin of the spleen (S). **B:** A prominent splenic lobule is noted extending off the anterior margin of the spleen (S).

combination of both splenorenal and gastrosplenic ligaments forms the deep margins of the lesser sac (79).

Splenic Lobulation

In light of this fairly complex development, it should not be surprising that the shape and position of the normal spleen vary considerably from one individual to another (110). Commonly, there is a bulge or lobule of splenic tissue that extends medially from the posterior portion of the spleen to lie anterior to the upper pole of the left kidney (Fig. 14-7) (121,162,236). This can simulate the appearance of a left renal or adrenal mass on excretory urography,

but is usually identifiable without difficulty by CT. Less commonly, a bulge from the anterior margin of the spleen also occurs and can simulate an intrasplenic mass. Occasionally, a lobule of splenic tissue can lie partially behind the left kidney and displace it anteriorly. Residual clefts between adjacent lobulations can be sharp and occasionally are as deep as 2 to 3 cm (Fig. 14-8). They tend to occur on the superior diaphragmatic portion of the spleen and may mimic lacerations (79).

The spleen is sufficiently soft and pliable in texture that left upper quadrant abdominal masses or organ enlargement can cause considerable displacement and deformity of its shape. When this happens, the spleen conforms to

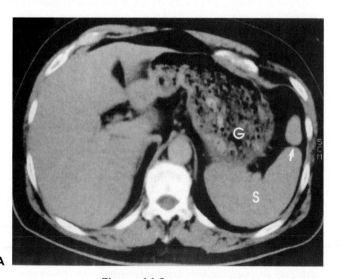
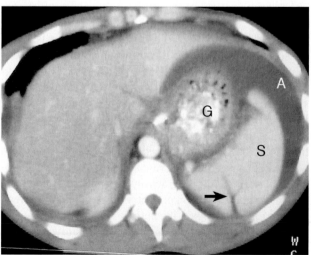

A

B

Figure 14-8 Prominent splenic clefts between adjacent splenic lobulations. This anatomic variation can simulate a splenic laceration. **A:** Prominent cleft (*arrow*) along the anterior margin of the spleen. **B:** Bifid splenic cleft (*arrow*) along the posterior splenic margin. S, spleen; G, stomach; A, ascites.

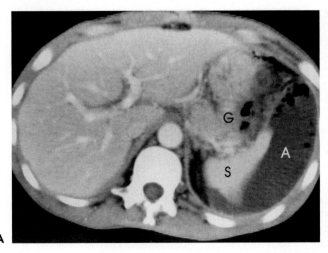
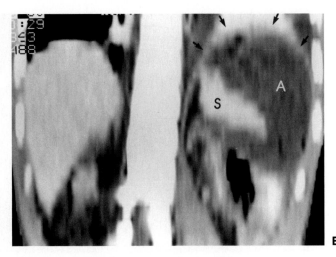

Figure 14-9   Marked alteration in splenic shape and position resulting from compression by a left subphrenic abscess (A). **A:** Axial slice. S, spleen; A, subphrenic abscess; G, stomach. **B:** Coronal reconstruction. S, spleen; A, subphrenic abscess, arrows, hemidiaphragm.

the shape of the adjacent mass, and the resulting deformity can be quite striking (Fig. 14-9). Likewise, changes in the position of the spleen occur when adjacent organs are surgically removed. This is particularly true in patients who have undergone left nephrectomy, in which case the spleen can occupy the left renal fossa. Occasionally, there is sufficient laxity in the ligamentous attachments of the spleen that it lies in an unusual position in the absence of an abdominal mass or previous operation. The upside-down spleen (69,357) is a variant in which the splenic hilum is directed superiorly toward the medial, or occasionally the lateral, portion of the left hemidiaphragm.

"Wandering" Spleen

The "wandering" spleen is another congenital variant that sometimes causes diagnostic difficulties. In this rare condition, most common in women, there is striking laxity of the suspensory splenic ligaments, which permits the spleen to move about in the abdomen (8,40). The CT findings consist of an abdominal soft-tissue-density "mass" with a size appropriate for the spleen, plus the absence of a spleen in the normal location (Fig. 14-10). It may be possible to recognize the characteristic shape of the spleen and splenic hila and to trace the splenic vasculature back to its origin. A whirled appearance to the vasculature may be seen if torsion is present (256). The density and pattern of enhancement after bolus injection of contrast material may also lend support to the diagnosis. When there is uncertainty whether the mass truly represents an ectopically located spleen, radionuclide imaging with technetium-99m (^{99m}Tc)-sulfur colloid can resolve the dilemma (8). The most common clinical presentation is that of a mass, with intermittent abdominal pain. Less commonly, an asymptomatic mass is discovered in the abdomen or pelvis (72). An acute abdominal presentation is least common but most worrisome and indicates torsion and compromise of the vascular supply (25,40,53–55, 256,275,287). With infarction, the radionuclide study can be falsely negative (287). Although splenic enhancement is absent with complete infarction, the remaining CT findings should still allow for a correct diagnosis (134,211). Ascites can also be present (134,287). If the pancreatic tail is involved in the torsion, CT can demonstrate a whorled appearance of the pancreatic tail and adjacent fat (228). A thick, enhancing pseudocapsule representing omental and peritoneal adhesions has been described in one case in which torsion and infarction were missed for several weeks (289).

Chronic torsion with venous congestion also has been reported to lead to the development of splenomegaly, hypersplenism, and gastric varices (40,114). Pancreatitis has also been reported as a consequence of torsion and the resultant obstruction of the pancreatic tail (60,114,206). Intestinal obstruction has also been reported as a complication secondary to ileal volvulus around the splenic pedicle (116).

Accessory Spleens

An accessory spleen is a common finding on CT and arises as a result of failure of fusion of some of the multiple buds of splenic tissue in the dorsal mesogastrium during embryonic life. In autopsy series, accessory spleens are noted in 10% to 20% of individuals (128,346). Although accessory spleens are usually single, approximately 10% of patients with one accessory spleen have a second focus. More than two deposits are seen infrequently (5%) (128,346). Studies on patients who have undergone splenectomy show an

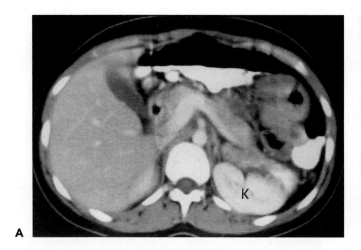

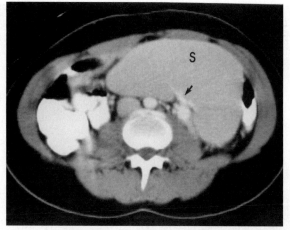

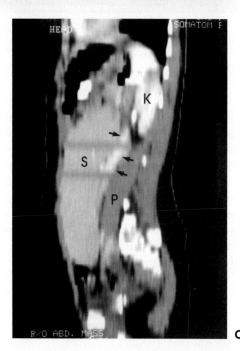

Figure 14-10 Wandering spleen. **A:** No splenic shadow is seen in the left upper abdomen. K, kidney. **B:** The spleen (S) is seen in the lower midabdomen and mimics the appearance of an abdominal tumor, Arrow, splenic hila. **C:** Sagittal reconstruction shows the splenic vein (*arrows*) running cephalad. Marked splenomegaly in this case is secondary to mononucleosis. K, kidney; P, psoas muscle.

increased prevalence of both single and multiple accessory spleens, probably because the underlying pathology necessitating splenectomy has made microscopic deposits clinically apparent (68,89).

Accessory spleens usually occur near the hilum of the spleen (Fig. 14-11), but they are sometimes found in its suspensory ligaments or in the tail of the pancreas (Fig. 14-12) (63,133,174,294). Rarely, they occur elsewhere in the abdomen or retroperitoneum (76,300,330). They vary in size from microscopic deposits that are not visible on CT or MRI, to nodules that are 2 to 3 cm in diameter (22,128, 346). In patients with pathologic splenic findings or those who have previously undergone splenectomy, accessory spleens can hypertrophy and reach a size of 5 cm or more (22). The typical accessory spleen has a smooth, round or

ovoid shape. Its blood supply is usually derived from the splenic artery with drainage occurring into the splenic vein.

In most patients, accessory spleens represent an incidental finding of no clinical significance. Occasionally, it is important to identify accessory splenic tissue, particularly when it is confused with a mass of another type. For instance, an accessory spleen can mimic the findings of a gastric (147), pancreatic (63,133,174,294), left adrenal (309, 330), hepatic (76), or other mass. Identification is particularly crucial in patients in whom a splenectomy was initially performed for a hematologic disorder resulting in hypersplenism. In these patients, the growth of accessory splenic tissue can lead to a return of splenic hyperactivity, with a resultant relapse (9). Torsion and infarction have also been reported involving an accessory spleen and can present as a

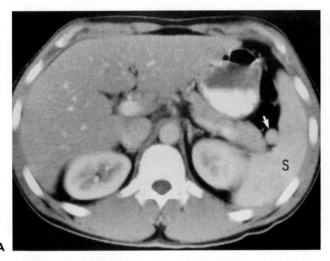
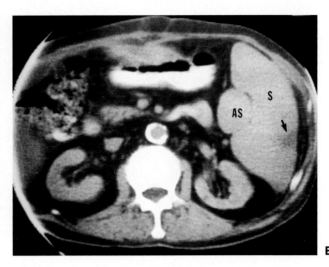

A   B

Figure 14-11 Accessory spleen **A:** Small accessory spleen (*arrow*) adjacent to the splenic hilum. S, spleen. **B:** Enlarged accessory spleen (AS) in a patient with myeloid metaplasia. S, spleen; arrow, small infarct.

painful abdominal mass (234,338). Spontaneous rupture has also been reported (67). Other splenic lesions, such as congenital cysts, have also been reported in accessory spleens and may complicate their identification (106).

When there is uncertainty whether a nodule seen on CT represents an accessory spleen, one can compare the CT attenuation number of the structure in question with that of the spleen before and after IV injection of contrast material. Accessory splenic tissue tends to exhibit the same pattern of contrast enhancement as does the spleen itself (117).

In problematic cases, a radionuclide study (^{99m}Tc sulfur colloid scan or heat-damaged tagged red blood cell study) may prove useful (22,131,223). Ultrasound (US) also has been used to document that the vessels supplying a presumed accessory spleen arise from the splenic artery and vein (312). In cases of torsion, the accessory spleen has appeared as a hypodense soft tissue mass with a thick hyperenhancing pseudocapsule that may be indistinguishable from other entities such as an abscess, pseudocyst, or torsed mesenteric cyst (338).

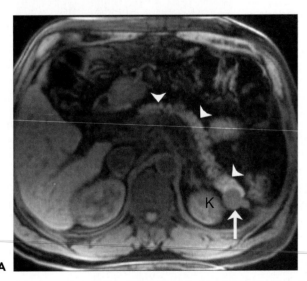
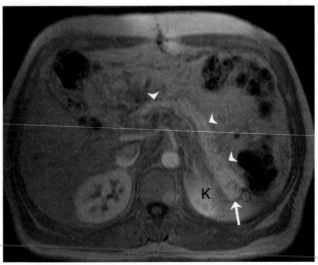

A   B

Figure 14-12 Intrapancreatic accessory spleen. **A:** T1-weighted fat-saturated fast low-angle shot (FLASH) image shows an intermediate-signal rounded mass in the tail of the pancreas. **B:** T1-weighted FLASH image performed during the early arterial phase of intravenous administration of gadolinium—diethylene-triamine penta-acetic acid shows early heterogeneous enhancement of the mass. Surgical removal revealed an accessory spleen. The patient had idiopathic thrombocytopenia and had undergone prior splenectomy.

Polysplenia

Polysplenia is a rare combination of congenital anomalies characterized by multiple aberrant splenic nodules and malformations in other organ systems. Although frequently referred to as left isomerism (bilateral left-sidedness), the associated abnormalities are complex and characterized by no single pathognomonic anomaly (Table 14-1) (233,363). In most cases, the spleen is divided into 2 to 16 masses of equal size. These are located in either the right or left upper quadrant along the greater curve of the stomach (Fig. 14-13). Less commonly, there are one or two large spleens along with several small splenules. Rarely, there may be only a single bilobed spleen (233). Anomalous positions of other abdominal viscera also can occur. In one study of 146 cases of polysplenia (233), a symmetric midline position of the liver was noted in 57%, with 21% having full situs inversus. In 65% of patients, interruption of the inferior vena cava with azygous continuation was noted. A short pancreas in which the body and tail are truncated also has been observed frequently (109,125,134). A semiannular pancreas (161) has also been noted. Abnormal rotation of the bowel was common and usually characterized as either reverse rotation or nonrotation of the midgut loop (109). A preduodenal portal vein was noted in seven of eight patients described in one series (109,161). Genitourinary tract anomalies, including renal agenesis or hypoplasia and multiple ureters, are also observed.

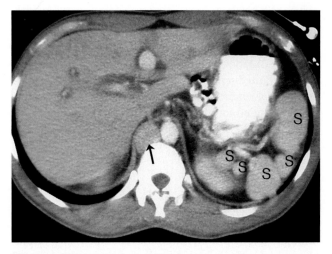

Figure 14-13 Polysplenia. Multiple splenules (S) are seen in the right upper quadrant. The azygos vein (*arrow*) is prominent, and the inferior vena cava is absent. Note that the patient has situs inversus, although the image is displayed reversed for viewing purposes.

Associated thoracic anomalies include bilateral morphologic left lungs (i.e., with two lobes and hyparterial bronchus) in 58% of cases. Bilateral superior vena cava, right-sided aortic arch, and partial anomalous pulmonary venous return occur in 40% to 50% of patients. Cardiac anomalies are common and are the usual cause of death, with half of patients succumbing before 6 months of age.

TABLE 14-1
SUMMARY OF ANOMALIES IN ASPLENIA AND POLYSPLENIA

Anomaly	Asplenia (right isomerism)	Polysplenia (left isomerism)
Lungs	Bilateral trilobed lungs (69%)	Bilateral bilobed lungs (58%)
Superior vena cava (SVC)	Bilateral SVC (53%)	Bilateral SVC (47%)
Inferior vena cava (IVC)	Normal IVC–atrial communication	Azygous continuation of IVC (65%)
Cardiac	Single atrioventricular valve (87%)	Atrial septal defect (78%)
	Absent coronary sinus (85%)	Ventricular septal defect (63%)
	Pulmonary stenosis or atresia (78%)	Right sided aortic arch (44%)
	Total anomalous pulmonary venous return (72%)	Partial anomalous pulmonary venous return (39%)
	Transposition of great vessels (72%)	Mal- or transposition of great vessels (31%)
	Atrial septal defect (66%)	Pulmonary valvular stenosis (23%)
	Single ventricle (44%)	Subaortic stenosis (8%)
Spleen	Absent	Multiple spleens
Gastrointestinal tract	Abdominal heterotaxia (38%)	Abdominal heterotaxia (57%)
	Situs inversus (15%)	Situs inversus (21%)
	Partial situs inversus (15%)	
	Situs solitus (31%)	Situs solitus (21%)
Genitourinary tract	Miscellaneous anomalies (15%)	Miscellaneous anomalies (17%)

Data from Peoples WM, Moller JH, Edwards JE. Polysplenia: a review of 146 cases. *Pediatr Cardiol* 1983;4:129–137 (polysplenia) and Rose V, Izukawa T, Moes CAF. Syndromes of asplenia and polysplenia: a review of cardiac and non-cardiac malformations in 60 cases with special reference to diagnosis and prognosis. *Br Heart J* 1975;37:840–852 (asplenia).

The most common cardiac anomalies are atrial septal defect, ventricular septal defect, malposition or transposition of the great vessels, and pulmonary stenosis or atresia (233). Although only 10% of patients survived to mid-adolescence in one reported series (233), it is important to note that the polysplenia syndrome occasionally can exist without significant cardiac anomalies and may be discovered as an incidental finding on CT (109,284,301,363). CT or MRI may be used to characterize the visceral anomalies (144,344).

Asplenia

The congenital asplenia syndrome (right isomerism or Ivemark syndrome) is characterized by an absent spleen and multiple anomalies in both the abdomen and thorax (Table 14-1). The inferior vena cava–right atrial communication is usually normal; however, abnormal visceral position is frequently observed. In one study of 39 cases of asplenia (267), total or partial situs inversus was noted in 31%, with abdominal heterotaxy seen in 38%. Associated intestinal malrotation is common (194), genitourinary tract anomalies are seen in 15% (267), and bilateral morphologic right lungs are noted in 69% of cases (267). The most serious associated anomalies are cardiovascular. These typically are more complex malformations than those seen with polysplenia. In the series of 39 patients cited (267), 87% had a single atrioventricular valve and a single ventricle was seen in 44%. Transposition of the great vessels and total anomalous pulmonary venous drainage were also common. These serious anomalies account for much of the high mortality, with 80% of patients dying by the end of their first year (267). Sepsis related to asplenia also contributes to this mortality figure.

Although the majority of patients with asplenia present with cyanosis or cardiorespiratory problems, a few present with bowel obstruction (194). In both groups, CT or MRI can be helpful in suggesting the diagnosis and fully characterizing the disorder (327).

Splenic–Gonadal Fusion

Splenic–gonadal fusion is a rare congenital anomaly in which functioning splenic tissue is located in close proximity to gonadal tissue. This entity is found predominantly in men, with a male:female ratio of 17:1 (46). The functioning splenic tissue, which usually appears as an encapsulated mass, may lie in the epididymis, along the spermatic cord, or within the tunica albuginea. It is hypothesized that this anomaly arises from adhesion between the developing gonadal primordia and the splenic anlage prior to gonadal descent. A fibrous band that can contain additional splenic tissue is found extending to the main spleen in slightly over half of patients. This "continuous" type of splenic–gonadal fusion is associated with other congenital anomalies, including limb defects, micrognathia, and cardiac defects (197). Hernia and undescended testis are associated in 15% to

20% of patients (46). The "discontinuous" type, in which there is no connection to the main spleen, is usually not associated with other congenital anomalies. Although the mass is usually asymptomatic, confusion with testicular malignancy or inflammation can occur if the mass is noted on routine physical exam or if the splenic tissue enlarges or becomes tender secondary to a systemic illness such as mononucleosis or malaria (23). Such confusion can lead to unnecessary orchiectomy (23,46). Bowel obstruction produced by the fibrous band present in the continuous type of fusion has also been reported (46). ^{99m}Tc-labeled sulfur colloid scan has been suggested as the best procedure to establish a diagnosis of splenic–gonadal fusion in cases in which a questionable mass has been identified with either US or CT (64,308). On CT, the splenic tissue has been described as a well-defined homogenous mass (145).

Splenorenal Fusion

Splenorenal fusion is a very rare congenital anomaly in which splenic tissue has fused with the kidney during embryologic development. The resultant mass can mimic renal neoplasia (368).

PATHOLOGIC CONDITIONS

Cysts

Three types of nonneoplastic cysts are known to arise in the spleen (70,108): hydatid cysts resulting from *Echinococcus granulosa* infection, congenital cysts, and posttraumatic pseudocysts.

Echinococcal Cysts

On a worldwide basis, echinococcal infection is thought to be responsible for two thirds of all splenic cysts (108). This is despite the fact that splenic involvement occurs in less than 2% to 3% of cases of echinococcosis (34,184,242). In greater than 70% of patients with echinococcal involvement of the spleen, other structures also are involved, the liver being the most common (103,343). In North America, echinococcal disease is unusual, with fewer than 200 cases diagnosed yearly. More than 90% of these are acquired on other continents (362). Patients are frequently asymptomatic (336). Symptoms, when present, are generally related to the large size of the cyst. Fever is not usually present unless secondary infection of a cyst has developed (362). When present, echinococcal cysts are well-circumscribed, low-density lesions that enlarge the spleen (Fig. 14-14A). Cyst wall calcification is common, occurring in approximately half of patients in two series (105,343). Multiple separate cysts were also seen frequently, although daughter cysts and collapsed membranes were less commonly identified. No enhancement of the lesions was observed on CT (105), although prior studies with angiography have shown

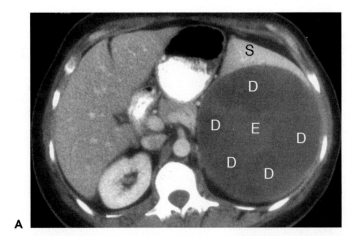

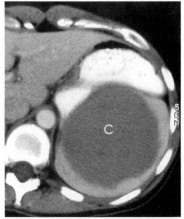

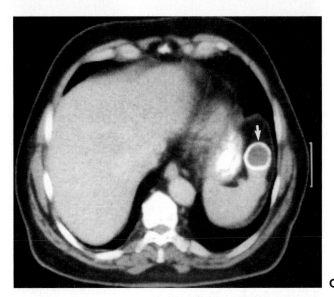

Figure 14-14 Splenic cysts. **A:** Echinococcal cyst. A large low-density lesion (E) is noted in the spleen (S). Note daughter cysts lining the lesion with slightly lower attenuation than the main cyst fluid. (Case courtesy of John K. McLarney, Armed Forces Institute of Pathology.) **B:** In another patient, a large unilocular low-density lesion is noted. Following removal, this was shown to be an epithelial cyst (C). **C:** This round and sharply circumscribed cyst (*arrow*) with a calcified rim was presumed to be secondary to trauma.

enhancement of the outer cyst wall (263). On MR, hydatid cysts are hypointense compared with liver parenchyma on T1-weighted images and hyperintense on T2-weighted images. In 75% of cases, the signal intensity is heterogeneous. Daughter cysts typically give a slightly lower signal than the main cyst on T1-weighted sequences. A continuous 4- to 5-mm-thick low-intensity rim surrounding the cyst usually is evident. This rim corresponds to a dense fibrous capsule encasing the parasitic membranes (185,342). Treatment is by surgical removal. Percutaneous aspiration should be avoided because of the risk of allergic reaction to cyst contents and spread of infection (86,146).

Congenital Cysts

Epithelial (also called epidermoid, mesothelial, primary, or true) cysts are congenital in origin (122,200). Pathologically, they are true cysts, with an epithelial lining thought to originate from peritoneal mesothelial cells that have become trapped within the splenic parenchyma during development (43,70,200,224). Grossly, they have a typical glistening white trabeculated surface (200). Epithelial cysts are said to make up approximately 20% of nonparasitic

splenic cysts. Some researchers have suggested, however, that this percentage is artificially low and reflects an incomplete evaluation of the cyst lining. Epithelial cysts are usually discovered in childhood or in the early adult years (70,88,108) and are more common in females than in males (70,200). Although the vast majority of cases are sporadic, familial occurrence has been reported (5,115, 142,255). Elevated serum and intracystic levels of several tumor markers [cancer antigen (CA) 19-9, CA 125, and carcinoembryonic antigen (CEA)] have also been reported in patients with large epithelial cysts (142,181). In 80% of cases, congenital splenic cysts are unilocular and solitary. On CT, they appear as spherical, sharply circumscribed, water-density lesions, that show no central or rim enhancement after IV administration of contrast material (70,293)(Fig. 14-14B). Although usually solitary, multiple lesions have been reported (115). CT may show cyst wall trabeculation or peripheral septation. The wall of an epidermoid cyst occasionally calcifies (70). The MR appearance is usually that of a fluid-containing cyst with increased T2 signal and intermediate or low T1 signal. Lobulation or trabeculation may also be visible (293).

Posttraumatic Cysts

Posttraumatic cysts are thought to represent a final stage in the evolution of splenic hematoma. Histologically, they lack a cellular lining and thus are referred to as pseudocysts (70,82,171). Grossly they have a shaggy hemorrhagic internal appearance. Most splenic cysts encountered in the United States are thought to be posttraumatic in origin, although this number has been recently challenged (70,108,200).

Like epithelial cysts, posttraumatic cysts appear on CT as sharply demarcated lesions. They are almost always unilocular, show no enhancement, and contain fluid of a density similar to or slightly above that of water (70). In one series, the average greatest dimension was 13 cm, with no significant size difference noted between pseudocysts and true cysts (70). CT-visible calcification was more common in pseudocysts than congenital cysts (50% versus 14%) (Fig. 14-14C). Cyst wall trabeculation or peripheral septation was more common in congenital cysts (86% versus 17%).

Although often asymptomatic, nonparasitic splenic cysts of either type may present as a left upper quadrant mass, causing a sense of epigastric fullness or intermittent dull pain (70,108). An acute abdominal presentation may occur with rupture or infection (70,255,258). Compression of the left kidney may lead to renal colic, or rarely, hypertension (249).

Other Cystic Lesions

The differential diagnosis of a splenic cyst includes abscess, acute hematoma, intrasplenic pancreatic pseudocyst (221), cystic neoplasm (lymphangioma or hemangioma), and cystic or necrotic metastasis (70,90,337).

Benign Splenic Tumors

Hemangiomas

Benign splenic tumors are uncommon. Hemangiomas and lymphangiomas are the two most frequent types, with hemangiomas seen in 0.01% to 0.14% of patients at autopsy (35,168,237,277). They are usually asymptomatic incidental findings (361). Less frequently, they present with an abdominal mass or pain. Rupture and hemorrhage are reported in up to 25% in some series (139). Anemia, thrombocytopenia, and a consumptive coagulopathy (Kasabach-Merritt syndrome) have been noted (226,285). Portal hypertension with esophageal varices also has been infrequently reported (240,316). Splenic hemangiomas can be multiple or occur with hemangiomas in other organs (Fig. 14-15 and 14-16). They have been described in association with Klippel-Trenaunay-Weber syndrome (cutaneous hemangioma, venous varicosities, soft tissue and bony hypertrophy of an extremity) (225). They range in size from a few millimeters to over 15 cm (266). In rare circumstances, diffuse hemangiomatosis may occur, in which the entire spleen may be replaced by hemangioma (204). This type of involvement is frequently accompanied by angiomas in other hematopoietic organs as well as by hematologic abnormalities (169).

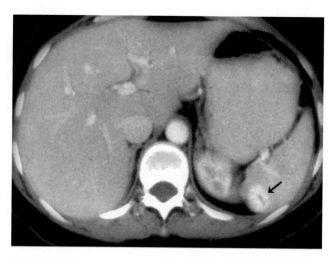

Figure 14-15 Splenic hemangioma. Contrast-enhanced computed tomography scan shows a solitary hyperenhancing lesion. (Case courtesy of John K. McLarney, Armed Forces Institute of Pathology.)

In the spleen, cavernous hemangiomas are more common than capillary-type hemangiomas (169,199).

The imaging characteristics of splenic hemangiomas are similar to those in the liver. On unenhanced CT, they appear as a well-defined hypodense mass that may contain cystic components. With contrast injection, most lesions enhance from the periphery with gradual fill in and persistence of contrast enhancement on delayed images. Some lesions, however, may remain hypodense, show diffuse enhancement, or show discrete mottled areas of density (85,95,204,225,232,250,266). Clearly defined peripheral discontinuous nodular enhancement seen with liver hemangioma is uncommon, occurring in only 2 of 22 patients in

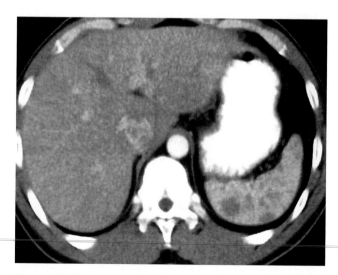

Figure 14-16 Splenic hemangiomatosis. Contrast-enhanced computed tomography scan shows multiple poorly defined hypodense splenic nodules. The patient was also noted to have a mediastinal hemangioma.

one series using MRI and gadolinium (257). Calcification can occur as scattered, punctate, curvilinear densities, or as dense rays radiating from a central point (127,225,266). On MR, these lesions appear hypointense or, less commonly, isointense with respect to the rest of the spleen on T1-weighted images and hyperintense on T2-weighted sequences. Heterogeneous signal is sometimes noted on T2-weighted images, reflecting the presence of cystic and solid components with varying amounts of fibrosis, necrosis, and hemorrhage (85,232,250,257). Injection of IV Gd-DTPA causes enhancement similar to that observed with iodinated contrast material on CT (257). ^{99m}Tc—labeled red blood cell (RBC) scintigraphy with early and delayed single photon emission computed tomography (SPECT) views has been used to confirm the suspected diagnosis of splenic hemangioma in a manner similar to its use with liver hemangioma (360).

Littoral Cell Angioma

Littoral cell angioma is an unusual vascular tumor unique to the spleen. It is thought to be derived from the lining (littoral) cells of the splenic red pulp sinuses and hence shows both endothelial and macrophage characteristics (91,169). The lesion has no age or sex predilection. Patients may be asymptomatic or present with splenomegaly. Hypersplenism with associated thrombocytopenia and anemia has been reported, as has fever of unknown origin and portal hypertension (91,306). Although the lesion itself is benign, an association with other malignancies has been reported (66). This association, however, may reflect the widespread use of CT in staging malignancy rather than a causative role (169,207). On CT, the lesions are usually multiple, ranging from 0.2 to 9 cm in diameter and of low attenuation (Fig. 14-17) (91,119,306).

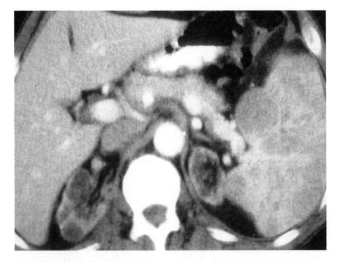

Figure 14-17 Littoral cell angioma. The patient had adenocarcinoma of the lung. Splenectomy performed to rule out metastatic disease or lymphoma involving the spleen revealed littoral cell angioma. Incidental note is made of renal atrophy secondary to Alport syndrome.

Lymphangiomas

Although most common in the neck and axilla, lymphangiomas occur rarely in the abdominal viscera. Disseminated lymphangiomatosis affecting multiple areas also has been reported (16,239,347). Lymphangiomas are categorized as capillary, cavernous, or cystic, depending on the size of the abnormal lymphatic channels. In the spleen, the cystic type is most common. Splenic lymphangiomas are usually asymptomatic or discovered as a left upper quadrant mass. Lymphangiomas can occur as single or multiple lesions (199,349). CT may demonstrate a well-defined, multilocular cyst or multiple, thin-walled, well-marginated cysts often in a subcapsular location. Diffuse involvement of the spleen with complete replacement of the normal splenic parenchyma has also been observed (20). No or only slight enhancement of the septations and cyst walls is noted after IV administration of contrast material. CT attenuation measurements from the cysts vary from 15 to 35 HU (30,239,247,299,332). Curvilinear calcifications have also been noted (239). Rarely, a solid lesion may be mimicked if the cysts are small (163). T2-weighted MR images display the typical high signal intensity of fluid with multiple hypointense septae usually well seen (141,299). T1-weighted images usually show hypointense cysts, although hyperintensity is occasionally seen if there has been prior hemorrhage or the cyst fluid is proteinaceous (30).

Splenic Hamartomas

Splenic hamartomas (also called splenomas or nodular hyperplasia of the spleen) are rare, benign splenic lesions (108,167,349). They are composed of an anomalous mixture of normal splenic elements with red pulp predominating. A mixture of red and white pulp, or white pulp predominating, occurs less commonly. Whether they represent a developmental anomaly, a neoplasm, or a post-traumatic lesion is uncertain (349). Hamartomas occur singly or, less commonly, as multiple nodules (307). Their diameter ranges from less than 1 cm to greater than 15 cm (198,307). Like most other benign splenic lesions, they are usually discovered incidentally or as a result of mass-related symptomatology. Thrombocytopenia and anemia have been reported rarely, as has spontaneous rupture (140,198,364). Splenic hamartomas are reported as a rare manifestation of tuberous sclerosis (73,339).

On CT, splenic hamartomas appear as well-circumscribed iso- or hypodense masses on precontrast images, with occasional lesions showing cystic components (36, 370). Calcification has been observed (323,370). They usually show slow enhancement and fill in after IV administration of contrast material (Fig. 14-18). Prolonged enhancement similar to that seen with hemangiomas is often noted and can serve to differentiate hamartomas from lymphomas (219). Lesions that are isodense to normal spleen on both pre- and postcontrast images also have been reported (215). On unenhanced MR images, the lesions are usually isointense on T1-weighted images and heterogeneously

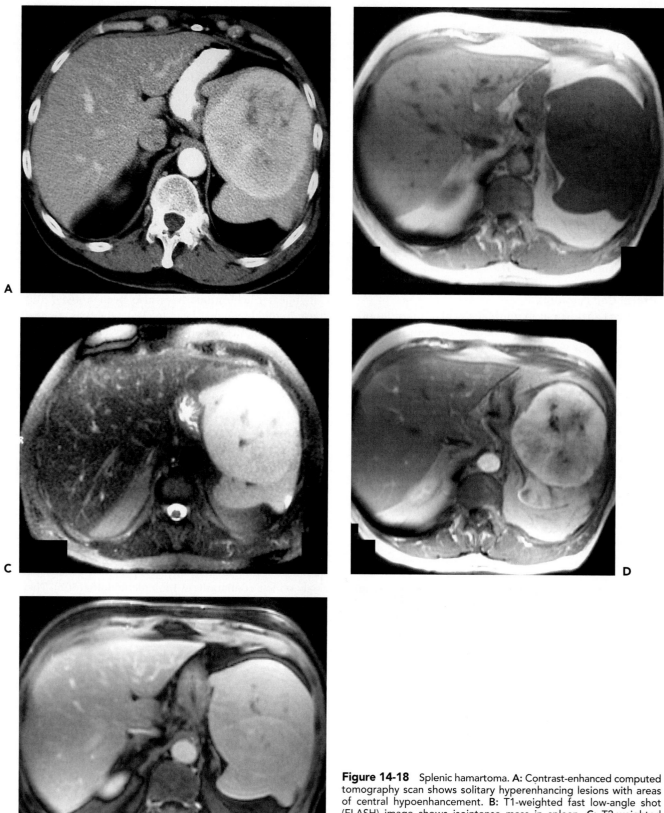

Figure 14-18 Splenic hamartoma. **A:** Contrast-enhanced computed tomography scan shows solitary hyperenhancing lesions with areas of central hypoenhancement. **B:** T1-weighted fast low-angle shot (FLASH) image shows isointense mass in spleen. **C:** T2-weighted half-Fourier acquisition single-shot turbo spin-echo image shows isointense mass in spleen. **D:** Early postgadolinium FLASH images show heterogeneously hyperenhancing mass in the spleen. **E:** On delayed FLASH images, lesion becomes isointense to the remainder of the spleen.

hyperintense on T2-weighted images relative to the background spleen (36,219,257) (see Fig. 14-18). Slow, diffuse, heterogeneous enhancement is noted following gadolinium injection. On delayed images, more uniform and persistent enhancement is noted, often greater than that of adjacent normal spleen. Occasional areas of hypointensity are noted on delayed images that appear to correspond to cystic areas of necrosis (257). Uptake on ^{99m}Tc colloid scintigraphy as well as on heat-treated chromium-51–labeled RBC studies has been reported (220, 320,323). This may be useful in establishing a noninvasive diagnosis, but such activity is not invariably present.

Inflammatory Pseudotumor

Inflammatory pseudotumors are rare, benign lesions consisting of a polymorphous inflammatory cell infiltrate with varying amounts of granulomatous reaction, fibrosis, and necrosis (272). They have been described in virtually every organ system, including lung, esophagus, liver, lymph nodes, and spleen (349). They can be asymptomatic or present as a mass accompanied by vague constitutional symptoms (e.g., fever, malaise). Their etiology is uncertain, although there has been speculation that they have an infectious or autoimmune origin. Most patients with splenic inflammatory pseudotumor are adults; however, the lesion has been described in children as young as 4 years of age (167,274). Although the lesion is benign, increase in size during observation has been noted (202). In the spleen, inflammatory pseudotumors appear as well-circumscribed, encapsulated masses. They usually are solitary, but multiple lesions have been reported in the liver and spleen (118,272). They range from 1.5 cm to more than 12 cm in diameter (195,272). On CT, they appear as a heterogeneous hypodense mass (104,272). Peripheral calcification has been described (104). After IV administration of contrast material, heterogeneous enhancement may occur, with the lesion being hypodense or isodense with the remainder of the spleen (104,202,359, 366). Persistent areas of hypodensity corresponding to regions of fibrosis are often noted (104,202,359,366). On MR, the lesions have been described as both slightly hyperintense and hypointense relative to normal spleen on T1-weighted images (118,202). On T2-weighted images, the lesions have been described as both hyperintense and hypointense relative to normal spleen (118,366). Mild-to-moderate enhancement is noted after IV administration of gadolinium (118). The variation in described appearances may reflect the underlying histologic heterogeneity of these lesions.

Extramedullary Hematopoiesis

Extramedullary hematopoiesis may also produce focal tumorlike lesions in the spleen, although it more commonly produces homogeneous enlargement (84,111). Although usually associated with significant underlying hematologic disease, they have been reported in patients with only mild anemia (84). On enhanced CT, focal extramedullary hematopoiesis appears as a hypodense mass relative to the

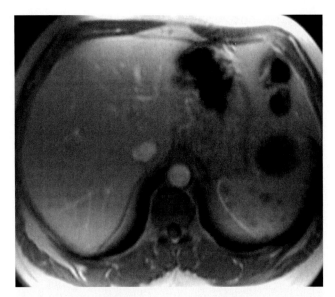

Figure 14-19 Extramedullary hematopoiesis. T1-weighted fast low-angle shot image after gadolinium administration shows multiple hypoenhancing splenic nodules of varying sizes.

remainder of the spleen (84,111). On MRI, lesions are slightly hypointense on T1-weighted imaging and hyperintense on T2-weighted images. The lesions showed progressive enhancement after bolus injection of gadolinium and went from hypointense relative to splenic parenchyma on early-phase gadolinium-enhanced images to isointense on late images (Fig. 14-19) (107). In one report, focal lesions of extramedullary hematopoiesis did not produce a defect on ^{99m}Tc-sulfur colloid scans (111). Successful diagnosis of focal splenic extramedullary hematopoiesis has been noted with fine needle aspiration (FNA) (13).

Other Benign Splenic Tumors

Other benign tumors are quite rare and include lipomas, fibromas, and angiomyolipomas (35,87,168,365). The latter have been observed both in patients with and without tuberous sclerosis (11,317). Both lipomas and angiomyolipomas are suggested on CT and MRI by the characteristic appearance of fat (Fig. 14-20).

Malignant Splenic Tumors

Lymphoma

Primary splenic lymphoma is rare and makes up less than 1% of all lymphomas (Fig. 14-21) (6,38,349). When it occurs, it is usually a non-Hodgkin lymphoma (NHL). Although small-cell lymphomas have been said to be the most common histologic type of primary splenic lymphoma (303,349), several studies have shown a diffuse large cell predominance (71,123,165). Left upper quadrant pain or discomfort was the most common presenting symptom. Systemic symptoms of weight loss, malaise, and fever were also frequently noted (6,71,349). Although splenic lymphoma

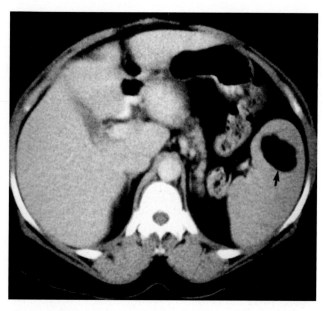

Figure 14-20 Splenic lipoma. Contrast-enhanced computed tomography scan shows a well-defined fat-density mass (*arrow*).

may be confined by the splenic capsule, local extension with invasion into adjoining structures has been reported (Fig. 14-22) (132,150). The majority of lesions were either solitary (and larger than 5 cm) or multiple masses of varying size (greater than 1 cm). On unenhanced CT, lesions were either slightly hypodense or isodense to adjacent spleen. Calcification was uncommon (71). Following IV administration of contrast, lesions remained hypodense relative to normal spleen. Very-low-density foci were not uncommonly noted, suggesting areas of necrosis or ischemia. Rim enhancement was rarely seen (71).

Secondary splenic involvement in both Hodgkin and non-Hodgkin lymphoma is frequent, with lymphomas as a group being the most common splenic malignancy. The spleen is frequently involved by Hodgkin and non-Hodgkin lymphoma at the time of diagnosis. The percentage varies according to cell type (349,365). Splenic involvement in lymphoma can take several forms: (a) homogeneous enlargement, (b) miliary nodules, (c) multifocal lesions greater than 1 cm, and (d) a single solitary mass (6,98,365)

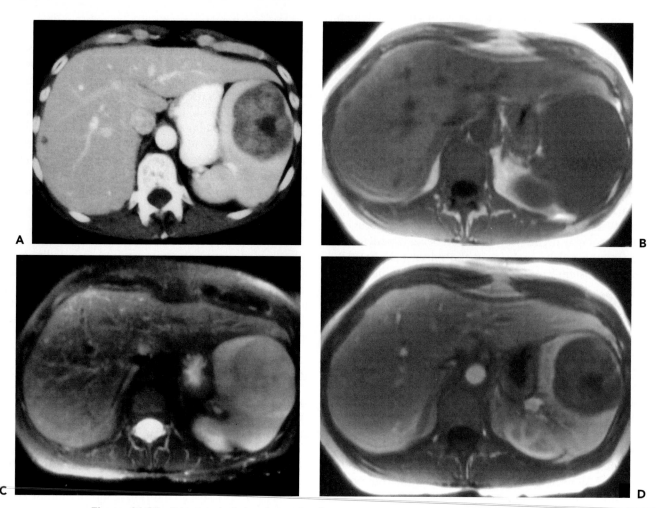

Figure 14-21 Primary splenic lymphoma, B cell type **A:** Contrast-enhanced computed tomography scan shows a heterogeneous hypoenhancing mass with central necrosis. **B:** On T1-weighted magnetic resonance (MR) image, the mass is isointense to the normal spleen. **C:** On T2-weighted MR image, the mass is slightly hypointense relative to the normal spleen. **D:** Following intravenous administration of gadolinium, the mass is heterogeneously hypointense.

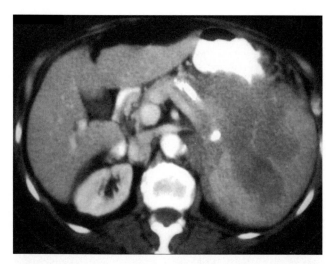

Figure 14-22 Intermediate-grade, large-cell lymphoma (B phenotype) with invasion into adjacent structures. Contrast-enhanced computed tomography scan shows homogeneous infiltrating mass.

(Figs. 14-23 to 14-25). As a general rule in non-Hodgkin lymphoma, large-cell lymphomas produce either solitary or multiple masses. Small cleaved and mixed cell types and intermediate lymphocytic lymphomas commonly produce a miliary pattern. Low-grade lymphomas with associated blood involvement typically cause homogeneous enlargement. Hodgkin disease can cause solitary or multiple masses or a miliary pattern (365). All types of Hodgkin disease may involve the spleen, although involvement with the lymphocyte-predominant form is least common (148,349,365).

On CT, focal lymphomatous lesions typically show lower attenuation than normal splenic parenchyma. Lesions are usually homogeneous, but necrosis of large lesions has been reported and can give an irregular cystic appearance (33,132). In a patient with lymphoma-associated

fever, this appearance may mimic a splenic abscess. Radiologically visible calcification is unusual but has been reported in aggressive lesions and after therapy (see Fig. 14-23) (186). On unenhanced MR, focal lesions are frequently isointense compared with splenic parenchyma on T1- and T2-weighted images. Occasionally, lesions are lower in signal than spleen on T2-weighted images—a feature that may be helpful in distinguishing lymphoma from metastasis (208). Portions of lesions can also have either increased or decreased signal intensity if necrosis, hemorrhage, fibrosis, and edema are present (126,217,218). The use of IV contrast material on MRI improves its ability to detect focal splenic lesions (193). Lesions are typically lower signal on postcontrast images than background spleen (208). Agents specific for reticuloendothelial tissue may be useful for MRI. Superparamagnetic iron oxide has been shown to improve significantly the ability of MRI to distinguish normal spleen from diffuse splenic lymphoma (356).

Although focal lesions can be seen with CT and MRI, neither modality is accurate for staging splenic lymphoma. On CT, involvement is often isodense with adjacent normal spleen, or lesions are below the resolving power of the technique. The reported accuracy of CT as a predictor of splenic involvement by lymphoma ranges from a low sensitivity and specificity of 30% and 71%, respectively (49,113,190), to a high sensitivity and specificity of approximately 90% (310,311). The lower figures are more in line with extensive clinical literature that demonstrates that normal-size spleens frequently show microscopic involvement and that mildly to moderately enlarged spleens are often uninvolved (94,130,148,155,365). However, markedly enlarged spleens almost always show lymphomatous involvement (50,270,340).

MRI has similarly not proved successful at staging splenic lymphoma. No significant change has been noted in T1 or T2 values for spleens involved with lymphoma

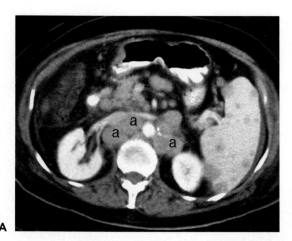

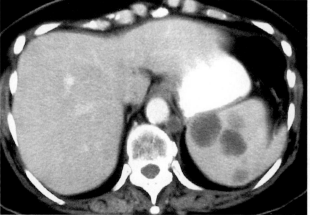

Figure 14-23 Non-Hodgkin lymphoma in two patients. **A:** Splenomegaly with multiple hypodense nodules and extensive retroperitoneal adenopathy (a) in a patient with small cleaved-cell lymphoma. **B:** Multiple larger hypodense nodules in a patient with mixed large- and small-cell lymphoma. Also noted is an enlarged left retrocrural lymph node.

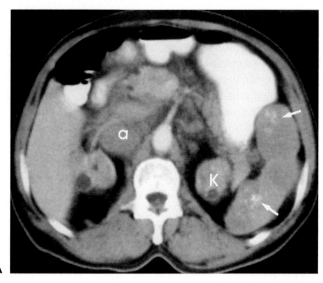 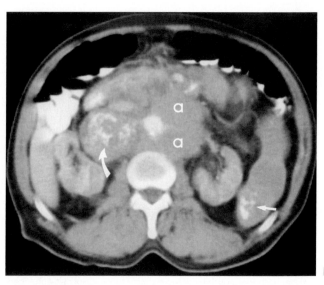

A B

Figure 14-24 Non-Hodgkin lymphoma. Faintly hypodense nodules with scattered punctate calcification (*arrows*) are noted in the spleen in a patient with untreated diffuse large-cell lymphoma. Note extensive retroperitoneal adenopathy (a), which also demonstrates calcification (curved arrow). K, Kidney. **A:** At the level of the superior mesenteric artery takeoff. **B:** At the level of the renal arteries.

(218,324,356). In a study comparing MRI, CT, and US for detecting splenic infiltration in patients with Hodgkin and non-Hodgkin lymphoma, MRI and US were better than CT in demonstrating infiltration in patients with Hodgkin lymphoma, although no major difference was noted with NHL. All three imaging techniques failed to detect the majority of cases of NHL infiltration (217).

Recently, the use of fluorodeoxyglucose positron emission tomography (FDG-PET) has been proposed for identifying lymphomatous involvement in the spleen. A small study comparing it with CT in seven patients showed improved accuracy with FDG-PET (100%, versus 57% for CT) (262). FDG-PET was also shown to have a higher accuracy (97% versus 78%) in predicting splenic involvement than

gallium-67 in a study involving 32 patients with Hodgkin Lymphoma (261).

Angiosarcomas

Malignancies arising from the mesenchymal components of the spleen occur but are quite rare (74,349,358). Most are tumors of vascular origin. *Angiosarcoma* (hemangiosarcoma, malignant hemangioendothelioma, endothelial sarcoma) refers to the frankly malignant variety, whereas *hemangioendothelioma* has been used to refer to vascular tumors of borderline malignant potential (212,349,365). Most patients with splenic angiosarcoma are older than 40 years. No sex predilection is noted. Symptoms include abdominal pain, left upper quadrant mass, fever, weight loss, anemia,

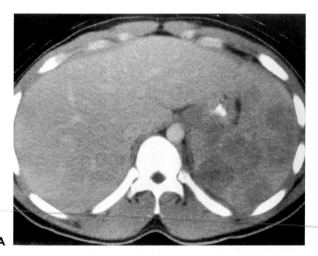 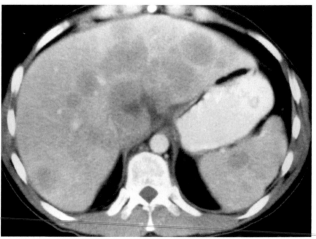

A B

Figure 14-25 Hodgkin disease. **A:** Splenomegaly with multiple hypodense splenic nodules in a patient with nodular sclerosing Hodgkin disease. **B:** Multiple hypodense nodules in the liver and spleen in a patient with advanced Hodgkin disease.

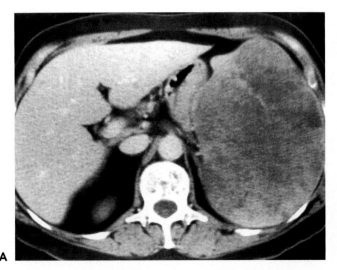
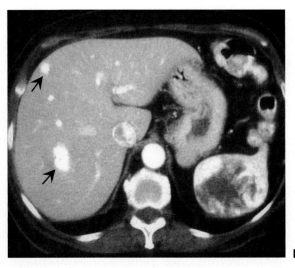

Figure 14-26 Splenic angiosarcoma in two patients. **A:** Large, partially enhanced angiosarcoma of the spleen. **B:** Irregular brightly enhancing splenic lesion with two metastases noted in the liver (*arrows*). (Case courtesy of Emil Balthazar, M.D., New York, NY)

and consumptive coagulopathy (92,349). The duration of symptoms is usually short (169). Distant metastases are common and the prognosis is poor (212,349). Splenomegaly is noted in the vast majority of patients and splenic rupture is reported to occur in approximately one quarter to one third of patients (14,92,212,296,358). On CT, such neoplasms generally appear as focal, rounded, or irregular areas of heterogeneous low attenuation (176,296, 326). Lesions range from 1 cm to as large as 18 cm in diameter (169). Cystic and necrotic areas may be evident within the mass. Acute hemorrhage and hemosiderin deposits may appear as areas of increased density (250). Extensive calcification has been reported in one case (158). Heterogeneous enhancement, which can be marked, has also been seen (Fig. 14-26) (158,250). On T2-weighted MR images, lesions have been described as heterogeneously hyperintense. T1-weighted images show hypointense tumor. Prior intratumoral hemorrhage may also produce increased T1 signal (158). Hemosiderin deposition may produce decreased T1 and T2 signals (250). At angiography, multiple vascular lakes have been observed, which may mimic the appearance of cavernous hemangiomata (159).

Angiosarcoma has been caused by exposure to Thorotrast, a colloidal suspension of thorium dioxide used until the 1950s as an angiographic contrast agent (176). In these patients, CT shows a striking increase in the attenuation of the splenic parenchyma resulting from chronic retention of the radiopaque material in reticuloendothelial cells of the spleen. Although Thorotrast-associated angiosarcoma has occurred much more commonly in the liver, a primary case in the spleen has been reported (176). Vinyl chloride and arsenic exposure, although associated with hepatic angiosarcoma, have not been shown to predispose to splenic angiosarcoma (32,259,365).

Other Malignant Splenic Tumors

Other primary mesenchymal malignancies that have been reported in the spleen include fibrosarcoma, leiomyosarcoma, malignant teratoma, and malignant fibrous histiocytoma (MFH) (199,349,358). The CT appearance of these lesions is not specific. MFH has been described as a large mass with extensive areas of necrosis (39). Mucinous cystadenocarcinoma also has been reported in the spleen and is thought to arise from either invaginated capsular mesothelium or embryonic rests of pancreatic or enteric tissue. On CT, mucinous cystadenocarcinoma has the appearance of a large multicystic mass. Calcification can be observed (201).

Metastatic Disease

Metastatic deposits in the spleen are unusual. They occur most commonly from hematogenous spread. Although they are almost always seen in patients with widespread carcinoma (i.e., metastasis to three or more organs), isolated splenic metastases have been reported (93,160,222,241, 350,355). In autopsy series, splenic metastases are noted in approximately 1% to 9% of patients with carcinoma (2,350). Of these, one third to one-half are found only on microscopic examination (26,187,350). The lack of afferent splenic lymphatics, periodic changes in spleen size, filtering of blood by liver and lung, and immune surveillance within the spleen have all been suggested to explain the relative infrequency of gross splenic metastasis (47,350). The most common primary sites of splenic metastases are breast and lung (26,187). Melanoma has the highest frequency of splenic involvement on a per primary basis, with 34% of melanoma patients showing splenic metastasis at autopsy (26). Splenic metastases most frequently appear as multiple nodules, although diffuse infiltration occurs in 8% to 10% of affected patients (187). The splenic deposits are usually asymptomatic.

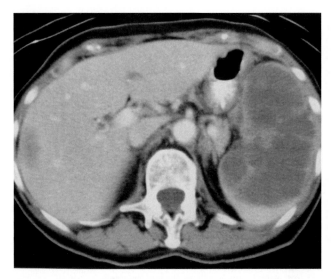

Figure 14-27 Endometrial carcinoma metastatic to the spleen. Contrast-enhanced computed tomography scan demonstrates a large, complex low-density metastasis.

On CT, nodular metastases appear as rounded, hypodense lesions (Fig. 14-27 and 14-28). Cystic lesions may occur with metastasis from ovary, breast, endometrium, and melanoma (47,99,166,241,250,337,355). Calcification is uncommon

but does occur in patients with serous or mucinous cystadenocarcinomas (47,250). Peritoneal implants in patients with an ovarian, gastrointestinal, or pancreatic cancer can cause scalloping of the capsular surface of the spleen (99). Direct splenic invasion is unusual but can occur from adjacent primaries in the stomach, colon, pancreas, or kidney (166,250). On MRI, metastases from colorectal carcinoma have been described as hypointense to isointense relative to normal spleen on T1-weighted images, hypointense on T2-weighted images, and hypoenhancing post gadolinium administration (355).

Splenic Infection

Splenic infection can occur either as a single focus or as part of a diffuse or miliary process. Although splenic infection is uncommon, the increasing prevalence of immunosuppression in cancer, transplant, and acquired immunodeficiency syndrome (AIDS) patients has placed a greater population at risk (48,209).

Splenic infection is usually the result of hematogenous dissemination, with predisposing primary infections occurring in 68% of patients in one series (62). In more recent reviews, this rate is significantly lower, probably because of more aggressive antibiotic use (209). Endocarditis was the

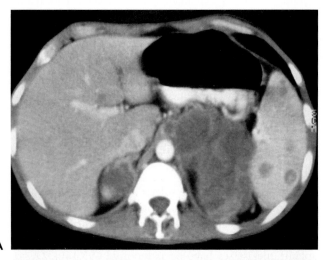

A

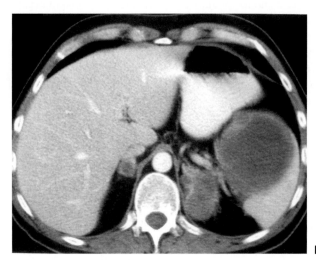

B

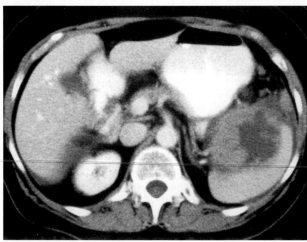

C

Figure 14-28 Carcinoma metastatic to the spleen. **A:** Small, low-density lesions in the spleen with bilateral adrenal metastases in a patient with squamous cell carcinoma of the lung. **B:** Hypodense mass within the spleen with bilateral adrenal masses in a patient with malignant melanoma. **C:** Complex mass in the splenic hilum in a patient with ovarian carcinoma.

most common associated infection, occurring in 12% of patients with splenic abscess. Conversely, splenic abscess is seen in about 5% of patients with endocarditis (264). Other associated infections included urinary tract infection, surgical wound infection, appendicitis, and pneumonia (62). Abscess in other organs occurs in 15% to 20% of patients (62,325). Direct spread of infection from adjacent organs has been reported in cases of gastric ulcer and carcinoma, carcinoma of the descending colon, and perihepatic abscess. Noninfectious predisposing factors include diabetes, immunosuppression, and sickle cell disease. Disruption of the normal splenic parenchyma by trauma or infarction also predisposes to subsequent infection (48,62).

Patients with splenic abscess present clinically with fever, leukocytosis, and pain. The latter can localize in either the left upper quadrant or left side of the chest, or can be referred to the shoulder (62,213). Although this presentation is typical for a solitary splenic abscess in a normal host, the immunosuppressed patient with multiple splenic abscesses often shows no localizing signs (48). Splenomegaly is noted on physical examination in about half of the patients with splenic abscess (62). The most common organisms are *Staphylococcus* and *Streptococcus*, each occurring in approximately 10% to 20% of patients. *Escherichia coli* and *Salmonella* are also frequent. Other reported organisms include *Klebsiella, Pseudomonas, Enterobacter,* and *Bartonella henselae* (265,325). Anaerobic organisms are noted in 5% to 17% of patients (62,209,213). Mycobacteria and *Pneumocystis carinii* infection also occur (59,231). With the increasing prevalence of immunosuppression, fungal infection has become more frequent, and in some series now causes approximately 25% of splenic abscesses (48,209).

On CT, a splenic abscess appears as a nonenhancing or hypoenhancing area of lower attenuation (Figs. 14-29 and 14-30). The rim of the abscess often is isodense to the surrounding spleen, but it may be enhanced when iodinated contrast material is injected IV (7,292). Although IV administration of contrast medium usually aids in demonstrating splenic abscesses, lesions that are more easily seen on unenhanced studies have been reported (229). Some authors recommend performance of both pre- and postcontrast scans, particularly when the miliary abscesses typical of fungal or mycobacterial infection are suspected (229). Size may vary from less than 1 cm, in the patient with a multifocal or miliary abscess, to 14 cm in diameter (7,19,48,325). Fungal and mycobacterial infection in the spleen is most likely to appear as a miliary, multifocal, or multilocular process (57,101,292) (Figs. 14-31 to 14-33). Whereas 64% of multilocular abscesses have a fungal etiology, unilocular abscesses have a bacterial etiology in 94% of cases (209). Gas occasionally is noted within splenic abscesses, but usually is absent. Calcification has been seen in treated *Candida* microabscess and in lesions caused by other fungi (most notably *Histoplasmosis*), mycobacteria, and *Pneumoocystis carinii* (96,97,179,291,292) (see Fig. 14-33). Intrasplenic psuedoaneurysms, infarcts, and hemorrhage have been reported

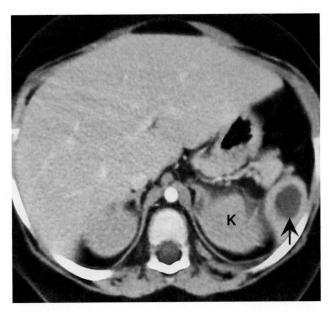

Figure 14-29 Splenic abscess. Computed tomography scan shows a hypodense mass without rim enhancement. Aspirate was positive for enterobacteria.

with murine typhus (a rickettsial infection), presumably as a manifestation of systemic vasculitis (252).

The overall sensitivity of CT for splenic abscess is significantly higher than that of US and radionuclide scintigraphy. It should be noted, however, that a CT scan without focal abnormality does not exclude the possibility of early infection, particularly in hematogenously disseminated fungal disease (292).

On MR, hepatosplenic candidiasis appears as low signal on T1-weighted and high signal on T2-weighted images relative to the normal splenic parenchyma (58,281). After IV administration of gadolinium, the lesions show no enhancement. T2-weighted fat-suppressed imaging as well as early postcontrast T1-weighted spoiled gradient echo imaging appear to be the most sensitive MRI sequences for detecting lesions, even more sensitive than contrast-enhanced CT (281,283).

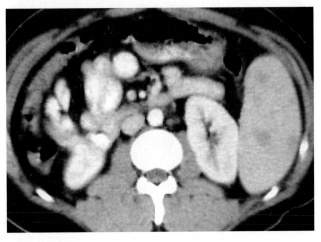

Figure 14-30 Splenomegaly with multiple small faintly visualized hypodense nodules in a patient with brucellosis.

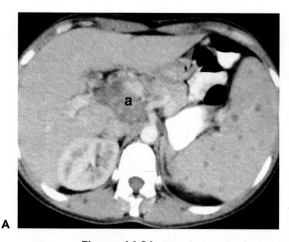
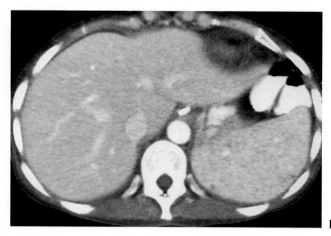

Figure 14-31 Mycobacterial infection in two patients. **A:** Computed tomography scan (CT) shows multiple small, hypodense nodules in a patient with tuberculosis. Note low-density portal adenopathy (a). **B:** CT scan shows innumerable tiny hypodensities in a patient with *Mycobacterium avium intracellulare complex* infection.

Splenic Trauma

Please refer to Chapter 21 (Thoracoabdominal Trauma) for a full discussion of splenic trauma.

Miscellaneous Splenic Disorders

Amyloidosis

Amyloidosis results from the deposition of extracellular fibrillar material in a wide variety of tissues and organs. It occurs commonly with multisystem involvement, although an unusual localized form is reported. Systemic amyloidosis can be divided into two main types based on the biochemistry of the amyloid fibril. In type AL (primary) amyloidosis, the amyloid protein is produced by a monoclonal population of plasma cells, either with or without clinical signs of multiple myeloma. In type AA, or secondary amyloidosis, amyloid deposition is secondary to chronic inflammatory disease, such as rheumatoid arthritis (37,156,170). Splenic involvement occurs in both types and usually is homogeneous and diffuse. Splenomegaly, however, is unusual, occurring in only 4% to 13% of patients (156). Focal tumorlike lesions in the spleen also have been reported and can occur as part of either systemic or localized disease (56,177). Splenic involvement is usually asymptomatic, although pain, infarction, and hyposplenism have been noted (154). Spontaneous splenic rupture has also been observed, even in normal-size spleens, and is felt to be secondary to vascular and/or splenic capsular fragility from amyloid deposition (124,138,154,318) (Fig. 14-34). Splenic rupture is frequently the initial manifestation of amyloidosis in these patients (164).

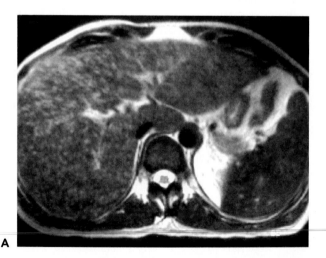
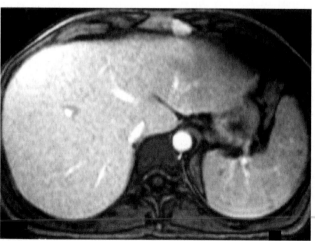

Figure 14-32 Hepatosplenic candidiasis. **A:** T2-weighted magnetic resonance (MR) image (repetition time, 3,800 ms; echo time, 90 ms) shows multiple, small high-signal-intensity lesions in liver and spleen. **B:** gadolinium–diethylene-triamine penta-acetic acid-enhanced T1-weighted MR image (repetition time, 130 ms; echo time, 4 ms; flip angle, 80 degrees). Abscesses appear as multiple, small hypointense lesions. (Case courtesy of Dr. Susan M. Ascher, Georgetown University.)

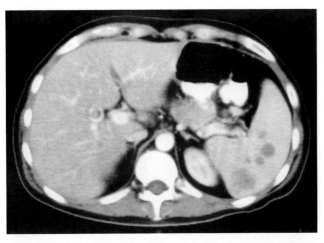
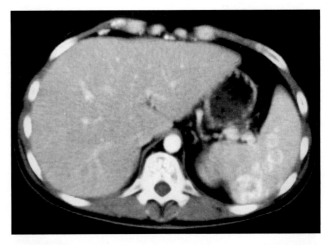

A **B**

Figure 14-33 *Pneumocystis carinii* infection. **A:** Lesions initially appear as multiple hypodense nodules. **B:** After 10 weeks of therapy, lesions show peripheral and some central calcification.

On CT, diffusely decreased splenic attenuation and enhancement have been observed (156,196,313). Focal masses are also hypodense and hypoenhancing with ill-defined margins (177,313). Extensive splenic calcification was reported in a case of primary amyloidosis (152). On MR, decreased signal intensity on T2-weighted images has been reported in cases of splenic amyloidosis (196,253). Decreased splenic uptake on ^{99m}Tc-sulfur colloid imaging has been seen frequently with amyloid, and although it does not always correlate with anatomic imaging, it is frequently accompanied by abnormal red cell morphology consistent with relative functional hyposplenism (244).

Gamna-Gandy Bodies

Gamna-Gandy bodies are small siderotic nodules in the spleen that contain varying amounts of hemosiderin, fibrous

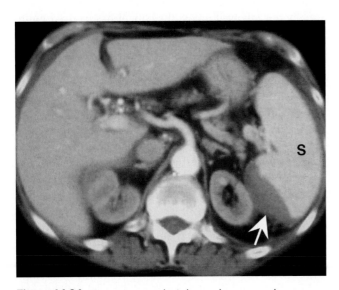

Figure 14-34 Spontaneous splenic hemorrhage secondary to amyloidosis. S, spleen; *arrow*, perisplenic hematoma.

tissue, and calcium. They occur following intraparenchymal petechial hemorrhage and are most commonly associated with portal hypertension (192). They are also reported with portal or splenic vein thrombosis, hemolytic anemia, secondary hemochromatosis, paroxysmal nocturnal hemoglobinuria, and following blood transfusions (78). They are typically not visualized with CT but are seen well with MRI secondary to the paramagnetic properties of the deposited iron (273). They appear on all pulse sequences as small foci of signal void scattered throughout the spleen (Fig. 14-35). They range in size from a few millimeters up to 1 cm in diameter (78).

Gaucher Disease

Gaucher disease is an autosomal recessive deficiency of the lysosomal enzyme glucocerebrosidase. Type 1 Gaucher disease accounts for almost all cases and has an approximate prevalence of 1 in 50,000. It is the most common lysosomal storage disease and results in the accumulation within macrophages of glucocerebroside (a breakdown product from cell membranes) (77). Accumulation of these lipid-laden macrophages (Gaucher cells) occurs most commonly in the liver, spleen, bone marrow, and to a lesser degree lung. Such accumulation results in splenomegaly, which can be marked. Thrombocytopenia, anemia, hepatic dysfunction, and bone infarcts and fractures are noted complications. The incidence of lymphoproliferative disease is also significantly increased (29). Focal nodules are reported in 20% to 30% of cases and correspond to areas of varying amounts of Gaucher cells, fibrosis, and areas of infarction (136,243,321).

On CT, focal lesions are described as hypodense and hypoenhancing in comparison to the remainder of the spleen. On MR, lesions have a varied appearance showing both areas of increased and decreased signal on T2-weighted images, with the majority of lesions being hypointense (136,243). A targetlike appearance, with a hypointense center and hyperintense rim, has also been reported on T2-weighted imaging (136). On T1-weighted images, lesions

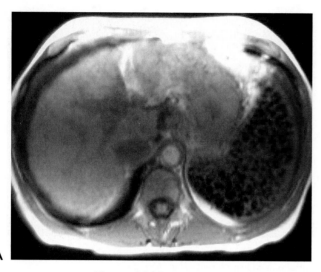
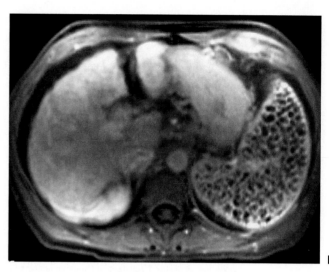

A   **B**

Figure 14-35   Gamna-Gandy bodies. **A:** T1- weighted image. **B:** T1-weighted fat-saturated post-gadolinium image shows multiple areas of signal void throughout the splenic parenchyma in this patient with cirrhosis.

were iso- or slightly hypointense and hypoenhancing after gadolinium administration (136,243,321).

Hemochromatosis

Hemochromatosis is categorized into primary and secondary forms. The latter form, usually seen in patients receiving multiple blood transfusions or in patients with diseases causing extravascular hemolysis (degradation of damaged or defective red cells by the reticuloendothelial system), such as hereditary spherocytosis or autoimmune hemolytic anemia, causes reticuloendothelial deposition of iron. This deposition is most readily seen on MRI, on which the paramagnetic properties of iron result in a marked decrease in signal intensity in the liver and spleen particularly on T2-weighted spin echo and gradient echo sequences (Fig. 14-36) (120,295,305).

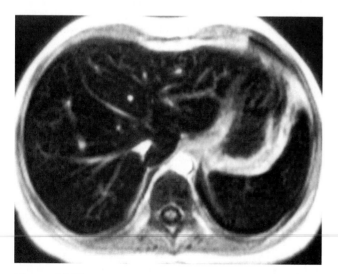

Figure 14-36   Secondary hemochromatosis. Iron deposition in the reticuloendothelial system has caused loss of signal in both liver and spleen on this T1-weighted magnetic resonance image (repetition time, 140 ms; echo time, 4 ms; flip angle, 80 degrees).

An increase in density on CT can occasionally be appreciated, although CT is much less sensitive in this regard (137,178). Primary hemochromatosis, caused by inappropriately high iron absorption from the gastrointestinal tract, results in parenchymal iron deposition in the liver, pancreas, heart, and other organs. In this setting, the spleen is not usually involved; however, primary hemochromatosis when severe, can occasionally result in reticuloendothelial involvement. Similarly when severe, secondary hemochromatosis can occasionally cause parenchymal iron deposition in other organs (137,178). Erythropoietic hemochromatosis, which may develop in patients with thalassemia major, also shows increased iron absorption and may mimic the iron distribution pattern seen with primary hemochromatosis (367). The intravascular hemolysis characteristic of paroxysmal nocturnal hemoglobinuria commonly results in iron deposition in the renal cortex, with the liver and spleen usually not involved unless the patient has received multiple transfusions (269).

Peliosis

Peliosis is a rare condition in which multiple, blood-filled spaces form in the liver, spleen, and, rarely, other parts of the reticuloendothelial system. It has been associated with the use of anabolic steroids and oral contraceptives. It is also seen in patients with human immunodeficiency virus infection or chronic wasting states, although it has also been noted in otherwise healthy patients (52,251,319,331). An association with bacillary angiomatosis as well as immunosuppression in organ transplantation is noted (254). Patients are usually asymptomatic, although splenic rupture has been reported in patients with peliosis (52,319,331).

On unenhanced CT, peliosis usually appears as small, hypodense lesions (189), which occasionally can coalesce to form large, multiloculated masses with well-defined septa (65). Enhancement varies, with some lesions becoming isodense and others demonstrating no enhancement (65,189,251). On MR, the lesions in peliosis have a variety of signal characteristics depending on the state of contained blood (189).

Sarcoid

Studies using percutaneous splenic aspiration have demonstrated splenic involvement in 24% to 59% of patients with sarcoidosis (279,314). Splenic sarcoidosis usually is asymptomatic. However, with marked involvement, abdominal discomfort, fever, malaise, hypersplenism, and even rupture may occur (157). The presentation and appearance of the spleen may also mimic lymphoma, resulting in unnecessary splenectomy. In one review of the CT findings in 59 patients with sarcoidosis (351), marked splenic enlargement was noted in 6% of patients, with mild to moderate splenomegaly seen in 27% (Fig. 14-37). Hypodense nodules, corresponding to aggregated granulomata, were seen in the spleen in 15% of patients (Fig. 14-38). No peripheral enhancement is usually seen with sarcoid nodules. Punctate calcifications are uncommon but have been reported (102). Coexistent abdominal lymphadenopathy is noted frequently in patients with splenomegaly. The chest radiograph, however, has been reported to be normal in 25% of patients with splenomegaly or discrete nodules (351). Sarcoid was noted to be a common cause of multiple splenic nodules in both the symptomatic and the asymptomatic patient in one study looking at all patients presenting with five or more splenic nodules (354). It should be noted, however, that this study may not be applicable to all populations because of the wide geographic variation in the prevalence of sarcoid. On follow-up examination, the presence of splenic nodules did not presage a worsening of the patient's pulmonary disease (353).

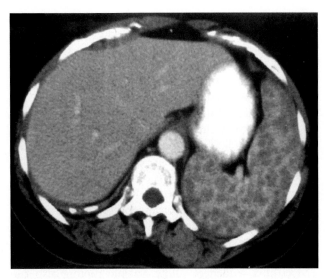

Figure 14-38 Sarcoidosis with splenomegaly and multiple hypodense nodules.

On MRI, splenic nodules caused by sarcoid are typically hypointense on all sequences and hypoenhancing relative to normal spleen. Lesions are best visualized on T2-weighted fat-suppressed or T1-weighted early gadolinium-enhanced images (352).

Sickle Cell Anemia

Patients with sickle cell anemia usually have repeated episodes of splenic infarction that eventually result in a shrunken spleen containing diffuse, microscopic deposits of calcium and iron (Fig. 14-39) (182) CT has been helpful in establishing that a focal area of uptake of ^{99m}Tc-diphosphonate seen in the left upper abdomen on radionuclide scintigraphy is the result of uptake in a calcified spleen rather than in a focus of osteomyelitis in the overlying rib (235). On CT, the spleen will typically be atrophic and may be densely

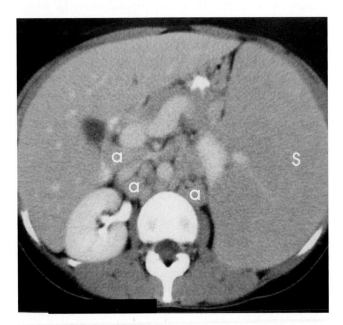

Figure 14-37 Sarcoidosis with marked splenomegaly (S), paraaortic, and portacaval adenopathy (a).

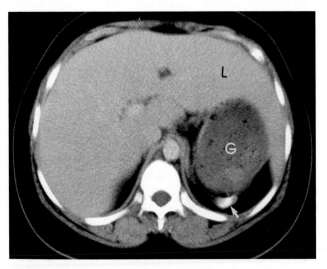

Figure 14-39 Tiny calcified infarcted spleen (*arrow*) in an adult with sickle cell anemia. G, stomach; L, liver.

calcified (183). MRI shows diminished T1 and T2 signal intensity consistent with hemosiderin and/or calcium deposition. Hyperintense areas may be noted on T1-weighted images if infarct and hemorrhage are present (4).

Acute splenic sequestration crisis occurs predominantly in children as a result of blood pooling in the spleen. The clinical presentation is varied from mild to massive splenomegaly with circulatory collapse. Although the diagnosis is usually made on clinical grounds with an abrupt drop in hematocrit and presence of splenomegaly, imaging studies may be requested. On contrast-enhanced CT, the spleen typically shows either multiple peripheral nonenhancing low-density areas or larger more diffuse areas of low density involving most of the spleen (288). These low-attenuation regions are thought to represent areas of subacute hemorrhage and show high signal on both T1- and T2-weighted sequences (268). Splenic rupture also can complicate sickle cell disease and can be readily diagnosed with CT (183).

Splenic Artery Aneurysm

Splenic artery aneurysm is the most common abdominal visceral artery aneurysm. Its incidence in autopsy series generally has been 0.01% to 0.2%, although when specifically looked for, they have been found in up to 10% of autopsies (24,44,278,302). This latter figure includes lesions less than 0.5 to 1 cm in diameter (24). Predisposing conditions include pregnancy and multiparity, systemic and portal hypertension, and arteriosclerotic disease (1,44,75,304, 329). Because of their association with pregnancy, splenic artery aneurysms are significantly more common in women, with only 15% to 20% being seen in men (1,329). Most aneurysms are saccular, and over 80% occur in the mid- and distal third of the splenic artery (286,329). Five percent to 40% are multiple. Size ranges from less than 1 cm to 30 cm, with a mean between 2 and 3 cm (1,329). Although the vast majority of patients are asymptomatic, the presence of a pulsatile mass, left upper quadrant pain, and rupture have been reported (1,44,304,329). Embolization or resection are recommended if the aneurysm is found in pregnant women or women of childbearing age, is symptomatic, is greater than 1.5 to 2.0 cm in diameter, or is increasing in size (1,5,17).

Occasionally, a specific cause can be cited for the development of splenic artery pseudoaneurysms. Acute and chronic pancreatitis, penetrating gastric ulcer, trauma, and septic emboli have all been implicated (42,44,188,227,304). Mycotic aneurysms involving the intrasplenic branches of the splenic artery also have been reported (15).

On unenhanced CT, a low-density lesion with peripheral calcification is observed along the course of the splenic artery. When large, there may be significant areas of heterogeneous attenuation corresponding to areas of clot and hemorrhage. On unenhanced MRI, heterogeneous signal can be observed on T1- and T2-weighted sequences, again representing areas of focal clot (151). A flow void is seen

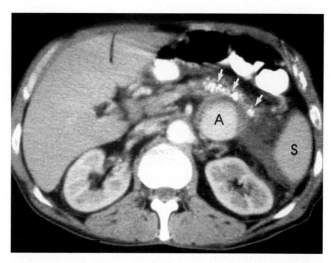

Figure 14-40 Splenic artery aneurysm (A) in a patient with a history of pancreatitis. Note pancreatic calcifications (*arrowheads*). S, spleen.

corresponding to the perfused lumen of the aneurysm. Following IV administration of contrast material, on both MRI and CT, bright enhancement is observed unless the lesion is thrombosed (Fig. 14-40) (42,151,334).

Splenic Involvement in Pancreatitis

The spleen is located adjacent to the pancreatic tail and is frequently involved in pancreatitis. In a study of 100 consecutive patients with pancreatitis, the most common splenic-associated abnormalities were perisplenic fluid collections (noted in 58%), splenic vein thrombosis (19%), splenic infarction (7%), and subcapsular hemorrhage (2%) (203). Pseudocysts arising in the tail of the pancreas adjacent to the splenic hilum occasionally extend beneath the splenic capsule or even into the splenic parenchyma (Fig. 14-41)

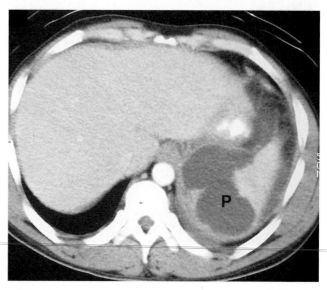

Figure 14-41 Pancreatic pseudocyst (P) extending into the splenic parenchyma.

(100,173,348). Although many of these collections will re-solve spontaneously or with percutaneous drainage, splenic rupture has been reported (3,271,328). Infarction, subcapsular hematoma, and splenic artery pseudoaneurysm have also been reported in patients with complicated pancreatitis (100,173,188,203,345). Transient splenic enlargement has been associated with acute pancreatitis, particularly in severe cases, presumably from stenosis or obstruction of the splenic vein (333).

DIAGNOSTIC ISSUES

Splenomegaly

Confusion sometimes arises as to whether a mass felt in the left upper abdomen truly represents an enlarged spleen. In such cases, CT, US, or MRI can provide a definite answer as to whether the spleen is enlarged or whether there is a separate abdominal mass. When the spleen is enlarged, its visceral surface often becomes convex as the spleen assumes a more globular shape.

When splenomegaly is present, there often are clinical or CT findings that indicate its cause. Neoplasm, abscess, or cyst may be seen within the spleen. Abdominal lymph node enlargement may suggest lymphoma or sarcoidosis. Cirrhotic patients with splenomegaly based on portal hypertension often show characteristic alterations in the size and shape of the liver and prominence of the venous structures in the splenic hilum and gastrohepatic ligament (see Chapter 12). The patient may have a clinical history of mononucleosis, sickle cell anemia, or idiopathic thrombocytopenic purpura. Rarely, the patient may show clinical symptoms of amyloid or Gaucher disease. In a study of 18 patients with splenomegaly of unknown etiology referred for splenectomy, 7 were diagnosed with lymphoma, 6 with benign hypersplenism, 4 with sarcoid, and 1 with Castleman disease (45).

Solitary Splenic Mass

Many of the entities discussed can produce a focal splenic mass. When the lesion is cystic or low density, the differential diagnosis includes congenital cysts as well as posttraumatic and pancreatic pseudocysts. Neoplasia, including lymphangioma and cystic or necrotic metastasis, are also considered. In the appropriate clinical setting, a solitary splenic abscess or echinococcal cyst would be listed. If a lesion is thought to be solid, the differential diagnosis includes hemangioma (the most common benign tumor), lymphoma (the most common malignant lesion), and more unusual tumors such as splenic hamartoma, angiosarcoma, and metastatic disease. In most cases, imaging findings are not sufficiently distinctive to allow a specific diagnosis, although some appearances can be quite suggestive, such as the bright enhancement associated with some angiosarcomas,

the classical appearance of hemangioma, or uptake on liver spleen scan seen with hamartoma. In other cases fine needle aspiration (discussed later) may be revealing.

Multiple Splenic Masses

The differential diagnosis for multiple splenic masses is fairly broad. In a study of patients having greater than five splenic nodules, the most common entities associated with a symptomatic patient were lymphoma, granulomatous infection, and sarcoid. In the asymptomatic patient, sarcoid, benign angiomatous tumor, and metastatic disease were most common (354). These results (from the southeastern United States) may vary in other geographic locations where endemic fungal infection is more common and sarcoid less frequent. Other rare entities associated with multiple splenic nodules include extramedullary hematopoiesis, amyloid, Gaucher disease, drug reaction to phenytoin, and peliosis.

Splenic Infarcts

Splenic infarction can occur with embolic disease of cardiac or atherosclerotic origin and in patients with arteritis, myeloproliferative disease, pancreatitis, pancreatic mass, and sickle cell anemia (18,143,214). If they are small, splenic infarcts are frequently asymptomatic. Large infarcts can cause left upper quadrant pain, fever, and diaphragmatic irritation. On CT, infarcts classically appear as sharply marginated, low-density regions that are wedge-shaped, with the base at the splenic capsule and the apex toward the hilum (Fig. 14-42) (18,290). Not uncommonly, however, infarcts appear as multiple, poorly marginated, hypodense lesions, indistinguishable from other forms of focal splenic

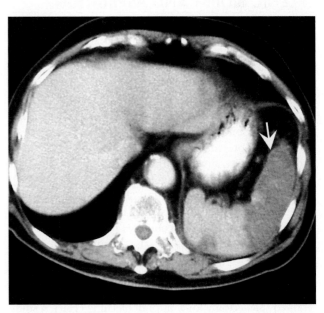

Figure 14-42 Splenic infarcts. Infarction involving more than half the spleen. Note preservation of some capsular enhancement (*arrow*).

pathology (18). When the entire spleen is infarcted, such as after occlusion or avulsion of the splenic artery, there is failure of contrast enhancement of all but the parenchyma immediately subjacent to the capsule. This peripheral enhancement, the so-called rim sign, is the result of persistent arterial supply from capsular vessels.

Diminished splenic parenchymal enhancement without infarction also occurs in the setting of profound hypotension (28). This can mimic splenic arterial disruption after blunt abdominal trauma. In the setting of massive splenic infarction, gas bubbles can appear, even in uninfected splenic parenchyma, and may cause confusion with splenic abscess formation (83). Splenic infarction also can be seen with MRI. Hemorrhagic infarcts have a high signal intensity on both T1- and T2-weighted images (135).

Spontaneous Splenic Rupture

Spontaneous splenic rupture has been associated with splenomegaly such as might occur with infection (e.g. malaria [31,260] or mononucleosis [12]) or with hematologic malignancy (e.g. leukemia or lymphoma [21,112]). Rupture has also been reported in normal-size spleens involved with amyloid (154,164) or malignancy (21). More focal processes can also cause splenic rupture, including infection (19,209), focal tumor involvement (199), sarcoidosis (216), and involvement by a pancreatic pseudocyst (3,328). Anticoagulation with low-molecular-weight heparin has also been reported to be associated with rupture (41,315). Although rare, splenic rupture has been reported in patients with pathologically unremarkable spleens (230), as well as in histologically normal accessory spleens (67).

SPLENIC BIOPSY AND ASPIRATION

Percutaneous diagnostic splenic needle aspiration and biopsy has been used in the evaluation of sarcoidosis and lymphoma and to evaluate focal lesions in the spleen (153,248,279,280,297,298,314,369). Diagnostic rates are generally high (80% to 90%), especially for focal lesions (153,180,205). The addition of flow cytometry to routine fine-needle aspiration (FNA) biopsy has been reported to be helpful in providing a definitive diagnosis in lymphoid and myeloproliferative disorders (369). The complication rate with FNA (20 to 22 gauge) is low (153,280,298,314). Core biopsy using a fine needle (22- or 21-gauge Surecut) has also been undertaken for staging of lymphoma, with no significant complications encountered in 46 patients (51). A retrospective review of 24 adult cases of splenic core biopsy (18-, 19- and 20-gauge needles) performed over a 10-year period showed two major complications, both of which occurred during FNA of a vascular tumor and both of which required splenectomy for control of bleeding (180). A study of 27 children who underwent US-guided core biopsies (18 to 21 gauge) showed no complications (205).

Multiple reports have shown that splenic abscess can be treated with aspiration or percutaneous drainage (27,61, 175,180,209,248,325). This procedure may aid in splenic salvage (322).

REFERENCES

1. Abbas MA, Stone WM, Fowl RJ, et al. Splenic artery aneurysms: two decades of experience at Mayo clinic. *Ann Vasc Surg* 2002; 16:442–449.
2. Abrams HL, Spiro R, Goldstein N. Metastases in carcinoma: analysis of 1000 autopsied cases. *Cancer* 1950;3:74–85.
3. Adelekan MO, Nasmyth DG, Joglekar VM. Acute pancreatitis presenting as a case of splenic rupture. *Hosp Med* 2003;64:432–433.
4. Adler DD, Glazer GM, Aisen AM. MRI of the spleen: normal appearance and findings in sickle-cell anemia. *AJR Am J Roentgenol* 1986;147:843–845.
5. Ahlgren LS, Beardmore HE. Solitary epidermoid splenic cysts: occurrence in sibs. *J Pediatr Surg* 1984;19:56–58.
6. Ahmann DL, Kiely JM, Harrison EG Jr, et al Malignant lymphoma of the spleen: a review of 49 cases in which the diagnosis was made at splenectomy. *Cancer* 1966;19:461–469.
7. Allal R, Kastler B, Gangi A, et al. Splenic abscesses in typhoid fever: US and CT studies. *J Comput Assist Tomogr* 1993;17:90–93.
8. Allen KB, Gay BB Jr, Skandalakis JE. Wandering spleen: anatomic and radiologic considerations. *South Med J* 1992;85:976–984.
9. Ambriz P, Munoz R, Quintanar E, et al. Accessory spleen compromising response to splenectomy for idiopathic thrombocytopenic purpura. *Radiology* 1985;155:793–796
10. Amenta PS, Amenta PS II. The anatomy of the spleen. In Bowdler AJ, ed. *The spleen: structure, function and clinical significance.* London: Chapman and Hall Medical; 1990:3–7.
11. Asayama Y, Fukuya T, Honda H, et al. Chronic expanding hematoma of the spleen caused by angiomyolipoma in a patient with tuberous sclerosis. *Abdom Imaging* 1998;23:527–530.
12. Asgari MM, Begos DG. Spontaneous splenic rupture in infectious mononucleosis: a review. *Yale J Biol Med* 1997;70:175–182.
13. Austin GE, Giltman LI, Varma V, et al. Myeloid metaplasia presenting as a splenic mass: report of a case with fine-needle aspiration cytology. *Diagn Cytopathol* 2000;23:359–361.
14. Autry JR, Weitzner S. Hemangiosarcoma of spleen with spontaneous rupture. *Cancer* 1975;35:534–539.
15. Avery GR, Wilsdon JB, Mitchell L. Case report: CT and angiographic appearances of intrasplenic mycotic aneurysm. *Clin Radiol* 1991;44:271–272.
16. Avigad S, Jaffe R, Frand M, et al. Lymphangiomatosis with splenic involvement. *JAMA* 1976;236:2315–2317.
17. Babb RR. Aneurysm of the splenic artery. *Arch Surg* 1976; 111:924–925.
18. Balcar I, Seltzer SE, Davis S, et al. CT patterns of splenic infarction: a clinical and experimental study. *Radiology* 1984;151:723–729.
19. Balthazar EJ, Hilton S, Naidich D, et al. CT of splenic and perisplenic abnormalities in septic patients. *AJR Am J Roentgenol* 1985;144:53–56.
20. Barrier A, Lacaine F, Callard P, et al. Lymphangiomatosis of the spleen and 2 accessory spleens. *Surgery* 2002;131:114–116.
21. Bauer TW, Haskins GE, Armitage JO. Splenic rupture in patients with hematologic malignancies. *Cancer* 1981;48:2729–2733.
22. Beahrs JR, Stephens DH. Enlarged accessory spleens: CT appearance in postsplenectomy patients. *AJR Am J Roentgenol* 1980; 135:483–486.
23. Bearss RW. Splenic-gonadal fusion. *Urology* 1980;16:277–279.
24. Bedford PD, Lodge B. Aneurysm of the splenic artery. *Gut* 1960;1:312–320.
25. Benfatto G, Catania G, D'Urso GM, et al. Acute abdomen due to wandering spleen infarction: a case report. *Chir Ital* 2003; 55:243–247.
26. Berge T. Splenic metastases: frequencies and patterns. *Acta Pathol Microbiol Scand* 1974;82:499–506.
27. Berkman WA, Harris SA Jr, Bernardino ME. Nonsurgical drainage of splenic abscess. *AJR Am J Roentgenol* 1983;141:395–396.
28. Berland LL, Van Dyke JA. Decreased splenic enhancement on CT in traumatized hypotensive patients. *Radiology* 1985;156:469–471.

29. Beutler E. Gaucher's Disease. *N Engl J Med* 1991;325:1354–1360.
30. Bezzi M, Spinelli A, Pierleoni M, et al. Cystic lymphangioma of the spleen: US-CT-MRI correlation. *Eur Radiol* 2001;11: 1187–1190.
31. Black SR, Trenholme GM, Racenstelm M, et al. Spontaneous rupture of the malarial spleen. *Am J Med* 2001;111:330–331.
32. Block JB. Angiosarcoma of the liver following vinyl chloride exposure. *JAMA* 1974;229:53–54.
33. Bloom RA, Freund U, Perkes EH, et al. Acute Hodgkin disease masquerading as splenic abscess. *J Surg Oncol* 1981;17:279–282.
34. Bonakdarpour A. Echinococcus disease: report of 112 cases from Iran and a review of 611 cases from the United States. *Am J Roentgenol Radium Ther Nucl Med* 1967;99:660–667.
35. Bostick WL. Primary splenic neoplasm. *Am J Pathol* 1945; 21:1143–1165.
36. Brinkley AA, Lee JK. Cystic hamartoma of the spleen: CT and sonographic findings. *J Clin Ultrasound* 1981:136–138.
37. Browning MJ, Banks RA, Tribe CR, et al. Ten years' experience of an amyloid clinica clinicopathological survey. *Q J Med* 1985; 54:213–227.
38. Brox A, Bishinsky JI, Berry G. Primary non-Hodgkin lymphoma of the spleen. *Am J Hematol* 1991;38:95–100.
39. Bruneton JN, Drouillard J, Rogopoulos A, et al. Extraretroperitoneal abdominal malignant fibrous histiocytoma. *Gastrointest Radiol* 1988;13:299–305.
40. Buehner M, Baker MS. The wandering spleen. *Surg Gynecol Obstet* 1992;175:373–387.
41. Burg MD, Dallara JJ. Rupture of a previously normal spleen in association with enoxaparin: an unusual cause of shock. *J Emerg Med* 2001;20:349–352.
42. Burke JW, Erickson SJ, Kellum CD, et al. Pseudoaneurysms complicating pancreatitis: detection by CT. *Radiology* 1986;161: 447–450.
43. Burrig KF. Epithelial (true) cysts: pathogenesis of the mesothelial and so-called epidermoid cyst of the spleen. *Am J Surg Pathol* 1988;12:275–281.
44. Busuttil RW, Brin BJ. The diagnosis and management of visceral artery aneurysms. *Surgery* 1980;88:619–624.
45. Carr JA, Shurafa M, Velanovich V. Surgical indications in idiopathic splenomegaly. *Arch Surg* 2002;137:64–68.
46. Carragher AM. One hundred years of splenogonadal fusion. *Urology* 1990;35:471–475.
47. Carrington BM, Thomas NB, Johnson RJ. Intrasplenic metastases from carcinoma of the ovary. *Clin Radiol* 1990;41:418–420.
48. Caslowitz PL, Labs JD, Fishman EK, et al. The changing spectrum of splenic abscess. *Clin Imaging* 1989;13:201–207.
49. Castellino RA, Hoppe RT, Blank N. Computed tomography, lymphography, and staging laparotomy: correlations in initial staging of Hodgkin disease. *AJR Am J Roentgenol* 1984;143:37–41.
50. Castellino RA. Hodgkin disease: practical concepts for the diagnostic radiologist. *Radiology* 1986;159:305–310.
51. Cavanna L, Civardi G, Fornari F, et al. Ultrasonically guided percutaneous splenic tissue core biopsy in patients with malignant lymphomas. *Cancer* 1992;69:2932–2936.
52. Celebrezze JP Jr, Cottrell DJ, Williams GB. Spontaneous splenic rupture due to isolated splenic peliosis. *South Med J* 1998; 91:763–764.
53. Chan KC, Chang YH. Acute abdomen due to torsion of a pelvic wandering spleen. *J Formos Med Assoc* 2002;101:577–580.
54. Chang YW, Kim Han BK, Yoon HK, et al. Multidetector-row CT appearance of acute torsion of wandering spleen in a child. *Acta Radiol* 2003;44:107.
55. Chawla S, Boal DK, Dillon PW, et al. Splenic torsion. *Radiographics* 2003;23:305–308.
56. Chen KT, Flam MS, Workman RD. Amyloid tumor of the spleen. *Am J Surg Pathol* 1987;11:723–725.
57. Chew FS, Smith PL, Barboriak D. Candidal splenic abscesses. *AJR Am J Roentgenol* 1991;156:474.
58. Cho J-S, Kim EE, Varma DGK, et al. MR imaging of hepatosplenic candidiasis superimposed on hemochromatosis. *J Comput Assist Tomogr* 1990;14:774–776.
59. Choi BI, Im J-G, Han MC, et al. Hepatosplenic tuberculosis with hypersplenism: CT evaluation. *Gastrointest Radiol* 1989;14: 265–267.
60. Choi YH, Menken FA, Jacobson IM, et al. Recurrent acute pancreatitis: an additional manifestation of the "wandering spleen" syndrome." *Am J Gastroenterol* 1996;91:1034–1038.
61. Chou Y-H, Hsu C-C, Tiu C-M, et al. Splenic abscess: sonographic diagnosis and percutaneous drainage or aspiration. *Gastrointest Radiol* 1992;17:262–266.
62. Chun CH, Raff MJ, Contreras L, et al. Splenic abscess. *Medicine (Baltimore)* 1980;59:50–65.
63. Churei H, Inoue H, Nakajo M. Intrapancreatic accessory spleen: case report. *Abdom Imaging* 1998;23:191–193.
64. Cochlin DL. Splenic-gonadal fusion—the ultrasound appearances. *Clin Radiol* 1992;45:290–291.
65. Cochrane LB, Freson M. Peliosis of the spleen. *Gastrointest Radiol* 1991;16:83–84.
66. Collins GL, Morgan MB, Taylor FM 3rd. Littoral cell angiomatosis with poorly differentiated adenocarcinoma of the lung. *Ann Diagn Pathol* 2003;7:54–59.
67. Coote JM, Eyers PS, Walker A, et al. Intra-abdominal bleeding caused by spontaneous rupture of an accessory spleen: the CT findings. *Clin Radiol* 1999;54:689–691.
68. Curtis GM, Movitz D. The surgical significance of the accessory spleen. *Ann Surg* 1946;123:276–298.
69. D'Altorio RA, Cano JY. Upside-down spleen as cause of suprarenal mass. *Urology* 1978;11:422–424.
70. Dachman AH, Ros PR, Murari PJ, et al. Nonparasitic splenic cysts: a report of 52 cases with radiologic-pathologic correlation. *AJR Am J Roentgenol* 1986;147:537–542.
71. Dachman AH, Buck JL, et al. Primary non-Hodgkin's splenic lymphoma. *Clin Radiol* 1997;53:137–142.
72. Dalpe C, Cunningham M. Wandering spleen as an asymptomatic pelvic mass. *Obstet Gynecol* 2003;101:1102–1104.
73. Darden JW, Teeslink R, Parrish A. Hamartoma of the spleen: a manifestation of tuberous sclerosis. *Am Surg* 1975;41: 564–566.
74. DasGupta T, Coombes B, Brasfield RD. Primary malignant neoplasms of the spleen. *Surg Gynecol Obstet* 1965;120:947–960.
75. Dave SP, Reis ED, Hossain A, et al. Splenic artery aneurysm in the 1990s. *Ann Vasc Surg* 2000;14:223–229.
76. Davidson LA, Reid IN. Intrahepatic splenic tissue. *J Clin Pathol* 1997;50:532–533.
77. de Fost M, Aerts JM, Hollak CE. Gaucher disease: from fundamental research to effective therapeutic interventions. *Neth J Med* 2003;61:3–8.
78. Dobritz M, Nomayr A, Bautz W, et al. Gamna-Gandy bodies of the spleen detected with MR imaging: a case report. *Magn Reson Imaging* 2001;19:1249–1251.
79. Dodds WJ, Taylor AJ, Erickson SJ, et al. Radiologic imaging of splenic anomalies. *AJR Am J Roentgenol* 1990;155:805–810.
80. Donnelly LF, Emery KH, Bove KE, et al. Normal changes in the MR appearance of the spleen during early childhood. *AJR Am J Roentgenol* 1996;166:635–639.
81. Donnelly LF, Foss JN, Frush DP, et al. Heterogeneous splenic enhancement patterns on spiral CT images in children: minimizing misinterpretation. *Radiology* 1999;210:493–497.
82. Dourthe O, Maquin P, Pradere B, et al. Splenic cyst: demonstration of the relationship between subcapsular hematoma and false cyst by imaging. *Br J Radiol* 1992;65:541–542.
83. Downer WR, Peterson MS. Massive splenic infarction and liquefactive necrosis complicating polycytemia vera. *AJR Am J Roentgenol* 1993;161:79–80.
84. Du E, Overstreet K, Zhou W, et al. Fine needle aspiration of splenic extramedullary hematopoiesis presenting as a solitary mass. A case report. *Acta Cytol* 2002;46:1138–1142.
85. Duddy MJ, Calder CJ. Cystic haemangioma of the spleen: findings on ultrasound and computed tomography. *Br J Radiol* 1989;62:180–182.
86. Durgun V, Kapan S, Kapan M, et al. Primary splenic hydatidosis. *Dig Surg* 2003;20:38–41.
87. Easler RE, Dowlin WM. Primary lipoma of the spleen. Report of a case. *Arch Pathol* 1969;88:557–559.
88. Ehrlich P, Jamieson CG. Nonparasitic splenic cysts: a case report and review. *Can J Surg* 1990;33:306–308.
89. Eraklis AJ, Filler RM. Splenectomy in childhood: review of 1413 cases. *J Pediatr Surg* 1972;7:382–388.

90. Faer MJ, Lynch RD, Lichtenstein JE, et al. Traumatic splenic cysts: radiologic-pathologic correlation from the Armed Forces Institute of Pathology. *Radiology* 1980;134:371–376.

91. Falk S, Stutte HJ, Frizzera G. Littoral cell angioma: a novel splenic vascular lesion demonstrating histiocytic differentiation. *Am J Surg Pathol* 1991;15:1023–1033

92. Falk S, Krishnan J, Meis JM. Primary angiosarcoma of the spleen. A clinicopathologic study of 40 cases. *Am J Surg Pathol* 1993; 17:959–970.

93. Farias-Eisner R, Braly P, Berek JS. Solitary recurrent metastasis of epithelial ovarian cancer in the spleen. *Gynecol Oncol* 1993;48:338–341.

94. Farrer-Brown G, Bennett MH, Harrison CV, et al. The diagnosis of Hodgkin's disease in surgically excised spleens. *J Clin Pathol* 1972;25:294–300.

95. Ferrozzi F, Bova D, Draghi F, et al. CT findings in primary vascular tumors of the spleen. *AJR Am J Roentgenol* 1996;166:1097–1101.

96. Feuerstein IM, Francis P, Raffeld M, et al. Widespread visceral calcifications in disseminated *Pneumocystis carinii* infection: CT characteristics. *J Comput Assist Tomogr* 1990;14:149–151.

97. Fishman EK, Magid D, Kuhlman JE. *Pneumocystis carinii* involvement of the liver and spleen: CT demonstration. *J Comput Assist Tomogr* 1990;14:146–148.

98. Fishman EK, Kuhlman JE, Jones RJ. CT of lymphoma: spectrum of disease. *Radiographics* 1991;11:647–669.

99. Fishman EK, Kawashima A. *Infections and diffuse diseases*. Baltimore: Mosby, 1993:138–170.

100. Fishman EK, Soyer P, Bliss DF, et al. Splenic involvement in pancreatitis: spectrum of CT findings. *AJR Am J Roentgenol* 1995; 164:631–635.

101. Fitzgerald EJ, Coblentz C. Fungal microabscesses in immunosuppressed patients—CT appearances. *Can Assoc Radiol J* 1988;39:10–12.

102. Folz SJ, Johnson CD, Swensen SJ. Abdominal manifestations of sarcoidosis in CT studies. *J Comput Assist Tomogr* 1995;19: 573–579.

103. Fowler RH. Collective review: Hydatid cysts of the spleen. *Int Abstr Surg* 1953;96:105–116.

104. Franquet T, Montes M, Aizcorbe M, et al. Inflammatory pseudotumor of the spleen: ultrasound and computed tomographic findings. *Gastrointest Radiol* 1989;14:181–183.

105. Franquet T, Montes M, Lecumberri FJ, et al. Hydatid disease of the spleen: imaging findings in nine patients. *AJR Am J Roentgenol* 1990;154:525–528.

106. Furukawa H, Kosuge T, Kanai Y, et al. Epidermoid cyst in an intrapancreatic accessory spleen: CT and pathologic findings. *AJR Am J Roentgenol* 1998;171:271.

107. Gabata T, Kadoya M, Mori A, et al. MR imaging of focal splenic extramedullary hematopoiesis in polycythemia vera: case report. *Abdom Imaging* 2000;25:514–516.

108. Garvin DF, King FM. Cysts and nonlymphomatous tumors of the spleen. *Pathol Annu* 1981;16:61–80.

109. Gayer G, Apter S, Jonas T, et al. Polysplenia syndrome detected in adulthood: report of eight cases and review of the literature. *Abdom Imaging* 1999;24:178–184.

110. Gayer G, Zissin R, Apter S, et al. CT findings in congenital anomalies of the spleen. *Br J Radiol* 2001;74:767–772.

111. Gellett LR, Williams MP, Vivian GC. Focal intrasplenic extramedullary hematopoiesis mimicking lymphoma: diagnosis made using liver-spleen scintigraphy. *Clin Nucl Med* 2001;26: 145–146.

112. Giagounidis AAN, Burk M, Meckenstock G, et al. Pathologic rupture of the spleen in hematologic malignancies: two additional cases. *Ann Hematol* 1996;73:297–302.

113. Gilbert T, Castellino RA. Critical review: the spleen in Hodgkin disease: diagnostic value of CT. *Invest Radiol* 1986;21:437–439.

114. Gilman RS, Thomas RL. Wandering spleen presenting as acute pancreatitis in pregnancy. *Obstet Gynecol* 2003;101:1100–1102.

115. Gilmartin D. Familial multiple epidermoid cyst of the spleen. *Conn Med* 1978;42:297–300.

116. Githaiga JW, Adwok JA. Wandering spleen presenting as a right hypochondrial mass and intestinal obstruction. *East Afr Med J* 2002;79:450–452.

117. Glazer GM, Axel L, Goldber HI, et al. Dynamic CT of the normal spleen. *AJR Am J Roentgenol* 1981;137:343–346.

118. Glazer M, Lally J, Kanzer M. Inflammatory pseudotumor of the spleen: MR findings. *J Comput Assist Tomogr* 1992;16:980–983.

119. Goldfeld M, Cohen I, Loberant N, et al. Littoral cell angioma of the spleen: appearance on sonography and CT. *J Clin Ultrasound* 2002;30:510–513.

120. Gomori JM, Grossman RI, Drott HR. MR relaxation times and iron content of thalassemic spleens: an in vitro study. *AJR Am J Roentgenol* 1998;150:567–569.

121. Gooding GAW. The ultrasonic and computed tomographic appearance of splenic lobulations: a consideration in the ultrasonic differential of masses adjacent to the left kidney. *Radiology* 1978;126:719–720.

122. Griscom NT, Hargreaves HK, Schwartz MZ, et al. Huge splenic cyst in a newborn: comparisons with 10 cases in later childhood and adolescence. *AJR Am J Roentgenol* 1977;129:889–891.

123. Grosskreutz C, Troy K, Cuttner J. Primary splenic lymphoma: report of 10 cases using the REAL classification. *Cancer Invest* 2002;20:749–753.

124. Gupta R, Singh G, Bose SM, et al. Spontaneous rupture of the amyloid spleen: a report of two cases. *J Clin Gastroenterol* 1998; 26:161.

125. Hadar H, Gadoth N, Herskovitz P, et al. Short pancreas in polysplenia syndrome. *Acta Radiol* 1991;32:299–301.

126. Hahn PF, Weissleder R, Stark DD, et al. MR imaging of focal splenic tumors. *AJR Am J Roentgenol* 1988;150:823–827.

127. Halgrimson CG, Rustad DG, Zeligman BE. Calcified hemangioma of the spleen. *JAMA* 1984;252:2959–2960.

128. Halpart B, Gyorkey F. Lesions observed in accessory spleens of 311 patients. *Am J Clin Pathol* 1959;31:165–168.

129. Halvorsen RA, Dunnick NR, Thompson WM. Contrast agent enhancement in abdominal computed tomography: ionic vs. nonionic agents. *Invest Radiol* 1984;19:S234–S243.

130. Hancock SL, Scidmore NS, Hopkins KL, et al. Computed tomography assessment of splenic size as a predictor of splenic weight and disease involvement in laparotomy staged Hodgkin's disease. *Int J Radiat Oncol Biol Phys* 1994;28:93–99.

131. Hansen S, Jarhult J. Accessory spleen imaging: Radionuclide, ultrasound and CT investigations in a patient with thrombocytopenia 25 yr after splenectomy for ITP. *Scand J Haematol* 1986;37:74–77.

132. Harris NL, Aisenberg AC, Meyer JE, et al. Diffuse large cell (histiocytic) lymphoma of the spleen: clinical and pathologic characteristics of ten cases. *Cancer* 1984;54:2460–2467.

133. Hayward I, Mindelzeun RE, Jeffrey RB. Intrapancreatic accessory spleen mimicking pancreatic mass on CT. *J Comput Assist Tomogr* 1992;16:984–985.

134. Herman TE, Siegel MJ. Polysplenia syndrome with congenital short pancreas. *AJR Am J Roentgenol* 1991;156:799–800.

135. Hess CF, Griebel J, Schmiedl U, et al. Focal lesions of the spleen: preliminary results with fast MR imaging at 1.5 T. *J Comput Assist Tomogr* 1988;12:569–574.

136. Hill SÇ, Damaska BM, Ling A, et al. Gaucher disease: abdominal MR imaging findings in 46 patients. *Radiology* 1992;184:561–566.

137. Housman JF, Chezmar JL, Nelson RC. Magnetic resonance imaging in hemochromatosis: extrahepatic iron deposition. *Gastrointest Radiol* 1989;14:59–60.

138. Hurd WW, Katholi RE. Acquired functional asplenia: association with spontaneous rupture of the spleen and fatal spontaneous rupture of the liver in amyloidosis. *Arch Intern Med* 1980;140: 844–845.

139. Husni EA. The clinical course of splenic hemangioma with emphasis on spontaneous rupture. *Arch Surg* 1961;83:681–688.

140. Iozzo RV, Haas JE, Chard RL. Symptomatic splenic hamartoma: a report of two cases and review of the literature. *Pediatrics* 1980; 66:261–265.

141. Ito K, Murata T, Nakanishi T. Cystic lymphangioma of the spleen: MR findings with pathologic correlation. *Abdom Imaging* 1995;20:82–84.

142. Ito Y, Shimizu E, Miyamoto T, et al. Epidermoid cysts of the spleen occurring in sisters. *Dig Dis Sci* 2002;47:619–623.

143. Iuliano L, Gurgo A, Gualdi G, et al. Succeeding onset of hepatic, splenic, and renal infarction in polyarteritis nodosa. *AJG Am J Roentgenol* 2000;:1837–1838.

144. Jelinek JS, Stuart PL, Done SL, et al. MRI of polysplenia syndrome. *Magn Reson Imaging* 1989;7:681–686.

145. Jequier S, Hanquinet S, Lironi A. Splenogonadal fusion. *Pediatr Radiol* 1998;28:526.

146. Jones TC. *Cestodes (Tapeworms)*, 3rd ed. New York: Churchill Livingston, 1990:2155–2156.

147. Joshi SN, Wolverson MK, Cusworth RB, et al. Complementary use of computerized tomography and technetium scanning in the diagnosis of accessory spleen. *Dig Dis Sci* 1980;25:888–892.

148. Kadin ME, Glatstein E, Dorfman RF. Clinicopathologic studies of 117 untreated patients subjected to laparotomy for the staging of Hodgkin's disease. *Cancer* 1971;27:1277–1294.

149. Kaneko J, Sugawara Y, Matsui Y, et al. Normal splenic volume in adults by computed tomography. *Hepatogastroenterology* 2002;49:1726–1727.

150. Karpeh MS Jr, Hicks DG, Torosian MH. Colon invasion by primary splenic lymphoma: a case report and review of the literature. *Surgery* 1992;111:224–227.

151. Kehagias DT, Tzalonikos MT, Moulopoulos LA, et al. MRI of a giant splenic artery aneurysm. *Br J Radiol* 1998;71:444–446.

152. Kennan N, Evans C. Case report: hepatic and splenic calcifications due to amyloid. *Clin Radiol* 1991;44:60–61.

153. Keogan MT, Freed KS, Paulson EK, et al. Imaging-guided percutaneous biopsy of focal splenic lesions: update on safety and effectiveness. *AJR Am J Roentgenol* 1999;172:933–937.

154. Khan AZ, Escofet X, Roberts KM, et al. Spontaneous splenic rupture—a rare complication of amyloidosis. *Swiss Surg* 2003;9:92–94.

155. Kim H, Dorfman RF. Morphological studies of 84 untreated patients subjected to laparotomy for the staging of non-Hodgkin's lymphomas. *Cancer* 1974;33:657–674.

156. Kim SH, Han JK, Lee KH, et al. Abdominal amyloidosis: spectrum of radiological findings. *Clin Radiol* 2003;58:610–620.

157. Kimbrell OC Jr. Sarcoidosis of the spleen. *N Engl J Med* 1957;257:128–131.

158. Kinoshita T, Ishii K, Yajima Y, et al. Splenic hemangiosarcoma with massive calcification. *Abdom Imaging* 1999;24:185–187.

159. Kishikawa T, Numaguchi Y, Tokunaga M, et al. Hemangiosarcoma of the spleen and liver metastases: angiographic manifestations. *Radiology* 1977;123:31–35.

160. Klein B, Stein M, Kuten A, et al. Splenomegaly and solitary spleen metastasis in solid tumors. *Cancer* 1987;60:100–102.

161. Kobayashi H, Kawamoto S, Tamaki T, et al. Polysplenia associated with semiannular pancreas. *Eur Radiol* 2001;11:1639–1641.

162. Koehler RE, Evens RG. *The spleen*. Philadelphia: WB Saunders, 1981:1064–1088.

163. Komatsuda T, Ishida H, Konno K, et al. Splenic lymphangioma: US and CT diagnosis and clinical manifestations. *Abdom Imaging* 1999;24:414–417.

164. Kozicky OJ, Brandt LJ, Lederman M, et al. Splenic amyloidosis: a case report of spontaneous splenic rupture with a review of the pertinent literature. *Am J Gastroenterol* 1987;82:582–587.

165. Kraus MD, Fleming MD, Vonderheide RH. The spleen as a diagnostic specimen: a review of 10 years' experience at two tertiary care institutions. *Cancer* 2001;91:2001–2009.

166. Krause R, Larsen CR, Scholz FJ. Gastrosplenic fistula: complication of adenocarcinoma of stomach. *Comput Med Imaging Graph* 1990;14:273–276.

167. Krishnan J, Frizzera G. Two splenic lesions in need of clarification: hamartoma and inflammatory pseudotumor. *Semin Diagn Pathol* 2003;20:94–104.

168. Krumbhaar EB. The incidence and nature of splenic neoplasm. *Ann Clin Med* 1927;5:833–860.

169. Kutok JL, Fletcher CDM. Splenic vascular tumors. *Sem Diagn Pathol* 2003;20:128–139.

170. Kyle RA, Gertz MA. Systemic amyloidosis. *Crit Rev Oncol Hematol* 1990;10:49–87.

171. Labruzzo C, Haritopoulos KN, El Tayar AR, et al. Posttraumatic cyst of the spleen: a case report and review of the literature. *Int Surg* 2002;87:152–156.

172. Lackner K, Brecht G, Janson R, et al. [The value of computer tomography in the staging of primary lymph node neoplasms (author transl).] *Rofo* 1980;132:21–30.

173. Lankisch PG. The spleen in inflammatory pancreatic disease. *Gastroenterology* 1990;98:509–516.

174. Lauffer JM, Baer HU, Maurer CA, et al. Intrapancreatic accessory spleen. A rare cause of pancreatic mass. *Int J Pancreatol* 1999;25:65–68.

175. Lerner RM, Spataro RF. Splenic abscess: percutaneous drainage. *Radiology* 1984;153:643–645.

176. Levy DW, Rindsberg S, Friedman AC, et al. Thorotrast-induced hepatosplenic neoplasia: CT identification. *AJR Am J Roentgenol* 1986;146:997–1004.

177. Liu T-Y, Chen S-C, Wang L-Y, et al. Systemic amyloidosis presenting as splenic tumor. *Gastrointest Radiol* 1991;16:137–138.

178. Long JA, Doppman JL, Nienhus AW, et al. Computed tomographic analysis of beta-thalassemic syndromes with hemochromatosis: pathologic findings with clinical and laboratory correlations. *J Comput Assist Tomogr* 1980;4:159–165.

179. Lubat E, Megibow AJ, Balthazar EJ, et al. Extrapulmonary *Pneumocystis carinii* infection in AIDS: CT findings. *Radiology* 1990;174:157–160.

180. Lucey BC, Boland GW, Maher MM, et al. Percutaneous nonvascular splenic intervention: a 10-year review. *AJR Am J Roentgenol* 2002;179:1591–1596.

181. Madia C, Lumachi F, Veroux M, et al. Giant splenic epithelial cyst with elevated serum markers CEA and CA 19-9 levels: an incidental association? *Anticancer Res* 2003;23:773–776.

182. Magid D, Fishman EK, Siegelman SS. Computed tomography of the spleen and liver in sickle cell disease. *AJR Am J Roentgenol* 1984;143:245–249.

183. Magid D, Fishman EK, Charache S, et al. Abdominal pain in sickle cell disease: the role of CT. *Radiology* 1987;163:325–328.

184. Manterola C, Vial M, Losada H, et al. Uncommon locations of abdominal hydatid disease. *Trop Doct* 2003;33:179–180.

185. Marani SA, Canossi GC, Nicoli FA, et al. Hydatid disease: MR imaging study. *Radiology* 1990;175:701–706.

186. Marti-Bonmati L, Ballesta A, Chirivella M. Unusual presentation of non-Hodgkin lymphoma of the spleen. *Can Assoc Radiol J* 1989;40:49–50.

187. Marymont JG Jr, Gross S. Patterns of metastatic cancer in the spleen. *Am J Clin Pathol* 1963;40:58–66.

188. Mauro MA, Schiebler ML, Parker LA, et al. The spleen and its vasculature in pancreatitis: CT findings. *Am Surg* 1993;59:155–159.

189. Maves CK, Caron KH, Bisset GS 3rd, et al. Splenic and hepatic peliosis: MR findings. *AJR Am J Roentgenol* 1992;158:75–76.

190. Mendenhall NP, Cantor AB, Williams JL, et al. With modern imaging techniques, is staging laparotomy necessary in pediatric Hodgkin's disease? A Pediatric Oncology Group study. *J Clin Oncol* 1993;11:2218–2225.

191. Miles KA, McPherson SJ, Hayball MP. Transient splenic inhomogeneity with contrast-enhanced CT: mechanism and effect of liver disease. *Radiology* 1995;194:91–95.

192. Minami M, Itai Y, Ohtomo K, et al. Siderotic nodules in the spleen: MR imaging of portal hypertension. *Radiology* 1989;172:681–684.

193. Mirowitz SA, Brown JJ, Lee J, et al. Dynamic gadolinium-enhanced MR imaging of the spleen: normal enhancement patterns and evaluation of splenic lesions. *Radiology* 1991;179:681–686.

194. Mishalany H, Mahnovski V, Woolley M. Congenital asplenia and anomalies of the gastrointestinal tract. *Surgery* 1982;91:38–41.

195. Monforte-Munoz H, Ro JY, Manning JT Jr, et al. Inflammatory pseudotumor of the spleen: report of two cases with a review of the literature. *Am J Clin Pathol* 1991;96:491–495.

196. Monzawa S, Tsukamoto T, Omata K, et al. A case with primary amyloidosis of the liver and spleen: radiologic findings. *Eur J Radiol* 2002;41:237–241.

197. Moore PJ, Hawkins EP, Galliani CA, et al. Splenogonadal fusion with limb deficiency and micrognathia. *South Med J* 1997;90:1152–1155.

198. Morgenstern L, McCafferty L, Rosenberg J, et al. Hamartomas of the spleen. *Arch Surg* 1984;119:1291–1293.

199. Morgenstern L, Rosenberg J, Geller SA. Tumors of the spleen. *World J Surg* 1985;9:468–476.

200. Morgenstern L. Nonparasitic splenic cysts: pathogenesis, classification, and treatment. *J Am Coll Surg* 2002;194:306–314.

201. Morinaga S, Ohyama R, Koizumi J. Low-grade mucinous cystadenocarcinoma in the spleen. *Am J Surg Pathol* 1992;16: 903–908.

202. Moriyama S, Inayoshi A, Kurano R. Inflammatory pseudotumor of the spleen: report of a case. *Surg Today* 2000;30:942–946.

203. Mortele KJ, Mergo PJ, Taylor HM, et al. Splenic and perisplenic involvement in acute pancreatitis: determination of prevalence and morphologic helical CT features. *J Comput Assist Tomogr* 2001;25:50–54.

204. Moss CN, Van Dyke JA, Koehler RE, et al. Multiple cavernous hemangiomas of the spleen: CT findings. *J Comput Assist Tomogr* 1986;10:338–340.

205. Muraca S, Chait PG, Connolly BL, et al. US-guided core biopsy of the spleen in children. *Radiology* 2001;218:200–206.

206. Murray KF, Morgan A, Christie DL. Pancreatitis caused by a wandering spleen. *J Pediatr Gastroenterol Nutr* 1994;18:486–489.

207. Musgrave NJ, Williamson RM, O'Rourke NA, et al. Test and teach. Incidentally discovered splenic vascular lesion. Littoral cell angioma of the spleen. *Pathology* 2002;34:579–581.

208. Nagase LL, Semelka RC, Armao D. Spleen. In: Semelka RC, ed. *Abdominal-pelvic MRI*. New York: Wiley-Liss, 2002:491–526.

209. Nelken N, Ignatius J, Skinner M, et al. Changing clinical spectrum of splenic abscess: a multicenter study and review of the literature. *Am J Surg* 1987;154:27–34.

210. Nelson RC, Chezmar JL, Peterson JE, et al. Contrast-enhanced CT of the liver and spleen: comparison of ionic and nonionic contrast agents. *AJR Am J Roentgenol* 1989;153:973–976.

211. Nemcek AA Jr, Miller FH, Fitzgerald SW. Acute torsion of a wandering spleen: diagnosis by CT and duplex Doppler and color flow sonography. *AJR Am J Roentgenol* 1991;157:307–309.

212. Neuhauser TS, Derringer GA, Thompson LDR, et al. Splenic angiosarcoma: a clinicopathologic and immunophenotypic study of 28 cases. *Mod Pathol* 2000;13:978–987.

213. Ng KK, Lee TY, Wan YL, et al. Splenic abscess: diagnosis and management. *Hepatogastroenterology* 2002;49:567–571.

214. Nguyen VD. A rare cause of splenic infarct and fleeting pulmonary infiltrates: polyarteritis nodosa. *Comput Med Imaging Graph* 1991;15:61–65.

215. Norowitz DG, Morehouse HT. Isodense splenic mass: hamartoma, a case report. *Comput Med Imaging Graph* 1989;13:347–350.

216. Nusair S, Kramer MR, Berkman N. Pleural effusion with splenic rupture as manifestations of recurrence of sarcoidosis following prolonged remission. *Respiration* 2003;70:114–117.

217. Nyman R, Rehn S, Glimelius B, et al. Magnetic resonance imaging, chest radiography, computed tomography, and ultrasonography in malignant lymphoma. *Acta Radiol* 1987;28:253–262.

218. Nyman R, Rhen S, Ericsson A, et al. An attempt to characterize malignant lymphoma in spleen, liver and lymph nodes with magnetic resonance imaging. *Acta Radiol* 1987;28:527–533.

219. Ohtomo K, Fukuda H, Mori K, et al. CT and MR appearances of splenic hamartoma. *J Comput Assist Tomogr* 1992;16:425–428.

220. Okada J, Yoshikawa K, Uno K, et al. Increased activity on radiocolloid scintigraphy in splenic hamartoma. *Clin Nucl Med* 1990;15:112–115.

221. Okuda K, Taguchi T, Ishihara K, et al. Intrasplenic pseudocyst of the pancreas. *J Clin Gastroenterol* 1981;3:37–41.

222. Okuyama T, Oya M, Ishikawa H. Isolated splenic metastasis of sigmoid colon cancer: a case report. *Jpn J Clin Oncol* 2001;31:341–345.

223. Ota T, Tei M, Yoshioka A, et al. Intrapancreatic accessory spleen diagnosed by technetium-99m heat-damaged red blood cell SPECT. *J Nucl Med* 1997;38:494–495.

224. Ough YD, Nash HR, Wood DA. Mesothelial cysts of the spleen with squamous metaplasia. *Am J Clin Pathol* 1981;76:666–669.

225. Pakter RL, Fishman EK, Nussbaum A, et al. CT findings in splenic hemangiomas in the Klippel-Trenaunay-Weber syndrome. *J Comput Assist Tomogr* 1987;11:88–91.

226. Pampin C, Devillers A, Treguier C, et al. Intratumoral consumption of indium-111-labeled platelets in a child with splenic hemangioma and thrombocytopenia. *J Pediatr Hematol Oncol* 2000;22:256–258.

227. Pantongrag-Brown L, Suwanwela N, Arjhansiri K, et al. Demonstration on computed tomography of two pseudoaneurysms complicating chronic pancreatitis. *Br J Radiol* 1991;64:754–757.

228. Parker LA, Mittelstaedt CA, Mauro MA, et al. Torsion of a wandering spleen: CT appearance. *J Comput Assist Tomogr* 1984;8:1201–1204.

229. Pastakia B, Shawker TH, Thaler M, et al. Hepatosplenic candidiasis: wheels within wheels. *Radiology* 1988;166:417–421.

230. Paulvannan S, Pye JK. Spontaneous rupture of a normal spleen. *Int J Clin Pract* 2003;57:245–246.

231. Pedro-Botet J, Maristany MT, Miralles R, et al. Splenic tuberculosis in patients with AIDS. *Rev Infect Dis* 1991;13:1069–1071.

232. Peene P, Wilms G, Stockx L, et al. Splenic hemangiomatosis: CT and MR features. *J Comput Assist Tomogr* 1991;15:1070–1072.

233. Peoples WM, Moller JH, Edwards JE. Polysplenia: a review of 146 cases. *Pediatr Cardiol* 1983;4:129–137.

234. Perez Fontan FJ, Soler R, Santos M, et al. Accessory spleen torsion: US, CT and MR findings. *Eur Radiol* 2001;11:509–512.

235. Perlmutter S, Jacobstein JG, Kazam E. Splenic uptake of 99mTc-diphosphonate in sickle cell disease associated with increased splenic density on computerized transaxial tomography. *Gastrointest Radiol* 1977;2:77–79.

236. Piekarski J, Federle MP, Moss AA, et al. CT of the spleen. *Radiology* 1980;135:683–689.

237. Pines B, Rabinovitch J. Hemangioma of the spleen. *Arch Pathol* 1942;33:487–503.

238. Pinkhas J, Djaldetti M, de Vries A, et al. Diffuse angiomatosis with hypersplenism: splenectomy followed by polycythemia. *Am J Med* 1968;45:795–801.

239. Pistoia F, Markowitz SK. Splenic lymphangiomatosis: CT diagnosis. *AJR Am J Roentgenol* 1988;150:121–122.

240. Pitlik S, Cohen L, Hadar H, et al. Portal hypertension and esophageal varices in hemangiomatosis of the spleen. *Gastroenterology* 1977;72:937–940.

241. Place RJ. Isolated colon cancer metastasis to the spleen. *Am Surg* 2001;67:454–457.

242. Polat P, Kantarci M, Alper F, et al. Hydatid disease from head to toe. *Radiographics* 2003;23:475–494; quiz 536–477.

243. Poll LW, Koch J-A, vom Dahl S, et al. Gaucher disease of the spleen: CT and MR findings. *Abdom Imaging* 2000;25:286–289.

244. Powsner RA, Simms RW, Chudnovsky A, et al. Scintigraphic functional hyposplenism in amyloidosis. *J Nucl Med* 1998;39:221–223.

245. Prassopoulos P, Cavouras D. CT assessment of normal splenic size in children. *Acta Radiol* 1994;35:152–154.

246. Prassopoulos P, Daskalogiannaki M, Raissaki M, et al. Determination of normal splenic volume on computed tomography in relation to age, gender and body habitus. *Eur Radiol* 1997;7:246–248.

247. Pyatt RS, Williams ED, Clark M, et al. CT diagnosis of splenic cystic lymphangiomatosis. *J Comput Assist Tomogr* 1981;5:446–448.

248. Quinn SF, vanSonnenberg E, Casola G, et al. Interventional radiology in the spleen. *Radiology* 1986;161:289–291.

249. Qureshi MA, Hafner CD. Clinical manifestations of splenic cysts: study of 75 cases. *Am Surg* 1965;31:605–608.

250. Rabushka LS, Kawashima A, Fishman EK. Imaging of the spleen: CT with supplemental MR examination. *Radiographics* 1994;14:307–332.

251. Radin DR, Kanel GC. Peliosis hepatis in a patient with human immunodeficiency virus infection. *AJR Am J Roentgenol* 1991;156 91–92.

252. Radin R, Hirbawi IA, Henderson RW. Splenic involvement in endemic (murine) typhus: CT findings. *Abdom Imaging* 2001;26:298–299.

253. Rafal RB, Jennis R, Kosovsky PA, et al. MRI of primary amyloidosis. *Gastrointest Radiol* 1990;15:199–201.

254. Raghavan R, Alley S, Tawfik O, et al. Splenic peliosis: a rare complication following liver transplantation. *Dig Dis Sci* 1999;44:1128–1131.

255. Ragozzino MW, Singletary H, Patrick R. Familial splenic epidermoid cyst. *AJR Am J Roentgenol* 1990;155:1233–1234.

256. Raissaki M, Prassopoulos P, Daskalogiannaki M, et al. Acute abdomen due to torsion of wandering spleen: CT diagnosis. *Eur Radiol* 1998;8:1409–1412.

257. Ramani M, Reinhold C, Semelka RC, et al. Splenic hemangiomas and hamartomas: MR imaging characteristics of 28 lesions. *Radiology* 1997;202:166–172.

258. Rathaus V, Zissin R, Goldberg E. Spontaneous rupture of an epidermoid cyst of spleen: preoperative ultrasonographic diagnosis. *J Clin Ultrasound* 1991;19:235–237.

259. Regelson W, Kim U, Ospina J, et al. Hemangioendothelial sarcoma of liver from chronic arsenic intoxication by Fowler's solution. *Cancer* 1968;21:514–522.

260. Ribordy V, Schaller MD, Martinet O, et al. Spontaneous rupture of the spleen during malaria treated with transcatheter coil embolization of the splenic artery. *Intensive Care Med* 2002;28:996.

261. Rini JN, Manalili EY, Hoffman MA, et al. F-18 FDG versus Ga-67 for detecting splenic involvement in Hodgkin's disease. *Clin Nucl Med* 2002;27:572–577.

262. Rini JN, Leonidas JC, Tomas MB, et al. 18F-FDG PET versus CT for evaluating the spleen during initial staging of lymphoma. *J Nucl Med* 2003;44:1072–1074.

263. Rizk GK, Tayyarah KA, Ghandur-Mnaymneh L. The angiographic changes in hydatid cysts of the liver and spleen. *Radiology* 1971;99:303–309.

264. Robinson SL, Saxe JM, Lucas CE, et al. Splenic abscess associated with endocarditis. *Surgery* 1992;112:781–786; discussion 786–787.

265. Rolain JM, Chanet V, Laurichesse H, et al. Cat scratch disease with lymphadenitis, vertebral osteomyelitis, and spleen abscesses. *Ann N Y Acad Sci* 2003;990:397–403.

266. Ros PR, Moser RP Jr, Dachman AH, et al. Hemangioma of the spleen: radiologic-pathologic correlation in ten cases. *Radiology* 1987;162:73–77.

267. Rose V, Izukawa T, Moes CAF. Syndromes of asplenia and polysplenia: a review of cardiac and non-cardiac malformations in 60 cases with special reference to diagnosis and prognosis. *Br Heart J* 1975;37:840–852.

268. Roshkow JE, Sanders LM. Acute splenic sequestration crisis in two adults with sickle cell disease: US, CT, and MR imaging findings. *Radiology* 1990;177:723–725.

269. Roubidoux MA. MR of the kidneys, liver, and spleen in paroxysmal nocturnal hemoglobinuria. *Abdom Imaging* 1994;19:168–173.

270. Rueffer U, Sieber M, Stemberg M, et al. Spleen involvement in Hodgkin's lymphoma: assessment and risk profile. *Ann Hematol* 2003;82:390–396.

271. Rypens F, Deviere J, Zalcman M, et al. Splenic parenchymal complications of pancreatitis: CT findings and natural history. *J Comput Assist Tomogr* 1997;21:89–93.

272. Safran D, Welch J, Rezuke W. Inflammatory pseudotumors of the spleen. *Arch Surg* 1991;126:904–908.

273. Sagoh T, Itoh K, Togashi K, et al. Gamna-Gandy bodies of the spleen: evaluation with MR imaging. *Radiology* 1989;172:685–687.

274. Sarker A, An C, Davis M, et al. Inflammatory pseudotumor of the spleen in a 6-year-old child: a clinicopathologic study. *Arch Pathol Lab Med* 2003;127:e127–e130.

275. Sayeed S, Koniaris LG, Kovach SJ, et al. Torsion of a wandering spleen. *Surgery* 2002;132:535–536.

276. Schlesinger AE, Hildebolt CF, Siegel MJ, et al. Splenic volume in children: simplified estimation at CT. *Radiology* 1994;193:578–580.

277. Schottenfeld LE, Wolfson WL. Cavernous hemangioma of the spleen. *Arch Surg* 1937;35:867–877.

278. Seids JV, Hauser H. Aneurysm of the splenic artery. Radiology 1941;36:171–180.

279. Selroos O. Fine-needle aspiration biopsy of the spleen in diagnosis of sarcoidosis. *Ann N Y Acad Sci* 1976;278:517–521.

280. Selroos O, Koivunen E. Usefulness of fine-needle aspiration biopsy of spleen in diagnosis of sarcoidosis. *Chest* 1983;83:193–195.

281. Semelka RC, Shoenut JP, Greenberg HM, et al. Detection of acute and treated lesions of hepatosplenic candidiasis: comparison of dynamic contrast-enhanced CT and MR imaging. *J Magn Reson Imaging* 1992;2:341–345.

282. Semelka RC, Shoenut JP, Lawrence PH, et al. Spleen: Dynamic enhancement patterns on gradient-echo MR images enhanced with gadopentetate dimeglumine. *Radiology* 1992;185:479–482.

283. Semelka RC, Kelekis NL, Sallah S, et al. Hepatosplenic fungal disease: diagnostic accuracy and spectrum of appearances on MR imaging. *AJR Am J Roentgenol* 1997;169:1311–1316.

284. Sener R, Alper H. Polysplenia syndrome: a case associated with transhepatic portal vein, short pancreas, and left inferior vena cava with hemiazygous continuation. *Abdom Imaging* 1994;19:64–66.

285. Shanberge JN, Tanaka K, Gruhl MC. Chronic consumptive coagulopathy due to hemangiomatous transformation of the spleen. *Am J Clin Pathol* 1971;56:723–729.

286. Shanley CJ, Shah NL, Messina LM. Common splanchnic artery aneurysms: splenic, hepatic, and celiac. *Ann Vasc Surg* 1996;10:315–322.

287. Sheflin JR, Lee CM, Kretchmar KA. Torsion of wandering spleen and distal pancreas. *AJR Am J Roentgenol* 1984;142:100–101.

288. Sheth S, Ruzal-Shapiro C, Piomelli S, et al. CT imaging of splenic sequestration in sickle cell disease. *Pediatr Radiol* 2000;30: 830–833.

289. Shiels WE, Johnson JF, Stephenson SR, et al. Chronic torsion of the wandering spleen. *Pediatr Radiol* 1989;19:465–467.

290. Shirkhoda A, Wallace S, Sokhandan M. Computed tomography and ultrasonography in splenic infarction. *J Can Assoc Radiol* 1985;36:29–33.

291. Shirkhoda A, Lopez-Berestein G, Holbert JM, et al. Hepatosplenic fungal infection: CT and pathologic evaluation after treatment with liposomal amphotericin B. *Radiology* 1986;159: 349–353.

292. Shirkhoda A. CT findings in hepatosplenic and renal candidiasis. *J Comput Assist Tomogr* 1987;11:795–798.

293. Shirkhoda A, Freeman J, Armin AR, et al. Imaging features of splenic epidermoid cyst with pathologic correlation. *Abdom Imaging* 1995;20:449–451.

294. Sica GT, Reed MF. Case 27: intrapancreatic accessory spleen. *Radiology* 2000;217:134–137.

295. Siegelman ES, Mitchell DG, Rubin R. Parenchymal versus reticuloendothelial iron overload in the liver: distinction with MR imaging. *Radiology* 1991;179:361–366.

296. Smith VC, Eisenberg BL, McDonald EC. Primary splenic angiosarcoma: case report and literature review. *Cancer* 1985;55:1625–1627.

297. Soderstrom N. How to use cytodiagnostic spleen puncture. *Acta Med Scand* 1976;199:1–5.

298. Solbiati L, Bossi MC, Bellotti E, et al. Focal lesions in the spleen: sonographic patterns and guided biopsy. *AJR Am J Roentgenol* 1983;140:59–65.

299. Solomou EG, Patriarheas GV, Mpadra FA, et al. Asymptomatic adult cystic lymphangioma of the spleen: case report and review of the literature. *Magn Reson Imaging* 2003;21:81–84.

300. Souparis A, Papaziogas B, Alexandrakis A, et al. An unusual case of retroperitoneal accessory spleen with vascular supply directly from the aorta. *Minerva Chir* 2002;57:513–515.

301. Spencer JA, Golding SJ. Case of the month: not another case of aortic dissection! *Br J Radiol* 1993;66:565–566.

302. Sperling L. Aneurysm of the splenic artery. *Surgery* 1940;8:633–638.

303. Spier CM, Kjeldsberg CR, Eyre HJ, et al. Malignant lymphoma with primary presentation in the spleen: a study of 20 patients. *Arch Pathol Lab Med* 1985;109:1076–1080.

304. Stanley JC, Fry WJ. Pathogenesis and clinical significance of splenic artery aneurysms. *Surgery* 1974;76:898–909.

305. Stark DD. Hepatic iron overload: Paramagnetic pathology. *Radiology* 1991;179:333–335.

306. Steensma DP, Morice WG. Littoral cell angioma associated with portal hypertension and resected colon cancer. *Acta Haematol* 2000;104:131–134.

307. Steinberg JJ, Suhrland MJ, Valensi QJ. The association of splenoma with disease. Lab Invest 1985;52:65A.

308. Steinmetz AP, Rappaport A, Nikolov G, et al. Splenogonadal fusion diagnosed by spleen scintigraphy. *J Nucl Med* 1997;38:1153–1155.

309. Stiris MG. Accessory spleen versus left adrenal tumor: computed tomographic and abdominal angiographic evaluation. *J Comput Assist Tomogr* 1980;4:534–544.

310. Strijk SP, Wagener DJ, Bogman MJ, et al. The spleen in Hodgkin disease: diagnostic value of CT. *Radiology* 1985;154:753–757.

311. Strijk SP, Boetes C, Bogman MJ, et al. The spleen in non-Hodgkin lymphoma. Diagnostic value of computed tomography. *Acta Radiol* 1987;28:139–144.

312. Subramanyam BR, Balthazar EJ, Horii SC. Sonography of the accessory spleen. *AJR Am J Roentgenol* 1984;143:47–49.

313. Suzuki S, Takizawa K, Nakajima Y, et al. CT findings in hepatic and splenic amyloidosis. *J Comput Assist Tomogr* 1986;10:332–334.

314. Taavitsainen M, Koivuniemi A, Helminen J, et al. Aspiration biopsy of the spleen in patients with sarcoidosis. *Acta Radiol* 1987;28:723–725.

315. Taccone FS, Starc JM, Sculier JP. Splenic spontaneous rupture (SSR) and hemoperitoneum associated with low molecular weight heparin: a case report. *Support Care Cancer* 2003;11:336–338.

316. Tada S, Shin M, Takashima T. Diffuse capillary hemangiomatosis of the spleen as a cause of portal hypertension. *Radiology* 1972;104:63–64.

317. Tang P, Alhindawi R, Farmer P. Case report: primary isolated angiomyolipoma of the spleen. *Ann Clin Lab Sci* 2001;31:405–410.

318. Tanno S, Ohsaki Y, Osanai S, et al. Spontaneous rupture of the amyloid spleen in a case of usual interstitial pneumonia. *Intern Med* 2001;40:428–431.

319. Taxy JB. Peliosis: a morphologic curiosity becomes an iatrogenic problem. *Hum Pathol* 1978;9:331–340.

320. Teates CD, Seale DL, Allen MS. Hamartoma of the spleen. *Am J Roentgenol Radium Ther Nucl Med* 1972;116:419–422.

321. Terk MR, Esplin J, Lee K, et al. MR imaging of patients with type 1 Gaucher's disease: relationship between bone and visceral changes. *AJR Am J Roentgenol* 1995;165:599–604.

322. Thanos L, Dailiana T, Papaioannou G, et al. Percutaneous CT-guided drainage of splenic abscess. *AJR Am J Roentgenol* 2002; 179:629–632.

323. Thompson SE, Walsh EA, Cramer BC, et al. Radiological features of a symptomatic splenic hamartoma. *Pediatr Radiol* 1996;26: 657–660.

324. Thomsen C, Josephsen P, Karle H, et al. Determination of T1 and T2 relaxation times in the spleen of patients with splenomegaly. *Magn Reson Imaging* 1990;8:39–42.

325. Tikkakoski T, Siniluoto T, Paivansalo M, et al. Splenic abscess: imaging and intervention. *Acta Radiol* 1992;33:561–565.

326. Tiu CM, Chou YH, Wang HT, et al. Epithelioid hemangioendothelioma of spleen with intrasplenic metastasis: ultrasound and computed-tomography appearance. *Comput Med Imaging Graph* 1992;16:287–290.

327. Tonkin ILD, Tonkin AK. Visceroatrial situs abnormalities: sonographic and computed tomographic appearance. *AJR Am J Roentgenol* 1982;138:509–515.

328. Torricelli P, Coriani C, Marchetti M, et al. Spontaneous rupture of the spleen: report of two cases. *Abdom Imaging* 2001;26:290–293.

329. Trastek VF, Pairolero PC, Joyce JW, et al. Splenic artery aneurysms. *Surgery* 1982;91:694–699.

330. Tsuchiya N, Sato K, Shimoda N, et al. An accessory spleen mimicking a nonfunctional adrenal tumor: a potential pitfall in the diagnosis of a left adrenal tumor. *Urol Int* 2000;65:226–228.

331. Tsuda K, Nakamura H, Murakami T, et al. Peliosis of the spleen with intraperitoneal hemorrhage. *Abdom Imaging* 1993; 18:283–285.

332. Tsurui N, Ishida H, Morikawa P, et al. Splenic lymphangioma: report of two cases. *J Clin Ultrasound* 1991;19:244–249.

333. Tsushima Y, Tamura T, Tomioka K, et al. Transient splenomegaly in acute pancreatitis. *Br J Radiol* 1999;72:637–643.

334. Ueda J, Kobayashi Y, Hara K, et al. Giant aneurysm of the splenic artery and huge varix. *Gastrointest Radiol* 1985;10:55–57.

335. Urban BA, Fishman EK. Helical CT of the spleen. *AJR Am J Roentgenol* 1998;170:997–1003.

336. Uriarte C, Pomares N, Martin M, et al. Splenic hydatidosis. *Am J Trop Med Hyg* 1991;44:420–423.

337. Urrutia M, Mergo PJ, Ros LH, et al. Cystic masses of the spleen: radiologic-pathologic correlation. *Radiographics* 1996;16:107–129.

338. Valls C, Mones L, Guma A, et al. Torsion of a wandering accessory spleen: CT findings. *Abdom Imaging* 1998;23:194–195.

339. Van Heerden JA, Longo MF, Cardoza F, et al. The abdominal mass in the patient with tuberous sclerosis. Surgical implications and report of a case. *Arch Surg* 1967;95:317–319.

340. Veronesi U, Musumeci R, Pizzetti F, et al. The value of staging laparotomy in non-Hodgkin's lymphomas (with emphasis on the histiocytic type). *Cancer* 1974;33:446–459.

341. Vibhakar SD, Bellon EM. The bare area of the spleen: a constant CT feature of the ascitic abdomen. *AJR Am J Roentgenol* 1984; 142:953–955.

342. von Sinner W, te Strake L, Clark D, et al. MR imaging in hydatid disease. *AJR Am J Roentgenol* 1991;157:741–745.

343. von Sinner WN, Stridbeck H. Hydatid disease of the spleen. Ultrasonography, CT and MR imaging. *Acta Radiol* 1992;33: 459–461.

344. Vossen PG, Van Hedent EF, Degryse HR, et al. Computed tomography of the polysplenia syndrome in the adult. *Gastrointest Radiol* 1987;12:209–211.345.

345. Vyborny CJ, Merrill TN, Reda J, et al. Subacute subcapsular hematoma of the spleen complicating pancreatitis: successful percutaneous drainage. *Radiology* 1988; 169:161–162.

346. Wadham BM, Adams PB, Johnson MA. Incidence and location of accessory spleens. *N Engl J Med* 1981;304:1111.

347. Wadsworth DT, Newman B, Abramson SJ, et al. Splenic lymphangiomatosis in children. *Radiology* 1997;202:173–176.

348. Wang SJ, Chen J-J, Changchien C-S, et al. Sequential invasions of pancreatic pseudocysts in pancreatic tail, hepatic left lobe, caudate lobe and spleen. *Pancreas* 1993;8:133–136.

349. Warnke RA, Weiss LM, Chan JKC, et al. *Tumors of the lymph nodes and spleen*, third ed. Washington, DC: Armed Forces Institute of Pathology, 1995.

350. Warren S, Davis AH. Studies on tumor metastasis: the metastases of carcinoma to the spleen. *Am J Cancer* 1981;21:517–533.

351. Warshauer DM, Dumbleton SA, Molina PL, et al. Abdominal CT findings in sarcoidosis: radiologic and clinical correlation. *Radiology* 1994;192:93–98.

352. Warshauer DM, Semelka RC, Ascher SM. Nodular sarcoidosis of the liver and spleen: appearance on MR images. *J Magn Reson Imaging* 1994;4:553–557.

353. Warshauer DM, Molina PL, Hamman SM, et al. Nodular sarcoidosis of the liver and spleen: analysis of 32 cases. *Radiology* 1995;195:757–762.

354. Warshauer DM, Molina PL, Worawattanakul S. The spotted spleen: CT and clinical correlation in a tertiary care center. *J Comput Assist Tomogr* 1998;22:694–702.

355. Weathers BK, Modesto VL, Gordon D. Isolated splenic metastasis from colorectal carcinoma: report of a case and review of the literature. *Dis Colon Rectum* 1999;42:1345–1348.

356. Weissleder R, Elizondo G, Stark DD, et al. The diagnosis of splenic lymphoma by MR imaging: value of superparamagnetic iron oxide. *AJR Am J Roentgenol* 1989;152:175–180.

357. Westcott JL, Krufky EL. The upside-down spleen. *Radiology* 1972;105:517–521.

358. Wick MR, Scheithauer BW, Smith SL, et al. Primary nonlymphoreticular malignant neoplasm of the spleen. *Am J Surg Pathol* 1982;6:229–242.

359. Wiernik PH, Rader M, Becker NH, et al. Inflammatory pseudotumor of spleen. *Cancer* 1990;66:597–600.

360. Wijaya J, Kapoor R, Roach P. Tc-99m-labeled RBC scintigraphy and splenic hemangioma. *Clin Nucl Med* 2001;26:1022–1023.

361. Willcox TM, Speer RW, Schlinkert RT, et al. Hemangioma of the spleen: presentation, diagnosis, and management. *J Gastrointest Surg* 2000;4:611–613.

362. Wilson ME. *A world guide to infections: disease, distribution, diagnosis*. New York: Oxford University Press, 1991.

363. Winer-Muram HT, Tonkin ILD, Gold RE. Polysplenia syndrome in the asymptomatic adult: computed tomography evaluation. *J Thorac Imaging* 1991;6:69–71.

364. Wirbel RJ, Uhlig U, Futterer KM. Case report: splenic hamartoma with hematologic disorders. *Am J Med Sci* 1996;311:243246.

365. Wolf BC, Neiman RS. *Disorders of the spleen*. Philadelphia: WB Saunders, 1989.

366. Yano H, Imasato M, Monden T, et al. Inflammatory pseudotumor of the spleen: report of two cases. *Surgery* 2003;133:349–350.

367. Yoon DY, Choi BI, Han MC, et al. MR findings of secondary hemochromatosis: transfusional vs erythropoietic. *J Comput Assist Tomogr* 1994;18:416–419.

368. Yuan S, Vaughan M, Agoff SN. Left-sided splenorenal fusion with marked extramedullary hematopoiesis and concurrent lithium toxicity. A case report and review of the literature. *Arch Pathol Lab Med* 2003;127:e1–e3.

369. Zeppa P, Picardi M, Marino G, et al. Fine-needle aspiration biopsy and flow cytometry immunophenotyping of lymphoid and myeloproliferative disorders of the spleen. *Cancer* 2003; 99:118–127.

370. Zissin R, Lishner M, Rathaus V. Case report: unusual presentation of splenic hamartoma; computed tomography and ultrasonic findings. *Clin Radiol* 1992;45:410–411.

The Pancreas

Desiree E. Morgan   Robert J. Stanley

PANCREAS

The past 5 years have seen remarkable changes in the performance of computed tomography (CT) for diseases of the pancreas. As with all abdominal visceral imaging, the majority of these changes involve multidetector or multislice (314) helical techniques. Because of multiple detector rows, helical multidetector CT (MDCT) units are much faster than helical single detector CT (SDCT) units (five to eight times) and have a higher z-axis resolution (283). Precise timing and rapid sequence acquisition allow multiple abdominal imaging passes during MDCT examinations to provide a combined angiographic and organ-directed study at precisely defined circulation phases (99). Multiplanar three-dimensional reformations generated with MDCT techniques allow precise evaluation of peripancreatic relationships in a variety of normal and disease states. However, the increased capabilities and applications of MDCT have led to critical consideration of issues once taken for granted. Most importantly, when thinner image slices are chosen for a MDCT data acquisition and the same signal to noise ratio as for thicker slices is desired, increased tube current and radiation dose result. With shorter temporal scan acquisitions the timing, method, and dose of intravenous (IV) contrast enhancement are crucial. Because high attenuation oral contrast results in degradation of nonaxial reconstructed images, water is used for oral contrast when CT angiography is to be performed. The large data sets generated during MDCT of the pancreas, often greater than 500 images per patient, make workstation use mandatory.

Contrast Issues

As helical CT techniques developed, a revolution in contrast timing for evaluation of the pancreas occurred. In 1996, Lu et al. (196) first described the pancreatic parenchymal phase of contrast enhancement (Fig. 15-1) as the period during which the pancreatic parenchyma is most markedly enhanced. This phase occurs between 40 to 70 seconds after IV injection of 150 cc low osmolar contrast medium at a rate of 3 cc per second. With SDCT, the breathhold required for thin-section coverage through the pancreas usually requires the majority of this period. However, with MDCT, the same z-axis coverage area through the pancreas may require only 8 to 12 seconds with a four-detector ring scanner. With newer 16- or 32-detector ring configurations, proportionately less time is required for the same anatomic coverage, making consideration of contrast issues pertinent to capabilities of individual scanners.

Comparison of earlier SDCT and MDCT reports in the literature is confusing due to variability in rates and doses of IV contrast injections, timing of scans, and technical parameters such as slice thickness, detector configuration, and even scan direction (49,85,141,170,212,340,342). It is quite likely that the end of the arterial phase in many SDCT examinations overlaps the pancreatic parenchymal phase in MDCT examinations. In general, the rate that IV contrast is administered determines when the pancreatic parenchymal phase occurs, and the dose administered determines how long the peak pancreatic enhancement lasts. Specifically, the faster the injection rate, the higher the peak pancreatic enhancement and the sooner it is reached. The larger the dose, the higher the peak and the more constant maintenance of the peak (170,340). The equation for determining when peak pancreatic enhancement occurs described by Tublin et al. (340) is helpful. The initial scanning delay for an individual patient can be calculated by adding 10 seconds (the aortic transfer time) to the injection duration (contrast medium volume divided by injection rate) and then subtracting one half the pancreatic scanning time. In general, three circulatory phases of contrast may aid in diagnosis of pancreatic disorders: true arterial phase

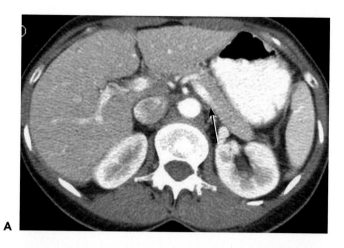

A

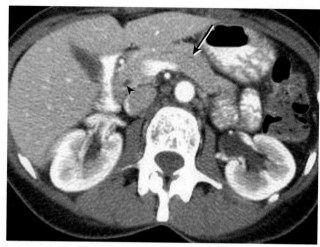

B

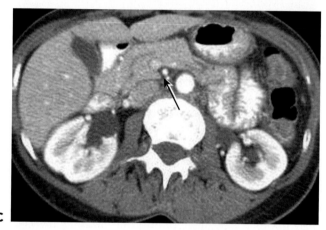

C

Figure 15-1 Normal pancreatic phase computed tomography (CT). **A:** A 5-mm pancreatic parenchymal phase CT image demonstrates normal pancreatic tail posterior to the stomach, extending towards the splenic hilum. Note splenic vein (*arrow*) coursing along dorsal aspect of the pancreas. **B:** Slightly more caudal image shows normal caliber main pancreatic duct (*arrow*) in the body. Note pancreatic parenchyma is thinnest in the neck, anterior to the portal confluence. Normal caliber distal common bile duct (*arrowhead*) lies within posterior portion of pancreatic head, bordered by second portion of duodenum to the right. **C:** Slightly more caudal image shows confluence of main pancreatic duct and distal common bile duct near ampulla. Note fat plane separating right border of superior mesenteric vein from pancreatic parenchyma and uncinate process (*arrow*) insinuating posterior to mesenteric vessels.

(Fig. 15-2), when there is bright enhancement within the aorta and visceral arteries prior to venous filling; pancreatic parenchymal phase, when maximal differences in normally enhancing pancreatic parenchyma versus hypovascular tumors (Fig. 15-3) or necrosis are best depicted; and portal venous phase, when the liver parenchyma (Fig. 15-4) and portomesenteric venous system are ideally enhanced. It is critical to evaluate the circulatory phases for abnormalities best depicted with a particular phase to avoid misinterpretation. For example, an underfilled hepatic vein segment may be diagnosed as a potential hepatic metastasis during the pancreatic parenchymal phase in a patient with pancreatic adenocarcinoma and should be confirmed only after viewing the portal venous phase images (Fig. 15-5). Because the desired goals for contrast enhancement now vary with the type of pancreatic disease suspected, more specific recommendations for SDCT and MDCT scan techniques are given in the sections to follow.

Computed Tomography Techniques

With respect to the evaluation of a known or suspected pancreatic mass, the goals of CT are to confirm the diagno-

sis by detecting and localizing the mass and to evaluate the extent of disease in anticipation of potential resection. In the case of pancreatic adenocarcinoma, exclusion of hepatic and peritoneal metastases and evaluation of local extension of tumor into the peripancreatic tissues, lymph nodes, and most importantly the critical arterial (superior mesenteric artery, celiac axis, hepatic artery) and venous (superior mesenteric vein, portal confluence, main portal vein) structures to predict resectability of the lesion are desired. With CT angiography (CTA), the goal of preoperative vascular mapping in patients who are potential candidates to undergo Whipple procedure is to clearly define the angiographic map with an accuracy equal to classic angiography and to depict the relationship of the mass to potentially invaded vessels, attempting to differentiate between abutment and invasion of vessels along their course. With axial images alone, narrowing or constriction of vessels may be difficult to judge (97). In addition to CTA, optimal techniques for mass detection now include thin section scanning in the pancreatic parenchymal phase, followed by scanning through the entire abdomen and pelvis in the portal venous phase. Generally, a precontrast study through the pancreas to localize the area to be studied after IV con-

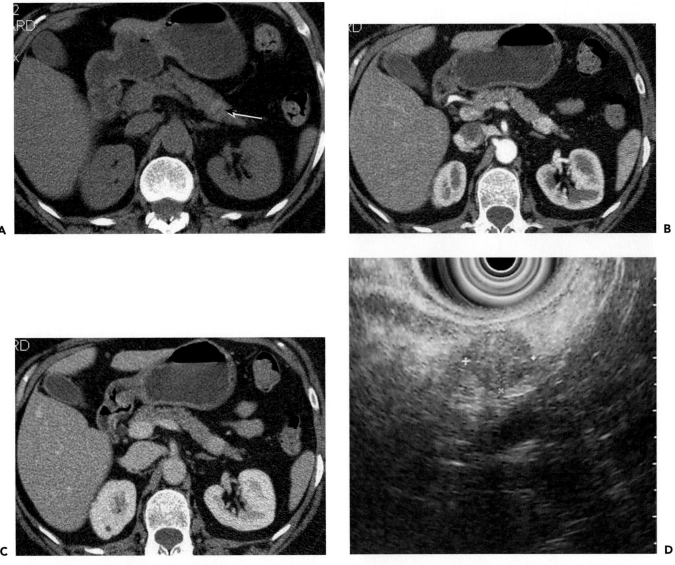

Figure 15-2 Insulinoma in a 61-year-old woman with hyperinsulinemia and negative outside computed tomography (CT) scan. **A:** Pre-intravenous 5-mm CT image demonstrates no contour altering mass; however, a slightly higher attenuation focus is visible (*arrow*). **B:** Arterial phase contrast-enhanced 3-mm CT image demonstrates a corresponding focal 1.2-cm hyperenhancing mass at the body/tail junction. **C:** Portal venous phase image demonstrates diminished conspicuity of the lesion. **D:** Endoscopic ultrasound (EUS) image shows well-defined hypoechoic round mass corresponding to CT image. (EUS image courtesy of Mohammed Eloubeidi, MD.)

trast enhancement is performed with thicker section images. In the case of functional neuroendocrine tumors of the pancreas, the arterial phase helps to identify hyperenhancing lesions, which may be multiple or located in a peripancreatic location. IV contrast must be given at a rate of at least 3 cc per second (ideally administered at a rate of 5 cc per second whenever possible), with most centers using 150 cc of a nonionic medium (300 mg of iodine per milliliter). Water is the oral contrast agent of choice when evaluating for pancreatic mass (Tables 15-1 and 15-2).

The advantages of multiple detector over SDCT hinge on the ability to image the pancreas in both the pancreatic and venous phases with an adequate number of thin slices during a comfortable breathhold. These high-quality volumetric data sets are then postprocessed using techniques such as volume rendering (VR), maximum intensity projections (MIPs), and curved planar reformations (CPRs) (Fig. 15-6). With four-slice MDCT scanners, the slice thickness is typically on the order of 1.00 to 1.50 mm but the pitch and gantry rotation times yield relatively slow table speeds, and as a result respiratory misregistration can be problematic. With six- to ten-slice scanners, the minimum slice thickness is still on the order of 1.00 to 1.50 mm but the table speeds are faster and the breathhold duration shorter. With 16-slice scanners, the minimum slice thickness is 0.50 to 0.75 mm yielding data sets that

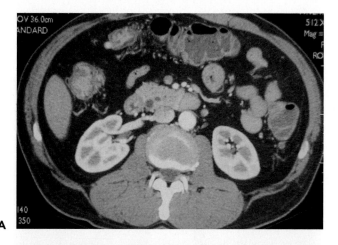

A

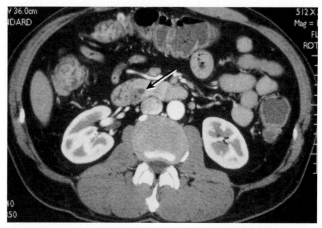

B

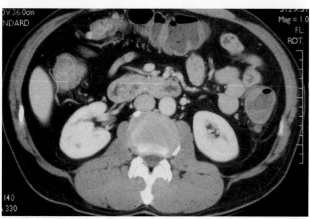

C

Figure 15-3 Small pancreatic adenocarcinoma in a 63-year-old man with abdominal pain and biliary enzyme elevation. **A:** Pancreatic parenchymal phase 2.5-mm computed tomography (CT) image through the pancreatic head demonstrates slight dilatation of the vertical portion of the main pancreatic duct and bile duct in the pancreatic head region, near the ampulla. **B:** More caudal pancreatic parenchymal phase 2.5-mm CT image demonstrates a fairly well-circumscribed 1-cm heterogeneous mass present at the abrupt termination of the dilated bile duct, seen immediately to the right and slightly posterior to the vertical pancreatic duct (*arrow*). **C:** Same slice portal venous phase 5-mm CT image demonstrates less conspicuity of the lesion obstructing the bile duct. The tumor was resectable.

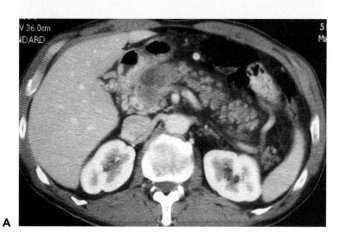

A

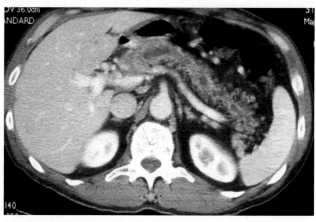

B

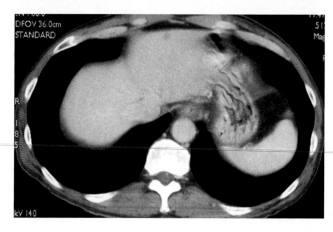

C

Figure 15-4 Small liver metastasis, and normal fatty infiltration of the pancreas, making solid pancreatic head adenocarcinoma more obvious. **A:** Contrast-enhanced portal venous phase 3-mm image demonstrates normal fatty replacement and lobularity of the tail and body. Heterogeneous low attenuation solid appearing mass in the superior head is readily apparent. **B:** Slightly superior image to A demonstrates dilated main pancreatic duct in the neck and body. Heterogeneous mass abuts portal confluence and hepatic artery. **C:** Portal venous phase computed tomography image through the superior liver reveals a focal 8-mm hypodense liver lesion consistent with a metastasis, indicating an inoperable tumor.

TABLE 15-1

MDCT FOR PANCREATIC MASS

Contrast: IV—150 mL 4/sec, Oral—750–1,000 mL water.

Arterial phase (AP): 20-sec delay from start of injection, FOV 20–25, 1.25 HS table speed of 1 cm/sec (7.5 mm/0.8 sec), cover from 1 cm above celiac axis to 3rd duodenum 3-D reformations using volume rendering and/or MIP, with curved planar reconstruction along major vessels.

Pancreatic parenchymal phase (PPP): 35-sec delay, 2.5 mm w/5 mm recon interval HQ, table speed 1 cm/sec (7.5 mm/0.8), same coverage area, both AP and PPP acquired during single breathhold. 3-D reformations using volume rendering and or curved planar reconstruction along ducts.

Portal venous phase (PVP): 60-sec delay, larger FOV, diaphragm to iliac crest, 5-mm collimation w/5 mm recon in HQ table speed of 1 cm/sec (7.5 mm/0.8 sec).

3-D, three-dimensional; FOV, field of view; HQ, high quality; HS, high speed; MDCT, multidetector computed tomography; MIP, maximum intensity projection.

TABLE 15-2

SDCT FOR PANCREATIC MASS[a]

Contrast: IV—150 mL 3/sec, Oral—750–1,000 mL water.

Pancreatic parenchymal phase (PPP): 35–40 sec delay, 2.5 mm with 1.5–1.8 pitch to cover 1 cm above celiac axis to 3rd duodenum during single breathhold, recon to 3 mm, with 3-D reformations using volume rendering and or curved planar reconstruction along ducts.

Portal venous phase (PVP): 70-sec delay, 7 mm from diaphragm to crest, if length of breathhold allows, narrow to 5 mm through pancreas, 1:1 pitch, larger FOV.

[a]Must select either PPP or arterial phase, to accompany PVP due to breathhold requirements for coverage and contrast timing issues.
3-D, three-dimensional; FOV, field of view; SDCT, single detector computed tomography.

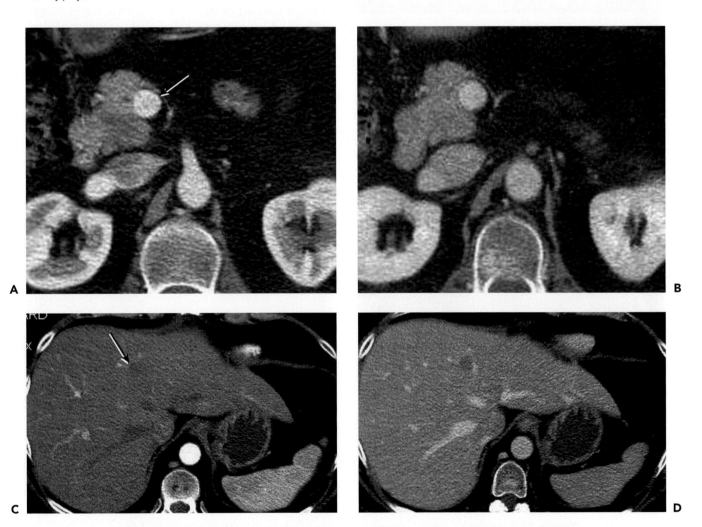

Figure 15-5 Small pancreatic adenocarcinoma in uncinate, best seen on pancreatic parenchymal phase. Liver metastases best depicted on portal venous phase. **A:** Pancreatic parenchymal phase 2.5-mm image demonstrates 1.2-cm mass in the medial aspect of the uncinate process. The mass abuts, but does not deform, the portal vein (*arrow*). **B:** Portal venous phase image, same level, demonstrates diminished conspicuity of the mass. **C:** Arterial phase through the superior liver demonstrates lack of opacification within the hepatic veins. Note rounded lesion similar in attenuation in the interlobar area (*arrow*). **D:** Portal venous phase same level demonstrates filling of the hepatic veins and greater conspicuity of the liver metastasis in this patient despite very small pancreatic mass at presentation.

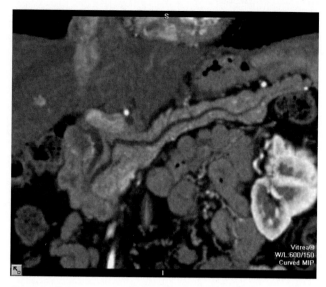

Figure 15-6 Curved planar reformatted image of normal pancreas. With cursor drawn along course of the main pancreatic duct, the entire gland is visualized, and the relationship of the pancreatic duct to distal common bile duct is well depicted.

are isotropic. Isotropic resolution occurs when the voxel dimensions are equal in the x-, y-, and z-axes. For example, when a data set is acquired with a display field-of-view of 360 mm, a matrix size of 512 × 512 and a 0.625-mm slice thickness, the voxel dimension are 360/512 = 0.703 mm in the x- and y-axes and 0.625 mm in the z-axis (plus some inherent slice broadening due to table motion). With 32- to 64-slice scanners, the minimum voxel dimensions are

still on the order of 0.50 to 0.75 mm but the table speeds are much faster.

Although scanners acquiring 16 or more slices per gantry rotation are capable of generating isotropic data sets, these small voxels may have an inherent and intolerable increase in image noise unless the tube current (and the corresponding radiation dose) is significantly boosted. When nonisotropic images are reconstructed from isotropic data sets (i.e., 2.50- to 5.00-mm axial slices or 2.00- to 3.00-mm coronal and sagittal images), the noise is reduced to a tolerable level. However, certain types of image reconstructions, such as VR and CPR, display individual voxels and as a result often demonstrate unacceptable levels of image noise. Therefore, many institutions have chosen to address this problem by acquiring data set of the pancreas (at least during the pancreatic phase of enhancement) with nonisotropic voxels on the order of 1.00 to 1.50 mm. Although the spatial resolution is lower, the ability to detect and characterize vascular encasement, ductal obstruction and peripancreatic lymph nodes remains. Artifacts resulting from more complex CPR techniques may be encountered (Fig. 15-7).

One of the main advantages of 32- to 64-slice scanners for the pancreas is the ability to perform a CT-perfusion study of the entire gland rather than at a single anatomic level. In the future, CT-perfusion information may be helpful for detecting pancreatic adenocarcinomas that are isodense to pancreatic parenchyma or for predicting which tumors are likely to respond to various treatment regimens (particularly chemotherapy).

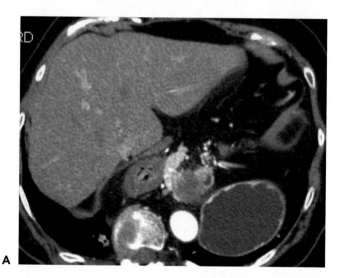

A

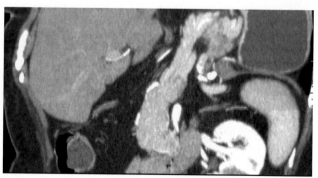

B

Figure 15-7 Pancreatic adenocarcinoma of body/tail junction, located in large hiatal hernia. **A:** Axial image through the upper abdomen/lower chest in pancreatic parenchymal phase demonstrates hypoattenuating mass in the body/tail of pancreas, located within a very large hiatal hernia. Peripancreatic stranding and upstream ductal dilatation are noted. Splenic artery is encased. **B:** Angled coronal volume rendered image through the upper abdomen demonstrates the normal appearing pancreatic parenchyma in the head, neck, and body, with hypoattenuating mass at the body/tail junction, ductal dilation/inflammatory changes involving the tail. (*continued*)

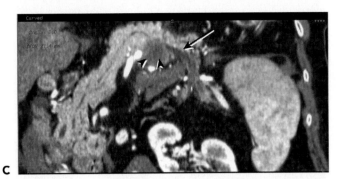

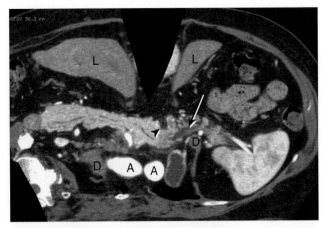

C

D

Figure 15-7 *(continued)* **C:** Coronal curved planar reformatted image aligned with the inverted U-shaped main pancreatic duct demonstrates termination of the upstream dilated duct *(arrow)* in the mass *(arrowhead)* at the tail/body junction, and normal appearing pancreatic duct in the remainder of the gland. **D:** Axial curved planar reformatted image aligned with the inverted U-shaped main pancreatic duct demonstrates termination of the upstream dilated duct *(arrow)* in the mass *(arrowhead)* at the tail/body junction and normal appearing pancreatic duct in the remainder of the gland. Note butterfly artifact due to two curved directions (superior-inferior and anterior-posterior) in this patient with marked pancreatic positional distortion due to the hiatal hernia. L, liver; D, diaphragmatic crus; A, aorta.

For the follow-up of pancreatic masses after surgical resection (Fig. 15-8), routine abdominal scanning is usually adequate. Surgical clips typically produce problematic artifacts in the surgical bed, limiting the quality of postprocessed images. If the patient has received radiation and/or chemotherapy after the initial diagnosis of a pancreatic mass, and posttreatment response is to be evaluated prior to consideration of surgical resection, the same protocol as used for the initial evaluation of the mass should be used.

When pancreatitis is a clinical concern, the goals of the CT examination are to confirm a suspected but uncertain clinical diagnosis and, more importantly, to evaluate for complications of pancreatitis such as pancreatic necrosis (Fig. 15-9), hemorrhage, infection, development of pan-

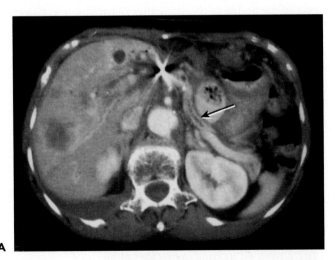

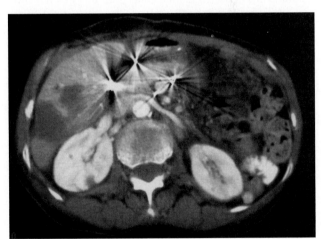

A

B

Figure 15-8 Recurrent pancreatic adenocarcinoma in a 74-year-old woman 8 months after Whipple resection with free margins. **A:** Pancreatic parenchymal phase 5-mm computed tomography image demonstrates atrophied pancreatic body and tail *(arrow)*. There is abnormal hypovascular soft tissue surrounding the celiac axis, posterior to the clip. Multiple hepatic metastases are present. **B:** 3.5 cm inferiorly, there is beam hardening artifact due to multiple surgical clips, a common finding in patients after Whipple. Liver metastases and abnormal soft tissue anterior to the left renal vein are clearly evident despite the artifact.

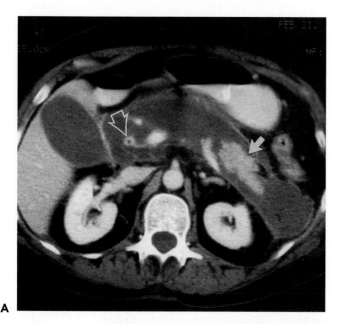
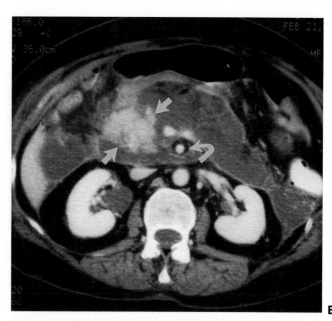

A   B

Figure 15-9 Two weeks post onset of gallstone pancreatitis with severe necrosis. **A:** Computed tomography scan through the level of the body of the pancreas shows enhancement in only a small portion of the tail of the pancreas (*arrows*). The skeletonized common bile duct (*open arrow*) courses through this loculated collection. **B:** Enhancement of the pancreatic head (*arrows*) is preserved. No other portions of the pancreas, in addition to the small portion of the tail, remained vascularized. Note the heterogeneous composition of the material within the distended anterior pararenal space, reflecting the process of necrosis. Note also the preservation of the sleeve of fat (*curved arrow*) surrounding the enhancing superior mesenteric artery. This patient remained severely symptomatic for an additional month before being successfully decompressed by an endoscopic method.

creatic fluid collections, or development of vascular complications such as venous thrombosis or pseudoaneurysm formation. As opposed to pancreatic mass evaluation, high-density oral contrast agent should be used to ideally define relationships of potential fluid collections to adjacent bowel and identify fistulae (99). CTA is not routinely used for this indication but can be used if vascular complications are suspected in particular (Tables 15-3 and 15-4).

For the follow-up of pancreatitis, routine abdominal scanning is usually adequate. If the patient's creatinine has become elevated, noncontrast helical CT may be used to follow-up the size of peripancreatic fluid collections (Fig. 15-10)

or the response of those fluid collections to percutaneous, surgical, or endoscopic drainage (Fig. 15-11).

Standard magnetic resonance imaging (MRI) techniques for evaluation of the pancreas mirror those of CT with respect to the timing of the scans after IV contrast injection of extracellular fluid contrast agents such as gadolinium chelates. For pancreatic mass evaluation, T1-weighted fat suppressed images may be obtained in the axial or coronal planes prior to IV gadolinium enhancement, 35 to 45 seconds after commencement of contrast for the pancreatic parenchymal phase and 70 seconds for the portal venous phase. These T1-weighted images are generally gradient refocused echo (GRE) sequences with breathhold technique (Fig. 15-12) (302). With the increasing use of power injectors for

TABLE 15-3
MDCT FOR ROUTINE ABDOMEN OR PANCREATITIS

Contrast: IV—150 mL 4/sec, Oral—720 mL 3% iodinated contrast medium.

Portal venous phase (PVP): 60-sec delay, large FOV, diaphragm to iliac crest, 5 mm collimation w/5 mm recon in HQ table speed of 1 cm/sec (7.5 mm/0.8 sec).

Consider acquiring: Pancreatic parenchymal phase (PPP): 35-sec delay, 2.5 mm w/5 mm recon interval HQ, table speed 1 cm/sec (7.5 mm/0.8), coverage through pancreas to evaluated necrosis in patients with severe acute pancreatitis.

FOV, field of view; HQ, high quality; MDCT, multidetector computed tomography.

TABLE 15-4
SDCT FOR ROUTINE ABDOMEN OR PANCREATITIS

Contrast: IV—150 mL 3/sec, Oral—720 mL 3% iodinated contrast medium.

Portal venous phase (PVP): 70-sec delay, 7 mm from diaphragm to crest, if length of breathhold allows, narrow to 5 mm through pancreas, 1:1 pitch, larger FOV.

FOV, field of view; SDCT, single detector computed tomography.

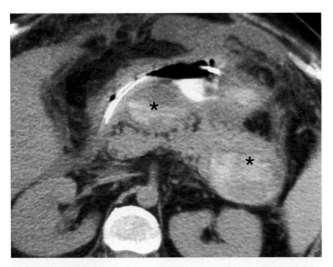

Figure 15-10 Hemorrhagic pancreatitis demonstrated with noncontrast computed tomography (CT) in a 38-year-old man with known pancreatitis and elevated creatinine, worsening clinically. A 5-mm oral-contrast-only CT image demonstrates two heterogeneous fluid collections (*), one located anterior to the neck, the other posterior to the tail; both contain high-density acute hemorrhage.

gadolinium administration, timing issues for ideal pancreatic and peripancreatic vascular enhancement are evolving as in MDCT. Kanematsu et al. (161) suggest that the best dual-phase method for dynamic breathhold GRE postgadolinium images to be obtained is to initiate imaging so that middle of the first acquisition occurs 15 seconds after initiation of contrast administration at 3 mL per second and to repeat the sequence at 45 seconds (middle of acquisition) for evaluation of peripancreatic veins and liver. T2-weighted imaging of the pancreas is not routinely used for mass evaluation but is used for evaluation of potential liver metastases. Fast spin echo or single shot fast spin echo techniques may be used. One advantage of MRI is the ability to perform magnetic resonance cholangiopancreatography (MRCP). When a pancreatic mass is suspected clinically,

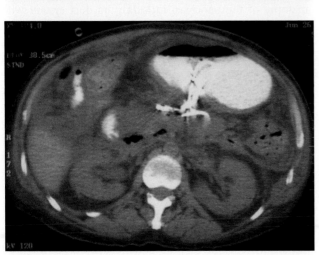

A

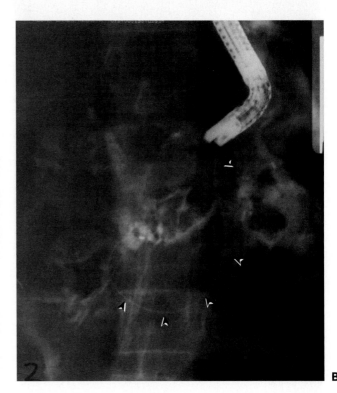

B

Figure 15-11 Infected pancreatic necrosis incompletely drained by percutaneous catheter in a 50-year-old man with onset of acute necrotizing pancreatitis 6 weeks earlier, transferred for failure to improve. **A:** A 7-mm portal venous phase computed tomography (CT) image demonstrates anterior percutaneous catheter entering a heterogeneous, gas containing, multiloculated fluid collection in the pancreatic bed. Small amount of enhancing gland is seen within the head region at this level. **B:** Spot radiograph during endoscopic drainage reveals portions of the percutaneous catheter (*arrow*). The endoscopic catheter (*arrowheads*) has been placed from the stomach into the collection, with injection demonstrating multiple large filling defects consistent with necrotic debris. **C:** Three months later after transgastric endoscopic drainage of the collection combined with the percutaneous catheter for irrigation, CT with oral-contrast-only shows near complete collapse of the cavity surrounding the intrapancreatic portions of the transgastric double J stents.

C

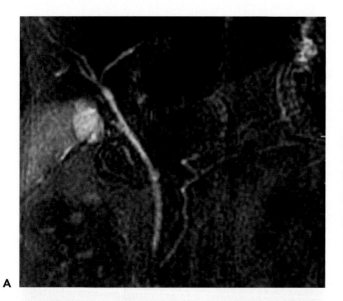

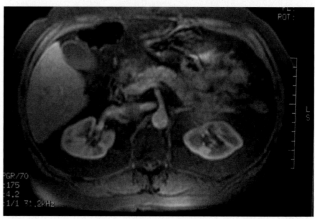

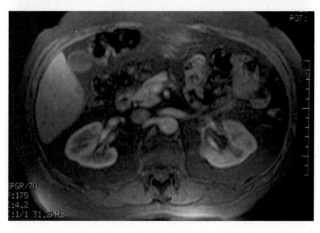

Figure 15-12 Normal pancreatic magnetic resonance imaging. **A:** Angled coronal 5-cm slab half-Fourier acquisition single-shot turbo spin echo (HASTE) magnetic resonance cholangiopancreatography demonstrates normal caliber biliary and pancreatic ducts, as well as the gallbladder. **B:** Intravenous gadolinium enhanced portal venous phase 5-mm T1-weighted fat suppressed fast spoiled gradient (FSPGR) breathhold image through the pancreatic body and tail demonstrates normal glandular contour. **C:** Same sequence through the pancreatic head shows normal contour and enhancement pattern.

MRCP may be the first sequence performed on a patient to localize the level of biliary or pancreatic duct obstruction for the remaining T1 fat suppressed and post IV gadolinium enhanced images. Newer MRI techniques using manganese based IV contrast media that is taken up by normal hepatic and pancreatic tissue have been used to define focal pancreatic lesions (294).

Normal Anatomy

Considerable variation exists in the size shape and location of the normal pancreas, depending on differences in body habitus as well as the normal or abnormal size and positioning of contiguous organs. In the most common normal configuration, the long axis of the body and tail the pancreas lies in an oblique orientation, extending from the hilum of the spleen at its lateral and most cephalad extent, toward the midline of the body, where it passes anterior to that portion of the portal vein formed by the confluence of the superior mesenteric vein and splenic vein (Fig. 15-13). At this point, the pancreas turns caudally in a more vertical orientation ending in the uncinate process, its most caudal extent. The main pancreatic duct in most people represents

the fusion of the dorsal duct (Santorini) and the ventral duct (Wirsung) and empties into the duodenum through the major papilla. In one third or slightly more of normal individuals, a separate drainage site for the continuation of the dorsal duct is located in the medial wall of the duodenum proximal to the major papilla. This is referred to as the minor papilla. High-quality CT and MRI can define the anatomy of the pancreas, including its duct system with great precision, affording information on the integrity of the pancreatic parenchyma, the caliber of the duct system, and the relationships of the pancreas to surrounding anatomic structures (Fig. 15-14). Modern CT and MRI consistently show that the thickness of the normal pancreatic parenchyma, measured perpendicular to its long axis on the cross-sectional view, varies depending on whether the head, neck, body, or tail is measured. The thickness of the head averages approximately 2.0 cm; the neck of the pancreas, just anterior to the portal vein, its thinnest portion, ranges in thickness from 0.5 to 1.0 cm. The body and tail range from 1.0 to 2.0 cm, with many normal glands tapering slightly towards the tail. The cephalocaudal dimension of the body and tail ranges from 3.0 to 4.0 cm in most individuals, whereas the cephalocaudal dimension of the head

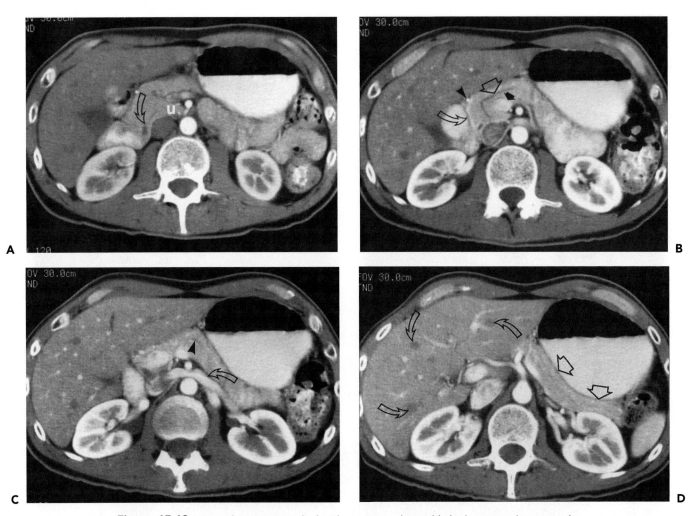

Figure 15-13 Normal pancreas studied with contrast-enhanced helical computed tomography. Because of the paucity of perivisceral fat, the surface of the pancreas has a smooth rather than lobular appearance. All portions of the pancreas are clearly defined in the early arterial and capillary phase of this dynamic study. **A:** At the level of the pancreatic head and uncinate process (u), the junction of the main pancreatic duct and common bile duct (*curved arrow*) is clearly defined. The brightly enhancing superior mesenteric artery lies directly anterior to the aorta and posterior to the junction of the neck and body of the pancreas. **B:** At the level of the neck of the pancreas, a normal caliber main pancreatic duct (*open arrow*) is visible over several centimeters of its length. The portal vein, only partially enhanced in this early phase (*black arrow*), lies immediately posterior to the neck of the pancreas and lateral to the superior mesenteric artery. The tissue plane separating the lateral surface of the pancreatic head and medial wall of the duodenum (*curved arrow*) is well seen at this level. *Arrowhead,* Anterior superior pancreaticoduodenal artery, which is also visible in Fig. 15-2A. **C:** More cephalad at the level of the body of the pancreas, a short segment of the main pancreatic duct (*arrowhead*) is visible. As the contrast reaches the early venous phase, the left renal vein (*curved arrow*) is well opacified. **D:** At this most cephalad level the body and tail of the pancreas are now seen to be uniformly enhanced and sharply defined by the posterior wall of the stomach (*arrows*). The hepatic veins (*curved arrows*) are not yet enhanced at this phase.

is more variable, and portions of the head can be seen over distances ranging from 3.0 cm to as much as 8.0 cm. With respect to size and shape, the most reliable indicator of a pancreatic mass has been the presence of an abrupt focal change rather than generalized variations from the range of normal dimensions. However, with the use of high-quality contrast-enhanced helical CT imaging subtle focal changes in the pancreatic parenchyma indicative of the presence of tumor, which do not change the size or shape of the pan-

creas, can be defined (196). CPRs aligned with the pancreatic duct may also aid in the identification of small, non-contour-altering adenocarcinomas (Fig. 15-15) and better define the relationships of intraductal papillary mucinous tumors (IPMTs) to the main pancreatic duct or side branches (242) (Fig. 15-16). Recent detailed analyses of normal variations in the lateral contour of the head and neck of the pancreas, obtained with helical CT examinations, have shown three general categories of variation from

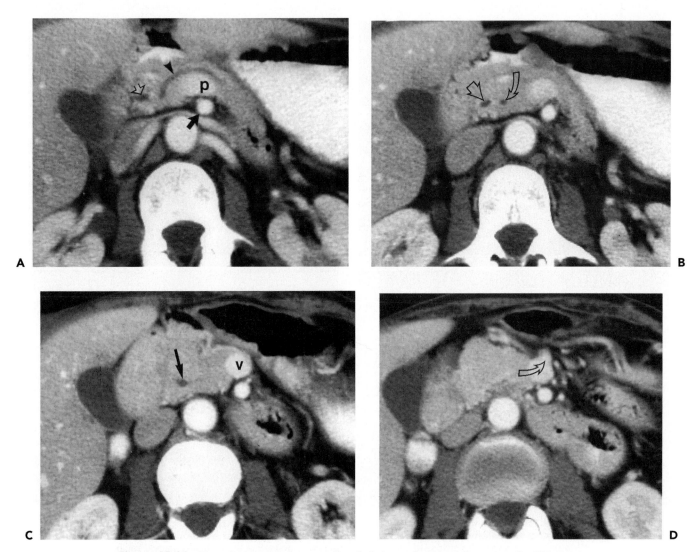

Figure 15-14 Normal pancreatic anatomy. Detailed views of computed tomography (CT) scans through the neck and head of the pancreas. **A:** The main pancreatic duct lies in the plane of the CT scan as it passes through the neck of the pancreas (*arrowhead*). The enhancing portal vein (p) lies immediately posterior to the neck. The superior mesenteric artery lies posterior to the portal vein at this level and anterior to the left renal vein (*black arrow*). The caliber of the main pancreatic duct at this level is approximately 2.5 mm. A normal caliber common bile duct (*open arrow*) lies lateral to the main pancreatic duct. **B:** At this level both the normal caliber common bile duct (*arrow*) and main pancreatic duct (*curved arrow*) are seen in cross-section as they approach the ampulla. **C:** 5 mm caudal, the main pancreatic duct and common bile duct have joined to form the ampulla (*arrow*). Note that in this patient, the head of the pancreas lies directly anterior to the aorta rather than to the right of it. The superior mesenteric artery lies posterior to the superior mesenteric vein (v). **D:** CT section just caudal to the entry of the ampulla into the major papilla. No ducts are visible at this level, which is through the most caudal portion of the head of the pancreas and uncinate process. Note the gastrocolic trunk (*curved arrow*) as it enters the anterior aspect of the superior mesenteric vein.

the normal flat interface of the lateral border of the head of pancreas to the medial wall of the duodenum, which could be misinterpreted as a focal mass (285). In each instance, the character of the enhancement of the focal variation was identical to the adjacent normal pancreatic parenchyma studied during the parenchymal phase, allowing a correct interpretation. Newer techniques of MRI also allow for detection of subtle lesions that do not alter the size or shape of the pancreas.

The surface contour of the pancreatic parenchyma can either be smooth or lobular, the latter being more frequently seen when there is abundant peripancreatic retroperitoneal fat. Although the pancreas is totally invested in fine connective tissue, it does not have a true fibrous capsule. Therefore, the lobular architecture of the pancreas is well defined by the interdigitated peripancreatic fat (Fig. 15-17). Fatty replacement of much of the pancreatic substance is a common degenerative process seen in the

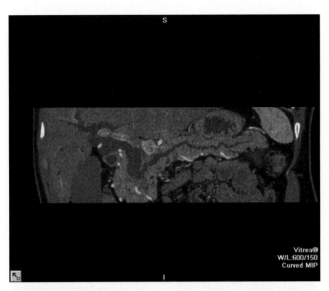

Figure 15-15 Small moderately differentiated adenocarcinoma arising from an IPMT of the head region. Curved planar reformation demonstrates noncontour-altering adenocarcinoma as it obstructs the upstream pancreatic and distal common bile ducts.

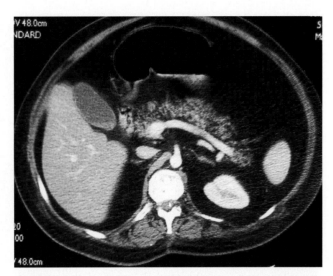

Figure 15-17 Normal fatty infiltration. Portal venous phase 5-mm computed tomography image through the level of the splenic vein and portal confluence shows low density fat interdigitating the normally enhancing pancreatic parenchyma.

elderly. However, marked interdigitation in the peripancreatic fat can simulate this late degenerative process in obese individuals. Fatty replacement may also be associated with alterations in pancreatic function and may be a late sequel to various forms of chronic pancreatitis.

Part or all of the normal main pancreatic duct can be seen in nearly all patients studied, if high detail CT technique is used. With such high-resolution, contrast-enhanced, thin section technique, the portion of the duct within the head of the pancreas, perpendicular to the plane of the slice, is most conspicuous (see Fig. 15-14). Such technique also greatly increases the chances of demonstrating that portion of the duct in the body and tail of the pancreas, which lies generally parallel to the plane of the CT image (see Figs. 15-1 and 15-13). A technique of projectional CT cholangiopancreatography developed by Raptopoulos et al. (269) uses minimum intensity projections of selected slab thickness tissue volumes to visualize the pancreatic and distal bile ducts. With this noninvasive technique, the authors found improved depiction of the duct compared with helical axial images alone, with good correlation to endoscopic retrograde cholangiopancreatography (ERCP). The use of this method is not widespread.

Anatomic Relationships

The splenic vein lies on the dorsal surface of the body and tail of the pancreas, caudal to the splenic artery (see Figs. 15-1A and 15-13D). In comparison with the more tortuous course of the splenic artery, the vein runs closely parallel to the longitudinal orientation of the pancreas. Depending on how much retroperitoneal fat is present, a thin fat plane may separate the anterior surface of the splenic vein from the posterior surface of the pancreatic parenchyma. The left adrenal gland lies posteromedial to the splenic vein and the pancreas at the junction of the body and tail.

The tail of the pancreas extends to the splenic hilum, entering the splenorenal ligament and becoming intraperitoneal for a short distance. Although generally located anterior to the splenic vein, the tail of pancreas is occasionally imaged in the same plane as, or even posterior to, the splenic vein or a tributary. The body and tail of the pancreas normally are located anterior or anterolateral to the left kidney. However, in a patient lacking a left kidney (surgically removed or congenitally absent), or in a patient with an ectopic

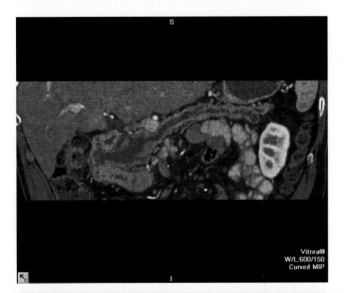

Figure 15-16 Moderately differentiated IPMT. Curved planar reformation demonstrates diffuse main pancreatic duct dilation, with the dilated papilla bulging into the duodenal lumen.

left kidney, the body and tail will be displaced posteromedially, lying adjacent to the spine and occupying the empty renal fossa. Usually there is an accompanying posteromedial rotation in the position of the spleen.

The body of the pancreas arches anteriorly over the superior mesenteric artery, close to its origin from the aorta, separated by distinct fat plane that encircles the superior mesenteric artery in all but the leanest individuals. The superior mesenteric vein runs parallel and to the right of the superior mesenteric artery and usually is larger in diameter. At the point where the superior mesenteric vein joins the splenic vein to form the portal vein, the neck of the pancreas is seen to pass immediately ventral to the portal vein. Generally, there is no intervening fat plane between the neck of the pancreas and the portal vein. The presence of a fat plane between the lateral surface of the superior mesenteric vein and the medial aspect of the uncinate process of the pancreatic head is variable.

The head of the pancreas lies medial to the second portion of the duodenum, to the right of the superior mesenteric vein, and anterior to the inferior vena cava. Generally, a thin, distinct fat plane separates the posterior surface of the head of the pancreas from the anterior surface of the inferior vena cava (IVC). The uncinate process of the pancreatic head is a curving, beaklike inferior and medial extension of the head that originates lateral to the superior mesenteric vein and curves posteriorly behind it, approximately at the level of the left renal vein.

With the improvement in technique supported by helical CT scanners, finer details of arterial and venous anatomy can be defined. The arterial and venous structures that lie anterior and posterior to the pancreatic head can now be identified in a significant percentage of patients. In 1992, Mori (231) first described the appearance of the normal gastrocolic trunk that courses over the anterior surface of the head of the pancreas. The gastrocolic trunk is formed by veins that lie in the transverse mesocolon, the right gastroepiploic vein, and the anterior pancreaticoduodenal vein. The authors reported being able to identify a normal gastrocolic trunk (2.6 to 4.7 mm diameter) in approximately half of the control group with CT scans obtained using 10-mm thick sections and in 90% of CT scans obtained using 5-mm thick sections. They also noted abnormal dilatation of the gastrocolic trunk in cases in which the superior mesenteric vein or portal vein, downstream from the junction of the gastrocolic trunk and superior mesenteric vein, were involved by disease resulting in stenosis, occlusion, or thrombosis (231) (Fig. 15-18). With the advent of even thinner section helical techniques, peripancreatic tributary veins emptying into the portomesenteric venous system including not only the gastrocolic trunk but also the right gastroepiploic vein, first jejunal branch, inferior mesenteric vein, left gastric vein, posterior superior pancreaticoduodenal vein, middle colic vein, right colic vein, and anterior superior pancreaticoduodenal vein may be seen in normal individuals.

Lack of visualization of these veins or identification of the inferior peripancreatic veins that in normal patients are frequently too small in caliber to detect with thin section helical CT, may indicate subtle invasion of the superior mesenteric vein (SMV) or portal confluence in patients with adenocarcinoma of the head of the pancreas (138,231,346,368). With MDCT, 3-D reformations help to create venous maps that more clearly depict involvement by tumor than axial images alone (97,137,186) (Fig. 15-18). CTA techniques for larger visceral arteries are well established. Although early reports suggested that the smaller peripancreatic arteries were not well depicted with thin section helical CT (160,313), Chong et al. (64) were able to demonstrate adequate arterial studies in 87 of 100 normal patients; using SDCT, all major abdominal arterial vessels were shown in all patients in addition to the dorsal pancreatic artery in 94%, pancreatica magna in 52%, caudal pancreatic in 39%, anterior arcade in 54%, and posterior arcade in 72%.

In a small percentage of patients, the head of the pancreas may lie in a position that is completely to the left of the aorta. Although this situation may develop because of an enlarging mass in the liver or peripancreatic area displacing the pancreas to the left, it has also been seen in patients with no relevant abdominal disease. In these instances, despite the fact that the head of the pancreas is completely to the left of the aorta, the pancreas still bears the normal relationship to the superior mesenteric vein and artery. It has been suggested that the left-sided pancreas may be an acquired positional variation due to increasing laxity of retroperitoneal tissues occurring with age as well as tortuosity of the abdominal aorta, causing it to swing farther to the right than usual. In one study, all of the patients who had a left-sided pancreas and no associated abdominal disease were older than 50 years (87).

The normal-sized common bile duct, varying in diameter from 3 to 6 mm, can be seen in cross-section within the head of the pancreas, close to its lateral and posterior surface, appearing as a circular or oval near water density structure. Its detectability is improved if the surrounding substance of the pancreatic parenchyma is enhanced by IV contrast material. Under optimal imaging conditions, the vertically oriented segment of the main pancreatic duct lying in the head can be seen running parallel and medial to the common bile duct (see Fig. 15-14C), ranging in diameter from 1 to 3 mm. The utility of thin section axial images in depicting isoattenuating or small pancreatic tumors obstructing the duct (99,265) and in determining the relationship of the side branches and main pancreatic duct in patients with intraductal papillary mucinous tumor (IPMT) (99,107) has been reported.

The pancreas lies in the anterior pararenal space and is related to the second segment of the duodenum along the lateral surface of the head and to the third and fourth segments of the duodenum along the inferior surface of the head, body, and tail. The stomach lies anterior to the

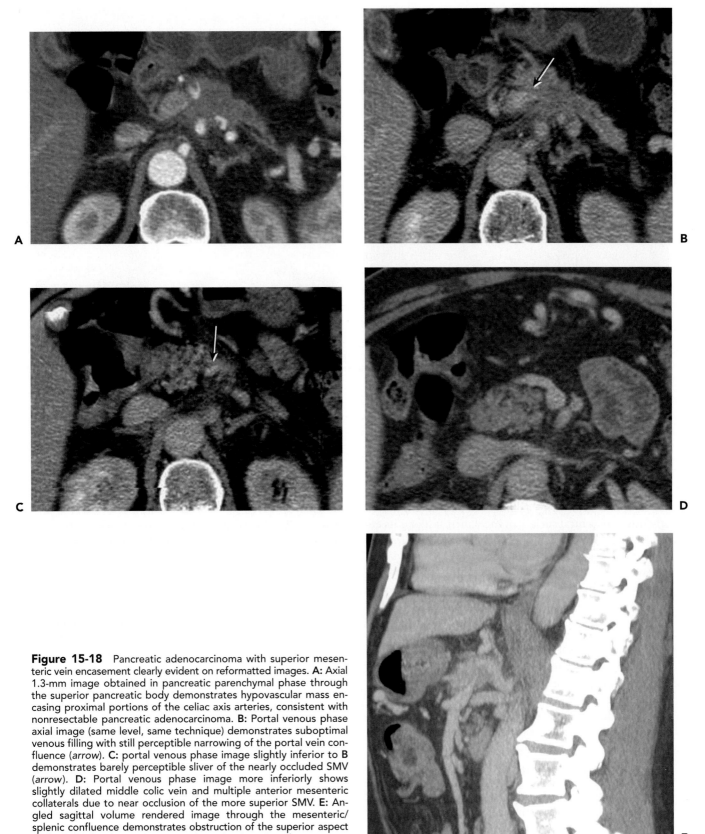

Figure 15-18 Pancreatic adenocarcinoma with superior mesenteric vein encasement clearly evident on reformatted images. **A:** Axial 1.3-mm image obtained in pancreatic parenchymal phase through the superior pancreatic body demonstrates hypovascular mass encasing proximal portions of the celiac axis arteries, consistent with nonresectable pancreatic adenocarcinoma. **B:** Portal venous phase axial image (same level, same technique) demonstrates suboptimal venous filling with still perceptible narrowing of the portal vein confluence (*arrow*). **C:** portal venous phase image slightly inferior to B demonstrates barely perceptible sliver of the nearly occluded SMV (*arrow*). **D:** Portal venous phase image more inferiorly shows slightly dilated middle colic vein and multiple anterior mesenteric collaterals due to near occlusion of the more superior SMV. **E:** Angled sagittal volume rendered image through the mesenteric/splenic confluence demonstrates obstruction of the superior aspect of the SMV, despite poor contrast dynamics. (*continued*)

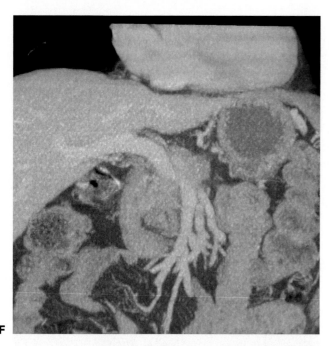
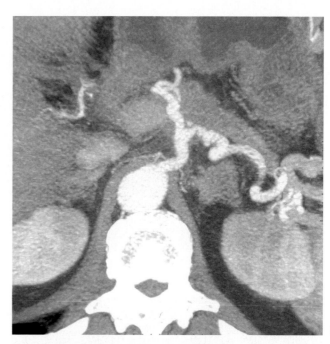

F   G

Figure 15-18 (*continued*) **F:** Angled coronal volume rendered image through the mesenteric/splenic confluence demonstrates obstruction of the superior aspect of the SMV. **G:** Axial maximum intensity projection image demonstrates arterial encasement of the celiac axis by the nonresectable tumor.

pancreas and is separated from it by the parietal peritoneum and the lesser sac, a potential intraperitoneal space. The transverse mesocolon, which forms the inferior boundary of lesser sac, is formed by the fusion of the parietal peritoneal leaves as they fuse and extend anteriorly from the ventral surface of the pancreas along its entire length. The significance of this anatomic relationship between the transverse colon and the pancreas via the transverse mesocolon becomes important in acute pancreatitis because this peritoneal communication serves as a pathway for the flow of inflammatory exudates associated with pancreatitis.

When retroperitoneal perivisceral fat is abundant, the pancreas will be well defined. However, even in lean patients, the pancreas can be accurately delineated by the use of ample quantities of water or high density oral contrast material to negatively or positively opacify the lumen of contiguous loops of bowel, and IV contrast material to delineate the intra- and peripancreatic vascular structures.

Developmental Variants and Anomalies

Pancreas divisum, the most common anatomic variant of the human pancreas, is defined as a completely separate pancreatic ductal system in a grossly undivided gland. It results from failure of fusion of the dorsal and ventral pancreatic ducts, which normally occurs in the second month in utero. The main portion of the pancreas, including the anterior part of the head, body, and tail, is drained by the dor-

sal pancreatic duct through the accessory papilla (Fig. 15-19). The posterior inferior part of the head and uncinate process are drained by the short, narrow, ventral pancreatic duct that joins the common bile duct in the ampulla. In autopsy series, pancreas divisum has an incidence of 5% to 10%. As an ERCP finding, the incidence is up to 4% (230,234). In a series of patients with pancreatitis, however, there was a 16% incidence of pancreas divisum, and the incidence of the abnormality increased to 25% in idiopathic pancreatitis (68). In a large ERCP series of 1,741 patients, 94 (5.5%) patients were discovered to have pancreas divisum; in those patients, pancreatitis was found in 54 (57%), with the majority of changes affecting the dorsal pancreatic duct (230). Therefore, it appears as though pancreas divisum is associated with pancreatitis.

The diagnosis of pancreas divisum can be suggested with high-detail CT and MRI when an isolated ventral duct is identified or when separate dorsal and ventral pancreatic moieties can be defined. With MRCP, pancreas divisum is routinely imaged (Fig. 15-20) (31,57,190). Although the overall size of the pancreas may be normal in this developmental variant, the craniocaudal extent or anteroposterior (AP) thickness of the pancreatic head may be increased. Additionally, the ventral and dorsal moieties may be distinctly visible, separated by fat plane (373).

Annular pancreas, a rare developmental anomaly with only three cases reported among 20,000 autopsies (149,273) may be suggested on CT by apparent thickening of the anterior, lateral, and posterior aspect of the descending duode-

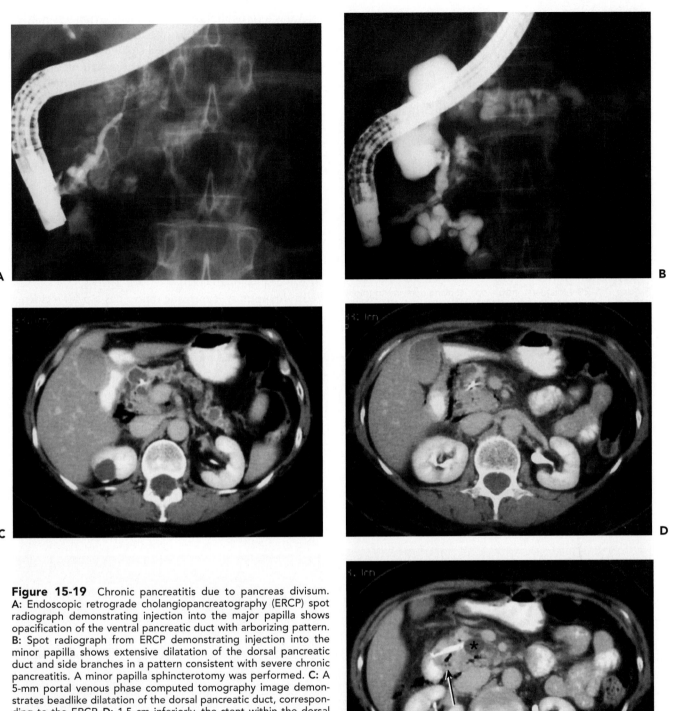

Figure 15-19 Chronic pancreatitis due to pancreas divisum. **A:** Endoscopic retrograde cholangiopancreatography (ERCP) spot radiograph demonstrating injection into the major papilla shows opacification of the ventral pancreatic duct with arborizing pattern. **B:** Spot radiograph from ERCP demonstrating injection into the minor papilla shows extensive dilatation of the dorsal pancreatic duct and side branches in a pattern consistent with severe chronic pancreatitis. A minor papilla sphincterotomy was performed. **C:** A 5-mm portal venous phase computed tomography image demonstrates beadlike dilatation of the dorsal pancreatic duct, corresponding to the ERCP. **D:** 1.5 cm inferiorly, the stent within the dorsal duct is seen in cross section, along with a small amount of retroperitoneal gas from limited perforation during the minor papilla sphincterotomy. Note the more normal appearance of ventral pancreatic parenchyma. **E:** Next caudal image shows path of minor papilla stent into the duodenum, anterior to the nondilated distal common bile duct (*arrow*). A dilated side branch of the dorsal ductal system (∗) is also apparent.

num caused by tissue having a density and enhancement characteristics identical to that of the pancreatic parenchyma (Fig. 15-21) (6,142,149). The diagnosis of annular pancreas on CT will be reinforced by typical changes on an upper gastrointestinal (GI) radiogram and confirmed by successful

demonstration of the portion of the pancreatic duct system within the annular component by ERCP or MRCP.

Agenesis of the dorsal pancreatic moiety has been reported (304). In this developmental anomaly, only the head of the pancreas is visible on CT. No pancreatic parenchyma can be

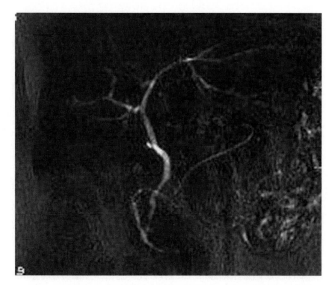

Figure 15-20 Magnetic resonance cholangiopancreatography (MRCP) pancreas divisum. A 5-cm slab half-Fourier acquisition single-shot turbo spin echo (HASTE) angled coronal image demonstrates the dorsal pancreatic duct (Santorini) extending to the medial duodenal wall through the minor papilla, superior to the exit of the distal common bile duct through the major papilla.

identified in the expected location of the neck, body, and tail. In contrast to pancreas divisum, dorsal pancreas agenesis is an extremely rare anomaly. Because most of the islet cells are located in the tail of the pancreas, the absence of the body and tail may contribute to the development of diabetes. Most of the reported cases of complete agenesis of the dorsal pancreas were in patients with diabetes mellitus (356).

Aplasia or hypoplasia of the uncinate process may be present in patients with intestinal nonrotation. In a small series, CT demonstrated a small or absent uncinate process in patients with intestinal nonrotation; in four of five patients, mesenteric inversion (superior mesenteric vein located to left of superior mesenteric artery) was also depicted (143).

Pathologic Conditions

Neoplasia

Adenocarcinoma

Cancer of the pancreas is currently the ninth most common malignancy but represents the fourth most common cause of cancer-related death (235,236,359). The National Cancer Institute has projected 31,860 new cases and 31,270 deaths for 2004 (8).

In this country, pancreatic cancer has a peak incidence in the seventh and eighth decades. Adenocarcinoma accounts for between 90% to 95% of all primary pancreatic malignant neoplasms (Table 15-5). With respect to risk factors, there is evidence to indicate an increased risk of pancreatic cancer associated with diabetes and cigarette smoking, but the relationship to alcohol intake and to chronic pancreatitis is less clear (50,100,113,194).

The signs and symptoms of pancreatic cancer are varied and nonspecific. Other diseases may cause features identical to those experienced by patients with pancreatic cancer. Weight loss and pain are common features for patients with pancreatic cancer, whether the tumor is located in the head, body, or tail. One distinguishing sign is the presence

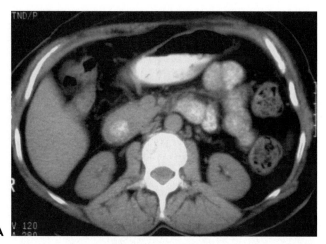
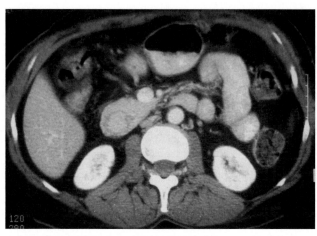

Figure 15-21 Annular pancreas in a 52-year-old woman with computed tomography (CT) for renal disease. **A:** A 10-mm CT image obtained after oral and before intravenous (IV) contrast demonstrates high-density contrast within the stomach and duodenum. Homogeneous soft tissue encircling the right lateral margin of the duodenum is the same attenuation as the pancreatic head, which lies medial to the duodenum. **B:** Same level after IV contrast administration, 5-mm portal venous phase CT image, demonstrates similar enhancement of the soft tissue surrounding the duodenum, indicating annular pancreas.

TABLE 15-5
PANCREATIC TUMOR CLASSIFICATION

I. Epithelial neoplasms
  A. Exocrine tumors
    1. Duct cell origin
      a. Adenocarcinoma
      b. Adenocarcinoma variants
        (1) Mucinous adenocarcinoma
        (2) Pleomorphic large cell carcinoma
        (3) Undifferentiated anaplastic carcinoma
        (4) Signet ring cell carcinoma
        (5) Adenosquamous carcinoma
        (6) Mixed ductal endocrine carcinoma
      c. Microcystic adenoma
      d. Mucinous cystic tumor
      e. Intraductal papillary mucinous tumor
    2. Acinar cell origin
    3. Uncertain histogenic origin
  B. Endocrine tumors
    1. Insulinoma
    2. Gastrinoma
    3. Glucagonoma
    4. VIPoma
    5. Somatostatinoma
    6. Polypeptidoma
    7. Carcinoid tumor
    8. Pheochromocytoma
    9. Small cell carcinoma
    10. Nonfunctioning tumor
II. Nonepithelial neoplasms
  A. Sarcoma
  B. Lymphoma
  C. Metastases

Reproduced from Demos TC, Posniak HV, Harmath C, et al. Cystic lesions of the pancreas. *AJR Am J Roentgenol* 2002;179:1375–1388, with permission.

of jaundice. Jaundice will be present in more than 80% of patients with a tumor in the head, whereas it is most un-usual in patients with body and tail neoplasms.

The majority (60% to 65%) of pancreatic carcinomas occur in the head, whereas approximately 20% and 10% occur in the body and tail, respectively. Between 5% and 10% affect the pancreas diffusely (67,104). Because of the pancreatic head's intimate involvement with the common bile duct and duodenum, tumors that arise there tend to present clinically at an earlier stage than those that occur in the body or tail. Consequently, tumors in the pancreatic head tend to be smaller at the time of discovery. On rare occasions, very large tumors arising in the head may be present without causing jaundice.

Five-year survival rates for pancreatic adenocarcinoma are as low as 2% to 3% (236). In patients with tumors less than 2 cm, improved survival rates up to 30% at 5 years have been observed (234,339). Therefore, if helical CT tech-niques are to affect survival it is necessary to accurately de-tect and stage these smaller cancers (Fig. 15-22). Because pancreatic cancer tends to be disseminated at the time of diagnosis in the majority of patients, the role of CT is to

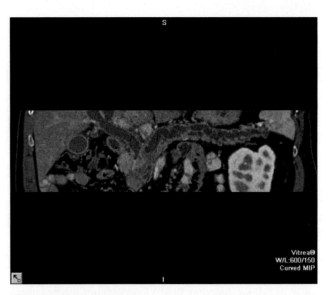

Figure 15-22 Resectable moderately differentiated pancreatic adenocarcinoma of the pancreatic head. Curved planar reformat-ted image shows very small tumor in line with the ductal struc-tures. Patient was successfully resected and is alive 4 years later with a single hepatic metastasis.

exclude those patients with distant metastases (Fig. 15-23) or local invasion (Fig. 15-24) from potential unnecessary laparotomies for surgical resection.

Most studies continue to support the view that CT should be the initial diagnostic procedure in any patient suspected of having a pancreatic neoplasm. The landmark report of the Radiology Diagnostic Oncology Group (RDOG), in which the relative values of CT versus MR imaging of pancreatic adeno-carcinoma were compared, concluded that CT is recom-mended for initial imaging assessment. (214). Although

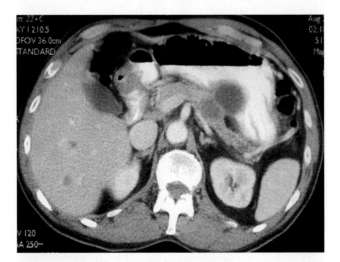

Figure 15-23 Small pancreatic adenocarcinoma with liver metas-tases in a 60-year-old man with abdominal pain. Contrast-enhanced portal venous phase image through the body of the pancreas demonstrates a 2.5-cm low-attenuation lesion expanding the pan-creas body, immediately adjacent to the splenic vein. Upstream pan-creatic duct dilatation is present in the tail. There is no dilatation of the duct in the neck and head. An adjacent 3-cm well-circumscribed pseudocyst is seen anterior to the mass. Also noted are two 1-cm liver lesions in the right hepatic lobe, indicating inoperability.

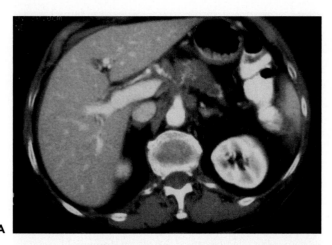
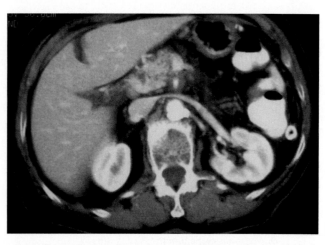

Figure 15-24 Nonresectable pancreatic adenocarcinoma with arterial encasement. **A:** Portal venous phase 7-mm computed tomography image demonstrates hypovascular mass extending superiorly from the pancreatic neck and body, producing classic encasement of the celiac axis and its branches. **B:** At 1.5 cm inferiorly, a cuff of neoplastic soft tissue is seen also surrounding the superior mesenteric artery in a pattern typical of neurovascular tracking of pancreatic adenocarcinoma.

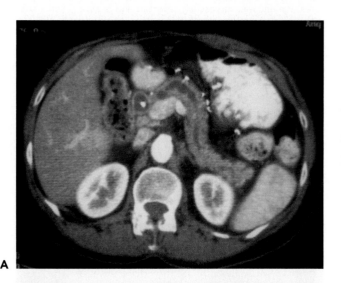
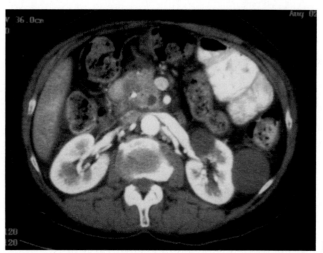
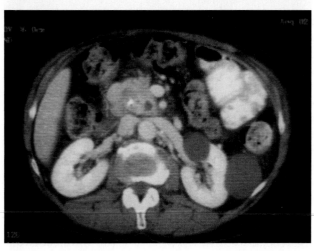

Figure 15-25 Computed tomography (CT) double duct sign with focal mass in a 63-year-old woman with jaundice and abdominal pain. **A:** Pancreatic parenchymal phase 3.75-mm CT image demonstrates dilatation of the main pancreatic duct in the neck, body, and tail. Common bile duct is also dilated and contains a biliary stent. **B:** Pancreatic parenchymal phase 3.75-mm CT image through the pancreatic head reveals a focal 2.0-cm hypoattenuating mass at the point of termination of the biliary ductal dilatation, surrounding the stent, consistent with a small adenocarcinoma. **C:** Portal venous phase 3.75-mm CT image through the same level as B reveals diminished but persistent conspicuity of the mass, which was resectable.

ultrasound (US) is widely used as an initial abdominal screening procedure, it has not been found to be as sensitive as CT in defining the entire constellation of important findings related to pancreatic malignancies including local nodal spread or involvement of the major arterial and venous structures. The relative merits and roles of endoscopic ultrasound (EUS) and MRI relating to evaluation of pancreatic pathology also continue to evolve.

Helical Computed Tomography Detection of Pancreatic Adenocarcinoma. Since the time of the RDOG study (214), CT imaging of pancreatic disease has changed dramatically with the advent of multidetector helical technique. The advantage of MDCT technique relates to its capacity for thin section volumetric imaging, performed in a single breathhold at a time of optimal pancreatic enhancement following IV contrast administration (46,49). Image reconstruction is possible with the volumetrically acquired data, allowing multiplanar viewing (46). This is particularly helpful for evaluation of the ductal structures (48) and vasculature. The two most important goals when performing CT for evaluation of pancreatic adenocarcinoma are detection of the tumor and assessment of resectability (46). Sensitivity for lesion detection is high, ranging from 93% to 100% (46,114,196,212). CT has a positive predictive value for tumor detection of greater than 90%. CT is excellent for determining nonresectability, with a positive predictive value approaching 100%. However, it is not as accurate in depicting resectable tumor. The negative predictive value is only 56% with uniphasic imaging and 79% with dual phase (212).

The CT appearance of pancreatic adenocarcinoma is variable. If IV contrast medium is not administered, the attenuation value of tumor generally is very similar to that of normal parenchyma, unless extensive necrosis or cystic change is present. Without IV contrast, tumors may be recognized only when they become large and alter the contour of the gland. When IV contrast medium is used, most adenocarcinomas will be hypoenhancing with respect to the surrounding uninvolved pancreatic parenchyma. If contrast dynamics are suboptimal, advanced tumors may often still be detected and diagnosed as nonresectable (158), but this is not necessarily true for small lesions. With good contrast dynamics, even small tumors that do not produce a contour alteration of the gland will be detectable as a focal area of diminished enhancement. The conspicuity of the tumor depends on the CT technique. Because most pancreatic tumors are hypovascular, they should exhibit greatest conspicuity when displayed in a maximally enhanced pancreas (49). However, performing helical CT during arterial injection of contrast medium does not improve detection over IV contrast techniques (109). Varying conclusions of recent reports reflect the dependence of tumor conspicuity on technique. Lu (196) first described that the tumor to pancreas contrast was greater in the pancreatic parenchymal phase (67 ± 19 Hounsfield units) compared with a true arterial phase

(39 ± 16 Hounsfield units) due to greater normal pancreatic parenchymal and less tumor enhancement at that particular circulatory time (Figs. 15-3, 15-5, and 15-25). This represents an average of 70% improvement in tumor to pancreas contrast. Although Diehl (85) concluded that the arterial phase produced improved tumor conspicuity over the portal venous phase, the arterial phase in that particular study began 36 seconds after initiation of contrast and likely resembled a pancreatic parenchymal phase. Imbriaco (141) found no difference in the detection and determination of resectability comparing arterial phase to a caudocranial portal venous phase beginning with a 50-second scan delay. Graf (114) showed that arterial phase images were inferior to portal venous phase images for tumor detection. Tumor to pancreas conspicuity was 31 ± 29 Hounsfield units in true arterial phase, and 54 ± 31 Hounsfield units in portal venous phase. Although tumor enhancement was significantly higher in portal venous phase, the difference between tumor and pancreatic enhancement was greater. Keogan (165) found no statistically significant difference in tumor attenuation subjectively between true arterial and portal venous phase images and concluded that the acquisition of arterial phase images does not result in improved detection of pancreatic malignancies. Using multidetector CT techniques, McNulty detected 27 of 28 adenocarcinomas and found that tumor to pancreas Hounsfield unit differences were significantly greater with pancreatic parenchymal phase and portal venous phase compared with arterial phase, but there was no significant difference in tumor conspicuity between the portal venous phase and pancreatic parenchymal phase. It is likely that the pancreatic parenchymal phase of prior SDCT studies (Lu and Boland) overlapped with the pancreatic parenchymal phase and early portal venous phase in McNulty's MDCT study.

Dynamic gadolinium-enhanced MRI of the pancreas using breathhold T1-weighted fat suppressed GRE techniques demonstrates similar lesion detection rates compared with CT (Fig. 15-26) (139,243,306,323). With combined thick slab MRCP, breathhold IV gadolinium enhanced MRA, and breathhold T1-weighted GRE dynamic postgadolinium imaging, Hanninen et al. (127) reported a 95% sensitivity for lesion detection, with an overall accuracy of 91%. In a recent comparison of SDCT and MRI using phased array torso coil and mangofodipir trisodium (formerly Mn-DPDP) as the IV contrast agent, tumor detection sensitivity in 26 cases was 100% for MRI and 94% (two small missed cancers) for CT (294). Because it is taken up by normal pancreatic parenchyma, manganese-based contrast agents may be better than gadolinium chelates in delineating pancreatic tumors (84,274,282,294). Diffusion-weighted MRI and MR spectroscopy of the pancreas may prove useful in cancer detection or aid in determining response to novel therapies in patients with pancreatic cancer.

The data pertaining to EUS detection of pancreatic masses and prediction of resectability has been variable.

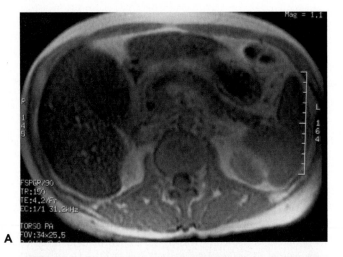

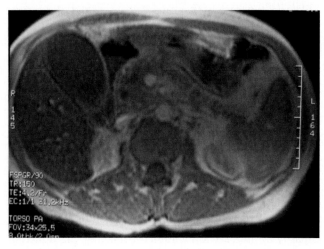

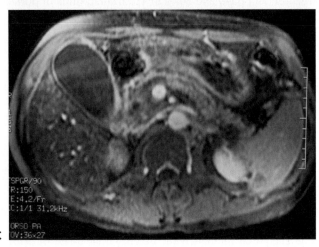

Figure 15-26   Pancreatic adenocarcinoma demonstrated by gadolinium enhanced T1-weighted fat suppressed fast spoiled gradient (FSPGR) breathhold magnetic resonance imaging (MRI). **A:** Precontrast T1-weighted FSPGR breathhold MR image through the pancreas demonstrates normal appearance of the gland without a focal mass evident. **B:** Initial FSPGR post intravenous (IV) gadolinium axial image demonstrates no differential enhancement, the lack of conspicuity exacerbated by lack of fat suppression. **C:** Dynamic post IV gadolinium pancreatic phase fat-suppressed T1-weighted FSPGR axial image through the pancreas shows normally enhancing pancreatic body and tail and heterogeneously hypoenhancing lower signal within the pancreatic head, surrounding but not narrowing the superior mesenteric vein. Note the better depiction of slightly dilated main pancreatic duct compared to A, and that the subtle difference in enhancement may be the only indication of tumor.

After initial reports indicating very high accuracies for EUS T stage (93% regardless of size) and resectability (93%), and resultant claims of supremacy over incremental and early SDCT (115), most studies now indicate that EUS is more sensitive than helical CT in detection of smaller (<2 cm) lesions in the pancreatic head and that CT is better for determining resectability (157,221,355). Because most patients undergo CT as the initial imaging study for the evaluation of potential pancreatic abnormalities, concerns regarding bias and inadequate blinding on comparisons of EUS and CT have been raised and investigated (215,284). In one study comparing single detector arterial and portal venous phase CT to EUS, using surgery as the gold standard, differences in tumor detection were found only for tumors smaller than 1.5 cm diameter, but this difference was not statistically significant (Fig. 15-27). Sensitivity for both techniques was 100% when tumors were between 15 and 35 mm and larger than 35 mm. EUS produced two false positives, whereas dual-phase CT found no false positives. When combined, EUS plus CT gave 100% accuracy for detection (184).

In addition to detecting a focal mass, several other signs on CT may indicate the presence of a neoplasm. First, because with aging the pancreas may become heterogeneous in its attenuation value due to diffuse fatty infiltration, a focal region of homogenous soft tissue density within such a gland (see Fig. 15-4) should be viewed with suspicion (352). Second, the presence of both a dilated common bile duct and dilated main pancreatic duct in the absence of an obstructing calculus suggests an ampullary or pancreatic head neoplasm (Figs. 15-25 and 15-28). This finding may also be seen in benign disease (180). Third, the finding of a dilated main pancreatic duct in the body and tail but not in the head or neck also sug-

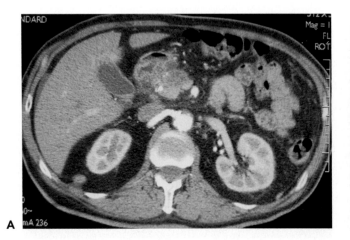

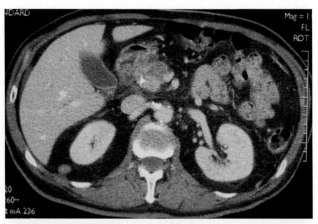

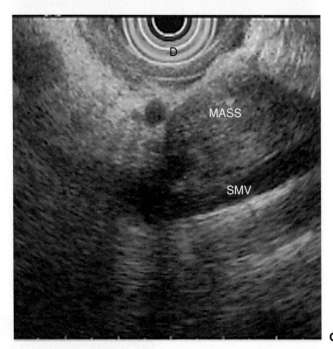

Figure 15-27 Nonresectable pancreatic adenocarcinoma due to SMV better seen on portal phase in a 74-year-old man with pain. **A:** Pancreatic parenchymal phase 3-mm computed tomography (CT) image through the superior pancreatic head demonstrates a heterogeneously enhancing hypovascular mass within the anterior portion of the pancreas at this level. The SMA appears uninvolved. The SMV is not opacified sufficiently to determine potential invasion. **B:** Portal venous phase CT image same level demonstrates 180 degrees abutment and transverse narrowing of the SMV, consistent with involvement. **C:** Coronal endoscopic ultrasound (EUS) image demonstrates heterogeneous, hypoechoic mass adjacent to and narrowing the superior SMV, with indistinct vessel wall. D, duodenal lumen; SMV, superior mesenteric vein; mass, pancreatic adenocarcinoma. (EUS image courtesy of Mohammed Eloubeidi, MD.)

gests the presence of a neoplasm (see Fig. 15-23). With MDCT, Prokesh et al. (266) reported that approximately 10% of patients had isoattenuating pancreatic lesions, best depicted with CPRs (Fig. 15-29) demonstrating focal interruption of the main pancreatic duct, dilated pancreatic and/or biliary ducts, atrophic distal pancreas, or convex contour abnormality. In this subset of patients, mean Hounsfield unit differences between pathologically proven isoattenuating tumors and remaining pancreas was 9.25 ± 11.3 Hounsfield units during the pancreatic phase and 4.15 ± 4.5 Hounsfield units during the portal venous phase. These secondary signs may be helpful in evaluating small tumors as well.

A carcinoma in the head or distal body of the pancreas may produce changes in the more proximal body and tail. In a patient without a history of pancreatitis, a dilated pancreatic duct implies the presence of a distal obstructing neoplasm. In addition to pancreatic duct dilation, typical changes of acute pancreatitis, cyst due to duct obstruction (Figs. 15-23 and 15-30) and atrophy may be demonstrated on CT when malignant obstruction is present. A dilated pancreatic duct is a sensitive indicator of pancreatic disease but is not specific for carcinoma; it may be seen in pancreatitis or duodenal inflammatory disease. (40,193,362). Smooth dilatation of the duct favors malignant obstruction, whereas irregular or beaded dilatation favors chronic

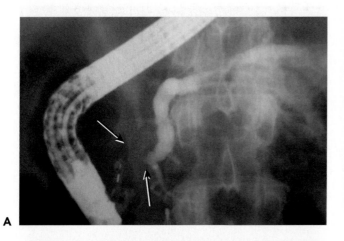

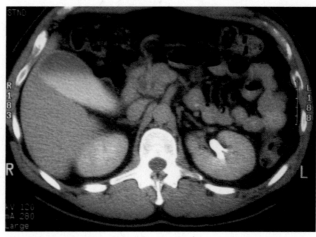

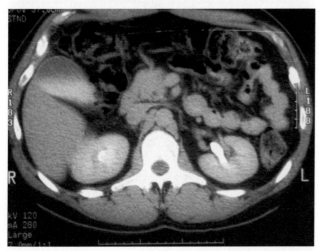

Figure 15-28 Double duct without identifiable mass (poor dynamics) in a 41-year-old man with jaundice and abdominal pain. **A:** Endoscopic retrograde cholangiopancreatography (ERCP) spot radiograph demonstrates moderate dilatation of biliary and pancreatic ducts down to adjacent focal, irregular strictures near the ampulla (*arrows*), suspicious for pancreatic neoplasm. **B:** Excretory phase 7-mm computed tomography (CT) images through the pancreatic head demonstrates dilatation of both ducts, corresponding to the double duct sign. **C:** Immediately inferior excretory phase 7-mm CT image through the point of termination of the dilated ducts reveals no mass. Because of the suspicious ERCP findings and positive ERCP brushings, the patient underwent operation, revealing adenocarcinoma.

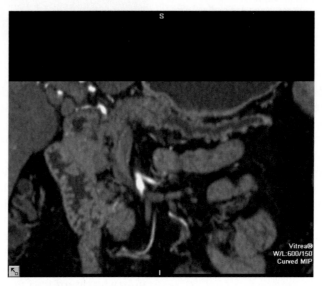

Figure 15-29 Isoattenuating, non-contour-altering pancreatic tumor. Curved planar reformation demonstrates focal obstruction of the main pancreatic duct in the midbody region, due to the tiny mass, a moderately well differentiated adenocarcinoma. The patient underwent successful resection with distal pancreatectomy.

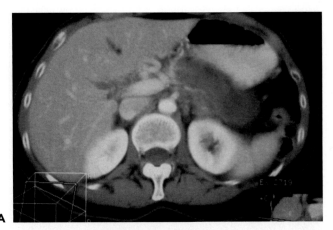
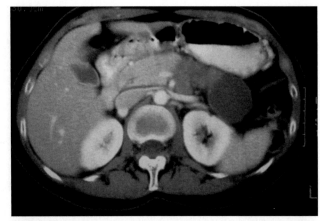

Figure 15-30 Pancreatic inflammation produced by carcinoma involving the body region. **A:** Angled axial computed tomography (CT) image reconstructed from pancreatic parenchymal phase demonstrates 4 × 2 cm low attenuation mass in the pancreatic neck and body producing encasement of the celiac axis and its branches. Focal pseudocyst is present extending from the tail, due to ductal obstruction by the tumor. **B:** Standard axial 7-mm pancreatic parenchymal phase CT image shows sharp demarcation between the mass and normal enhancement of the pancreatic head region.

pancreatitis (Fig. 15-31). In addition, when the ratio of pancreatic duct diameter to pancreatic gland width is greater than 0.5, the presence of carcinoma is favored (Fig. 15-32). In one study, carcinoma was present approximately 90% of the time when this ratio exceeded 0.5 (162). The contour of duct termination can help in distinguishing malignant from inflammatory obstruction. Abrupt termination of either the main pancreatic duct or distal common bile duct favors the presence of neoplasm (Fig. 15-33). In a series of patients with isoattenuating tumors, the interrupted duct is a critical secondary sign. Using MDCT with CPRs aligned with the pancreatic duct, the entire length of the dilated pancreatic duct may be seen on one image, making identification of the interrupted duct sign easier to identify (266). In one large series, gradual smooth tapering of the distal bile duct was present in 80% of patients with benign disease (Fig. 15-34) and in none of the patients with malignant disease in the pancreatic head (32).

That portion of the pancreas which is proximal to an obstructing cancer may show similar secondary changes on MRI including increased fluid content, changes of acute or chronic pancreatitis, duct dilatation, and atrophy. MRCP may aid in detection of tumors by demonstrating the level of duct obstruction and help direct gadolinium enhanced T1-weighted GRE images for mass detection. Using widely available thick-slab breath-hold techniques of half Fourier acquisition single-shot turbo spin echo (HASTE) with fat saturation, the ductal structures are well seen, but the surrounding soft tissues are not. In a series of

32 patients with malignant biliary obstruction, a technique using single shot fast spin echo (SSFSE) images with intermediate TE and no fat saturation enabled visualization of the level as well as the cause of obstruction in a single breathhold (297). The contour and scope of duct dilation may aid in diagnosis. With MRCP, visualization of dilated side branches along with the main pancreatic duct was more often seen in patients with pancreatic adenocarcinoma compared with other periampullary neoplasms (169).

Positron emission tomography (PET) is a useful and sensitive technique in identifying a variety of neoplasms. For pancreatic cancer, sensitivity and specificity range from 85% to 100% and 67% to 88%, respectively (76,134,375). Unfortunately, chronic pancreatitis is a cause of false-positive findings on PET (166,328). In a series of 39 patients suspected with pancreatic carcinoma based on CT and ERCP, PET was positive in 22 of 24 patients with proven adenocarcinoma, including four of five patients with indeterminate CT findings. This series also found three false negatives, and the authors concluded that PET was particularly useful in cases in which the CT findings were equivocal but clinical suspicion was strong (166). Authors of a recent review of PET and CT in evaluating pancreatic tumors concluded that cross-sectional imaging with either CT or MRI provides anatomic information regarding local tumor invasion and surgical resectability that cannot be gained from PET. However, when the metabolic information of PET is combined with the structural resolution of CT, a re-

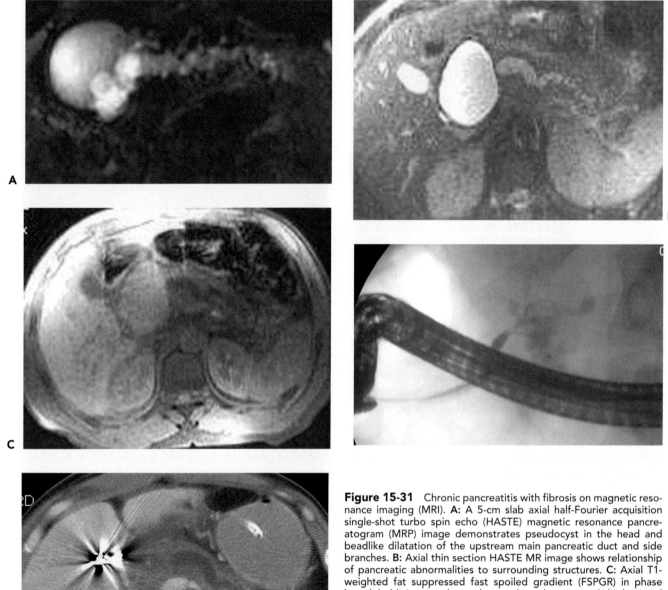

Figure 15-31 Chronic pancreatitis with fibrosis on magnetic resonance imaging (MRI). **A:** A 5-cm slab axial half-Fourier acquisition single-shot turbo spin echo (HASTE) magnetic resonance pancreatogram (MRP) image demonstrates pseudocyst in the head and beadlike dilatation of the upstream main pancreatic duct and side branches. **B:** Axial thin section HASTE MR image shows relationship of pancreatic abnormalities to surrounding structures. **C:** Axial T1-weighted fat suppressed fast spoiled gradient (FSPGR) in phase breath-hold image shows low rather than normal high signal throughout the pancreatic parenchyma, consistent with fibrosis seen in chronic pancreatitis. **D:** Endoscopic retrograde cholangiopancreatography spot radiograph showing obstruction of the pancreatic duct in the head, without visualization of the pseudocyst or upstream duct better depicted on MRP. **E:** After pseudocyst drainage and cholecystectomy, patient returned three months later for abdominal pain evaluation. A 5-mm portal venous phase computed tomography image shows diffuse low attenuation in the parenchyma, and ductal dilatation with a ratio of less than 0.5 gland width, similar to the MRI and consistent with chronic pancreatitis.

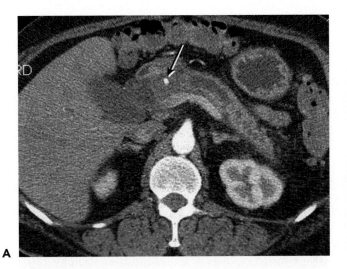

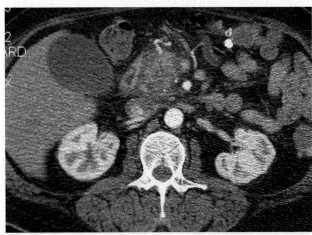

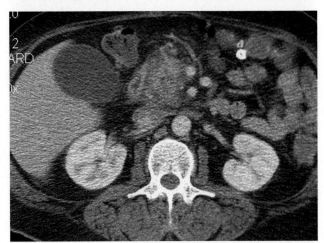

Figure 15-32 Pancreatic ductal width greater than 0.5 width of gland. **A:** A 3-mm pancreatic parenchymal phase computed tomography (CT) image demonstrates dilation of the main pancreatic duct to greater than 0.5 the width of the gland through the body level. There is abrupt termination of the pancreatic duct into a large hypoattenuating mass in the head, surrounding the gastroduodenal artery (*arrow*) and abutting the portal confluence. **B:** A 3-mm pancreatic parenchymal phase CT image inferiorly shows hypovascular mass abutting the superior mesenteric artery. The vein is not evident, but at this phase is not yet filled. **C:** A 5-mm portal venous phase CT image through same level as B demonstrates lack of visualization of the superior mesenteric vein indicating occlusion and nonresectability.

liable method of differentiating recurrent or residual tumor from inflammatory or scar tissue, detecting unsuspected metastases and evaluating pancreatic masses with equivocal CT findings results (159) (Table 15-6).

Although a focal mass is the primary CT finding of pancreatic adenocarcinoma, not all masses are neoplastic; pancreatitis can present as a focal mass (Fig. 15-35) (32,155,162,171,275,363). Differentiating between carcinoma and inflammatory disease occasionally can be difficult because the pancreas may be diffusely enlarged by an extensive cystic and necrotic tumor or a carcinoma- induced pancreatitis. Less extensive focal pancreatitis may also mimic small pancreatic adenocarcinomas on CT (171,294,332) and MRI (127,155,294), even with state of the art techniques; this is problematic given the extensive surgery required for attempted cure of pancreatic neoplasm. The abundant fibrosis in both pathologic conditions likely accounts for their similar imaging appearance (155,332). Newer US techniques including pulse inversion harmonic imaging after IV Levovist (microbubble) enhancement has

been proposed as a means of differentiating between neoplastic and inflammatory pancreatic masses (177,252). Although now commercially available, the use of this technology is not widespread in the United States. Some signs previously depended on to elucidate the difference between inflammatory masses and neoplasm have been challenged. For example, Baker (20) and Schulte (296) demonstrated that acute and chronic inflammatory processes may result in infiltration of the fat surrounding the superior mesenteric artery, whereas in the past this finding was reserved solely for pancreatic carcinoma. With CT, secondary signs of pancreatic carcinoma when present permit the distinction to be made. These include hepatic, peritoneal, and lymph node metastases; contiguous organ invasion; and vascular encasement (22,32,275,363). It is also these features which determine potential for surgical resection, or resectability, on CT.

Resectability of Pancreatic Tumors

Adenocarcinoma of the pancreas is the tumor most likely to be spread beyond the organ of origin at diagno-

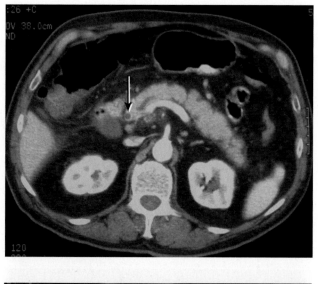

A

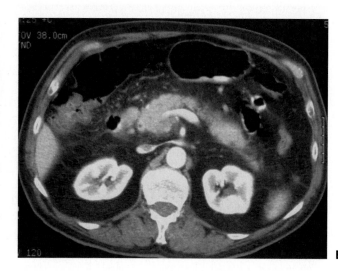

B

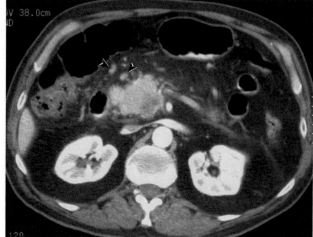

C

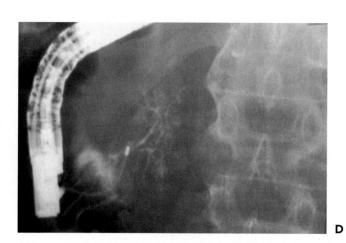

D

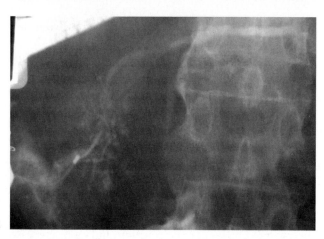

E

Figure 15-33 Pancreatic adenocarcinoma producing abrupt duct termination, also with superior mesenteric vein thrombosis/occlusion in a 68-year-old without jaundice. **A:** Contrast-enhanced portal-venous phase 5-mm image through the pancreatic neck demonstrates mild dilatation of the main pancreatic duct to 5 mm. Note the normal caliber bile duct (*arrow*). **B:** Next caudal portal-venous phase image demonstrates termination of the pancreatic duct dilatation by a heterogeneous, low-attenuation mass measuring 4.2 × 4.0 cm replacing the pancreatic head. Note absence of enhancement in the expected location of the superior mesenteric vein, which normally lies just to the right of the superior mesenteric artery, and enlarged peripancreatic lymph nodes (*arrowheads*). **D, E:** Two spot radiographs from same patient's ERCP reveals pseudodivisum. In **D**, filling of branching structures in the pancreatic head is present without dorsal duct opacification; however, with further injection (**E**), filling of the slightly dilated dorsal portion of the main pancreatic duct is noted. There is an irregular stricture within the superior pancreatic head produced by the tumor, which was not resectable because of venous invasion.

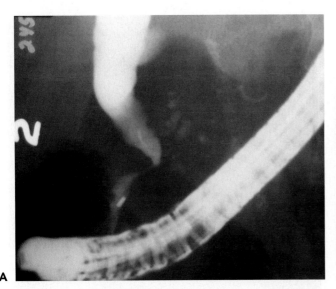
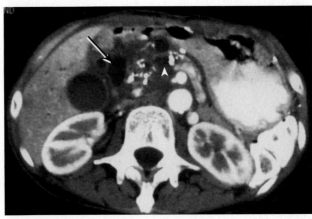

A   B

Figure 15-34   Chronic pancreatitis with tapered distal common bile duct stricture. **A:** Spot radiograph during endoscopic retrograde cholangiopancreatography (ERCP) injection demonstrates conical narrowing of the distal common bile duct through the pancreatic head. Numerous calcifications are noted to the left of the duct, within the pancreatic parenchyma. **B:** Axial 5-mm pancreatic parenchymal phase image through the pancreatic head demonstrates dilatation of the tapering common bile duct (*arrow*), dilation of the pancreatic duct (*arrowhead*), diffuse low attenuation within the parenchyma, and several large calcifications, consistent with chronic pancreatitis. On successively more caudal computed tomography images, there was smooth concentric narrowing as the bile duct approached the ampulla, similar to the ERCP appearance, which helps to differentiate inflammatory from neoplastic strictures.

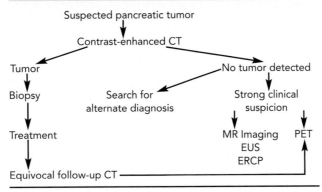

TABLE 15-6
PANCREATIC PROTON EMISSION TOMOGRAPHY ALGORITHM

CT, computed tomography; ERCP, endoscopic retrograde cholangiopancreatography; EUS, endoscopic ultrasound; MR, magnetic resonance; PET, positron emission tomography.

Reproduced from Kalra MK, Maher MM, Boland GW, et al. Correlation of positron emission tomography and CT in evaluating pancreatic tumors: technical and clinical implications. *AJR Am J Roentgenol* 2003;181:387–393, with permission.

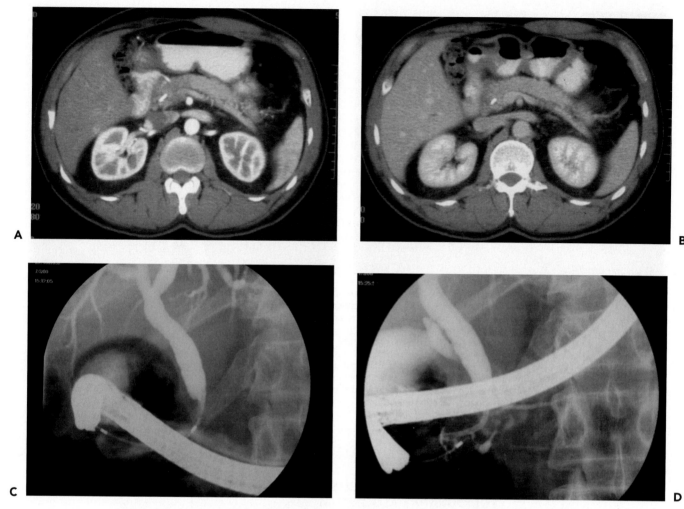

Figure 15-35   Chronic pancreatitis mimicking pancreatic adenocarcinoma. **A:** Pancreatic parenchymal phase 5-mm computed tomography (CT) image demonstrates differential enhancement of the head of the pancreas compared to the body and tail, with the hypoattenuating area surrounding the stent within the distal common bile duct. **B:** Portal venous phase 5-mm CT image same level demonstrates decreased conspicuity of the mass in the pancreatic head. **C:** Endoscopic retrograde cholangiopancreatography (ERCP) spot radiograph demonstrates eccentric shelf like narrowing of the distal 1.5 cm of bile duct, corresponding to the site of abnormal enhancement on the CT. **D:** ERCP spot radiograph during pancreatic duct injection reveals irregularity of the distal most main pancreatic duct near the ampulla. Because of the combined findings, the patient underwent Whipple resection, with focal chronic pancreatitis diagnosed histologically. No tumor was present.

sis (Fig. 15-36) (158). The most common sites of metastases, in order of decreasing frequency, are liver, regional lymph nodes, other retroperitoneal and intraperitoneal structures (Fig. 15-37), and lungs. The only chance for cure in the small number of patients without obvious spread is surgical resection, most commonly a Whipple procedure or Whipple variant. These procedures carry up to a 25% mortality rate (Fig. 15-38), decreasing to 5% in experienced hands (158).

Evidence of the distant tumor metastases, particularly liver metastases, and detection of local or peripancreatic spread of tumor including invasion of critical vascular structures determines potential for resectability (46). Positive predictive values for nonresectability have been excellent with helical CT, ranging between 89% and 100% (43,104, 195,212,214). Although helical CT is highly specific for the determination of nonresectability when it enables identification of tumor extension into the adjacent peripancreatic structures, the accuracy for predicting resectability is between 70% and 80%, in part because of its lower specificity (43,85,212). In other words, a substantial number of patients identified by CT as potentially resectable have been found to have inoperable tumor at laparotomy (Fig. 15-39) (197). CT has a relatively poor performance in the detection of small peritoneal implants and small hepatic surface and parenchymal metastases (85,342). Lymph node metastases in normal size nodes are another source for inaccuracy in predicting resectability (43,85,212,279). Sensitivity for vas-

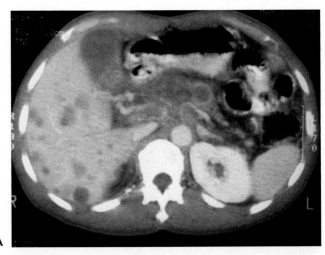
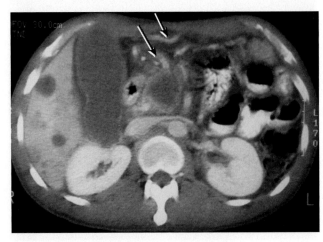

A   B

Figure 15-36 Widely metastatic inoperable pancreatic adenocarcinoma in a 51-year-old man with cachexia and abdominal pain. **A:** Portal venous phase 7-mm computed tomography (CT) image through the superior pancreas demonstrates a 5 × 7 cm heterogeneously enhancing hypovascular mass producing encasement of the celiac axis as well as occlusion of the main portal vein. Numerous low-attenuation hepatic metastases are present. **B:** Portal venous phase 7-mm CT image 3 cm inferiorly demonstrates necrotic, low-attenuation tumor in pancreatic head. Large venous collaterals can be seen anteriorly (*arrows*), due to the obstruction of the superior mesenteric vein at this level and portal confluence more superiorly.

cular invasion with helical CT (detection of unresectable disease) is 50% to 70% (43,214). The accuracy of CT in staging small pancreatic adenocarcinomas is 70%, due to the inability to stage locally invasive disease (43). According to Lu (195), much of the problem has been the difficulty in detecting more subtle, yet real, invasion of the peripancreatic vessels because of the inherent small size of the vessels relative to slice width (5 to 10 mm).

Opacification of arteries is best on arterial phase or pancreatic parenchymal phase and veins on portal venous phase images (114,165,315). The smaller peripancreatic arteries traditionally evaluated with conventional angiography for assessment of resectability are seen well with helical SDCT arterial phase techniques (64). This is also true with multidetector techniques (212), which also lend themselves to better multiplanar and 3-D reconstructions

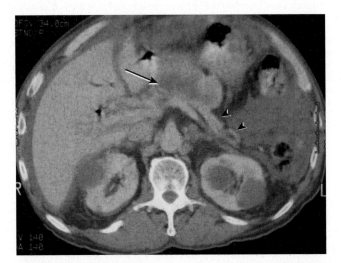

Figure 15-37 Pancreatic adenocarcinoma with peritoneal carcinomatosis. Contrast-enhanced 5-mm computed tomography image demonstrates lobular, centrally necrotic 7- × 3-cm mass (*arrow*) extending anteriorly from the pancreatic neck and body region and pancreatic tail atrophy (*arrowheads*). Soft tissue density within the greater omentum, ascites, and nodular thickening of the peritoneum are present, consistent with peritoneal carcinomatosis due to pancreatic adenocarcinoma.

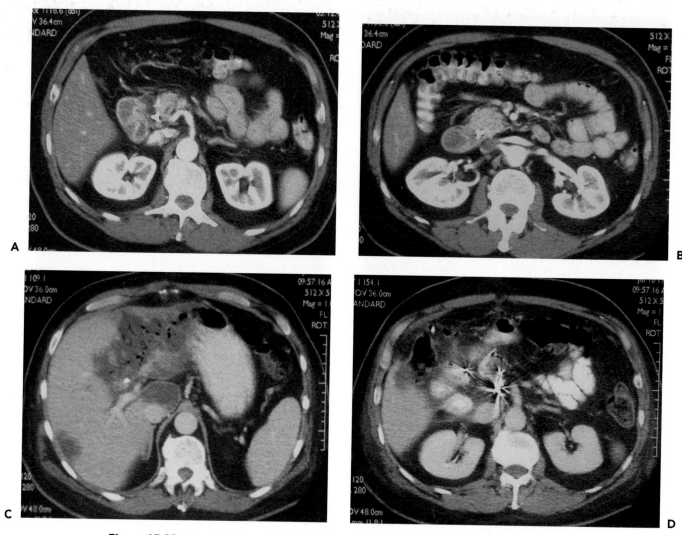

Figure 15-38 Hepatic infarction after Whipple resection. **A:** Preoperative pancreatic phase 5-mm image through the superior pancreatic head region demonstrates minimal dilatation of the main pancreatic duct, biliary stent in place, and replaced hepatic artery to the superior mesenteric artery. **B:** Subtle decreased attenuation in the anterior aspect of the inferior pancreatic head adjacent to the biliary stent is consistent with 2.7-cm pancreatic adenocarcinoma. There is a clean fat plane separating the lesion and the mesenteric artery and vein. **C:** Contrast-enhanced portal venous phase computed tomography (CT) through the level of the porta 48 hours after pylorus sparing Whipple procedure demonstrates low attenuation within the caudate and majority of left hepatic lobe. Intraparenchymal gas is also seen, as well as focal infarct involving the peripheral right hepatic lobe. Proximal end of a biliary stent (hepaticojejunostomy stent) is seen. **D:** Portal venous phase CT image at level of superior mesenteric artery origin demonstrates clips near the replaced common hepatic artery takeoff.

(Figs. 15-18, 15-30, and 15-40). Although several authors concluded that critical venous structures were best seen on the pancreatic parenchymal phase rather than the portal venous phase (46,195,346), because of the relatively slower z-axis transit of the SDCT techniques in these earlier studies, it is likely that the mesenteric veins were actually imaged in the early portal phase (60 to 70 seconds).

Encasement of 100% of an adjacent vessel has long been known to indicate nonresectable tumor (195). Using SDCT, Lu et al. (196) set out to determine the criteria for nonresectability of major splanchnic vessels, grading the celiac axis, hepatic artery, superior mesenteric artery (SMA), portal vein, and SMV on a scale of 1 to 4 for vessel involvement by tumor. Grade 1 equals tumor contiguous to less than 25% vessel circumference, grade 2 equals tumor contiguous to 25% to 50% vessel circumference, grade 3 equals tumor contiguous to 50% to 75% vessel circumference, and grade 4 equals more than 75% tumor contiguous to vessel circumference or any vasoconstriction. Cut off between grade 2, representing a resectable lesion, and grade 3, representing an unresectable lesion, yielded the lowest number of false negatives and acceptable false positives, with sensitivity and specificity for unresectability reaching 84% and 98%, and positive predictive value and negative predictive value reaching 95% and 93%. As a general rule, involvement of any vessel by tumor exceeding 50%, or 180 degrees of the

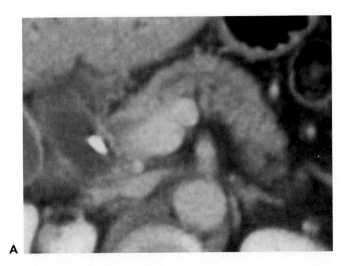

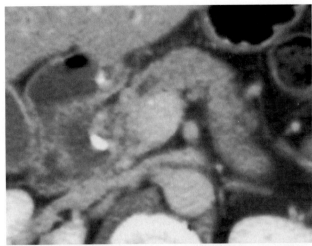

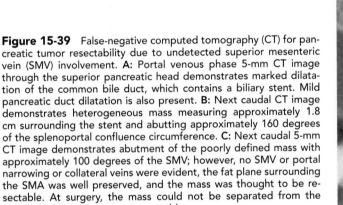

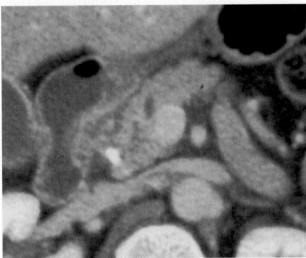

Figure 15-39 False-negative computed tomography (CT) for pancreatic tumor resectability due to undetected superior mesenteric vein (SMV) involvement. **A:** Portal venous phase 5-mm CT image through the superior pancreatic head demonstrates marked dilatation of the common bile duct, which contains a biliary stent. Mild pancreatic duct dilatation is also present. **B:** Next caudal CT image demonstrates heterogeneous mass measuring approximately 1.8 cm surrounding the stent and abutting approximately 160 degrees of the splenoportal confluence circumference. **C:** Next caudal 5-mm CT image demonstrates abutment of the poorly defined mass with approximately 100 degrees of the SMV; however, no SMV or portal narrowing or collateral veins were evident, the fat plane surrounding the SMA was well preserved, and the mass was thought to be resectable. At surgery, the mass could not be separated from the SMV, and the patient was unresectable.

circumference is highly specific for unresectable tumor. This is especially true of the arteries (Fig. 15-41). Parameters for unresectable venous involvement are more variable. In some studies, alteration of vein lumen shape (see Figs. 15-27 and 15-40), obliteration of the vein (see Figs. 15-18 and 15-41), and thrombosis, rather than contiguity of more than 50% circumference, are required before the tumor is deemed unresectable (342). There is more room for false positives in predicting significant venous involvement because some surgeons more aggressively resect and graft the superior mesenteric vein (Fig. 15-42) and portal confluence in an attempt to cure the patient.

In attempts to better define significant venous involvement (which would preclude successful resection), several authors have studied the smaller peripancreatic veins (173,346). The anterior- and posterior-superior pancreaticoduodenal veins and gastrocolic trunk are routinely imaged in normal individuals. In patients with pancreatic cancer involving the larger splanchnic veins, dilation of these smaller veins may indicate nonresectability. In a study of 30 patients with pancreatic cancer, only 1 of 11 patients with dilation of the superior peripancreatic veins was resectable (346). However, the size threshold for dila-

tion is not well established. On the contrary, the inferior pancreaticoduodenal veins are generally not seen in normal individuals, even with the latest thin section MDCT techniques. Visualization of the anterior or posterior inferior pancreaticoduodenal veins in patients with pancreatic cancer indicates a high likelihood of central splanchnic vein involvement (see Fig. 15-41) (368). Compromise of the lumen of the SMV or portal vein may have effects further downstream within the liver due to the homeostatic relationship between portal venous and hepatic arterial flow. Sheiman et al. (305) described increased hepatic enhancement in the arterial phase and lower enhancement in the portal venous phase in pancreatic cancer patients with greater than 120 degrees circumference contiguity or flattening of the SMV, compared with normals and pancreatic cancer patients without venous luminal narrowing.

Using CTA techniques in the assessment of vascular invasion has great potential; however, early reports using SDCT techniques found greater intra- and interobserver variability in interpreting these reformatted images, suggesting that interpretation along with the helical images is mandatory (18,85). However, axial images are not optimal for visualizing the course of peripancreatic arteries that run perpendicu-

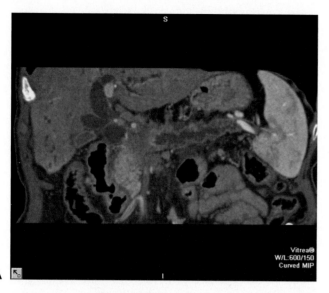
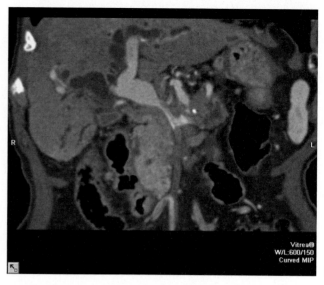

Figure 15-40 Unresectable pancreatic adenocarcinoma of the neck. **A:** Curved planar reformation aligned with the main pancreatic duct demonstrates the hypovascular mass at the point of duct obstruction in the neck region. **B:** Curved planar reformation aligned with the superior mesenteric vein/portal confluence shows circumferential venous encasement in this nonresectable patient.

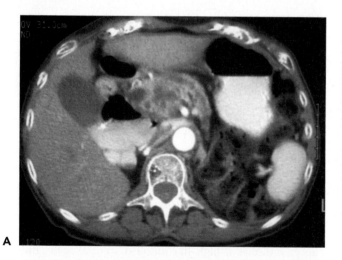
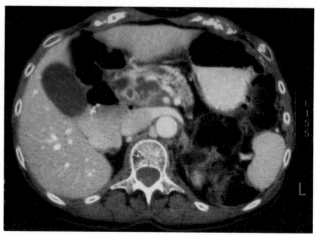

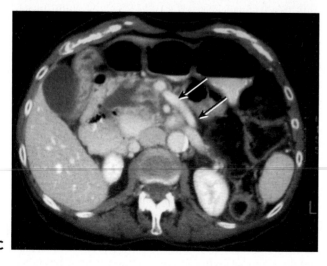

Figure 15-41 Nonresectable pancreatic adenocarcinoma due to arterial encasement in an 81-year-old woman with 36 pound weight loss over 2 years and left abdominal pain. **A:** Pancreatic phase 5-mm computed tomography (CT) demonstrates a heterogeneous, partially necrotic 5-cm mass in the superior pancreatic head, with main pancreatic duct dilatation and atrophy of the body and tail. The left margin of the mass abuts approximately 90 degrees of the superior mesenteric artery. The superior mesenteric vein is not visible. **B:** Portal venous phase 5-mm CT image through the same level demonstrates the heterogeneity of the infiltrating mass, with more apparent near circumferential encasement of the superior mesenteric artery. The superior mesenteric vein is absent, and more inferiorly on **C**, a dilated collateral vessel, likely representing first jejunal branch, is present (*arrows*).

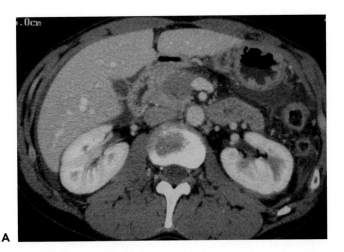

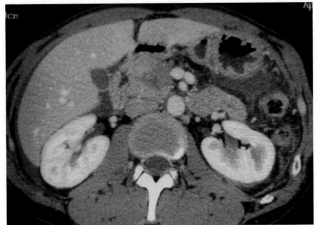

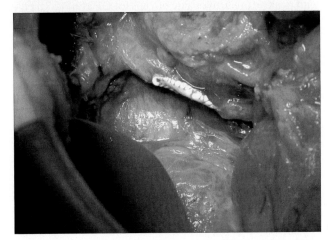

Figure 15-42 Vein graft for limited superior mesenteric vein (SMV) involvement. **A:** A 2.5-mm portal venous phase computed tomography (CT) image demonstrates a hypovascular 2-cm mass within the medial pancreatic head abutting the SMV over 150 degrees. **B:** Next caudal image shows decreasing contact with the SMV and no venous collaterals; the tumor was thought to be resectable by CT. **C:** Photograph obtained during surgery reveals successful graft repairing defect where SMV was focally invaded. (Surgical photograph courtesy of Martin J. Heslin, MD.)

lar to the imaging plane (136). The ideal type and angle of reformation display depends on the vessel being evaluated. MIP provides a global perspective in cases of vessel occlusion and collateralization. Volume-rendered techniques are particularly helpful in the abdomen (97). One potential advantage to volume-rendered display is the detection of vessel narrowing and invasion, rather than depicting simply the effect of tumor surrounding a vessel (136). Optimal display of the portal vein is coronal oblique with settings optimized to view soft tissue mass effect. Tumor involvement will appear as circumferential encasement and narrowing of the vessel, focal invasion, or complete occlusion (136) (see Fig. 15-40).

The object of sophisticated vascular display techniques is improved accuracy in resectability. Raptopoulos (270) found that CTA was more accurate than review of axial images alone for evaluation of peripancreatic arteries, with negative predictive value of 96% when CTA interpretation was added to interpretation of transverse images, compared with 70% for interpretation of transverse images alone. On the other hand, Lepanto et al. (186) found that CTA significantly increases the ability to detect venous invasion compared with axial images alone, but arterial invasion accuracy was not improved. With MDCT, the number of sections through the pancreas is increased by a factor of 2 or 3 compared with the number acquired in the best SDCT exam. With its increased

data sampling and higher resolution MDCT may prove better than SDCT for defining key vascular structures even if only axial images are reviewed. In a recent study using MDCT techniques, there was no difference in accuracy for tumor detection and assessment of resectability between interpretations of 3-D curved planar reformatted images (created by trained technologists specializing in 3-D reformations) alone compared with transverse images alone (266). The authors surmised that, although radiologists would tend to interpret from transverse images, CPRs were most helpful for concise presentation to referring clinicians. No matter which method is used to evaluate the peripancreatic vessels in efforts to determine resectability, one must remember that the lower spatial resolution in the z-axis may produce indistinct vessel margins that should not be interpreted as tumor ingrowth. In addition, the presence of soft tissue in contact with a vein wall may be due to tumor desmoplastic inflammatory reaction (371) leading to false-positive interpretations of nonresectability. Subtle venous abnormalities should not preclude surgery, so as to not disallow surgery for potentially curable patients.

The initial report of the RDOG found that dynamic CT was better than non-breathhold MRI for assessment of resectability (214). However, newer breathhold MRI using a phased array body coil with MR angiography (MRA) techniques may provide an accurate noninvasive screen for non-resectability (110,111,139). With two-dimensional (2-D) time of flight techniques evaluating portal venous involvement, McFarland et al. (210) correctly identified 11 of 11 resectable and 5 of 9 nonresectable patients with pancreatic cancer. However, the significant number of false negatives indicates that unnecessary laparotomies in cases of nonresectable lesions would not be eliminated. Timing the gadolinium-enhanced breathhold fast multiplanar spoiled gradient recalled echo (FMPSPGR) T1 sequences to correspond to the pancreatic parenchymal phase may also help to better evaluate the peripancreatic vessels (161). Using a definition of vascular involvement greater than 180 degrees indicating nonresectability, MRI may be more accurate than CT for predicting resectability (positive predictive value of 86.5%, compared with positive predictive value of 76% for CT) (306). The use of a phased array torso coil is mandatory when performing MRA in the assessment of resectability (317).

Identification of small hepatic metastases may be improved with newer MRI techniques, but this remains to be proven. For example, more small hepatic metastases were detected with mangofodipir trisodium as the MR contrast agent compared with biphasic SDCT in a recent prospective comparison. Although the numbers in this series were too small to achieve statistical significance, the nonresectability sensitivity of 90% with this MR technique compared favorably to the sensitivity of 80% with SDCT (294). Because manganese-based MR contrast agents are taken up by the pancreatic parenchyma, vascular staging is not improved by their use (294).

The role of EUS in patients with pancreatic cancer is to detect small tumors not identified on dual-phase helical CT in the setting of a strong clinical suspicion for cancer. Difficulties in staging with EUS have been encountered, with recent reviews suggesting that resectability should be determined with CT (157,221,284,355). One study comparing tumor staging with EUS to single detector arterial and portal venous phase CT found that overall accuracy for EUS was 90%, (one overstaged and one understaged), and for CT was 86% (one overstaged, two understaged). Although EUS detected 86% of lymph nodes compared with 77% for CT, EUS missed liver metastases in three patients. All had T3 lesions that are unresectable in any case (184). Conventional transabdominal sonography may detect vascular involvement by tumors (12), but EUS is markedly better (374). The contribution of laparoscopy and laparoscopic US to information gained from preoperative imaging may improve evaluation of resectability prior to formal Whipple attempts and alter management in a significant number of patients (126).

Because of the pancreas' rich vascular supply and lack of a fibrous capsule, metastasis to regional lymph nodes tends to occur early. Involvement of peripancreatic nodes (Figs. 15-33 and 15-43) will not preclude surgical resection in most cases but may have an impact on survival (279). Not uncommonly, enlarged contiguous peripancreatic lymph nodes may be indistinguishable from the substance of the pancreas itself and appear as a large pancreatic mass. This could result in upstaging in the TMN classification. Nonmalignant lymph node enlargement can occur in patients with pancreatitis, recent biliary stent placement, or unrelated conditions such as active hepatitis, resulting in overstaging of tumors. In one study comparing dual arterial and portal venous phase CT to EUS, lymph node staging was correct in 86% of 30 patients with EUS and in 77% with CT. CT understaged in three patients and overstaged in two using short axis size greater than or equal to 1 cm as the sole criterion for metastatic involvement (184). Although one recent study reported an overall accuracy of 73% for

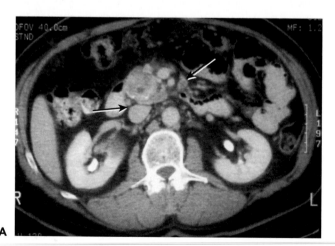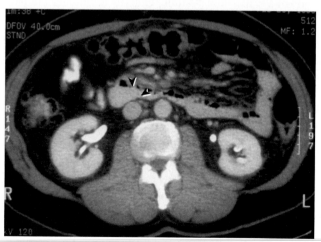

A   **B**

Figure 15-43 Resectable pancreatic adenocarcinoma in a 57-year-old man with abdominal pain, history of chronic pancreatitis, and remote history of pancreatic tail resection for pseudocyst. **A:** Excretory phase 5-mm computed tomography (CT) image through the inferior pancreatic head demonstrates a heterogeneously enhancing hypodense round 3-cm mass. Although several low attenuation peripancreatic lymph nodes are present (*arrow*), there was no CT evidence of vascular involvement or distant metastases. **B:** 1.5 cm more caudal image demonstrates the mass eroding into the third portion of the duodenum, and regional node. Note calcifications (*arrowheads*) within the pancreatic parenchyma, due to chronic pancreatitis.

MDCT staging of lymph nodes in patients with pancreatic adenocarcinoma, if short axis diameter of greater than 1 cm is considered the sole criterion for positivity, sensitivity was only 14% (279). Many histologically positive nodes may be smaller than 1 cm (279). In fact, although histologic analysis may be negative for pancreatic adenocarcinoma, identification of mutant K-ras oncogene has been reported in surgically resected lymph nodes (79). Architectural features described as helpful in EUS studies (253), such as ovoid shape, clustering, and absence of fatty hilum, may not be helpful on CT evaluation. If a patient is considered otherwise resectable, depiction of peripancreatic nodes should not prevent attempted resection (279).

The use of adjuvant chemotherapy and chemoradiation after resection has been investigated in several large trials, with some protocols showing a survival benefit with chemoradiation (258,320) and others with chemotherapy alone (238) even in the presence of microscopic margin involvement by tumor (239). Others have not discovered survival advantage compared with surgical resection alone (327) and believe that adjuvant therapy should be used judiciously because its benefit is confined to only a fraction of patients (65). The survival benefit (median survival time) of adjuvant chemotherapy or radiochemotherapy has been demonstrated to be 6 to 10 months (37). Likewise, the benefit of neoadjuvant chemoradiation prior to surgical excision in patients with pancreatic carcinoma is under investigation but has thus far shown limited success, with conversion from locally aggressive nonresectable tumor to resectable lesion ranging from 3% to 13% (9,91,168), and as yet there are no firm conclusions regarding survival benefits (37,168). Serial CT performed during preoperative chemotherapy or chemoradiotherapy is used to assess response, both locally (Fig. 15-44) and for metastatic disease;

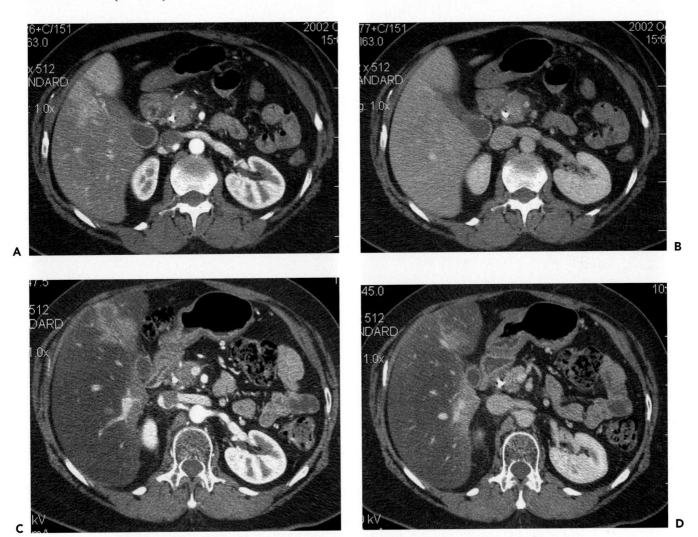

Figure 15-44 Locally aggressive pancreatic adenocarcinoma converted to resectable after neoadjuvant chemoradiation. **A:** Pancreatic parenchymal phase computed tomography (CT) image shows a poorly defined hypoattenuating mass surrounding the stent in the distal common bile duct. **B:** Portal venous phase CT image same level demonstrates the mass surrounding nearly the entire superior mesenteric vein (SMV) circumference, with narrowing of the lumen. **C:** Six months later after chemoradiation, the mass is no longer measurable on pancreatic phase CT image. **D:** Portal venous phase image same study date shows contact of normally enhancing tissue with 180 degrees of the SMV, now normal in caliber. Note worsening of fatty infiltration of the liver compared to **B.**

CT technique for preoperative reassessment should be dual phase (see Tables 15-1 and 15-2) (Fig. 15-45).

When it is not possible to distinguish between malignant disease and focal inflammation, follow up studies should be performed to confirm that resolution occurs. In equivocal, nonresolving, or indeterminate cases in which strong suspicion for neoplasm precludes follow-up imaging as an option, percutaneous biopsy, EUS-guided biopsy, or ERCP-directed brushings may aid in diagnosis. Percutaneous biopsy of the pancreas is safe and effective, with CT success rates of 50% to 94% (77,93), and US success rates of 67% to 97% (56,123,124) reported in the literature. In a large retrospective review of percutaneous imaging–guided (CT and US) pancreatic biopsies in 211 patients, a combined accuracy of 93% for diagnosis of malignancy was found. In this study, there were 33 false–negative find-

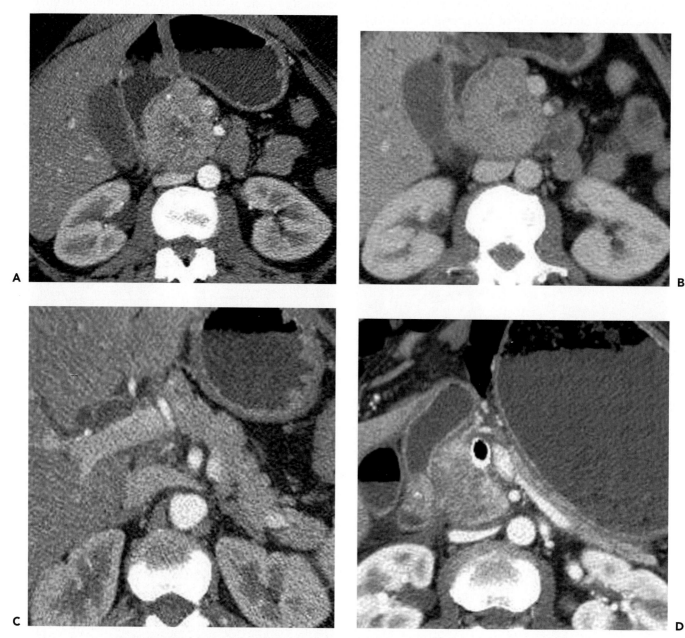

Figure 15-45   Postchemoradiation changes of the pancreas in patient with neuroendocrine tumor of the head with vascular invasion. **A:** Axial pancreatic parenchymal phase image through the head of pancreas demonstrates a large, heterogeneously enhancing mass with probable superior mesenteric vein (SMV) involvement and superior mesenteric artery abutment. **B:** Axial portal venous phase image through same level demonstrates better filling of the SMV, which appears slightly flattened at this level and was clearly narrowed more superiorly. **C:** Axial pancreatic parenchymal phase image through main portion of the gland reveals little upstream pancreatic duct dilation or glandular atrophy present at the time of diagnosis. **D:** Following chemoradiation, the mass in the head may be slightly smaller, but there is continued involvement of the SMV. Marked glandular atrophy has developed in the 3-month interval during chemoradiation trial.

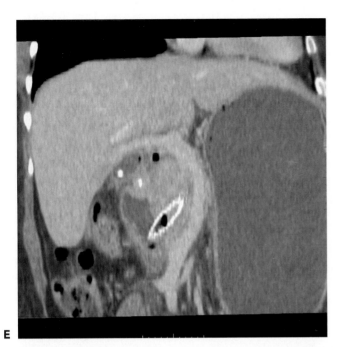

E

Figure 15-45 (continued) E: Volume-rendered angled coronal image following chemoradiation demonstrates persistent narrowing and irregularity of SMV involved by tumor. A metallic stent is seen in the distal common bile duct.

ings in 269 biopsy procedures for a negative biopsy rate of 12%; in 31 patients with initially negative biopsy results, repeat biopsy resulted in diagnosis in half (54). EUS-guided fine needle aspirate (EUSFNA) biopsy of the pancreas or peripancreatic lymph nodes is safe and reliable in early and advanced pancreatic cancer, with sensitivities ranging from 82% to 93% (272,308,355), specificity of 100% (308,355), and complication rate of 2% to 7% (116,135,272). As with CT- or US-guided techniques, negative or nondiagnostic cases require further workup with repeat biopsy by EUS or CT in cases in which clinical or radiographic findings do not correlate with fine needle aspiration (FNA) results (308). Recently, a study of quantitative mutant K-ras oncogene combined with standard cytology in EUSFNA specimens showed improved sensitivities up to 88% compared with cytology alone (62%). More important, the same study showed absent or low level mutant K-ras oncogenes despite suspicious cytology in patients with benign chronic pancreatitis mass lesions (330).

Other potentially useful aids for distinguishing between neoplastic and inflammatory disease are recently developed tumor markers including the monoclonal antibodies CA-19-9 and CA-125 (254). In the detection of pancreatic cancer, both had approximately the same sensitivity, about 75%, somewhat better than carcinoembryonic antigen (CEA) which ranges from 25% to 62% (277). However, CA-19-9 may be positive in the presence of other GI neoplasms and has a false–positive rate of 11% in patients with pancreatitis and 2% of normals. The summary of the National Cancer Institute Tumor Marker Conference concluded that serum tumor markers might be useful in con-

firming a diagnosis of pancreatic cancer and might be helpful in distinguishing between benign and malignant disease. However, the lack of tumor specificity and pancreas organ specificity makes these unreliable when used by themselves (219). This is an active area of research because of the need to diagnose pancreatic adenocarcinomas at a size that has a significant impact on survival rates (53). Ultimately tumor markers may be a promising approach for early detection.

At this time, MDCT helical technique with dual (pancreatic parenchymal and portal venous) phase images probably represents the most widely available and best first test for patients suspected of having pancreatic adenocarcinoma. If the tumor is found to be unresectable, the imaging workup is stopped, and clinical decisions regarding palliative treatment can be made. With the larger number of images generated per examination using MDCT, workstation rather than film interpretation of reconstructed images will become the norm. If optimal CT technique fails to demonstrate a mass, but pancreatic neoplasm is suspected, EUS with guided biopsy may be beneficial in detecting and further characterizing small lesions not seen on CT. MRI may also help to further define the mass and especially provide additional information regarding liver metastases if small indeterminate lesions are detected in that region on CT. If a strong clinical suspicion or indeterminate workup persists, PET scanning with positive findings may also be of benefit in continuing the workup, possibly with serum tumor markers for confirmation.

Cystic Pancreatic Neoplasms

The most common cystic lesion of the pancreas is a pseudocyst. When the diagnosis of pancreatitis is confidently excluded, cystic neoplasms must be considered. Traditionally, cystic neoplasms have been classified as serous or mucinous cystadenomas or cystadenocarcinomas; newer nomenclature is addressed in specific sections to follow. Occasionally, pancreatic neuroendocrine tumors or adenocarcinomas may appear cystic due to tumor necrosis. In addition, with the increasing use of water as oral contrast for CT, duodenal diverticula may also mimic cystic neoplasms (200). The natural history of incidentally discovered pancreatic cysts has recently been described. With improved spatial resolution of CT these small cystic lesions are being found with increasing frequency. When under 2 cm, observation of simple pancreatic cysts may be a safe management option, because morbidity and mortality of these cysts is very unlikely (125). A recent review of these lesions by the cooperative pancreatic cyst study has been reported (59).

Mucinous Carcinoma

Mucinous (colloid) carcinoma is an uncommon variant of typical pancreatic adenocarcinoma. This neoplasm produces a large volume of mucin that results in a cystic appearance on imaging studies (3,353), and may lead to inspissated mucin obstructing the pancreatic or bile ducts. Pseudomyxoma peritonei and tumoral calcifications have been reported in association with this tumor, which shares the same poor prognosis as typical pancreatic adenocarcinoma (80).

Intraductal Papillary Mucinous Tumor. IPMT of the pancreas is the unifying name for mucin-producing pancreatic neoplasms that arise from the ducts. These tumors have previously been referred to as mucinous ductal ectasia, ductectatic tumor, ductectatic cystadenoma or cystadeno carcinoma, mucin-secreting tumor, mucinous villous adenomatosis, and intraductal papillary neoplasm (35,118). IPMT have low, but definite, potential for malignancy, grow slowly, and rarely metastasize or recur, with overall 5-year survival rate approximating 60% (2). They are usually discovered in men (2:1 male-to-female ratio) between the ages of 60 and 80 years and produce nonspecific symptoms of epigastric pain, occasionally accompanied by diabetes, weight loss, and palpable mass when large. Histologically, dysplastic tall mucin-producing columnar cells lining the pancreatic ducts proliferate and form papillary projections that protrude into the lumen of an expanded duct (313). Mucin plugs may produce main or branch ductal obstruction that mimics chronic pancreatitis when extensive. IPMT of the pancreas are divided into two types: those affecting the main pancreatic duct and those arising within a side branch. Symptoms, potential for malignancy, prognosis, and imaging features vary according to the subtype of tumor. Ohhashi (249) first described the endoscopic features of this lesion in 1982, and Itai (148) described the findings on CT shortly thereafter.

On CT, side branch type IPMT typically appears as a cystic mass 1.0 to 6.0 cm diameter, located within the uncinate portion or head of the pancreas (Fig. 15-46). The cyst may appear unilocular or as a grapelike cluster of small cysts (107,118,145). Irregularity of the wall, mural nodules, or papillary excrescences suggest malignancy (145,251,329). Thin section helical CT may reveal multiple tubes and arcs within the lesion, representing the dilated side branch lumen and walls cut obliquely (118). Even with side branch type tumors, the main pancreatic duct may be dilated due to mucin production (Fig. 15-47) (118,192,263). As with main duct type tumors, a bulging papilla and dilated duct (>10 mm) are more common with malignant lesions. (107). Larger size may also suggest malignancy, with lesions greater than 3 cm more often being malignant (145). Communication of the cystic lesion with the main pancreatic duct may be demonstrated on SDCT in 70% of patients (107). The communication of the mass to the main duct is particularly well depicted on thin section coronal MRCP source images (251). Koito (176) found that detection of cystic dilated branches was significantly better with MRCP than with ERCP and that MRCP allowed simultaneous visualization of the main pancreatic duct and cystic side branch lesion.

Main pancreatic duct IPMT produces diffuse dilation of the main pancreatic duct, often with atrophy of the gland to

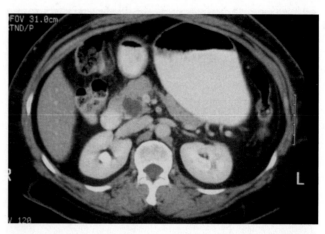

Figure 15-46 Side branch intraductal papillary mucinous tumor (IPMT) of uncinate in a 52-year-old asymptomatic woman. Portal venous phase 5-mm computed tomography image demonstrates a 2.0-cm, partially septated low attenuation mass within the uncinate process that is typical of small side branch IPMT. Note absence of main pancreatic duct dilation.

a thin rim of tissue surrounding the duct (118) (see Fig. 15-16). Occasionally, dysmorphic calcifications may be present within the duct (313). On CT, these features may mimic chronic pancreatitis, and this is an important differential diagnosis to consider, because abdominal pain and diabetes may also be present in both kinds of patients (35) (Fig. 15-48). In general, patients with main duct IPMT present at a later age than patients with chronic pancreatitis (35). Unlike typical chronic pancreatitis patients, patients with IPMT have mucin distending the distal duct, which on CT often results in an enlarged, bulging papilla projecting into the duodenal lumen (313). Formerly, ERCP with visualization of abundant mucin exiting the papilla was considered the gold standard for diagnosing IPMT (192). However, MRI with MRCP is now recognized as superior to ERCP because of its ability to reveal the full extent of ductal involvement, oftentimes prevented on ERCP when mucin obstructs the main pancreatic duct or side branches (176,313). In addition to MRCP, standard T1- and T2-weighted images can be used to look for evidence of local spread. Imaging features that suggest malignancy include a duct diameter greater than 15 mm and the presence of large filling defects within the dilated duct (145,313). Irie et al. (145) found with MRCP that in patients with main duct type tumors, greater mean duct dilation (20 mm compared with 11 mm), diffuse rather than segmental main pancreatic duct expansion, and intraductal filling defects were associated with malignancy. The absence of nodules does not ensure benignancy however (145). Although main duct type tumors are more likely than side branch type to be malignant, the presence and degree of invasion cannot be reliably determined with CT or MRI (313) or on clinical grounds. Because they are all considered premalignant, resection is the rule for main duct type IMPT (35). A recent study of 49 patients with IPMT using EUS and intraductal sonography showed a high accuracy rate in determining in-

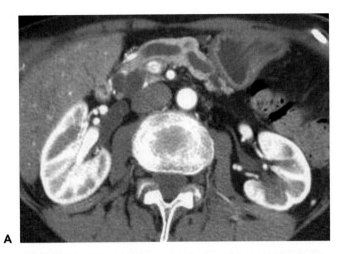

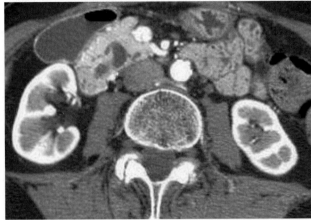

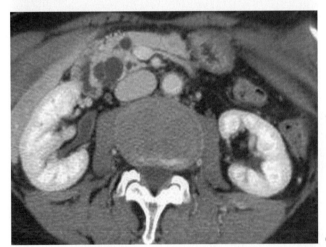

Figure 15-47 Side branch intraductal papillary mucinous tumor (IPMT) in a 77-year-old woman with abdominal pain. **A:** Contrast-enhanced portal venous phase image through the pancreatic body demonstrates dilatation of the main pancreatic duct. No intraductal calculi are evident. **B:** Portal venous phase image through the pancreatic head demonstrates connection of dilated side branch cystic lesion to the main pancreatic duct. **C:** A 2.4-cm cystic mass in the posterior aspect of the pancreatic head is consistent with the side branch tumor, proven at surgery. Histologically, the tumor did not extend into the main duct, which was dilated due to increased mucin production.

vasive IPMT from noninvasive lesions, reporting a sensitivity of 55%, specificity of 97%, and accuracy of 88% (369); however, intraductal sonography is not widely available.

Mucinous Cystic Neoplasm. This cystic pancreatic lesion has been previously known as macrocystic adenoma, mucinous cystadenoma or cystadenocarcinoma, and mucin hypersecreting carcinoma (118). As with IPMT, the mucinous cystic neoplasm cavity is filled with mucinous material and may have papillary projections and nodules. Unlike IPMT however, no communication with the pancreatic ductal system should be present. Also unlike IMPT, these tumors are more common in females (9:1 female-to-male ratio) in the fifth to sixth decade and are typically located in the body or tail of the pancreas. Bounded by a thick fibrous capsule, the epithelial lining of this tumor contains a variable population of abnormal cells ranging from benign to dysplastic to malignant. Although the minority of these tumors are frankly malignant at the time of diagnosis, all are considered potentially malignant and are resected.

CT demonstrates a near water density unilocular or multilocular cystic mass, usually 6 to 10 cm in diameter, although some tumors may grow as large as 30 cm (118).

This tumor is typically located within the pancreatic body or tail (Fig. 15-49). The cyst walls may be irregular and contain nodular excrescences or septations that are best demonstrated after IV contrast administration (Fig. 15-50). Although the presence of enhancing nodules and septations correlates well with malignancy, their absence does not preclude malignancy. Curvilinear calcifications may be present within the peripheral capsule or cyst walls. In a recent review, the presence of peripheral tumoral calcification was the only statistically significant finding associated with identifying mucinous tumors compared with other cystic pancreatic lesions (72). When multilocular, individual cysts tend to be greater than 2 cm diameter and fewer than six in number (156). Both MRI and US may depict the features of septations and cyst wall excrescences in these lesions (61,80,118,298), but the peripheral calcifications are easier to see on CT than on MRI (80).

Mucinous cystic neoplasm may be mistaken for a variety of benign pancreatic lesions (72,80,264,298). Although mucinous cystic neoplasm should be considered when a cystic pancreatic mass is discovered, only 5% to 15% of cystic masses are neoplastic (357). When unilocular, mucinous cystic neoplasm may mimic an inflammatory pancreatic cystic lesion (pseudocyst). The absence of CT features

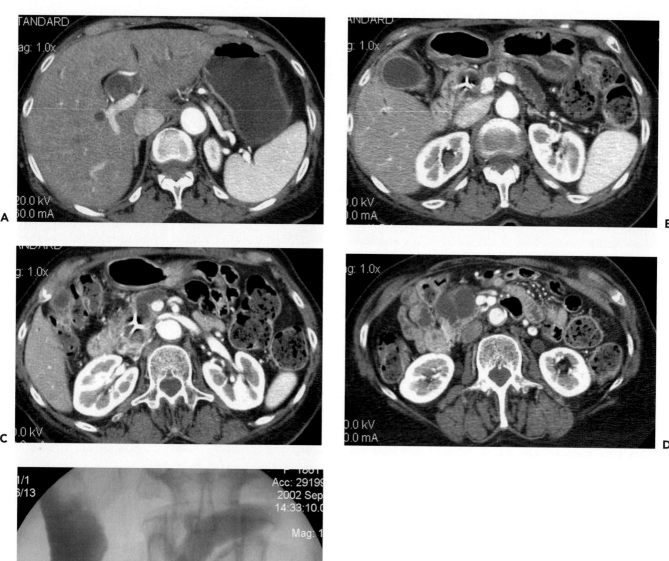

Figure 15-48 Sphincter of Oddi dysfunction with soft biliary calculi and pancreatic duct dilation mimicking intraductal papillary mucinous tumor. **A:** Contrast-enhanced portal venous phase computed tomography at the level of common hepatic duct demonstrates high density, noncalcified stone within markedly dilated duct. **B:** Portal venous phase image through the body of the pancreas demonstrates main duct dilation. No intraductal calculi are evident. **C:** Portal venous phase image through the pancreatic head demonstrates a stent within the dilated bile duct, adjacent to vertical portion of main pancreatic duct. **D:** Portal venous phase image through the pancreatic head slightly inferiorly demonstrates cystic lesion anteriorly. **E:** Endoscopic retrograde cholangiopancreatography spot radiograph shows dilated ducts and common duct stones. At surgery, no malignancy was found, and the cystic lesion was consistent with pseudocyst.

of peripancreatic inflammation and lack of change over time, in addition to lack of clinical history or laboratory evidence of pancreatitis, aid in differentiating a unilocular lesion (Fig. 15-51) from the much more common pseudocyst. Differentiating cystic neoplasms from pseudocysts can almost always be accomplished by clinical and radiologic means, but in doubtful cases, when observation is contemplated, or when it is important to determine preoperatively the type of cystic neoplasm, cyst fluid analysis is useful (see later) and can be obtained with EUS aspiration (94,188).

The more serious problem is misdiagnosing a mucinous cystic tumor as a benign neoplasm, the microcystic adenoma. Microcystic adenomas are characterized by mul-

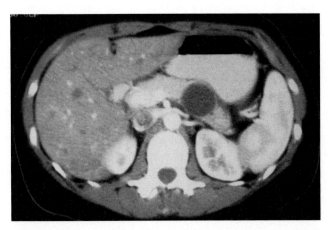

Figure 15-49 Unilocular mucinous cystic neoplasm. Pancreatic parenchymal phase 5-mm computed tomography image demonstrates a 3-cm well-circumscribed low-attenuation lesion at the pancreatic body tail junction, consistent with unilocular mucinous cystic neoplasm; benign histology was noted in the resected specimen. Low attenuation foci in liver are unopacified hepatic vein branches.

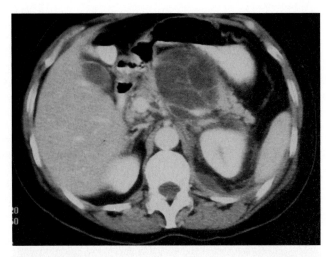

Figure 15-50 Mucinous cystic neoplasm in a 47-year-old woman with nausea. Portal venous phase 7-mm computed tomography image demonstrates a 7-cm low attenuation mass within the pancreatic body. The mass contains multiple enhancing septations, slightly irregular wall, and mild nodularity of the wall and septa. At resection, hyperplasia but no malignancy was found.

tiple cysts smaller than 2 cm diameter, but some may contain larger cysts, making their distinction from mucinous cystic neoplasm difficult. In selected patients percutaneous aspiration biopsy or EUSFNA may be used to identify mucin, which is not present in pseudocysts or microcystic adenomas (69,370), or to confirm the presence of glycogen, found in microcystic adenomas. Complications such as inadvertent spillage of potentially malignant fluid into the peritoneum must be considered (72). In general, even in experienced hands, CT is an insensitive tool for differentiating these tumors when cysts greater than 2 cm are present (72,80,167). This difficulty is not limited to CT. In a recent review of sonographic features considered typical for microcystic adenoma, Yeh et al. (370) found that if the diagnosis is based on US findings alone, many malignant tumors

will be misdiagnosed as microcystic adenomas. Morphologic characteristics of cystic masses on EUS cannot differentiate between benign and malignant lesions (5). Neither MRI nor US has been successful at differentiating subtypes of cystic pancreatic masses (217).

Microcystic Adenoma. Microcystic adenoma, also known as serous cystadenoma or glycogen-rich adenoma, is a benign cystic neoplasm of the pancreas that is more common in females (female-to-male ratio 2:1), occurs most frequently in the seventh decade, and usually is not associated with symptoms unless large. It is well documented that microcystic neoplasms have no malignant potential, and thus they are resected only when symptomatic (72,179). On CT, microcystic adenomas can be

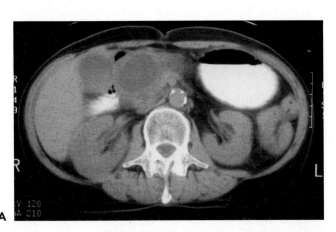

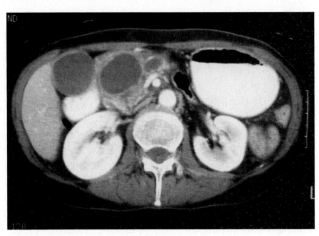

A   B

Figure 15-51 Unilocular mucinous cystic neoplasm. **A:** Preintravenous contrast 10-mm computed tomography (CT) image demonstrates a round, low attenuation lesion expanding the anterosuperior pancreatic head. **B:** Pancreatic parenchymal phase 5-mm CT image demonstrates a unilocular cystic mass with a perceptible, slightly irregular wall. No peripancreatic stranding is seen; however, the main pancreatic duct is dilated. In the absence of a history of pancreatitis or prior unexplained abdominal pain, finding is suspicious for mucinous cystic neoplasm, confirmed at surgery.

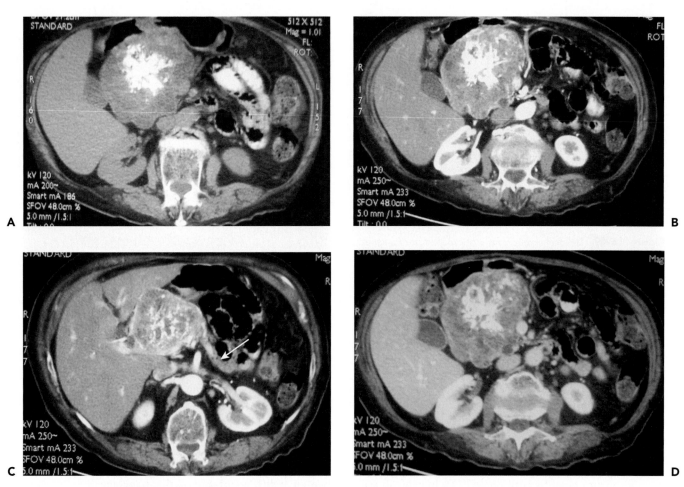

Figure 15-52 Microcystic adenoma in a 72-year-old woman with vague abdominal pain. **A:** Pre-intravenous contrast 5-mm computed tomography (CT) image demonstrates heterogeneous lobular 13 cm mass extending superiorly from the pancreatic head and neck. Note central branching calcifications. **B:** Pancreatic parenchymal phase 5-mm CT image same level demonstrates enhancement of the capsule and numerous very fine septa within the lesion. **C:** Pancreatic parenchymal phase CT image slightly more cephalad reveals atrophy of the body and tail (*arrow*). Note absence of biliary ductal dilatation despite large size of tumor. **D:** Portal venous phase 5-mm CT image through the lesion reveals the better opacification of the septa with two cysts measuring up to 1 cm. The CT appearance suggests a cut surface of a natural sponge, in this classic microcystic adenoma.

water, soft tissue, or heterogeneous mixed density and are usually made up of multiple small cysts (147). The cut edge of this tumor has been described as similar to the cut surface of a sponge (Fig. 15-52). Within the mass, individual cysts are typically smaller than 2 cm, but some lesions contain cysts that are larger, making differentiation from mucinous cystic neoplasm difficult on the basis of imaging alone (Fig. 15-53) (72,80,118,167). Enhancement of the cyst walls is variable after IV contrast administration; some cysts may be apparent only after IV contrast enhancement (80). A characteristic feature of this lesion, although seen in the minority of cases, is a central stellate scar that may contain calcification (see Fig. 15-52). MRI shows similar features as CT, with generalized low signal on T1 and high signal on T2, septations, and central scar. US depicts the cyst walls and septa well; the mass may appear echogenic or solid on US when the cysts are very small (80,199). Microcystic adenoma is one of the pancreatic lesions found in patients with von Hippel-Lindau (VHL) disease (Fig. 15-54). Rarely, microcystic adenomas may produce a unilocular macrocystic appearance on CT and therefore be mistaken for unilocular mucinous cystic tumors or pseudocysts. A recent study found that combined features of location in the pancreatic head, lobulated contour, absence of wall enhancement, and thin capsule could help to distinguish these lesions; when two of four criteria were used, a specificity of 83% was achieved, and when three of four were present, specificity of 100% was achieved (68). Because the cells of microcystic adenomas are rich in cytoplasmic glycogen and contain no mucin, percutaneous aspiration may aid in the diagnosis of this lesion if the imaging appearance is not typical (69). EUS-guided aspiration of suspected microcystic lesions with larger individual cysts may provide glycogen-rich epithelial cells to allow the diagnosis of a benign lesion (10).

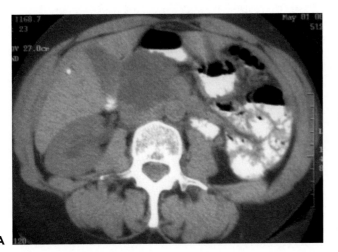

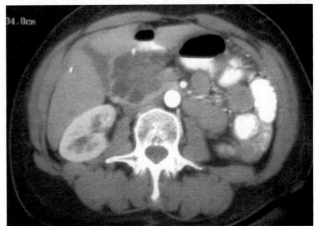

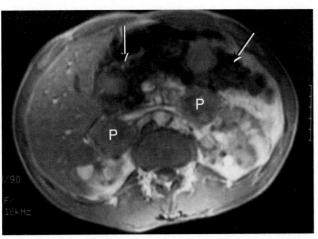

Figure 15-53 Microcystic adenoma with large cysts. **A:** Pre-intravenous contrast 5-mm computed tomography (CT) image demonstrates a lobular low attenuation mass in the pancreatic neck. **B:** Pancreatic parenchymal phase 5-mm CT image reveals multiloculated cystic mass. Individual cysts measure up to 2.0 cm diameter. **C:** Portal venous phase 5-mm CT image shows the mass abutting the right margin of the superior mesenteric vein, without narrowing, and a thin rim of normally enhancing pancreatic parenchyma posteriorly. The imaging appearance suggests a mucinous cystic neoplasm, likely resectable. Histologic evaluation after resection demonstrated microcystic adenoma with several large cysts.

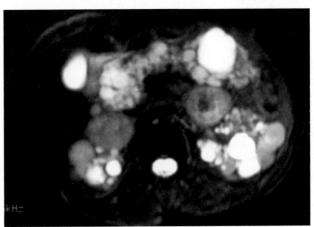

Figure 15-54 Von Hippel-Lindau patient with numerous pancreatic cysts. **A:** Postgadolinium portal venous phase T1-weighted fast multiplanar spoiled gradient recalled echo (FMPSPGR) breath-hold image through the pancreas demonstrates near total replacement of the pancreatic glandular tissue by low signal cysts (*arrows*). Larger higher signal intensity cystic lesion is seen in the tail, likely representing a protein containing cyst. Also noted are two enhancing soft tissue adrenal masses, consistent with pheochromocytomas (P). **B:** Feridex-enhanced T2-weighted magnetic resonance image through the same level demonstrates markedly diminished signal intensity within the liver due to the iron containing contrast agent. Note varied fluid signal within the cysts replacing both the pancreas and the kidneys. Once again, soft tissue adrenal masses consistent with pheochromocytomas are seen.

Pancreatic Neuroendocrine Tumors (Islet Cell Tumors)

Pancreatic neuroendocrine tumors are uncommon, having a prevalence of less than 10 per million population (140,152,222,307). Although most neuroendocrine tumors appear sporadically, an increased prevalence of these tumors is seen in patients with VHL syndrome and in those affected by multiple endocrine neoplasia type I (MEN I) (206,307). Despite their rarity, these tumors are important because they have a high rate of malignancy, ranging from 60% to 92% (89). Neuroendocrine tumors are classified as functioning (those that secrete various hormones) or nonfunctioning. Functioning neuroendocrine tumors are named for the main hormone produced. The diagnosis of functioning neuroendocrine tumors is almost always established biochemically when the lesion is small and easier to resect (7), whereas nonfunctioning neuroendocrine tumors are typically diagnosed when the lesions are large and produce symptoms because of mass effect. Insulinomas and gastrinomas are the most common of these rare tumors, whereas glucagonomas, VIPomas, and somatostatinomas are much rarer. GRFomas (tumors that secrete growth hormone releasing factor) are exceedingly rare. PPomas, which secrete pancreatic polypeptide, have no known symptoms due to hypersecretion and are much like nonfunctioning or hormonally quiescent pancreatic endocrine tumors. In surgical studies, nonfunctioning pancreatic endocrine tumors are reported to compose 15% to 20% of all pancreatic endocrine tumors removed (58). In a large surgical pathology series, the nonfunctioning tumors accounted for 36% of all pancreatic endocrine tumors (175).

Although commonly referred to as islet cell tumors, the bulk of evidence suggests a non-islet cell duct tumor origin (78). The tumors are thought to originate from cells that are part of the diffuse neuroendocrine cell system (117). These neuroendocrine cells share cytochemical properties and, together with pheochromocytomas, melanomas, carcinoid tumors, and medullary carcinoma of the thyroid, have been called APUDomas. APUD is an acronym for amine precursor uptake and decarboxylation. This would account for several different hormones, not present in normal islet cells, being present in the various tumors under this category. The benign or malignant nature of these tumors is sometimes difficult to establish unless metastatic tumor has been documented. To establish that one of these tumors is benign, long-term follow-up is required. In general, 5% to 10% of insulinomas are reported as malignant, whereas in various series 50% to 90% of the other tumors are reported as malignant (44,71,131,151).

Nonfunctioning pancreatic neuroendocrine tumors are clinically silent until they cause symptoms due to their size or to metastases. As a consequence, they are usually large at the time of discovery (Fig. 15-55), ranging in size from 3 to 24 cm in diameter and 30% are larger than 10 cm (90,245). It is important to differentiate between nonfunctioning neuroendocrine tumors of the pancreas and ductal adenocarcinomas because patients with endocrine tumors

often respond favorably to surgery and specific chemotherapy and consequently have a better prognosis than patients with adenocarcinomas (152). When a nonfunctioning neuroendocrine tumor is encountered on CT, three features that aid in differentiation from an adenocarcinoma are the presence of calcification, the lack of vascular encasement, and the absence of central necrosis or cystic degeneration when small. When larger, cystic degeneration or necrosis may be present (307). Rarely, both functioning and nonfunctioning islet cell tumors may appear completely cystic (80,191). Approximately 20% of pancreatic neuroendocrine tumors contain calcification, whereas less than 2% of adenocarcinomas do. Notably, calcification is more common in malignant than in benign islet cell tumors (55,364).

Encasement of the celiac artery or superior mesenteric artery, which is commonly seen in adenocarcinomas (see Fig. 15-55), is rarely seen in the neuroendocrine tumors; however, encasement of the superior mesenteric vein or portal vein has been reported (45,90). Pancreatic neuroendocrine tumors, even when large, may not undergo central necrosis or cystic degeneration because of the rich vascularity, which continues to grow as the mass grows (335). Although 60% of pancreatic neuroendocrine tumors occur in the body and tail, location is not useful as a differentiating feature in individual cases. In summary, the diagnosis of a nonfunctioning or hormonally quiescent neuroendocrine tumor should be considered when a large, nonuniformly enhancing, calcified pancreatic mass without cystic areas and with hyperdense areas is identified on a contrast-enhanced CT examination (90).

The presenting symptoms of a functioning neuroendocrine tumor depend on the hormone secreted. Insulinomas are the most common functioning neuroendocrine tumor, with patients presenting with symptoms of intractable hypoglycemia, low blood levels of glucose, and high circulating plasma insulin. These lesions are essentially always confined to the pancreas and are small (see Fig. 15-2), with 50% measuring less than 1.3 cm (257). Gastrinomas are the second most common functioning neuroendocrine tumor, with patients presenting with peptic ulcer disease, diarrhea, abdominal pain, and elevated serum gastrin levels. They occur most frequently in the general vicinity of the head of pancreas, including the pancreatic head itself, the wall of the duodenum and stomach, and lymph nodes in an area termed the "gastrinoma triangle" (Fig. 15-56). Ninety percent of the extrapancreatic gastrinomas occur in this area bounded by the junction of the cystic and common hepatic duct superiorly, the second and third portions of the duodenum inferiorly and the junction between the neck and body of the pancreas medially (233,324). Similar to insulinomas, gastrinomas usually are small (90% are less than 2 cm in diameter), and both tumors may be multiple (gastrinomas and insulinomas are multiple 60% and 10% of the time, respectively) (120,121,152,262,335). VIPomas (Fig. 15-57), glucagonomas, and somatostatino-

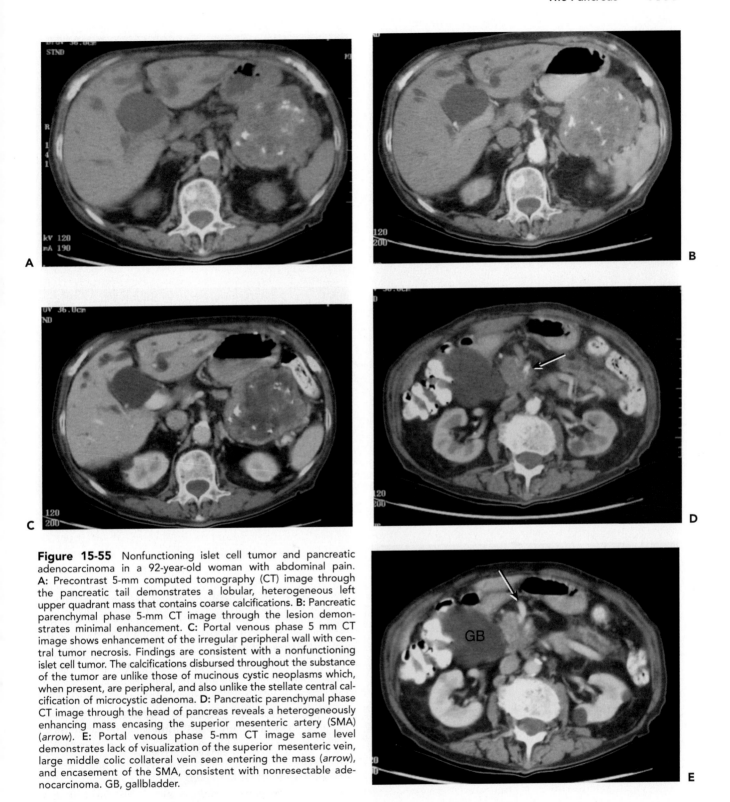

Figure 15-55 Nonfunctioning islet cell tumor and pancreatic adenocarcinoma in a 92-year-old woman with abdominal pain. **A:** Precontrast 5-mm computed tomography (CT) image through the pancreatic tail demonstrates a lobular, heterogeneous left upper quadrant mass that contains coarse calcifications. **B:** Pancreatic parenchymal phase 5-mm CT image through the lesion demonstrates minimal enhancement. **C:** Portal venous phase 5 mm CT image shows enhancement of the irregular peripheral wall with central tumor necrosis. Findings are consistent with a nonfunctioning islet cell tumor. The calcifications disbursed throughout the substance of the tumor are unlike those of mucinous cystic neoplasms which, when present, are peripheral, and also unlike the stellate central calcification of microcystic adenoma. **D:** Pancreatic parenchymal phase CT image through the head of pancreas reveals a heterogeneously enhancing mass encasing the superior mesenteric artery (SMA) (*arrow*). **E:** Portal venous phase 5-mm CT image same level demonstrates lack of visualization of the superior mesenteric vein, large middle colic collateral vein seen entering the mass (*arrow*), and encasement of the SMA, consistent with nonresectable adenocarcinoma. GB, gallbladder.

mas are frequently larger, many being greater than 5 cm in diameter, due to the nonspecificity of their symptoms and resultant delay in diagnosis (44,151,347).

The reported sensitivity of CT in localizing functioning neuroendocrine tumors varies from 30% in early studies (86) to 71% to 82% with dual-phase helical techniques

(140,307). Because of the typically small size of insulinomas and gastrinomas, they seldom alter the contour of the pancreas. Generally, neuroendocrine tumors of the pancreas enhance to a greater degree than normal pancreatic parenchyma during arterial and capillary phases of bolus contrast administration and are typically hyperattenuating

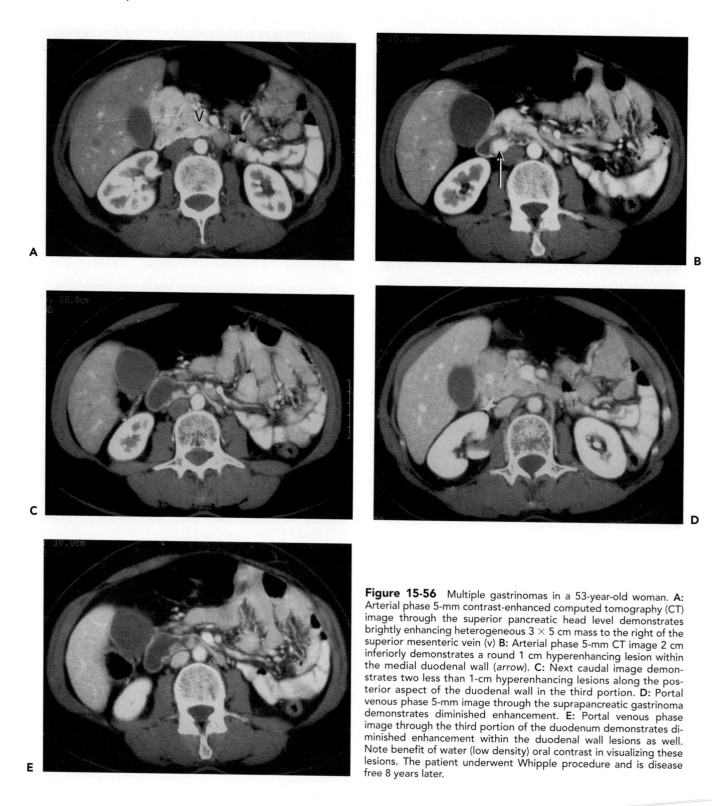

Figure 15-56 Multiple gastrinomas in a 53-year-old woman. **A:** Arterial phase 5-mm contrast-enhanced computed tomography (CT) image through the superior pancreatic head level demonstrates brightly enhancing heterogeneous 3 × 5 cm mass to the right of the superior mesenteric vein (v) **B:** Arterial phase 5-mm CT image 2 cm inferiorly demonstrates a round 1 cm hyperenhancing lesion within the medial duodenal wall (*arrow*). **C:** Next caudal image demonstrates two less than 1-cm hyperenhancing lesions along the posterior aspect of the duodenal wall in the third portion. **D:** Portal venous phase 5-mm image through the suprapancreatic gastrinoma demonstrates diminished enhancement. **E:** Portal venous phase image through the third portion of the duodenum demonstrates diminished enhancement within the duodenal wall lesions as well. Note benefit of water (low density) oral contrast in visualizing these lesions. The patient underwent Whipple procedure and is disease free 8 years later.

in both the arterial and portal venous phases (140,172, 307,343,360). Occasionally, the smaller tumors are best or only seen on portal venous phase images (140,325,343) and may mimic arterial structures on arterial phase images when in a peripancreatic location (307). The use of water as a negative oral contrast agent will improve the con-

spicuity of the tumors when located in the duodenal wall (see Fig. 15-56) (360).

Because US and CT are readily available, these imaging methods may be used initially for the detection and localization of functioning endocrine tumors of the pancreas. However, there is evidence to show that MRI is at least as

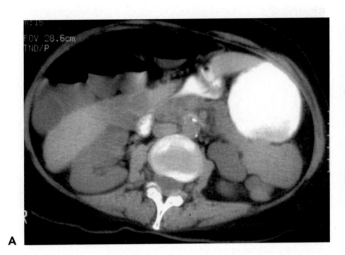

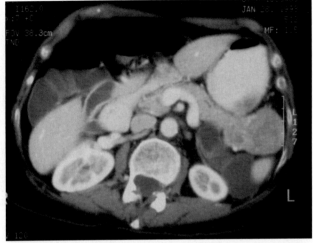

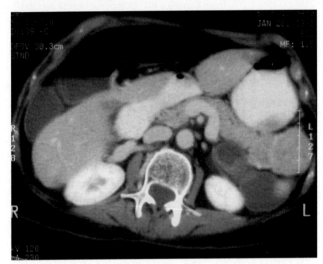

Figure 15-57 VIPoma in a 67-year-old woman with unexplained diarrhea for 1 year. **A:** Pre-intravenous contrast computed tomography (CT) image demonstrates isoattenuating expansion of the pancreatic tail region. **B:** Early portal venous phase 5-mm CT image demonstrates heterogeneous hyperenhancing mass in the tail of pancreas. The mass contains several large vascular channels, and appears clearly separate from the fluid filled adjacent jejunal loops. **C:** Portal venous phase 5-mm CT image demonstrates diminished, but persistent, enhancement within the mass, which now appears more isoattenuating with the remainder of the pancreas.

effective as CT (140). In the MRI evaluation of pancreatic neuroendocrine tumors, T1 fat-suppressed (T1FS) immediate postgadolinium spoiled GRE images and T2 fat-suppressed (T2FS) images may be useful (226,300,301). The tumors are low in signal intensity on precontrast T1FS images, demonstrate homogeneous or ring enhancement on immediate postgadolinium spoiled GRE and are high in signal intensity on T2FS images. The MRI features that distinguish neuroendocrine tumors from ductal adenocarcinomas include high signal intensity on T2FS, increased homogeneous enhancement on immediate postgadolinium images, and hypervascular liver metastases. Morphologic features include lack of vascular encasement and absence of central necrosis in large tumors as is similarly shown on CT examinations. MR imaging is particularly helpful in the evaluation of neuroendocrine tumors of the pancreas in patients with VHL syndrome, a tumor-prone group with renal disease for whom a limitation of

both ionizing radiation and iodinated contrast is desirable. In this population, most tumors are benign, small, located in the pancreatic head, and associated with more pheochromocytomas and fewer pancreatic cystic lesions (microcystic adenomas) than VHL patients without neuroendocrine tumors (206).

The literature provides conflicting information on the relative merits of MRI, transabdominal US, CT, and angiography in the evaluation of neuroendocrine tumors. One study demonstrated that MRI was more sensitive than the other imaging methods for detecting metastatic disease to the liver (Fig. 15-58), but the role of MRI remains unclear for detecting primary pancreatic endocrine tumors with the same study cited previously demonstrating that it has a low sensitivity (22%), equal to that of US and CT, and less than that of angiography (259). Another study reported that MRI with gadolinium enhancement and fat suppression techniques demonstrated 91% of all primary pancreatic

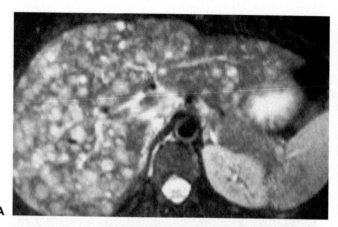
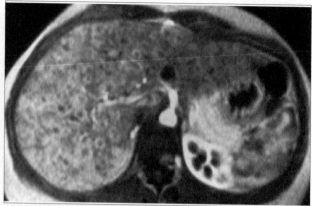

Figure 15-58 Gastrinoma liver metastases. T2FS **A:** and immediately postgadolinium spoiled gradient echo (SGE) **B:** images demonstrate well-defined small metastases that are high in signal on T2FS (**A**) and possess distinct ring enhancement immediately following contrast (**B**). (Reproduced from Semelka RC, Cumming MJ, Shoenut JP, et al. Islet cell tumors: comparison of dynamic contrast-enhanced CT and MR imaging with dynamic gadolinium enhancement and fat suppression. *Radiology* 1993;186: 799–802, with permission.)

neuroendocrine tumors (301). The striking difference in sensitivity in these two studies largely reflects differences in MR technique; however, it may also reflect the size of the primary tumors. In the latter study, 90% of the tumors were at least 2 cm in diameter. It appears that the ability of the various imaging methods to detect pancreatic neuroendocrine tumors depends on the size of the tumor. Using any of the above standard imaging methods, less than 10% of tumors smaller than 1 cm, 30% to 40% of tumors 1 to 3 cm, and 70% to 80% of tumors larger than 3 cm were detected (16,17,106,152,207,259). Recommended imaging algorithms for evaluation of patients with functioning neuroendocrine tumors are controversial because of the variety of modalities available. In addition to CT, MRI, and US, other techniques such as somatostatin receptor scintigraphy, angiography, and arterial stimulation with venous hormone sampling have been used in these patients, each with unique advantages and limitations (96).

Before the availability of EUS, selective portal venous sampling for localization of hormone gradients and intraoperative US were the techniques having the greatest sensitivity for detection of functioning neuroendocrine tumors, with detection rates superior to standard imaging methods (244,246). Nowadays, EUS is a highly accurate technique for visualization of small functioning neuroendocrine tumors (see Fig. 15-2) not evident on CT and for identification of patients with multiple lesions. In a series of 82 patients with mean tumor size of 1.5 cm (71% of tumors ≤2 cm), EUS demonstrated a sensitivity of 93% and specificity of 95% (11) but was not reliable in detecting extrapancreatic disease. In a population of 10 patients with suspected functioning neuroendocrine tumors, EUS identified 14 tumors (mean size 1.2 cm) in 10 patients; CT did not demonstrate the tumor or missed at least one of multiple lesions

in 9 of 10 patients (112). EUSFNA may readily provide cytologic confirmation of the lesions (112,153). Another EUS study designed as a retrospective review of 12 patients with surgically proven insulinomas reported an 83% sensitivity for EUS detection and 16% sensitivity for helical CT (15). These very low sensitivities were found using varied CT techniques. A recent study of multiphase helical CT in 30 patients with proven insulinomas reported an overall sensitivity of 83%. Most tumors were hyperdense on at least one phase, usually the pancreatic parenchymal phase, and false negatives were most commonly due to tumor location adjacent to vessels, pedunculated morphology, or nonhyperattenuating lesions (95). Insulinomas are perhaps the most difficult neuroendocrine tumor to image because of their notoriously small size. Nonetheless, because of the wide availability of high-quality CT compared with EUS, it appears that dual-phase helical CT will remain the mainstay of imaging in these patients initially, with EUS reserved for patients clinically suspected of having a functioning neuroendocrine tumor not detected on CT.

Other Neoplastic Lesions

The solid pseudopapillary tumor of the pancreas (formerly referred to as solid and papillary epithelial neoplasm, papillary cystic neoplasm, solid cystic papillary tumor, etc.) is an uncommon low-grade malignant tumor that occurs chiefly in young women (mean age 25 years) (60,62). These tumors are generally large, with a mean transverse diameter of 9 cm and, although predominating in the tail, can be found in any portion of pancreas (Fig. 15-59). CT and MRI of solid pseudopapillary tumors will commonly show hemorrhage with typical fluid–debris level indicating blood products in areas of cystic degeneration and necrosis. In a review of six patients with these tumors studied with

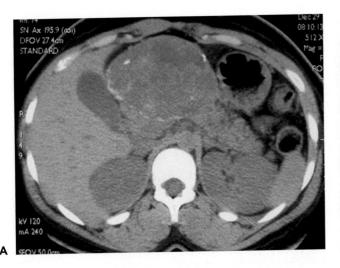

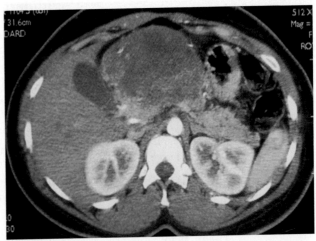

Figure 15-59 Solid pseudopapillary tumor in a 27-year-old woman undergoing evaluation as potential renal donor. **A:** Pre-intravenous contrast 3.8-mm computed tomography (CT) image through the superior pancreatic head region demonstrates a heterogeneous 7 × 9 cm mass extending anteriorly from the neck. There are focal calcifications along the periphery and within the substance of the mass. **B:** Pancreatic parenchymal phase 2.5-mm CT image through the same level demonstrates heterogeneous enhancement within the lesion. **C:** Portal venous phase 3.8-mm CT image through the same level demonstrates progressive enhancement from the periphery of the mass. There is displacement of the vascular structures posteriorly. The lesion was resectable.

MRI, the authors found that all tumors were well-demarcated lesions containing central high signal intensity on T1-weighted images consistent with hemorrhagic necrosis (250). In a more recent study, 5 of 19 patients with proven solid pseudopapillary tumors did not have high T1 signal within the lesion and thus concluded that the absence of this finding should not exclude the diagnosis (62). The same authors reported early peripheral enhancement with progressive fill in of the mass on gadolinium-enhanced dynamic images, which may aid in differentiating this tumor from cystic neoplasms and neuroendocrine tumors of the pancreas (62), diagnoses with which it has been previously compared (27,60,105,173,288).

Pleomorphic carcinoma is an uncommon malignant neoplasm that has a fulminant clinical course. It metastasizes early to the liver, lung, adrenal, kidney, thyroid, and bone. This tumor shows irregular enhancement after IV contrast administration and may be cystic, with thick irregular walls and a lobulated contour. The presence of extensive retroperitoneal lymphadenopathy helps to differentiate from adenocarcinoma (365).

Acinar cell carcinoma is a rare exocrine pancreatic tumor, making up only 1% of exocrine pancreatic tumors despite the fact that the majority of pancreatic parenchyma is made up of acinar cells. These tumors are less aggressive than typical pancreatic adenocarcinoma. On contrast-enhanced CT acinar cell carcinomas may be located anywhere in the pancreas and tend to be well marginated, exophytic, hypoenhancing, and large (333). A variety of other rare neoplasms of the pancreas have been reported including malignant giant cell tumor, sarcoma, plasmacytoma, lipoma, oncocytoma, and small cell carcinoma (82,83,228,248,299,358).

Pancreatic tumors are rare in infants and children. The CT, MRI, and US imaging characteristics of pancreatoblastomas, a rare pancreatic tumor of acinar cell origin in children between ages of 1 and 8, have been reported (150,198,326).

Although lymphoma (Fig. 15-60) can involve pancreas and peripancreatic lymph nodes and can be confused with a primary pancreatic neoplasm, usually it is a systemic disease with retroperitoneal and mesenteric lymphadenopathy

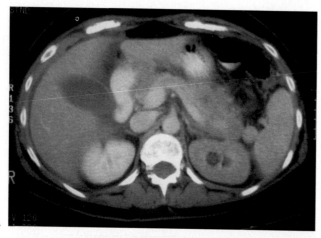
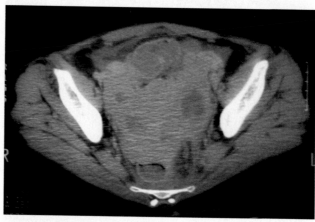

Figure 15-60 Pancreatic involvement by systemic lymphoma in a 36-year-old woman with abdominal pain. **A:** Portal venous phase 7-mm computed tomography (CT) image through the pancreatic body and tail demonstrates heterogeneously enhancing expansion of this region. Note obstruction of left renal collecting system. **B:** Delayed 5-mm CT image through the pelvis demonstrates bulky lymphadenopathy filling the deep pelvis. At pathology, high grade B-cell lymphoma with some features of Burkitt's was found.

also present (261,309,350). On MRI, intermediate signal intensity peripancreatic lymph nodes are readily distinguished from high signal intensity pancreatic parenchyma on the T1 fat suppressed images. Invasion of the pancreas is shown by loss of the usual signal intensity of the pancreatic parenchyma on the T1 fat-suppressed images. When primary pancreatic lymphoma is present, the mass is often larger than a typical adenocarcinoma. In one study, it was reported that no adenocarcinoma was larger than 10 cm, and 60% were between 4 and 6 cm (334). Because lymphoma does not require surgical staging or palliative Whipple procedure before chemotherapy or radiation therapy, dif-

ferentiating pancreatic lymphoma from adenocarcinoma is important. Two findings that may help are the absence of pancreatic ductal dilatation despite large mass size, and the presence of retroperitoneal adenopathy located below the level of the left renal vein (218). Rarer tumors such as malignant fibrous histiocytoma (Fig. 15-61) may also arise in the pancreas; typically, the diagnosis is made with evaluation of the surgical specimen.

Pancreatic metastases, which are rarely diagnosed clinically, most commonly arise from melanoma and carcinomas of the breast (Fig. 15-62), lung, kidney, prostate, and GI tract (Fig. 15-63). Isolated metastases to the pancreas from

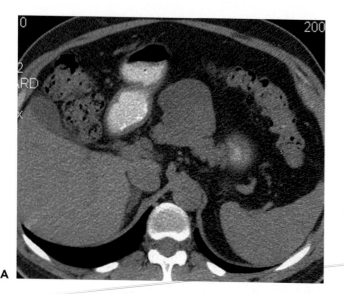
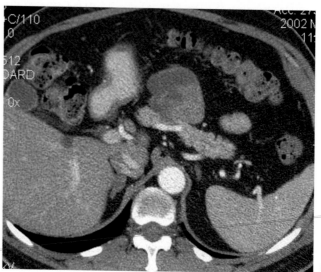

Figure 15-61 Pancreatic malignant fibrous histiocytoma (MFH). **A:** Pre-intravenous contrast computed tomography (CT) image demonstrates a well circumscribed smooth low attenuation mass extending anteriorly from the body. **B:** Pancreatic parenchymal phase CT image same level shows cystic and hypovascular solid components of the lesion. Note focal intrapancreatic low attenuation tumor and normal enhancement of remainder of pancreas.

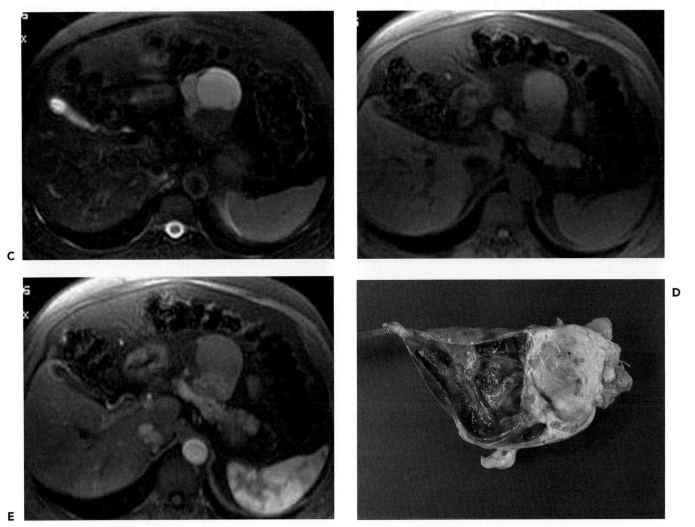

Figure 15-61 (*continued*) **C:** T2 fat suppressed magnetic resonance (MR) image demonstrates fluid signal within the cystic component. **D:** T1 fat suppressed MR image reveals high signal intensity within the cystic component, indicating proteinaceous or hemorrhagic material. Note normal high signal within the normal pancreatic parenchyma, and focal low signal in the body indicating the intrapancreatic tumor. **E:** T1 fat-suppressed gadolinium-enhanced MR image shows hyperenhancement of the solid component of the tumor, more so than on CT. **F:** Surgical specimen cut open to reveal hemorrhagic cystic and yellow-tan solid portions of tumor, completely resected with extended distal pancreatectomy and splenectomy. (Surgical photograph courtesy of Martin J. Heslin, MD.)

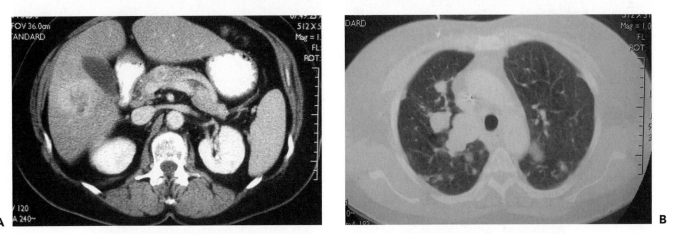

Figure 15-62 Pancreatic metastases from breast carcinoma. **A:** Early portal venous phase 5-mm computed tomography image demonstrates a focal, round, 1-cm heterogeneously enhancing mass in the pancreatic neck. Similar enhancement can be seen within a mass located in the right hepatic lobe. Multiple lung nodules are also present on **B,** 5-mm image through inferior chest filmed at lung windows. Findings are consistent with metastases in this patient with known primary breast cancer.

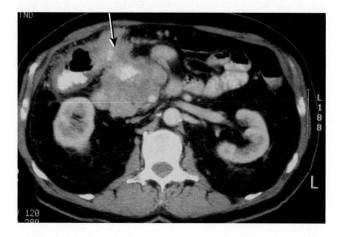

Figure 15-63 Colon carcinoma with contiguous spread into the pancreatic head in a 77-year-old man with abdominal pain. Portal venous phase 5-mm computed tomography image demonstrates heterogeneous, lobular soft tissue mass replacing the pancreatic head and neck, in direct contact with a similar appearing mass of the proximal transverse colon (*arrow*). Calcification is seen within the substance of the mass, proven to be mucinous colon carcinoma with contiguous spread through the transverse mesocolon to involve the pancreatic head.

primary bone tumors have also been reported (286). When multiple masses are present in the pancreas in a patient with a known primary carcinoma, metastases can be presumed; however, when solitary, it may be indistinguishable from primary pancreatic carcinoma (287). On CT, the pattern of

a single, localized mass is the most common presentation of pancreatic metastasis (293). The interval from diagnosis of an extrapancreatic primary tumor to subsequent detection of a pancreatic metastasis is variable, usually ranging from 1 to 3 years (293), but in the case of renal carcinomas metastases may occur many years after primary tumor diagnosis. Identifying renal carcinoma metastases to the pancreas, best detected during the early phases of helical CT, is potentially important because aggressive surgical resection may be beneficial (240). MRI may be useful in the evaluation of pancreatic metastases by showing features such as increased vascularity in the context of a hypervascular primary malignancy (164). The majority of metastases are low signal on a background of high-signal pancreas on T1 fat-suppressed images. Melanoma has a typically high signal intensity on T1-weighted images due to the paramagnetic properties of melanin.

Periampullary tumors arise within 2 cm of the major papilla, and because of their similar clinical features and location may be difficult to differentiate from pancreatic adenocarcinomas. Although often treated with Whipple resection, the long-term outcomes for this diverse group of tumors are generally more favorable due to inherent differences in tumor biology. Ampullary villous adenomas (Fig. 15-64) and ampullary adenocarcinomas (Fig. 15-65) may cause isolated biliary or combined biliary and pancreatic duct dilation and frequently produce a mass bulging into the duodenal lumen. Duodenal adenocarcinomas less frequently result in ductal dilatation and may be polypoid,

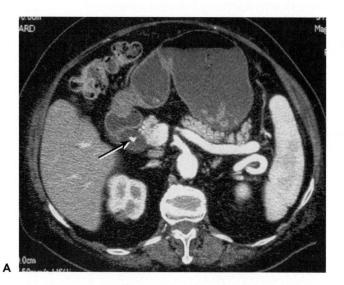

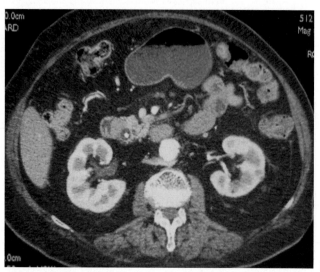

A

B

Figure 15-64 Ampullary mass in a 70-year-old woman with 2-week history of painless jaundice. A: Pancreatic parenchymal phase computed tomography (CT) image through the superior pancreas demonstrates marked common bile ductal dilatation, with biliary endoprosthesis in place (*arrow*). B: 2 cm inferiorly, a focal 2-cm hypoattenuating mass is seen between the dilated bile duct and medial duodenal wall. (*continued*)

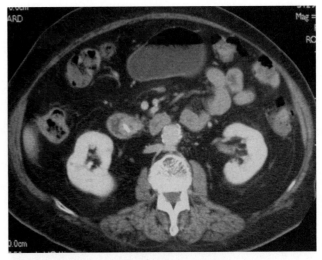

Figure 15-64 (*continued*) **C:** Next caudal CT image shows heterogeneous hypoattenuating mass surrounding the distal common bile duct at the ampulla. **D:** Same level portal venous phase image demonstrates decreased demarcation of the mass compared to the normal sleeve of pancreatic tissue seen medially on the pancreatic parenchymal phase images. At Whipple resection, a 3.0-cm villous adenoma with high grade dysplasia was found at the ampulla.

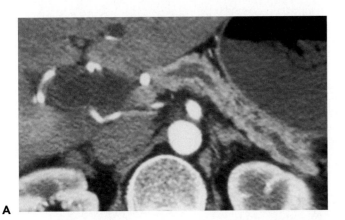

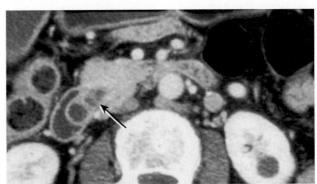

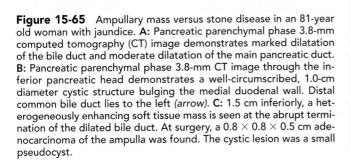

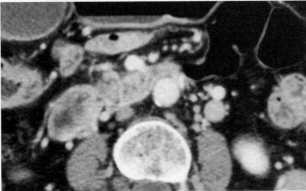

Figure 15-65 Ampullary mass versus stone disease in an 81-year old woman with jaundice. **A:** Pancreatic parenchymal phase 3.8-mm computed tomography (CT) image demonstrates marked dilatation of the bile duct and moderate dilatation of the main pancreatic duct. **B:** Pancreatic parenchymal phase 3.8-mm CT image through the inferior pancreatic head demonstrates a well-circumscribed, 1.0-cm diameter cystic structure bulging the medial duodenal wall. Distal common bile duct lies to the left (*arrow*). **C:** 1.5 cm inferiorly, a heterogeneously enhancing soft tissue mass is seen at the abrupt termination of the dilated bile duct. At surgery, a 0.8 × 0.8 × 0.5 cm adenocarcinoma of the ampulla was found. The cystic lesion was a small pseudocyst.

ulcerating, or annular lesions that on CT arise to the right of the distal common bile duct. Distal bile duct adenocarcinomas produce obliteration of the duct lumen and when advanced invade the adjacent pancreatic parenchyma; these may be most difficult to distinguish from pancreatic adenocarcinomas with imaging. Occasionally, chronic inflammation (Fig. 15-66), squamous carcinomas (Fig. 15-67), or rare lesions such as duodenal gastrointestinal stromal tumor (GIST) (Fig. 15-68) may be present in a periampullary location. MRCP and sectional MRI may be useful in determining the origins of periampullary lesions (169).

Inflammatory Diseases

Acute Pancreatitis

Acute pancreatitis is most commonly associated with choledocholithiasis and ethanol abuse, with other etiologic factors such as metabolic disorders (hypercalcemia and hyperlipidemia), trauma including ERCP-induced pancreatitis (Fig. 15-69), medications (azathioprine, sulfonamides), and structural abnormalities such as pancreas divisum and tumors (70,193) (Fig. 15-70) being much less common. Most patients present with nausea, vomiting, and abdominal

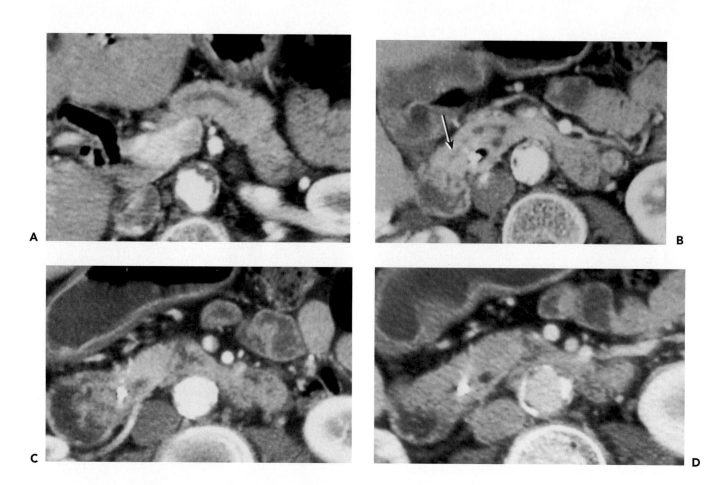

Figure 15-66 Ampullary mass. **A:** Pancreatic parenchymal phase 5-mm computed tomography (CT) image through the porta demonstrates air within the biliary tree in this patient with recent biliary stent placement. Note dilatation of the main pancreatic duct in the neck and body. **B:** Next caudal 5-mm pancreatic parenchymal phase CT image demonstrates emptying of the duct of Santorini to the medial duodenal wall (*arrow*) with biliary endoprosthesis seen within the nondilated distal common bile duct. **C:** 1.5 cm inferiorly, there is a heterogeneously enhancing hypoattenuating mass surrounding the distal common bile duct stent, and extending into the duodenal lumen. **D:** Portal venous phase CT image, same level as **C** demonstrates poor demarcation between the mass and remaining normal pancreas. Specimen from Whipple resection showed chronic inflammation and no neoplasm.

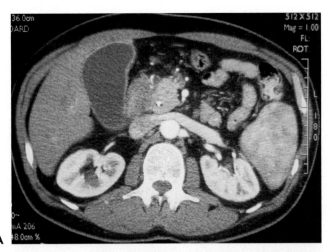
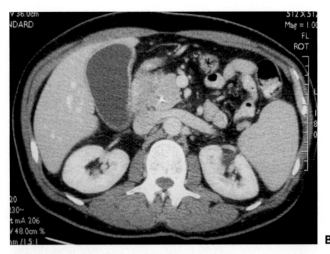

Figure 15-67   Squamous carcinoma of pancreatic head in a 52-year-old man with 2-week history of painless jaundice. **A:** Pancreatic parenchymal phase 3-mm computed tomography (CT) image through the pancreatic head demonstrates common bile duct stent in place through a nondilated duct. There is hypoattenuating soft tissue located to the right, but not surrounding, the distal common bile duct as well as narrowing of the duodenal lumen. Note gastroduodenal artery coursing through lesion. **B:** Portal venous phase 3-mm CT image same level demonstrates isoattenuation of the soft tissue mass compared to the normal pancreatic head parenchyma. After Whipple resection, pathologic and histologic evaluation revealed that the majority of the squamous carcinoma was within the pancreatic parenchyma, with islands of tumor extending into but not through the intact columnar lining of the bile duct.

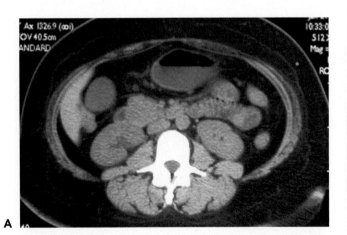
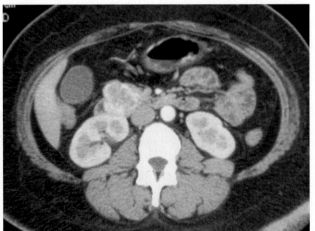
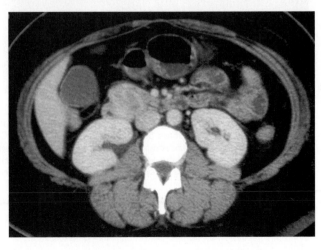

Figure 15-68   Ampullary mass. **A:** Pre-intravenous contrast 5-mm computed tomography (CT) image through the inferior pancreatic head demonstrates moderate lobularity and relative expansion of the head compared to the remainder of the gland. **B:** Pancreatic parenchymal phase 2.5-mm CT image through the same level demonstrates a hyperenhancing heterogeneous 2.3-cm mass. **C:** Portal venous phase 5-mm CT image through the same level demonstrates diminished but persistently heterogeneous enhancement through the same region. At surgery, a gastrointestinal stromal tumor (GIST) of the medial duodenal wall was found.

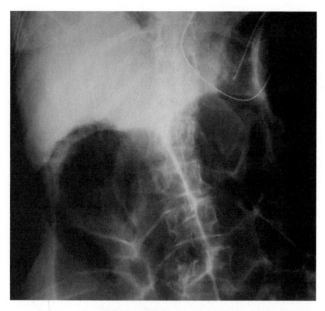

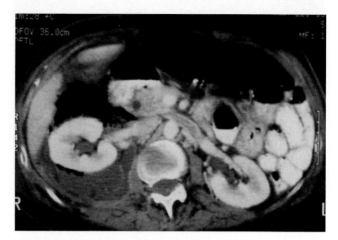

Figure 15-69   Endoscopic retrograde cholangiopancreatography (ERCP) perforation with pancreatitis in a 61-year-old woman. **A:** Abdominal radiograph demonstrates retroperitoneal mottled air in the right abdomen. Gaseous distention of the bowel is due to recent endoscopic procedure. **B:** Contrast-enhanced computed tomography of the abdomen 2 days later demonstrates persistent retroperitoneal air anterior to the right kidney with a moderate amount of retroperitoneal fluid. Pancreatitis associated with ERCP perforation resulted in prolonged recovery in this patient.

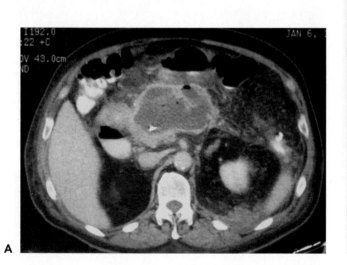

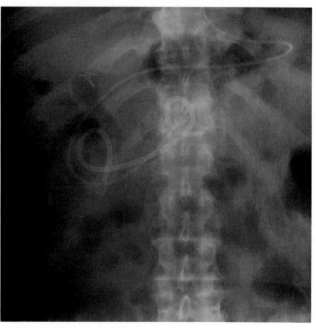

A

B

Figure 15-70   Subacute necrotizing pancreatitis, initial episode in an 82-year-old man. **A:** Portal venous phase 5-mm computed tomography (CT) image demonstrates a heterogeneous, gas containing collection replacing portions of the head and neck. A transpapillary endoprosthesis is in place without adequate drainage of the collection. **B:** Endoscopic transduodenal naso-pancreatic irrigation catheter and double J stent were placed. (*continued*)

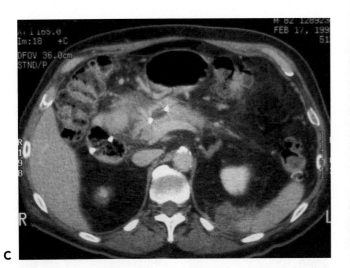

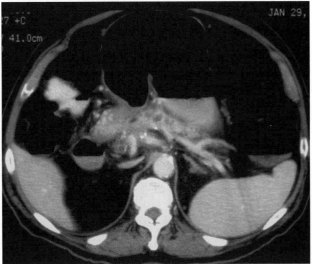

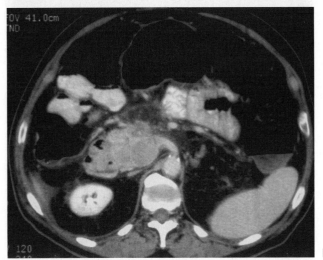

Figure 15-70 (*continued*) **C:** Approximately 5 weeks later, CT demonstrates complete collapse of the necrotic collection. **D:** Two years later, portal venous phase 5-mm CT image through the superior pancreatic head region reveals focal defect produced by necrotizing pancreatitis. Upstream main pancreatic duct dilatation and atrophy are present. **E:** 3 cm caudally, there is a lobular, heterogeneously enhancing mass within the uncinate, which represents biopsy proven nonfunctioning neuroendocrine tumor. In retrospect, the lesion could not be seen 2 years earlier during the episode of acute necrotizing pancreatitis, but tumors should always be sought in elderly patients presenting with a first episode of acute pancreatitis.

pain; occasionally, the symptoms are indirectly related to pancreatic inflammation (Fig. 15-71). Once the diagnosis of acute pancreatitis is established, the treatment of patients is based on the early assessment of disease severity. Seventy percent to 80% of patients with acute pancreatitis have mild disease (Fig. 15-72), and 20% to 30% have severe attacks. Early assessment is critical for predicting which patients are likely to suffer lethal attacks, which occur in 2% to 10% of cases (4,21,28,30,38,39,51,81,204). The increased frequency of death in acute pancreatitis is directly correlated with the development and extent of pancreatic necrosis (Fig. 15-73) (4,21,28,30,38,39,51,81,204). In addition to clinically based numeric disease severity grading systems such as the Ranson score (267) and Acute Physiology and Chronic Health Eval-

uation (APACHE) II assessment (182), both of which are indicators of generalized systemic disease, IV contrast-enhanced CT is essential in the evaluation of patients with severe acute pancreatitis, because it is used to evaluate local pancreatic morphology, most importantly to identify and quantitate pancreatic glandular necrosis (21). Although various laboratory assays of enzymes and proteins released during episodes of severe acute pancreatitis have been studied clinically, including serum trypsinogen, urinary trypsinogen-activated peptide, methemalbumin, cytokines Il-6 and phospholipase A2, C reactive protein and polymorphonuclear cell elastase, direct correlation of these chemicals with the presence and extent of pancreatic necrosis, and thus their clinical utility, have yet to be proven (21).

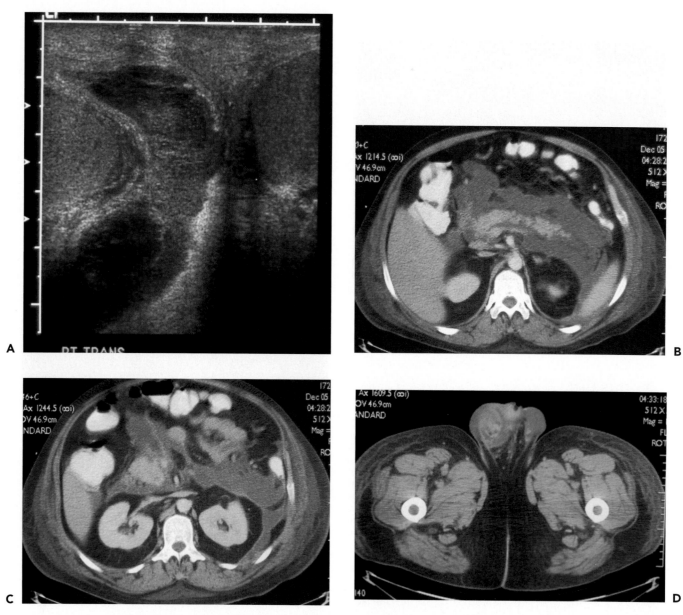

Figure 15-71 Scrotal inflammation as the presenting sign of acute pancreatitis in a 35-year-old man admitted to urology service for abdominal pain and swollen scrotum. **A:** Transverse sonographic image through the superior scrotum demonstrates a large amount of heterogeneous, partially septated fluid surrounding the right testicle; findings led to computed tomography (CT) evaluation. **B:** Contrast-enhanced portal venous phase 5-mm CT image through the pancreas demonstrates a moderate amount of retroperitoneal fluid, which appears partially organized. **C:** Slightly more inferior portal venous phase 5-mm CT image demonstrates fluid tracking into the mesenteric root and left anterior pararenal space. **D:** Transverse 5-mm CT image through the groin demonstrates heterogeneous fluid surrounding the right testicle. Findings are consistent with acute pancreatitis, Grade E, no glandular necrosis, CT severity index (CTSI) of 6, with dissection of fluid into the scrotum.

Mild Acute Pancreatitis

Most patients with acute pancreatitis have clinically mild disease, also called interstitial or edematous pancreatitis. This is a self-limited disease with uneventful recovery, minimal organ dysfunction, and no significant complications. If acute pancreatitis is suspected and is mild by clinical criteria, cross-sectional imaging is not immediately necessary to specifically evaluate the pancreas but may be helpful if the cause of abdominal pain is uncertain. No radiologic evaluation is necessary if the patient's clinical course improves. However, investigation of radiographically detectable potential causes of acute pancreatitis such as cholelithiasis (Fig. 15-74) should commence as soon as clinically feasible. Specifically, prompt identification of gallstones is beneficial, as studies have shown that the morbidity of gallstone pancreatitis is reduced dramatically the sooner cholecystectomy is performed (154). US is the most readily accessible and sensitive imaging test for identifying gallstones,

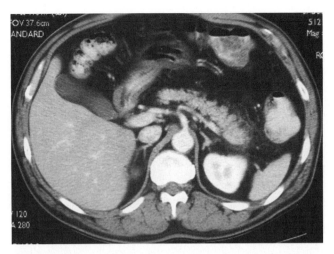

Figure 15-72 Mild acute pancreatitis in a 57-year-old man. Contrast-enhanced portal venous phase 5-mm image through the tail of pancreas demonstrates a small amount of the peripancreatic inflammatory stranding, consistent with grade C pancreatitis. No glandular necrosis is evident, for CT severity index (CTSI) of 4.

ing peripancreatic fat may often appear normal, or there may be mild glandular low attenuation indicating interstitial edema (Fig. 15-75). The pancreas is either normal appearing or minimally enlarged.

Severe Acute Pancreatitis

On the other hand, CECT is the mainstay of imaging in patients with severe acute pancreatitis, which frequently produces local retroperitoneal complications as well as shock, hypoxemia, respiratory failure, renal failure, GI bleeding, and metabolic abnormalities. Severe acute pancreatitis is most often a clinical expression of pancreatic glandular necrosis, which occurs within 24 to 48 hours from the onset of symptoms (21,38,146). Dynamic incremental or helical contrast-enhanced CT with imaging of the pancreas at peak perfusion (23,28,51,174) is the gold standard for the clinical diagnosis of pancreatic necrosis, with an accuracy of 80% to 90%. As with mild pancreatitis, the CECT findings in patients with severe acute pancreatitis mirror the pathology. In severe acute pancreatitis, confluent zones of acinar cell and vascular necrosis with microscopic and sometimes macroscopic ductal disruption are seen, in addition to extensive intra- and extrapancreatic fat necrosis. Turbid, hemorrhagic fluid may enter the retroperitoneal and peritoneal cavities (23).

CT Severity Index in Patients with Acute Pancreatitis

Balthazar et al. (25) first attempted in 1985 to correlate CT findings in patients with acute pancreatitis to clinical follow-up, morbidity, and mortality (25). In those patients whose initial CT demonstrated one or more peripancreatic fluid collections (Balthazar Grade D and E, respectively), a

which may not be seen on contrast enhanced CT (CECT) due to the similar density of gallstones and surrounding bile. MRCP is a very sensitive test for biliary stone detection (31,276) but is more expensive and not as readily available to emergently evaluate patients with acute pancreatitis. With mild acute pancreatitis pathologically, there is minimal interstitial edema with occasional microscopic acinar cell necrosis. No macroscopic acinar cell necrosis occurs, but necrosis of intra- and extrapancreatic adipose tissue may occur (23,28,51). Imaging findings reflect this pathology. Should contrast-enhanced CT be performed on patients with mild pancreatitis, the pancreas and surround-

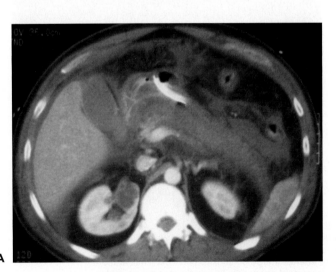 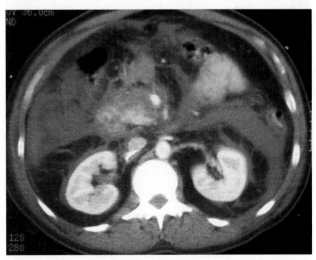

A B

Figure 15-73 Severe acute pancreatitis secondary to ethanol abuse in a 37-year-old man. A: Contrast-enhanced portal venous phase 7-mm computed tomography image demonstrates absence of enhancement throughout the majority of the pancreas involving the neck, body, and tail. B: Portal venous phase image 3.5 cm inferiorly demonstrates a minimal amount of enhancing pancreatic glandular tissue in the head region. Acute fluid collection is seen within the left and right anterior pararenal space, and extends into the transverse mesocolon. Findings are consistent with greater than 50% gland necrosis, greater than two fluid collections, (Balthazar E) for CT severity index (CTSI) of 10.

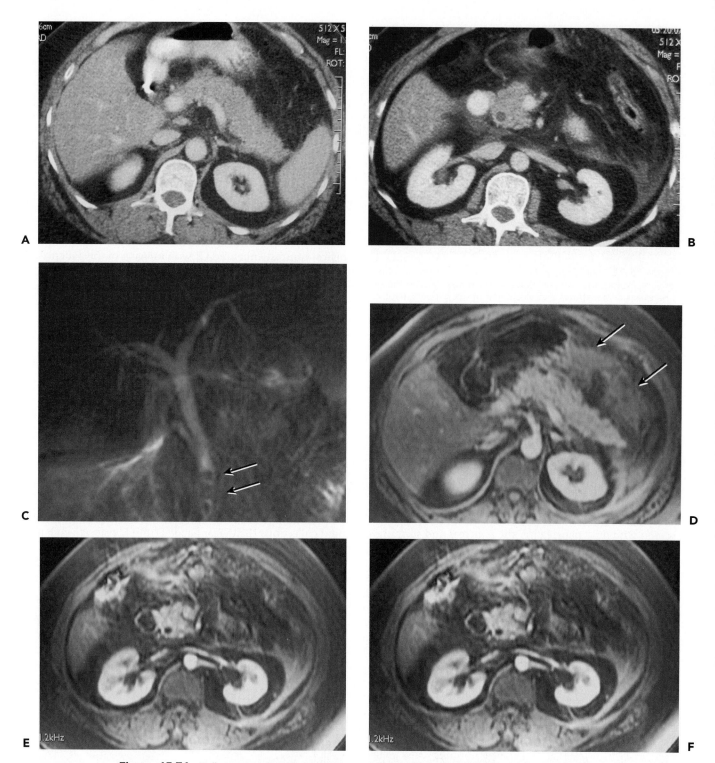

Figure 15-74 Gallstone pancreatitis with increasing severity in a 48-year-old woman. **A:** Contrast-enhanced portal venous phase 5-mm computed tomography (CT) image through the pancreatic body and tail demonstrates a small amount of inflammatory stranding surrounding the pancreatic head region superiorly and pancreatic tail posteriorly. **B:** More inferior image on same day shows small amount of inflammatory fluid tracking into the left anterior pararenal space. **C:** Magnetic resonance cholangiopancreatography (MRCP) 5-cm slab angled coronal image next day demonstrates multifaceted low signal distal common bile duct stones (*arrows*) and mild biliary dilatation. **D:** Axial intravenous gadolinium-enhanced fat-suppressed spoiled gradient echo (SPGR) image shows normal enhancement of the pancreatic body and tail, and fluid tracking anteriorly within the retroperitoneal fat (*arrows*). Slightly inferior image **E:** shows fluid within the retroperitoneum tracking into the left anterior pararenal space. **F:** One week later, portal venous phase contrast-enhanced CT through the body and tail region demonstrates increasing fluid, similar to that seen on the axial MR images.

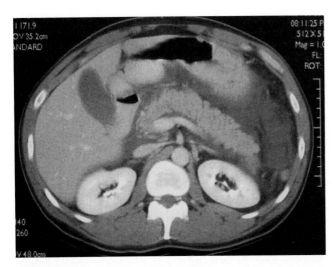

Figure 15-75 Mild acute pancreatitis in a 34-year-old man with ethanol abuse. Contrast-enhanced portal venous phase 5-mm image through the pancreas demonstrates normal pancreatic glandular enhancement throughout, with low attenuation fluid surrounding the pancreas and extending into the left anterior pararenal space. Findings are consistent with grade D pancreatitis, no necrosis, and CT severity index (CTSI) of 5.

CT evaluation of pancreatitis severity was achieved when Kivisaari et al. (174) reported that areas of diminished CT attenuation values identified on IV contrast-enhanced incremental dynamic CT correlated with surgically proven areas of pancreatic glandular necrosis. Subsequent authors confirmed the correlation, demonstrating that CT has an overall sensitivity of 100% for the detection of extensive pancreatic necrosis and a sensitivity of 50% if only minor necrotic areas were present at surgery (21). The extent of pancreatic necrosis is the most important indicator of disease severity. Patients with less than 30% glandular necrosis (Fig. 15-77) exhibited no mortality and a 48% morbidity rate, whereas those with larger areas of necrosis (30% to 50% and more than 50%) were associated with a morbidity rate of 75% to 100% and a mortality rate of 11% to 25% (26). A CT scoring system combining the pancreatitis grade and amount of necrosis was developed by Balthazar et al. (21,26) in 1990 in an effort to provide a more accurate imaging prognosticator of disease severity. On a scale of 1 to 10, patients were assigned 0 to 4 points for grade of pancreatitis A to E, and to this, 2, 4, or 6 points were added, corresponding to less than 30%, 30% to 50%, or more than 50% gland necrosis, respectively. A CT severity index (CTSI) score of 7 to 10 yielded a mortality rate of 17% and a complication rate of 92%. Recently, modifications of the CTSI were suggested to incorporate imaging evidence of extrapancreatic disease in patients with acute pancreatitis. This simplified method of assessment correlated more closely with outcome parameters such as length of hospital stay and need for drainage procedures, with a similar interobserver variability in calculation compared with the original CTSI (232).

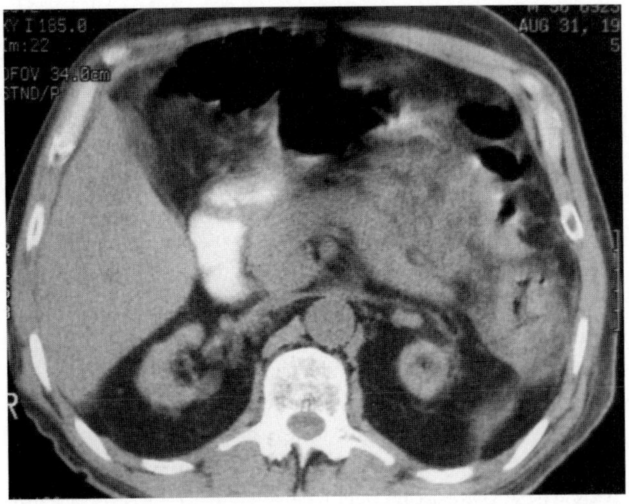

morbidity rate of 54% and a mortality rate of 14% were documented, compared with those patients with a normal or mildly enlarged pancreas (grades A and B) and those with mild peripancreatic inflammatory stranding (grade C), who, combined, had no mortality and only a 4% morbidity rate. This evaluation was and still today may be performed without IV contrast enhancement, but if performed in this way it renders no information about the presence of pancreatic necrosis (Fig. 15-76). A major improvement in the

Figure 15-76 Noncontrast pancreatitis evaluation in a 56-year-old man with renal failure who presents with abdominal pain. A 5-mm oral-contrast-only computed tomography image through the pancreas demonstrates heterogeneous fluid extending in the left retroperitoneum anteriorly from the pancreas, surrounding the descending colon in the left anterior pararenal space. Findings are consistent with grade D pancreatitis. No assessment of necrosis can be made without intravenous contrast in this patient.

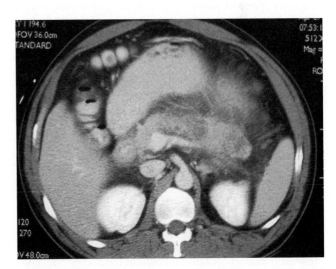

Figure 15-77 Acute pancreatitis with focal, less than 30% gland necrosis. Portal venous phase 5-mm image through the pancreatic body demonstrates focal 2 cm area of decreased enhancement at the body tail junction. Strandy acute fluid is seen within the retroperitoneal fat, and extends inferiorly into the mesenteric root. Findings are consistent with grade D pancreatitis and limited necrosis for a CT severity index (CTSI) of 5.

Recommendations for imaging patients with acute pancreatitis include an initial CECT obtained on presentation or early in the workup of the following patients: those in whom the diagnosis is in doubt, those with hyperamylasemia and severe clinical pancreatitis, defined as a patient with Ranson's score greater than 3 or APACHE II score greater than 8, those with no demonstrable clinical improvement after 72 hours of conservative therapy, and those patients who initially improved but then suffered clinical deterioration (23). Follow-up CECT is recommended every 7 to 10 days in patients with severe acute pancreatitis or more frequently for clinical deterioration or failure to show clinical improvement. Complications such as hemorrhage into the collection (see Fig. 15-10), splenic artery pseudoaneurysm formation, or colonic necrosis are readily depicted by CECT. In addition, CECT at the time of hospital discharge may be useful to confirm reasonable resolution of the inflammation and to establish baseline acute fluid collections. If the patient is unable to receive IV iodinated contrast, a CT using high-density oral contrast may help define the degree of acute fluid accumulation but it will not render any information regarding the presence of pancreatic necrosis. To reiterate, the need for IV contrast during follow-up CT is not as critical and studies performed with oral but no IV contrast may be adequate to follow the size of a pancreatic collection once the diagnosis of necrosis has been established (203,354).

The effects of IV iodinated contrast required for CECT on the human pancreas are not precisely known. Investigators have demonstrated deleterious effects of IV contrast material on the pancreas in rats (98,295,349). These authors showed that iodinated contrast produces decreased total capillary flow within the pancreas in rats with experimentally induced pancreatitis and concluded that IV contrast media may convert borderline pancreatic ischemia to irreversible necrosis. To date there have been no prospective studies of these effects in humans. However, a retrospective clinical study on patients with severe pancreatitis showed that the length of hospitalization and severity of pancreatitis was worse in patients who had received IV contrast medium during CT versus those who had no CT or who had CT without IV contrast (211). Saifudden et al. (290) first suggested that IV gadolinium-enhanced MRI may have the potential for demonstrating the presence of necrosis when the patient is scanned early in the clinical course of pancreatitis. More recently, in a study comparing interobserver agreement and correlation of contrast-enhanced CT, nonenhanced MRI, and enhanced MRI of the pancreas in patients with acute pancreatitis, better linear correlation between findings on MRI and patient morbidity rate, compared with contrast-enhanced CT, was demonstrated (183). The authors of this study suggested that because of the potential risk of iodinated IV contrast to humans, MRI may be a more prudent means of imaging all patients with severe acute pancreatitis, especially during follow-up of fluid collections associated with necrosis. Unless specif-

ically contraindicated due to severe allergic history or acutely elevated serum creatinine, we continue to use nonionic iodinated IV contrast medium in all patients being evaluated for severe acute pancreatitis. We also feel that the more widely accepted and available means of follow-up in patients with renal dysfunction, once the initial contrast-enhanced CT has been obtained, is unenhanced CT. In patients with renal dysfunction or other contraindication to iodinated contrast, MRI is appropriate for evaluation any time during the course of the patient's illness.

International Symposium on Acute Pancreatitis

A clinically based classification system for acute pancreatitis was established during the International Symposium on Acute Pancreatitis held in Atlanta, Georgia in 1992 (Atlanta Symposium). To facilitate improved clinical care of individual patients with acute pancreatic inflammation and to guide academicians seeking to compare populations with this complex disease, experts in surgery, gastroenterology, pathology, internal medicine, anatomy, and radiology from around the world met and created standard definitions for findings in patients with mild and severe acute pancreatitis. Although other radiologic examinations may demonstrate abnormalities in patients with acute pancreatitis, such as pleural effusion on chest radiograph or a diffusely enlarged and hypoechoic gland on transabdominal sonography, IV contrast-enhanced CT has greatly improved and changed the clinical management of this condition because of its ability to consistently and accurately depict the extent of local pancreatic injury (21). A monophasic single or multidetector acquisition of 5-mm thick images obtained through the abdomen and pelvis in the portal venous phase, using high-density oral contrast, is appropriate for evaluation in patients suspected of having acute pancreatitis. For staging purposes, more reliable results are obtained when the CT is performed 48 to 72 hours after the onset of an acute attack. The contrast-enhanced CT findings in patients with acute pancreatitis and the specific types of pancreatic and peripancreatic abnormalities defined by the Atlanta Symposium (23,28,51) are now described in further detail.

Acute Fluid Collections

An acute fluid collection attributable to acute pancreatitis is defined as a collection of enzyme-rich pancreatic juice that usually develops in the periphery of the gland, lacks a well-defined wall, and may dissect throughout the retroperitoneum, usually into the anterior pararenal spaces (left greater than right), transverse mesocolon, and mesenteric root. These collections occur early (within 48 hours) in the course of pancreatitis in 30% to 50% of patients and resolve spontaneously 50% of the time (Fig. 15-78). Conversely, the remainder of these acute fluid collections may evolve over time and contribute to the formation of pseudocysts, abscesses, or necrotic collections (Fig. 15-79). In severe acute pancreatitis, the acute fluid collection may be turbid and hemorrhagic. The extension of the collections to the anterior

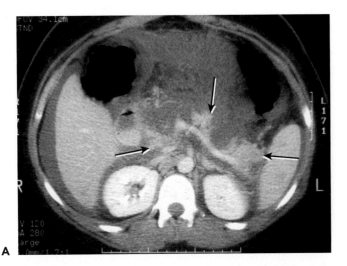

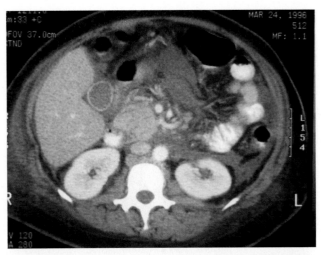

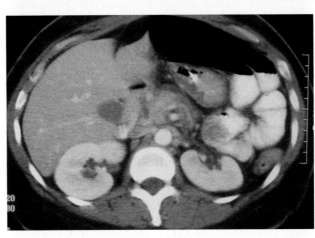

Figure 15-78 Acute fluid collection associated with severe acute pancreatitis in a 38-year-old woman with gallstone pancreatitis; spontaneous resolution. **A:** Contrast-enhanced portal venous phase 5-mm image through the pancreatic neck, body, and tail demonstrates a large amount of low attenuation fluid within the pancreatic bed, extending into the left anterior pararenal space, as well as the peritoneal cavity. Small wisps of enhancing residual pancreatic parenchyma are evident (*arrows*), but extensive necrosis of the body and tail is seen. **B:** The fluid dissected into the mesenteric root inferiorly, where there is some enhancement within the pancreatic head. Findings are consistent with Balthazar grade E pancreatitis, and greater than 50% necrosis, for CT severity index (CTSI) of 10. **C:** Contrast-enhanced portal venous phase 7-mm scan 6 months later demonstrates resolution of acute inflammation with enhancement of the residual pancreas in the superior head region. The pancreas in the body and tail region was no longer evident.

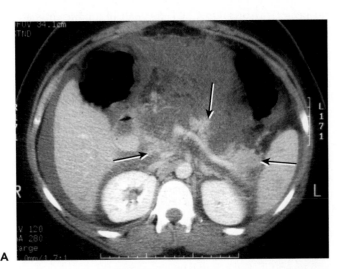

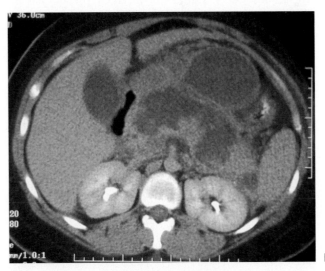

Figure 15-79 Severe acute pancreatitis with necrosis evolving over a 6-month period in a 23-year-old woman with gallstone pancreatitis. **A:** Initial contrast-enhanced portal venous phase 5-mm image demonstrates low density retroperitoneal fluid collection replacing portions of the pancreatic head anteriorly, with fluid extending into the transverse mesocolon, right and left anterior pararenal spaces, and peritoneum. Focal areas of residual enhancing pancreas in the posterior head, tail, and body regions are present (arrows). **B:** One week later, excretory phase contrast-enhanced computed tomography (CT) demonstrates partial organization of the collection with multiple septations. (*continued*)

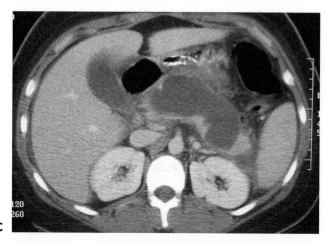

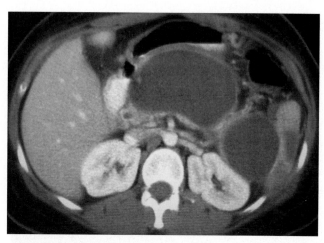

C D

Figure 15-79 (*continued*) **C:** Two weeks later, contrast-enhanced portal venous phase 7-mm image demonstrates a more homogeneous appearing fluid collection within the retroperitoneum, replacing portions of the pancreas that underwent necrosis on the initial CT. The patient remained clinically stable. **D:** Contrast-enhanced portal venous phase CT 7 months later demonstrates well demarcated fluid collections replacing the pancreatic body anteriorly and extending laterally from the tail. At endoscopic drainage, components were completely liquefied.

pararenal space may produce the Grey Turner's sign, flank ecchymosis, and the tracking of fluid into the gastrohepatic and subsequently the falciform ligament may result in Cullen's sign, periumbilical ecchymosis (220); these are classic clinical signs of severe acute pancreatitis.

Acute Pseudocyst

An acute pseudocyst is defined as a collection of pancreatic juice confined by a nonepithelialized wall of granulation tissue. An acute pseudocyst occurs as a result of acute pancreatitis or trauma, and requires at least four weeks to form (Fig. 15-80). On IV contrast-enhanced CT, pseudocysts ap-

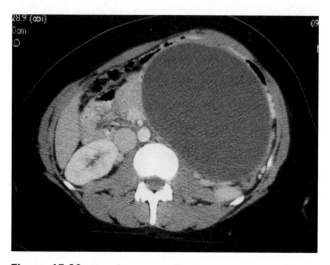

Figure 15-80 Pseudocyst complicating acute pancreatitis in a 27-year-old woman 3 months after gallstone pancreatitis. Contrast-enhanced portal venous phase 5-mm image through the midabdomen demonstrates a homogeneous 14 × 11 cm fluid collection extending inferiorly from the pancreatic tail region. Displacement of the stomach superiorly, left kidney posteriorly, and the bowel to the right is noted.

pear as well circumscribed, thin-walled, homogeneously low-attenuation collections adjacent to, or occasionally within, an otherwise normal appearing pancreas. Pseudocysts may produce symptoms due to gastric outlet or biliary obstruction (Fig. 15-81).

Pancreatic Abscess

A pancreatic abscess is defined as a circumscribed intraabdominal collection of pus in close proximity to the pancreas (Fig. 15-82), resulting from an episode of acute pancreatitis or trauma. Like acute pseudocysts, these collections require at least 4 weeks to form and typically have little or no necrotic debris. On CECT, the wall of a pancreatic abscess may appear thicker or more irregular than the well delineated but thin wall of the pseudocyst, and both collections have a homogeneously low attenuation center.

Pancreatic Necrosis

According to the symposium, pancreatic necrosis is defined as diffuse or focal area(s) of nonviable pancreatic parenchyma, which is typically associated with peripancreatic fat necrosis. Because dynamic IV contrast-enhanced CT was at the time (and remains today) the gold standard for the clinical diagnosis of pancreatic necrosis, the definition was also given in terms of imaging. Pancreatic necrosis is present when there are one or more focal areas of nonenhancing pancreatic parenchyma comprising greater than 30% of the gland, as demonstrated by dynamic contrast-enhanced CT. The nonenhancing areas correspond to nonviable pancreatic tissue (168). As the degree of necrosis increases, so does the specificity and sensitivity of CECT for its detection (21,23,51,354). Although CT scans performed to evaluate acute pancreatitis typically do not include unenhanced images through the pancreas, a homogeneous increase to Hounsfield numbers of 100 to 150 should be seen

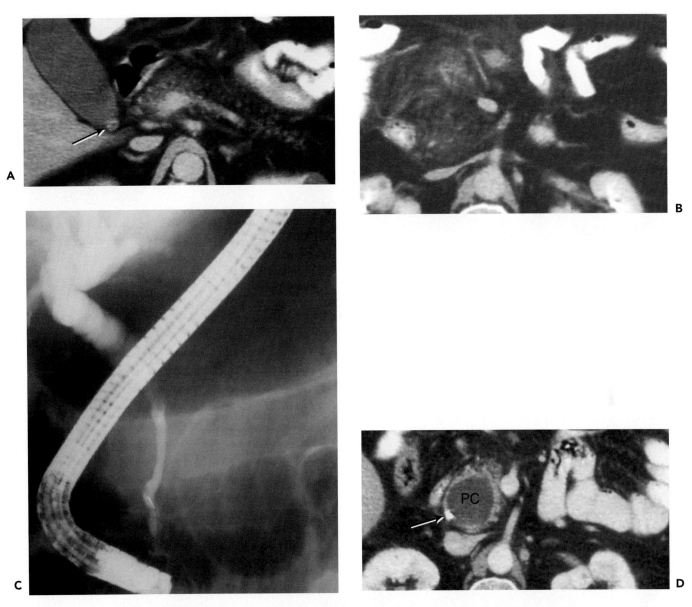

Figure 15-81 Pseudocyst complicating acute pancreatitis, leading to obstruction of the common bile duct. **A:** Late portal venous phase computed tomography (CT) image through the pancreas demonstrates normal fatty infiltration of tail and body region. Note blurred appearance of the interdigitating fat of the head and neck due to acute inflammation, and gallstone (*arrow*) in the gallbladder neck. **B:** 3 cm inferiorly, inflammatory stranding is seen extending from the inferior pancreatic head region into the mesenteric root, Grade C pancreatitis. **C:** Eight weeks later, patient had persistent elevated bilirubin. Endoscopic retrograde cholangiopancreatography spot radiograph with injection into the distal common bile duct demonstrates smooth narrowing of the lower half of the bile duct through the superior pancreatic head and suprapancreatic regions. The transition from smoothly narrowed to dilated proximal duct occurs at the level of the scope. Faintly seen pancreatic duct appears normal. **D:** Portal venous phase CT image after endoscopic biliary stent (*arrow*) placement demonstrates smooth round 3.5-cm pseudocyst (PC) within the pancreatic head, which was responsible for the mass effect on the distal duct.

in normal glands. Any area of the pancreas with Hounsfield numbers of ≤30 indicates decreased blood perfusion (ischemia) and correlates with the development of necrosis (21). If Hounsfield unit measurements are not possible, an estimate of pancreatic enhancement may be made by comparing the attenuation of the gland to the spleen. In the absence of pancreatic necrosis, the pancreas and spleen should be similar in attenuation on portal venous phase images (see Fig. 15-72). Potential pitfalls in the identification of pancreatic necrosis include apparent diminished enhancement value in patients with normal fatty infiltration of the gland as well as in patients with diffuse parenchymal edema in less severe, interstitial pancreatitis. Small intrapancreatic focal fluid collections are sometimes

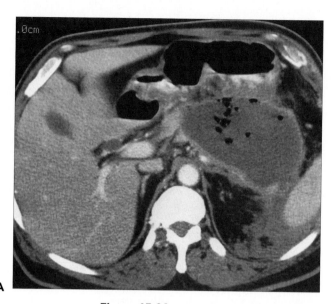
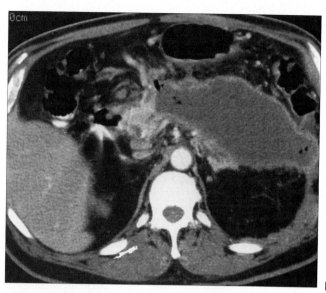

Figure 15-82 Pancreatic abscess. **A** and **B**: Two scans at a level inferior to the body and tail of the pancreas show a well-defined fluid collection with typical changes of an abscess. Gas bubbles are noted throughout the high-viscosity pus, which was subsequently drained percutaneously successfully.

seen in patients with acute pancreatitis and should not be mistaken for focal areas of necrosis; this distinction may not be possible unless previous or follow up CT images are available for comparison (21). Pancreatic necrosis typically is accompanied by gross peripancreatic fat necrosis, but the reverse is not true. This phenomenon probably explains the 22% incidence of local complications in patients without pancreatic necrosis but with peripancreatic fluid collections (201). The greater the amount of pancreatic necrosis, the more likely the pancreatic duct will be disrupted (256), contributing to increased morbidity and mortality. Necrosis involving the neck and body of the gland, central cavitary necrosis (29) is frequently associated with duct disruption (Fig. 15-83) (28,103,256). Between 20% and 30% of all patients with severe acute pancreatitis have necrotizing pancreatitis (51). Review of autopsy and surgical series indicate that pancreatic necrosis and its complications account for 70% to 86% of deaths from acute pancreatitis (256).

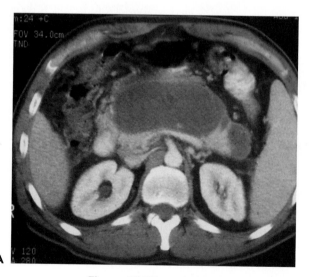
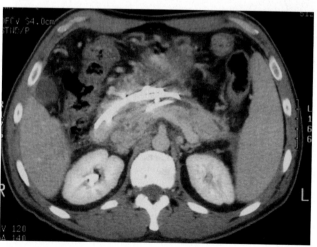

Figure 15-83 Transduodenal endoscopic drainage of organized pancreatic necrosis. **A**: A 7-mm portal venous phase computed tomography (CT) image demonstrates organized, slightly heterogeneous collection replacing portions of the pancreatic neck, body, and tail. Note adjacent relationship of the right border of the collection with the second portion of the duodenum, ideal for transduodenal drainage. **B**: Six weeks later, 5-mm excretory phase CT image demonstrates collapse of the cavity around the transduodenal double J stents. A transpapillary stent is also in place.

Infected Pancreatic Necrosis

Infected necrosis is defined as culture positivity of infected pancreatic and/or peripancreatic necrotic tissue. Infection of pancreatic necrosis occurs in 36% to 71% of all patients with pancreatic necrosis (36,52,271) usually occurring in the second to third week following the onset of acute pancreatitis (Fig. 15-84); the infection is typically polymicrobial (36). The devitalized pancreatic parenchyma is an ideal medium for infection and abscess formation (256). Gas bubbles within the collection suggest spontaneous infection, but the absence of gas does not exclude infection of the necrosis. Likewise, spontaneous fistulization to bowel may introduce air into a previously sterile necrotic collection (Fig. 15-85). Percutaneous aspiration of the necrotic collection for Gram stain and culture using sonographic or CT guidance (Fig. 15-86) is often necessary to distinguish between infected and sterile pancreatic necrosis. This procedure is safe and accurate, with a sensitivity of 96% and a specificity of 99% (23), and is recommended in patients with necrotizing pancreatitis who clinically deteriorate or fail to improve, because it may be impossible to distinguish these two entities clinically. In a recent study evaluating the role of gallium single photon emission computed tomography (SPECT) imaging in a population of patients with severe acute pancreatitis, uptake was seen in 18 of 18 patients with infected pancreatic collections (infected necrosis or abscesses), and in none of 5 patients with sterile pancreatic collections. No correlation between the presence or absence of necrosis and gallium avidity was found. The authors of this study suggest that gallium SPECT may be a useful adjunct to CT in the evaluation of patients with severe acute pancreatitis, especially to help guide intervention (351).

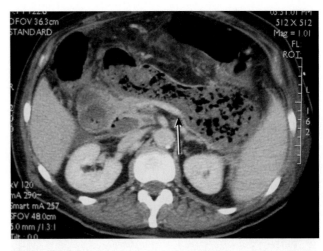

Figure 15-84 Infected pancreatic necrosis in a 60-year-old man with 1 week hospitalization for severe acute pancreatitis. Portal venous phase 5-mm computed tomography image demonstrates a 12 × 7 cm heterogeneous, gas containing collection replacing the pancreas anterior to the splenic vein (*arrow*), consistent with infected pancreatic necrosis.

The treatment of patients with acute necrotizing pancreatitis continues to evolve since the Atlanta Symposium. As conservative medical management of patients with pancreatic necrosis has gained popularity over the past decade, more patients who survive the acute event of severe necrotizing pancreatitis and require no immediate therapeutic surgical or radiologic interventions, frequently undergo repeat imaging. The serial CECTs in these patients demonstrate evolution of the acute pancreatic necrosis and acute fluid collections to a more organized, partially encapsulated, multiseptate state (see Fig. 15-79) (33,256). After the initial CECT, necrosis (whether sterile or infected)

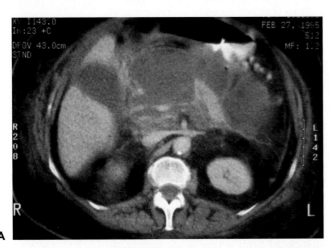

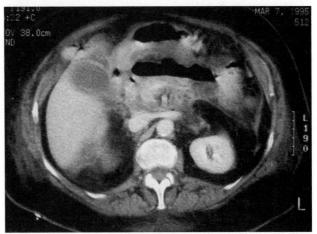

A   **B**

Figure 15-85 Severe subacute pancreatitis with spontaneous gas in a 79-year-old woman. **A:** Contrast-enhanced portal venous phase computed tomography (CT) image through the pancreas reveals a focal segment of enhancing pancreatic body, with a partially septated heterogeneous fluid collection replacing the neck and superior head region. Findings are consistent with subacute necrotic collection, pancreatitis grade D, with 30% to 50% necrosis, indicating CT severity index (CTSI) of 7. **B:** Contrast-enhanced portal venous phase 8 days later, without drainage therapy, demonstrates marked reduction in size of collection, which now contains an air–fluid level. This likely represents spontaneous fistulization to bowel and partial evacuation.

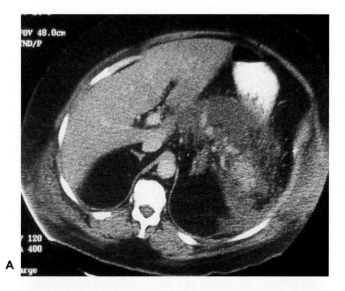

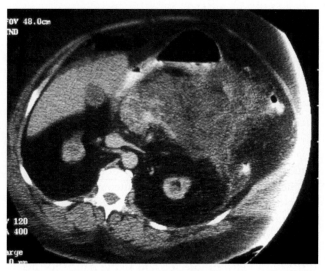

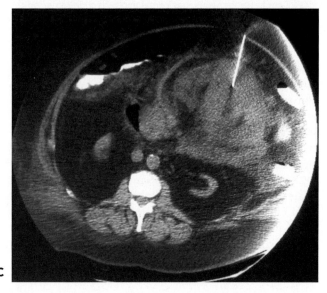

Figure 15-86 Computed tomography (CT) guided needle aspiration for potential infected pancreatic necrosis. **A:** Late portal venous phase 7-mm CT image demonstrates acute fluid collection, with little enhancement of the pancreatic body and tail. **B:** More caudal image at the level of the splenic vein and portal confluence reveals larger heterogeneous acute fluid collection with minimal enhancement of the pancreatic head. Findings are consistent with grade D pancreatitis, greater than 50% necrosis, CT severity index (CTSI) of 9. **C:** Three weeks later on supportive therapy, the patient's condition deteriorated. A 10-mm axial CT image demonstrates the tip of a spinal needle within the collection, with material aspirated for Gram stain and culture.

most commonly produces a low attenuation or near fluid density collection replacing a portion of the pancreas. The collections occupy and expand within the pancreatic bed and, rather than being located in a peripancreatic location, replace portions of the gland which initially demonstrated necrosis (Figs. 15-83 and 15-87). The low attenuation of the collections on these later CECTs may often be misleading in that extensive residual solid necrotic debris may not be discernible until nonsurgical drainage is undertaken, and the liquefied portion of the collection is removed.

The distinction between this subacute type of necrotic collection, referred to as organized pancreatic necrosis by Baron et al., and pseudocysts is important, regardless of title. Near universal failure of drainage (including endoscopic, percutaneous, and even closed surgical drainage) occurs when partially liquefied necrotic collections are mistaken for typical acute pseudocysts (34,128,185,203). This is due to the inability to remove solid debris through

standard drainage catheters. Thus, before labeling a low-attenuation pancreatic collection as a pseudocyst, a diligent search for evidence of pancreatic necrosis should be made and often requires evaluation of prior scans. The presence of necrosis is established by decreased enhancement of the pancreas on the initial CECT, and subsequent evolution of acute fluid collections and nonenhancing pancreas to a better defined low-attenuation (often homogeneous) collection *replacing* the pancreas. Morgan et al. demonstrated that MRI was more accurate than CECT for demonstrating the complex nature of "fluid" collections associated with severe acute pancreatitis (229). Fat suppressed T2-weighted spin echo MR images depict the gross solid and liquefied components of pancreatic necrosis in the subacute setting, and require no contrast (Figs. 15-87 and 15-88). MRI may be most helpful as an adjunct to CECT in patients in whom necrosis is suspected and drainage is contemplated.

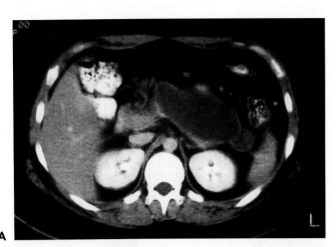
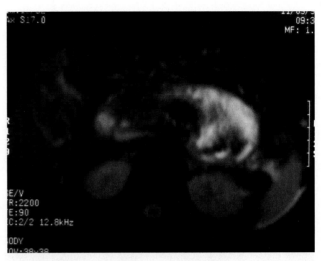

A   B

Figure 15-87 Organized pancreatic necrosis in a 21-year-old woman with gallstone pancreatitis, referred for "pseudocyst drainage." **A:** Contrast-enhanced computed tomography of the abdomen approximately 8 weeks after onset of pancreatitis demonstrates a homogeneous well encapsulated fluid collection anterior to the splenic vein. **B:** Prior to drainage, T2-weighted fat suppressed magnetic resonance image of the same region demonstrates marked heterogeneity within the collection, with high signal fluid as well as large areas of low signal soft tissue consistent with persistent solid debris.

Pancreatic Hemorrhage

Pancreatic necrosis is often hemorrhagic because of leakage from small veins (256). CT will demonstrate areas of increased attenuation within the pancreatic or peripancreatic collection (see Fig. 15-10). Pseudoaneurysms may form when arterial walls are affected by necrosis or autodigestive enzymes. Catastrophic bleeding may occur, leading to death.

Computed Tomography Guidance for Pancreatic Interventions

In addition to delineating a pathway for percutaneous needle aspiration of necrotic collections or abscesses for Gram stain and culture, CT may be used before, during, and after pancreatic interventions. Drainage of the variety of collections that may arise from acute pancreatitis may be performed percutaneously, endoscopically, surgically, or by a combination of approaches. A meaningful discussion of pancreatic interventional options is beyond the scope of this chapter, but several informative references are available (1,23,30,33,34,38,52,88,103,185,271,344,345). Prior to drainage, CT readily demonstrates the location, size, and relationship of the collection to adjacent critical structures. In the case of percutaneous drainage, CT guidance may be used during placement of one or more catheters. When endoscopic drainage is used CT is critical in demonstrating the approximation of the collection to the intestinal lumen (gastric or duodenal) through which catheters may be placed (see Fig. 15-83). The presence of loculations, septations, and solid debris when depicted on CT immediately prior to catheter placement may alter how many and what caliber catheters and or stents are used (see Fig. 15-88). Again, in the case of necrotic collections, CT may underesti-

mate the complexity of the collections, and when a patient's original CT demonstrates significant unenhanced pancreatic glandular tissue, the physician performing the drainage must be made aware that the potential for solid debris is present. Over time, as liquefaction occurs the relative amount of solid debris within the collection decreases. Historically, surgeons performing necrosectomies attempted to wait 4 to 6 weeks after onset of necrotizing pancreatitis, if clinically possible, to allow necrotic tissues to undergo liquefactive necrosis (Fig. 15-89) and make the distinction between dead and viable tissue more apparent at operation.

Once a drainage procedure has been performed, follow-up CT is critical in assessing the success of the procedure. The presence of residual solid debris may prompt more aggressive irrigation of the cavity, additional percutaneous or endoscopic procedures, or surgery. Complete evacuation of the collection may be confirmed once drain output diminishes. Reaccumulation of fluid demonstrated on CT after catheters have been removed may suggest ductal communication with the collection, a condition that renders cure by percutaneous methods difficult (256). In general, the development of a persistent pancreaticocutaneous fistula after percutaneous drainage of pancreatic fluid collections correlates with the severity of the pancreatitis initially (101). Frequency and length for follow-up CT after interventions depend on the type of collection. Collections such as typical pseudocysts may be completely evacuated within days (185), whereas necrotic collections may require drainage intervals of several months' duration (103). Focal parenchymal defects, fistulae, and pseudoaneurysm formation (Fig. 15-90) are well depicted on CT after the acute episode subsides.

Magnetic Resonance Imaging in Acute Pancreatitis

The diagnosis of acute pancreatitis on MR images relies on the presence of morphologic changes, much the same as CT (300). In mild cases, the pancreas may appear normal or slightly enlarged. Homogeneous high signal is present throughout the gland on T1 fat-suppressed images. Strandy peripancreatic fluid may be demonstrated as low signal intensity on a background of high-intensity retroperitoneal fat on noncontrast spoiled GRE images, or conversely as high signal intensity strands of fluid surrounding the low signal pancreas on a background of low signal intensity retroperitoneal fat on T2 fat suppressed images (see Fig. 15-74). In cases of severe acute pancreatitis, the presence of fluid is similarly demonstrated. In addition, pancreatic necrosis may be evaluated with dynamic IV gadolinium-enhanced T1 fast spoiled gradient images, with areas of nonenhancement corresponding to areas of gland necrosis (183,290,348).

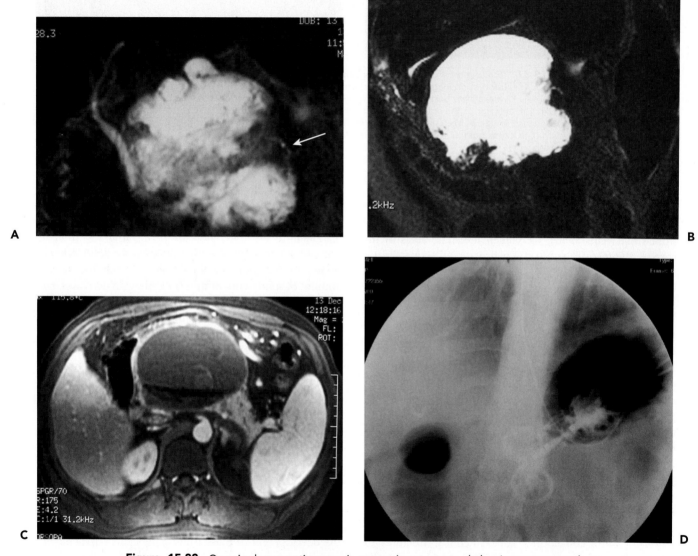

Figure 15-88 Organized pancreatic necrosis magnetic resonance cholangiopancreatography (MRCP) in a 42-year-old man, 8 weeks after onset acute pancreatitis, with failure to thrive. **A:** A 2.5-cm angled coronal half-Fourier acquisition single-shot turbo spin echo (HASTE) MRCP image demonstrates an 8 × 10 cm heterogeneous fluid signal collection in midline, to the right of the slightly dilated common bile duct. A portion of normal caliber pancreatic duct in the tail is evident *(arrow)*. Heterogeneous nature of the collection is consistent with fluid and residual necrotic debris. **B:** Thin section HASTE angled coronal image shows relationship of pancreatic duct in the tail to the collection, and more irregularity of the solid debris along the inferior margin. **C:** Axial intravenous gadolinium enhanced fast spoiled gradient (FSPGR) fat-suppressed T1-weighted gradient breath-hold image demonstrates organized pancreatic necrotic collection replacing the superior pancreatic head, neck, and body, with residual normal pancreatic tissue seen in the tail. **D:** Spot radiograph during endoscopic drainage shows two double J transgastric stents and nasal pancreatic irrigation catheter, typically used for endoscopic drainage of complex collections associated with pancreatic necrosis.

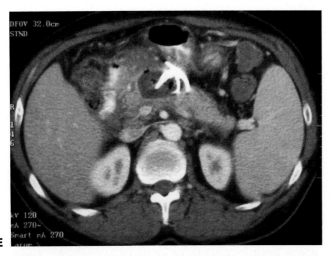

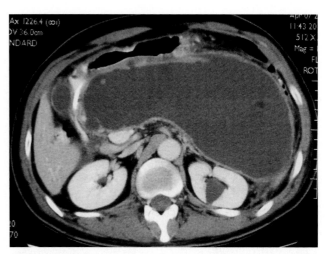

Figure 15-88 (*continued*) **E:** One month later after transgastric endoscopic drainage, the size of the collection has been markedly reduced with only a small amount of fluid seen surrounding the pancreatic portion of the double J stents.

Figure 15-89 Organized pancreatic necrosis in a 48-year-old man 8 weeks after onset severe acute pancreatitis with failure to thrive. A 5-mm portal venous phase computed tomography image demonstrates very large predominantly low attenuation collection replacing the pancreas. Note the low attenuation retroperitoneal fat and faintly visible residual pancreas within the collection. There is marked narrowing of the gastric outlet, but oral contrast does pass into the bowel. Because of the patient's symptoms, limited surgical necrosectomy through the posterior gastric wall was performed; approximately 1000 cc dark liquid and several grams of necrotic debris were removed.

More recently, Lecesne et al. (183) reported excellent correlation of necrosis diagnosed on contrast-enhanced MR compared with contrast-enhanced CT. Interestingly, in this same study, nonenhanced MR images with focal areas of necrosis defined as well-marginated areas of signal intensity different from the signal intensity of the normal pancreas also correlated well with areas of necrosis seen on CT and contrast-enhanced MR images. The calculation of severity based on pancreatic fluid and necrosis (in a method similar to the Balthazar CTSI) was reproducible on MRI and, as previously mentioned, correlated with patient outcome more closely than the CTSI. Heterogeneity of acute fluid collections manifesting as high signal on both T1- and T2-weighted images may be due to proteina-

ceous material or hemorrhage (34,183). The complexity of necrotic pancreatic fluid collections in the acute and subacute stages is much better demonstrated with MRI compared with CT (see Figs. 15-86 and 15-87) (229). Key advantages to MRI in the evaluation of acute pancreatitis include the lack of radiation and potential benefit of lack of nephrotoxicity in these patients, who are often young and may require multiple scans (224).

Ductal structures are excellently depicted with MRCP techniques (31,119,276,311) and may be useful for the

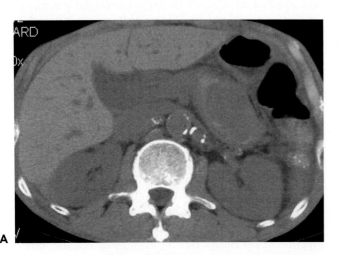

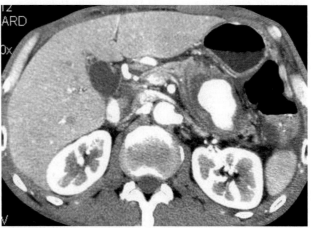

Figure 15-90 Post pancreatitis splenic artery pseudoaneurysm. **A:** Well-circumscribed, ovoid, 4 × 2 cm structure is seen anterior to the body of the pancreas on precontrast computed tomography (CT). The curvilinear high density within the right aspect of the lesion represents fresh clot. **B:** Contrast-enhanced CT through the same level demonstrates enhancement of blood within the lumen of the pseudoaneurysm, surrounded by clot.

identification of choledocholithiasis in cases of gallstone pancreatitis (see Fig. 15-74) or identification of structural anomalies in patients with pancreas divisum. With secretin stimulation, thin, normal main pancreatic ducts and side branches may be visualized. IV secretin injection stimulates the exocrine pancreas to secrete fluid and bicarbonate, resulting in a transient increase in main pancreatic duct diameter, improving visualization. The distension of normal ducts is helpful in identifying pancreas divisum (108,129,205). MRCP using single-shot half-Fourier rapid acquisition relaxation enhancement (RARE) techniques (108) is ideally carried out during the first 5 minutes after secretin injection. Beyond this time, the high signal of fluid entering the duodenum from the pancreatic duct on the heavily T2-weighted images may obscure the ductal structures. The degree of filling of the duodenum with fluid has been used to estimate pancreatic exocrine function (205,208).

Chronic Pancreatitis

Chronic pancreatitis is a disease of prolonged pancreatic inflammation and fibrosis characterized by irreversible morphologic and/or functional abnormalities (292,316). The histologic changes include fibrosis and atrophy of glandular elements. According to the revised classification of pancreatitis from the Marseilles symposium of 1984, acute and chronic pancreatitis are very different diseases and only rarely does acute pancreatitis lead to chronic pancreatitis.

There is a strong association between alcohol abuse and chronic pancreatitis. It is postulated that when the first bout of clinical pancreatitis occurs in patients who are alcoholics of 6 years duration or greater, the pancreas is already diffusely scarred, and the initial bout of alcoholic pancreatitis actually heralds the onset of chronic pancreatitis (189,268,291).

In addition to chronic alcoholic pancreatitis, chronic pancreatitis is found with familial occurrence in kindred with hyperlipidemia, hyperparathyroidism, cystic fibrosis (CF), and cholelithiasis (163). Additionally, there is a familial form of pancreatitis termed hereditary pancreatitis that is thought to be inherited in an autosomal dominant fashion with variable penetrance. The typical clinical features include an early age of onset, with varying degrees of abdominal pain and disability. Complications of endocrine and exocrine pancreatic insufficiency, pseudocyst formation, and adenocarcinoma of the pancreas may develop. The hallmark finding in this form of pancreatitis is the presence of very large calculi within dilated pancreatic ducts, visible on plain radiographs of the abdomen in childhood (163,281). Chronic pancreatitis caused by hyperparathyroidism and pancreas divisum (230) may also be associated with intraductal calculi. Other causes of pancreatitis, including gallstones, drugs, trauma, and viruses, do not characteristically cause pancreatic calcifications (187).

The pathognomonic features on CT in patients with chronic pancreatitis are scattered glandular and ductal calcifications and ductal dilatation (Figs. 15-91 and 15-92). The intraductal calcifications arise from proteinaceous plugs that accumulate calcium carbonate and range in size from microscopic (Fig. 15-93) to greater than 1 cm (187). In a retrospective analysis of 56 patients with documented chronic pancreatitis studied with contrast-enhanced CT examinations, dilatation of the main pancreatic duct was seen in 68% of cases, parenchymal atrophy in 54%, pancreatic calcifications in 50%, fluid collections in 30%, focal pancreatic enlargement in 30%, biliary ductal dilatation in 29%, and alterations in peripancreatic fat or fascia in 16%. In only 7% of the patients were no abnormalities detected (197).

As stated previously, smooth or beaded dilatation of the main pancreatic duct is most commonly associated with carcinoma, whereas irregular dilatation is more frequently seen in chronic pancreatitis. Furthermore, a ratio of duct width to total gland width of less than 0.5 favors the diagnosis of chronic pancreatitis (see Fig. 15-31) (162). Morphologic changes frequently result in a shrunken and atrophic gland surrounding the dilated duct. However, the pancreas is occasionally enlarged, and chronic pancreatitis can even present as a focal, noncalcified mass that by all CT criteria would be indistinguishable from a carcinoma (see Fig. 15-35) (180,237). In a recent study correlating CT and MRI features in patients with chronic pancreatitis presenting as a focal mass, four of seven patients had isoattenuation of the focal mass and the remaining pancreatic tissue on all helical CT sequences, including unenhanced, dynamic pancreatic phase and portal venous phase images. Pathologic evaluation of the mass and the remaining nonenlarged pancreatic parenchyma revealed a similar degree of fibrosis in both areas of the gland. In the same study, three of seven patients had focal masses that were visibly demarcated as hypoattenuating on the pancreatic phase images and similar in density to the remainder of the pancreas on portal venous phase images. In these patients, pathologic evaluation revealed no fibrosis in the nonenlarged portion of the pancreas and typical fibrosis, infiltration of lymphocytes, and reduction in glandular elements in the masslike portion (171). EUS may aid in differentiating focal masses due to pancreatitis from cancer. EUS is equivalent to ERCP in identifying advanced chronic pancreatitis and is more sensitive than ERCP in early stages because it detects parenchymal changes not visible by other techniques (157), including morphologic features of echo-intense septa/ echo-reduced foci (pseudolobularity), ductal irregularities, and calcifications [sensitivity 97%, specificity 60%, positive predictive value (PPV) 94%, negative predictive value (NPV) 75%—with EUS-fine needle biopsy, NPV increases to 100% (135)].

Chronic pancreatitis also can be associated with obstruction of the biliary tree. In most instances, the lumen of the obstructed bile duct tapers gradually (see Fig. 15-34), in contrast to an abrupt transition commonly associated with neoplasm. In an analysis of 51 patients with chronic alcoholic pancreatitis and common duct obstruction, an

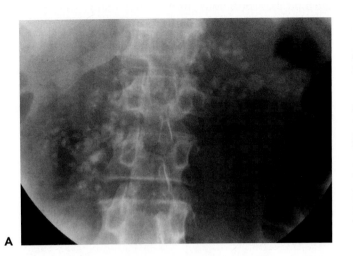

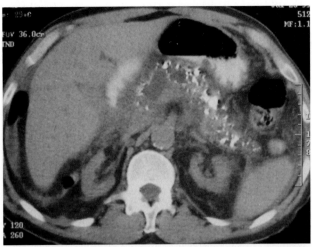

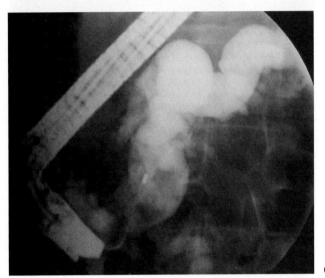

Figure 15-91 Classic severe chronic pancreatitis. **A:** Spot radiograph prior to endoscopic retrograde cholangiopancreatography demonstrates multiple coarse calcifications in the midline upper abdomen, in a distribution consistent with pancreatic calcifications and chronic pancreatitis. **B:** A 5-mm oral-contrast-only computed tomography image demonstrates marked dilatation of the main pancreatic duct in the neck and numerous large calcifications throughout the gland. **C:** Spot radiograph during injection of the pancreatic duct demonstrates severe dilatation of the main duct and side branches with focal filling defects near the ampulla consistent with intraductal calculi.

elevated serum alkaline phosphatase level was the most common abnormal laboratory finding (14). The elevation in serum bilirubin level was never progressive; a rising and falling pattern was most often encountered. A combination of CT evaluation showing a gradually diminishing duct diameter on successive images towards the ampulla, and cholangiography by either ERCP or MRCP, correlated with the clinical laboratory findings, generally will permit differentiation of this type of bile duct obstruction secondary to pancreatitis from that due to neoplasm.

Pseudocysts can occur in both acute pancreatitis and chronic pancreatitis (Fig. 15-94), but have very different origins. When pseudocysts are found in association with ductal dilatation and intraductal calcification, chronic pancreatitis is the underlying disease (Fig. 15-95). Along with hemorrhage and superinfection, another major complication of pseudocyst formation is spontaneous rupture. Pseudocysts may rupture into the peritoneal cavity (with the development of ascites), the extraperitoneal spaces, the pleural cavity, or the GI tract. Pancreatico-pleural fistulas

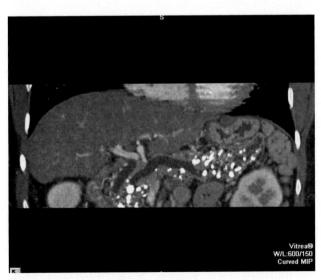

Figure 15-92 Chronic pancreatitis with obstructing stone. Curved planar reformatted image aligned with the main pancreatic duct shows the large obstructing calculus within the duct in the neck region.

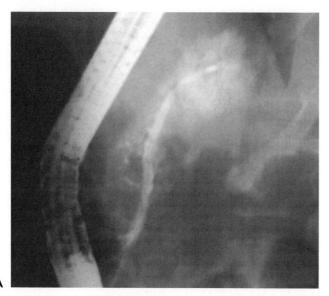

A

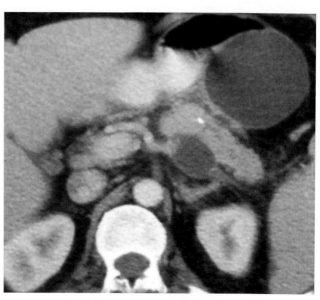

B

Figure 15-93 Less severe chronic pancreatitis in a 51-year-old man. **A:** Spot radiograph during endoscopic retrograde cholangiopancreatography (ERCP) with injection into the pancreatic duct reveals acinarization of the head and neck with abrupt termination of the pancreatic duct in the body. There is irregularity of the main pancreatic duct, dilatation and irregularity of the side branches. However, the abrupt termination of the duct could be due to chronic pancreatitis stricture or mass. **B:** A 7-mm portal venous phase computed tomography image demonstrates a 3-mm focal calcification in the pancreatic body, corresponding to the site of duct cut off on ERCP. Note dilatation of the main pancreatic duct in the tail, upstream from the calcification. Peripancreatic pseudocysts (PC) are also present.

(Fig. 15-96) are most often associated with chronic alcoholic pancreatitis, and in these cases the patients present more often with chest symptoms than with abdominal symptoms. Endoscopic retrograde pancreatography combined with CT can generally delineate the cause for the recurrent pleural effusion (209,280,341) or even a much

rarer complication, pancreaticobronchial fistula (74). When communication with the lumen of the bowel is established, gas may be seen within the pseudocyst and will not necessarily be an indication of a gas forming infection (216,337).

Pseudocysts can be confused with cystic or necrotic tumors, a markedly dilated and tortuous pancreatic duct (see Fig. 15-95), or a true or false aneurysm of an intrapancreatic or peripancreatic artery. Cystic tumors usually occur in patients without a history of pancreatitis and may show characteristic CT findings, as previously described. Necrotic tumors generally have thick and irregular walls that rarely calcify, compared with the uniform and occasionally calcified walls of pseudocyst. Aneurysms or false aneurysms characteristically will be enhanced following an IV bolus of contrast material. Even prior to administration of contrast material, the similarity between the density of the fluid in the false aneurysm and the density of the blood in the aorta or vena cava will be a clue to its nature. Aneurysms or false aneurysms can also be diagnosed by MRI and pulsed Doppler US without the use of IV contrast agents.

Chronic pancreatitis may be associated with splenic and portal venous obstruction (Fig. 15-97). In a review of 266 patients with chronic pancreatitis who were followed up for a mean time of 8.2 years, splenic and portal venous obstruction was found in 35 patients (13.2%) but was symptomatic in only two. Obstruction involved the splenic vein in 22 patients, the portal vein in 10, and the superior mesenteric vein in 3. The authors concluded that

Figure 15-94 Chronic pancreatitis with pseudocyst dissecting into the superior recess lesser sac. A 7-mm portal venous phase computed tomography image demonstrates well-defined focal fluid collection within the potential space of the peritoneal folds creating the superior recess of the lesser sac, producing some adjacent mass effect on the hepatic parenchyma.

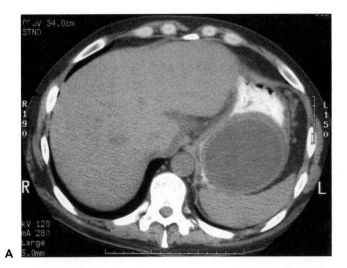

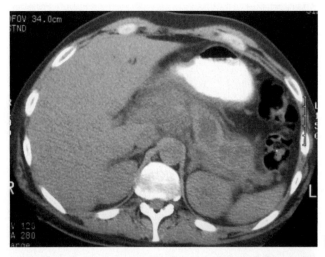

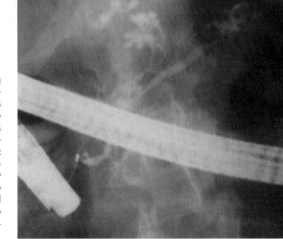

Figure 15-95 Chronic pancreatitis with pseudocyst dissecting into wall of stomach. **A:** A 5-mm oral-contrast-only computed tomography (CT) image through the upper abdomen demonstrates well-circumscribed 8 × 7 cm fluid collection dissecting within the posterior gastric wall. **B:** 4 cm inferiorly, inflammatory change is seen surrounding the superior pancreatic body, which contains several low attenuation collections representing either intrapancreatic pseudocysts or dilated duct. No calcifications are noted. **C:** Spot radiograph from endoscopic retrograde cholangiopancreatography (ERCP) with injection into the major papilla shows irregularity of the nondilated main pancreatic duct with several focal strictures and two areas of extravasation into complex tracks, likely leading to the pseudocysts seen on CT. By Cambridge classification, this represents severe chronic pancreatitis.

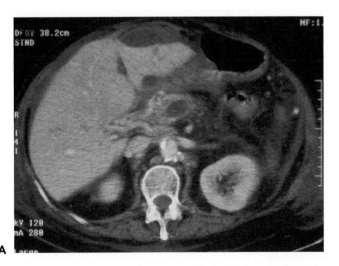

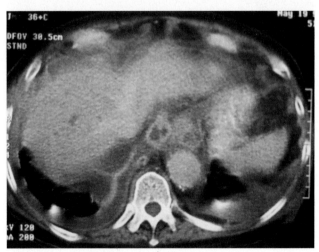

Figure 15-96 Chronic pancreatitis with pancreatico-pleural fistula. **A:** A 7-mm portal venous phase computed tomography (CT) image through the superior pancreatic head level demonstrates an ovoid 2.5 (1.5 cm fluid collection in the pancreatic neck. Note fluid also dissecting around the left hepatic lobe. **B:** A 7-mm CT image located 8 cm superior to the pancreatic neck demonstrates well-defined track of fluid in the posterior mediastinum. (*continued*)

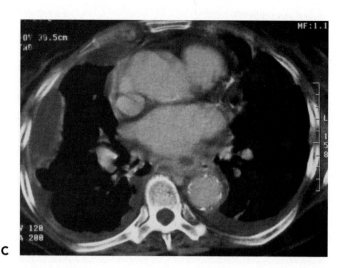

C

Figure 15-96 (*continued*) **C:** 15 cm superiorly to **A**, focal tubular fluid collections in the posterior mediastinum have tracked further into the chest. Note partial loculation of pleural fluid within the right hemithorax. Communication between the pancreatic duct, retroperitoneal and posterior mediastinal fluid tracks, and right pleural space was demonstrated on subsequent endoscopic retrograde cholangiopancreatography.

in chronic pancreatitis, splenic and portal venous obstruction should be systematically sought in patients with acute problems or pseudocysts, especially if therapeutic decisions would be modified by a diagnosis of venous obstruction. The data also showed that the risk of GI variceal bleeding was lower than previously reported (41). Splenic vein interruption and gastroepiploic varices are easily depicted with CT.

Chronic pancreatitis frequently results in pancreatic insufficiency of both the exocrine and endocrine functions.

On the contrary, if a patient recovers from severe acute necrotizing pancreatitis, exocrine function is generally preserved although it may diminish over time (13). Some patients with no significant past medical history may initially present in a state of pancreatic insufficiency without clear cause; in this population, CT was found to be a key diagnostic tool in understanding the cause of the problem (310). Previously undiagnosed pancreatic carcinoma, classic changes of chronic pancreatitis, confirmation of complete surgical removal, and evidence of complete idiopathic atrophy were some of the diagnostic findings described.

In theory, MRI may be better suited to detect the fibrosis of chronic pancreatitis than CT. In the presence of fibrosis, MRI will show a diminished signal intensity of the gland on T1 fat-suppressed images and diminished heterogeneous enhancement on immediate postgadolinium-spoiled GRE images (303). In a report on 22 patients, including 13 with chronic calcifying pancreatitis and 9 with presumed acute recurrent pancreatitis, differences between these groups were observed on T1 fat-suppressed (see Fig. 15-31) and immediate postgadolinium MRI images. All patients with pancreatic calcifications had a diminished signal intensity of the pancreatic parenchyma on T1 fat-suppressed and abnormally low percent contrast enhancement on postgadolinium images. In patients with acute recurrent pancreatitis the involved pancreas had signal intensity comparable to normal pancreatic parenchyma. Because fibrosis may precede the development of calcification, MRI may be capable of detecting the onset of fibrosis in chronic pancreatitis earlier than CT. However, CT is much more sensitive than MRI in detecting calcifications. The diagnosis of chronic pancreatitis on MRI is based on signal intensity and enhancement as well as morphologic changes of the pancreatic and bile ducts depicted with MRCP (225).

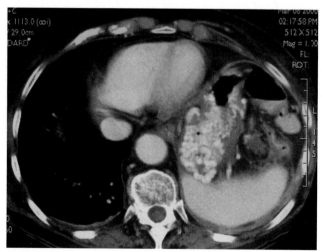

A   **B**

Figure 15-97 Chronic pancreatitis with chronic splenic vein thrombosis. **A:** A 5-mm portal venous phase computed tomography image demonstrates atrophy of the pancreatic body and tail with 1 cm calcification, possibly within the main pancreatic duct. Note patency of splenic vein to the tail/body junction. Upstream to this level, no normal splenic vein could be seen coursing towards the hilum. **B:** 5 cm cephalad, extensive varices of the posterior gastric wall in the gastroepiploic distribution are noted due to chronic thrombosis of the splenic vein near the hilum.

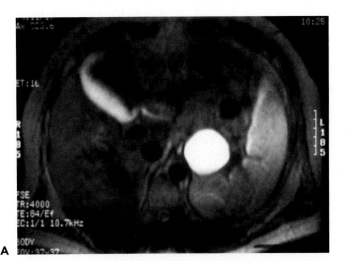
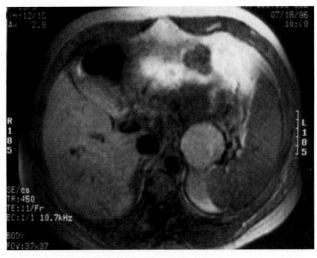

A

B

Figure 15-98 Proteinaceous pseudocyst on magnetic resonance imaging. **A:** A 8-mm axial T2-weighted fat suppressed fast spin echo image through the upper abdomen demonstrates a smooth, 4-cm fluid signal collection superior to the pancreatic body-tail junction, consistent with a pseudocyst. No internal debris is seen. **B:** A 6-mm T1-weighted fat suppressed spin echo axial image similar level demonstrates moderately high, homogeneous signal within the collection compared to the low signal cerebrospinal fluid.

In cases in which the differential diagnosis is between pancreatic cancer and focal chronic pancreatitis, MRI may be capable of showing diffuse low signal intensity of the entire pancreas, including the area of focal enlargement on T1 fat-suppressed and immediate postgadolinium spoiled GRE images, lending support for a diagnosis of chronic pancreatitis. Johnson and Outwater (155) found that both masslike chronic pancreatitis and pancreatic carcinoma showed more gradual progressive enhancement on dynamic MRI than did normal pancreatic parenchyma and were not distinguishable on the basis of degree and time of enhancement. Interestingly, nontumorous pancreas in patients with carcinoma showed gradual enhancement that was significantly different from that of normal parenchyma. In a recent study correlating CT and MRI features in patients with chronic pancreatitis presenting as a focal mass, four of seven patients had isointensity of the focal mass and the remaining pancreatic tissue on all MR sequences, including dynamic parenchymal phase, portal venous phase, and delayed T1-weighted images. Similar to the previously described findings in patients whose CT demonstrated no difference in attenuation, pathologic evaluation of the mass and the remaining pancreatic parenchyma revealed a similar degree of fibrosis. When focal masses were detectable on MRI, pathologic evaluation revealed no fibrosis in the nonenlarged portion of the pancreas, and typical changes of chronic pancreatitis in the masslike portion. Small pseudocysts are well shown on gadolinium-enhanced T1 fat-suppressed images and T2-weighted sequences. High T1 signal within the pseudocyst may be due to hemorrhage or proteinaceous material (Fig. 15-98). EUS may be helpful in evaluating patients with focal chronic pancre-

atitis versus pancreatic adenocarcinoma, especially when endoscopic biopsy is used (331).

Depiction of the main pancreatic duct and side branches with MRCP has improved dramatically with newer techniques including single shot RARE (half-Fourier rapid acquisition with relaxation enhancement) or HASTE images (Fig. 15-99) without or with secretin stimulation. The evaluation of branch ducts is important and is essential for diagnosing pancreatic abnormalities such as chronic pancreatitis

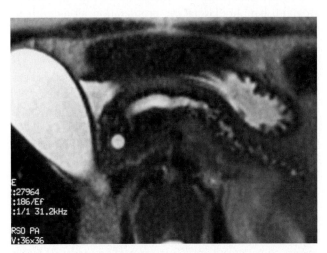

Figure 15-99 Chronic pancreatitis magnetic resonance cholangiopancreatography. A 5.0-cm thick axial slab half-Fourier acquisition single-shot turbo spin echo (HASTE) image demonstrates moderate dilatation of the main pancreatic duct through the neck, body, and tail, up to 8 mm, with several abnormally dilated side branches in the tail region. No intraductal filling defects are identified. Common bile duct is noted in the pancreatic head and is slightly prominent in caliber. The pattern of ductal dilatation is consistent with moderate chronic pancreatitis.

or IPMT (108). However, the segments of duct affected by chronic desmoplastic pancreatitis may not be able to dilate (108,129). Hellerhof et al. (108) found that visualization of side branches was significantly improved in patients with chronic pancreatitis, but only if a dominant stricture of the main duct was not present. This particular study found an improvement in the sensitivity for detection of chronic pancreatitis from 77% to 89%. In patients with severely stenotic portions of the main pancreatic duct, secretin stimulation corrects overestimation of the length of strictures on standard MRCP, likely attributable to improved visualization of the duct downstream from the stricture. Hellerhoff et al. reported alteration in the primary diagnosis in 15 (16%) of 95 patients after the addition of dynamic secretin stimulation images to routine MRCP; better visualization of side branches and/or small ducts allowed the authors to detect additional cases of chronic pancreatitis and pancreas divisum. In addition to improved visualization of the pancreatic ductal system during secretin stimulation MRCP, quantitative assessment of pancreatic exocrine function may be estimated noninvasively (63,129,208).

Autoimmune Pancreatitis

The recently described phenomenon of autoimmune pancreatitis (372), although considered a form of chronic pancreatitis, is different in that steroid therapy is effective in reversing both morphologic and functional pancreatic abnormalities. Response to steroid therapy is one of the criteria for diagnosing this rare condition, also supported by the following: elevation of serum gamma globulin and IgG, autoantibodies to pancreatic antigens, impaired pancreatic exocrine function, diffuse irregular narrowing of the main pancreatic duct on endoscopic retrograde pancreatogram, lymphoplasmacytic proliferation along with fibrosis on biopsy, absence of acute attacks of pancreatitis, and occasional association with other autoimmune disease. The CT features of autoimmune pancreatitis are diffuse or focal pancreatic enlargement, diffuse delayed enhancement on dynamic studies, and a capsule-like low-density rim surrounding the pancreas (Fig. 15-100) (144). In addition, there is minimal or no peripancreatic inflammation and no vascular encasement (289). Recognition of this disease is clinically important because it is reversible when diagnosed and treated correctly (144).

Pancreatic Changes in Cystic Fibrosis

CF is a dysfunction of exocrine glands characterized by chronic bronchopulmonary infections, malabsorption secondary to pancreatic insufficiency, and an increased sweat sodium concentration. Complete fatty replacement of the pancreatic parenchyma has been shown by both CT and US to occur in CF (Fig. 15-101) (73,255). The amount of fatty replacement correlates with the degree of pancreatic exocrine, but not endocrine, dysfunction, and also correlates directly with the degree of pulmonary dysfunction (322). MRI has been able to demonstrate similar changes in the pancreas, and lack of ionizing radiation may be of value in this young patient population. Three patterns of pancreatic abnormality have been described on MRI: lobulated enlarged pancreas with complete fatty replacement, small atrophic pancreas with partial fatty replacement, and diffusely atrophic pancreas without fatty replacement (338). Fatty replacement is well shown on T1-weighted images as high signal intensity tissue. The fatty nature of the tissue may be confirmed with T1 fat-suppressed images, by demonstrating suppression of the signal from the gland. A less common manifestation of CF has been complete replacement of the pancreas by multiple macroscopic cysts. This form of pancreatic cystosis is considered a process in which complete cystic transformation of the pancreas occurs, possibly related to ductal protein hyperconcentration, inspissation, and ductal ectasia (66,132).

The Schwachman-Diamond syndrome, which occurs 100 times less commonly than CF, is considered second only to CF as a cause of exocrine pancreatic insufficiency in children. The absence of abnormal sweat electrolytes and the tendency to improvement distinguishes this disease from CF. On CT examination in this disease, the pancreas commonly is totally replaced by fat. Lipomatosis of the pancreas is the typical pathologic feature of the syndrome (278).

The Johansen-Blizzard syndrome, which consists of congenital aplasia of the alae nasi, deafness, hypothyroidism, dwarfism, absent permanent teeth, and malabsorption, presents with pancreatic insufficiency as a nearly uniform finding, and the severe degree of malabsorption is often fatal in infancy. If enzyme supplements successfully correct the malabsorption, the affected individuals can reach adulthood. Total lack of a normal pancreas and fatty replacement of pancreatic bed is the characteristic CT finding. In contrast to the Schwachman-Diamond syndrome, in which the pancreatic defect is restricted to exocrine dysfunction, diabetes mellitus will develop in patients with the Johansen-Blizzard syndrome (338).

Primary Hemochromatosis

Primary hemochromatosis is a hereditary disease in which iron is deposited in the parenchyma of various organs. Liver, pancreas, and heart are primarily affected. On MR images, the iron deposition results in loss of signal on T2-weighted sequences. Iron deposition is predominantly in the liver. Deposition of iron in the pancreas tends to occur later, after liver damage is irreversible (Fig. 15-102) (312).

Pancreatic Trauma

Because of its relatively fixed extraperitoneal location just anterior to the spine, the pancreas occasionally is affected in blunt upper abdominal trauma. Pancreatic injuries occur in 2% to 12% of patients with blunt abdominal trauma (321). Either blunt or penetrating abdominal trauma may cause pancreatic ductal disruption, with subsequent escape of pancreatic enzymes and the potential for development

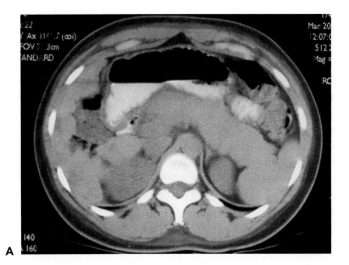

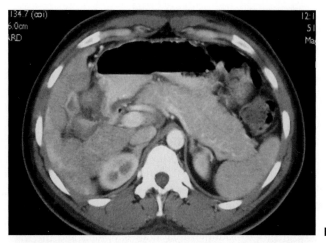

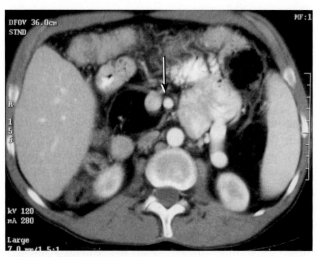

Figure 15-100   Autoimmune pancreatitis in a 27-year-old woman with autoimmune hepatitis. **A:** Pre-intravenous contrast 5-mm image demonstrates global enlargement of the pancreas. **B:** Portal venous phase 5-mm computed tomography image demonstrates homogeneous enhancement with several large vascular channels seen in the grossly enlarged pancreas. **C:** Diffuse enlargement included the pancreatic head, which is smooth in contour, normal and homogeneous in attenuation, and without evidence of ductal dilatation. No low attenuation peripheral capsule is seen, as has been reported in some patients with autoimmune pancreatitis. Note incidental jejunal intussusception (✱).

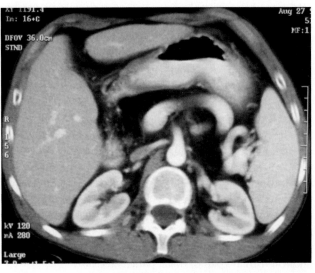

Figure 15-101   Fatty replacement of the pancreas in a 35-year-old man with cystic fibrosis. **A:** Portal venous phase 7-mm computed tomography image at the level of the splenic vein portal confluence demonstrates slightly heterogeneous fat replacing the superior head, neck, and body of the pancreas. **B:** 3 cm inferiorly, faint soft tissue capsule is seen surrounding the fat replacing the pancreatic head, normally located to the right of the superior mesenteric vessels (*arrow*).

of the entire spectrum of acute pancreatitis. The appearances of traumatic pancreatitis on CT are the same as with a nontraumatic cause (336). One study of 10 patients with surgical or autopsy proved pancreatic injury after blunt abdominal trauma who were all evaluated with CT scan showed the presence of fluid interdigitating between the splenic vein and the pancreatic parenchyma in nine patients. The authors concluded that this was a very helpful CT finding for the diagnosis of traumatic pancreatic injury (181). Complete transection of the pancreas (Fig. 15-103) can be diagnosed by CT. The two ends of the transected gland generally are separated by a variable quantity of low-density fluid that will remain relatively confined to the anterior pararenal space in the immediate postinjury period (19,319). When little fluid is present and the fractured segments are minimally separated, the hypoattenuating fracture line may be difficult to detect. Other appearances of pancreatic trauma on well-performed dynamic helical CT (see Tables 15-3 and 15-4) include diffuse gland enlargement with pancreatitis, peripancreatic hematoma, and large peripancreatic fluid collection (321) or in less severe injury, focal gland enlargement, contour irregularity, or small intra- or peripancreatic fluid accumulation (Fig. 15-104) (177, 247). Determination of duct integrity in cases of pancreatic trauma historically required endoscopic retrograde pancreatography. Occasionally, the pancreas may have almost normal morphologic features on CT despite the presence of duct disruption (367). A recent study found that MR pancreatography is an adequate noninvasive test for the detection of complete traumatic disruptions of the main pancreatic duct (321). MRI also depicts fluid occupying the space between fractured portions of the gland. Intraoperative injury of the pancreas occasionally will be seen following splenectomy. The diagnosis can be established by CT in the early postoperative period (24,361).

Pancreatic Infections

Opportunistic infections that have been reported to affect the pancreas in patients with acquired immunodeficiency syndrome (AIDS) include cytomegalovirus, *Mycobacterium tuberculosis,* and *Pneumocystis carinii.* Most often, pancreatic involvement by an infectious agent or neoplasm such as Kaposi sarcoma or lymphoma is overshadowed by symptoms related to the disease manifested elsewhere in the body (47,223). Extrapulmonary *Pneumocystis* infection of the pancreas can present on CT as punctuate calcifications dispersed throughout the gland. With other infections, the pancreas may appear normal, or show typical changes of acute pancreatitis produced by other etiologies. Pancreatic tuberculosis features on MRI have been recently described in a very small case series and include focal or diffuse disease with hypointensity on fat-suppressed T1 sequences and heterogeneous high signal on T2-weighted images (75). Drugs such as pentamidine and trimethoprim-sulfamethoxazole often used in AIDS patients may produce acute pancreatitis as well (223).

Peripancreatic lymph node enlargement due to mycobacterial infections or lymphoma is frequently evident.

Postoperative Evaluation

In patients who have either partial or total pancreatectomy, most often for neoplastic disease, frequently it is difficult to opacify with oral contrast material the segments of bowel used for the anastomosis to the biliary tree or remaining segment of pancreas because of the direction of flow in these Roux-en-Y loops. Administration of glucagon prior to CT imaging facilitates opacification of the afferent jejunal loop with oral contrast material, thus helping to define the structures in the right upper quadrant and to distinguish the unopacified loop of bowel from possible recurrent tumor in the region of the surgical bed formerly occupied by the head of pancreas (130). In postoperative patients, the lymph node–bearing region between the aorta and the SMV and SMA, previously occupied by the uncinate process of the pancreas, is an important area to evaluate for tumor recurrence (see Fig. 15-8). Because radical pancreatectomy usually leaves this area free of tissue having the attenuation value of either pancreatic tissue or lymph nodes, tumor recurrence will be readily detectable by CT. Whether the Whipple is done in a standard fashion or with a pylorus-sparing technique, where the duodenal bulb apex is anastomosed end-to-side to the Roux-en-Y jejunal loop, the appearance on CT is quite similar. Often after surgery, metallic clips produce beam-hardening artifact, making evaluation of the region even more challenging than simply understanding the postoperative anatomy. The evaluation of pancreatic function in patients after pancreaticoduodenectomy is important, because many may become diabetic following resection. Secretin stimulation during MR pancreatography not only helps in visualization of the main pancreatic duct and pancreaticojejunal anastomosis in these patients but also may show reduced jejunal filling in patients with diminished pancreatic remnant function (227).

After endoscopic, percutaneous, or surgical drainage of fluid collections associated with acute pancreatitis, CT may demonstrate a variety of abnormalities, including adhesions (Fig. 15-105), varices (Fig. 15-106), and fistulae (Fig. 15-107). With transgastric endoscopic therapy, adhesions between the posterior gastric wall and pancreatic region are readily depicted, particularly when gastric distension is good. A focal fluid collection tracking along the course of a previously pulled percutaneous catheter or dissecting within the retroperitoneum in a patient with history of acute necrotizing pancreatitis may indicate disruption of the pancreatic duct (disconnected duct syndrome); identification of this finding on CT may prompt further interventions including surgical fistula repair or distal pancreatectomy.

With surgery performed for chronic pancreatitis, such as the Puestow procedure (side-to-side pancreaticojejunostomy), the postsurgical anatomy is often complex, and adequate history is necessary to properly interpret the scan.

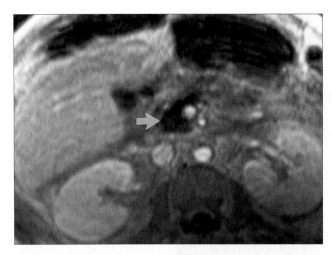

Figure 15-102 Pancreas in primary hemochromatosis. The pancreas *(arrow)* is near signal void on 90-second postgadolinium FLASH image consistent with iron deposition in the pancreas. The liver appears more normal in signal because it is a transplanted liver.

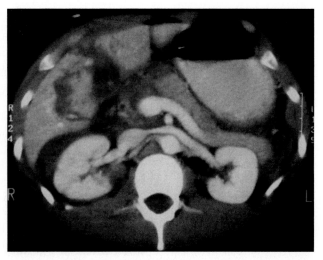

Figure 15-103 Traumatic pancreatic laceration in a 23-year-old man involved in a motor vehicle collision. Contrast-enhanced computed tomography through the level of the portal confluence demonstrates abrupt discontinuity of pancreatic enhancement at the junction of the neck and head, consistent with pancreas laceration. Fluid is seen tracking into the anterior pararenal space bilaterally. Large stellate hepatic laceration with active extravasation is also noted. The pattern of small bowel and adrenal enhancement is consistent with shock (hypotension and hypovolemia).

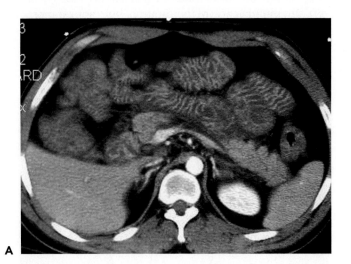

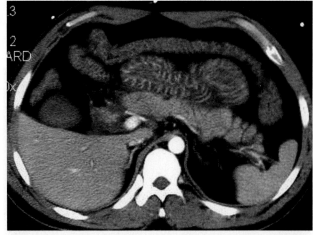

Figure 15-104 Pancreatic injury without laceration in an 18-year-old male pedestrian struck by motor vehicle, with hypovolemia due to scalp laceration hemorrhage. **A:** Contrast-enhanced computed tomography through the level of the pancreatic tail demonstrates normal lobularity. No focal lacerations are noted, but there is fluid within the retroperitoneal fat anterior to the pancreatic head. **B:** Image 2.5-mm caudal to A reveals fluid surrounding the pancreatic head. **C:** Fluid from the pancreatic injury tracks inferiorly into the mesenteric root.

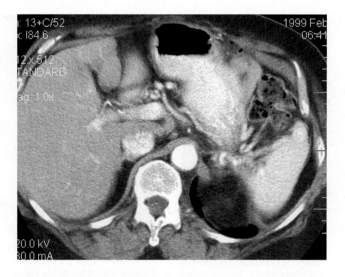

Figure 15-105   Adhesions following transgastric endodrainage. A 7-mm portal venous phase computed tomography image demonstrates tenting of the posterior gastric wall towards the pancreatic tail region with several collateral vessels. Similar findings may be noted after surgical drainage.

CT may be the first test performed after duodenal perforation during ERCP, most often associated with endoscopic sphincterotomy. Generally, a large amount of retroperitoneal air (Fig. 15-108), and sometimes intraperitoneal air are present, along with a variable amount of fluid in the anterior pararenal space, especially when there is superimposed ERCP-induced pancreatitis (see Fig. 15-69). In the absence of perforation, the appearance of ERCP-induced pancreatitis is similar to acute pancreatitis produced by other etiologies.

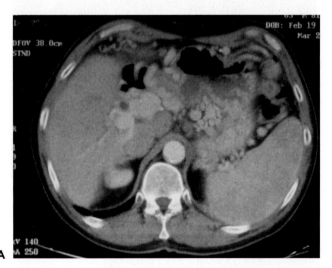
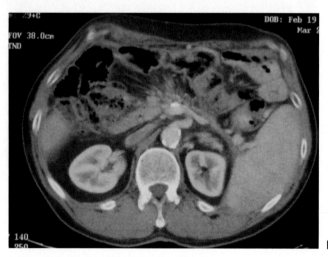

A   B

Figure 15-106   Venous collateral formation after necrosectomy for severe acute pancreatitis in a 63-year-old man with history of surgery 17 years previously. **A:** Portal venous phase computed tomography image demonstrates numerous collaterals in the gastrohepatic ligament and porta due to portal confluence obstruction. Gastroepiploic collaterals are also present due to splenic vein occlusion. **B:** Necrosectomy bed anterior to splenic vein and portal confluence demonstrates absence of normal pancreatic tissue and scarring of the retroperitoneum. No main portal vein or splenic vein were identifiable superior to this level.

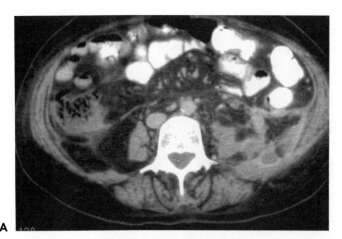

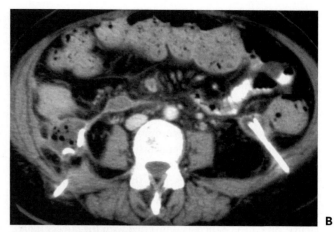

A

B

Figure 15-107 Left flank fistula 26 months after combined endoscopic and percutaneous drainage of pancreatic necrosis. **A:** The patient presented with focal redness and swelling of the left flank. Contrast-enhanced computed tomography (CT) image reveals heterogeneous peripherally enhancing complex fluid collection in the left anterior pararenal space, consistent with fistula formation. **B:** Contrast-enhanced CT image during acute drainage of necrotic pancreatic collection 26 months earlier shows bilateral anterior pararenal space percutaneous catheters in place. The patient required distal pancreatectomy for disconnected duct with residual functioning tissue in the tail (same patient as Figure 15-6).

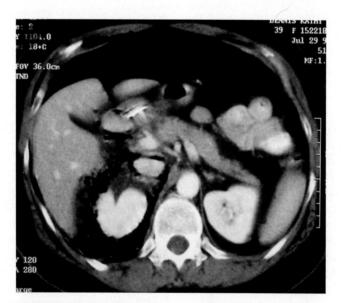

Figure 15-108 Endoscopic retrograde cholangiopancreatography perforation in a 39-year-old woman undergoing sphincterotomy. Contrast-enhanced computed tomography demonstrates air dissecting around the right kidney, right border of the pancreatic head, and inferior vena cava. The patient recovered uneventfully and was discharged to home 2 days later.

PANCREAS TRANSPLANTATION

The majority of pancreatic transplants are combined with renal transplants in patients with end stage renal disease due to severe type 1 diabetes mellitus. Higher pancreatic graft survival rates occur in patients with a combined procedure, rather than pancreatic transplant alone (241,260,318). The surgical techniques for pancreatic transplantation continue to evolve. The most common method of pancreatic transplantation places the graft in an intraperitoneal location of the iliac fossa opposite the renal transplant, with the vascular pedicle anastomosed to the common or external iliac vessels, and the accompanying cuff of duodenum anastomosed to the dome of the urinary bladder (Fig. 15-109). Hence, on CT the pancreas is inverted with the tail cephalad, and the head adjacent to the urinary bladder. Undesirable peripheral hyperinsulinemia and urinary complications due to discharge of exocrine secretions into the bladder have led to the development of a different surgical method of pancreas transplantation. With the newer procedure, the portal-enteric technique, the duodenal cuff is anastomosed side to side with the recipient jejunum, and the venous drainage of the graft is anastomosed to the recipient superior mesenteric vein. On CT, the head of the pancreas is cephalad, and the graft is located in a near-midline right paramedian position.

The normal postoperative findings of both transplant methods are well depicted with high-resolution 3-D MRA (122).

CT has not been particularly valuable in determining the presence or absence of pancreas transplant rejection (202), which has been reported in up to 60% of cases (178). Doppler sonography (241,366) and more recently contrast-enhanced MRI (172) are both useful techniques in evaluating pancreas transplants, with sonographic signs of rejection including diffuse allograft enlargement, loss of marginal definition, resistive index greater than 0.7 (366). Although these signs are reasonably specific, they have low sensitivity and percutaneous biopsy of the pancreas transplant may be needed to determine rejection in ambiguous cases. The finding of a diminished mean percentage of parenchymal enhancement indicates rejection on dynamic gadolinium-enhanced MRI and has a greater sensitivity for acute rejection (96%) (178).

In addition to rejection, the graft may be lost in the immediate perioperative period, most commonly due to vascular thrombosis, reported from 2% to 19% (92), and less commonly due to infection, pancreatitis, bleeding, and anastomotic leaks. CT is helpful in evaluating postoperative complications such as anastomotic leaks (42), hemorrhage or other peripancreatic fluid collections, or graft pancreatitis, and with CTA techniques has the potential to identify vascular thrombosis. Vascular thrombosis is detectable with Doppler US (102,241) and MRI (92,122). In particular, CT may aid in differentiating between acute rejection and pancreatitis, which may appear similar on US (241) and can readily identify gas in patients with emphysematous pancre-

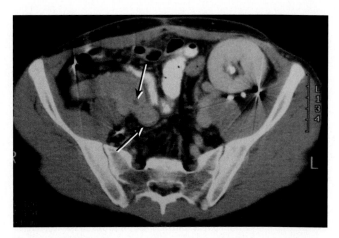

Figure 15-109 Normal renal pancreas transplant in a 27-year-old man. Contrast-enhanced computed tomography through the pelvis demonstrates renal allograft in the left iliac fossa. Anterior to the right psoas muscles and external iliac vessels lies the inferior portion of the pancreas transplant with a small ductal structure evident in the head (*arrow*). Duodenal cuff (*long arrow*) lies immediately posterior and on lower images communicates with the bladder dome.

atitis of the graft, due either to infection or major vascular thrombosis. A recently described feasibility study evaluating secretin-augmented MR pancreatography in transplant patients showed diminished exocrine secretion volumes in patients with pancreatic allograft dysfunction compared with patients with normal function. When combined with MR perfusion measurement techniques, this method may be of value in evaluation of graft function (133).

CT is also useful in identifying posttransplantation lymphoproliferative disorder (PTLD), which in one study (213) occurred in 2.4% of 337 pancreas-kidney transplant recipients at a mean of 137 days after transplantation. On CT, diffuse enlargement of the allograft was the most common finding, making differentiation from pancreatitis or rejection difficult, but in other cases focal mass in the allograft, or focal intra- and extraallograft masses suggested the diagnosis of PTLD (213). However, the concerns for renal dysfunction in this particular patient population are great, and it is likely that the role of CT as a first-line imaging method in the evaluation of pancreas transplants will be limited.

CT remains the workhorse of pancreatic imaging. Advances in volumetric abdominal imaging hold the promise of improved accuracy for CT evaluation of common pancreatic pathology such as acute and chronic pancreatitis, trauma, and pancreatic carcinoma. Technology changes today and in the future will require careful attention to contrast timing and administration techniques on a disease-specific basis. Gadolinium-enhanced MRI is useful when iodinated contrast for CT is contraindicated due to allergy or impaired renal function and for problem solving when standard imaging leaves clinically important questions unanswered. MRCP is an ideal method to noninvasively study pancreatic ductal structures, and is useful as an adjunct to CT. The emerging role of EUS in the evaluation of pancreatic disorders has yet to be defined; the operator dependency and limited availability of this modality relegate the use of EUS to a problem-solving imaging technique. Likewise, the role of PET imaging for pancreatic disorders will likely increase as the need for combined physiologic and anatomic information becomes more critical.

REFERENCES

1. Adkisson KW, Baron TH, Morgan DE. Pancreatic fluid collections: diagnosis and endoscopic management. *Semin Gastrointest Dis* 1998;9:61–72.
2. Adsay NV, Longnecker DS, Klimstra DS. Pancreatic tumors with cystic dilatation of the ducts: intraductal papillary mucinous neoplasms and intraductal oncocytic papillary neoplasms. *Semin Diagn Pathol* 2000;17:16–30.
3. Adsay NV, Pierson C, Sarkar F, et al. Colloid (mucinous noncystic) carcinoma of the pancreas. *Am J Surg Pathol* 2001;25:26–42.
4. Agarwal N, Pitchumoni CS. Assessment of severity in acute pancreatitis. *Am J Gastroenterol* 1991;86:1385–1391.
5. Ahmad NA, Kochman ML, Lewis JD, Ginsberg GG. Can EUS alone differentiate between malignant and benign cystic lesions of the pancreas? *Am J Gastroenterol* 2001;96:3295–300.
6. Ahmed A, Chan KF, Song IS. Annular pancreas. *J Comput Assist Tomogr* 1982;6:409–411.
7. Akerstrom G, Hellman P, Hessman O, Osmak L. Surgical treatment of endocrine pancreatic tumours. *Neuroendocrinology* 2004;80:62–66.
8. American Cancer Society. *Cancer facts and figures 2004: year surveillance research from the American Cancer Society.* Bethesda MD: American Cancer Society, 2004.
9. Ammori JB, Colletti LM, Zalupski MM, et al. Surgical resection following radiation therapy with concurrent gemcitabine in patients with previously unresectable adenocarcinoma of the pancreas. *J Gastrointest Surg* 2003;7:766–772.
10. Anderson MA, Scheiman JM. Nonmucinous cystic pancreatic neoplasms. *Gastrointest Endosc Clin North Am* 2002;12:769–79.
11. Anderson MA, Carpenter S, Thompson NW, et al. Endoscopic ultrasound is highly accurate and directs management in patients with neuroendocrine tumors of the pancreas. *Am J Gastroenterol* 2000;95:2271–2277.
12. Angeli E, Venturini M, Vanzulli A, et al. Color Doppler imaging in the assessment of vascular involvement by pancreatic carcinoma. *AJR Am J Roentgenol* 1997;168:193–197.
13. Angelini G, Pederzoli P, Caliari S, et al. Long-term outcome of acute necrohemorrhagic pancreatitis: a 4-year follow-up. *Digestion* 1984;30:131–137.
14. Aranha GV, Prinz RA, Freeark RJ, Greenlee HB. The spectrum of biliary tract obstruction from chronic pancreatitis. *Arch Surg* 1984;119:595–600.
15. Ardengh JC, Rosenbaum P, Ganc AJ, et al. Role of EUS in the preoperative localization of insulinomas compared with spiral CT. *Gastrointest Endosc* 2000;51:552–555.
16. Aspestrand F, Kolmannskog F. CT compared to angiography for staging of tumors of the pancreatic head. *Acta Radiol* 1992;33:556–560.
17. Aspestrand F, Kolmannskog F, Jacobsen M. CT, MR imaging and angiography in pancreatic apudomas. *Acta Radiol* 1993;34:468–473.
18. Baek SY, Sheafor DH, Keogan MT, et al. Two-dimensional multiplanar and three dimensional volume-rendered vascular CT in pancreatic carcinoma: interobserver agreement and comparison with standard helical techniques. *AJR Am J Roentgenol* 2001;176:1467–1473.
19. Baker LP, Wagner EJ, Brotman S, Whitley NO. Transection of the pancreas. *J Comput Assist Tomogr* 1982;6:411–412.
20. Baker ME. Pancreatic adenocarcinoma: are there pathognomonic changes in the fat surrounding the superior mesenteric artery? *Radiology* 1991;180:613–614.
21. Balthazar EJ. Acute pancreatitis: assessment of severity with clinical and CT evaluation. *Radiology* 2002;223:603–613.
22. Balthazar EJ, Chako AC. Computed tomography of pancreatic masses. *Am J Gastroenterol* 1990;85:343–349.
23. Balthazar EJ, Freeny PC, vanSonnenberg E. Imaging and intervention in acute pancreatitis. *Radiology* 1994;193:297–306.
24. Balthazar EJ, Megibow A, Rothberg M, Lefleur RS. CT evaluation of pancreatic injury following splenectomy. *Gastrointest Radiol* 1985;10:139–144.
25. Balthazar EJ, Ranson JHC, Naidich DP, et al. Acute pancreatitis: prognostic value of CT. *Radiology* 1985;156:767–772.
26. Balthazar EJ, Robinson DL, Megibow AJ, Ranson JHC. Acute pancreatitis: value of CT in establishing prognosis. *Radiology* 1990;174:331–336.
27. Balthazar EJ, Subramanyam BR, Lefleur RS, Barone CM. Solid and papillary epithelial neoplasm of the pancreas: radiographic, CT, sonographic, and angiographic features. *Radiology* 1984;150: 39–40.
28. Banks PA. Acute pancreatitis: medical and surgical management. *Am J Gastroenterol* 1994;89:S78–S85.
29. Banks PA. Central cavitary necrosis. *Pancreas* 1993;8:141–145.
30. Banks PA. Practice guidelines in acute pancreatitis. *Am J Gastroenterol* 1997;92:377–386.
31. Barish MA, Soto JA. MR cholangiopancreatography: techniques and clinical applications. *AJR Am J Roentgenol* 1997;169: 1295–1303.
32. Baron RL, Stanley RJ, Lee JKT, et al. Computed tomographic features of biliary obstruction. *AJR Am J Roentgenol* 1983;140: 1173–1178.
33. Baron TH, Morgan DE. Current concepts: acute necrotizing pancreatitis. *N Engl J Med* 1999;340:1412–1417.
34. Baron TH, Thaggard WG, Morgan DE, Stanley RJ. Endoscopic therapy of organized pancreatic necrosis. *Gastroenterology* 1996; 111: 755–764.
35. Bassi C, Procacci C, Zamboni G, et al. Intraductal papillary mucinous tumors of the pancreas: where are we now? *Int J Pancreatol* 2000;27:181–193.
36. Beger HG, Krautzberger W, Bittner R, et al. Results of surgical treatment of necrotizing pancreatitis. *World J Surg* 1985;9: 972–979.
37. Beger HG, Rau B, Gansauge F, et al. Treatment of pancreatic cancer: challenge of the facts. *World J Surg* 2003;D:1075–1084.
38. Beger H, Rau B, Mayer J, et al. Natural course of acute pancreatitis. *World J Surg* 1997;21:130–135.
39. Berk JE. The Management of acute pancreatitis: a critical assessment as Dr. Bockus would have wished. *Am J Gastroenterol* 1995;90:696–703.
40. Berland LL, Lawson TL, Foley WD, et al. Computed tomography of the normal and abnormal pancreatic duct: correlation with pancreatic ductography. *Radiology* 1981;141:715–724.
41. Bernades P, Baetz A, Levy P, et al. Splenic and portal venous obstruction in chronic pancreatitis. A prospective longitudinal study of a medical-surgical series of 266 patients. *Dig Dis Sci* 1992;37:340–346.
42. Bischof TP, Thoeni RF, Melzer JS. Diagnosis of duodenal leaks from kidney-pancreas transplants in patients with duodenovesical anastomoses: value of CT cystography. *AJR Am J Roentgenol* 1995;165:349–354.
43. Bluemke DA, Cameron JL, Hruban RH, et al. Potentially resectable pancreatic adenocarcinoma: spiral CT assessment with surgical and pathologic correlation. *Radiology* 1995;197:381–385.
44. Boden G. Glucagonomas and insulinomas. *Gastroenterol Clin North Am* 1989;18:831–845.
45. Bok EJ, Cho KJ, Williams DM, et al. Venous involvement in islet cell tumors of the pancreas. *AJR Am J Roentgenol* 1984;142: 319–322.
46. Boland GW, O'Malley ME, Saez M, et al. Pancreatic-phase versus portal vein-phase helical CT of the pancreas: optimal temporal window for evaluation of pancreatic adenocarcinoma. *AJR Am J Roentgenol* 1999;172:605–608.
47. Bonacini M. Pancreatic involvement in human immunodeficiency virus infection. *J Clin Gastroenterol* 1991;13:58–64.
48. Bonaldi VM, Bret PM, Atri M, Reinhold C. Helical CT of the pancreas: a comparison of cine display and film-based viewing. *AJR Am J Roentgenol* 1998;170:373–376.
49. Bonaldi VM, Bret PM, Atri M, et al. A comparison of two injection protocols using helical and dynamic acquisitions in CT examinations of the pancreas. *AJR Am J Roentgenol* 1996;167: 49–55.

50. Boyle P, Hsieh CC, Maisonneuve P, et al. Epidemiology of pancreas cancer (1988). *Int J Pancreatol* 1989;5:327–346.

51. Bradley EL. A clinically based classification system for acute pancreatitis. *Arch Surg* 1993;128:586–590.

52. Bradley EL, Allen K. A prospective longitudinal study of observation versus surgical intervention in the management of necrotizing pancreatitis. *Am J Surg* 1991;161:19–25.

53. Brand R. The diagnosis of pancreatic cancer. *Cancer J* 2001;7: 287–297.

54. Brandt KR, Charboneau JW, Stephens DH, et al. CT and US guided biopsy of the pancreas. *Radiology* 1993;187:99–104.

55. Breatnach ES, Han SY, Rahatzad MT, Stanley RJ. CT evaluation of glucagonomas. *J Comput Assist Tomogr* 1985;9:25–29.

56. Bret PM, Nicolet V, Labadie M. Percutaneous fine-needle aspiration biopsy of the pancreas. *Diagn Cytopathol* 1986;2:221–222.

57. Bret PM, Reinhold C, Taourel P, et al. Pancreas divisum: evaluation with MR cholangiopancreatography. *Radiology* 1996;100: 99–103.

58. Broughan TA, Leslie JD, Soto JM, Hermann RE. Pancreatic islet cell tumors. *Surgery* 1986;99:671–678.

59. Brugge WR, Lewandrowski K, Lee-Lewandrowski E, et al. Diagnosis of pancreatic cystic neoplasms: a report of the cooperative pancreatic cyst study. *Gastroenterology* 2004;126:1330–1336.

60. Buetow PC, Buck JL, Pantongrag-Brown L, et al. Solid and papillary epithelial neoplasm of the pancreas: imaging-pathologic correlation in 56 cases. *Radiology* 1996;199:707–711.

61. Beutow PC, Rao P, Thompson LD. Mucinous cystic neoplasms of the pancreas. *Radiographics* 1998;18:433–449.

62. Cantisani V, Mortele KJ, Levy A, et al. MR imaging features of solid pseudopapillary tumor of the pancreas in adult and pediatric patients. *AJR Am J Roentgenol* 2003;181:395–401.

63. Cappeliez O, Delhaye M, Deviere J, et al. Chronic pancreatitis: evaluation of pancreatic exocrine function with MR pancreatography after secretin stimulation. *Radiology* 2000;215:358–364.

64. Chong N, Freeny PC, Schmiedl UP. Pancreatic arterial anatomy: depiction with dual-phase helical CT. *Radiology* 1998;208: 537–542.

65. Chu QD, Khushalani N, Javle MM, et al. Should adjuvant therapy remain the standard of care for patients with resected adenocarcinoma of the pancreas? *Ann Surg Oncol.* 2003;10:539–45.

66. Churchill RJ, Cunningham DG, Henkin RE, Reynes CJ. Macroscopic cysts of the pancreas in cystic fibrosis demonstrated by multiple radiological modalities. *JAMA* 1981;245:72–74.

67. Clark LR, Jaffe MH, Choyke PL, et al. Pancreatic imaging. *Radiol Clin North Am* 1985;23:489-501.

68. Cohen-Scali F, Vilgrin V, Brancatelli G, et al. Discrimination of unilocular macrocystic serous cystadenoma from pancreatic pseudocyst and mucinous cystadenoma with CT: initial observations. *Radiology* 2003;228:727–733.

69. Compton C. Serous cystic tumors of the pancreas. *Semin Diagn Pathol* 2000;17:43–55.

70. Cotton PB. Congenital anomaly of pancreas divisum as cause of obstructive pain and pancreatitis. *Gut* 1980;21:105–114.

71. Creutzfeldt W. Endocrine tumors of the pancreas. In: Volk BW, Arquilla ER, eds. *The diabetic pancreas,* 2nd ed. New York: Plenum, 1985:543–586.

72. Curry CA, Eng J, Horton KM, et al. CT of primary cystic pancreatic neoplasms; can CT be used for patient triage and treatment? *AJR Am J Roentgenol* 2000;175:99–103.

73. Daneman A, Gaskin K, Martin DJ, Cutz E. Pancreatic changes in cystic fibrosis: CT and sonographic appearances. *AJR Am J Roentgenol* 1983;141:653–655.

74. Davidian M, Koo A. Pancreatobronchial fistula diagnosed by combined ERP and CT. *AJR Am J Roentgenol* 1996;166:53–54.

75. DeBacker AI, Mortele KJ, Bomans P, et al. Tuberculosis of the pancreas: MRI features. *AJR Am J Roentgenol* 2005;184:50–54.

76. Delbeke D, Rose DM, Chapman WC, et al. Optimal interpretation of FDG PET in the diagnosis, staging, and management of pancreatic carcinoma. *J Nucl Med* 1999;40:1784–1791.

77. Del Maschio A, Vanzulli A, Sironi S, et al. Pancreatic cancer versus chronic pancreatitis: diagnosis with CA 19-9 assessment, US, CT and CT-guided fine needle biopsy. *Radiology* 1991;178:178: 95–99.

78. Delvalle J, Yamada T. Secretory tumors of the pancreas. In: Sleisenger MH, Fordtran JS, eds. *Gastrointestinal disease: pathophysiology, diagnosis, management,* 4th ed. Philadelphia: Saunders, 1990:1884–1900.

79. Demeure MJ, Doffek KM, Komorowski RA, et al. Molecular metastases in stage 1 pancreatic cancer: improved survival with adjuvant chemoradiation. *Surgery* 1998;124:663–669.

80. Demos TC, Posniak HV, Harmath C, et al. Cystic lesions of the pancreas. *AJR Am J Roentgenol* 2002;179:1375–1388.

81. Dervenis C, Johnson CD, Bassi C, et al. Diagnosis, objective assessment of severity, and management of acute pancreatitis. *Int J Pancreatol* 1999;25:195–210.

82. Di Maggio EM, Solcia M, Dore R, et al. Intrapancreatic lipoma: first case diagnosed with CT. *AJR Am J Roentgenol* 1996;167: 56–57.

83. di Sant'Agnese PA. Acinar cell carcinoma of the pancreas. *Ultrstruct Pathol* 1991;15:573–577.

84. Diehl SJ, Lehmann KJ, Gaa J, et al. MR imaging of pancreatic lesions: comparison of manganese-DPDP and gadolinium chelate. *Invest Radiol* 1999;34:589–595.

85. Diehl SJ, Lehmann KJ, Sadick M, et al. Pancreatic cancer: value of dual-phase helical CT in assessing resectability. *Radiology* 1998; 206:373–378.

86. Doppman JL, Shawker TH, Miller DL. Localization of islet cell tumors. *Gastroenterol Clin North Am* 1989;18:793–804.

87. Dunn GD, Gibson RN. The left-sided pancreas. *Radiology* 1986;159:713–714.

88. Echenique AM, Sleeman D, Yrizarry J, et al. Percutaneous catheter-directed debridement of infected pancreatic necrosis: results in 20 patients. *J Vasc Interv Radiol* 1998;9:565–571.

89. Eckhauser FE, Cheung PS, Vinik AI, et al. Nonfunctioning malignant neuroendocrine tumors of the pancreas. *Surgery* 1986;100: 978–988.

90. Eelkema EA, Stephens DH, Ward EM, Sheedy PF II. CT features of nonfunctioning islet cell carcinoma. *AJR Am J Roentgenol* 1984;143:943–948.

91. El-Rayes BF, Zalupski MM, Shields AF, et al. Phase II study of gemcitabine, cisplatin, and infusional fluorouracil in advanced pancreatic cancer. *J Clin Oncol* 2003;21:2920–2925.

92. Eubank WB, Schmiedl UP, Levy AE, Marsh CL. Venous thrombosis and occlusion after pancreas transplantation: evaluation with breath-hold gadolinium-enhanced three-dimensional MR imaging. *AJR Am J Roentgenol* 2000;175:381–385.

93. Fekete PS, Nunez C, Pitlik DA. Fine-needle aspiration biopsy of the pancreas: a study of 61 cases. *Diagn Cytopathol* 1986;2: 301–306.

94. Fernandez-del Castillo C, Warshaw AL. Cystic neoplasms of the pancreas. *Pancreatology* 2001;1:641–647.

95. Fidler JL, Fletcher JG, Reading CC, et al. Preoperative detection of pancreatic insulinomas on multiphasic helical CT. *AJR Am J Roentgenol* 2003;181:775–780.

96. Fidler Jl, Johnson CD. Imaging of neuroendocrine tumors of the pancreas. *Int J Gastrointest Cancer* 2001;30:73–85.

97. Fishman EK. CT angiography: clinical applications in the abdomen. *Radiographics* 2001;21:S3–S16.

98. Foitzik T, Bassi D, Schmidt J, et al. Intravenous contrast medium accentuates the severity of acute necrotizing pancreatitis in the rat. *Gastroenterology* 1994;106:207–214.

99. Foley WD. Multidetector CT: abdominal visceral imaging. *Radiographics* 2002;22:701–719.

100. Fontham ET, Correa P. Epidemiology of pancreatic cancer. *Surg Clin North Am* 1989;69:551–567.

101. Fotoohi M, D'Agostino HB, Wollman B, et al. Persistent pancreatocutaneous fistula after percutaneous drainage of pancreatic fluid collections: role of cause and severity of pancreatitis. *Radiology* 1999;213:573–578.

102. Foshager MC, Hedlund LJ, Troppman C, et al. Venous thrombosis of pancreatic transplants: diagnosis by duplex sonography. *AJR Am J Roentgenol* 1997;169:1269–1273.

103. Freeny PC, Hauptmann E, Althaus SJ, et al. Percutaneous CT-guided catheter drainage of infected acute necrotizing pancreatitis: techniques and results. *AJR Am J Roentgenol* 1998;170: 969–975.

104. Freeny PC, Traverso LW, Ryan JA. Diagnosis and staging of pancreatic adenocarcinoma with dynamic computed tomography. *Am J Surg* 1993;165:600–606.

105. Friedman AC, Lichtenstein JE, Fishman EK, et al. Solid and papillary epithelial neoplasm of the pancreas. *Radiology* 1985;154: 333–337.

106. Frucht H, Doppman JL, Norton JA, et al. Gastrinomas: comparison of MR imaging with CT, angiography, and US. *Radiology* 1989;171:713–717.

107. Fukukura Y, Fujiyoshi F, Sasaki M, et al. Intraductal papillary mucinous tumors of the pancreas: thin-section helical CT findings. *AJR Am J Roentgenol* 2000;174:441–447.

108. Fukukura Y, Fujiyoshi F, Sasaki M, Nakajo M. Pancreatic duct: morphologic evaluation with MR cholangiopancreatography after secretin stimulation. *Radiology* 2002;222: 674–680.

109. Furukawa H, Iwata R, Moriyama N, Kosuge T. Selective intraarterial contrast-enhanced CT of pancreaticoduodenal tumors: early clinical experience in evaluating blood supply and detectability. *AJR Am J Roentgenol* 2000;175:91–97.

110. Gabata T, Masui S, Kadoya M, et al. Small pancreatic adenocarcinomas: efficacy of MR imaging with fat suppression and gadolinium enhancement. *Radiology* 1994; 193:683–688.

111. Ghode SC, Toth J, Krestin GP, Debatin JF. Dynamic contrast-enhanced FMPSPGR of the pancreas: impact on diagnostic performance. *AJR Am J Roentgenol* 1997;168:689–696.

112. Gines A, Vasquez-Sequeiros E, Soria MT, et al. Usefulness of EUS-guided fine needle aspiration (EUS-FNA) in the diagnosis of functioning neuroendocrine tumors. *Gastrointest Endosc* 2002; 56:291–296.

113. Gold EB, Cameron JL. Chronic pancreatitis and pancreatic cancer. *N Engl J Med* 1993;328:1485–1486.

114. Graf O, Boland GW, Warshaw AL, et al. Arterial versus portal venous phase helical CT for revealing pancreatic adenocarcinoma: conspicuity of tumor and critical vascular anatomy. *AJR Am J Roentgenol* 1997;169:119–123.

115. Gress FG, Hawes RH, Savides TJ, et al. Role of EUS in the preoperative staging of pancreatic cancer: a large single-center experience. *Gastrointest Endosc* 1999;50:786–791.

116. Gress F, Michael H, Gelrud D, et al. EUS-guided fine-needle aspiration of the pancreas: evaluation of pancreatitis as a complication. *Gastrointest Endosc* 2002;56:864–867.

117. Grizzle WE. Use of silver staining methods to identify cells of the dispersed neuroendocrine system. *J Histotechnol* 1996;19: 225–234.

118. Grogan JR, Saeian K, Taylor AJ, et al. Making sense of mucin-producing pancreatic tumors. *AJR Am J Roentgenol* 2001;176: 921–929.

119. Guiband L, Bret PM, Reinhold C, et al. Diagnosis of choledocholithiasis: value of MR Cholangiopancreatography. *AJR Am J Roentgenol* 1994;163:847–850.

120. Günther RW, Klose KJ, Rückert K, et al. Localization of small islet-cell tumors. Preoperative and intraoperative ultrasound, computed tomography, arteriography, digital subtraction angiography, and pancreatic venous sampling. *Gastrointest Radiol* 1985;10:145–152.

121. Günther RW, Klose KJ, Rückert K, et al. Islet-cell tumors: detection of small lesions with computed tomography and ultrasound. *Radiology* 1983;148:485–488.

122. Hagspiel KD, Nandalur K, Burkholder B, et al. Contrast-enhanced MR angiography after pancreas transplantation: normal appearance and vascular complications. *AJR Am J Roentgenol* 2005; 184:465–473.

123. Hajdu ED, Kamari-Subaiya S, Phillips G. Ultrasonically guided percutaneous aspiration biopsy of the pancreas. *Semin Diagn Pathol* 1986;3:166–175.

124. Hall-Craggs, MA, Lees WR. Fine needle aspiration biopsy: pancreatic and biliary tumors. *AJR Am J Roentgenol* 1986;147: 399–403.

125. Handrich SJ, Hough DM, Fletcher JG, Sarr MG. The natural history of the incidentally discovered simple pancreatic cyst: long-term follow up and clinical implications. *AJR Am J Roentgenol* 2005;184:20–23.

126. Hann LE, Conlon KC, Dougherty EC, et al. Laparoscopic sonography of peripancreatic tumors: preliminary experience. *AJR Am J Roentgenol* 1997;169:1257–1262.

127. Hanninen EL, Amthauer H, Hosten N, et al. Prospective evaluation of pancreatic tumors: accuracy of MR imaging with MR Cholangiopancreatography and MR angiography. *Radiology* 2002; 224:34–41.

128. Hariri M, Slivka A, Carr-Locke DL, Banks PA. Pseudocyst drainage predisposes to infection when pancreatic necrosis is unrecognized. *Am J Gastroenterol* 1994;89:1781–1784.

129. Hellerhof K, Hekmberger H, Rosch T, et al. Dynamic MR pancreatography after secretin administration: image quality and diagnostic accuracy. *AJR Am J Roentgenol* 2002;179;121–129.

130. Heiken JP, Balfe DM, Picus D, Scharp DW. Radical pancreatectomy: postoperative evaluation by CT. *Radiology* 1984;153: 211–215.

131. Heitz PU, Kasper M, Polak JM, Kloppel G. Pancreatic endocrine tumors. *Hum Pathol* 1982;13:263–271.

132. Hernanz-Schulman M, Teele RL, Perez-Atayde A, et al. Pancreatic cystosis in cystic fibrosis. *Radiology* 1986;158:629–631.

133. Heverhagen JT, Wagner HJ, Ebel H, et al. Pancreatic transplants: noninvasive evaluation with secretin-augmented MR pancreatography and MR perfusion measurements—preliminary results. *Radiology* 2004;233:273–280.

134. Ho CL , Dehdashti F, Griffeth LK, et al. FDG-PET evaluation of indeterminate pancreatic masses. *J Comput Assist Tomogr* 1996;20: 363–369

135. Hollerbach S, Klamann A, Topalidis T, Schmiegel WH. Endoscopic ultrasonography (EUS) and fine-needle aspiration (FNA) cytology for diagnosis of chronic pancreatitis. *Endoscopy* 2001;33: 824–831.

136. Horton KM, Fishman EK. Multidetector CT angiography of pancreatic carcinoma: part 1, evaluation of arterial involvement. *AJR Am J Roentgenol* 2002;178:827–831.

137. Horton KM, Fishman EK. Multidetector CT angiography of pancreatic carcinoma: part 2, evaluation of arterial involvement. *AJR Am J Roentgenol* 2002;178:833–836.

138. Ibukuro K, Tsukiyama T, Mori K, Inoue Y. Peripancreatic veins on thin-section (3mm) helical CT. *AJR Am J Roentgenol* 1996;167:1003–1008.

139. Ichikawa T, Haradome H, Hachiya J, et al. Pancreatic ductal adenocarcinoma: preoperative assessment with helical CT versus dynamic MR imaging. *Radiology* 1997;202:655–662.

140. Ichikawa T, Peterson MS, Federle MP, et al. Islet cell tumor of the pancreas: biphasic CT versus MR Imaging in tumor detection. *Radiology* 2000;216:163–171.

141. Imbriaco M, Megibow AJ, Camera L, et al. Dual phase versus single phase helical CT to detect and assess resectability of pancreatic carcinoma. *AJR Am J Roentgenol* 2002;178:1473–1479.

142. Inamoto K, Ishikawa Y, Itoh N. CT demonstration of annular pancreas: case report. *Gastrointest Radiol* 1983;8:143–144.

143. Inoue Y, Nakamura H. Aplasia or hypoplasia of the pancreatic uncinate process: comparison in patients with and patients without intestinal nonrotation. *Radiology* 1997;205:531–533.

144. Irie H, Honda H, Baba S, et al. Autoimmune pancreatitis: CT and MR characteristics. *AJR Am J Roentgenol* 1998;179:1323–1327.

145. Irie H, Honda H, Aibe H, et al. MR cholangiopancreatographic differentiation of benign and malignant intraductal mucin-producing tumors of the pancreas. *AJR Am J Roentgenol* 2000;174:1403–1408.

146. Isenmann R, Buchler M, Uhl W, et al. Pancreatic necrosis: an early finding in severe acute pancreatitis. *Pancreas* 1993;8: 358–361.

147. Itai Y, Ohhashi K, Furui S, et al. Microcystic adenoma of the pancreas: spectrum of computed tomographic findings. *J Comput Assist Tomogr* 1988;12:797–803.

148. Itai Y, Ohhashi K, Nagai H, et al. "Ductectatic" mucinous cystadenoma and cystadenocarcinoma of the pancreas. *Radiology* 1986;161:697–700.

149. Itoh Y, Hada T, Terano A, et al. Pancreatitis in the annulus of annular pancreas demonstrated by the combined use of computed tomography and endoscopic retrograde cholangiopancreatography. *Am J Gastroenterol* 1989;84:961–964.

150. Jaksic T, Yaman M, Thorner P, et al. A 20-year review of pediatric pancreatic tumors. *J Pediatr Surg* 1992;27:1315–1317.

151. Jensen RT, Gardner JD. Gastrinoma. In: Go VW, DiMagno EP, Gardner JD, et al, eds. *The pancreas: biology, pathobiology and disease,* 2nd ed. New York: Raven Press, 1993:931–978.

152. Jensen RT, Norton JA. Endocrine neoplasms of the pancreas. In: Yamada T, ed. *Textbook of gastroenterology,* 2nd ed., vol. 2. Philadelphia: JB Lippincott, 1995:2131–2160.

153. Jhala D, Eloubeidi M, Chieng DC, et al. Fine needle aspiration biopsy of the islet cell tumor of the pancreas: a comparison between computerized axial tomography and endoscopic ultrasound-guided fine needle aspiration biopsy. *Ann Diag Pathol* 2002;6:106–112.

154. Johnson CD. Timing of intervention in acute pancreatitis. *Postgrad Med J* 1993;69:509–515.

155. Johnson PT, Outwater EK. Pancreatic carcinoma versus chronic pancreatitis: dynamic MR imaging. *Radiology* 1999;212: 213–218.

156. Johnson CD, Stephens DH, Charboneau JW, et al. Cystic pancreatic tumors: CT and sonographic assessment. *AJR Am J Roentgenol* 1988;151:1133–1138.

157. Kahl S, Glasbrenner B, Zimmermann S, Malfertheiner P. Endoscopic ultrasound in pancreatic diseases. *Dig Dis* 2002;20(2): 120–126.

158. Kalbhen CL, Yetter EM, Olson MC, et al. Assessing the resectability of pancreatic carcinoma: the value of reinterpreting abdominal CT performed at other institutions. *AJR Am J Roentgenol* 1998;171:1571–1576.

159. Kalra MK, Maher MM, Boland GW, et al. Correlation of positron emission tomography and CT in evaluating pancreatic tumors: technical and clinical implications. *AJR Am J Roentgenol* 2003;181: 387–393.

160. Kaneko K, Honda H, Hayashi T, et al. Helical CT evaluation of arterial invasion in pancreatic tumors: comparison with angiography. *Abdom Imaging* 1997;22:204–207.

161. Kanematsu M, Shiratori Y, Hoshi H, et al. Pancreas and peripancreatic vessels: effect of gadolinium enhancement at dynamic gradient-recalled-echo MR imaging. *Radiology* 2000;215: 95–102.

162. Karasawa E, Goldberg HI, Moss AA, et al. CT pancreatogram in carcinoma of the pancreas and chronic pancreatitis. *Radiology* 1983;148:489–493.

163. Kattwinkel J, Lapey A, di Sant'Agnese PA, et al. Hereditary pancreatitis: three new kindreds and a critical review of the literature. *Pediatrics* 1973;51:55–69.

164. Kelekis NL, Smelka RC, Siegelman ES. MRI of pancreatic metastases from renal cancer. *J Comput Assist Tomogr* 1996;20: 249–253.

165. Keogan MT, McDermott VG, Paulson EK, et al. Pancreatic malignancy: effect of dual-phase helical CT in tumor detection and vascular opacification. *Radiology* 1997;205:513–518.

166. Keogan MT, Tyler D, Clark L, et al. Diagnosis of pancreatic carcinoma: role of FDG PET. *AJR Am J Roentgenol* 1998;171: 1565–1570.

167. Khurana B, Mortele KJ, Glickman J, et al. Macrocystic serous adenoma of the pancreas: radiologic-pathologic correlation. *AJR Am J Roentgenol* 2003;181:119–123.

168. Kim HJ, Czischke K, Brennan MF, Conlon KC. Does neoadjuvant chemoradiation downstage locally advanced pancreatic cancer? *J Gastrointest Surg* 2002;5:763–769.

169. Kim JH, Kim MJ, Chung JJ, et al. Differential diagnosis of periampullary carcinomas at MR imaging. *Radiographics* 2002;22: 1335–1352.

170. Kim T, Murakami T, Takahashi S, et al. Pancreatic CT imaging: effects of different injection rates and doses of contrast media. *Radiology* 1999;212:219–225.

171. Kim T, Murakami T, Takamua M, et al. Pancreatic mass due to chronic pancreatitis: correlation of CT and MR imaging features with pathologic findings. *AJR Am J Roentgenol* 2001;177:367–371.

172. King AD, Ko GTC, Yeung VTF, et al. Dual phase spiral CT in the detection of small insulinomas of the pancreas. *Br J Radiol* 1998;71:20–23.

173. Kingsnorth AN, Galloway SW, Lewis-Jones H, et al. Papillary cystic neoplasm of the pancreas: presentation and natural history in two cases. *Gut* 1992;33:421–423.

174. Kivisaari L, Somer K, Standertskjold-Nordenstam CG, et al. A new method for the diagnosis of acute hemorrhagic-necrotizing pancreatitis using contrast enhanced CT. *Gastrointest Radiol* 1984;9:27–30.

175. Kloppel G, Heitz PU. Pancreatic endocrine tumors. *Pathol Res Pract* 1988;183:155–168.

176. Koito K, Namieno T, Ichimura T, et al. Mucin-producing pancreatic tumors: comparison of MR cholangiopancreatography with endoscopic retrograde cholangiopancreatography. *Radiology* 1998; 208:231–237.

177. Koito K, Namieno T, Nagakawa T, et al. Inflammatory pancreatic masses; differentiation from ductal carcinomas with contrast-enhanced sonography using carbon dioxide microbubbles. *AJR Am J Roentgenol* 1997;169:1263–1267.

178. Krebs TL, Daly B, Wong JJ, et al. Acute pancreatic transplant rejection: evaluation with dynamic contrast-enhanced MR imaging compared with histopathologic analysis. *Radiology* 1999;210: 437–442.

179. Lal A, Bourtsos EP, DeFrias DV, et al. Microcystic adenoma of the pancreas: clinical, radiologic, and cytologic features. *Cancer* 2004;102:288–294.

180. Lammer J, Herlinger H, Zalaudek G, Hofler H. Pseudotumorous pancreatitis. *Gastrointest Radiol* 1985;10:59–67.

181. Lane MJ, Mindelzun RE, Sandhu JS, et al. CT diagnosis of blunt pancreatic trauma: importance of detecting fluid between the pancreas and the splenic vein. *AJR Am J Roentgenol* 1994;163: 833–835.

182. Larvin M Mc Mahon MJ. APACHE II score for assessment and monitoring of acute pancreatitis. *Lancet* 1989;ii;201–204.

183. Lecesne R, Taourel P, Bret PM, et al. Acute pancreatitis: interobserver agreement and correlation of CT and MR cholangiopancreatography with outcome. *Radiology* 1999;211:727–735.

184. Legmann P, Vignaux O, Dousset B, et al. Pancreatic tumors: comparison of dual-phase helical CT and endoscopic sonography. *AJR Am J Roentgenol* 1998;170:1315–1322.

185. Lehman GA. Endoscopic management of pancreatic pseudocysts continues to evolve. *Gastrointest Endosc* 1995;42: 273–275.

186. Lepanto L, Arzoumanian Y, Gianfelice D, et al. Helical CT with CT angiography in assessing periampullary neoplasms: identification of vascular invasion. *Radiology* 2002;347–352.

187. Lesniak RJ, Hohenwalter MD, Taylor AJ. Spectrum of causes of pancreatic calcifications. *AJR Am J Roentgenol* 2002;178:79–86.

188. Levy MJ, Clain JE. Evaluation and management of cystic pancreatic tumors: emphasis on the role of EUS FNA. *Clin Gastroenterol Hepatol* 2004;8:639–653.

189. Levy P, Mathurin P, Roqueplo A, et al. A multidimensional case-control study of dietary, alcohol, and tobacco habits in alcoholic men with chronic pancreatitis. *Pancreas* 1995;10:231–238.

190. Leyendecker JR, Elsayes KM, Gratz BI, Brown JJ. MR cholangiopancreatography: spectrum of pancreatic duct abnormalities. *AJR Am J Roentgenol* 2002;179:1465–1471.

191. Ligneau B, Lombard-Bohas C, Partensky C, et al. Cystic endocrine tumors of the pancreas: clinical, radiologic and histopathologic features in 13 cases. *Am J Surg Pathol* 2001;25: 752–760.

192. Lim JH, Lee G, Oh YL. Radiologic spectrum of intraductal papillary mucinous tumors of the pancreas. *Radiographics* 2001: 21-232–340.

193. Lin A, Feller ER. Pancreatic carcinoma as a cause of unexplained pancreatitis: report of ten cases. *Ann Intern Med* 1990;113: 166–167.

194. Lowenfels AB, Maisonneuve P, Cavallini G, et al. Pancreatitis and the risk of pancreatic cancer. International Pancreatitis Study Group. *N Engl J Med* 1993;328:1433–1437.

195. Lu DSK, Reber HA, Krasny RM, et al. Local staging of pancreatic cancer: criteria for unresectability of major vessels as revealed by pancreatic-phase thin- section helical CT. *AJR Am J Roentgenol* 1997;168:1439–1443.

196. Lu DSK, Vedantham S, Krasny RM, et al. Two phase helical CT for pancreatic tumors: pancreatic versus hepatic phase enhancement of tumor, pancreas and vascular structures. *Radiology* 1996;199:697–701.

197. Luetmer PH, Stephens DH, Ward EM. Chronic pancreatitis: re-assessment with current CT. *Radiology* 1989;171:353–357.

198. Lumkin B, Anderson MW, Ablin DS, McGahan JP. CT, MRI, and color Doppler ultrasound correlation of pancreatoblastoma: a case report. *Pediatr Radiol* 1993;23:61–62.

199. Lundstet C, Dawiskiba S. Serous and mucinous cystadenomas/cystadenocarcinomas of the pancreas. *Abdom Imaging* 2000;25:201–206.

200. Macari M, Lazarus D, Israel G, Megibow A. Duodenal diverticula mimicking cystic neoplasm of the pancreas: CT and MR imaging findings in seven patients. *AJR Am J Roentgenol* 2003;180:195–199.

201. Maier W. Early objective diagnosis and staging of acute pancreatitis by contrast enhanced CT. In: Beger H, Buchler M, eds. *Acute pancreatitis*. Berlin: Springer-Verlag, 1987:132–140.

202. Maile CW, Crass JR, Frick MP, et al. CT of pancreas transplantation. *Invest Radiol* 1985;20:609–612.

203. Mainwaring R, Kern J, Schenk WG, Rudolf LE. Differentiating pancreatic pseudocyst and pancreatitis necrosis using computerized tomography. *Ann Surg* 1989;209:562–568.

204. Malfertheiner P, Dominguez-Munoz JE. Prognostic factors in acute pancreatitis. *Int J Pancreatol* 1993;14:1–8.

205. Manfredi R, Costamagna G, Brizi MG, et al. Severe chronic pancreatitis versus suspected pancreatic disease: dynamic MR cholangiopancreatography after secretin stimulation. *Radiology* 2000;215:358–364.

206. Marcos HB, Libutti SK, Alexander HR, et al. Neuroendocrine tumors of the pancreas in von Hippel-Lindau disease: spectrum of appearances at CT and MR imaging with histopathologic correlation. *Radiology* 2002;225:751–758.

207. Maton PN, Miller DL, Doppman JL, et al. Role of selective angiography in the management of patients with Zollinger-Ellison syndrome. *Gastroenterology* 1987;92:913–918.

208. Matos C, Metens T, Deviere J, et al. Pancreatic duct: morphologic and functional evaluation with dynamic MR pancreatography after secretin stimulation. *Radiology* 1997;203:435–441.

209. McCarthy S, Pellegrini CA, Moss AA, Way LW. Pleuropancreatic fistula: endoscopic retrograde cholangiopancreatography and computed tomography. *AJR Am J Roentgenol* 1984;142:1151–1154.

210. McFarland EG, Kaufman JA, Saini S, et al. Preoperative staging of cancer of the pancreas: value of MR angiography versus conventional angiography in detecting portal venous invasion. *AJR Am J Roentgenol* 1996;166:37–43.

211. McMenamin DA, Gates LK. A retrospective analysis of the effect of contrast enhanced CT on the outcome of acute pancreatitis. *Am J Gastroenterol* 1996;91:1384–1387.

212. McNulty NJ, Francis IR, Platt JF, et al. Multi-detector row helical CT of the pancreas: effect of contrast-enhanced multiphasic imaging on enhancement of the pancreas, peripancreatic vasculature, and pancreatic adenocarcinoma. *Radiology* 2001;220:97–102.

213. Meador TL, Krebs TL, Wong JJ, et al. Imaging features of post-transplantation lymphoproliferative disorder in pancreas transplant recipients. *AJR Am J Roentgenol* 2000;174:121–124.

214. Megibow AJ, Zhou XH, Rotterdam H, et al. Pancreatic adenocarcinoma: CT versus MR imaging in the evaluation of resectability-report of the Radiology Diagnostic Oncology Group. *Radiology* 1995;195:327–332.

215. Meining A, Dittler HJ, Wolf A, et al. You get what you expect? A critical appraisal of imaging methodology in endosonographic cancer staging. *Gut* 2002;50:599–603.

216. Mendez G Jr, Isikoff MB. Significance of intrapancreatic gas demonstrated by CT: a review of nine cases. *AJR Am J Roentgenol* 1979;132:59–62.

217. Mergo P, Helmberger T, Buetow PC, et al. Pancreatic neoplasms: MR imaging and pathologic correlation. *Radiographics* 1997;17:281–301.

218. Merkle EM, Bender G, Brambs HJ. Imaging findings in pancreatic lymphoma: differential aspects. *AJR Am J Roentgenol* 2000;174:671–675.

219. Metzgar RS, Asch HL. Antigens of human pancreatic adenocarcinomas: their role in diagnosis and therapy. *Pancreas* 1988;3:352.

220. Meyers MA, Feldberg MA, Oliphant M. Grey Turner's sign and Cullen's sign in acute pancreatitis. *Gastrointest Radiol* 1989;14:31–37.

221. Midwinter MJ, Beveridge CJ, Wilsdon JB, et al. Correlation between spiral computed tomography, endoscopic ultrasonography and findings at operation in pancreatic and ampullary tumours. *Br J Surg* 1999;86:189–193.

222. Miller DL. Islet cell tumors of the pancreas: diagnosis and localization. In: Freeny PC, Stevenson GW eds. *Margulis and Burhenne's alimentary tract radiology*, vol. 2. St. Louis: Mosby-Year Book, 1994:1167–1196.

223. Miller FH, Gore RM, Nemcek AA, Fitzgeral SW. Pancreaticobiliary manifestations of AIDS. *AJR Am J Roentgenol* 1996;166:1269–1274.

224. Miller FH, Keppe AL, Dalal K, et al. MRI of pancreatitis and its complications: part I, acute pancreatitis. *AJR Am J Roentgenol* 2004;183:1645–1652.

225. Miller FH, Keppe AL, Wadhwa A, et al. MRI of pancreatitis and its complications: part II, chronic pancreatitis. *AJR Am J Roentgenol* 2004;183:1645–1652.

226. Mitchell DG, Cruvella M, Eschelman DJ, et al. MRI of pancreatic gastrinomas. *J Comput Assist Tomogr* 1992;16:583–585.

227. Monill J, Pernas J, Clavero J, et al. Pancreatic duct after pancreatoduodenectomy: Morphologic and functional evaluation with secretin-stimulated MR pancreatography. *AJR Am J Roentgenol* 2004;183:1267–1274.

228. Morant R, Bruckner HW. Complete remission of refractory small cell carcinoma of the pancreas with cisplatin and etoposide. *Cancer* 1989;64:2007–2009.

229. Morgan DE, Baron TH, Sith JK, et al. Pancreatic fluid collection prior to intervention: evaluation with MR imaging compared with CT and US. *Radiology* 1997;203:773–778.

230. Morgan DE, Logan K, Baron TB, et al. Pancreas divisum: implications for diagnostic and therapeutic pancreatography. *AJR Am J Roentgenol* 1999;173:193–198.

231. Mori H, McGrath FP, Malone DE, Stevenson GW. The gastrocolic trunk and its tributaries: CT evaluation. *Radiology* 1992;182:871–877.

232. Mortele KJ, Weisner W, Intriere L, et al. A modified CT Severity Index for evaluating acute pancreatitis: improved correlation with patient outcome. *AJR Am J Roentgenol* 2004;183:1261–1265.

233. Mozell E, Stenzel P, Woltering EA, et al. Functional endocrine tumors of the pancreas: clinical presentation, diagnosis, and treatment. *Curr Probl Surg* 1990;27:301–386.

234. Mulholland MW, Moossa AR, Liddle RA. Pancreas: anatomy and structural anomalies. In: Yamada T, ed. *Textbook of gastroenterology*, 2nd ed., vol. 2. Philadelphia: JB Lippincott, 1995:2051–2064.

235. Murr MM, Sarr MG, Oishi AJ, van Heerden JA. Pancreatic cancer. *Ca Cancer J Clin* 1994;44:304–318.

236. National Cancer Institute. Annual cancer statistics review: 1975-1988. Bethesda, MD: US Department of Health and Human Services;1991. NIH Publication 91-1789.

237. Neff CC, Simeone JF, Wittenberg J, et al. Inflammatory pancreatic masses: problems in differentiating focal pancreatitis from carcinoma. *Radiology* 1984;150:35–38.

238. Neoptolemos JP, Dunn JA, Stocken DD, et al. European Study Group for Pancreatic Cancer. Adjuvant chemoradiotherapy and chemotherapy in resectable pancreatic cancer: a randomised controlled trial. *Lancet* 2001;358:1576–1585.

239. Neoptolemos JP, Stocken DD, Dunn JA, et al. European Study Group for Pancreatic Cancer. Influence of resection margins on survival for patients with pancreatic cancer treated by adjuvant chemoradiation and/or chemotherapy in the ESPAC-1 randomized controlled trial. *Ann Surg* 2001;234:758–768.

240. Ng CS, Loyer EM, Iyer RB, et al. Metastases to the pancreas from renal cell carcinoma: findings on three-phase contrast-enhanced helical CT. *AJR Am J Roentgenol* 1999;172:1555–1559.

241. Nikolaides P, Amin RS, Hwang C, et al. Role of sonography on pancreatic transplantation. *Radiographics* 2003;23:939–949.

242. Nino-Murcia M, Jeffrey RB, Beaulieu, et al. Multidetector CT of the pancreas and bile duct system: value of curved planar reformations. *AJR Am J Roentgenol* 2001;176:689–693.

243. Nishiharu T, Yamashita Y, Abe Y, et al Local extension of pancreatic carcinoma: assessment with thin section helical CT versus with breath-hold fast MR imaging-ROC analysis. *Radiology* 1999; 212:445–452.

244. Norton JA, Cromack DT, Shawker TH, et al. Intraoperative ultrasonographic localization of islet cell tumors: a prospective comparison to palpation. *Ann Surg* 1988;207:160–168.

245. Norton JA, Levin B, Jensen RT. Cancer of the endocrine system. In: DeVita VT Jr, Hellman S, Rosenberg SA, eds. *Cancer: principles and practice of oncology*, vol 2, 4th ed. Philadelphia: JB Lippincott, 1993:1333–1435.

246. Norton JA, Shawker TH, Doppman JL, et al. Localization and surgical treatment of occult insulinomas. *Ann Surgery* 1990;212:615–620.

247. Novelline R, Rhea JT, Bell T. Helical CT of abdominal trauma. *Radiol Clin North Am* 1999;37:591–612.

248. Nozawa Y, Abe M, Sakuma H, et al. A case of pancreatic oncocytic tumor. *Acta Pathol Jpn* 1990;40:367–370.

249. Ohhashi K, Murakami F, Maruyama K, et al. Four cases of "mucin-producing" cancer of the pancreas. *Prog Dig Endosc* 1982;20:348–351.

250. Ohtomo K, Furui S, Onoue M, et al. Solid and papillary epithelial neoplasm of the pancreas: MR imaging and pathologic correlation. *Radiology* 1992;184:567–570.

251. Onaya H, Itai Y, Niitsu M, Chiba T, et al. Duct ectatic mucinous cystic neoplasms of the pancreas: evaluation with MR Cholangiopancreatography. *AJR Am J Roentgenol* 1998;171:171–177.

252. Oshikawa O, Tanaka S, Ioka T, et al. Dynamic sonography of pancreatic tumors; comparison with dynamic CT. *AJR Am J Roentgenol* 2002;178:1133–1137.

253. Palazzo,L, Roseau G, Gayet B, et al. Endoscopic ultrasonography in the diagnosis and staging of pancreatic adenocarcinoma. *Endoscopy* 1993;25:143–150.

254. Pasanen PA, Eskelinen M, Partanen K, et al. A prospective study of the value of imaging, serum markers and their combination in the diagnosis of pancreatic carcinoma in symptomatic patients. *Anticancer Res* 1992;12:2309–2314.

255. Patel S, Bellon EM, Haaga J. Fat replacement of the exocrine pancreas. *AJR Am J Roentgenol* 1980;135:843–845.

256. Paulson EK, Vitellas KM, Keogan MT, et al. Acute pancreatitis complicated by gland necrosis: spectrum of findings on contrast-enhanced CT. *AJR Am J Roentgenol* 1999;172:609–613.

257. Phan GQ, Yeo CJ, Hruban RH, Lillemore KD, et al. Surgical experience with pancreatic and peripancreatic neuroendocrine tumors: review of 125 patients. *J Gastroinest Surg* 1998;2:472–482.

258. Picozzi VJ, Kozarek RA, Traverso LW. Interferon-based adjuvant chemoradiation therapy after pancreaticoduodenectomy for pancreatic adenocarcinoma. *Am J Surg* 2003;185:476–480.

259. Pisegna JR, Doppman JL, Norton JA, et al. Prospective comparative study of ability of MR imaging and other imaging modalities to localize tumors in patients with Zollinger-Ellison syndrome. *Dig Dis Sci* 1993;38:1318–1328.

260. Pozniak MA, Propeck PA, Kelcz F, Sollinger H. Imaging of pancreas transplants. *Radiol Clin North Am* 1995;33:581–594.

261. Prayer L, Schurawitzki H, Mallek R, Mostbeck G. CT in pancreatic involvement of non-Hodgkin lymphoma. *Acta Radiol* 1992;33:123–127.

262. Price J, Cockram CS, McGuire LJ, et al. Uptake of 99mTc-methylene diphosphonate by pancreatic insulinoma. *AJR Am J Roentgenol* 1987;149:69–70.

263. Procacci C, Graziani R, Bicego E, et al. Intraductal mucin-producing tumors of the pancreas: imaging findings. *Radiology* 1996;198:249–257.

264. Procacci C, Biastiutti C, Carbognin G, et al. Characterization of cystic tumors of the pancreas: CT accuracy. *J Comput Assist Tomogr* 1999;23:906–912.

265. Prokesh RW, Chow LC, Beaulieu C, et al. Isoattenuating pancreatic adenocarcinoma at multi-detector row CT: secondary signs. *Radiology* 2002;224:746–768.

266. Prokesh RW, Chow, LC, Beaulieu CF, et al. Local staging of pancreatic carcinoma with multi-detector row CT: use of curved planar reformations- initial experience. *Radiology* 2002;225:759–765.

267. Ranson JHC, Rifkind KM, Roses DF, et al. Objective early identification of severe acute pancreatitis. *Am J Gastroenterol* 1974;61:443–451.

268. Ranson JH. Acute pancreatitis—where are we? *Surg Clin North Am* 1981;61:55–70.

269. Raptopoulos V, Prassopoulos P, Chuttani R, et al. Multiplanar CT pancreatography and distal cholangiography with minimum intensity projections. *Radiology* 1998;207:317–324.

270. Raptopoulos V, Steer ML, Sheiman RG, et al. The use of helical CT and CT angiography to predict vascular involvement from pancreatic cancer: correlation with findings at surgery. *AJR Am J Roentgenol* 1997;168:971–977.

271. Rattner DW, Legermate DA, Lee MJ, et al. Early surgical debridement of symptomatic pancreatic necrosis is beneficial irrespective of infection. *Am J Surg* 1992;163:105–110.

272. Raut CP, Grau AM, Staerkel GA, et al. Diagnostic accuracy of endoscopic ultrasound-guided fine-needle aspiration in patients with presumed pancreatic cancer. *J Gastroinest Surg* 2003;7(1):118–128.

273. Ravitch MM, Woods AC. Annular pancreas. *Ann Surg* 1950;132:1116–1127.

274. Rieber A, Tomczak R, Nussle K, et al. MRI with mangofodipir trisodium in the detection of pancreatic tumours: comparison with helical CT. *Br J Radiol* 2000;73:1165–1169.

275. Reiman TH, Balfe DM, Weyman PJ. Suprapancreatic biliary obstruction: CT evaluation. *Radiology* 1987;163:49–56.

276. Reinhold C, Bret PM. Current status of MR cholangiopancreatography. *AJR Am J Roentgenol* 1996;166:1285–1290.

277. Ritts R Jr, Klug T, Jacobsen D, et al. Multiple tumor marker tests enhance sensitivity of pancreatic carcinoma detection. *Cancer Detect Prev* 1984;7:459.

278. Robberecht E, Nachtegaele P, Van Rattinghe R, et al. Pancreatic lipomatosis in the Shwachman-Diamond syndrome: identification by sonography and CT scan. *Pediatr Radiol* 1985;15:348–349.

279. Roche CJ, Hughes ML, Garvey CJ, et al. CT and pathological assessment of prospective nodal staging inpatients with ductal adenocarcinoma of the head of the pancreas. *AJR Am J Roentgenol* 2003;180:475–480.

280. Rockey DC, Cello JP. Pancreaticopleural fistula. Report of 7 patients and review of the literature. *Medicine* 1990;69:332–344.

281. Rohrmann CA, Surawicz CM, Hutchinson D, et al. The diagnosis of hereditary pancreatitis by pancreatography. *Gastrointest Endosc* 1981;27:168–173.

282. Romijn MG, Stoker J, van Eijck CHJ, et al. MRI with mangofodipir trisodium in the detection and staging of pancreatic cancer. *J Magn Reson Imaging* 2000;12:261–268.

283. Ros PR, Hoon J. Multisection (multidetector) CT: applications in the abdomen. *Radiographics* 2002;22:697–700.

284. Rosch T, Dittler HJ, Strobel K, et al. Endoscopic ultrasound criteria for vascular invasion in the staging of cancer of the head of the pancreas: a blind reevaluation of videotapes. *Gastrointest Endosc* 2000;52:469–477.

285. Ross BA, Jeffrey RB Jr, Mindelzun RE. Normal variations in the lateral contour of the head and neck of the pancreas mimicking neoplasm: evaluation with dual-phase helical CT. *AJR Am J Roentgenol* 1996;166:799–801.

286. Rubin E, Dunham WK, Stanley RJ. Pancreatic metastases in bone sarcomas: CT demonstration. *J Comput Assist Tomogr* 1985;9:886–888.

287. Rumancik WM, Megibow AJ, Bosniak MA, Hilton S. Metastatic disease to the pancreas: evaluation by computed tomography. *J Comput Assist Tomogr* 1984;8:829–834.

288. Rustin RB, Broughan TA, Hermann RE, et al. Papillary cystic epithelial neoplasms of the pancreas: a clinical study of four cases. *Arch Surg* 1986;121:1073–1076.

289. Sahani DV, Kalva SP, Farrell J, et al. Autoimmune pancreatitis: imaging features. *Radiology* 2004;233:345–352.

290. Saifuddin A, Ward J, Ridgway J, Chalmers AG. Comparison of MR and CT scanning in severe acute pancreatitis: initial experiences. *Clin Radiol* 1993;48:111–116.

291. Sarles H. Chronic calcifying pancreatitis—chronic alcoholic pancreatitis. *Gastroenterology* 1974;66:604–616.

292. Sarner M. Pancreatitis: definitions and classification. In: Go VLW, ed. *The exocrine pancreas: biology, pathobiology, and diseases.* New York: Raven, 1986:459–464.

293. Scatarige JC, Horton KM, Sheth S, Fishman EK. Pancreatic parenchymal metastases: observation on helical CT. *AJR Am J Roentgenol* 2001;176:695–699.

294. Schima W, Fugger R, Schober E, et al. Diagnosis and staging of pancreatic cancer: comparison of mangofodipir trisodium-enhanced MR imaging and contrast-enhanced helical hydro CT. *AJR Am J Roentgenol* 2002;179:717–724.

295. Schmidt J, Hotz H, Foitzik T, et al. Intravenous contrast medium aggravates the impairment of pancreatic microcirculation in necrotizing pancreatitis in the rat. *Ann Surg* 1995;221:257–264.

296. Schulte SH, Baron RL, Freeny PC, et al. Root of the superior mesenteric artery in pancreatitis and pancreatic carcinoma: evaluation with CT. *Radiology* 1991;180:659–662.

297. Schwartz LH, Coakley FV, Sun Y, et al. Neoplastic pancreaticobiliary duct obstruction: evaluation with breathhold MR cholangiopancreatography. *AJR Am J Roentgenol* 1998;170:1491–1495.

298. Scott J, Martin I, Redhead D, et al. Mucinous cystic neoplasms of the pancreas: imaging features and diagnostic difficulties. *Clin Radiol* 2000;55:187–192.

299. Scott R, Jersky J, Hariparsad G. Case report: malignant giant cell tumour of the pancreas presenting as a large pancreatic cyst. *Br J Radiol* 1993;66:1055–1057.

300. Semelka RC, Ascher SM. MR imaging of the pancreas. *Radiology* 1993;188:593–602.

301. Semelka RC, Cumming MJ, Shoenut JP, et al. Islet cell tumors: comparison of dynamic contrast-enhanced CT and MR imaging with dynamic gadolinium enhancement and fat suppression. *Radiology* 1993;186:799–802.

302. Semelka RC, Kroeker MA, Shoenut JP, et al. Pancreatic disease: prospective comparison of CT, ERCP, and 1.5-T MR imaging with dynamic gadolinium enhancement and fat suppression. *Radiology* 1991;181:785–791.

303. Semelka RC, Shoenut JP, Kroeker MA, Micflikier AB. Chronic pancreatitis: MR imaging features before and after administration of gadopentetate dimeglumine. *J Magn Reson Imaging* 1993; 3:79–82.

304. Shah KK, DeRidder PH, Schwab RE, Alexander TJ. CT diagnosis of dorsal pancreas agenesis. *J Comput Assist Tomogr* 1987;11:170–171.

305. Sheiman RG, Reynolds K, Raptopoulos V. Alterations in hepatic perfusion resulting from splanchnic venous luminal compromise caused by pancreatic carcinoma. *AJR Am J Roentgenol* 2000; 175:105–108.

306. Sheridan MB, Ward J, Guthrie JA, et al. Dynamic contrast enhanced MR imaging and dual phase helical CT in the preoperative assessment of suspected pancreatic cancer: a comparative study with receiver operating characteristic analysis: *AJR Am J Roentgenol* 1999;173:583–590.

307. Sheth S, Hruban RK, Fishman EK. Helical CT of islet cell tumors of the pancreas: typical and atypical manifestations. *AJR Am J Roentgenol* 2002;179:724–730.

308. Shin HJ, Lahoti S, Sneige N. Endoscopic ultrasound-guided fine-needle aspiration in 179 cases: the M. D. Anderson Cancer Center experience. *Cancer* 2002;96:174–180.

309. Shtamler B, Bickel A, Manor E, et al. Primary lymphoma of the head of the pancreas. *J Surg Oncol* 1988;38:48–51.

310. Shuman WP, Carter SJ, Montana MA, et al. Pancreatic insufficiency: role of CT evaluation. *Radiology* 1986;158:625–627.

311. Sica GT, Braver J, Cooney MJ, et al. Comparison of endoscopic retrograde cholangiopancreatography with MR cholangiopancreatography in patients with pancreatitis. *Radiology* 1999;210:605–610.

312. Siegelman ES, Mitchell DG, Outwater E, et al. Idiopathic hemochromatosis: MR imaging findings in cirrhotic and precirrhotic patients. *Radiology* 1993;188:637–641.

313. Silas AM, Morrin MM, Raptopoulos V, Keogan MT. Intraductal papillary mucinous tumors of the pancreas. *AJR Am J Roentgenol* 2001;176:179–185.

314. Silverman PM, Kalender WA, Hazle JD. Common terminology for single and multislice helical CT. *AJR Am J Roentgenol* 2001; 176:1135–1136.

315. Sim JS, Choi BS, Han JK, et al. Helical CT anatomy of the pancreatic arteries. *Abdom Imaging* 1996;21:517–521.

316. Singer MV, Gyr K, Sarles H. Revised classification of pancreatitis. Report of the Second International Symposium on the Classification of Pancreatitis in Marseille, France, March 28-30, 1984. *Gastroenterology* 1985;89:683–685.

317. Sironi S, DeCobelli F, Zerbi A, et al. Pancreatic adenocarcinoma: assessment of vascular invasion with high-field MR imaging and a phased-array coil. *AJR Am J Roentgenol* 1996;167:997–1001.

318. Smets YFC, Westendorp RG, Van der Pijl JW, et al. Effect of simultaneous pancreas-kidney transplantation on mortality of patients with type-1 diabetes mellitus and end-stage renal disease. *Lancet* 1999;353:1915–1919.

319. Smith DR, Stanley RJ, Rue LW III. Delayed diagnosis of pancreatic transection after blunt abdominal trauma. *J Trauma* 1996;40: 1009–1013.

320. Sohn TA, Yeo CJ, Cameron JL, et al. Resected adenocarcinoma of the pancreas-616 patients: results, outcomes, and prognostic indicators. *J Gastrointest Surg* 2000;4:567–579.

321. Soto JA, Alvarez O, Munera F, et al. Traumatic disruption of the pancreatic duct: diagnosis with MR pancreatography. *AJR Am J Roentgenol* 2001;176:175–178.

322. Soyer P, Spelle L, Pelage JP, et al. Cystic fibrosis in adolescents and adults: fatty replacement of the pancreas-CT evaluation and functional correlation. *Radiology* 1999;210:611–615.

323. Spencer JA, Ward J, Guthrie JA, et al. Assessment of resectability of pancreatic cancer with dynamic contrast-enhanced MR imaging: technique, surgical correlation, and patient outcome. *Eur Radiol* 1998;8:23–29.

324. Stabile BE, Morrow DJ, Passaro E Jr. The gastrinoma triangle: operative implications. *Am J Surg* 1984;147:25–31.

325. Stafford-Johnson DB, Francis IR, Eckhauser FE, et al. Dual-phase helical CT of nonfunctioning islet cell tumors. *J Comput Assist Tomogr* 1998;22:335–339.

326. Stephenson CA, Kletzel M, Seibert JJ, Glasier CM. Pancreatoblastoma: MR appearance. *J Comput Assist Tomogr* 1990;14: 492–493.

327. Stojadinovic A, Brooks A, Hoos A, et al. An evidence-based approach to the surgical management of resectable pancreatic adenocarcinoma. *J Am Coll Surg* 2003;196:954–964.

328. Stollfuss JC, Glatting G, Friess H, et al. 2-(Fluorine-18)-fluoro-2-deoxy-D-glucose PET in detection of pancreatic cancer: value of quantitative image interpretation. *Radiology* 1995;195: 339–344.

329. Sugiyama M, Atomi Y, Hachiya J. Intraductal papillary tumors of the pancreas: evaluation with magnetic resonance cholangiopancreatography. *Am J Gastroenterol* 1998;93:156–159.

330. Tada M, Komatsu Y, Kawabe T, et al. Quantitative analysis of K-ras gene mutation in pancreatic tissue obtained by endoscopic ultrasonography-guided fine needle aspiration: clinical utility for diagnosis of pancreatic tumor. *Am J Gastroenterol* 2002 97: 2263–2270.

331. Takahashi K, Yamao K, Okubo K, et al. Differential diagnosis of pancreatic cancer and focal pancreatitis by using EUS-guided FNA. *Gastrointest Endosc* 2005;61:76–79.

332. Tamm EP, Silverman PM, Charnsangavej C, Evans DB. Imaging in oncology from the University of Texas MD Anderson Cancer Center. Diagnosis, staging, and surveillance of pancreatic cancer. *AJR Am J Roentgenol* 2003;180:1311–1323.

333. Tatli S, Mortele KJ, Levy AD, et al. CT and MRI features of pure acinar cell carcinoma of the pancreas in adults. *AJR Am J Roentgenol* 2005;184:511–519.

334. Teefey SA, Stephens DH, Sheedy PF II. CT appearance of primary pancreatitis lymphoma. *Gastrointest Radiol* 1986;11:41–43.

335. Thompson NW, Eckhauser FE, Vinik AI, et al. Cystic neuroendocrine neoplasms of the pancreas and liver. *Ann Surg* 1984;199: 158–164.

336. Toombs BD, Lester RG, Ben-Menachem Y, Sandler CM. Computed tomography in blunt trauma. *Radiol Clin North Am* 1981;19: 17–35.

337. Torres WE, Clements JL, Sones PJ, Knopf DR. Gas in the pancreatic bed without abscess. *AJR Am J Roentgenol* 1981;137: 1131–1133.

338. Trellis DR, Clouse RE. Johanson-Blizzard syndrome. Progression of pancreatic involvement in adulthood. *Dig Dis Sci* 1991;36: 365–369.

339. Tsuchiya R, Noda T, Harada N. et al. Collective review of small carcinomas of the pancreas. *Ann Surg* 1986;203:77–81.

340. Tublin ME, Tessler FN, Cheng SL, et al. Effect of injection rate of contrast medium n pancreatic and hepatic helical CT. *Radiology* 1999;210:97–101.

341. Uchiyama T, Suzuki T, Adachi A, et al. Pancreatic pleural effusion: case report and review of 113 cases in Japan. *Am J Gastroenterol* 1992;87:387–391.

342. Valls C, Andia E, Sanchez A, et al. Dual phase helical CT of pancreatic adenocarcinoma: assessment of resectability before surgery. *AJR Am J Roentgenol* 2002;178:821–826.

343. Van Hoe L, Gryspeerdt S, Marchal G, et al. Helical CT for the preoperative localization of islet cell tumors of the pancreas: Value of arterial and parenchymal phase images. *AJR Am J Roentgenol* 1995;165:1437–1439.

344. vanSonnenberg E, Wittich GR, Casola G, et al. Percutaneous drainage of infected and noninfected pancreatic pseudocysts: experience in 101 cases. *Radiology* 1989;170:757–761.

345. vanSonnenberg E, Wittich GR, Chon KS, et al. Percutaneous radiologic drainage of pancreatic abscesses. *AJR Am J Roentgenol* 1997;168:979–984.

346. Vedantham S, Lu DSK, Reber HA, Kadell B. Small peripancreatic veins: improved assessment in pancreatic cancer patients using thin-section pancreatic phase helical CT. *AJR Am J Roentgenol* 1998;170:377–383.

347. Vinik AI, Strodel WE, Eckhauser FE, et al. Somatostatinomas, PPomas, neurotensinomas. *Semin Oncol* 1987;14:263–281.

348. Ward J, Chalmers AG, Guthrie AJ, et al. T2 weighted and dynamic enhanced MRI in acute pancreatitis: comparison with contrast enhanced CT. *Clin Radiol* 1997;52:109–114.

349. Warshaw AL, Rattner DW, Fernandez-del-castillo C. Intravenous contrast does aggravate experimental pancreatitis. *Gastroenterology* 1994;107:320–321.

350. Webb TH, Lillemoe KD, Pitt HA, et al. Pancreatic lymphoma. Is surgery mandatory for diagnosis or treatment? *Ann Surg* 1989;209:25–30.

351. West JH, Vogel SB, Drane WE. Gallium uptake in complicated pancreatitis: a predictor of infection. *AJR Am J Roentgenol* 2002; 178:841–846.

352. Weyman PJ, Stanley RJ, Levitt RG. Computed tomography in evaluation of the pancreas. *Semin Roentgenol* 1981;16:301–311.

353. Whang EE, Danial T, Dunn JC, et al. The spectrum of mucin-producing adenocarcinoma of the pancreas. *Pancreas* 2001;21: 147–151.

354. White EM, Wittenberg J, Mueller PR, et al. Pancreatic necrosis: CT manifestations. *Radiology* 1986;158:343–346.

355. Wiersema MJ. Accuracy of endoscopic ultrasound in diagnosing and staging pancreatic carcinoma. *Pancreatology* 2001;1:625–632.

356. Wildling R, Schnedl WJ, Reisinger EC, et al. Agenesis of the dorsal pancreas in a woman with diabetes mellitus and in both of her sons. *Gastroenterology* 1993;104:1182–1186.

357. Wilentz RE, Albores-Saavedra J, Hruban RH. Mucinous cystic neoplasms of the pancreas. *Semin Diagn Pathol* 2000;17: 31–42.

358. Wilson TE, Korobkin M, Francis IR. Pancreatic plasmacytoma: CT findings. *AJR Am J Roentgenol* 1989;152:1227–1228.

359. Wingo PA, Tong T, Bolden S. Cancer statistics, 1995. *Ca Cancer J Clin* 1995;45:8–30.

360. Winter TC, Freeny PC, Nghiem HV. Extrapancreatic gastrinoma localization: value of arterial-phase helical CT with water as an oral contrast agent. *AJR Am J Roentgenol* 1996;166:51–52.

361. Winsett MZ, Kumar R, Balachandran S, et al. Pseudocyst following splenectomy: impact of CT and ultrasound on its diagnosis and management. *Gastrointest Radiol* 1988;13:177–179.

362. Wise RH Jr, Stanley RJ. Carcinoma of the ampulla of Vater presenting as acute pancreatitis. *J Comput Assist Tomogr* 1984;8: 158–161.

363. Wittenberg J, Simone JF, Ferrucci JT Jr, et al. Non-focal enlargement in pancreatic carcinoma. *Radiology* 1982;144:131–135.

364. Wolf EL, Sprayregen S, Frager D, et al. Calcification in an insulinoma of the pancreas. *Am J Gastroenterol* 1984;79:559–561.

365. Wolfman NT, Karstaedt N, Kawamoto EH. Pleomorphic carcinoma of the pancreas: computed-tomographic, sonographic, and pathologic findings. *Radiology* 1985;154:329–332.

366. Wong JJ, Krebs TL, Klassen DK, et al. Sonographic evaluation of acute pancreatic transplant rejection: morphology-Doppler analysis versus guided percutaneous biopsy. *AJR Am J Roentgenol* 1996;166:803–807.

367. Wong Yc, Wang LJ,Lin BC, et al. CT grading of pancreatic injuries: prediction of ductal disruption and surgical correlation. *J Comput Assist Tomogr* 1997;21:246–250.

368. Yamada Y, Mori H, Kiyosue H, et al. CT assessment of the inferior peripancreatic veins: clinical significance. *AJR Am J Roentgenol* 2000;174:677–684.

369. Yamao K, Ohashi K, Nakamura T, et al. Evaluation of various imaging methods in the differential diagnosis of intraductal papillary-mucinous tumor (IPMT) of the pancreas. *Hepatogastroenterology* 2001;48:962–966.

370. Yeh HC, Stancato-Pasik A, Shapiro RS. Microcystic features at US: a nonspecific sign for microcystic adenomas of the pancreas. *Radiographics* 2001;21:1455–1461.

371. Yeo CS, Cameron JL. Pancreatic cancer. *Curr Probl Surg* 1999; 36:57–152.

372. Yoshida K, Toki F, Takeuchi T, et al. Chronic pancreatitis caused by an autoimmune abnormality: proposal of the concept of autoimmune pancreatitis. *Dig Dis Sci* 1995;40:1561–1568.

373. Zeman RK, McVay L, Silverman PM, et al. Thin section CT of pancreas divisum. In: *Syllabus of the Society of Gastrointestinal Radiologists*, Seventeenth Annual Meeting and Postgraduate Course, January 16-20, 1988, Nassau, Bahamas, p. 31(abst).

374. Zerby AL, Lee MJ, Brugge WR, Mueller PR. Endoscopic sonography of the upper gastrointestinal tract and pancreas. *AJR Am J Roentgenol* 1996;166:45–50.

375. Zimny M, Bares R, Fass J, et al. Fluorine-18 fluorodeoxyglucose positron emission tomography in the differential diagnosis of pancreatic carcinoma: a report of 106 cases. *Eur J Nucl Med* 1997;24:678–682.

Abdominal Wall and Peritoneal Cavity

16

Jay P. Heiken   Christine O. Menias   Khaled Elsayes

ABDOMINAL WALL

Anatomy

The normal anatomy of the abdominal wall is discussed in Chapter 10.

Pathology

Hernias

Although the diagnosis of hernia usually can be established clinically, computed tomography (CT) may be useful in select instances in differentiating between a hernia and a mass within the abdominal cavity or abdominal wall (219). CT also can demonstrate symptomatic incisional hernias in patients who are difficult to examine, such as obese individuals, those in the early postoperative period, and those with abdominal wall scars. In addition, CT may reveal clinically unsuspected incisional hernias in patients undergoing postoperative CT examinations and may show ventral hernias in patients who have sustained blunt or penetrating abdominal trauma (84,155,224). CT is useful in demonstrating the size of the hernia sac and the underlying fascial defect, as well as the hernia content and any associated complications such as bowel obstruction, ischemia, or infarction. Acquiring the CT images while the patient performs the Valsalva maneuver to increase intra-abdominal pressure can aid in demonstrating some hernias, particularly those involving the ventral abdominal wall (68,116,121,127). A ventral hernia is produced when the linea alba is disrupted and fat and/or

bowel herniate anteriorly through the defect (Fig. 16-1). An incisional hernia can occur at any abdominal wall surgical incision site, including a laparoscopic port site (Fig. 16-2). A Spigelian hernia results from weakness in the internal oblique and transversus aponeuroses, allowing peritoneal contents to herniate beneath an intact external oblique muscle. CT can establish the diagnosis by demonstrating a peritoneal and muscular defect at the lateral border of the rectus sheath (18) (Figs. 16-3 and 16-4). Lumbar hernias can occur at two weak points in the posterolateral abdominal wall (15,153). The lower of the two weak points, called the *inferior lumbar triangle*, or *Petit's triangle*, lies just above the iliac crest between the external oblique and latissimus dorsi muscles (15,153). The larger point is called the *superior lumbar triangle*, or *Grynfelt's triangle*, and is bounded by the 12th rib, the serratus posticus muscle, the internal oblique muscle, and the erector spinae muscles. These rare posterior abdominal wall hernias may contain intraperitoneal or extraperitoneal contents.

The indirect inguinal hernia, the most common type of external abdominal hernia, results from herniation of peritoneal contents through the deep inguinal ring (Fig. 16-5). If sufficiently large, the hernia sac may extend into the scrotum in men or into the labium majorum in women. A femoral hernia results when peritoneal contents enter the femoral canal adjacent to the femoral artery and vein. In this type of hernia, the sac protrudes lateral to the inguinal canal between the external oblique muscle insertion on the superior pubic ramus and the superior pubic ramus itself (265). It is often difficult to distinguish small inguinal and femoral hernias radiographically (3,328). The most

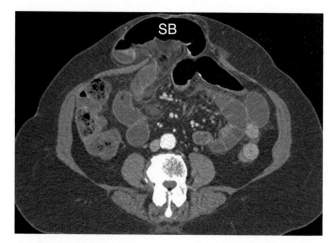

Figure 16-1 Ventral hernia. A small bowel loop (SB) has herniated anteriorly through a wide defect in the linea alba; note edema of the small bowel mesentery.

common type of obturator hernia results when intraperitoneal or extraperitoneal contents protrude between the pectineus and external obturator muscles (Fig. 16-6) (189). Less commonly, herniation occurs between the external and internal obturator muscles (Fig. 16-7) or between the fasciculi of the external obturator muscle.

Masses: Hematoma

Abdominal wall hematomas occur most commonly within the sheath of the rectus abdominis muscle and are most often secondary to anticoagulant therapy, although they may occur with various disease states, abdominal wall trauma, and severe exertion (25,77,240). Clinical findings

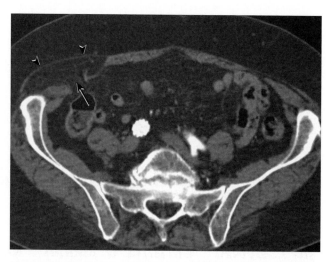

Figure 16-3 Spigelian hernia. Omental fat protrudes through a defect in the right linea semilunaris (*arrow*) but is contained by an intact external oblique muscle (*arrowheads*). The hernia sac may be confused with an abdominal wall lipoma if the muscular defect is not recognized.

that suggest an abdominal wall hematoma include acute onset of abdominal pain in association with a palpable mass, discoloration of the skin overlying the mass, and a decreasing hematocrit. Often the clinical presentation is one of acute abdominal pain alone, and CT can establish the diagnosis of hematoma, excluding other intraperitoneal etiologies. CT may accurately assess the extent of hematoma and determine if a concomitant intra-abdominal or retroperitoneal hematoma is present.

The CT appearance of abdominal wall hematoma is that of an abnormal mass, often elliptical or spindle-

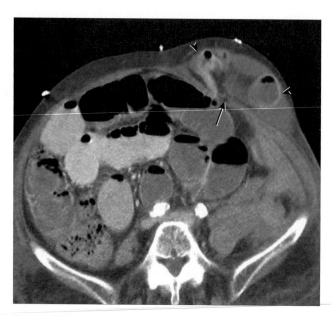

Figure 16-2 Laparoscopic port site hernia. Herniation of a small bowel loop (*arrowheads*) through a fascial defect (*arrow*) just lateral to the rectus abdominis muscle has resulted in small bowel obstruction.

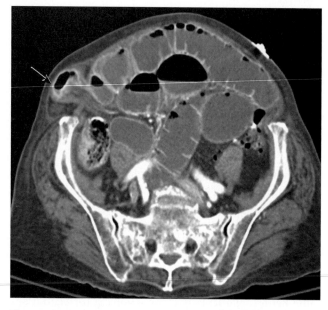

Figure 16-4 Spigelian hernia with small bowel obstruction. Herniation of a small bowel loop (*arrow*) through a defect in the right linea semilunaris has resulted in a high-grade small bowel obstruction.

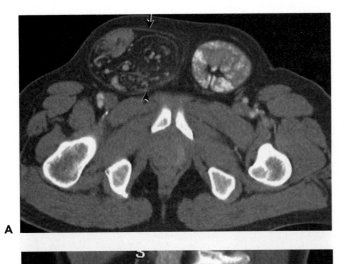

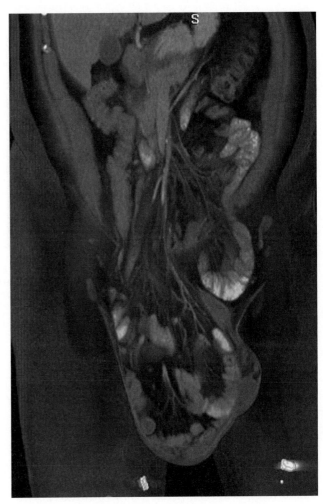

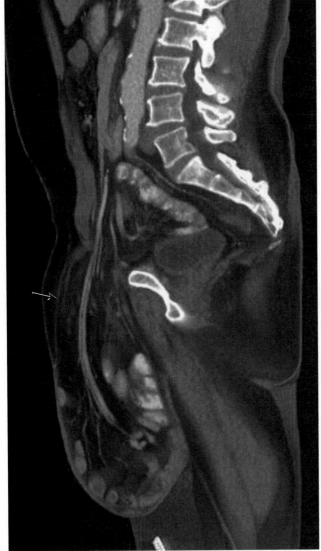

Figure 16-5 Bilateral inguinal hernias. Transaxial pelvic computed tomography **(A)** and volume-rendered coronal **(B)** and sagittal **(C)** reformatted images show small bowel loops and small bowel mesentery herniated through bilateral fascial defects. The aponeurosis of the external oblique muscle (*arrow*) forms the anterior wall and the aponeurosis of the transversus muscle (*arrowhead*) forms the posterior wall of the canal.

shaped, in one or more layers of the abdominal wall, enlarging, obliterating, or displacing normal structures (Fig. 16-8A). Rectus sheath hematomas are usually limited to one side of the abdomen by the linea alba. Large

hematomas may, however, dissect inferiorly along fascial planes and extend into the pelvis, compressing viscera and crossing to the contralateral side (221). An acute abdominal wall hematoma has a density equal to or greater

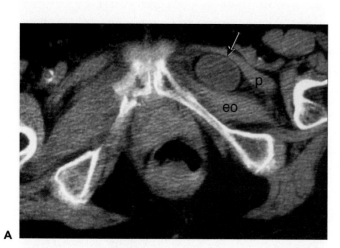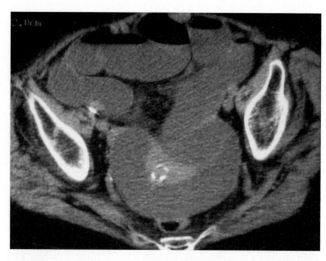

A

B

Figure 16-6 Obturator hernia causing small bowel obstruction. **A:** A loop of small bowel (*arrow*) has herniated between the pectineus (p) and external obturator (eo) muscles. **B:** A more cephalad image shows dilated, obstructed small bowel loops.

than the density of the abdominal muscles because of the high protein content of hemoglobin. Of all body wall hematomas scanned within the first 2 weeks after hemorrhage, 75% are hyperdense and often heterogeneous (288). On occasion, a fluid–fluid level can be seen as a result of the settling of cellular elements within the hematoma ("the hematocrit effect") (Fig. 16-8B). As the hematoma matures, the progressive breakdown and removal of protein within red blood cells reduces the attenuation value of the hematoma (203). The process of clot lysis often occurs in a centripetal fashion, producing a low-attenuation halo at the periphery that widens as lysis progresses. By 2 to 4 weeks after the initial bleeding episode, the density of the hematoma may approach that of serum (20 to 30 HU) and then remains serum density for the duration of its existence. With time a fibroblastic and vascular membrane (pseudocapsule) grows around the hematoma, producing a dense rim on CT images. On occasion, the periphery of a chronic hematoma (seroma) may calcify.

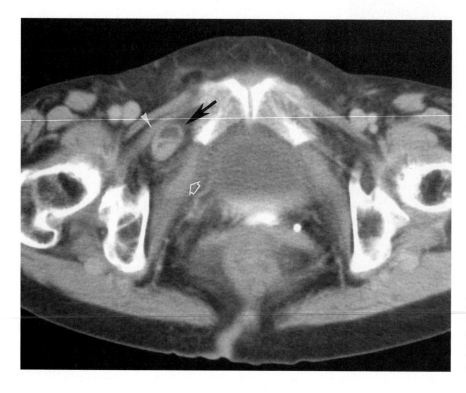

Figure 16-7 Obturator hernia causing small bowel obstruction. **A:** In this patient the hernia sac, which contains a small bowel loop (*arrow*), passes between the external (*arrowhead*) and internal (*open arrow*) obturator muscles, a less common form of obturator hernia than that seen in Figure 16-6.

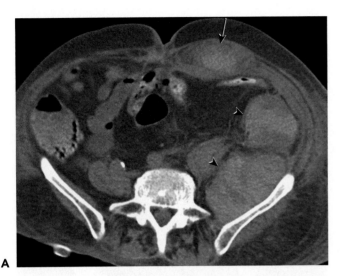
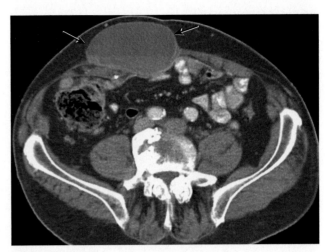

A   B

Figure 16-8 Abdominal wall hematomas. **A:** Unenhanced computed tomography shows spindle shaped enlargement and high attenuation (*arrow*) in the left rectus abdominis muscle. Note the extraperitoneal hemorrhage (*arrowheads*) in the left side of the pelvis. **B:** A contrast-enhanced image in another patient demonstrates an oval fluid collection (*arrows*) with a hematocrit level in the right rectus abdominis muscle sheath.

The MRI appearance of abdominal wall hematoma undergoes an evolution similar to that seen on CT. In addition to age, the MRI appearance of a hematoma depends on the magnetic field strength at which it is imaged and the pulse sequence used. When examined at high magnetic field strength (1.5 T), an acute hematoma has a signal intensity similar to that of muscle on longitudinal relaxation time (T1)-weighted images with marked hypointensity on transverse relaxation time (T2)-weighted images (252). The prominent hypointensity on T2-weighted images implies preferential T2 proton relaxation enhancement (89). It has been proposed that the high concentration of Fe^{2+}-deoxyhemoglobin inside intact red blood cells in acute hematomas creates local heterogeneity of magnetic susceptibility, resulting in preferential T2 proton relaxation enhancement (89). This T2-shortening effect is more pronounced with a gradient-echo sequence than with a spin-echo technique. Large acute hematomas may demonstrate a fluid–fluid level on MR images, similar to that seen on CT. On CT, the dependent portion of the hematoma is high in attenuation. On T1-weighted MR images, the dependent portion is hyperintense compared with the supernatant, whereas on T2-weighted images this signal intensity relationship is reversed (102).

Subacute hematomas (older than 1 week) have a more characteristic MRI appearance on T1-weighted images, consisting of a medium-signal-intensity (slightly greater than muscle) central area corresponding to the high-attenuation area on CT, surrounded by a high-intensity ring corresponding to the area of low attenuation on CT, which in turn is surrounded by a thin rim of very low signal intensity (102,252,297). On T2-weighted images, the signal intensity of the central core is similar to that of the peripheral zone. The thin outer rim remains very low in signal intensity. The high signal intensity of subacute hematomas is a result of T1 shortening caused by the presence of extracellular methemoglobin resulting from oxidative denaturation of hemoglobin (28).

Inflammation/Infection

Inflammation in the abdominal wall is most often the result of infection, most commonly postoperative wound infection (323). Other less common causes include trauma, direct extension from intra-abdominal inflammatory processes, and altered host defense (266). Clinical diagnosis of an abdominal wall infection is often difficult, especially in early postoperative or obese patients. The extent of tissue involvement is often underestimated by physical examination. CT can be useful in differentiating abscess from cellulitis, diagnosing or excluding infection in patients with postoperative wound tenderness, delineating the size and extent of an abscess when present, and determining whether or not the peritoneal cavity is involved.

The CT findings of abdominal wall inflammation are nonspecific and include streaky soft tissue densities, loss of normal intermuscular fat planes, enlargement of abdominal wall muscles, localized masses of varying density, and masses that dissect along fascial planes. An abdominal wall abscess appears as an abnormal mass that usually has a low-attenuation central zone (Fig. 16-9). The peripheral zone or wall of the abscess may enhance after administration of intravenous iodinated contrast material. Occasionally, gas, resulting from gas-producing organisms, may be present in an abdominal wall abscess. However, the presence of gas within the abdominal wall is not a specific sign of abscess because gas in a partially open abdominal wound or gas in a fistula connecting bowel to the skin surface

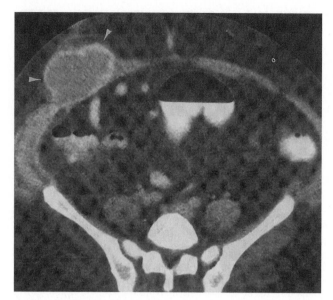

Figure 16-9 Abdominal wall abscess. The right rectus abdominis muscle contains a low attenuation fluid collection with an enhancing wall (*arrowheads*).

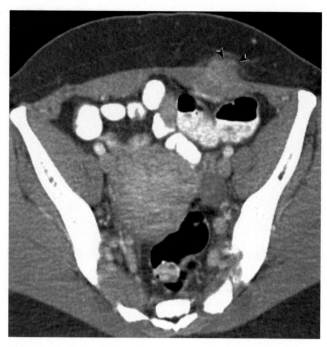

Figure 16-10 Abdominal wall endometrioma. Pelvic computed tomography shows a small enhancing soft tissue mass (*arrowheads*) within the left rectus abdominis muscle in this patient who previously had undergone laparoscopy for endometriosis.

may appear similar. Because the CT appearance of abscess is not specific, needle aspiration may be necessary to confirm the diagnosis. Both MRI and CT are effective in demonstrating and characterizing abdominal wall infections. The multiplanar capability of CT and MRI can be of particular help in defining intraperitoneal extension and in surgical planning (113,266).

Other Nonneoplastic Entities

Endometrial implants in the abdominal wall can occur in laparotomy incisions or in the tracts of instrument ports from laparoscopy (Figs. 16-10 and 16-11). Although these implants usually result from procedures that expose the endometrial cavity, such as cesarean section (317), seeding also can occur from adnexal or peritoneal endometriosis. CT may demonstrate a soft tissue attenuation mass that is difficult to differentiate from the adjacent abdominal wall musculature. MRI may show high signal intensity on T1- and T2-weighted images resulting from hemorrhage (Fig. 16-12).

Heterotopic ossification, a form of myositis ossificans traumatica, can occur in midline abdominal surgical incisions. The osseous, cartilaginous, and, less commonly, marrow elements are responsible for the predictable CT appearance of soft tissue, bone, and sometimes fat attenuation components. Recognition of this lesion allows distinction from other entities such as postoperative hematoma or infection, retained foreign body, and primary or metastatic malignancy (125). Exuberant scar formation in an abdominal wall wound (keloid), appears as a superficial soft tissue mass centered within the skin overlying an incision site. On MR images, it demonstrates low signal intensity on both T1- and T2-weighted images.

Diffuse lipomatosis of the abdominal wall is a benign condition that may be impossible to differentiate from a well-differentiated liposarcoma with CT or MRI, requiring histologic diagnosis (53).

Neoplasms

Both primary and secondary neoplasms can involve the abdominal wall. Although large masses generally are discovered by inspection and palpation, small tumors may be difficult to detect clinically, particularly in obese patients or in those with surgical scars or indurated tissue. CT is capable of demonstrating small abdominal wall tumors and may be valuable in defining the extent of palpable lesions for the purpose of placing radiotherapy ports and assessing the effectiveness of chemotherapy. CT is also helpful in detecting tumor recurrence after surgical excision (66).

Lipomas are common, benign tumors that can be found throughout the body, including the subcutaneous fat or muscle layers of the abdominal wall. They are well-defined, homogeneous, fat attenuation (-40 to -100 HU) masses that may contain thin soft tissue septa and vessels.

Desmoid tumors are locally aggressive, benign fibrous tissue neoplasms that occur most commonly in the musculoaponeurotic fascia of the anterior abdominal wall, usually in the rectus abdominis and internal oblique muscles and their fascial coverings. Approximately three fourths of abdominal wall desmoids occur in women, predominantly during the childbearing years (29). On precontrast CT images, desmoid tumors have an attenuation value similar to

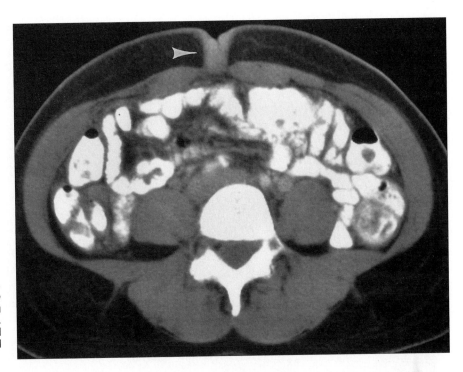

Figure 16-11 Umbilical endometriosis. Soft tissue attenuation prominence of the umbilicus (*arrowhead*) represents seeding of a laparoscopy tract by endometriosis. This patient experienced cyclic umbilical bleeding, corresponding to her menstrual cycle.

that of muscle, but they may enhance after contrast medium administration to become hyperdense relative to muscle (Fig. 16-13) (117). On MR images, desmoid tumors commonly appear isointense to muscle on T1-weighted images, variable in signal intensity on T2-weighted images, and demonstrate diffuse enhancement after intravenous administration of gadolinium (246). Extensive fibrosis is suggested by areas of low signal intensity on both T1- and T2-weighted images (122). These MR signal characteristics are nonspecific, but suggestive in the proper clinical setting. The multiplanar capability of MRI and multidetector CT is helpful in defining the connection of the mass to the abdominal wall muscle or fascia (122).

Neurofibromas, seen most commonly in patients with neurofibromatosis, often appear as homogeneous soft tissue masses of varying size involving the skin and subcutaneous fat (Fig. 16-14). The attenuation of abdominal wall neurofibromas is usually similar to that of skeletal muscle.

The most common primary malignant neoplasms of the abdominal wall are sarcomas (Fig. 16-15), followed in frequency by lymphomas. Hematogenously spread metastases may involve either the abdominal wall muscles (Fig. 16-16) or the subcutaneous fat. Metastatic involvement of muscle produces enlargement of the muscle, often with an associated alteration in normal attenuation value. Subcutaneous metastases usually are nodular, and are readily demonstrated at CT as soft tissue attenuation masses in the lower attenuation subcutaneous fat (222). Direct spread to the abdominal wall by an intra-abdominal neoplasm appears as a thickening of the muscles with loss of the intermuscular and perimuscular fat planes (219). Malignant neoplasms that spread intraperitoneally, such as ovarian and gastrointestinal tract carcinomas, have a tendency to involve the umbili-

cal region, producing periumbilical masses. Such periumbilical metastases are sometimes referred to as *Sister Mary Joseph nodules*, named after the first assistant to Dr. William Mayo, who while preparing patients' abdomens prior to surgery in the early days of the Mayo Clinic, observed that patients with advanced intra-abdominal malignancy often had umbilical nodules (52). Abdominal wall metastases of colon, ovarian, gastric, and gallbladder carcinoma have been reported in incisions and port sites after laparoscopy (Fig. 16-17) (23,33,48,86,126,129,306). Differentiation of abdominal wall neoplasm from abscess or hematoma may not be possible using CT criteria alone and clinical correlation is often necessary. Percutaneous needle biopsy under ultrasound or CT guidance may be required to differentiate among these entities.

PERITONEAL CAVITY

Anatomy

The peritoneal cavity contains a series of communicating but compartmentalized potential spaces that are not visualized on CT unless they are distended by fluid. Knowledge of the anatomy of these spaces and of the ligaments that define them is important in the understanding of pathologic processes involving the peritoneal cavity.

The walls of the peritoneal cavity, as well as the abdominal and pelvic organs contained within, are lined with peritoneum, an areolar membrane covered by a single row of mesothelial cells (93). Folds of peritoneum, called *ligaments*, connect and provide support for structures within this cavity. The name of a particular ligament usually reflects the two major structures that it joins (e.g., the gastrocolic

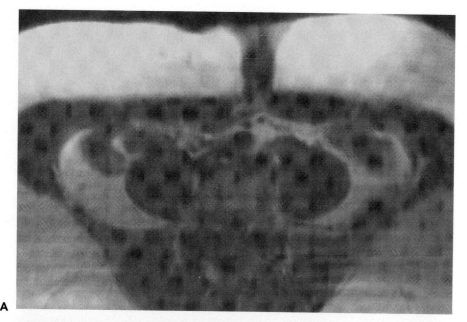

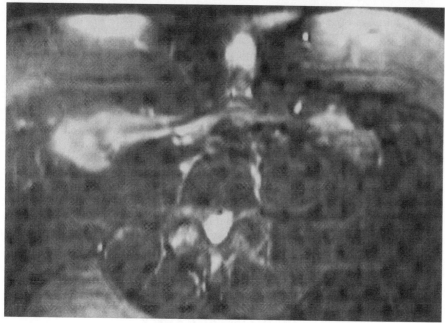

Figure 16-12 Umbilical endometriosis. Magnetic resonance imaging demonstrates thickening of the umbilicus which is intermediate in signal intensity on T1-weighted (**A**) and high in signal intensity on T2-weighted (**B**) images.

ligament extends between the greater curvature of the stomach and the transverse colon). A ligament that connects the stomach to other structures is called an *omentum*. The greater omentum joins the greater curvature of the stomach to the colon and then continues downward anterior to the small bowel. The lesser omentum (also called the *gastrohepatic ligament*) joins the lesser curvature of the stomach to the liver. A mesentery is a fold of peritoneum connecting either the small bowel or portions of the colon to the posterior abdominal wall. Normally, these peritoneal folds are not directly imaged by CT, but fat, lymph nodes, and vessels contained within them can be identified (273). When the peritoneal folds become thickened by edema, inflammation, or neoplastic infiltration, they can be directly visualized on CT. Ligaments, omenta, and

mesenteries can serve as routes of spread of benign and malignant pathologic processes within the peritoneal cavity, as well as between the peritoneum and the retroperitoneum (9,62,185,217). The mode of spread can be by direct extension or via the lymphatics, vessels, or nerves in the areolar tissue enclosed by peritoneum (9,62,41,42,185, 213–217), referred to by some authors as the *subperitoneal space* (185,216). Knowledge of these structures is important in image interpretation.

The major barrier dividing the peritoneal cavity is the transverse mesocolon, which separates the cavity into supramesocolic and inframesocolic compartments (181). An understanding of the anatomy of the supramesocolic compartment is aided by familiarity with the embryologic development of this space (discussed in Chapter 10).

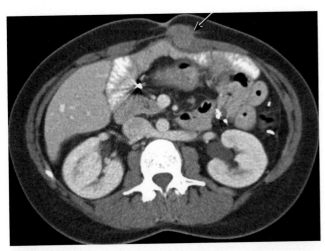

Figure 16-13 Desmoid tumor. Contrast-enhanced computed tomography shows a homogeneously enhancing mass (*arrow*) involving the left rectus abdominis muscle in this patient, who has undergone a colectomy for familial adenomatous polyposis.

Supramesocolic Compartment

In the following discussion, the left and right peritoneal spaces are arbitrarily divided into a number of subspaces. Although these spaces freely communicate, they often become separated by fibrous adhesions when inflammatory or neoplastic processes cause fluid to collect in these spaces. (For a complete discussion of the anatomy of the peritoneal spaces, see Chapter 10.)

Left Peritoneal Space

The left peritoneal space can be divided into anterior and posterior perihepatic and anterior and posterior subphrenic spaces. The left anterior perihepatic space can be affected by pathology emanating from the left lobe of the liver or the anterior wall of the body and antrum of the stomach (Fig. 16-18). In addition, it may be involved by extension of pathologic processes from other portions of the left peritoneal space (Fig. 16-19).

The left posterior perihepatic space is also referred to as the *gastrohepatic recess*. This space may be affected by pathologic processes arising in any of the structures to which it is closely related, including the left lobe of the liver, the lesser curvature of the stomach, the anterior wall of the duodenal bulb, and the anterior wall of the gallbladder (307).

The *left anterior subphrenic space* is in direct continuity with the left anterior perihepatic space inferomedially and with the left posterior subphrenic space dorsally (117,283) (Figs. 16-20, 16-21, and 16-22). Fluid collections in this region may result from perforation of the splenic flexure of the colon or of the fundus or upper body of the stomach. In addition, left anterior subphrenic space collections may result from extension of disease processes involving the left perihepatic spaces or the left posterior subphrenic space.

The *left posterior subphrenic (perisplenic) space* is the posterior continuation of the anterior subphrenic space (see Fig. 16-21). Common sources of pathology involving the left posterior subphrenic space include splenic surgery (i.e., postoperative abscess or hematoma), splenic trauma, and extension of disease processes involving the anterior subphrenic space. In addition, pathology involving the tail of the pancreas can affect the left subphrenic space. Uncommonly, disease processes arising in retroperitoneal organs such as the left kidney or left adrenal gland can extend into this peritoneal space.

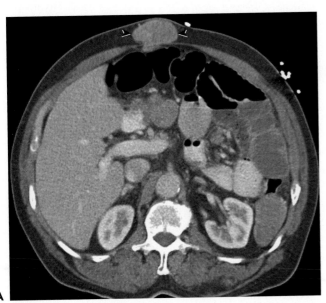

A

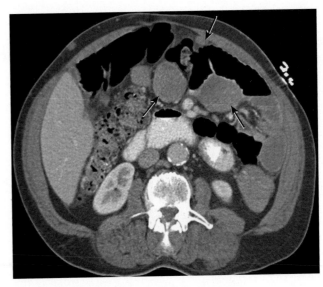

B

Figure 16-14 Neurofibromatosis type 1. **A** and **B**: Computed tomography shows homogeneous soft tissue attenuation masses within the subcutaneous fat (*arrowheads*) and the mesenteric and omental fat (*arrows*).

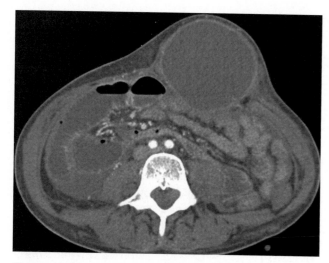

Figure 16-15 Abdominal wall neurofibrosarcoma. Computed tomography shows a large cystic mass within the left rectus abdominis muscle in this patient with metastatic neurofibrosarcoma.

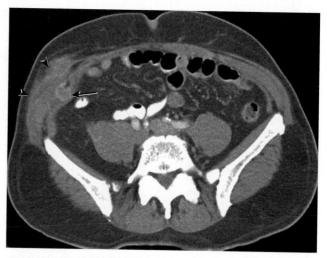

Figure 16-16 Metastatic colon carcinoma. Computed tomography demonstrates thickening of the right abdominal wall muscles (*arrowheads*) with loss of the intermuscular fat planes. A discrete enhancing tumor nodule (*arrow*) involves the transversus abdominis and internal oblique muscles.

Right Peritoneal Space

The right peritoneal space includes both the lesser sac and the right portion of the greater peritoneal space surrounding the liver (i.e., the right perihepatic space). These two spaces communicate via the epiploic foramen (foramen of Winslow).

Right Perihepatic Space

The right perihepatic space consists of a subphrenic and a subhepatic space (see Figs. 16-23 and 16-24), which are partially separated by the right coronary ligaments. The posterior subhepatic space projects cephalad into the recess between the liver and the right kidney (see Fig. 16-23B). This recess, known as the *hepatorenal fossa* or *Morison's*

pouch, is the most dependent part of the subhepatic space when the body is in the supine position and is therefore important in the spread and localization of intraperitoneal fluid collections. Common sources of pathology causing fluid collections in the right perihepatic space include the gallbladder, the descending portion of the duodenum (Figs. 16-25 to 16-27), the right lobe of the liver, and the right colon. Another important cause of a right perihepatic fluid collection is cephalad extension of pelvic fluid via the right paracolic gutter. Occasionally, retroperitoneal disease processes arising in the right kidney, right adrenal gland, head of pancreas, or duodenum can extend into the right perihepatic space.

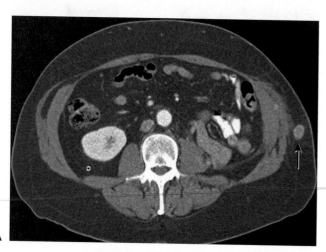

A

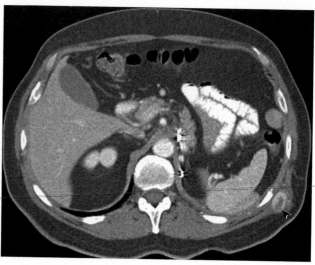

B

Figure 16-17 Renal cell carcinoma involving abdominal wall. **A** and **B**: Computed tomography shows enhancing masses within the subcutaneous fat (*arrow*) and abdominal wall muscles (*arrowhead*) in a patient who underwent left nephrectomy for renal cell carcinoma.

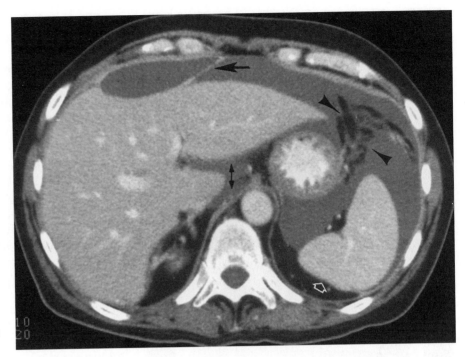

Figure 16-18 Malignant ascites in a woman with metastatic ovarian carcinoma. Anteriorly the falciform ligament (*arrow*) separates the right and left peritoneal spaces. Fat in the gastrocolic ligament (*arrowheads*) defines the left margin of the left anterior perihepatic space. A small amount of fluid is present in the lesser sac (*double arrow*). Along the posterior border of the spleen, fluid is limited medially by the spleen's peritoneal reflection (the bare area of the spleen) (*open arrow*).

Lesser Sac

The lesser sac communicates with the remainder of the right peritoneal space through a narrow inlet between the inferior vena cava and the free margin of the hepatoduodenal ligament called the *epiploic foramen* (or *foramen of Winslow*). In patients with intraperitoneal inflammation, this foramen may seal, separating the lesser sac from the greater peritoneal cavity (181). A prominent fold of peritoneum, elevated from the posterior abdominal wall by the left gastric artery, divides the lesser sac into two compartments—a large lateral compartment on the left and a smaller medial compartment on the right (181) (Fig. 16-28). The medial compartment contains a superior recess that wraps around the caudate lobe of the liver (Fig. 16-29).

Disease processes producing generalized ascites or those involving the pancreas, transverse colon, posterior wall of the stomach, posterior wall of the duodenum, and caudate lobe of the liver can produce pathologic changes in the lesser sac. The most common lesser sac collection is ascites (65). Whereas patients with benign, transudative

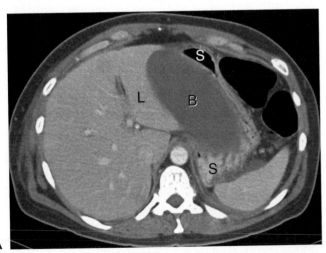

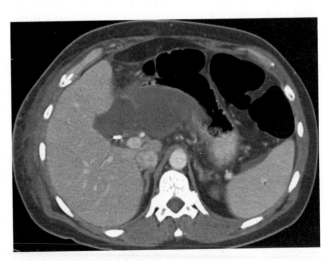

Figure 16-19 Biloma. **A:** A fluid collection (B) in the left anterior perihepatic space compresses the body of the stomach (S) and the left lobe of the liver (L). **B:** A more caudal image demonstrates communication of the collection with the gallbladder fossa in this patient who had undergone recent laparoscopic cholecystectomy.

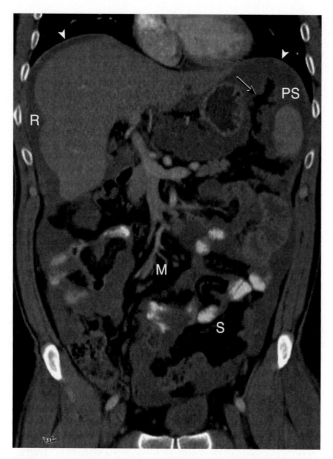

Figure 16-20 Pseudomyxoma peritonei. Coronal volume-rendered image shows diffuse peritoneal involvement with confluent low attenuation masses, which outline the small bowel mesentery (M) and sigmoid mesocolon (S). Involvement of the right and left subphrenic spaces is shown (*arrowheads*). The perisplenic space (PS) and right perihepatic space (R) are noted. The gastrosplenic ligament is seen (*arrow*).

ascites tend to have large greater sac collections with little fluid in the lesser sac, patients with peritoneal carcinomatosis often have proportional fluid volumes in the two spaces (91). The largest fluid collections to occupy the lesser sac occur in patients with disease processes involving organs directly bordering this space. Although pancreatitic fluid collections located anterior to the pancreas are generally considered to be within the lesser sac, an anatomic study has shown that such collections are more likely located within retroperitoneal fascial planes (193). Fluid collections involving the lateral compartment of the lesser sac displace the stomach anteriorly (see Fig. 16-23) and sometimes medially, whereas medial compartment collections may cause lateral displacement of the stomach. Collections extending below the level of the pancreatic body displace the transverse colon and mesocolon caudally. Less commonly, a lesser sac collection may extend ventral and caudal to the transverse colon due to a persistent inferior lesser sac recess in the leaves of the greater omentum (65). Occasionally, inflammation or neoplasm involving the medial compartment may extend via the aortic or diaphragmatic hiatus into the lower mediastinum (65).

Inframesocolic Compartment

The inframesocolic compartment is divided into two unequal spaces by the obliquely oriented small bowel mesentery (Fig. 16-30). The smaller right inframesocolic space is restricted inferiorly by the junction of the distal small bowel mesentery with the cecum, whereas the larger left inframesocolic space is open to the pelvis inferiorly except where it is bounded by the sigmoid mesocolon.

The paracolic gutters are located lateral to the attachments of the peritoneal reflections of the ascending and descending colon. The right paracolic gutter is continuous superiorly with the right perihepatic space. On the left, however, the phrenicocolic ligament forms a partial barrier between the left paracolic gutter and the left subphrenic space. The most dependent portion of the peritoneal cavity in both the erect and supine positions is in the pelvis and consists of lateral paravesical spaces and the midline pouch of Douglas (rectovaginal space in women, rectovesical space in men).

The natural flow of intraperitoneal fluid is directed by gravity and variations in intraabdominal pressure due to respiration along pathways determined by the anatomic compartmentalization of the peritoneal cavity (181) (see Fig. 16-30). Abscesses usually form and metastases usually grow in sites where natural flow permits pooling of infected fluid or malignant ascites. The most common sites of pooling of infected peritoneal fluid and thus for abscess formation are the pelvis, right subhepatic space, and right subphrenic space (181). Similarly, the most common sites for pooling of malignant ascites and subsequent fixation and growth of peritoneal metastases are the pouch of Douglas, the lower small bowel mesentery near the ileocecal junction, the sigmoid mesocolon, and the right paracolic gutter (182). Fluid in the inframesocolic compartment rapidly seeks the pelvis, where it first fills the pouch of Douglas and then the lateral paravesical fossae. Fluid in the right infracolic space flows along the recesses of the small bowel mesentery until it pools at the confluence of the mesentery with the colon near the ileocecal junction, with subsequent overflow into the pouch of Douglas. Fluid in the left infracolic space is frequently arrested by the sigmoid mesocolon before descending into the pelvis. From the pelvis, fluid can ascend both paracolic gutters with changes in intraabdominal pressure during respiration. Flow along the left paracolic gutter is slow and weak, and cephalad extension is usually limited by the phrenicocolic ligament (187,188). The major flow is along the right paracolic gutter into the right subhepatic space, particularly the posterior extension of this space, the Morison pouch (187). From the right subhepatic space, fluid may ascend further into the right subphrenic space. Direct spread from the right subphrenic space across the midline to the left subphrenic space is prevented by the falciform ligament.

A

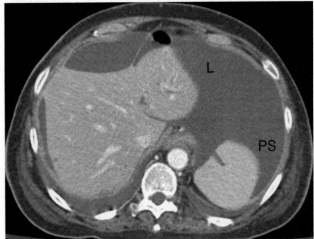

B

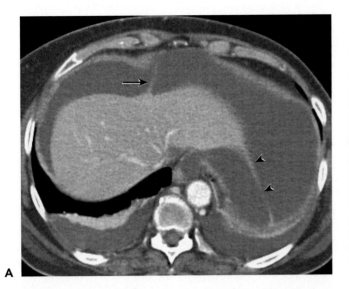

C

Figure 16-21 Malignant ascites in a patient with metastatic ovarian carcinoma. **A:** Peritoneal fluid outlines the falciform (*arrow*) and left triangular (*arrowheads*) ligaments. **B:** The left perihepatic spaces (L) are in continuity with the perisplenic space (PS). **C:** The gastrohepatic ligament (*open arrow*) separates fluid in the superior recess of the lesser sac (∗) posteriorly from fluid in the greater peritoneal space (G) anteriorly.

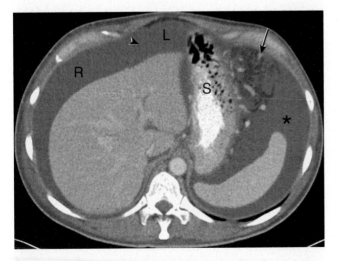

Figure 16-22 Ascites. Computed tomography demonstrates ascites in the right (R) and left (L) anterior perihepatic spaces, separated by the barely perceptible falciform ligament (*arrowhead*). In this patient, the left anterior perihepatic space is separated from the perisplenic space (∗) by the stomach (S) and gastrocolic ligament (*arrow*).

Pathology

Ascites

Ascites is the accumulation of fluid in the peritoneal cavity resulting from either increased fluid production or impaired removal. The etiologies of ascites include congestive heart failure, hypoalbuminemia, cirrhosis, venous or lymphatic obstruction, inflammation, and neoplasm. CT can accurately demonstrate and localize even small amounts of free peritoneal fluid. Localized collections of ascites are frequently seen in the right perihepatic space, the Morison pouch, or the pouch of Douglas (280). Peritoneal fluid in the paracolic gutter is easily distinguished from retroperitoneal fluid by the preservation of the retroperitoneal fat posterior to the ascending or descending colon (103,130). When a large amount of ascites is present, the small bowel loops usually are located centrally within the abdomen and fluid often accumulates in triangular configurations within the leaves of the small bowel mesentery or adjacent to bowel loops (253) (Fig. 16-31). Loculated ascites, secondary

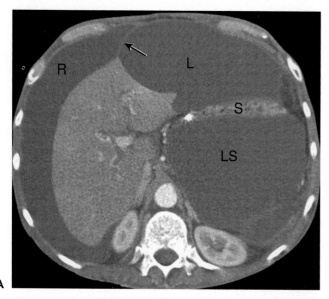
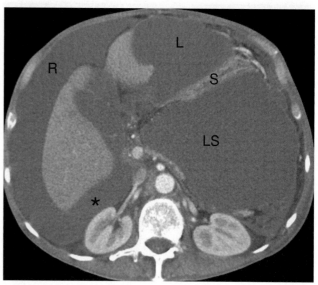

Figure 16-23   Malignant ascites. A and B: Large collections of ascites distend the right (R) and left (L) portions of the greater peritoneal space and the lesser sac (LS), compressing the left lobe of the liver and the stomach (S). The right perihepatic space is continuous with the right subhepatic space inferiorly. The falciform ligament (*arrow*) and Morison's pouch (*) are shown.

to postoperative, inflammatory, or neoplastic adhesions, may appear as a well-defined fluid attenuation mass that displaces adjacent structures (Fig. 16-32). Occasionally, peritoneal fluid collections can become loculated within the four normal or accessory fissures of the liver and can mimic intrahepatic cysts, abscesses, or hematomas (12). Peritoneal metastases in these locations also can be mistaken for intrahepatic lesions (Fig. 16-33) (12).

The attenuation value of ascitic fluid generally ranges from 0 to 30 HU but may be higher in cases of exudative ascites, with the density of the fluid increasing with increasing protein content (36). However, attenuation values of ascitic fluid are nonspecific, and infected or malignant ascites cannot reliably be distinguished from uncomplicated transudative ascites based on the attenuation value alone. Relatively acute intraperitoneal hemorrhage often

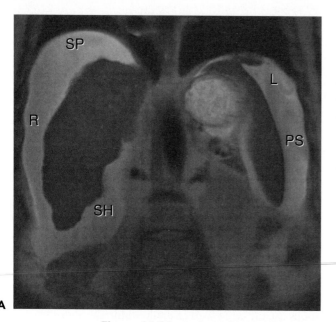
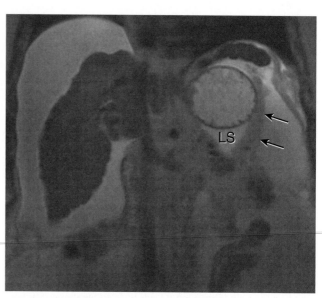

Figure 16-24   A: Coronal T2-weighted magnetic resonance image demonstrates ascitic fluid in the right subphrenic (SP), perihepatic (R), subhepatic (SH), left subphrenic (L), and perisplenic (PS) spaces. B: A more posterior image shows a small amount of fluid in the lesser sac (LS). The gastro-splenic ligament is noted (*arrows*).

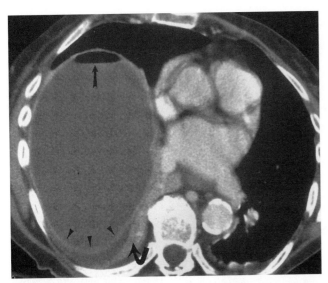

Figure 16-25 Right subphrenic abscess after gastrojejunostomy. A large fluid collection with an air–fluid level (*arrow*) fills the right subphrenic space. The diaphragm (*arrowheads*) separates the abscess from a right pleural effusion posteriorly. Atelectatic lung (*curved arrow*) is shown.

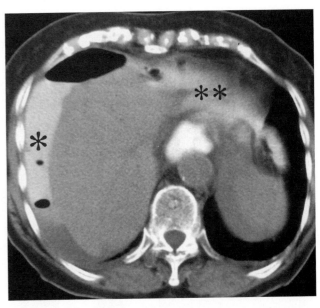

Figure 16-27 Perforated duodenal ulcer. Fluid, air, and high-density oral contrast material (*) fill the right perihepatic space. Air and oral contrast material are also identified in the left peritoneal space (**).

can be distinguished from other fluid collections because it results in peritoneal fluid with an attenuation value of more than 30 HU (74). However, acute traumatic hemoperitoneum can commonly have attenuation values of less than 20 HU and should not be assumed to be ascites in the proper clinical setting (157). Conversely, ascitic fluid may show enhancement on delayed intravenous

contrast-enhanced CT or MRI (8,55). This increase in the attenuation value of ascites on delayed postcontrast images is a nonspecific finding that should not be confused with high-attenuation fluid resulting from hemorrhage or perforation of the gastrointestinal or urinary tract.

The distribution of ascitic fluid in the peritoneal cavity may suggest the nature of the fluid. Patients with benign

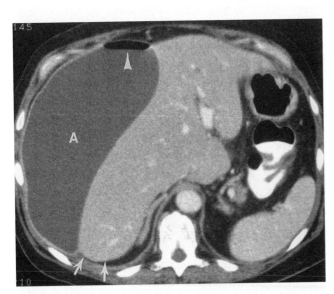

Figure 16-26 Abscess in right perihepatic space secondary to perforated duodenal ulcer. A near-water-density collection (A) with an air–fluid level (*arrowhead*) in the right perihepatic (subphrenic) space is limited posteriorly by the bare area of the liver (*arrows*).

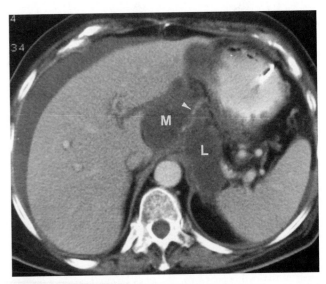

Figure 16-28 Ascites in the lesser sac. The lateral (L) and medial (M) compartments of the lesser sac are divided by a fold of peritoneum through which passes the left gastric artery (*arrowhead*). Ascites is also present in the left and right greater peritoneal spaces.

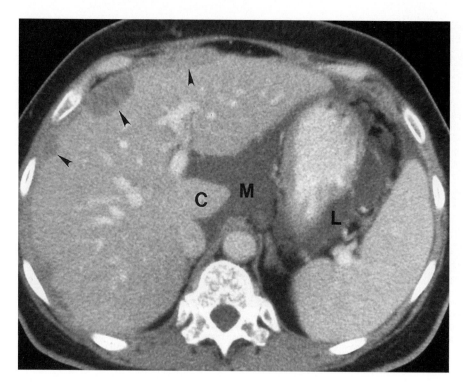

Figure 16-29 Metastatic ovarian carcinoma. Malignant ascites fills the medial (M) and lateral (L) compartments of the lesser sac. The superior recess of the medial compartment wraps around the caudate lobe of the liver (C). Perihepatic serosal metastatic implants (*arrowheads*) are present.

transudative ascites tend to have large greater sac collections with little fluid in the lesser sac, whereas patients with malignant ascites often have proportional volumes of fluid in these peritoneal spaces (50) (see Fig. 16-23). Large lesser sac collections may be seen in patients with disease processes in organs that border this space (91). However, these CT features are not specific and needle aspiration may be necessary to differentiate transudative from exudative ascites.

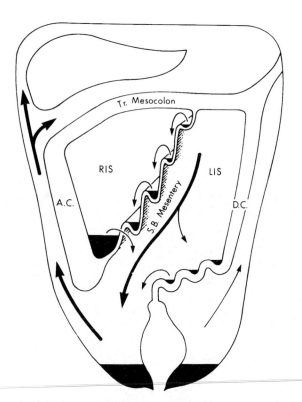

Figure 16-30 Schematic diagram of the inframesocolic compartment of the peritoneal cavity. The small bowel mesentery divides the inframesocolic compartment into two unequal spaces. The arrows indicate the natural flow of ascites within the peritoneal cavity. Right infracolic space (RIS); left infracolic space (LIS); ascending colon (AC); and descending colon (DC) are marked.

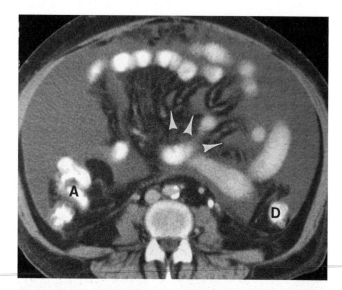

Figure 16-31 Massive ascites. The small bowel loops are located centrally within the abdomen. The pleated nature of the small bowel mesentery can be appreciated as fluid outlines several of the mesenteric leaves. Fluid accumulating between leaves of the mesentery takes on a triangular configuration (*arrowheads*). Note that the retroperitoneal fat posterior to the ascending (A) and descending (D) colon is preserved.

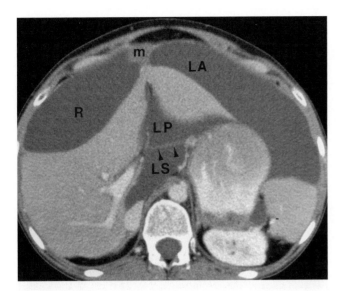

Figure 16-32 Ovarian carcinoma. A metastatic implant (m) on the falciform ligament separates malignant ascites in the right perihepatic (R) and left anterior (LA) perihepatic spaces. The right perihepatic fluid is loculated and deforms the liver margin. The gastrohepatic ligament (*arrowheads*) separates ascites in the left posterior perihepatic space (LP) and the medial compartment of the lesser sac (LS).

MRI also can be used to evaluate intraabdominal fluid collections. A recommended technique for peritoneal imaging is a breath-hold gadolinium-enhanced, T1-weighted gradient echo acquisition with fat suppression, obtained after administration of a large volume of dilute oral barium. Immediate and delayed postcontrast images are acquired, after acquiring T2-weighted images (168).

Transudative ascites appears low in signal intensity on T1-weighted images and high in signal intensity on T2-weighted images because of its long T1 and T2 relaxation (50,309) (Fig. 16-34). The T1 relaxation of fluid collections

decreases with increasing protein concentration (294). Thus exudative fluid collections demonstrate intermediate to short T1 and long T2 values. Both transudative and exudative fluid collections are well seen on contrast-enhanced T1-weighted images where they appear low in signal intensity and on T2-weighted images where they appear high in signal intensity. Delayed enhancement of ascitic fluid on images obtained 15 to 20 minutes after gadolinium chelate administration is indicative of an exudative ascitic fluid collection (8).

Intraperitoneal Abscess

The epidemiology of intraabdominal abscess has changed in recent decades. In the first half of the 20th century, perforated ulcer, appendicitis, and biliary tract disease were the most common causes (72,211). However, during the past several decades, intraabdominal abscess has occurred most commonly after surgery, particularly surgery involving the stomach, biliary tract, and colon (104,256,267,310). Despite advances in surgical technique and antimicrobial therapy, intraabdominal abscess remains a serious diagnostic and therapeutic problem. Even with treatment, mortality rates can reach 30% (229).

Although most patients present with fever, leukocytosis, and abdominal pain, patients with chronic, walled-off abscesses may present with few overt clinical signs or symptoms. Furthermore, some symptoms may be masked by the administration of antibiotics or corticosteroids (8).

CT is the most accurate single imaging test for diagnosing intra-abdominal abscess (64). When examining a patient for a suspected abscess, careful attention to technique is crucial for correct diagnosis. The entire abdomen from the diaphragm to the pubic symphysis should be scanned and adequate oral contrast material should be administered. Although a neutral contrast agent (water, methylcellulose or very low attenuation value barium solution) is

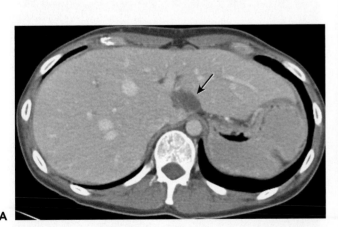

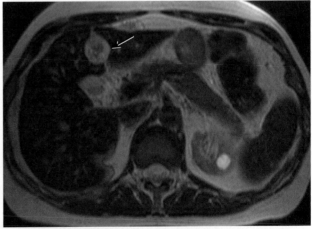

A   B

Figure 16-33 Peritoneal metastases simulating intrahepatic masses. **A:** Computed tomography shows a low attenuation peritoneal mass (*arrow*) within the fissure for the ligamentum venosum in a patient with colon carcinoma. **B:** T2-weighted magnetic resonance imaging demonstrates a hyperintense mass (*arrow*) within the fissure for the ligamentum teres in a patient with appendiceal carcinoma.

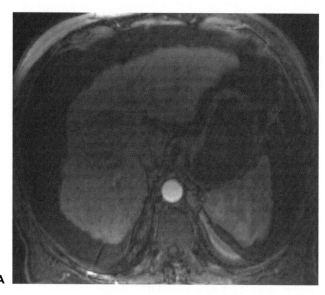

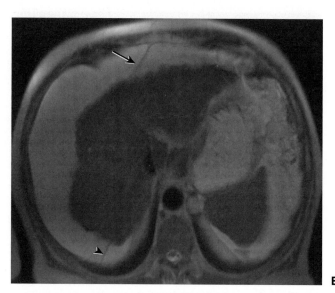

A   **B**

Figure 16-34   Ascites. Because of its long T1 and T2 relaxation, ascites appears low in signal intensity on T1-weighted (**A**) and high in signal intensity on T2-weighted (**B**) magnetic resonance images. Falciform ligament (*arrow*) and right triangular ligament (*arrowhead*) are noted.

useful for most abdominal and pelvic multi-detector CT applications, a water-soluble positive oral contrast agent (iodine solution) is preferable when an abscess is suspected to avoid mistaking a fluid-filled bowel loop for an abscess, or vice versa.

The CT appearance of an abscess is variable depending on its age and location. In its earliest stage, an abscess consists of a focal accumulation of neutrophils in a tissue or organ seeded by bacteria and thus appears as a mass with an attenuation value near that of soft tissue. As the abscess matures, it undergoes liquefactive necrosis. At the same time, highly vascularized connective tissue proliferates at the periphery of the necrotic region. At this stage, the abscess has a central region of near-water attenuation surrounded by a higher attenuation rim that usually enhances after administration of intravenous contrast material (10) (Fig. 16-35). Approximately one third of abscesses contain variable amounts of gas, appearing on CT as either multiple small bubbles or a gas–fluid level (10,37,103,128,148, 319) (Figs. 16-36 and 16-37). The presence of a long gas–fluid level suggests communication with the gastrointestinal tract (128). Postoperative packing materials used for hemostasis, such as oxidized cellulose (Surgicel) and gelatin bioabsorbable sponge, can mimic a gas-containing abscess. Findings that may help differentiate a hemostatic agent from an abscess are a linear arrangement of tightly packed gas bubbles, an unchanged appearance on subsequent examinations, and lack of either a gas–fluid level or an enhancing wall (257,327). Ancillary findings of an abscess include displacement of surrounding structures, thickening or obliteration of adjacent fascial planes, and increased density of adjacent mesenteric fat. Whereas most abscesses are round or oval in shape, those adjacent

to solid organs, such as the liver, may have a crescentic or lenticular configuration.

In some cases, the CT appearance of an abscess can suggest its etiology. A low-density right lower quadrant mass containing a round calcific density is highly suggestive of

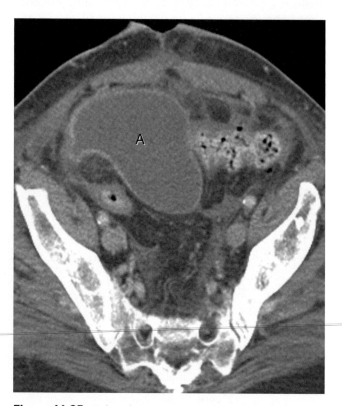

Figure 16-35   Pelvic abscess. Computed tomography in a postoperative patient shows a loculated fluid collection (**A**) with an enhancing rim.

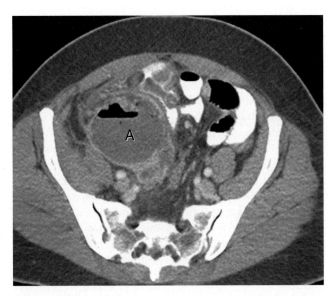

Figure 16-36 Pelvic abscess secondary to acute diverticulitis. Computed tomography shows a gas containing fluid collection (A) with rim enhancement.

an appendiceal abscess with an appendicolith. Elsewhere in the abdomen, a low-density mass containing a high-density object suggests a foreign body abscess. One of the more common causes of a foreign body abscess is a retained surgical sponge (called a *gossypiboma*) (269) (Fig. 16-38).

Although the CT findings previously discussed are highly suggestive of abscess, they are not specific. Other masses that can have a central low attenuation value include a cyst, pseudocyst, hematoma, urinoma, lymphocele, biloma,

loculated ascites, thrombosed aneurysm, and necrotic neoplasm. In addition, normal structures such as unopacified bladder, stomach, and bowel can mimic the appearance of an abscess (Fig. 16-39). Thickening of adjacent fascial planes is also nonspecific and can be seen with intraabdominal hematoma and neoplastic infiltration. Even the presence of gas within a mass is nonspecific for abscess because a necrotic noninfected neoplasm and a mass that communicates with bowel can also contain gas. Because a specific diagnosis of abscess based on CT findings alone is not possible, correlation with clinical history is important. Percutaneous needle aspiration may be necessary to make a definitive diagnosis. In this regard, CT can be very helpful in identifying a plane of access for aspiration that is both safe and free of contamination from bowel. The presence or absence of an abscess can be established by obtaining a specimen for Gram stain and culture. In most instances, if an abscess is present, a catheter can be inserted percutaneously for definitive drainage (279,303). Percutaneous abscess drainage has proven to be a safe and effective approach to the diagnosis and treatment of intraabdominal abscess (259,302). Although it was originally thought that only well-defined, unilocular abscesses with safe drainage routes should be drained percutaneously, the criteria for percutaneous drainage have been expanded to include ill-defined and multiseptated abscesses, as well as those communicating with the gastrointestinal tract or located deep to major abdominal organs (83,196). Even potentially complicated abscesses such as appendiceal, diverticular, and interloop abscesses secondary to Crohn disease can be drained without complications (20,131,202,208,255,304). In the

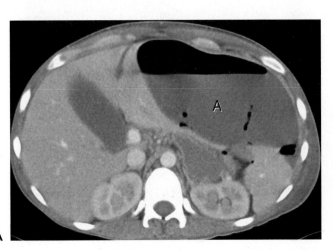

A

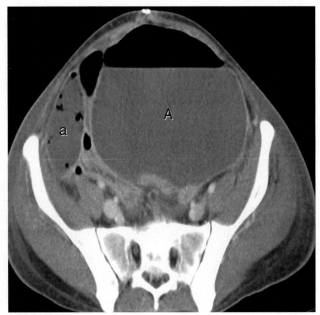

B

Figure 16-37 Peritoneal abscess. **A:** Contrast-enhanced computed tomography shows a large fluid collection (A) with a gas–fluid level and deeper foci of gas involving the left anterior perihepatic space. **B:** The abscess (A) extends into the pelvis, and a smaller gas-containing abscess (a) is seen in the right side of the pelvis.

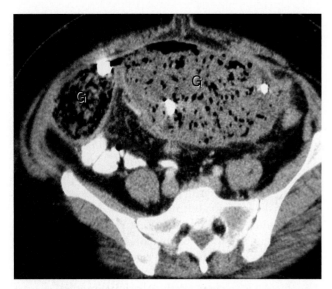

Figure 16-38 Gossypiboma. Transaxial computed tomography shows several high density foci within two large walled-off masses of mottled gas and soft tissue density (G) corresponding to the inflammatory reaction in this patient who had five retained surgical sponges from a recent laparotomy.

case of periappendiceal abscesses, percutaneous drainage may completely eliminate the need for surgery (20,131,207, 304), whereas percutaneous drainage of diverticular abscesses often converts complex two- or three-stage surgical procedures to safer one-stage colonic resections (202). Two abscess characteristics have been found to be valuable in predicting the eventual outcome of percutaneous drainage: the location of the abscess and the distribution of gas within the fluid collection. Subphrenic and hepatic abscesses are

more likely to have a successful outcome than those in other locations (128). In addition, abscesses with superficial gas (superficial bubbles or a gas-fluid level) are more likely to be drained completely than those with deep gas bubbles (96% versus 62%) (118). Because no specific CT feature of an abscess predicts that it cannot be drained successfully, all intraabdominal abscesses should be considered candidates for percutaneous drainage (83,128). The technical details of CT-guided abscess drainage are described in Chapter 3.

The MRI appearance of intraabdominal abscess is also nonspecific. Therefore, MRI does not eliminate the need for aspiration in establishing a diagnosis. Because of its intermediate T1 and long T2, an abscess demonstrates low to intermediate signal intensity on T1-weighted images and homogeneous or heterogeneous high signal intensity on T2-weighted images (204,261). It is usually best demonstrated on gadolinium-enhanced T1-weighted fat-suppressed images as a well defined fluid collection with peripheral rim enhancement and enhancement of adjacent tissues (204,261). In a study of percutaneously obtained normal and abnormal body fluids, the mean T1 value of abscess contents was found to be significantly shorter and the mean T2 value significantly longer than those of bile, ascitic fluid, urine collections, cysts and pseudocyst fluid, and pleural fluid (32).

The accuracy of CT and MRI in detecting intraabdominal abscess is approximately 95% (10,100,103,147,148,149, 150,204,260,319). Most false–positive diagnoses are a result of mistaking unopacified fluid-filled stomach, bowel, or bladder for an abscess or mistaking a sterile fluid collection for an abscess. If a question exists as to the nature of a fluid-filled structure, additional oral, rectal, or intra-

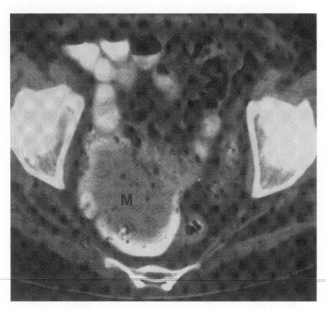

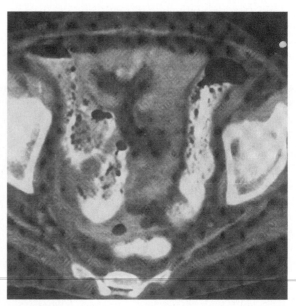

A

B

Figure 16-39 Fluid-filled cecum simulating an abscess. A: Initial computed tomography examination demonstrates a low-attenuation pelvic mass (M) with multiple gas bubbles simulating an abscess. B: Follow-up examination 1 day later demonstrates marked change in appearance of the now less-distended cecum containing stool and oral contrast material.

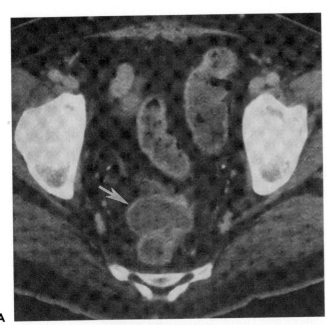

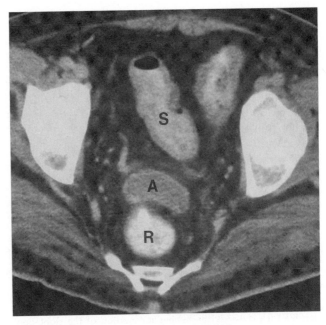

A   B

Figure 16-40   Cul-de-sac abscess after cholecystectomy. **A:** A small fluid collection (*arrow*) with enhancing rim is difficult to distinguish from unopacified adjacent rectum and sigmoid colon. **B:** After administration of rectal contrast material, the abscess (A) is easily distinguishable from the now opacified rectum (R) and sigmoid colon (S).

venous contrast material can be administered and a limited rescan performed (Fig. 16-40).

Other Intraperitoneal Fluid Collections

Intraperitoneal hemorrhage may result from over-anticoagulation; bleeding diathesis; trauma to the liver, spleen, or mesentery; spontaneous rupture of a vascular neoplasm; hemorrhagic cyst or ectopic pregnancy; perforation of a duodenal ulcer; or acute mesenteric ischemia. In addition, intraperitoneal blood is frequently seen after abdominal surgery. CT has been shown to be highly sensitive and specific for diagnosing hemoperitoneum (74), with the diagnosis being based on the high attenuation value of the peritoneal fluid (Figs. 16-41 and 16-42). However, it is important to keep in mind that acute hemoperitoneum can have attenuation values of less than 20 HU (157). The CT appearance of intraperitoneal hemorrhage depends on the location, age, and extent of the bleeding. Immediately after hemorrhage, intraperitoneal blood has the same attenuation as circulating blood. Within hours, however, the attenuation increases as hemoglobin is concentrated during clot formation (203,205). In most cases, the attenuation begins to decrease within several days as clot lysis takes place (24). The attenuation value decreases steadily with time and often approaches that of water (0 to 20 HU) after 2 to 4 weeks (150). During the hyperdense phase, the attenuation value of intraperitoneal blood ranges from 20 to 90 HU (74,161,289,318). In one large study, all patients with a less than 48-hour history of hemoperitoneum had fluid collections containing areas of attenuation more than 30 HU (74). The morphologic characteristics of re-

cent intraperitoneal hemorrhage are variable. The fluid collection may be homogeneously hyperdense or may be heterogeneous with nodular or linear areas of high attenuation surrounded by lower attenuation fluid. The heterogeneity may result from irregular clot resorption or intermittent bleeding (318). In most cases, intraperitoneal blood contains focal areas of clot that are higher in attenuation than the free intraperitoneal blood (see Fig. 16-42). These localized clots are helpful in determining the bleeding site because they usually form adjacent to the organ from which the hemorrhage originated (74). Occasionally, fresh blood within a hematoma or confined within a

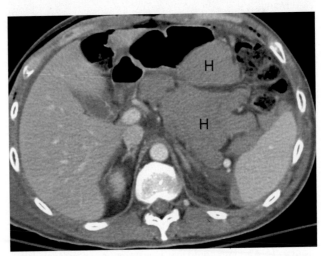

Figure 16-41   Hemoperitoneum. High attenuation fluid (H) involves the gastrosplenic ligament in a patient who had undergone a Nissen fundoplication.

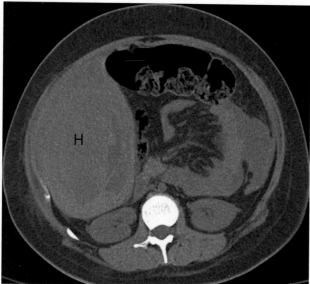

Figure 16-42   Hemoperitoneum. Heterogeneous high attenuation fluid (H) distends the subhepatic portion of the right peritoneal space in a patient who had a hepatic injury.

peritoneal space may show a hematocrit effect with sedimented erythrocytes producing a dependent layer of high attenuation (Fig. 16-43). The most common site of blood accumulation on CT after upper abdominal trauma is Morison's pouch (74,173). The right paracolic gutter is another common site of blood collection, even in cases of splenic trauma. With extensive hemorrhage, large collections of blood may fill the pelvis with little blood in upper abdominal sites. Therefore, it is important to include the pelvis in any CT examination performed for suspected intraabdominal hemorrhage, particularly in patients who

have sustained blunt abdominal trauma (74). Before beginning the examination, adequate oral contrast material should be administered to opacify all abdominal and pelvic bowel loops.

If a CT examination without intravenous contrast material has been obtained, viewing the images with a narrow window width is helpful to accentuate the density difference between the fresh blood and the adjacent soft tissues. In most cases however, a precontrast CT examination is unnecessary and one can begin the study with intravenous contrast material administered as a bolus. The contrast enhancement helps to demonstrate injuries to the liver, spleen, and kidneys and makes intraperitoneal fluid collections more apparent by increasing the density of the surrounding tissues. Extravasation of intravenous contrast material, resulting in an area of fluid with an attenuation higher than the remainder of the acute hemoperitoneum, is an indicator of significant active bleeding (277).

MRI also can be used to demonstrate intraperitoneal hemorrhage. However, many patients referred for suspected intraabdominal hemorrhage are unstable and require extensive monitoring and supportive equipment, making MRI less practical. A hematoma less than 48 hours old may have a nonspecific signal intensity (297). Intraabdominal hematoma more than 3 weeks old can have a specific appearance, referred to as the *concentric ring sign*, in which a thin peripheral rim that is dark on all sequences surrounds a bright inner ring that is most distinctive on T1-weighted images (102). A hematocrit effect occasionally can be seen on MRI also. On T1-weighted images, the dependent portion of the hemorrhagic collection is hyperintense compared with the supernatant, whereas on T2-weighted images the signal intensity relationship is reversed (Fig. 16-44).

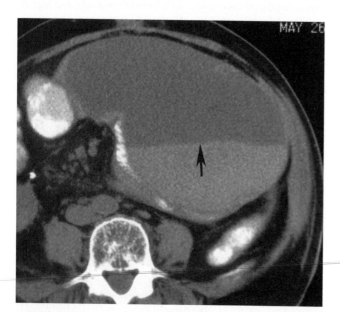

Figure 16-43   Intraperitoneal hematoma in an anticoagulated patient. Unenhanced computed tomography examination demonstrates a large fluid collection containing a hematocrit level (*arrow*) with higher attenuation erythrocytes layering dependently.

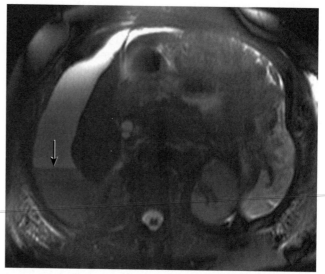

Figure 16-44   Hemoperitoneum. T2-weighted magnetic resonance image with fat suppression shows a large right perihepatic space fluid collection with a hematocrit level (*arrow*).

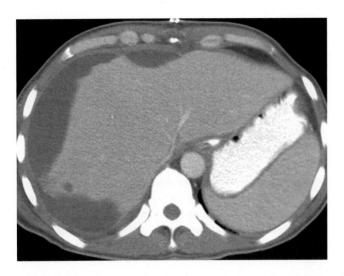

Figure 16-45 Biloma. Computed tomography shows intraperitoneal bile collections loculated in the right perihepatic space in this patient who had undergone laparoscopic cholecystectomy.

Intraperitoneal bile accumulation (biloma) is caused by iatrogenic, traumatic, or spontaneous rupture of the biliary tract (Fig. 16-45) (305). The bile elicits a low-grade inflammatory response that generally walls off the collection by the formation of a thin capsule or inflammatory adhesions within the mesentery and omentum (165,305). Most bilomas appear round or oval and have attenuation values of less than 20 HU. Those complicated by hemorrhage or infection may be higher in density. Bilomas are usually confined to the upper abdomen. Although most are located in the right upper quadrant, left upper quadrant bilomas are not uncommon, occurring in approximately 30% of cases (see Fig. 16-19) (197,305). Because the CT appearance is not specific, biloma cannot be distinguished from other abdominal fluid collections and either needle aspiration or hepatobiliary scintigraphy is usually required to establish the diagnosis. Most bilomas can be treated successfully with percutaneous catheter drainage (197,305).

Intraabdominal collections of urine may result from urinary tract obstruction or from surgery or trauma involving the kidney, ureter, or bladder. Free intraperitoneal urine usually results from traumatic rupture of the bladder dome. CT examination of patients with intraperitoneal bladder rupture performed after cystography or intravenous contrast material administration shows high-density fluid freely filling the peritoneal spaces. Although localized collections of urine (urinomas) usually occur within the retroperitoneal space, an intraperitoneal urinoma can occur if the anatomic boundaries of the retroperitoneum have been disrupted by trauma or prior surgery (112). On CT images obtained without intravenous contrast material, the attenuation value of a urinoma is less than 20 HU. After administration of intravenous contrast medium, however, the attenuation value can increase as a result of accumulation of opacified urine in the fluid collection. Thus, delayed

CT imaging may be helpful in establishing the diagnosis of urinoma.

Lymphoceles are abnormal accumulations of lymphatic fluid usually resulting from operative disruption of lymphatic vessels. The most common procedures to cause lymphoceles are renal transplantation and retroperitoneal lymph node dissection. Although most lymphoceles are confined to the retroperitoneum, intraperitoneal lymphoceles do occur. The more common manifestation of intraperitoneal lymph leakage is chylous ascites, usually resulting from lymphatic obstruction by tumor (232). A lymphocele has a nonspecific appearance and cannot be distinguished from other abdominal fluid collections by its CT or MRI features alone. The diagnosis can be established by percutaneous aspiration (232,313). Chylous ascites usually is indistinguishable from other types of ascitic fluid. Occasionally, however, the diagnosis may be suggested if negative Hounsfield numbers, caused by the high fat content of lymph, are detected. The rare finding of a fat–fluid level in ascitic fluid is pathognomonic of chylous ascites (114).

THE MESENTERIES AND GREATER OMENTUM

Anatomy

The small bowel mesentery is a broad, fan-shaped fold of peritoneum that connects the jejunum and ileum to the posterior abdominal wall (93). It originates at the duodenojejunal flexure just to the left of the spine and extends obliquely to the ileocecal junction. The root of the small bowel mesentery is contiguous superiorly with the hepatoduodenal ligament, anteriorly with the transverse mesocolon, and posterolaterally with the ascending and descending mesocolons (212). Within the two fused layers of the small bowel mesentery are contained the intestinal branches of the superior mesenteric artery and vein, lymphatic vessels, lymph nodes, nerves, and variable amounts of fat. On CT, the mesentery appears as a fat-containing area central to the small bowel loops within which the jejunal and ileal vessels can be identified as distinct, round, or linear densities (273). Normal lymph nodes less than 1 cm in diameter usually can be identified, particularly with multidetector row CT (170). The normal mesenteric fat is similar in attenuation to the subcutaneous fat (−100 to −160 HU) (272). In patients with a large amount of ascites, the pleated nature of the mesentery can be appreciated as fluid outlines the mesenteric folds.

The transverse mesocolon, which extends from the anterior surface of the pancreas to the transverse colon, contains the middle colic arteries and veins. On the right, the root of the mesocolon is continuous with the duodenocolic ligament and thus the posterior aspect of the hepatic flexure. Medially it crosses the descending duodenum and head of pancreas extending along the lower anterior edge of the body and tail of the pancreas. On the left it is continuous with the phrenicocolic and splenorenal ligaments (185). In most patients, the transverse mesocolon is readily identified on CT as a fat-containing area extending from the pancreas, particularly at the level of the uncinate process, to the margin of the colonic wall (133). In thin patients, the transverse mesocolon may be difficult to identify because of the lack of mesenteric fat and the steeply oblique orientation of the mesentery in such patients. Nevertheless, the middle colic branches of the transverse mesocolon can be identified in nearly all patients (273). The root of the small bowel mesentery at its origin near the duodenojejunal flexure is continuous with the root of the transverse mesocolon (182). The sigmoid mesocolon, extending from the posterior pelvic wall and containing the sigmoid and hemorrhoidal vessels, can usually be identified deep within the pelvis.

The greater omentum consists of a double layer of peritoneum that extends inferiorly from the greater curvature of the stomach, turns superiorly on itself draping over the transverse colon, and extends to the pancreas within the retroperitoneum (278). The vascular supply to the greater omentum is largely through the right and left gastroepiploic arteries. On CT and MRI, the greater omentum appears as a band of fatty tissue of variable thickness just deep to the anterior peritoneal fascia, extending from the antrum of the stomach superiorly to the pelvis inferiorly. It contains small vessels and is located just anterior to the transverse colon and the small bowel loops of the lower abdomen.

Pathology of the Mesenteries, Omentum, and Peritoneum

Mesenteric abnormalities are readily identified on CT in all but the leanest patients because of the abundance of fat present within the normal mesentery. Various pathologic processes, both benign and malignant, may infiltrate the mesentery causing an increase in attenuation of the mesenteric fat, distortion of the mesenteric architecture, and loss of definition of the mesenteric vessels (191). Some of these processes may also cause thickening of the peritoneal lining. Detection of mesenteric abnormalities requires rigorous attention to CT technique. It is particularly important to opacify the gastrointestinal tract with oral contrast material so that unopacifed bowel is not mistaken for a mesenteric mass. Conversely, a small mesenteric mass can be obscured if surrounded by unopacified bowel loops. At least 500 mL of an oral contrast agent should be given 30 to 45 minutes prior to the examination to opacify the distal small bowel. Another 500 mL of contrast material should be given 15 minutes before the examination to opacify the stomach and proximal small bowel. If bowel cannot confidently be distinguished from a mesenteric mass, additional images through the suspicious area can be acquired after additional oral contrast material has been administered or after delay allows transit of more proximal contrast material. Occasionally, it is helpful to opacify the colon per rectum with a dilute contrast solution or air to differentiate a redundant sigmoid colon from a pelvic mass.

MRI also can be used to detect, characterize, and delineate mesenteric abnormalities. T1-weighted gradient-echo images with fat suppression after intravenous gadolinium-chelate administration demonstrate mesenteric pathology well. Because of the longer image acquisition time of MRI, peristaltic and respiratory motion artifacts sometimes degrade MR images and limit spatial resolution in the region of the mesentery. Administration of a hypotonic bowel agent, such as glucagon intramuscularly or subcutaneously, can help limit peristaltic motion. As with CT, opacification of the abdominal and pelvic bowel loops is important when evaluating the abdominal mesenteries with MRI. A large volume of a dilute oral barium solution is useful for this purpose (166,167).

Edema

Diffuse mesenteric edema is most commonly the result of hypoalbuminemia, usually caused by cirrhosis (45,296). The nephrotic syndrome, heart failure, mesenteric ischemia, vasculitis and mesenteric venous or lymphatic obstruction are less common causes. The CT findings characteristic of mesenteric edema include increased density of the mesenteric fat, poor definition of segmental mesenteric vessels, and relative sparing of the retroperitoneal fat (191,272). Mesenteric edema secondary to a systemic disease often coexists with subcutaneous edema and ascites (212). Bowel wall thickening also is present in some patients. Whenever mesenteric edema is identified, the root of the mesentery should be carefully evaluated to exclude a focal tumor mass obstructing mesenteric vessels and creating secondary edema (272). Although diffuse infiltration of the mesentery by metastatic tumor may have an appearance similar to that of mesenteric edema, it can sometimes be distinguished from edema by the rigidity of the mesenteric leaves. Imaging with the patient in the lateral decubitus or prone position may be helpful in demonstrating the mesenteric fixation.

Pancreatitis

CT has established roles in the initial diagnosis, assessment of prognosis, evaluation of complications, direction of image-guided intervention, and follow-up of pancreatitis (16,19). The transverse mesocolon can be affected by dissection of pancreatic enzymes in patients with severe acute pancreatitis (180,274). In patients with fulminant pancreatitis, the mesocolon is involved in approximately one third of cases (133). The small bowel mesentery is involved much less commonly. The main CT finding in patients with mesenteric inflammation related to pancreatitis is streaky or confluent increased density of the mesenteric fat. MRI may demonstrate low signal intensity mesenteric stranding on T1-weighted images and either normal or high signal intensity in the mesenteric fat on T2-weighted images. Increased signal intensity within the peripancreatic fat on fat-suppressed T1-weighted images is associated with poor outcome in patients with acute pancreatitis (174). Dissection by pancreatic enzymes along the mesenteric leaves can result in formation of abscesses, pseudocysts, hemorrhage, enteric fistulae, and late bowel stenoses (133). The presence of gas bubbles in a mesenteric fluid collection may be caused by an abscess, necrosis without infection, or communication with the gastrointestinal tract and is better demonstrated on CT than MRI. Patients with mesenteric involvement demonstrated by CT have a higher morbidity and mortality than patients without CT evidence of mesenteric spread (133).

Crohn Disease

Crohn disease is a chronic granulomatous disease of the alimentary tract that most commonly involves the small intestine or colon. A major benefit of CT in patients with Crohn disease is to identify and characterize the extramucosal abnormalities, many of which cause separation of bowel loops on barium studies (88). Most important, CT is helpful in differentiating mesenteric abscess from fibrofatty proliferation or diffuse inflammatory reaction of the mesentery (Fig. 16-46). Bowel wall thickening and mesenteric lymphadenopathy are also well demonstrated (169,200). Fibrofatty mesenteric proliferation, the most common cause of bowel loop separation, is characterized by increased density of the fat between the separated loops (−70 to −90 HU) and lack of a soft tissue mass or fluid collection in the affected region (76,88). Diffuse inflammatory reaction of the mesentery produces a similar increase in density of the mesenteric fat but has no clearly defined borders. An abscess can be confidently diagnosed when a well-marginated near-water density mass is identified. Occasionally the mass may contain gas and oral contrast material, indicating communication with bowel (88,142). CT also can be helpful in identifying and defining the extent of sinus tracts and fistulae. In cases in which a mesenteric mass has an attenuation value near that of soft tissue, it may be

difficult to differentiate an abscess from an inflammatory mass (142). Occasionally, the identification of fibrofatty proliferation of the mesentery on CT can be helpful in establishing a diagnosis of Crohn disease when a patient's inflammatory bowel disease is difficult to classify clinically because mesenteric fat proliferation is not a common feature of ulcerative colitis (92). Fibrofatty proliferation and increased blood flow are responsible for the CT appearance of vascular dilation and tortuosity, as well as wide spacing and prominence of the vasa recta ("comb sign") seen in association with affected bowel segments (234) (Fig. 16-47). MRI also can demonstrate the mesenteric findings of Crohn disease. A disadvantage of MRI, however, is its insensitivity for demonstrating a small amount of extraluminal gas, which is an important sign of bowel perforation.

Diverticulitis

Although for many years the fluoroscopic contrast enema examination served as the primary imaging test for diagnosing diverticulitis, it is limited in that it does not delineate the extracolonic extent of disease. The advantage of CT is that it clearly delineates the extracolonic extent of disease, while not requiring direct distention of the colon with contrast material.

The most common CT finding in patients with diverticulitis is inflammation of the pericolonic fat, characterized by poorly defined soft tissue density and fine linear strands in the fat adjacent to the involved colon (119,148, 164) (Fig. 16-48). Accumulation of fluid within the root of the sigmoid mesentery is a frequent finding in left-sided diverticulitis (223). Other CT findings include colon wall thickening, engorged pericolonic mesenteric vessels, intramural sinus tracts, mural or extramural abscesses, fistulae, and peritonitis (239,271,290). The sensitivity of CT for the diagnosis of diverticulitis has been reported to be higher than that of contrast enema (7,164). In addition, CT is more accurate than contrast enema in demonstrating the extracolonic extent and complications of diverticulitis (7, 67,164,284), which include bladder involvement, ureteral obstruction, and distant abscesses. The presence of an abscess or an extraintestinal gas pocket larger than 5 mm is associated with an increased rate of nonoperative treatment failure (136,164,230). The combination of colonic wall thickening and pericolonic inflammatory changes is not pathognomonic of diverticulitis and can be mimicked by perforated colon carcinoma, pelvic inflammatory disease, appendicitis, epiploic appendagitis, endometriosis, Crohn disease, and other forms of colitis.

Epiploic Appendagitis

The appendices epiploicae are elongated adipose structures that arise from the serosal surface of the colon (228). They generally are not visible on CT images because their fat density merges with that of the surrounding pericolonic fat. However, these appendices can be identified in patients

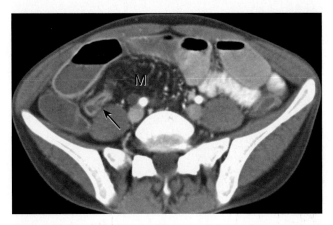

Figure 16-46 Fibrofatty proliferation of the small bowel mesentery in a patient with Crohn disease. The small bowel mesentery (M) adjacent to the thickened terminal ileum (*arrow*) is enlarged and compresses surrounding dilated bowel loops.

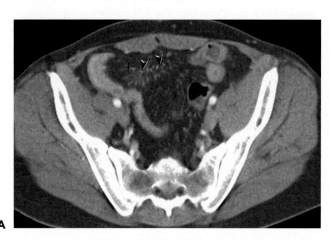

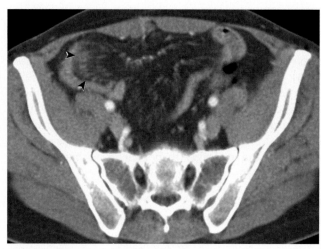

Figure 16-47 Comb sign in a patient with Crohn disease. **A, B:** Two computed tomography images demonstrate prominent vasa recta (arrowheads) coursing through the proliferative mesenteric fat to supply inflamed bowel.

with a large amount of ascites (Fig. 16-49). The epiploic appendages are supplied by end arteries of the vasa recta longa of the colon and are drained by a vein passing through their narrow pedicles. Torsion or venous thrombosis of an epiploic appendage can cause ischemic or hemorrhagic infarction, leading to a localized inflammatory process termed *epiploic appendagitis*, which mimics diverticulitis or appendicitis clinically (85,299). The CT appearance is that of a pericolonic oval of higher than normal fat attenuation, which represents the infarcted epiploic appendage, surrounded by a hyperattenuating rim, which corresponds to the inflamed visceral peritoneal lining (Fig. 16-50) (238,258,275). In some patients a central high-attenuation dot, indicative of an engorged or thrombosed vein or a central area of hemorrhage, can be identified in addition to localized colonic wall thickening (223,238, 275). Thickening of adjacent parietal peritoneum may also be identified (238,258,298). Occasionally, an infarcted appendage may develop peripheral dystrophic calcification

(226). On T1- and T2-weighted MR images, the pericolonic oval is high in signal intensity with a low signal intensity rim (276). On postgadolinium-chelate enhanced T1-weighted fat suppressed images, the rim demonstrates enhancement. A hypointense central dot also can be identified in some patients (276).

Peritonitis

Peritonitis is an inflammation of the peritoneum that can result from numerous causes and can be either localized or diffuse. The major types of peritonitis include bacterial,

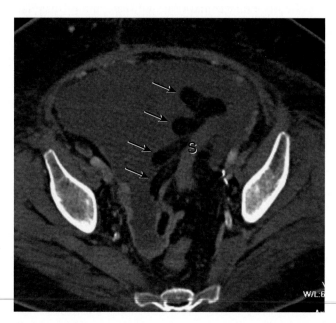

Figure 16-49 Appendages epiploicae. Computed tomography in a patient with a large amount of ascites demonstrates the normal appendices epiploicae (*arrows*) of the sigmoid colon (S), which appear as finger-like projections of pericolic fat floating within the ascites.

Figure 16-48 Diverticulitis. Pelvic computed tomography demonstrates thickening of the sigmoid colon with increased density of the adjacent sigmoid mesocolon (*arrows*).

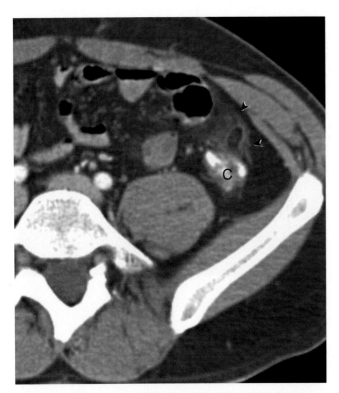

Figure 16-50 Epiploic appendagitis. Contrast-enhanced computed tomography shows an oval fat-density mass surrounded by a high attenuation rim (*arrowheads*) anterior to the descending colon (C). The mass contains a central high attenuation structure, which most likely represents thrombosed central vessels.

granulomatous, and chemical (229). Although bacterial peritonitis is sometimes primary, it usually results secondarily from perforation of an abdominal viscus. Common etiologies include appendicitis, diverticulitis, perforated ulcer, perforated carcinoma, acute cholecystitis, pancreatitis, salpingoopheritis, and abdominal surgery (229). With diffuse peritonitis, the CT findings consist of thickening of the peritoneum, omentum and mesentery, increased density of the mesenteric fat, and ascites (314). This CT appearance is nonspecific and can also be seen in patients with metastatic cancer or peritoneal mesothelioma.

Tuberculous peritonitis has become a relatively uncommon disease but remains a persistent problem in endemic areas or in immunocompromised patients (99). It is believed to occur by direct extension (ruptured lymph nodes or perforation of a tuberculous lesion in the gastrointestinal or genitourinary tract) or by lymphatic or hematogenous spread (295). The CT appearance of tuberculous peritonitis is varied. The most common CT feature is lymphadenopathy, predominantly in the mesenteric and peripancreatic areas (4,120) (Fig. 16-51). Central low density within the enlarged lymph nodes, presumably caused by caseation necrosis, is seen in approximately 40% of patients (70,120). Disseminated *Mycobacterium tuberculosis* infection is found in approximately three fourths of HIV-infected patients who have enlarged low-attenuation lymph nodes, whereas *Mycobacterium avium-intracellulare*

infection more often results in soft tissue attenuation lymphadenopathy (234). High-density ascites (20 to 45 HU) is another characteristic feature of tuberculous peritonitis, the increased density being related to the high protein content of the fluid (Fig. 16-51) (59,70,108,120). Additional CT findings include thickening and nodularity of peritoneal surfaces, mesentery, and omentum (59,70,120) (Figs. 16-51 and 16-52). Although these CT features are highly suggestive of tuberculous peritonitis, they are not pathognomonic, and other diseases, such as nontuberculous peritonitis, lymphoma, metastatic carcinoma, peritoneal mesothelioma, and pseudomyxoma peritonei, should be included in the differential diagnosis. The presence of mesenteric changes, soft tissue nodules with a diameter of at least 5 mm and peritoneal masses with low-attenuation center favors tuberculous peritonitis (see Fig. 16-52) over metastatic carcinoma, which more commonly has more prominent omental involvement (99). In addition, the peritoneal thickening in tuberculous peritonitis tends to be minimal and smooth with marked enhancement, whereas irregular peritoneal thickening is more common in peritoneal carcinomatosis (247).

Sclerosing peritonitis is a serious complication of chronic ambulatory peritoneal dialysis, which results in thickening of the peritoneum that encloses some or all of the small intestine. The main CT findings are diffuse peritoneal thickening and sheet-like calcification, loculated fluid collections and small bowel tethering (2,282). A rare form of peritonitis, called *sclerosing encapsulating peritonitis*, is characterized by a fibrotic membrane that encases the small bowel, forming a sac with internal adhesions ("abdominal cocoon"), resulting in small bowel obstruction (98). The cause of sclerosing encapsulating peritonitis is uncertain.

Rare parasitic infections of the peritoneum including *Echinococcus multilocularis*, *Paragonimus westermani*, *Sparganum mansoni*, and *Fasciola hepatica* result in multiple septated cystic masses in the peritoneal cavity, often associated with hazy omental soft tissue stranding and increased density (244,289). As with many of the entities discussed above, the appearances are nonspecific.

Sclerosing Mesenteritis

Sclerosing mesenteritis is an uncommon condition of unknown etiology characterized by chronic inflammation (115,254). It can be categorized into three subgroups based on the stage of the pathologic process and its predominant pathology. *Mesenteric panniculitis* is characterized by chronic inflammation, *mesenteric lipodystrophy* by fat necrosis, and *retractile mesenteritis* by fibrosis (69,152,175). Although the cause of the disorder is unknown, it often is associated with other idiopathic inflammatory disorders such as retroperitoneal fibrosis, sclerosing cholangitis, Riedel thyroiditis, and orbital pseudotumor (115). In one study, 69% of patients with sclerosisng mesenteritis had a coexisting malignancy (61). Patients may present with abdominal discomfort, but sclerosing

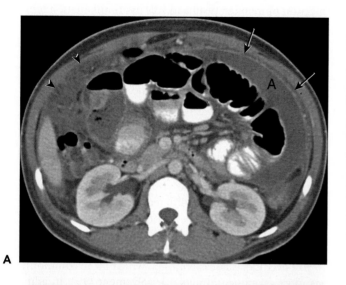

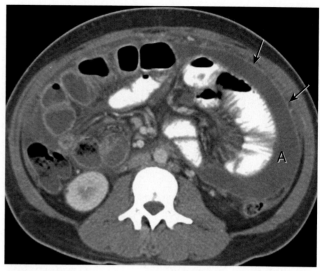

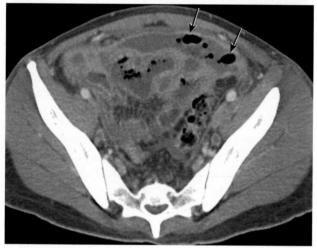

Figure 16-51 Tuberculous peritonitis. **A, B:** Computed tomography demonstrates enhancing thickened peritoneum (*arrows*) and omentum (*arrowheads*) in association with high attenuation ascites (A). **C:** The intraperitoneal gas (*open arrows*) is due to ileal perforation.

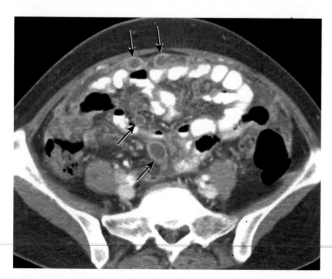

Figure 16-52 Tuberculous peritonitis. Computed tomography demonstrates extensive nodular thickening of the peritoneum and small bowel mesentery. Multiple low attenuation mesenteric and omental masses (*arrows*) can be identified.

mesenteritis often is discovered incidentally in asymptomatic patients (61). The CT appearance varies from a subtle diffuse increase in attenuation of the mesenteric fat (Fig. 16-53) to a solid mesenteric soft tissue mass (Fig. 16-54) (115,254). The inflamed mesentery may demonstrate regional mass effect with displacement of adjacent small bowel loops (300). Enlarged mesenteric lymph nodes may also be present (see Fig. 16-53). In some patients the normal low attenuation of the fat immediately surrounding the central mesenteric vessels is preserved ("fat ring" sign) (254). Rarely, the mesenteric inflammatory process may have a multicystic appearance, likely caused by lymphatic obstruction (134,138). When a solid mass is present within the mesentery, it sometimes contains calcification, which may be related to central fat necrosis (see Fig. 16-54) (110).

The CT appearance of sclerosing mesenteritis overlaps with that of other benign and malignant disorders. Entities that can mimic sclerosing mesenteritis include mesenteric edema or hemorrhage, mesenteric inflammation secondary to pancreatitis, fibrofatty mesenteric proliferation related to

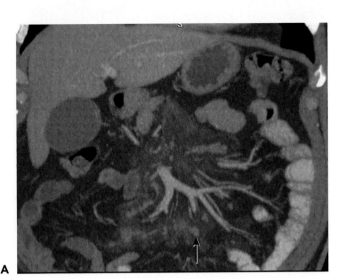

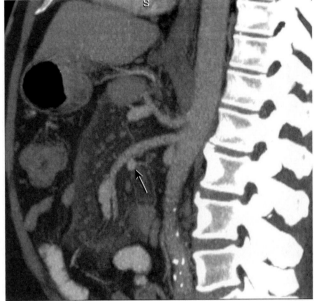

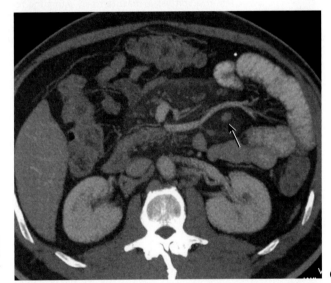

Figure 16-53 Mesenteric panniculitis. Coronal (**A**), sagittal (**B**) and transaxial (**C**) volume-rendered computed tomography shows diffusely increased attenuation of the central small bowel mesenteric fat. Note the enlarged mesenteric lymph nodes (*arrows*).

Crohn disease, lymphoma (particularly after chemotherapy), primary mesenteric neoplasms (e.g., desmoid, mesenteric cyst, or lipomatous tumors), peritoneal mesothelioma, and metastatic neoplasms, particularly carcinoid tumor (115,254, 300). Careful review of the entire CT examination, prior imaging studies, and the patient's clinical history are helpful in suggesting the correct diagnosis. Nevertheless, when sclerosing mesenteritis is suspected, biopsy is often necessary to establish the diagnosis and exclude infection or malignancy.

The association of fat necrosis and acute pancreatitis is well recognized (81). Fat necrosis, which can affect the mesentery, omentum, or retroperitoneum, can also be caused by infection, recent surgery, or a foreign body (137). The CT appearance varies from soft tissue attenuation mesenteric infiltration to nodular masses with soft tissue and/or fat attenuation (152,175) (Fig. 16-55). Calcifica-

tion in the necrotic central portion may also be detected (110). Cystic components may be seen, representing dilated lymphatics due to lymphatic and/or venous obstruction (138). In some cases, when fat attenuation is present, the CT appearance may be indistinguishable from that of a liposarcoma or a fat-containing teratoma (see Fig. 16-55). When soft tissue attenuation nodules are present, differential diagnostic considerations include carcinoid, desmoid tumor, mesenteric lymphoma, and metastatic carcinoma. The MRI appearance varies, with signal characteristics suggesting fluid or inflammation (low on T1, high on T2), fat (high on T1, low on T2), or fibrosis (low on T1 and T2) (152).

Segmental infarction of the greater omentum can result in a mass-like area of streaky increased attenuation within the omental fat (Figs. 16-56 and 16-57) (17,233,298). The infarction typically occurs on the right side, possibly because of an embryologic variant of the blood supply of the

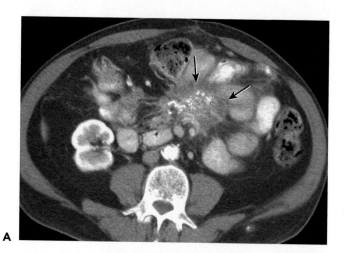

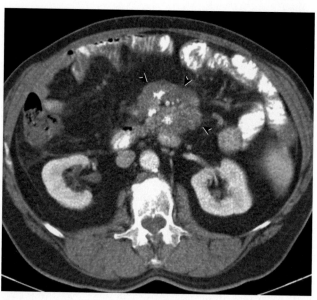

Figure 16-54 Two patients with sclerosing mesenteritis. **A:** Computed tomography shows an infiltrative soft tissue mass (*arrows*) within the root of the small bowel mesentery. The mass contains central calcifications and is associated with surrounding desmoplasia. The appearance is indistinguishable from that of a carcinoid tumor. **B:** In another patient a lobulated mesenteric soft tissue mass (*arrowheads*) with central calcifications is better circumscribed.

right side of the omentum, which predisposes it to venous thrombosis (71). Patients with omental infarction present with acute onset of right sided abdominal pain, which can mimic acute appendicitis or cholecystitis. Recognition on the CT examination that the abnormality is centered in the omentum with only minimal if any associated bowel or gall bladder wall thickening, enables the correct diagnosis. Omental infarction can be idiopathic or associated with adhesions, prior surgery, trauma, or omental torsion (17,40). Torsion of the greater omentum sometimes results in a characteristic CT appearance consisting of fibrous and fatty folds in a converging radial pattern (40).

Mesenteric Cyst (Lymphangioma)

A large variety of benign and malignant entities can present as cystic mesenteric or omental masses. These include lymphangioma, enteric duplication cyst, mesothelial cyst, ovarian cyst, nonpancreatic pseudocyst, cystic mesothelioma, cystic mesenchymal tumor, cystic teratoma and echinococcal cyst. Although CT findings may suggest a specific diagnosis in some cases, histologic diagnosis is often needed (249,285).

Mesenteric cysts (or lymphangiomas) are benign masses of vascular origin that show lymphatic differentiation (160). They originate most commonly in the small bowel mesentery, less commonly in the omentum, mesocolon and retroperitoneum (107,264). They contain either serous or chylous fluid (301). Clinically, mesenteric cysts usually are discovered incidentally as an asymptomatic abdominal mass, but they can cause chronic abdominal pain or acute pain secondary to a complication such as torsion, rupture, hemorrhage, or gastrointestinal obstruction. Mesenteric cysts appear on CT as well-defined, near-water attenuation, abdominal masses that sometimes contain higher density septa (Fig. 16-58) (107). When numerous thick septa are present, the mass may have an overall attenuation greater than that of water (Fig. 16-59). In some cases a thin wall can be identified peripherally. Chylous cysts occasionally have a pathognomonic fat–fluid layer, demonstrable with CT,

Figure 16-55 Fat necrosis. A large, well-defined mass (M) contains mixed soft tissue and fat attenuation components. The mass arose within the transverse mesocolon after partial pancreatectomy for pancreatic cancer.

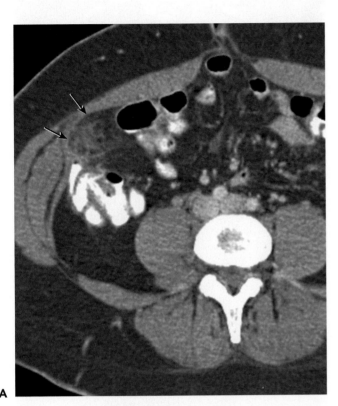

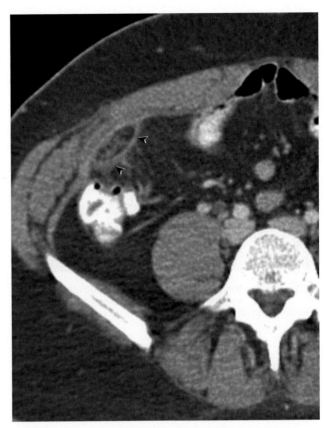

A   B

Figure 16-56 Segmental infarction of the greater omentum. **A:** Computed tomography demonstrates an ill-defined area of increased attenuation (*arrows*) within the omental fat anterior to the ascending colon. **B:** Follow-up examination 5 days later shows typical evolution of the abnormality, with a linear band of increased attenuation (*arrowheads*) surrounding the affected area.

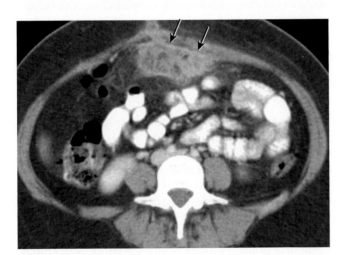

Figure 16-57 Segmental infarction of the greater omentum. Contrast-enhanced computed tomography demonstrates a mass-like area heterogeneous increased attenuation within the greater omentum (*arrows*). Follow-up examination (*not shown*) showed complete resolution. (Courtesy of Alvaro Huete, MD.)

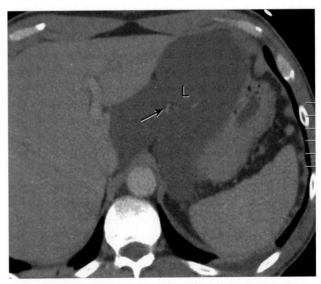

Figure 16-58 Lymphangioma. A large homogeneous water attenuation mass (L) arising from the gastrohepatic ligament surrounds the left gastric vessels (*arrow*) and displaces the stomach to the left.

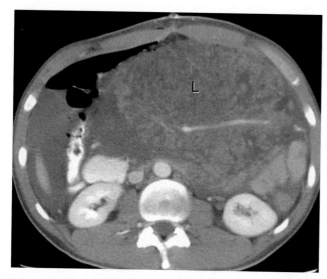

Figure 16-59 Mesenteric lymphangioma. A large mass (L) arising from the small bowel mesentery contains numerous thick septations. Courtesy of Alvaro Huete, M.D.

MRI, or ultrasound. The cysts are usually single, but can be multiple and vary widely in size. In children the cysts may fill most of the abdomen (107). Although the cyst content is usually water attenuation, cysts containing mucinous fluid or hemorrhage can have higher attenuation values (314). Mesenteric cysts have signal intensity characteristics similar to those of fluid, low on T1-weighted images and high on T2-weighted images (160). Negative CT attenuation values or shortened T1 signal intensity characteristics on MRI may indicate the presence of fat (285).

Other Nonneoplastic Processes of the Mesentery

Mesenteric hemorrhage, similar to hemorrhage elsewhere in the peritoneum, has a varied appearance depending on the age and extent of the bleeding. Acute mesenteric hemorrhage may produce localized, well-defined, soft tissue masses adjacent to bowel loops or larger "cake-like" masses that displace the bowel loops (314). When presenting as a focal mass, mesenteric hematoma can be mistaken for a primary or metastatic mesenteric tumor, an exophytic tumor of the bowel, or a mesenteric cyst with hemorrhage (235). With diffuse involvement the mesenteric fat is obliterated (Fig. 16-60). The attenuation of the hematoma is initially high with a gradual decrease in attenuation during a period of weeks followed by gradual resorption of the remaining seroma. After complete resorption, the mesentery may appear to return to normal or may contain residual fibrosis (314).

The term *pseudotumoral lipomatosis of the mesentery* refers to the excessive proliferation of normal mesenteric fat. This benign condition can be idiopathic or can be seen in association with obesity, Cushing syndrome, or steroid therapy (162). On contrast studies of the gastrointestinal

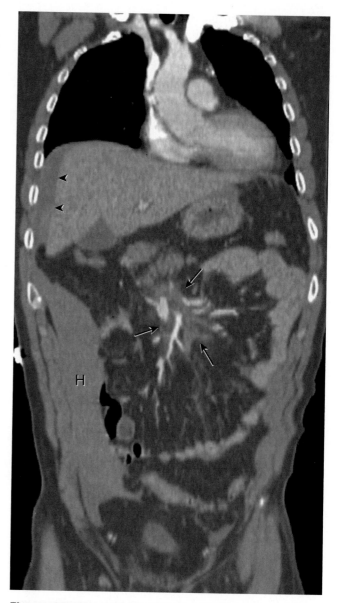

Figure 16-60 Mesenteric hemorrhage. Coronal computed tomography demonstrates an irregularly shaped collection of fluid (arrows) that contains areas of high attenuation, surrounding the vessels at the root of the small bowel mesentery. Note the blood in the right perihepatic space (*arrowheads*) and in the right paracolic gutter (H).

tract, mesenteric lipomatosis may displace bowel loops, simulating an abdominal mass or ascites. CT can exclude the presence of neoplasm by showing that the displacement is caused by either diffuse or focal accumulation of normal fat (51,162,270).

Systemic amyloidosis is characterized by diffuse extracellular tissue deposition of an amorphous eosinophilic protein-polysaccharide complex (57). Amyloidosis can occur as a primary process or in association with chronic inflammatory disease or multiple myeloma. Involvement of the mesentery, when extensive, is easily demonstrated by CT (5). The CT appearance, consisting of increased density of mesenteric fat with encasement of mesenteric vessels, is indistinguishable from other disease processes causing diffuse mesenteric infiltration including peritonitis, metastatic carcinoma, and peritoneal mesothelioma (56). Additional rare causes of mesenteric infiltration that can have a similar appearance are extramedullary hematopoiesis (96,226) and sarcoidosis (226).

The most commonly recognized radiographic manifestation of Whipple disease is thickening of the valvulae conniventes of the small bowel. However, CT is capable of demonstrating some of the less well-recognized extraintestinal manifestations of the disease including low-density retroperitoneal and mesenteric lymphadenopathy, and sacroiliitis (163,245). The enlarged lymph nodes in Whipple disease may be low in attenuation secondary to deposition of neutral fat and fatty acids within the nodes (163).

Mesenteric venous thrombosis is responsible for 5% to 15% of cases of intestinal ischemia (95). The superior mesenteric vein (SMV), which is involved in 95% of these cases, is easily imaged by CT. The typical appearance of chronic SMV thrombosis consists of enlargement of the vein with central low density surrounded by a higher density wall (250) (Fig. 16-61). The wall of the vein enhances after administration of intravenous contrast material, possibly due to enhancement of the arterially supplied vasa vasorum (329). The thrombus may be higher in attenuation than soft tissue when SMV thrombosis is acute. Associated portal venous or splenic venous thrombosis may be seen (250). In some cases, mesenteric venous thrombosis is associated with increased density of the mesenteric fat and poor definition of segmental mesenteric vessels, due to mesenteric edema (272). Thickening of the bowel wall may also be present. If the mesenteric ischemia is severe enough to cause bowel infarction, intramural, portal vein,

or mesenteric vein gas may also be identified (73). These associated findings are usually absent when the thrombus is nonocclusive.

Endometriosis can diffusely involve the peritoneum with cystic, solid, or mixed masses throughout the omentum, mesentery, and peritoneal surfaces. High-attenuation ascites may also be present. Although the CT appearance is nonspecific, this diagnosis should be considered in women of childbearing age. Differential diagnostic considerations include peritoneal carcinomatosis, pseudomyxoma peritonei, lymphoma, and tuberculous peritonitis. In most cases however, peritoneal endometrial implants are too small to be identified at CT. On MR images, large endometriomas appear as high signal intensity masses on T1-weighted images and low signal intensity masses with areas of high signal intensity on T2-weighted images (27). Endometriosis may also appear as multiple small cysts that are hyperintense on T1-weighted images with variable signal intensity on T2-weighted images (11,27). Most endometriomas remain bright on gadolinium-chelate enhanced T1-weighted images, and enhancement of adjacent peritoneal surfaces is also frequently seen (11). Although MR imaging is superior to CT in demonstrating peritoneal endometriosis, MR also is limited in demonstrating small peritoneal implants (94). In one study, gadolinium-enhanced T1-weighted fat-suppressed MR demonstrated 27% of endometrial implants with a positive predictive value of 64% (11).

Castleman disease is an idiopathic, benign entity characterized by proliferation of lymphoid tissue into tumoral masses. It is most often seen as a solitary mediastinal mass but can occur as solitary or widespread mesenteric disease (Fig. 16-62) (75,80). Classically, marked enhancement is seen on CT (75,80).

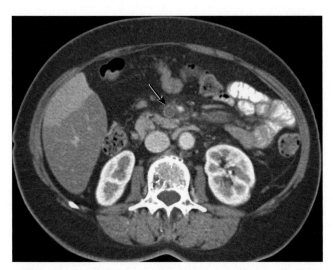

Figure 16-61 Superior mesenteric vein (SMV) thrombosis. The SMV (*arrow*) is enlarged and contains central low attenuation surrounded by a higher density wall.

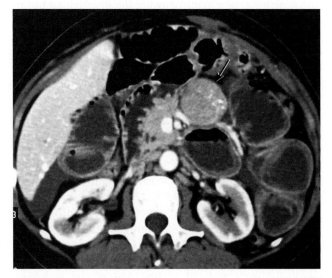

Figure 16-62 Castleman disease. A homogeneously enhancing mass (*arrow*) at the root of the small bowel mesentery has produced small bowel obstruction. The mass contains a small amount of calcification.

Primary Neoplasms of the Peritoneum

Cystic mesothelioma (also called *multicystic mesothelioma, benign cystic mesothelioma* and *multilocular peritoneal inclusion cyst*) is a rare neoplasm of peritoneal origin. It occurs predominantly in women of child-bearing age (210,311). Whether it is a true neoplasm is controversial. Cystic mesothelioma is considered by some researchers to be a benign neoplasm (210) and by others to be an intermediate grade neoplasm, between benign adenomatoid tumor of the peritoneum and malignant peritoneal mesothelioma (311). Still others consider it to represent nonneoplastic mesothelial proliferation rather than a true neoplasm (251). On CT, cystic mesothelioma appears as a multilocular cystic mass that may exert mass effect on adjacent anatomic structures but shows no signs of invasion (101,218). On MRI, the cysts are low in signal intensity on T1-weighted images and intermediate or high signal intensity on T2-weighted images (210,218,320). The imaging appearance of cystic mesothelioma may be identical to that of lymphangioma and overlaps with that of other cystic peritoneal masses. Therefore, diagnosis requires histologic evaluation (320).

Inflammatory pseudotumor, also known as *myofibroblastic tumor*, is a rare reactive lesion that can involve the peritoneum. It usually occurs in young individuals and can appear as an infiltrative mass or as multiple well-defined peritoneal masses (226).

Primary serous papillary carcinoma of the peritoneum is a rare primary neoplasm of the peritoneum that occurs primarily in postmenopausal women (141). It is characterized by abdominal carcinomatosis and no involvement or only surface involvement of the ovaries (78). The clinical and histopathologic features of primary serous papillary carcinoma of the peritoneum are indistinguishable from those of metastatic ovarian carcinoma (190). On imaging studies, the presence of ascites and extensive peritoneal and omental tumor involvement in the absence of an ovarian mass or evidence of a primary tumor in the gastrointestinal tract should suggest the diagnosis (44,46,78,141, 281,330). Peritoneal calcifications and lymph node enlargement may also be seen.

Mesothelioma is a rare malignant neoplasm arising from the mesothelial cells lining the pleura, peritoneum, and pericardium. Peritoneal involvement may occur, either alone or in combination with pleural involvement. The CT findings correlate with the two major clinical types of peritoneal mesothelioma. In the "wet" type, ascites is associated with peritoneal, mesenteric and omental thickening that may appear irregular or nodular (97,242,286,316) (Figs. 16-63 and 16-64). The mesenteric involvement may produce a "stellate" appearance due to thickening of the perivascular bundles by tumor (Fig. 16-65) (316). In the "dry-painful" type, CT demonstrates multiple small masses or a single dominant mass isolated to one part of the abdomen (140,286). In advanced cases, solid tumor with areas of cystic degeneration may fill the entire abdomen. The CT appearance of peritoneal mesothelioma may be indistin-

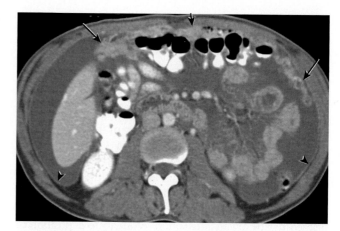

Figure 16-63 Primary peritoneal mesothelioma. Contrast-enhanced computed tomography shows ascites and diffuse thickening of the peritoneum (*arrowheads*) and omentum (*arrows*). The appearance is indistinguishable from that of peritoneal carcinomatosis.

guishable from peritoneal carcinomatosis, lymphoma, and benign disease processes such as tuberculous peritonitis. The amount of ascites relative to the soft tissue component of mesothelioma may be disproportionately small as compared with peritoneal carcinomatosis in which ascites is usually a prominent feature (242).

Desmoplastic round cell tumor of the abdomen is a rare aggressive malignant neoplasm that occurs in adolescents and young adults (mean age, 20 to 25 years) (47,82,227, 292). The CT findings range from one or more large lobulated peritoneal masses to diffuse irregular peritoneal thickening without discrete masses (47,227,292). The masses may contain areas of central low attenuation or punctuate calcification. On MRI, the masses demonstrate low signal intensity on T1-weighted images, high signal intensity on T2-weighted images, and heterogeneous contrast en-

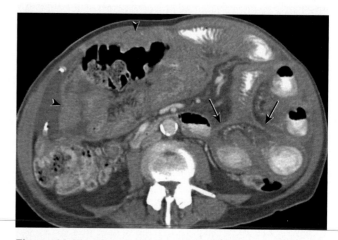

Figure 16-64 Primary peritoneal mesothelioma. Contrast-enhanced computed tomography shows diffuse thickening of the greater omentum (*arrowheads*) and the leaves of the small bowel mesentery (*arrows*). A drainage catheter is present within the ascites on the right side of the abdomen.

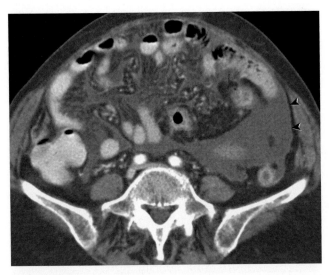

Figure 16-65 Primary peritoneal mesothelioma. Contrast-enhanced computed tomography demonstrates ascites, thickening of the small bowel mesentery, and mild thickening and enhancement of the peritoneal lining (*arrowheads*).

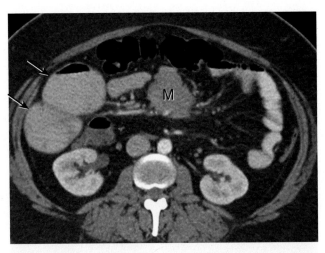

Figure 16-66 Desmoid tumor. Contrast-enhanced computed tomography shows a homogeneously enhancing soft tissue mass (M) with irregular margins within the small bowel mesentery. The mass has resulted in small bowel obstruction. Note the dilated, fluid-filled small bowel loops (*arrows*).

hancement with central hypointensity, indicative of necrosis (292). Fluid-fluid levels may be seen on T2-weighted images, corresponding to intratumoral hemorrhage (292). Ascites and abdominal or pelvic lymphadenopathy may also be present. Metastases most commonly involve the liver, less commonly the thorax and bones (47,227,292).

Primary Neoplasms of the Mesentery and Omentum

Primary neoplasms of the mesenteries and greater omentum are rare and generally of mesenchymal origin (268). The mesenteric desmoid tumor is a nonencapsulated, locally invasive form of fibromatosis (201). It occurs sporadically but is particularly common in patients with Gardner syndrome, especially in those who have undergone abdominal surgery (21,172,201). On CT, a desmoid tumor appears as a soft tissue mass displacing adjacent visceral structures (21) (Figs. 16-66 and 16-67). Although the mass may appear well circumscribed, it often has irregular margins extending into the mesenteric fat, reflecting its infiltrative nature (see Figs. 16-67). Less commonly the mass may have a "whorled" appearance (13,31). Mesenteric desmoid tumors demonstrate contrast enhancement, which may be homogeneous or heterogeneous. Other neoplasms such as mesenteric metastases and lymphoma can have a similar CT appearance. On MRI desmoid tumors appear hypo- or isointense relative to muscle on T1-weighted images, with variable signal intensity on T2-weighted images, reflecting their relative cellularity and fibrous content (13,39,111). High T2 signal intensity and marked enhancement after intravenous contrast medium administration are indicative of high tumor cellularity, which is predictive of rapid tumor growth (111).

Lipomatous tumors, which occur predominantly in the retroperitoneum, rarely involve the peritoneal cavity. Benign lipomas consist predominantly of fat, which is reflected in their CT attenuation and MR signal characteristics. Myolipoma is a rare benign mass that contains fat and soft tissue density and can simulate a liposarcoma (Fig. 16-68). Multiple histologic subtypes of liposarcoma exist, each with corresponding CT and MR characteristics. Well-differentiated liposarcoma can be of lipomatous or sclerosing type, with CT and MR appearance of fat or muscle, respectively. Myxoid liposarcoma has an appearance on unenhanced CT that is similar to water, with reticular enhancement after administration of intravenous contrast material. Round cell and pleiomorphic liposarcomas are nonfatty tumors with nonspecific soft tissue appearance on CT and MRI (Fig. 16-69) (144).

Benign or malignant primary peritoneal mesenteric and omental tumors other than desmoid and lipomatous tumors are extremely rare but can arise from any of the mesenchymal tissue elements (106,123,124,151,156,179, 198,199,236) (Figs. 16-70 and 16-71). Primary omental and mesenteric gastrointestinal stromal tumors are indistinguishable from other sarcomas arising from these structures (143). Primary mesenteric and omental teratomas have also been reported (106,312). Because both benign and malignant primary mesenteric and omental tumors may demonstrate cystic, solid, and complex features, histologic diagnosis is usually required.

Secondary Neoplasms

The most common malignant neoplasms involving the peritoneum are metastatic carcinoma and lymphoma. Metastases usually arise from the stomach, colon, or ovary

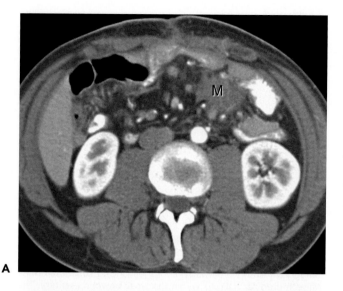

A

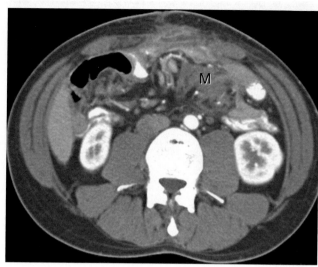

B

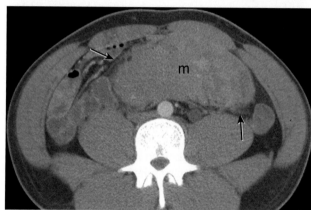

C

Figure 16-67 Mesenteric desmoid tumor in two patients with Gardner syndrome. **A, B:** An enhancing soft tissue mass with irregular margins (M) infiltrates the small bowel mesentery, encasing mesenteric vessels and displacing small bowel loops. **C:** A large mass (m) within the small bowel mesentery shows mild heterogeneous enhancement. Note the irregularity along the left posterior and right lateral borders (*arrows*) Both patients had undergone total colectomy.

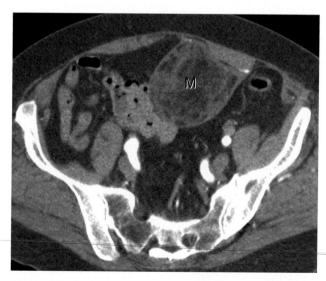

Figure 16-68 Myolipoma. Contrast-enhanced computed tomography shows an encapsulated heterogeneous fat-containing mass (M) within the greater omentum. The appearance is indistinguishable from that of mass-like fat necrosis or liposarcoma.

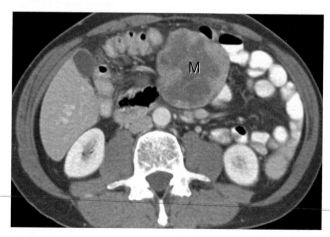

Figure 16-69 Pleiomorphic liposarcoma. Contrast-enhanced computed tomography demonstrates a large heterogeneously enhancing mass (M) in the small bowel mesentery.

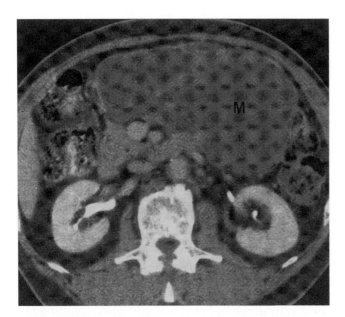

Figure 16-70 Primary angiosarcoma of the omentum. Large mass (M) in the greater omentum containing near-water attenuation and enhancing soft tissue attenuation components.

and less commonly from the pancreas, biliary tract, or uterus (1,60). Renal cell carcinoma, transitional cell carcinoma of the bladder and gastrointestinal leiomyosarcoma are reported as rare sites of origin (225,243,291). Very rarely, a late recurrence of malignant melanoma may present with peritoneal involvement (154). Prior to the availability of CT, peritoneal metastases were not detectable radiographically until they were large enough to displace adjacent organs or cause intestinal obstruction. Now with the routine use of multidetector-row CT, peritoneal metas-

tases less than 5 mm in diameter can be detected, although the sensitivity of CT for demonstrating subcentimeter metastases remains limited. A study using single-detector row CT to evaluate patients with ovarian cancer preoperatively demonstrated a sensitivity of 25% to 50% for metastases less than 1 cm in diameter, although the overall sensitivity for peritoneal metastases was 85% to 93% (49). MRI using breath-hold T1-weighted gradient echo imaging with fat suppression and gadolinium-chelate enhancement is also an excellent technique for demonstrating peritoneal tumors, with reported sensitivities of 84% to 95% (166,167,262,293). A multi-institutional study comparing CT, MRI, and ultrasound for the staging of patients with advanced ovarian cancer found no statistically significant difference between MRI and CT for demonstrating peritoneal metastases (95% and 92%, respectively) (293). In that study, both CT and MRI were superior to ultrasound (sensitivity, 69%).

Rigorous attention to technique is important in detecting small mesenteric and omental tumor implants. Administration of intraperitoneal air or iodinated contrast material may improve the detection of implants in some intraperitoneal compartments (38,105), but such techniques are not practical for routine imaging.

In patients with a large amount of ascites, ultrasound is capable of demonstrating superficial peritoneal and omental tumor nodules as small as 2 to 3 mm because of the acoustic window provided by the peritoneal fluid (325). However, it is difficult to detect peritoneal masses with ultrasound in patients with little or no ascites. Furthermore, centrally located tumors are poorly imaged by ultrasound because of the acoustic impedance of bowel gas and mesenteric fat (30).

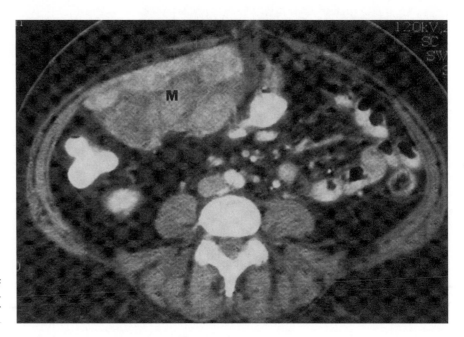

Figure 16-71 Spindle cell sarcoma of the omentum. Large heterogeneously enhancing, vascular mass (M) in the greater omentum displaces adjacent bowel.

Metastatic neoplasm can disseminate through the peritoneal cavity by four pathways: direct spread along mesenteric and ligamentous attachments, intraperitoneal seeding, lymphatic extension, and embolic hematogenous dissemination (184). Many neoplasms metastasize predominantly by one particular route producing characteristic CT findings (158).

Direct Spread Along Peritoneal Surfaces

Malignant neoplasms of the ovary, stomach, colon, and pancreas that have penetrated beyond the borders of these organs can spread directly along the adjacent visceral peritoneal surfaces to involve other peritoneal structures. Neoplastic spread along peritoneal pathways can also involve bowel at some distance from the primary tumor. The transverse mesocolon serves as a major route of spread from the stomach, colon, and pancreas. The gastrocolic ligament (greater omentum) is another important pathway between stomach and colon. Gastric malignancies can also extend along the gastrosplenic ligament to the spleen, whereas neoplasms in the tail of the pancreas may spread via the phrenicocolic ligament to involve the anatomic splenic

flexure of the colon (185). Biliary neoplasms often spread along the gastrohepatic and hepatoduodenal ligaments. Ovarian carcinoma spreads diffusely along all adjacent mesothelial surfaces. The CT appearance of direct peritoneal extension of tumor depends on the degree of spread. Early peritoneal infiltration produces an increase in the density of the fat adjacent to the neoplasm. More advanced spread results in a mass that is contiguous with the primary neoplasm and often extends along the expected course of the ligamentous attachment to involve adjacent organs (217). Because of their continuity with the retroperitoneum, the peritoneal ligaments, in addition to serving as the avenues of intraperitoneal tumor spread, also serve as conduits of disease spread between the peritoneum and retroperitoneum (185).

Neoplastic infiltration of the greater omentum can produce a distinctive CT or MR imaging appearance ranging from small nodules or strands of soft tissue that increase the density of the fat anterior to the colon or small intestine (Figs. 16-72 and 16-73) to large masses that separate the colon or small intestine from the anterior abdominal wall ("omental cakes") (54,159) (Figs. 16-74 and 16-75).

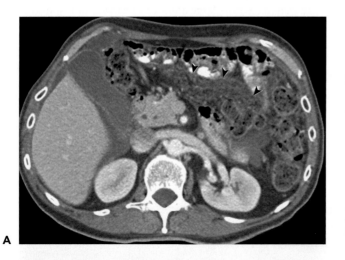

A

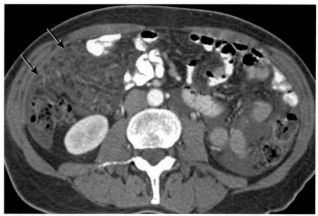

B

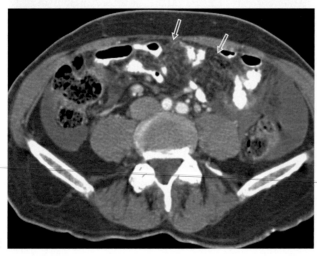

C

Figure 16-72 Peritoneal carcinomatosis in a patient with gastric adenocarcinoma. **A, B, C:** The transverse mesocolon (*arrowheads*), greater omentum (*arrows*), and small bowel mesentery (*open arrows*) are infiltrated with innumerable tiny soft tissue nodules.

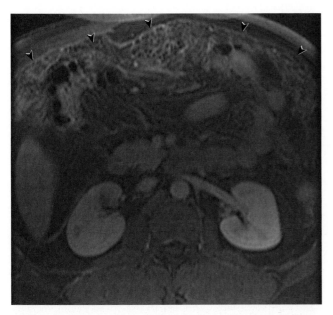

Figure 16-73 Omental metastases. T1-weighted gradient-echo image with fat suppression acquired after intravenous administration of gadolinium-chelate shows enhancement of the greater omentum (*arrowheads*), which is diffusely infiltrated with metastases from ovarian carcinoma.

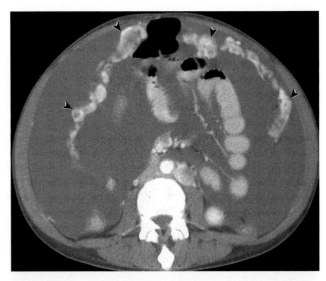

Figure 16-75 Metastatic colon carcinoma. Contrast-enhanced computed tomography demonstrates massive ascites with enhancing metastases that involve the greater omentum diffusely (*arrowheads*).

Extensive neoplastic infiltration of the omentum is produced most frequently by metastatic ovarian carcinoma but can occur with other neoplasms. Occasionally omental or other peritoneal metastases from ovarian carcinoma calcify (Fig. 16-76). This is most commonly seen with serous papillary cystadenocarcinoma in which psammomatous calcifications are seen histologically (192). Inflammatory thickening of the omentum, such as that produced by

peritonitis, may be indistinguishable from neoplastic infiltration of the omentum (54).

Involvement of the small bowel mesentery by carcinoid tumor often produces a characteristic CT appearance. The triad of calcification within a mesenteric mass, radiating soft tissue strands due to reactive desmoplasia around the mass, and mural thickening of an adjacent bowel loop is highly suggestive of this diagnosis (220,321) (Figs. 16-77 and 16-78). Calcification may be detected in up to 70% of cases (220) (Figs. 16-77 and 16-79). Moderate contrast

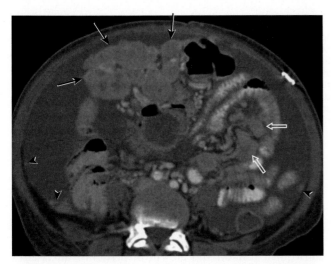

Figure 16-74 Metastatic ovarian carcinoma. Contrast-enhanced computed tomography shows a large amount of ascites associated with a conglomerate soft tissue mass involving the greater omentum (*arrows*). Also note multiple smaller masses involving the small bowel mesentery (*open arrows*) and peritoneum (*arrowheads*).

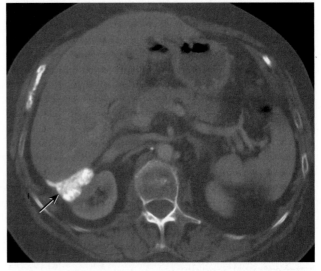

Figure 16-76 Calcified metastasis in a patient with ovarian carcinoma. Computed tomography with bone window settings demonstrates a calcium attenuation metastasis in Morison's pouch (*arrow*).

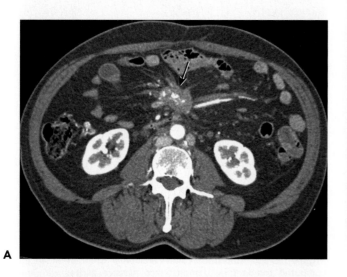

A

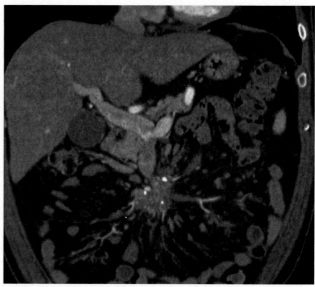

B

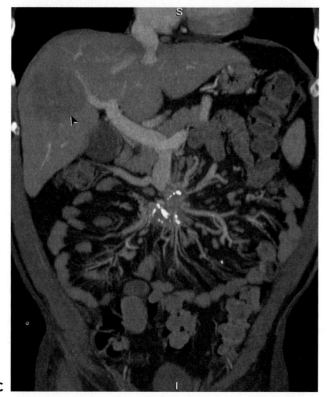

C

Figure 16-77 Metastatic carcinoid tumor. **A:** Transaxial computed tomography shows a lobulated soft tissue mass (*arrow*) with punctate central calcifications at the root of the small bowel mesentery. Strands of soft tissue density radiating from the mass toward the small bowel loops are indicative of desmoplastic response to the tumor. **B:** Coronal image also demonstrates the characteristic features of the mass. **C:** Coronal maximum intensity projection (MIP) image shows engorgement of the mesenteric veins due to partial obstruction by the mass. Note the large hepatic metastasis (*arrowhead*).

enhancement of the mesenteric mass is typical on both CT and MR examinations (14). Mesenteric venous congestion may be present secondary to obstruction of mesenteric veins by the mass (see Figs. 16-77C and 16-78B). Many patients have liver metastases at the time of diagnosis.

Intraperitoneal Seeding
Intraperitoneal seeding of neoplasm depends on the natural flow of fluid within the peritoneal cavity, which is governed by the compartmentalization of the peritoneal spaces in combination with the effects of gravity and changes in intraabdominal pressure caused by respiration (186). The most common sites of pooling of ascites and subsequent fixation and growth of peritoneal metastases are the pouch of Douglas (Figs. 16-79 and 16-80), the lower small bowel mesentery near the ileocecal junction, the sigmoid mesocolon, and the right paracolic gutter (186). The primary neoplasms that most commonly spread

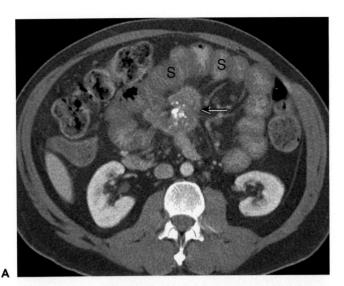
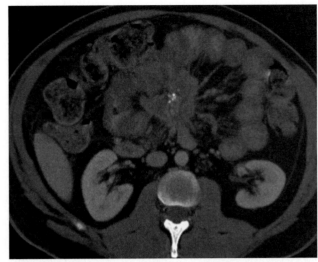

Figure 16-78 Metastatic carcinoid tumor. **A:** Computed tomography shows a soft tissue mass (*arrow*) with central calcifications in the root of the small bowel mesentery. Note the wall thickening of the adjacent loop of small bowel (S). **B:** Volume-rendered image demonstrates the desmoplastic reaction within the mesenteric fat and engorgement of the mesenteric veins.

by this route are adenocarcinoma of the ovary, colon, stomach, and pancreas. Approximately 70% of patients with ovarian carcinoma have peritoneal involvement at the time of diagnosis (322). On CT, seeded metastases appear as soft tissue masses, frequently associated with ascites, at one or more of the sites of normal pooling (Fig. 16-81) (132). In some cases the peritoneum is diffusely thickened. If a moderate amount of ascites is present, peritoneal implants less than 5 mm in diameter can be identified. If the metastases are very small, ascites may be the only sign of intraperitoneal seeding. When little or no ascites is present, the only CT manifestation of intraabdominal carcinomatosis may be replacement of the normal mesenteric fat density with soft tissue density.

The small bowel mesentery and the greater omentum are frequently involved by intraperitoneally disseminated tumor. Four general CT patterns of mesenteric involvement have been described: rounded masses, cake-like masses, ill-defined masses, and a stellate pattern (315). Rounded masses are seen most commonly with non-Hodgkin lymphoma (resulting primarily from lymphadenopathy rather than intraperitoneal seeding) (26,315) (Figs. 16-82 and 16-83) but can also be seen with other metastatic tumors (Figs. 16-84 and 16-85). Irregular ill-defined and cake-like masses are seen most often with ovarian carcinoma, although non-Hodgkin lymphoma and other metastatic carcinomas can produce a similar appearance. Cystic mesenteric masses are an occasional manifestation of ovarian carcinoma. The stellate pattern, consisting of a radiating pattern of the mesenteric leaves, can be produced by a number of metastatic carcinomas, including ovarian, pancreatic, colonic, and breast (Fig. 16-86). This pattern results from diffuse

mesenteric tumor infiltration causing thickening and rigidity of the perivascular bundles (159). These mesenteric patterns, although characteristic of metastatic involvement, are by no means specific and can be mimicked by primary peritoneal neoplasms such as mesothelioma (see Fig. 16-65) and by inflammatory processes such as pancreatitis and tuberculous peritonitis.

A distinctive CT appearance is produced by pseudomyxoma peritonei in which the peritoneal surfaces become diffusely involved with large amounts of mucinous material. Although there is continued debate regarding the site of origin of pseudomyxoma peritonei, clinicopathologic studies suggest that the vast majority of cases arise from primary mucinous adenomas of the appendix, with the ovaries being secondarily involved (79,231,248,326). Although a more benign form (disseminated peritoneal adenomucinosis) and a more malignant form (peritoneal mucinous carcinomatosis) of the disease have been described, the imaging findings of the two forms overlap (22). CT findings include low-attenuation masses with discrete walls or diffuse intraperitoneal low-attenuation material that may contain septations and often causes scalloping of the hepatic, splenic and mesenteric margins (58,177,206,263, 287,308,324) (Figs. 16-87 to 16-89). Calcifications are not uncommon in patients with large volume disease (177), particularly after chemotherapy (176,287). If the walls of the cystic masses are thin, the CT appearance may be similar to that produced by loculated ascites. Scalloping of the liver, spleen and mesenteric margins by extrinsic pressure of the gelatinous masses and failure of the bowel loops to "float" to the anterior abdominal wall may be useful in differentiating pseudomyxoma peritonei from ascites

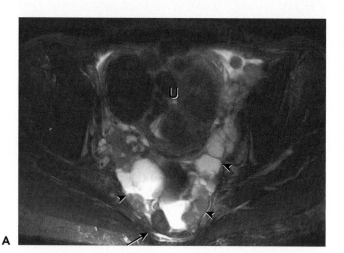

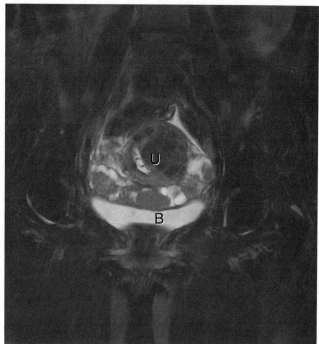

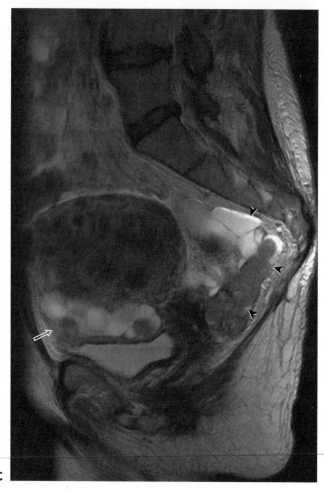

Figure 16-79 Metastatic ovarian carcinoma. **A:** Transaxial T2-weighted magnetic resonance image with fat suppression shows cystic and solid metastases involving the cul-de-sac (*arrowheads*). Myomatous uterus (U) and rectum (*arrow*) are noted. **B:** Coronal T2-weighted image with fat suppression shows metastases between the uterus (U) and urinary bladder (B). **C:** Sagittal T2-weighted image demonstrates numerous metastases in the cul-de-sac (*arrowheads*) and in the vesico-uterine space (*open arrow*).

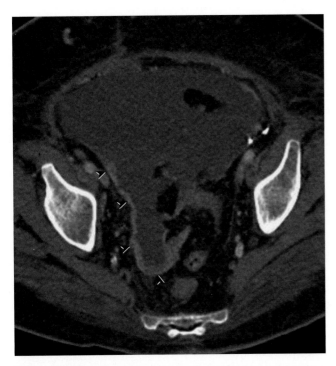

Figure 16-80 Metastatic colon carcinoma. Pelvic computed tomography demonstrates ascites with peritoneal thickening and enhancement in the cul-de-sac (*arrowheads*).

(263). MRI demonstrates morphologic changes similar to those seen on CT (Fig. 16-90) (35).

Lymphatic Dissemination

Lymphatic extension plays a minor role in the intraperitoneal dissemination of metastatic carcinoma (181) but is the primary mode of spread of lymphoma to mesenteric lymph nodes. At the time of presentation, approximately 50% of patients with non-Hodgkin lymphoma have mesenteric lymph node involvement, whereas only 5% of patients with Hodgkin's disease have mesenteric disease at presentation (87). Identification of mesenteric lymph node disease is extremely important as it almost always indicates the need for chemotherapy, sometimes in combination with radiation therapy (158). American Burkitt lymphoma is a B-cell lymphoma, primarily affecting children and young adults, that usually produces bulky extranodal tumors in the abdomen (90).

On CT the appearance of mesenteric lymph node involvement by lymphoma ranges from small round or oval masses within the mesenteric fat to large confluent masses displacing adjacent bowel loops (26,159,315) (Fig. 16-91). Large confluent masses of lymphomatous nodes may surround the superior mesenteric artery and veins, producing a "sandwich-like" appearance (109,195) (Fig. 16-92). After radiation or combined radiation and chemotherapy

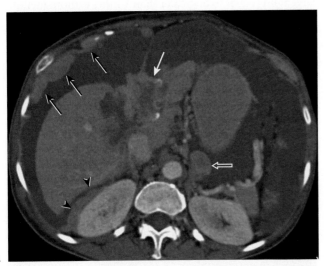

A

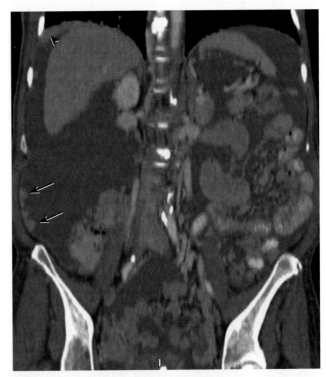

B

Figure 16-81 Metastatic ovarian carcinoma. **A:** Transaxial computed tomography shows ascites with nodular thickening of the peritoneum (*arrows*) and tumor implants in the Morison pouch (*arrowheads*), the lesser sac (*open arrow*), and along the falciform ligament (*white arrow*). **B:** Coronal reformatted image shows tumor implants in the right paracolic gutter (*arrows*) and along the peritoneal surface of the diaphragm (*arrowhead*).

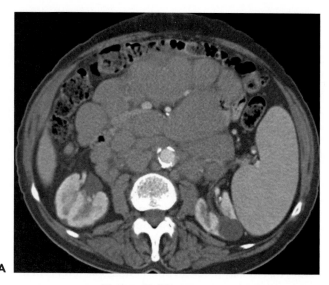

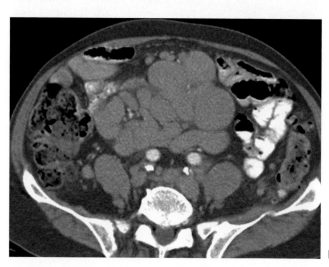

A   B

Figure 16-82 Mesenteric lymphadenopathy in a patient with chronic lymphocytic leukemia. **A, B:** Contrast-enhanced computed tomography shows multiple large discrete mesenteric masses that surround the superior mesenteric vessels. Note splenic enlargement.

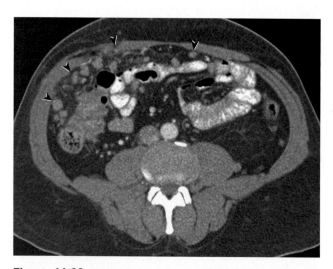

Figure 16-83 Peritoneal lymphoma. Multiple soft tissue nodules involve the greater omentum (*arrowheads*) in this patient with non-Hodgkin lymphoma.

treatment of non-Hodgkin lymphoma, peripheral curvilinear calcifications may be seen in the mesenteric masses (43). When lymphoma disseminates to peritoneal surfaces other than the mesentery (peritoneal lymphomatosis), the CT appearance may be indistinguishable from that of metastatic carcinoma (145) (Fig. 16-93). Patients with AIDS-related lymphoma often present with more advanced disease (209). Occasionally, the earliest CT sign of mesenteric lymphoma is an increased number of normal size (less than 1 cm) lymph nodes within the mesentery. However, mild mesenteric lymphadenopathy is a nonspecific finding and does not always represent lymphoma. Primary mesenteric adenitis consists of right sided mesenteric lymph node enlargement (equal to or greater than 5 mm) without identifiable acute inflammatory process or with only mild wall thickening of the terminal ileum (171,237) (Fig. 16-94).

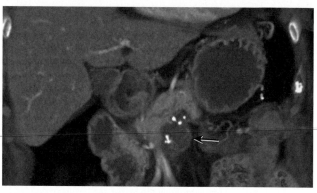

A   B

Figure 16-84 Two patients with metastatic colon carcinoma. Transaxial computed tomography image **(A)** and volume rendered coronal image **(B)** show a low attenuation mass (*arrow*) with punctuate calcifications at the root of the small bowel mesentery that encases the superior mesenteric artery (*arrowhead*).

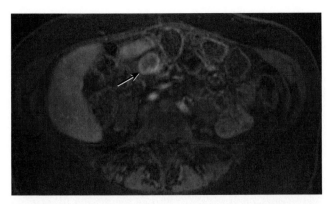

Figure 16-85   Mesenteric metastasis. T1-weighted gradient echo magnetic resonance image with fat suppression acquired after intravenous administration of gadolinium-chelate shows a rim-enhancing mass (*arrow*) in this patient with colon carcinoma.

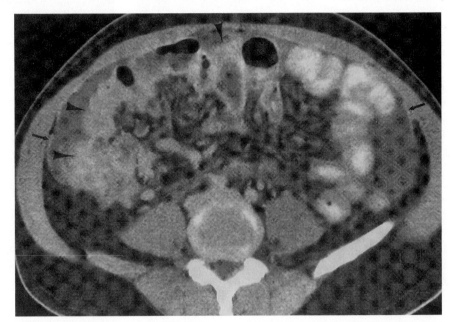

Figure 16-86   Peritoneal and mesenteric metastases from colon carcinoma. Contrast-enhanced computed tomography demonstrates ascites with diffuse peritoneal thickening (*arrows*), omental implants (*arrowheads*), and mesenteric infiltration. The mesenteric vascular bundles are thickened, and the mesentery has a rigid appearance.

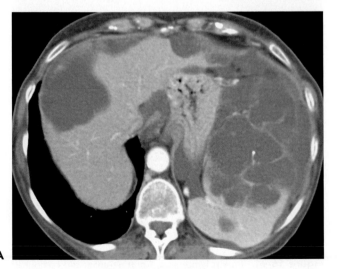

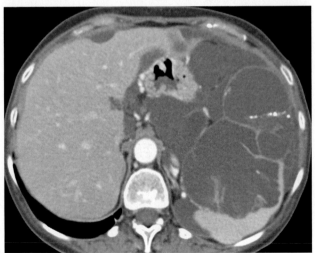

Figure 16-87   Pseudomyxoma peritonei. **A, B:** Contrast-enhanced computed tomography shows large confluent septated cystic masses that cause scalloping of the margins of the liver and spleen. Several of the masses contain punctuate calcifications.

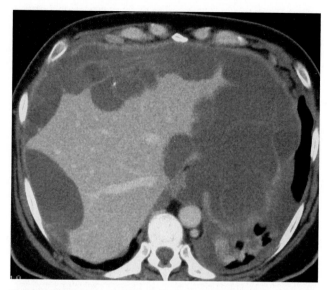

Figure 16-88 Pseudomyxoma peritonei. Contrast-enhanced computed tomography image shows extensive peritoneal involvement by septate cystic masses that scallop the liver margin.

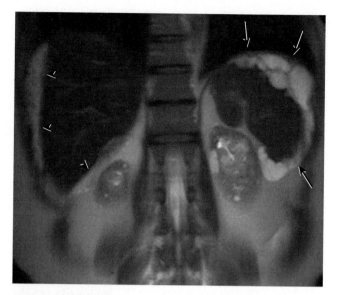

Figure 16-90 Pseudomyxoma peritonei. Coronal T2-weighted magnetic resonance image demonstrates multiple confluent high signal intensity perisplenic cystic masses (*arrows*) that cause scalloping of the splenic margin. Also note the perihepatic and subhepatic tumor implants (*arrowheads*).

Other nonneoplastic causes of mesenteric lymphadenopathy include infiltrative and inflammatory disease such as Crohn disease (63), sarcoidosis, Whipple disease (163,245), celiac disease (135), giardiasis, tuberculous peritonitis (120), *Mycobacterium avium-intracellulare* infection (208), mastocytosis (63), and acquired immune deficiency syndrome (AIDS) (194,208). Rarely, mesenteric lymph nodes associated with celiac disease can undergo cavitation and appear as fluid or fat attenuation mesenteric masses ("mesenteric cavitary lymph node syndrome") (34). Identification of enlarged mesenteric lymph nodes containing fat-fluid levels allows an imaging-specific diagnosis (226,241).

Embolic Metastases

Tumor emboli may be spread via the mesenteric arteries to the antimesenteric border of bowel where the cells implant and subsequently grow into intramural tumor nodules (184). On CT, these embolic metastases may produce thickening of the mesenteric leaves or focal bowel wall thickening, occasionally with recognizable ulceration. The most common neoplasms to spread in this manner are melanoma (139,178) and carcinoma of the breast or lung (Fig. 16-95).

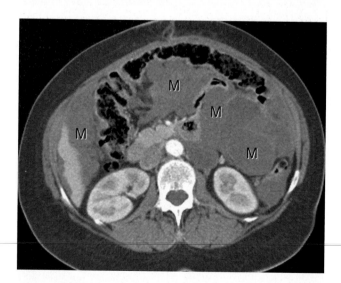

Figure 16-89 Pseudomyxoma peritonei. Confluent low-attenuation septated masses (M) scallop the liver margin and displace bowel.

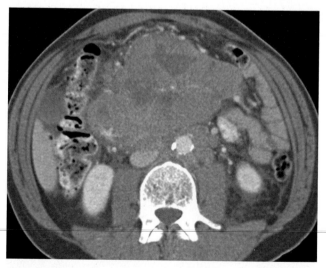

Figure 16-91 Burkitt lymphoma. Contrast-enhanced computed tomography shows a large confluent lymph node mass within the small bowel mesentery encasing the mesenteric vessels.

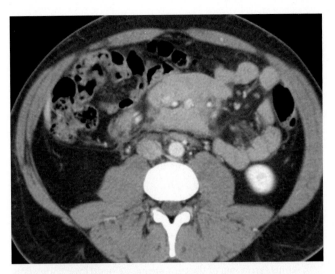

Figure 16-92   Non-Hodgkin lymphoma.. Large confluent mesenteric lymph node masses surround the superior mesenteric vessels producing a "sandwich-like" appearance.

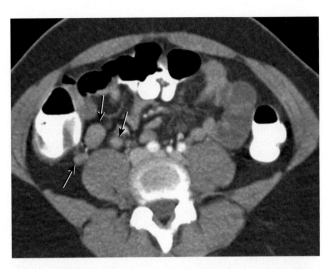

Figure 16-94   Mesenteric adenitis. Computed tomography shows several enlarged lymph nodes in the ileocolic region of the mesentery (*arrows*). A normal appendix was seen on lower pelvic images.

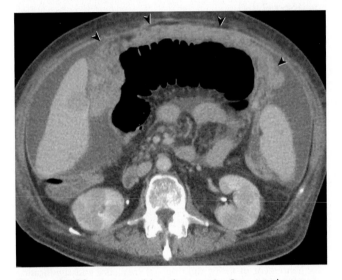

Figure 16-93   Peritoneal lymphomatosis. Computed tomography shows ascites and diffuse infiltration of the greater omentum (arrowheads) producing an "omental cake." Note the low attenuation hepatic mass and bilateral renal masses in this patient with diffuse dissemination of non-Hodgkin lymphoma.

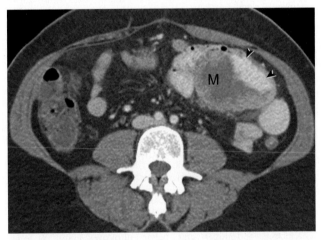

Figure 16-95   Metastatic breast carcinoma. Computed tomography image shows a large mass (M) involving the wall of a small bowel loop (*arrowheads*).

REFERENCES

1. Ackerman L. *Atlas of tumor pathology. Fascicles 23 and 24: Tumors of the retroperitoneum mesentery and omentum.* Washington, DC: Armed Forces Institute of Pathology; 1954.
2. Agarwal A, Yeh BM, Breiman RS, et al. Peritoneal calcification: causes and distinguishing features on CT. *AJR Am J Roentgenol.* 2004;182:441–445.
3. Aguirre D, Casola G, Sirlin C. Abdominal wall hernias: MDCT findings. *AJR Am J Roentgenol.* 2004;183:681–690.
4. Akhan O, Pringot J. Imaging of abdominal tuberculosis. *Eur Radiol.* 2002;12:312–323.
5. Allen HA 3rd, Vick CW, Messmer JM, et al. Diffuse mesenteric amyloidosis: CT, sonographic, and pathologic findings. *J Comput Assist Tomogr.* 1985;9:196–198.
6. Altemeier WA, Culbertson WR, Fullen WD, Shook CD. Intra-abdominal abscesses. *Am J Surg.* 1973;125:70–79.
7. Ambrosetti P, Jenny A, Becker C, et al. Acute left colonic diverticulitis–compared performance of computed tomography and water-soluble contrast enema: prospective evaluation of 420 patients. *Dis Colon Rectum.* 2000;43:1363–1367.
8. Arai K, Makino H, Morioka T, et al. Enhancement of ascites on MRI following intravenous administration of Gd-DTPA. *J Comput Assist Tomogr.* 1993;17:617–622.
9. Arenas AP, Sanchez LV, Albillos JM, et al. Direct dissemination of pathologic abdominal processes through perihepatic ligaments: identification with CT. *Radiographics* 1994;14:515–528.
10. Aronberg DJ, Stanley RJ, Levitt RG, et al. Evaluation of abdominal abscess with computed tomography. *J Comput Assist Tomogr.* 1978;2:384–387.
11. Ascher SM, Agrawal R, Bis KG, et al. Endometriosis: appearance and detection with conventional and contrast-enhanced fat-suppressed spin-echo techniques. *J Magn Reson Imaging.* 1995;5:251–257.

12. Auh YH, Lim JH, Kim KW, et al. Loculated fluid collections in hepatic fissures and recesses: CT appearance and potential pitfalls. *Radiographics* 1994;14:529–540.

13. Azizi L, Balu M, Belkacem A, et al. MRI features of mesenteric desmoid tumors in familial adenomatous polyposis. *AJR Am J Roentgenol.* 2005;184(4):1128–1235.

14. Bader TR, Semelka RC, Chiu VC, et al. MRI of carcinoid tumors: spectrum of appearances in the gastrointestinal tract and liver. *J Magn Reson Imaging.* 2001;14:261–269.

15. Baker ME, Weinerth JL, Andriani RT, et al. Lumbar hernia: diagnosis by CT. *AJR Am J Roentgenol.* 1987;148:565–567.

16. Balthazar EJ, Freeny PC, vanSonnenberg E. Imaging and intervention in acute pancreatitis. *Radiology* 1994;193:297–306.

17. Balthazar EJ, Lefkowitz RA. Left-sided omental infarction with associated omental abscess: CT diagnosis. *J Comput Assist Tomogr.* 1993;17:379–381.

18. Balthazar EJ, Subramanyam BR, Megibow A. Spigelian hernia: CT and ultrasonography diagnosis. *Gastrointest Radiol.* 1984;9:81–84.

19. Balthazar EJ. CT diagnosis and staging of acute pancreatitis. *Radiol Clin North Am.* 1989;27:19–37.

20. Barakos JA, Jeffrey RB Jr, Federle MP, et al. CT in the management of periappendiceal abscess. *AJR Am J Roentgenol.* 1986;146:1161–1164.

21. Baron RL, Lee JK. Mesenteric desmoid tumors: sonographic and computed-tomographic appearance. *Radiology* 1981;140:777–779.

22. Bechtold RE, Chen MY, Loggie BW, et al. CT appearance of disseminated peritoneal adenomucinosis. *Abdom Imaging.* 2001;26:406–410.

23. Becker G, Hess CF, Grund KE, et al. Abdominal wall metastasis following percutaneous endoscopic gastrostomy. *Support Care Cancer.* 1995;3:313–316.

24. Bergstrom M, Ericson K, Levander B, et al. Variation with time of the attenuation values of intracranial hematomas. *J Comput Assist Tomogr.* 1977;1:57–63.

25. Berna JD, Garcia-Medina V, Guirao J, et al. Rectus sheath hematoma: diagnostic classification by CT. *Abdom Imaging.* 1996;21:62–64.

26. Bernardino ME, Jing BS, Wallace S. Computed tomography diagnosis of mesenteric masses. *AJR Am J Roentgenol.* 1979;132:33–36.

27. Bis KG, Vrachliotis TG, Agrawal R, et al. Pelvic endometriosis: MR imaging spectrum with laparoscopic correlation and diagnostic pitfalls. *Radiographics* 1997;17:639–655.

28. Bradley WG, Jr, Schmidt PG. Effect of methemoglobin formation on the MR appearance of subarachnoid hemorrhage. *Radiology* 1985;156:99–103.

29. Brasfield RD, Das Gupta TK. Desmoid tumors of the anterior abdominal wall. *Surgery* 1969;65:241–246.

30. Bree RL, Schwab RE. Contribution of mesenteric fat to unsatisfactory abdominal and pelvic ultrasonography. *Radiology* 1981;140:773–776.

31. Brooks AP, Reznek RH, Nugent K, et al. CT appearances of desmoid tumours in familial adenomatous polyposis: further observations. *Clin Radiol.* 1994;49:601–607.

32. Brown JJ, vanSonnenberg E, Gerber KH, et al. Magnetic resonance relaxation times of percutaneously obtained normal and abnormal body fluids. *Radiology* 1985;154:727–731.

33. Buhr J, Hurtgen M, Heinrichs CM, et al. [Implantation metastases following laparoscopic cholecystectomy in gallbladder carcinoma]. *Dtsch Med Wochenschr.* 1996;121:57–61; discussion 61–62.

34. Burrell HC, Trescoli C, Chow K, et al. Case report: mesenteric lymph node cavitation, an unusual complication of coeliac disease. *Br J Radiol.* 1994;67:1139–1140.

35. Buy JN, Malbec L, Ghossain MA, et al. Magnetic resonance imaging of pseudomyxoma peritonei. *Eur J Radiol.* 1989;9:115–118.

36. Bydder GM, Kreel L. Attenuation values of fluid collections within the abdomen. *J Comput Assist Tomogr.* 1980;4:145–150.

37. Callen PW. Computed tomographic evaluation of abdominal and pelvic abscesses. *Radiology* 1979;131:171–175.

38. Caseiro-Alves F, Goncalo M, Abraul E, et al. Induced pneumoperitoneum in CT evaluation of peritoneal carcinomatosis. *Abdom Imaging.* 1995;20(1):52–55; discussion 6–7.

39. Casillas J, Sais GJ, Greve JL, et al. Imaging of intra- and extraabdominal desmoid tumors. *Radiographics* 1991;11:959–968.

40. Ceuterick L, Baert AL, Marchal G, et al. CT diagnosis of primary torsion of greater omentum. *J Comput Assist Tomogr.* 1987;11:1083–1084.

41. Charnsangavej C, DuBrow RA, Varma DG, et al. CT of the mesocolon. Part 1. Anatomic considerations. *Radiographics* 1993;13:1035–1045.

42. Charnsangavej C, Dubrow RA, Varma DG, et al. CT of the mesocolon. Part 2. Pathologic considerations. *Radiographics* 1993;13:1309–1322.

43. Cheng J, Castellino RA. Post-treatment calcification of mesenteric non-Hodgkin lymphoma: CT findings. *J Comput Assist Tomogr.* 1989;13:64–66.

44. Chiou SY, Sheu MH, Wang JH, et al. Peritoneal serous papillary carcinoma: a reappraisal of CT imaging features and literature review. *Abdom Imaging.* 2003;28:815–819.

45. Chopra S, Dodd GD 3rd, Chintapalli KN, et al. Mesenteric, omental, and retroperitoneal edema in cirrhosis: frequency and spectrum of CT findings. *Radiology* 1999;211:737–342.

46. Chopra S, Laurie LR, Chintapalli KN, et al. Primary papillary serous carcinoma of the peritoneum: CT-pathologic correlation. *J Comput Assist Tomogr.* 2000;24:395–399.

47. Chouli M, Viala J, Dromain C, et al. Intra-abdominal desmoplastic small round cell tumors: CT findings and clinicopathological correlations in 13 cases. *Eur J Radiol.* 2005;54:438–442.[D7]

48. Cirocco WC, Schwartzman A, Golub RW. Abdominal wall recurrence after laparoscopic colectomy for colon cancer. *Surgery* 1994;116:842–846.

49. Coakley FV, Choi PH, Gougoutas CA, et al. Peritoneal metastases: detection with spiral CT in patients with ovarian cancer. *Radiology* 2002;223:495–499.

50. Cohen JM, Weinreb JC, Maravilla KR. Fluid collections in the intraperitoneal and extraperitoneal spaces: comparison of MR and CT. *Radiology* 1985;155:705–708.

51. Cohen WN, Seidelmann FE, Bryan PJ. Computed tomography of localized adipose deposits presenting as tumor masses. *AJR Am J Roentgenol.* 1977;128:1007–1111.

52. Coll DM, Meyer JM, Mader M, et al. Imaging appearances of Sister Mary Joseph nodule. *Br J Radiol.* 1999;72(864):1230–1233.

53. Coode PE, McGuinness FE, Rawas MM, et al. Diffuse lipomatosis involving the thoracic and abdominal wall: CT features. *J Comput Assist Tomogr.* 1991;15:341–343.

54. Cooper C, Jeffrey RB, Silverman PM, et al. Computed tomography of omental pathology. *J Comput Assist Tomogr.* 1986;10:62–66.

55. Cooper C, Silverman PM, Davros WJ, et al. Delayed contrast enhancement of ascitic fluid on CT: frequency and significance. *AJR Am J Roentgenol.* 1993;161:787–790.

56. Coumbaras M, Chopier J, Massiani MA, et al. Diffuse mesenteric and omental infiltration by amyloidosis with omental calcification mimicking abdominal carcinomatosis. *Clin Radiol.* 2001;56:674–676.

57. Cryer PE, Kissane J. Infiltrative gastrointestinal disease. *Am J Med.* 1974;57:127–134.

58. Dachman AH, Lichtenstein JE, Friedman AC. Mucocele of the appendix and pseudomyxoma peritonei. *AJR Am J Roentgenol.* 1985;144:923–999.

59. Dahlene DH Jr, Stanley RJ, Koehler RE, et al. Abdominal tuberculosis: CT findings. *J Comput Assist Tomogr.* 1984;8:443–445.

60. Daniel O. The differential diagnosis of malignant disease of the peritoneum. *Br J Surg.* 1951;39:147–156.

61. Daskalogiannaki M, Voloudaki A, Prassopoulos P, et al. CT evaluation of mesenteric panniculitis: prevalence and associated diseases. *AJR Am J Roentgenol.* 2000;174:427–431.

62. DeMeo JH, Fulcher AS, Austin RF Jr. Anatomic CT demonstration of the peritoneal spaces, ligaments, and mesenteries: normal and pathologic processes. *Radiographics* 1995;15:755–770.

63. Deutch SJ, Sandler MA, Alpern MB. Abdominal lymphadenopathy in benign diseases: CT detection. *Radiology* 1987;163:335–338.

64. Dobrin PB, Gully PH, Greenlee HB, et al. Radiologic diagnosis of an intra-abdominal abscess. Do multiple tests help? *Arch Surg.* 1986;121:41–46.

65. Dodds WJ, Foley WD, Lawson TL, et al. Anatomy and imaging of the lesser peritoneal sac. *AJR Am J Roentgenol.* 1985;144: 567–575.
66. Dooms GC, Fisher MR, Hricak H, et al. MR imaging of intramuscular hemorrhage. *J Comput Assist Tomogr.* 1985;9:908–913.
67. Eggesbo HB, Jacobsen T, Kolmannskog F, et al. Diagnosis of acute left-sided colonic diverticulitis by three radiological modalities. *Acta Radiol.* 1998;39:315–321.
68. Emby D, Aoun G. CT technique for suspected anterior abdominal wall hernia. *AJR Am J Roentgenol.* 2003;181:431–433.
69. Emory TS, Monihan JM, Carr NJ, et al. Sclerosing mesenteritis, mesenteric panniculitis and mesenteric lipodystrophy: a single entity? *Am J Surg Pathol.* 1997;21:392–398.
70. Epstein BM, Mann JH. CT of abdominal tuberculosis. *AJR Am J Roentgenol.* 1982;139:861–866.
71. Epstein LI, Lempke RE. Primary idiopathic segmental infarction of the greater omentum: case report and collective review of the literature. *Ann Surg.* 1968;167:437–443.
72. Faxon H. Subphrenic abscess. *N Engl J Med.* 1940;222:289–299.
73. Federle MP, Chun G, Jeffrey RB, Rayor R. Computed tomographic findings in bowel infarction. *AJR Am J Roentgenol.* 1984;142:91–95.
74. Federle MP, Jeffrey RB Jr. Hemoperitoneum studied by computed tomography. *Radiology* 1983;148:187–192.
75. Ferreiros J, Gomez Leon N, Mata MI, et al. Computed tomography in abdominal Castleman's disease. *J Comput Assist Tomogr.* 1989;13:433–436.
76. Frager DH, Goldman M, Beneventano TC. Computed tomography in Crohn disease. *J Comput Assist Tomogr.* 1983;7:819–824.
77. Fukuda T, Sakamoto I, Kohzaki S, et al. Spontaneous rectus sheath hematomas: clinical and radiological features. *Abdom Imaging.* 1996;21:58–61.
78. Furukawa T, Ueda J, Takahashi S, et al. Peritoneal serous papillary carcinoma: radiological appearance. *Abdom Imaging.* 1999;24: 78–81.
79. Galani E, Marx GM, Steer CB, et al. Pseudomyxoma peritonei: the 'controversial' disease. *Int J Gynecol Cancer.* 2003;13:413–418.
80. Garber SJ, Shaw DG. Case report: the ultrasound and computed tomography appearance of mesenteric Castleman disease. *Clin Radiol.* 1991;43:429–430.
81. Gedgaudas RK, Rice RP. Radiological evaluation of complicated pancreatitis. *Crit Rev Diagn Imaging.* 1981;15:319–367.
82. Gerald WL, Miller HK, Battifora H, et al. Intra-abdominal desmoplastic small round-cell tumor. Report of 19 cases of a distinctive type of high-grade polyphenotypic malignancy affecting young individuals. *Am J Surg Pathol.* 1991;15:499–513.
83. Gerzof SG, Johnson WC, Robbins AH, et al. Expanded criteria for percutaneous abscess drainage. *Arch Surg.* 1985;120:227–232.
84. Ghahremani GG, Jimenez MA, Rosenfeld M, et al. CT diagnosis of occult incisional hernias. *AJR Am J Roentgenol.* 1987;148: 139–142.
85. Ghahremani GG, White EM, Hoff F, et al. Appendices epiploicae of the colon: radiologic and pathologic features. *Radiographics* 1992;12:59–77.
86. Gleeson NC, Nicosia SV, Mark JE, et al. Abdominal wall metastases from ovarian cancer after laparoscopy. *Am J Obstet Gynecol.* 1993;169:522–523.
87. Goffinet DR, Castellino RA, Kim H, et al. Staging laparotomies in unselected previously untreated patients with non-Hodgkin's lymphomas. *Cancer* 1973;32:672–681.
88. Goldberg HI, Gore RM, Margulis AR, et al. Computed tomography in the evaluation of Crohn disease. *AJR Am J Roentgenol.* 1983;140: 277–282.
89. Gomori JM, Grossman RI, Goldberg HI, et al. Intracranial hematomas: imaging by high-field MR. *Radiology* 1985;157:87–93.
90. Goodman P, Raval B. CT of the abdominal wall. *AJR Am J Roentgenol.* 1990;154:1207–1211.
91. Gore RM, Callen PW, Filly RA. Lesser sac fluid in predicting the etiology of ascites: CT findings. *AJR Am J Roentgenol.* 1982;139:71–74.
92. Gore RM, Marn CS, Kirby DF, et al. CT findings in ulcerative, granulomatous, and indeterminate colitis. *AJR Am J Roentgenol.* 1984;143:279–284.
93. Goss C. *Gray's Anatomy of the Human Body.* 29th American ed. Philadelphia: Lea and Febiger; 1973.
94. Gougoutas CA, Siegelman ES, Hunt J, et al. Pelvic endometriosis: various manifestations and MR imaging findings. *AJR Am J Roentgenol.* 2000;175:353–358.
95. Grendell JH, Ockner RK. Mesenteric venous thrombosis. *Gastroenterology* 1982;82:358–372.
96. Guermazi A, de Kerviler E, Cazals-Hatem D, et al. Imaging findings in patients with myelofibrosis. *Eur Radiol.* 1999;9:1366–1375.
97. Guest PJ, Reznek RH, Selleslag D, et al. Peritoneal mesothelioma: the role of computed tomography in diagnosis and follow up. *Clin Radiol.* 1992;45:79–84.
98. Gupta S, Shirahatti RG, Anand J. CT findings of an abdominal cocoon. *AJR Am J Roentgenol.* 2004;183:1658–1660.
99. Ha HK, Jung JI, Lee MS, et al. CT differentiation of tuberculous peritonitis and peritoneal carcinomatosis. *AJR Am J Roentgenol.* 1996;167:743–748.
100. Haaga JR, Alfidi RJ, Havrilla TR, et al. CT detection and aspiration of abdominal abscesses. *AJR Am J Roentgenol.* 1977;128:465–474.
101. Hafner M, Novacek G, Herbst F, et al. Giant benign cystic mesothelioma: a case report and review of literature. *Eur J Gastroenterol Hepatol.* 2002;14:77–80.
102. Hahn PF, Saini S, Stark DD, et al. Intraabdominal hematoma: the concentric-ring sign in MR imaging. *AJR Am J Roentgenol.* 1987;148:115–119.
103. Halber MD, Daffner RH, Morgan CL, et al. Intraabdominal abscess: current concepts in radiologic evaluation. *AJR Am J Roentgenol.* 1979;133:9–13.
104. Halliday P, Halliday JH. Subphrenic abscess: a study of 241 patients at the Royal Prince Edward Hospital, 1950–73. *Br J Surg.* 1976;63:352–366.
105. Halvorsen RA Jr, Panushka C, Oakley GJ, et al. Intraperitoneal contrast material improves the CT detection of peritoneal metastases. *AJR Am J Roentgenol.* 1991;157:37–40.
106. Hamrick-Turner JE, Chiechi MV, Abbitt PL, et al. Neoplastic and inflammatory processes of the peritoneum, omentum, and mesentery: diagnosis with CT. *Radiographics* 1992;12:1051–1068.
107. Haney PJ, Whitley NO. CT of benign cystic abdominal masses in children. *AJR Am J Roentgenol.* 1984;142:1279–1281.
108. Hanson RD, Hunter TB. Tuberculous peritonitis: CT appearance. *AJR Am J Roentgenol.* 1985;144:931–932.
109. Hardy SM. The sandwich sign. *Radiology* 2003;226:651–652.
110. Hayashi S, Oyama K, Hirakawa K, et al. [Mesenteric panniculitis—case report and its radiological diagnosis including CT (author's translation)]. *Rinsho Hoshasen.* 1982;27:143–146.
111. Healy JC, Reznek RH, Clark SK, et al. MR appearances of desmoid tumors in familial adenomatous polyposis. *AJR Am J Roentgenol.* 1997;169:465–472.
112. Healy ME, Teng SS, Moss AA. Uriniferous pseudocyst: computed tomographic findings. *Radiology* 1984;153:757–762.
113. Heiken JP, Brink JA, Sagel SS. Helical CT: abdominal applications. *Radiographics* 1994;14:919–924.
114. Hibbeln JF, Wehmueller MD, Wilbur AC. Chylous ascites: CT and ultrasound appearance. *Abdom Imaging.* 1995;20:138–140.
115. Horton KM, Lawler LP, Fishman EK. CT findings in sclerosing mesenteritis (panniculitis): spectrum of disease. *Radiographics* 2003;23:1561–1567.
116. Houer A, Rygaard H, Jess P. CT in the diagnosis of abdominal wall hernias: a preliminary study. *Eur Radiol.* 1997;7:1416–1418.
117. Hudson TM, Vandergriend RA, Springfield DS, et al. Aggressive fibromatosis: evaluation by computed tomography and angiography. *Radiology* 1984;150:495–501.
118. Hui GC, Amaral J, Stephens D, et al. Gas distribution in intraabdominal and pelvic abscesses on CT is associated with drainability. *AJR Am J Roentgenol.* 2005;184:915–919.
119. Hulnick DH, Megibow AJ, Balthazar EJ, Naidich DP, Bosniak MA. Computed tomography in the evaluation of diverticulitis. *Radiology* 1984;152:491–495.
120. Hulnick DH, Megibow AJ, Naidich DP, et al. Abdominal tuberculosis: CT evaluation. *Radiology* 1985;157:199–204.
121. Ianora A, Midiri M, Vinci R, et al. Abdominal wall hernias: imaging with spiral CT. *Eur Radiol.* 2000;10:914–919.

122. Ichikawa T, Koyama A, Fujimoto H, et al. Abdominal wall desmoid mimicking intra-abdominal mass: MR features. *Magn Reson Imaging.* 1994;12:541–544.

123. Ishida H, Ishida J. Primary tumours of the greater omentum. *Eur Radiol.* 1998;8:1598–601.

124. Ishida J, Ishida H, Konno K, et al. Primary leiomyosarcoma of the greater omentum. *J Clin Gastroenterol.* 1999;28:167–170.

125. Jacobs JE, Birnbaum BA, Siegelman ES. Heterotopic ossification of midline abdominal incisions: CT and MR imaging findings. *AJR Am J Roentgenol.* 1996;166:579–584.

126. Jacquet P, Averbach AM, Jacquet N. Abdominal wall metastasis and peritoneal carcinomatosis after laparoscopic-assisted colectomy for colon cancer. *Eur J Surg Oncol.* 1995;21:568–570.

127. Jaffe T, O'Connell M, Harris J, et al. MDCT of abdominal wall hernias: is there a role for Valsalva's maneuver? *AJR Am J Roentgenol.* 2005;184:847–851.

128. Jaques P, Mauro M, Safrit H, et al. CT features of intraabdominal abscesses: prediction of successful percutaneous drainage. *AJR Am J Roentgenol.* 1986;146:1041–1045.

129. Jatzko G, Lisborg P, Horn M, et al. [Abdominal wall implantation metastasis 2 years after apparently uneventful laparoscopic cholecystectomy]. *Chirurg* 1994;65:812–814.

130. Jeffrey R. Computed tomography of the peritoneal cavity and mesentery. In: Moss AA, Gansu G, Genant HK, eds. *Computed tomography of the body.* Philadelphia: WB Saunders; 1983.

131. Jeffrey RB Jr, Tolentino CS, Federle MP, et al. Percutaneous drainage of periappendiceal abscesses: review of 20 patients. *AJR Am J Roentgenol.* 1987;149:59–62.

132. Jeffrey RB Jr. CT demonstration of peritoneal implants. *AJR Am J Roentgenol.* 1980;135:323–326.

133. Jeffrey RB, Federle MP, Laing FC. Computed tomography of mesenteric involvement in fulminant pancreatitis. *Radiology* 1983;147:185–188.

134. Johnson LA, Longacre TA, Wharton KA Jr, et al. Multiple mesenteric lymphatic cysts: an unusual feature of mesenteric panniculitis (sclerosing mesenteritis). *J Comput Assist Tomogr.* 1997;21:103–105.

135. Jones B, Bayless TM, Fishman EK, et al. Lymphadenopathy in celiac disease: computed tomographic observations. *AJR Am J Roentgenol.* 1984;142:1127–1132.

136. Kaiser AM, Jiang JK, Lake JP, et al. The management of complicated diverticulitis and the role of computed tomography. *Am J Gastroenterol.* 2005;100:910–917.

137. Katz ME, Heiken JP, Glazer HS, et al. Intraabdominal panniculitis: clinical, radiographic, and CT features. *AJR Am J Roentgenol.* 1985;145:293–296.

138. Kawashima A, Fishman EK, Hruban RH, et al. Mesenteric panniculitis presenting as a multilocular cystic mesenteric mass: CT and MR evaluation. *Clin Imaging.* 1993;17:112–116.

139. Kawashima A, Fishman EK, Kuhlman JE, et al. CT of malignant melanoma: patterns of small bowel and mesenteric involvement. *J Comput Assist Tomogr.* 1991;15:570–574.

140. Kebapci M, Vardareli E, Adapinar B, et al. CT findings and serum ca 125 levels in malignant peritoneal mesothelioma: report of 11 new cases and review of the literature. *Eur Radiol.* 2003;13:2620–2626.

141. Kebapci M, Yalcin OT, Dundar E, et al. Computed tomography findings of primary serous papillary carcinoma of the peritoneum in women. *Eur J Gynaecol Oncol.* 2003;24:552–556.

142. Kerber GW, Greenberg M, Rubin JM. Computed tomography evaluation of local and extraintestinal complications of Crohn's disease. *Gastrointest Radiol.* 1984;9:143–148.

143. Kim HC, Lee JM, Kim SH, et al. Primary gastrointestinal stromal tumors in the omentum and mesentery: CT findings and pathologic correlations. *AJR Am J Roentgenol.* 2004;182:1463–1467.

144. Kim T, Murakami T, Oi H, et al. CT and MR imaging of abdominal liposarcoma. *AJR Am J Roentgenol.* 1996;166:829–833.

145. Kim Y, Cho O, Song S, et al. Peritoneal lymphomatosis: CT findings. *Abdom Imaging.* 1998;23:87–90.

146. Kircher MF, Rhea JT, Kihiczak D, et al. Frequency, sensitivity, and specificity of individual signs of diverticulitis on thin-section helical CT with colonic contrast material: experience with 312 cases. *AJR Am J Roentgenol.* 2002;178:1313–1318.

147. Knochel JQ, Koehler PR, Lee TG, et al. Diagnosis of abdominal abscesses with computed tomography, ultrasound, and 111In leukocyte scans. *Radiology* 1980;137:425–432.

148. Koehler PR, Moss AA. Diagnosis of intra-abdominal and pelvic abscesses by computerized tomography. *JAMA* 1980;244:49–52.

149. Korobkin M, Callen PW, Filly RA, et al. Comparison of computed tomography, ultrasonography, and gallium-67 scanning in the evaluation of suspected abdominal abscess. *Radiology* 1978;129:89–93.

150. Korobkin M, Moss AA, Callen PW, et al. Computed tomography of subcapsular splenic hematoma. Clinical and experimental studies. *Radiology* 1978;129:44144–44155.

151. Kosucu P, Ahmetoglu A, Cobanoglu U, et al. Mesenteric involvement in neurofibromatosis type 1: CT and MRI findings in two cases. *Abdom Imaging.* 2003;28:822–826.

152. Kronthal AJ, Kang YS, Fishman EK, et al. MR imaging in sclerosing mesenteritis. *AJR Am J Roentgenol.* 1991;156:517–519.

153. Lawdahl RB, Moss CN, Van Dyke JA. Inferior lumbar (Petit's) hernia. *AJR Am J Roentgenol.* 1986;147:744–745.

154. Lee EY, Heiken JP, Huettner PC. Late recurrence of malignant melanoma presenting as peritoneal "carcinomatosis." *Abdom Imaging.* 2003;28:284–286.

155. Lee GH, Cohen AJ. CT imaging of abdominal hernias. *AJR Am J Roentgenol.* 1993;161:1209–1213.

156. Lee JT, Kim MJ, Yoo KS, et al. Primary leiomyosarcoma of the greater omentum: CT findings. *J Comput Assist Tomogr.* 1991;15:92–94.

157. Levine CD, Patel UJ, Silverman PM, Wachsberg RH. Low attenuation of acute traumatic hemoperitoneum on CT scans. *AJR Am J Roentgenol.* 1996;166:1089–1093.

158. Levitt R. Abdominal wall and peritoneal cavity. In: Sagel SS, Stanley RJ, eds. *Computed body tomography.* New York: Raven Press; 1983.

159. Levitt RG, Sagel SS, Stanley RJ. Detection of neoplastic involvement of the mesentery and omentum by computed tomography. *AJR Am J Roentgenol.* 1978;131:835–838.

160. Levy AD, Cantisani V, Miettinen M. Abdominal lymphangiomas: imaging features with pathologic correlation. *AJR Am J Roentgenol.* 2004;182:1485–1491.

161. Lewin JR, Patterson EA. CT recognition of spontaneous intraperitoneal hemorrhage complicating anticoagulant therapy. *AJR Am J Roentgenol.* 1980;134:1271–1272.

162. Lewis VL, Shaffer HA Jr, Williamson BR. Pseudotumoral lipomatosis of the abdomen. *J Comput Assist Tomogr.* 1982;6:79–82.

163. Li DK, Rennie CS. Abdominal computed tomography in Whipple's disease. *J Comput Assist Tomogr.* 1981;5:249–252.

164. Lieberman JM, Haaga JR. Computed tomography of diverticulitis. *J Comput Assist Tomogr.* 1983;7:431–433.

165. Lorenz R, Beyer D, Peters PE. Detection of intraperitoneal bile accumulations: significance of ultrasonography, CT, and cholescintigraphy. *Gastrointest Radiol.* 1984;9:213–217.

166. Low R, Alzate G, Sigeti J, et al. Double-contrast MR imaging of peritoneal tumors with dilute barium oral contrast, intravenous gadolinium, and breath-hold FMPSPGR imaging. *Radiology* 1996;201:252.

167. Low R, Barone R, Lacey C, et al. Peritoneal tumor: MR imaging with dilute oral barium and intravenous Gadolinium-containing contrast agents compared with unenhanced MR imaging and CT. *Radiology* 1997;204:513–520.

168. Low RN. Gadolinium-enhanced MR imaging of liver capsule and peritoneum. *Magn Reson Imaging Clin N Am.* 2001;9:803–819, vii.

169. Lubat E, Balthazar EJ. The current role of computerized tomography in inflammatory disease of the bowel. *Am J Gastroenterol.* 1988;83:107–113.

170. Lucey BC, Stuhlfaut JW, Soto JA. Mesenteric lymph nodes: detection and significance on MDCT. *AJR Am J Roentgenol.* 2005;184:41–44.

171. Macari M, Hines J, Balthazar E, et al. Mesenteric adenitis: CT diagnosis of primary versus secondary causes, incidence, and clinical significance in pediatric and adult patients. *AJR Am J Roentgenol.* 2002;178:853–888.

172. Magid D, Fishman EK, Jones B, et al. Desmoid tumors in Gardner syndrome: use of computed tomography. *AJR Am J Roentgenol.* 1984;142:1141–1145.

173. Mall JC, Kaiser JA. CT diagnosis of splenic laceration. *AJR Am J Roentgenol.* 1980;134:265–269.

174. Martin DR, Karabulut N, Yang M, et al. High signal peripancreatic fat on fat-suppressed spoiled gradient echo imaging in acute pancreatitis: preliminary evaluation of the prognostic significance. *J Magn Reson Imaging.* 2003;18:49–58.

175. Mata JM, Inaraja L, Martin J, et al. CT features of mesenteric panniculitis. *J Comput Assist Tomogr.* 1987;11:1021–1023.

176. Matsuoka Y, Ohtomo K, Itai Y, et al. Pseudomyxoma peritonei with progressive calcifications: CT findings. *Gastrointest Radiol.* 1992;17:16–18.

177. Mayes GB, Chuang VP, Fisher RG. CT of pseudomyxoma peritonei. *AJR Am J Roentgenol.* 1981;136:807–808U.

178. McDermott VG, Low VH, Keogan MT, et al. Malignant melanoma metastatic to the gastrointestinal tract. *AJR Am J Roentgenol.* 1996;166:809–813.

179. McDonnell CH 3rd, McLeod M, Baker ME. Primary peritoneal neuroblastoma: computed tomography findings. *Clin Imaging.* 1990;14:41–43.

180. Mendez G, Jr, Isikoff MB, Hill MC. CT of acute pancreatitis: interim assessment. *AJR Am J Roentgenol.* 1980;135:463–469.

181. Meyers M. *Dynamic Radiology of the Abdomen: Normal and Pathologic Anatomy.* 2nd ed. New York: Springer-Verlag; 1982.

182. Meyers MA, Evans JA. Effects of pancreatitis on the small bowel and colon: spread along mesenteric planes. *Am J Roentgenol Radium Ther Nucl Med.* 1973;119:151–165.

183. Meyers MA, McGuire PV. Spiral CT demonstration of hypervascularity in Crohn disease: "vascular jejunization of the ileum" or the "comb sign". *Abdom Imaging.* 1995;20:327–332.

184. Meyers MA, McSweeney J. Secondary neoplasms of the bowel. *Radiology* 1972;105:1–11.

185. Meyers MA, Oliphant M, Berne AS, et al. The peritoneal ligaments and mesenteries: pathways of intraabdominal spread of disease. *Radiology* 1987;163:593–604.

186. Meyers MA. Distribution of intra–abdominal malignant seeding: dependency on dynamics of flow of ascitic fluid. *Am J Roentgenol Radium Ther Nucl Med.* 1973;119:198–206.

187. Meyers MA. Roentgen significance of the phrenicocolic ligament. *Radiology* 1970;95:539–545.

188. Meyers MA. The spread and localization of acute intraperitoneal effusions. *Radiology* 1970;95:547–554.

189. Meziane MA, Fishman EK, Siegelman SS. Computed tomographic diagnosis of obturator foramen hernia. *Gastrointest Radiol.* 1983;8:375–377.

190. Mills SE, Andersen WA, Fechner RE, et al. Serous surface papillary carcinoma. A clinicopathologic study of 10 cases and comparison with stage III–IV ovarian serous carcinoma. *Am J Surg Pathol.* 1988;12:827–834.

191. Mindelzun RE, Jeffrey RB Jr, Lane MJ, et al. The misty mesentery on CT: differential diagnosis. *AJR Am J Roentgenol.* 1996;167:61–65.

192. Mitchell DG, Hill MC, Hill S, et al. Serous carcinoma of the ovary: CT identification of metastatic calcified implants. *Radiology* 1986;158:649–652.

193. Molmenti EP, Balfe DM, Kanterman RY, et al. Anatomy of the retroperitoneum: observations of the distribution of pathologic fluid collections. *Radiology* 1996;200:95–103.

194. Moon KL Jr, Federle MP, Abrams DI, et al. Kaposi sarcoma and lymphadenopathy syndrome: limitations of abdominal CT in acquired immunodeficiency syndrome. *Radiology* 1984;150:479–483.

195. Mueller PR, Ferrucci JT Jr, Harbin WP, et al. Appearance of lymphomatous involvement of the mesentery by ultrasonography and body computed tomography: the "sandwich sign." *Radiology* 1980;134:467–473.

196. Mueller PR, Ferrucci JT Jr, Simeone JF, et al. Lesser sac abscesses and fluid collections: drainage by transhepatic approach. *Radiology* 1985;155:615–618.

197. Mueller PR, Ferrucci JT, Jr, Simeone JF, et al. Detection and drainage of bilomas: special considerations. *AJR Am J Roentgenol.* 1983;140:715–720.

198. Munk PL, Lee MJ, Poon PY, et al. Computed tomography of retroperitoneal and mesenteric sarcomas: a pictorial essay. *Can Assoc Radiol J.* 1996;47:335–341.

199. Murakami R, Tajima H, Kobayashi Y, et al. Mesenteric schwannoma. *Eur Radiol.* 1998;8:277–279.

200. Nanakawa S, Takahashi M, Takagi K, et al. The role of computed tomography in management of patients with Crohn disease. *Clin Imaging.* 1993;17:193–198.

201. Naylor EW, Gardner EJ, Richards RC. Desmoid tumors and mesenteric fibromatosis in Gardner's syndrome: report of kindred 109. *Arch Surg.* 1979;114:1181–1185.

202. Neff CC, vanSonnenberg E, Casola G, et al. Diverticular abscesses: percutaneous drainage. *Radiology* 1987;163:15–18.

203. New PF, Aronow S. Attenuation measurements of whole blood and blood fractions in computed tomography. *Radiology* 1976;121: 635–640.

204. Noone TC, Semelka RC, Worawattanakul S, et al. Intraperitoneal abscesses: diagnostic accuracy of and appearances at MR imaging. *Radiology* 1998;208:525–528.

205. Norman D, Price D, Boyd D, et al. Quantitative aspects of computed tomography of the blood and cerebrospinal fluid. *Radiology* 1977;123:335–338.

206. Novetsky GJ, Berlin L, Epstein AJ, et al. Case report. Pseudomyxoma peritonei. *J Comput Assist Tomogr.* 1982;6:398–399.

207. Nunez D, Jr, Huber JS, Yrizarry JM, et al. Nonsurgical drainage of appendiceal abscesses. *AJR Am J Roentgenol.* 1986;146: 587–589.

208. Nyberg DA, Federle MP, Jeffrey RB, et al. Abdominal CT findings of disseminated Mycobacterium avium-intracellulare in AIDS. *AJR Am J Roentgenol.* 1985;145:297–299.

209. Nyberg DA, Jeffrey RB Jr, Federle MP, et al. AIDS-related lymphomas: evaluation by abdominal CT. *Radiology* 1986;159: 59–63.

210. O'Neil JD, Ros PR, Storm BL, et al. Cystic mesothelioma of the peritoneum. *Radiology* 1989;170:333–337.

211. Ochsner A, Graves A. Subphrenic abscess: an analysis of 3372 collected and personal cases. *Ann Surg.* 1933;98:961–990.

212. Okino Y, Kiyosue H, Mori H, et al. Root of the small-bowel mesentery: correlative anatomy and CT features of pathologic conditions. *Radiographics* 2001;21:1475–1490.

213. Oliphant M, Berne AS, Meyers MA. Bidirectional spread of disease via the subperitoneal space: the lower abdomen and left pelvis. *Abdom Imaging.* 1993;18:117–125.

214. Oliphant M, Berne AS, Meyers MA. Direct spread of subperitoneal disease into solid organs: radiologic diagnosis. *Abdom Imaging.* 1995;20:141–147; discussion 147–148.

215. Oliphant M, Berne AS, Meyers MA. Imaging the direct bidirectional spread of disease between the abdomen and the female pelvis via the subperitoneal space. *Gastrointest Radiol.* 1988;13: 285–298.

216. Oliphant M, Berne AS, Meyers MA. Spread of disease via the subperitoneal space: the small bowel mesentery. *Abdom Imaging.* 1993;18:109–116.

217. Oliphant M, Berne AS. Computed tomography of the subperitoneal space: demonstration of direct spread of intraabdominal disease. *J Comput Assist Tomogr.* 1982;6:1127–1237.

218. Ozgen A, Akata D, Akhan O, et al. Giant benign cystic peritoneal mesothelioma: US, CT, and MRI findings. *Abdom Imaging.* 1998;23:502–504.

219. Pandolfo I, Blandino A, Gaeta M, et al. CT findings in palpable lesions of the anterior abdominal wall. *J Comput Assist Tomogr.* 1986;10:629–633.

220. Pantongrag-Brown L, Buetow PC, Carr NJ, et al. Calcification and fibrosis in mesenteric carcinoid tumor: CT findings and pathologic correlation. *AJR Am J Roentgenol.* 1995;164: 387–391.

221. Pastakia B, Horvath K, Kurtz D, et al. Giant rectus sheath hematomas of the pelvis complicating anticoagulant therapy: CT findings. *J Comput Assist Tomogr.* 1984;8(6):1120–1123.

222. Patten RM, Shuman WP, Teefey S. Subcutaneous metastases from malignant melanoma: prevalence and findings on CT. *AJR Am J Roentgenol.* 1989;152:1009–1012.

223. Pereira JM, Sirlin CB, Pinto PS, et al. CT and MR imaging of extrahepatic fatty masses of the abdomen and pelvis: techniques, diagnosis, differential diagnosis, and pitfalls. *Radiographics* 2005;25: 69–85.

224. Peters J, Reinertson J, Polansky, SM, et al. CT demonstration of traumatic ventral hernia. *J Comput Assist Tomogr.* 1988;12: 710–711.

225. Pevarski DJ, Mergo PJ, Ros PR. Peritoneal carcinomatosis due to transitional cell carcinoma of the bladder: CT findings in two patients. *AJR Am J Roentgenol.* 1995;164:929–930.

226. Pickhardt PJ, Bhalla S. Unusual nonneoplastic peritoneal and subperitoneal conditions: CT findings. *Radiographics* 2005;25: 719–730.

227. Pickhardt PJ, Fisher AJ, Balfe DM, et al. Desmoplastic small round cell tumor of the abdomen: radiologic-histopathologic correlation. *Radiology* 1999;210:633–638.

228. Pines B, Rabinovitch J, Biller SB. Primary torsion and infarction of the appendices epiploica. *Arch Surg.* 1941;42:775–787.

229. Pitt H. Peritonitis, intraabdominal abscess, and retroperitoneal abscess. In: *Surgery of the alimentary tract,* 2nd ed. Philadelphia: WB Saunders; 1986.

230. Poletti PA, Platon A, Rutschmann O, et al. Acute left colonic diverticulitis: can CT findings be used to predict recurrence? *AJR Am J Roentgenol.* 2004;182:1159–1165.

231. Prayson RA, Hart WR, Petras RE. Pseudomyxoma peritonei. A clinicopathologic study of 19 cases with emphasis on site of origin and nature of associated ovarian tumors. *Am J Surg Pathol.* 1994;18:591–603.

232. Press OW, Press NO, Kaufman SD. Evaluation and management of chylous ascites. *Ann Intern Med.* 1982;96:358–364.

233. Puylaert JB. Right-sided segmental infarction of the omentum: clinical, US, and CT findings. *Radiology* 1992;185:169–172.

234. Radin R. HIV infection: analysis in 259 consecutive patients with abnormal abdominal CT findings. *Radiology* 1995;197: 712–722.

235. Raghavendra BN, Grieco AJ, Balthazar EJ, et al. Diagnostic utility of sonography and computed tomography in spontaneous mesenteric hematoma. *Am J Gastroenterol.* 1982;77:570–573.

236. Ramboer K, Moons P, DeBreuck Y, et al. Benign mesenteric schwannoma: MRI findings. *J Belge Radiol.* 1998;81:3–4.

237. Rao PM, Rhea JT, Novelline RA. CT diagnosis of mesenteric adenitis. *Radiology* 1997;202:145–149.

238. Rao PM, Wittenberg J, Lawrason JN. Primary epiploic appendagitis: evolutionary changes in CT appearance. *Radiology* 1997;204:713–717.

239. Rao PM. CT of diverticulitis and alternative conditions. *Semin Ultrasound CT MR.* 1999;20:86–93.

240. Ray CE Jr, Wilbur AC. CT diagnosis of concurrent hematomas of the psoas muscle and rectus sheath: case reports and review of anatomy, pathogenesis, and imaging. *Clin Imaging.* 1993;17: 22–26.

241. Reddy D, Salomon C, Demos TC, et al. Mesenteric lymph node cavitation in celiac disease. *AJR Am J Roentgenol.* 2002;178):247.

242. Reuter K, Raptopoulos V, Reale F, et al. Diagnosis of peritoneal mesothelioma: computed tomography, sonography, and fine-needle aspiration biopsy. *AJR Am J Roentgenol.* 1983;140: 1189–1194.

243. Rha SE, Ha HK, Kim AY, et al. Peritoneal leiomyosarcomatosis originating from gastrointestinal leiomyosarcomas: CT features. *Radiology* 2003;227:385–390.

244. Rha SE, Ha HK, Kim JG, et al. CT features of intraperitoneal manifestations of parasitic infestation. *AJR Am J Roentgenol.* 1999;172:1289–1292.

245. Rijke AM, Falke TH, de Vries RR. Computed tomography in Whipple disease. *J Comput Assist Tomogr.* 1983;7:1101–1102.

246. Rodrigues A, Whitten C. Roentgenologic clinical pathologic case. *Invest Radiol.* 1993;28:260–262.

247. Rodriguez E, Pombo F. Peritoneal tuberculosis versus peritoneal carcinomatosis: distinction based on CT findings. *J Comput Assist Tomogr.* 1996;20:269–272.

248. Ronnett BM, Kurman RJ, Zahn CM, et al. Pseudomyxoma peritonei in women: a clinicopathologic analysis of 30 cases with emphasis on site of origin, prognosis, and relationship to ovarian mucinous tumors of low malignant potential. *Hum Pathol.* 1995;26:509–524.

249. Ros PR, Olmsted WW, Moser RP Jr, et al. Mesenteric and omental cysts: histologic classification with imaging correlation. *Radiology* 1987;164:327–332.

250. Rosen A, Korobkin M, Silverman PM, et al. Mesenteric vein thrombosis: CT identification. *AJR Am J Roentgenol.* 1984;143: 83–86.

251. Ross MJ, Welch WR, Scully RE. Multilocular peritoneal inclusion cysts (so-called cystic mesotheliomas). *Cancer* 1989;64: 1336–1346.

252. Rubin JI, Gomori JM, Grossman RI, et al. High-field MR imaging of extracranial hematomas. *AJR Am J Roentgenol.* 1987;148: 813–817.

253. Rust RJ, Kopecky KK, Holden RW. The triangle sign: a CT sign of intraperitoneal fluid. *Gastrointest Radiol.* 1984;9:107–113.

254. Sabate JM, Torrubia S, Maideu J, et al. Sclerosing mesenteritis: imaging findings in 17 patients. *AJR Am J Roentgenol.* 1999;172: 625–629.

255. Safrit HD, Mauro MA, Jaques PF. Percutaneous abscess drainage in Crohn's disease. *AJR Am J Roentgenol.* 1987;148:859–862.

256. Sanders RC. The changing epidemiology of subphrenic abscess and its clinical and radiological consequences. *Br J Surg.* 1970; 57:449–455.

257. Sandrasegaran K, Lall C, Rajesh A, et al. Distinguishing gelatin bioabsorbable sponge and postoperative abdominal abscess on CT. *AJR Am J Roentgenol* 2005;184:475–480.

258. Sandrasegaran K, Maglinte DD, Rajesh A, et al. Primary epiploic appendagitis: CT diagnosis. *Emerg Radiol.* 2004;11:9–14.

259. Schechter S, Eisenstat TE, Oliver GC, et al. Computerized tomographic scan-guided drainage of intra-abdominal abscesses. Preoperative and postoperative modalities in colon and rectal surgery. *Dis Colon Rectum.* 1994;37:984–988.

260. Schneekloth G, Terrier F, Fuchs WA. Computed tomography of intraperitoneal abscesses. *Gastrointest Radiol.* 1982;7:35–41.

261. Semelka RC, John G, Kelekis NL, et al. Bowel-related abscesses: MR demonstration preliminary results. *Magn Reson Imaging.* 1998;16(8):855–861.

262. Semelka RC, Lawrence PH, Shoenut JP, et al. Primary ovarian cancer: prospective comparison of contrast-enhanced CT and pre- and postcontrast, fat-suppressed MR imaging, with histologic correlation. *J Magn Reson Imaging.* 1993;3(1):99–106.

263. Seshul MB, Coulam CM. Pseudomyxoma peritonei: computed tomography and sonography. *AJR Am J Roentgenol.* 1981;136: 803–806.

264. Shackelford GD, McAlister WH. Cysts of the omentum. *Pediatr Radiol.* 1975;3:152–155.

265. Shackelford R, Grose W. Groin hernia. 5 In: Shackelford RT, Zuidema GD, eds *Surgery of the alimentary tract,* 2nd ed Philadelphia: WB Saunders, 1986.

266. Sharif HS, Clark DC, Aabed MY, et al. MR imaging of thoracic and abdominal wall infections: comparison with other imaging procedures. *AJR Am J Roentgenol.* 1990;154(5):989–995.

267. Sherman NJ, Davis JR, Jesseph JE. Subphrenic abscess. A continuing hazard. *Am J Surg.* 1969;117:117–123.

268. Sheth S, Horton KM, Garland MR, et al. Mesenteric neoplasms: CT appearances of primary and secondary tumors and differential diagnosis. *Radiographics* 2003;23:457–473; quiz 535–536.

269. Sheward SE, Williams AG Jr, Mettler FA Jr, et al. CT appearance of a surgically retained towel (gossypiboma). *J Comput Assist Tomogr.* 1986;10:343–345.

270. Shin MS, Ferrucci JT Jr, Wittenberg J. Computed tomographic diagnosis of pseudoascites (floating viscera syndrome). *J Comput Assist Tomogr.* 1978;2:594–597.

271. Siewert B, Raptopoulos V. CT of the acute abdomen: findings and impact on diagnosis and treatment. *AJR Am J Roentgenol.* 1994;163:1317–1324.

272. Silverman PM, Baker ME, Cooper C, et al. CT appearance of diffuse mesenteric edema. *J Comput Assist Tomogr.* 1986;10:67–70.

273. Silverman PM, Kelvin FM, Korobkin M, et al. Computed tomography of the normal mesentery. *AJR Am J Roentgenol.* 1984;143: 953–957.

274. Silverstein W, Isikoff MB, Hill MC, et al. Diagnostic imaging of acute pancreatitis: prospective study using CT and sonography. *AJR Am J Roentgenol.* 1981;137:497–502.

275. Singh AK, Gervais DA, Hahn PF, et al. CT appearance of acute appendicitis. *AJR Am J Roentgenol.* 2004;183:1303–1307.

276. Sirvanci M, Balci NC, Karaman K, Duran C, et al. Primary epiploic appendagitis: MRI findings. *Magn Reson Imaging.* 2002;20: 137–139.

277. Sivit CJ, Peclet MH, Taylor GA. Life-threatening intraperitoneal bleeding: demonstration with CT. *Radiology* 1989;171:430.

278. Sompayrac SW, Mindelzun RE, Silverman PM, et al. The greater omentum. *AJR Am J Roentgenol.* 1997;168:683–687.

279. Sones PJ. Percutaneous drainage of abdominal abscesses. *AJR Am J Roentgenol.* 1984;142:35–39.

280. Srinualnad N, Dixon AK. Right anterior subphrenic space: an important site for the early detection of intraperitoneal fluid on abdominal CT. *Abdom Imaging.* 1999;24:614–617.

281. Stafford-Johnson DB, Bree RL, Francis IR, et al. CT appearance of primary papillary serous carcinoma of the peritoneum. *AJR Am J Roentgenol.* 1998;171:687–689.

282. Stafford-Johnson DB, Wilson TE, Francis IR, et al. CT appearance of sclerosing peritonitis in patients on chronic ambulatory peritoneal dialysis. *J Comput Assist Tomogr.* 1998;22:295–299.

283. Steck WD, Helwig EB. Cutaneous endometriosis. *Clin Obstet Gynecol.* 1966;9:373–383.

284. Stefansson T, Nyman R, Nilsson S, et al. Diverticulitis of the sigmoid colon. A comparison of CT, colonic enema and laparoscopy. *Acta Radiol.* 1997;38:313–319.

285. Stoupis C, Ros PR, Abbitt PL, et al. Bubbles in the belly: imaging of cystic mesenteric or omental masses. *Radiographics* 1994;14:729–737.

286. Sugarbaker PH, Acherman YI, Gonzalez-Moreno S, et al. Diagnosis and treatment of peritoneal mesothelioma: The Washington Cancer Institute experience. *Semin Oncol.* 2002;29:51–61.

287. Sulkin TV, O'Neill H, Amin AI, et al. CT in pseudomyxoma peritonei: a review of 17 cases. *Clin Radiol.* 2002;57:608–613.

288. Swensen SJ, McLeod RA, Stephens DH. CT of extracranial hemorrhage and hematomas. *AJR Am J Roentgenol.* 1984;143:907–912.

289. Taneja K, Gothi R, Kumar K, et al. Peritoneal Echinococcus multilocularis infection: CT appearance. *J Comput Assist Tomogr.* 1990;14:493–494.

290. Taourel P, Pradel J, Fabre JM, et al. Role of CT in the acute nontraumatic abdomen. *Semin Ultrasound CT MR.* 1995;16:151–164.

291. Tartar VM, Heiken JP, McClennan BL. Renal cell carcinoma presenting with diffuse peritoneal metastases: CT findings. *J Comput Assist Tomogr.* 1991;15:450–453.

292. Tateishi U, Hasegawa T, Kusumoto M, et al. Desmoplastic small round cell tumor: imaging findings associated with clinicopathologic features. *J Comput Assist Tomogr.* 2002;26:579–583.

293. Tempany CM, Zou KH, Silverman SG, et al. Staging of advanced ovarian cancer: comparison of imaging modalities—report from the Radiological Diagnostic Oncology Group. *Radiology* 2000;215:761–777.

294. Terrier F, Revel D, Pajannen H, et al. MR imaging of body fluid collections. *J Comput Assist Tomogr.* 1986;10:953–962.

295. Thoeni RF, Margulis AR. Gastrointestinal tuberculosis. *Semin Roentgenol.* 1979;14:283–294.

296. Tyrrel RT, Montemayor KA, Bernardino ME. CT density of mesenteric, retroperitoneal, and subcutaneous fat in cirrhotic patients: comparison with control subjects. *AJR Am J Roentgenol.* 1990;155:73–75.

297. Unger EC, Glazer HS, Lee JK, et al. MRI of extracranial hematomas: preliminary observations. *AJR Am J Roentgenol.* 1986;146:403–407.

298. van Breda Vriesman AC, de Mol van Otterloo AJ, et al. Epiploic appendagitis and omental infarction. *Eur J Surg.* 2001;167:723–727.

299. van Breda Vriesman AC, Lohle PN, Coerkamp EG, Puylaert JB. Infarction of omentum and epiploic appendage: diagnosis, epidemiology and natural history. *Eur Radiol.* 1999;9:1886–1892.

300. van Breda Vriesman AC, Schuttevaer HM, Coerkamp EG, et al. Mesenteric panniculitis: US and CT features. *Eur Radiol.* 2004;14:2242–2248.

301. Vanek VW, Phillips AK. Retroperitoneal, mesenteric, and omental cysts. *Arch Surg.* 1984;119:838–482.

302. vanSonnenberg E, D'Agostino HB, Casola G, et al. Percutaneous abscess drainage: current concepts. *Radiology* 1991;181:617–626.

303. vanSonnenberg E, Mueller PR, Ferrucci JT Jr. Percutaneous drainage of 250 abdominal abscesses and fluid collections. Part I: Results, failures, and complications. *Radiology* 1984;151:337–341.

304. vanSonnenberg E, Wittich GR, Casola G, et al. Periappendiceal abscesses: percutaneous drainage. *Radiology* 1987;163:23–26.

305. Vazquez JL, Thorsen MK, Dodds WJ, et al. Evaluation and treatment of intraabdominal bilomas. *AJR Am J Roentgenol.* 1985;144:933–938.

306. Viala J, Morice P, Pautier P, et al. CT findings in two cases of port-site metastasis after laparoscopy for ovarian cancer. *Eur J Gynec Oncol.* 2002;4:293–294.

307. Vincent LM, Mauro MA, Mittelstaedt CA. The lesser sac and gastrohepatic recess: sonographic appearance and differentiation of fluid collections. *Radiology* 1984;150:515–519.

308. Walensky RP, Venbrux AC, Prescott CA, et al. Pseudomyxoma peritonei. *AJR Am J Roentgenol.* 1996;167:471–474.

309. Wall SD, Hricak H, Bailey GD, et al. MR imaging of pathologic abdominal fluid collections. *J Comput Assist Tomogr* 1986;10:746–750.

310. Wang SM, Wilson SE. Subphrenic abscess. The new epidemiology. *Arch Surg.* 1977;112(8):934–936.

311. Weiss SW, Tavassoli FA. Multicystic mesothelioma. An analysis of pathologic findings and biologic behavior in 37 cases. *Am J Surg Pathol.* 1988;12:737–746.

312. Whang SH, Lee KS, Kim PN, et al. Omental teratoma in an adult: a case report. *Gastrointest Radiol.* 1990;15:301–302.

313. White M, Mueller PR, Ferrucci JT Jr, et al. Percutaneous drainage of postoperative abdominal and pelvic lymphoceles. *AJR Am J Roentgenol.* 1985;145:1065–1069.

314. Whitley N. Mesenteric disease. In: Meyers MA, ed. *Computed tomography of the gastrointestinal tract.* New York: Springer-Verlag. 1986.

315. Whitley NO, Bohlman ME, Baker LP. CT patterns of mesenteric disease. *J Comput Assist Tomogr.* 1982;6:490–496.

316. Whitley NO, Brenner DE, Antman KH, et al. CT of peritoneal mesothelioma: analysis of eight cases. *AJR Am J Roentgenol.* 1982;138:531–535.

317. Wolf GC, Kopecky KK. MR imaging of endometriosis arising in cesarean section scar. *J Comput Assist Tomogr.* 1989;13:150–152.

318. Wolverson MK, Crepps LF, Sundaram M, et al. Hyperdensity of recent hemorrhage at body computed tomography: incidence and morphologic variation. *Radiology* 1983;148:779–784.

319. Wolverson MK, Jagannadharao B, Sundaram M, et al. CT as a primary diagnostic method in evaluating intraabdominal abscess. *AJR Am J Roentgenol.* 1979;133:1089–1095.

320. Wong WL, Johns TA, Herlihy WG, et al. Best cases from the AFIP: multicystic mesothelioma. *Radiographics* 2004;24:247–250.

321. Woodard PK, Feldman JM, Paine SS, et al. Midgut carcinoid tumors: CT findings and biochemical profiles. *J Comput Assist Tomogr.* 1995;19:400–405.

322. Woodward PJ, Hosseinzadeh K, Saenger JS. From the archives of the AFIP: radiologic staging of ovarian carcinoma with pathologic correlation. *Radiographics* 2004;24:225–246.

323. Yeh HC, Rabinowitz JG. Ultrasonography and computed tomography of inflammatory abdominal wall lesions. *Radiology* 1982;144:859–863.

324. Yeh HC, Shafir MK, Slater G, et al. Ultrasonography and computed tomography in pseudomyxoma peritonei. *Radiology* 1984;153:507–510.

325. Yeh HC. Ultrasonography of peritoneal tumors. *Radiology* 1979;133(2):419–24.

326. Young RH, Gilks CB, Scully RE. Mucinous tumors of the appendix associated with mucinous tumors of the ovary and pseudomyxoma peritonei. A clinicopathological analysis of 22 cases supporting an origin in the appendix. *Am J Surg Pathol.* 1991;15:415–429.

327. Young ST, Paulson EK, McCann RL, Baker ME. Appearance of oxidized cellulose (Surgicel) on postoperative CT scans: similarity to postoperative abscess. *AJR Am J Roentgenol.* 1993;160:275–277.

328. Zarvan NP, Lee FT Jr, Yandow DR, et al. Abdominal hernias: CT findings. *AJR Am J Roentgenol.* 1995;164:1391–1395.

329. Zerhouni EA, Barth KH, Siegelman SS. Demonstration of venous thrombosis by computed tomography. *AJR Am J Roentgenol.* 1980;134:753–758.

330. Zissin R, Hertz M, Shapiro-Feinberg M, et al. Primary serous papillary carcinoma of the peritoneum: CT findings. *Clin Radiol.* 2001;56:740–745.

Retroperitoneum

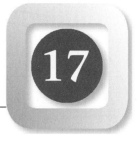

David M. Warshauer   *Joseph K. T. Lee*   *Harish Patel*

The retroperitoneum is bounded anteriorly by the parietal peritoneum and medially, posteriorly, and laterally by fascia covering the psoas, quadratus lumborum, and transversus abdominus musculature, respectively. It extends from the diaphragm superiorly to the level of the pelvic viscera inferiorly. At the level of the kidneys, the retroperitoneal space is divided into three discreet compartments—the perirenal space surrounded by the anterior and posterior pararenal spaces (Figs. 17-1 and 17-2) (25,164,209).

The perirenal space surrounds the kidney and adrenal and is bounded anteriorly by the anterior renal fascia (Gerota's) and posteriorly by the posterior renal fascia (Zuckerkandl's). The perirenal spaces can communicate across the midline, although this is inconstant, suggesting a partial or fenestrated barrier in the region anterior to the aorta and inferior vena cava (IVC) (265,317). The perirenal spaces also may infrequently communicate inferiorly with the infrarenal space and pelvic extraperitoneal spaces and superiorly with the diaphragmatic surface and bare area of the liver (189,211).

The anterior pararenal space contains the ascending and descending colon as well as the duodenum and pancreas. It is bordered anteriorly by the posterior peritoneum, posteriorly by the anterior renal fascia, and laterally by the lateral conal fascia representing the fusion of the anterior and posterior renal fascia. The posterior pararenal space contains only fat. Both the anterior and posterior pararenal spaces communicate inferiorly with the infrarenal space and extraperitoneal pelvic space and communicate superiorly with the extraperitoneal subdiaphragmatic space.

Additional potential retroperitoneal spaces exist within the fascial planes that separate the perirenal and pararenal spaces. These fascia, originally formed by fusion of two embryologic fascial planes, may be split by and contain pathologic fluid collections. A potential retromesenteric (or anterior interfascial) space exists within the anterior renal fascia, with a similar potential retrorenal (or posterior interfascial) space existing in the posterior renal fascia and a lateroconal space occurring in the lateroconal fascia. These potential fascial spaces also allow the extension of fluid collections from the retroperitoneum to the extraperitoneal pelvis (216).

Two types of viscera exist in the retroperitoneal space: the true embryonic retroperitoneal organs (i.e., the adrenal glands, kidneys, ureters, and gonads) and those structures closely attached to the posterior abdominal wall and only partly covered by the peritoneum and fascia (i.e., aorta, IVC, pancreas, portions of the duodenum, colon, lymph nodes, and nerves). In this chapter, discussion is limited to diseases involving the great vessels, lymph nodes, and psoas musculature, as well as primary retroperitoneal neoplasms. Diseases related to other solid retroperitoneal organs, such as the kidneys, the adrenals, and the pancreas, are covered in other chapters.

The diagnosis of retroperitoneal pathology has historically presented a challenge to physicians. The signs and symptoms of retroperitoneal diseases are myriad and often subtle. Because computed tomography (CT) and magnetic resonance imaging (MRI) allow direct, noninvasive demonstration of normal and pathologic retroperitoneal anatomy with a high level of clarity, both methods are now used routinely for evaluating retroperitoneal diseases. With current technology, diagnostic images can be obtained even in very emaciated and critically ill patients (Fig. 17-3).

TECHNIQUE

Computed Tomography

As in other parts of the body, careful patient preparation and attention to technical details are essential to the optimal conduct of CT evaluation of the retroperitoneum. The exact

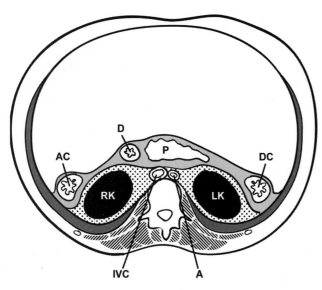

Figure 17-1 Retroperitoneal spaces (axial image). The anterior pararenal space (*light grey*) is bounded anteriorly by the peritoneum and posteriorly by the anterior renal fascia and contains the ascending (AC) and descending (DC) colon, duodenum (D), and pancreas (P). The perirenal space (*dotted*) is bordered by the anterior and posterior perirenal fascia and contains the left (LK) and right (RK) kidneys and great vessels: IVC, inferior vena cava; A, aorta. The posterior pararenal space (*dark grey*) is bordered anteriorly by the posterior perirenal fascia, lateral conal fascia, and peritoneum (from medial to lateral) and posteriorly by the transversalis fascia.

study protocol varies depending on the type of scanner available, the indication(s) of the examination, and the area to be imaged. For a survey examination of the retroperitoneum 5- to 7-mm-thick slices are obtained if a single detector row

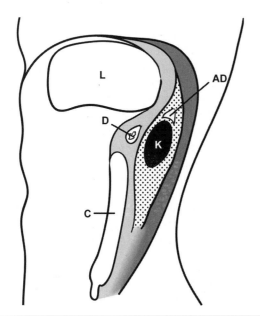

Figure 17-2 Retroperitoneal spaces (sagittal image): Anterior pararenal space (*light grey*), perirenal space (*dotted*), and posterior pararenal space (*dark grey*). Although closed at their superior ends, the retroperitoneal spaces may communicate inferiorly with the pelvic extraperitoneal space. L, liver; AD, adrenal; K, kidney; D, duodenum; C, colon.

helical CT scanner is used. If a 4- to 16-slice multidetector row CT (MDCT) scanner is used, a 5-mm-thick slice is routine using 1- to 2-mm detector collimation. For angiographic evaluation of the aorta and its major branches, thinner collimation (0.5 to 0.7 mm) is routinely used on the MDCT scanner (Fig. 17-4). Images may be reconstructed at 1- to 2-mm intervals in any defined plane; these images can be printed either on hard copy films or sent to a picture archiving and communication system (PACS) viewing station for interpretation. Alternatively, the entire data set may be viewed interactively on a dedicated computer workstation.

Except in emergency situations in which the CT examination must be performed without delay (e.g., in patients with suspected ruptured abdominal aortic aneurysms), retroperitoneal CT should be done only after the patient has ingested oral contrast media. Approximately 1,000 mL of oral contrast material (dilute barium suspension or iodinated water-soluble contrast material) is given to the patient at least 1 hour before the examination to opacify the colon and distal small bowel loops. An additional 300 to 500 mL of contrast is given approximately 15 minutes before the study to opacify the stomach and proximal small bowel loops. If the pelvis is to be included, a contrast material enema (200 mL) occasionally may be necessary to expedite opacification of the rectosigmoid and descending colon.

Although the retroperitoneum can be adequately studied without the use of intravenous contrast material, most retroperitoneal CT studies are performed with intravenous contrast material to allow distinction between vascular and nonvascular structures, to determine the vascularity of a retroperitoneal mass and its effect on the urinary tract and to maximize detection of focal lesions in solid abdominal organs. A dose of 150 mL of 60% iodine solution is administered intravenously on examinations performed on single-slice helical CT scanners; a reduced amount (80 to 120 mL) followed by 30 mL of saline can produce near equivalent opacification with MDCT (290). Intravenous contrast material is administered via a power injector as a bolus at a rate of 2 to 3 mL per second for routine survey examinations and 3 to 5 mL per second for CT angiography. Images are obtained 25 seconds after the initiation of contrast delivery for CT angiography; a longer delay (60 to 70 seconds) is used for all other retroperitoneal studies. Although these fixed scan delays work well for most patients, a different scan delay is required in patients with altered circulation time (e.g., patients with decreased left ventricular function). Computer software programs are available to assure more consistent vessel opacification by triggering scanning only after a selected area (e.g., proximal descending aorta) reaches a predetermined attenuation value.

Magnetic Resonance Imaging

The retroperitoneum can likewise be successfully examined with MRI. Transverse images are obtained in all patients, usually with 8- to 10-mm collimation at 10- to 12-mm

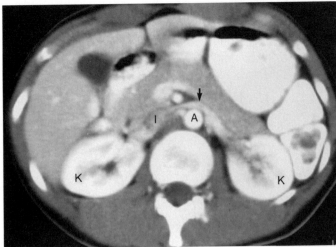

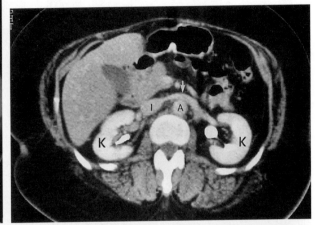

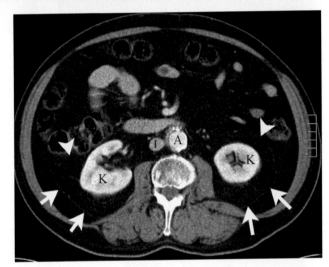

Figure 17-3 Computed tomography images of the normal retroperitoneum in patients with variations in body habitus. **A:** Thin patient with little body fat. **B:** Relative paucity of retroperitoneal and mesenteric fat compared with subcutaneous fat, a pattern common in women. **C:** Relative prominence of retroperitoneal and mesenteric fat compared with subcutaneous fat, a pattern common in men. Note anterior pararenal fascia (*arrowheads*), posterior pararenal fascia (*arrows*). A, aorta; I, inferior vena cava; K, kidney; *arrow*, left renal vein.

intervals. In addition, coronal and sagittal images often are performed to better define abnormalities of the aorta, IVC, and psoas muscle. The use of a 2-mm interslice gap reduces "crosstalk" between consecutive sections.

Both T1- and T2-weighted sequences are required for lesion detection and characterization. T1-weighted imaging can be achieved with either a breath-hold gradient echo (GRE) sequence [e.g., fast low-angle shot (FLASH) or spoiled gradient recalled acquisition in steady state (GRASS)] or a conventional spin-echo (SE) sequence [repetition time (TR) 300 to 1,000 msec, echo time (TE) as short as possible]. Although an SE sequence is less affected by magnetic susceptibility artifact, we prefer GRE for the T1-weighted sequence because it allows multiple sections to be obtained within a single breath-hold, resulting in high-quality images without respiratory-related artifacts and with minimal artifacts from bowel peristalsis. At 1.5 Tesla (T), with a TR of 130 msec, TE of 4 msec, flip angle of 80 degrees, and one excitation, a total of 14 sections can be obtained in 19 seconds. The short acquisition time of a GRE sequence also allows serial dynamic imaging after intravenous administration of a gadolinium contrast agent. T2-weighted

imaging (TR greater than 1,500 msec, TE greater than 70 msec) can be achieved with a conventional SE or a rapid SE (e.g., fast spin echo or turbo spin echo) technique. The advantage of rapid SE over conventional SE sequences is a substantial reduction in data acquisition time. The reduced acquisition time can be used to improve spatial resolution (by increasing imaging matrix elements) or obtain stronger T2 weighting (by increasing TR and obtaining later echoes) without significantly prolonging the total imaging time. Single-shot echo-train SE sequence [e.g., half Fourier snap shot turbo spin echo (HASTE) or single shot fast spin echo (SSFSE)] is a breathing-independent T2-weighted sequence that allows acquisition of high-quality abdominal T2-weighted images even in critically ill patients. Although rapid SE provides better image quality and contrast-to-noise ratio (CNR) for cystic abdominal lesions than does conventional SE, the qualitative conspicuousness and CNR of solid abdominal lesions are decreased (46). Both T1- and T2-weighted sequences can be combined with fat suppression. Fat saturation reduces ghosting artifacts and increases the contrast range of non-fatty tissues.

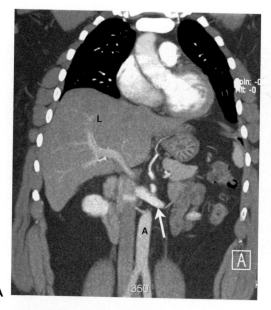

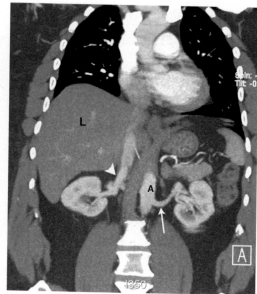

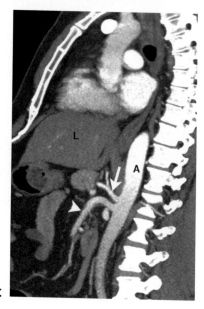

Figure 17-4 Multidetector row computed tomography. **A:** Coronal image of the abdomen shows aorta (A), with left renal vein (*arrow*). **B:** Coronal image posterior to **(A)** shows left renal artery (*arrow*), with right renal vein (*arrowhead*) running into the inferior vena cava. **C:** Sagittal image shows origin of celiac axis (*arrow*) and superior mesenteric artery (*arrowhead*). A, aorta; L, liver.

As in the case of CT, an MR oral contrast agent can aid in the differentiation of bowel from other normal or pathologic tissue. A variety of positive and negative gastrointestinal contrast agents, such as barium, perfluorooctylbromide, iron compound, and water, have been proposed to opacify the gastrointestinal tract. However, none of them has received widespread acceptance because of the high cost of the contrast materials, inconsistency in distending the bowel loops, and increased susceptibility artifact on the commonly used GRE sequences. Intravenous gadolinium chelate–based contrast is routinely used in MRI for evaluation of the retroperitoneum. It is given by bolus injection at 2 mL per second. T1-weighted FLASH images are then obtained immediately and 45 seconds after injection. An additional FLASH sequence at 90 seconds

after the injection is done with fat saturation to complete the evaluation.

To assess the vascular system, various MR angiographic (MRA) methods have been employed. Data can be acquired using a GRE sequence or its variant (e.g., turbo GRE) based on either a time-of-flight (TOF) or phase-contrast (PC) technique (142,154). Although the two-dimensional (2D) TOF technique is relatively accurate and requires less time, in-plane flow saturation of tortuous vessels and vessels with slow flow often lead to suboptimal images. Although the PC method is more sensitive to slow flow, it is more time consuming and is significantly affected by signal loss in areas of local turbulence (142). Three-dimensional (3D) gadolinium-enhanced GRE MRA technique does not rely on TOF effects but rather on the T1 shortening provided by

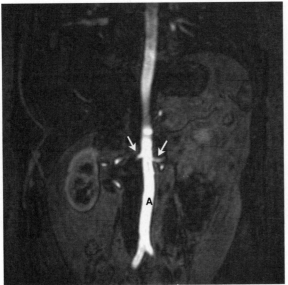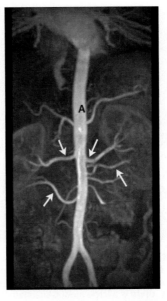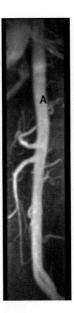

A, B

C

Figure 17-5 Magnetic resonance angiography. **A:** Thin-section gadolinium-enhanced T1-weighted coronal image that, when taken with adjoining slices and reconstructed as maximum-intensity projection (MIP), yields three-dimensional views, two of which are shown here. **B:** Coronal MIP. Note duplicated renal arteries bilaterally. **C:** Sagittal MIP. A, aorta; *arrow*, renal arteries.

gadolinium. This technique overcomes the disadvantages associated with 2D TOF and PC techniques and is our preferred technique. MR angiograms obtained using 3D gadolinium-enhanced GRE and reconstructed with maximum intensity projection (MIP) rendering technique allow exquisite display of the entire retroperitoneal arterial and/or venous system in multiple projections (97,107,254) (Fig. 17-5). For MRA, 0.1 to 0.2 mmol/kg body weight of gadolinium is administered into an anticubital vein using a power injector at a rate of 2 to 3 mL per second, followed by 15 mL of saline to clear lines and veins. A slower infusion technique may be used when visualization of lower extremity vessels is required. As in the case of CT, computer software programs exist that trigger the imaging sequence when the intraluminal aorta signal intensity reaches a preselected level.

AORTA

Normal Anatomy

The abdominal aorta begins at the hiatus of the diaphragm and usually extends along the ventral aspect of the lumbar spine to the level of the fourth lumbar vertebra, where it divides into the two common iliac arteries. The caliber of the abdominal aorta decreases as it progresses distally toward the bifurcation. Men usually have larger diameter vessels than age-matched women, and aortic diameter gradually increases with age in both sexes (126) . CT measurements of the normal aortic diameter at the level of the renal hila vary from a mean of 1.53 cm in women in their fourth decade to 2.10 cm in men in their eighth decade.

Normal infrarenal aortic dimensions (just proximal to the bifurcation) are smaller, averaging 1.43 cm and 1.96 cm, respectively, in these two groups of patients. An aortic diameter less than 12 mm at the level of the renal arteries should raise the possibility of hypovolemic shock (Fig. 17-6) (293).

The major branches arising from the abdominal aorta—the celiac trunk, the superior mesentery artery, renal arteries, and the inferior mesenteric artery—are well appreciated on both CT and MRI (355). Small accessory renal arteries likewise can be demonstrated on CT and MR angiograms when data are acquired with thin collimation (107,249).

The noncalcified aortic wall cannot be distinguished from intraluminal blood on noncontrast CT scans except in anemic patients. Whereas the attenuation value of the blood in the aortic lumen ranges from 50 to 70 Hounsfeld units (HU) in normal subjects, it is considerably less in patients with a markedly reduced hematocrit. Thus, a visible, noncalcified aortic wall is a clue to the presence of anemia. After bolus intravenous administration of water-soluble iodinated contrast medium, the attenuation value of the aortic lumen can rise to as high as +400 HU.

Flowing blood has an appearance on MR images that is distinct from that of stationary tissue. Depending upon the imaging technique used, blood may be bright or dark. In general, blood flowing at normal velocities (greater than 10 cm per second) usually produces no signal on SE sequences (especially at long TEs) and bright signal on GRE sequences (especially at short TEs) due to TOF phenomenon. Therefore, the aorta and its major branches appear as areas of signal void on SE images, but as bright foci on GRE images. With either technique, these arteries can be distinguished easily from the surrounding retroperitoneal

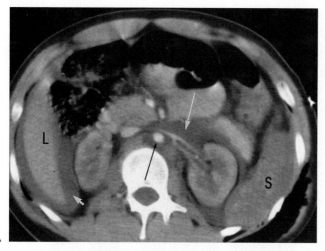 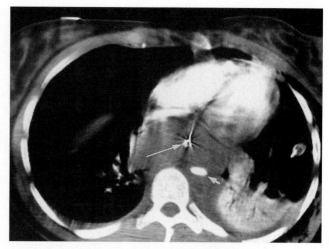

Figure 17-6 Small aorta in a 17-year-old woman in shock after a motor vehicle accident. **A:** Contrast-enhanced computed tomography scan shows a 7-mm diameter aorta (*long black arrow*) associated with intraperitoneal (*short white arrow*) and retroperitoneal (*long white arrow*) hemorrhage. **B:** 7 cm superiorly, there is a large mediastinal hematoma surrounding the aorta (*short arrow*) and esophagus (*long arrow*), which has artifact from a nasogastric tube. At surgery, thoracic aortic transection was found with dissection of hemorrhage into the retroperitoneum and peritoneal cavity. L, liver, S, spleen.

structures. However, the thin wall of the normal aorta usually is not clearly identified as a separate structure on either SE or GRE images. When transaxial images are obtained with a multislice SE technique, the aorta often demonstrates signal in the most cranial slice of the imaged volume because of a flow-related enhancement effect. Placement of a presaturation band above the imaging volume eliminates this effect and ensures that flowing blood remains black (68).

AORTA–PATHOLOGIC CONDITIONS

Atherosclerosis

Atherosclerotic changes of the aorta can be detected on CT scans. These include calcification in the wall, mild ectasia, and tortuosity (Fig. 17-7). Although the aorta usually is located in a prevertebral position, it may lie to the side of the spine

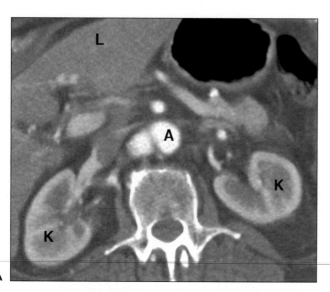 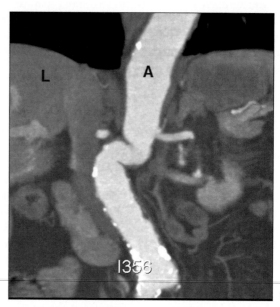

Figure 17-7 Aortic tortuosity may mimic dissection or focal aneurysm on axial images. **A:** Axial contrast-enhanced multidetector row computed tomography scan of the upper abdomen. **B:** Coronal reconstruction of the volume data shows aortic tortuosity. A, Aorta; L, liver; K, kidney.

and flowing blood is accentuated on postgadolinium GRE images.

Penetrating Atherosclerotic Ulcer and Intramural Hematoma

Penetrating atherosclerotic ulcers (PAUs) form when an atherosclerotic lesion erodes through the internal elastic lamina into the media. A focal craterlike outpouching or saccular aneurysm is created (116,197). Intramural hematoma or a localized dissection can then develop. Distinguishing this from primary aortic dissection may be difficult. The identification of a contrast-filled crater communicating with the aortic lumen, an irregular thick intimal flap, and the limited extent of dissection are helpful in distinguishing a penetrating ulcer from a primary aortic dissection (347). Most penetrating ulcers occur in the descending thoracic aorta; however, abdominal aortic involvement has been reported (219). The typical clinical presentation is that of an elderly patient with chest or back pain and hypertension. The prognosis in cases of penetrating ulcer is unclear (51,110,116,151). Incidentally discovered lesions may progress slowly with a low prevalence of rupture. Patients with persistent pain or with larger lesions often have a worse prognosis, with rapid enlargement, aneurysm formation, and rupture.

Intramural hematoma may occur either secondary to a PAU or as a spontaneous bleed from vasa vasorum usually in a hypertensive patient (197). As with PAU, intramural hematoma is more common in the thoracic aorta and may lead to aortic rupture or dissection (328). PAU with intramural hematoma is felt to have a worse prognosis with expansion of the hematoma and rupture, than intramural hematoma alone (85,198).

CT angiography (CTA) is useful in full evaluation of these lesions. Multiplanar reconstructions demonstrate the extent of the ulcer cavity in PAU and accompanying intramural hematoma. Although intramural hematoma is hyperdense on noncontrast exams, it cannot be distinguished from chronic thrombus by density alone but is indicated by inward displacement of intimal calcification (151). Intramural hematoma also produces smooth eccentric wall thickening that extends smoothly in a longitudinal direction, unlike the more irregular atherosclerotic plaque. MRA has also been advocated for evaluation of these lesions. Although acute intramural hematoma (within the first 7 days) may have intermediate signal intensity similar to that of muscle, subacute hemorrhage has increased T1 and T2 signals (198). Atherosclerotic plaque and chronic thrombus exhibit low to intermediate signal on both T1 and T2 sequences (368).

Stenosis and Occlusion

Occlusion and stenosis of the aorta or its primary branches is most commonly due to atherosclerotic change, although an arteritis such as Takayasu arteritis can also produce dramatic changes.

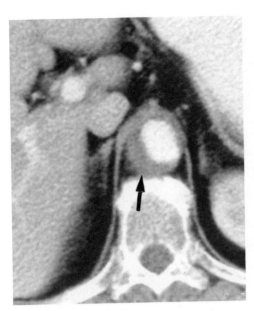

Figure 17-8 Atheromatous plaque in a normal-size aorta. The atheroma (*arrow*) has a lower attenuation value and is clearly differentiated from the aortic lumen on this contrast-enhanced computed tomography image.

in patients with severe atherosclerosis. Atheromatous plaque and chronic mural thrombus may be lower in attenuation value than flowing blood, but are best appreciated on postcontrast scans (Fig. 17-8). Occlusion of a vessel likewise is best demonstrated on postcontrast scans (Fig. 17-9).

Atherosclerotic changes of the aorta also can be seen on MR images. Calcification of the aortic wall appears as an arc or circumferential rim of low signal intensity. On SE images, atheromatous plaques and thrombi produce intraluminal signals of various intensities. Whereas organized thrombi have low signal intensities on both T1- and T2-weighted SE images, fresh unorganized thrombi have high signal intensities on T1- and T2-weighted images (45). A fibrous cap over the thrombus typically has uniform increased signal on T2-weighted imaging and shows enhancement on delayed postgadolinium T1-weighted images (167). Atheromatous plaques and thrombi can be differentiated easily from the aortic lumen, which usually appears as an area of signal void. However, slow blood flow may result in intraluminal signal. The signal from slow flow can be distinguished from that of atheromatous plaques and thrombus by comparing the signal intensities on first and second echo images. Slow flow may show an increase in the absolute signal intensity on the second or even echo, whereas the signal produced by thrombus and the atheromatous plaque decreases in intensity on the second echo. This increase in signal strength in blood vessels with slow flow has been described as an even-echo rephasing effect (31). On GRE images, atheromatous plaque and thrombi usually are less intense than flowing blood. The signal difference between atheromatous plaque/thrombus

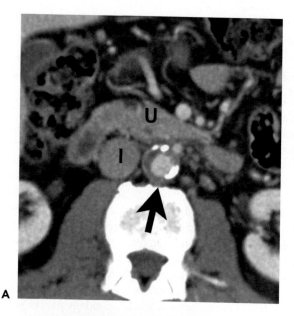

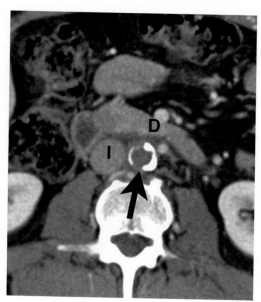

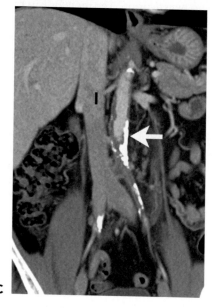

Figure 17-9 Atherosclerosis with occlusion of the distal aorta. **A:** Axial contrast-enhanced computed tomography scan shows atherosclerosis with plaque and thrombus in the abdominal aorta. **B:** Complete occlusion occurs at the level of the crossing duodenum. **C:** Coronal reconstruction. I, inferior vena cava; U, uncinate process of pancreas; D, duodenum; *arrow*, aorta.

Luminal narrowing of the aorta and its branch vessels can be well seen on helical CT angiograms using MIP and volume-rendering techniques (VRTs) (see Fig. 17-9). In one study performed with a single-detector row CT scanner (283), CTA depicted all main and accessory renal arteries that were seen with conventional arteriography. CTA was also 92% sensitive and 83% specific for the detection of renal artery stenosis when the stenosis was greater than or equal to 70%. In another study performed with an MDCT scanner, CTA was 92% sensitive and 99% specific for the detection of hemodynamically significant stenosis of aortoiliac and renal arteries (355). Underestimation or overestimation of arterial stenosis may occur on CT angiograms due to vessel wall calcifications (283,355). This problem is exacerbated on MIP images, which display only the voxels with the highest signal intensity along parallel rays, thereby obscuring the true arterial lumen. The use of multiple MIP images generated about both *x* and *z* axes is needed to ensure that the true lumen is appreciated (283). The use of a wide window width (window width, 2,000 HU) and a high window level (center level, 500 HU) for evaluating all arterial segments containing calcium is also suggested to minimize the "blooming" effect from the calcium (355).

Stenosis of the aorta, iliac vessels, and renal arteries can also be depicted on either noncontrast- or gadolinium-enhanced MR angiograms with a high degree of accuracy. Because it overcomes the inherent problems of TOF and phase-contrast techniques, gadolinium-enhanced MRA has become our technique of choice (142). Sensitivities and specificities between 90% and 100% have been achieved with contrast-enhanced 3D MRA for the detection of hemodynamically significant stenosis of aortoiliac and renal arteries (107,308,355)

Both MRI and CT can show the vessel wall thickening characteristic of Takayasu arteritis (159,204).

Aortic Aneurysm

In general, the abdominal aorta is considered aneurysmally dilated if it exceeds 3 to 3.5 cm in maximal diameter or if the infrarenal aorta is at least 5 mm larger than the renal aorta or if a localized dilation of the aorta is present (126,297). Abdominal aortic aneurysms (AAAs) greater than or equal to 29 mm in maximal diameter are found in approximately 6% of men and 1% of women age 55 to 65 years and increase in prevalence by about 6% per decade thereafter in men and 1.5% per decade in women (297). Aneurysms greater than 3.9 cm in diameter occur in 1% of men and in 0.1% of women from 55 to 64 years of age and increase by 3% to 4% per decade thereafter in men and 0.3% to 0.6% per decade in women (297). The incidence of AAA has increased in the last 50 years, likely a result, in part, of improved detection rates with the advent of modern imaging modalities. Smoking history is the strongest risk factor in the development of AAA with an odds ratio of from 1.4 to 8, depending on the duration of smoking (177,297).

In the United States, AAAs are mostly to the result of atherosclerosis (Fig. 17-10). Infectious (mycotic, syphilitic), inflammatory (e.g., Takayasu arteritis), congenital (e.g., Marfan syndrome), or traumatic causes are uncommon. The vast majority of AAAs are infrarenal in location. The applied pressure load in this location is greater because of the tapering geometry of the aorta and reflected pressure waves from the aortic bifurcation (62). Following LaPlace's law, in which wall tension increases geometrically with radius, larger aneurysms tend to grow at a more rapid rate than smaller ones. In one study (190), the annual growth rates for aneurysms less than 4 cm, between 4 and 5 cm, and greater than 5 cm in diameter were 5.3 mm, 6.9 mm, and 7.4 mm, respectively. Similarly, the incidence of rupture varies directly with the size of the aneurysm. Whereas the incidence of rupture is negligible for aneurysms less than 3.9 cm in diameter, the risk exceeds 20% annually for aneurysms larger than 5 cm in diameter (190). It is important to note that, for a given diameter, the risk of rupture is four times higher in women than in men, perhaps reflecting the generally smaller initial diameter of the aorta in women. Hence, the threshold for intervention in women should be somewhat lower than for men (244,253). Computer modeling of 3D shape and calculation of wall stress may also have a role in the prediction of rupture, but at present this technique is still experimental (77,78).

Accepted indications for repair of AAAs include size greater than 5 to 5.5 cm, rapid rate of aneurysm expansion

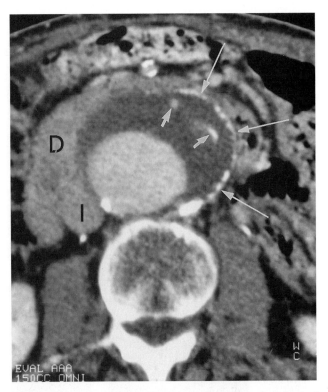

Figure 17-10 Mural thrombus with calcification in an abdominal aortic aneurysm. Contrast-enhanced computed tomography scan shows a 7-cm-diameter abdominal aortic aneurysm. Within the mural thrombus, there are calcifications (*short arrows*) that are distinct from the intact rim of intimal calcification (*long arrows*). This is in contradistinction to the displaced intimal calcification that may be seen in aortic dissection, in which case the peripheral rim of intimal calcification is disrupted or distorted. I, inferior vena cava; D, duodenum.

(increase of 5 mm or more in 6 months), known mycotic aneurysm, pain, concomitant occlusive disease, iliac or femoral artery aneurysms, and peripheral emboli (34,244,295).

AAAs can be detected and differentiated from a tortuous aorta by CT. Measurements of aortic diameter obtained on CT correlate well with those found at surgery (239). CT measurements are fairly reproducible. In one study, absolute intraobserver variation in measurements of maximal infrarenal aortic diameter was 2 mm or less in 94% of cases. Interobserver variation was somewhat greater but was still 2 mm or less in 82% (298). Although not large, these figures suggest that when assessing change in aortic diameter, prior CT scans should be reviewed contemporaneously with the new study to reduce interobserver error (298). The origin and the length of an aneurysm as well as its relationship to renal and iliac arteries can be traced on both serial axial scans and reconstructed images with MIP and VRT projectional CT angiograms (Fig. 17-11). When 10-mm sections are used, volume averaging of a tortuous juxtarenal aneurysm may produce an appearance suggesting involvement of the main renal arteries when in fact these vessels are actually uninvolved. However, with 2- to 5-mm sections, the overall accuracy of helical CT in predicting aneurysmal location with respect to the renal arteries is

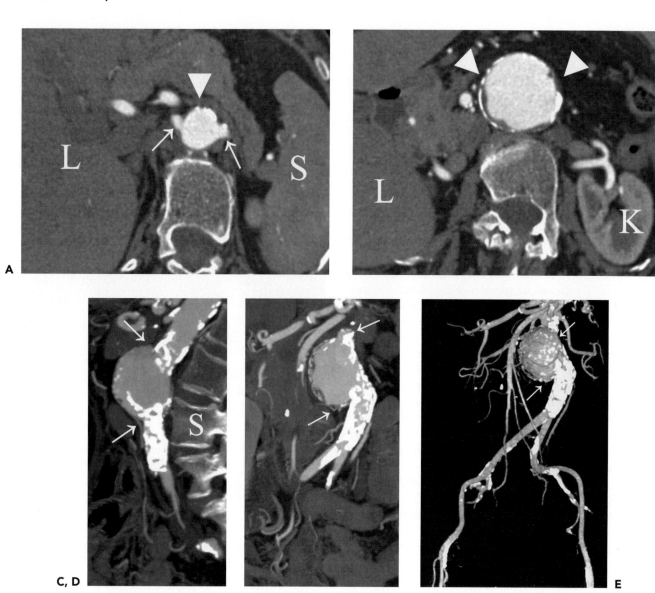

Figure 17-11 Infrarenal aortic aneurysm. **A:** Contrast-enhanced axial image shows normal caliber of aorta (*arrowhead*) at the level of the unusually high origin of the renal arteries (*arrows*). L, liver; S, spleen. **B:** Aneurysm is shown at the infrarenal level with atherosclerotic changes (*arrowheads*). L, liver; K, kidney. **C:** Sagittal maximum-intensity projection (MIP) image shows tortuous aorta with aneurysm and atherosclerotic changes (*arrows*). S, spine. **D:** Coronal MIP image shows tortuous aorta and aneurysm. **E:** Coronal volume-rendered image shows infrarenal aneurysm (*arrows*).

quite high (256,332). The ability to identify renal artery stenosis of greater than 70% has also improved significantly with the use of thin collimation helical CT technique (256,332). CT angiograms obtained on MDCT now provide all the information required for the planning of repair of an AAA.

MRI using conventional T1- and T2-weighted SE or GRE sequences is also an accurate method for demonstrating AAAs. It can accurately depict the size of an aneurysm and the aortic lumen, its relationship to the origin of the renal arteries, and the status of the iliac arteries. However, these noncontrast techniques do not reliably detect accessory renal arteries or depict associated occlusive disease of aortic branch vessels, knowledge of which is important for aneurysm repair. Contrast-enhanced 3D MRA performed in a breath-hold provides precise information regarding the aortic lumen as well as its relationship to aortic branch vessels (Fig. 17-12). Several studies have shown that contrast-enhanced 3D MRA has a high sensitivity and specificity for detection of hemodynamically significant stenosis of renal and iliac arteries (142,355).

Although both CT and MRI can detect the presence and the size of aortic aneurysms and their internal character with a high degree of accuracy, ultrasound (US) remains

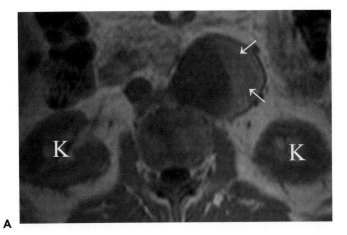

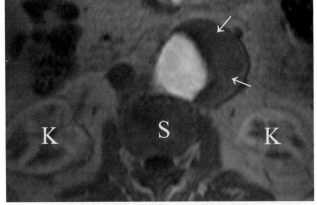

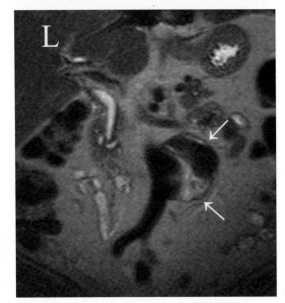

Figure 17-12 Infrarenal aortic aneurysm. **A:** Precontrast axial T1-weighted magnetic resonance image (MRI) shows thrombus (*arrow*) in the aortic aneurysm. K, kidneys. **B:** Postcontrast axial T1-weighted MRI shows nonopacification of the thrombus (*arrows*) in the aortic aneurysm. K, kidneys; S, spine. **C:** Coronal half Fourier snap shot turbo spin echo MRI of abdomen shows aortic aneurysm (*arrows*). L, liver.

the procedure of choice in patients with suspected AAA because of its ease of performance, lack of ionizing radiation, lower cost, and portability (43,357). In patients who have had an unsuccessful or equivocal sonographic examination because of postsurgical scar tissue, obesity, or abundant bowel gas, or in patients needing complete preoperative assessment, either a CT or an MRI study may be performed. In most cases, we prefer CT to MRI because of its better spatial resolution and ease of performance. Optimal CT evaluation of the abdominal aorta, however, requires intravenous contrast material, for example, to differentiate a pseudoaneurysm from periaortic lymphadenopathy. Thus, in patients who have a contraindication to the use of iodinated contrast material, it is advantageous to perform MRI rather than a CT examination.

Inflammatory AAA

Inflammatory AAA (IAAA) is diagnosed when a dense fibrotic and frequently highly vascular reaction is noted surrounding an AAA (Fig. 17-13). These changes may infiltrate surrounding structures such as the duodenum, IVC, left

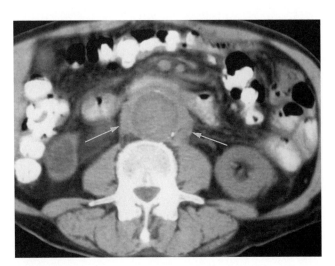

Figure 17-13 Perianeurysmal fibrosis. Noncontrast computed tomography scan shows an infrarenal abdominal aortic aneurysm associated with a sharply marginated rind of fibrotic soft tissue (*arrows*).

renal vein, ureters, mesentery, and small bowel. Approximately 3% to 15% of all AAAs are complicated by inflammatory change. IAAAs occur more commonly in men than in women and typically present at a younger age than noninflammatory AAAs. Symptoms are usually present and include abdominal or back pain, weight loss, and an elevated erythrocyte sedimentation rate (132,206,228,266). Although the pathogenesis of IAAA is unclear, an immune response to some component of the arterial wall or atherosclerotic plaque has been suggested. The time necessary for the development of the inflammatory response is also uncertain; however, the development of an inflammatory AAA from an uncomplicated aneurysm over a period of 6½ months has been documented by CT (176). In many cases, a decrease in the amount of fibrosis occurs following aneurysm repair (228,248,305).

CT has been reported to have variable sensitivity and specificity for the detection of IAAAs, ranging from approximately 50% to 80% (132,316). IAAAs usually appear as an AAA surrounded by a symmetric soft tissue mass or wall thickening with relative sparing of the posterior aortic wall (132). The mass is usually well defined, although a more infiltrative appearance is occasionally seen (14). The mass/wall thickening will demonstrate late phase contrast enhancement on both CT and MRI. On contrast-enhanced MRI, a low-intensity internal rim with no enhancement has been noted and is thought to represent thickened intima between inflammatory mass and the aortic lumen (115). Three or more alternating layers of high and low signal have also been noted in the inflammatory tissue on MRI. These changes were most prominent on noncontrast short tau inversion recovery (STIR) sequences but were also noted on T1-weighted sequences (315). Other authors have reported only an intermediate signal on T1-weighted sequences with poor distinction from an intraluminal thrombus (342).

Mycotic Aneurysm

Mycotic aneurysms form as a result of infectious inflammation causing weakening or necrosis of the aortic wall. The infection may occur from direct seeding of the roughened atherosclerotic surface, by septic emboli to the vasa vasorum, or from contiguous spread from an adjacent extravascular source such as a vertebral osteomyelitis or discitis. About half of patients in one series had a history of recent infection, which presumably acted as a bacteremic source (231). Immunocompromised patients also are more susceptible to the development of mycotic aneurysms (221,231). Typical presentation includes pain, fever, leukocytosis, and a positive blood culture. Bacteria cause most mycotic aneurysms, with *Staphylococcus aureus* being the most common agent. *Salmonella* and *Streptococcus* species and *Escherichia coli* are also frequent (221,231). Unlike atherosclerotic aneurysms, 85% of which involve the infrarenal aorta, mycotic aneurysms are more evenly distributed with approximately 35% to 40% being infrarenal (196).

A mycotic aneurysm usually is saccular and has a lobulated contour (Figs. 17-14 and 17-15). A periaortic soft tissue mass or stranding and/or fluid is frequently present. Gas is present infrequently, but when seen, is virtually pathognomic for infection (Fig. 17-16). Calcification can occur in mycotic aneurysms, but this is less common than in atherosclerotic aneurysms (196). Similarly, the absence of atherosclerotic change in other vessels points to a mycotic etiology. Rapid development or enlargement of a mycotic aneurysm may be noted if sequential scans are performed (196,366). Erosion of the adjacent vertebral body may also be seen but is infrequent (196).

Nonaneurysmal bacterial aortitis has also been described and can lead to rupture. A hazy periaortic density containing gas is the characteristic CT finding and should prompt aggressive management (201).

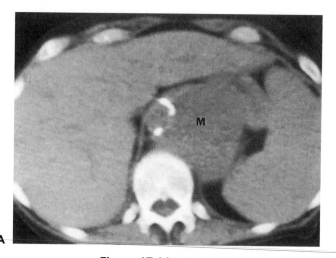
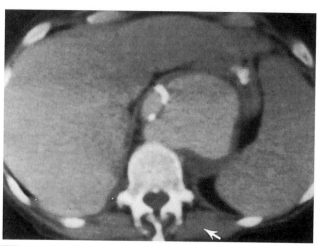

Figure 17-14 Mycotic aortic aneurysm: **A:** Noncontrast–enhanced computed tomography (CT) image shows a large soft tissue mass (M) adjacent to the calcified descending aorta. This could be confused with lymphadenopathy. **B:** Contrast-enhanced CT scan demonstrates enhancement of this mass to the same degree as the aorta, thus establishing its vascular nature.

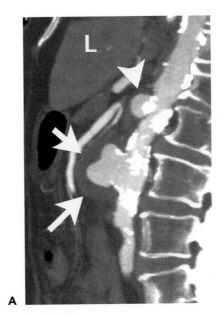

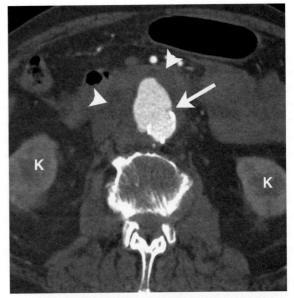

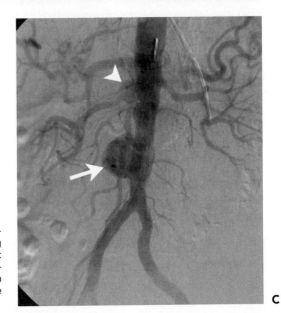

Figure 17-15 Mycotic aneurysm. **A:** Contrast-enhanced computed tomography (CT), sagittal reconstruction, shows a saccular aneurysm (*arrows*) coming off the infrarenal aorta with a second aneurysm arising at the level of the right renal artery (*arrowhead*). **B:** Axial CT image shows the break in intimal calcification (*arrow*) with saccular aneurysm (*arrowheads*). **C:** Angiogram shows a lobular infrarenal aneurysm (*arrow*) with a smaller aneurysm adjacent to the origin of the right renal artery (*arrowhead*).

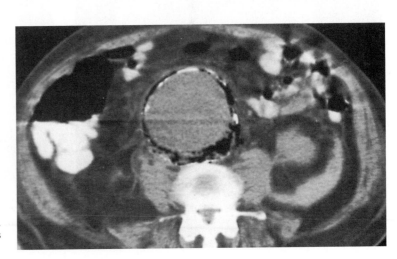

Figure 17-16 Infected atherosclerotic aortic aneurysm. Numerous air bubbles are seen within the wall of this fusiform aneurysm.

Ruptured AAA

Ruptured AAA can be a difficult clinical diagnosis. Less than one third of patients with ruptured AAAs present with the classic triad of abdominal pain, back pain, and a pulsatile mass (202). Over half of patients in one series were initially misdiagnosed (2). Conversely, up to two thirds of hemodynamically stable patients with known AAAs and abdominal pain do not turn out to have a ruptured aneurysm (173). The clinical presentation of renal colic, diverticulitis, bowel ischemia, cholecystitis, peptic ulcer disease, and acute myocardial infarction have all been shown both to mimic and to be mimicked by ruptured AAA (2,173,202). CT is a useful and effective imaging study for evaluating hemodynamically stable patients with suspected leaking AAAs. In this group of patients, the delay imposed by obtaining a preoperative CT study usually does not adversely affect patient outcome, and the information obtained from the CT study can both make an alternative diagnosis or confirm a diagnosis and aid substantially in both preoperative and intraoperative management (53,173,295).

The CT diagnosis of ruptured AAA is based on demonstration of irregular, high-density material corresponding to blood (approximately +70 HU on noncontrast scans) infiltrating the periaortic fat and extending into the adjacent perirenal and less commonly pararenal spaces (Fig. 17-17). The aorta may be anteriorly displaced by the mass or collection. Although intravenous contrast material is not required for the diagnosis of ruptured AAA, contrast-enhanced CT may document active arterial extravasation either as a focal high density area (attenuation values 80 to 130 HU) surrounded by a large hematoma or as a diffuse area of high density (140) (Figs. 17-17 and 17-18). Additional findings include anterior displacement of the kidney by the hematoma and enlargement or obscuration of the psoas muscle. A focally indistinct aortic margin on contrast-enhanced scans and focal discontinuity of a circumferentially calcified rim may indicate the site of rupture, but neither sign is specific (84,296) (Figs. 17-19 and 17-20). Rupture location is most commonly posterolateral, although this may not always be identifiable if there is a large amount of hemorrhage present (79). Occasionally blood from a ruptured AAA may extend into the peritoneal cavity. Free fluid with attenuation value greater than 30 HU and the presence of a hematocrit effect suggest a hemoperitoneum (27).

False–positive CT diagnoses of ruptured AAAs are uncommon; however, a variety of retroperitoneal masses, such as an opacified duodenum, lymphadenopathy, perianeurysmal fibrosis, and masses in the psoas muscle are occasionally seen in patients with AAAs and may be confused with areas of rupture. Retroperitoneal hemorrhage may also occur for reasons unconnected to the AAA, such as anticoagulation or neoplasm. Such unrelated hemorrhage may be suspected if the aortic wall is intact, well visualized, and has an intact periaortic fat plane (295).

Although false–negative CT diagnoses are uncommon, it should be noted that patients with impending or contained rupture may present with pain but show no obvious hemorrhage. Because of this, patients with large AAAs and unexplained abdominal or back pain should be admitted and consideration given to semielective repair (98,295).

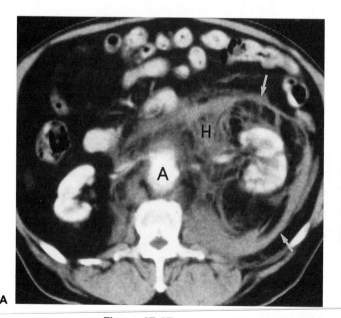
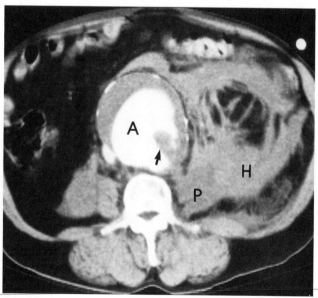

Figure 17-17   Ruptured abdominal aortic aneurysm. **A:** Contrast-enhanced computed tomography scan shows irregular soft tissue strands representing acute hemorrhage (H) extending from the aneurysm (A) into the left perirenal space. Note the thickened perirenal fascia (*arrows*). **B:** 5 cm caudad, acute hemorrhage (H) is hyperdense compared with psoas muscle (P). Note the irregular intraluminal thrombus (*arrow*) within the aorta.

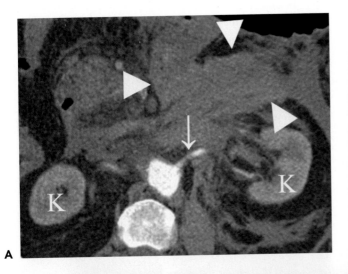

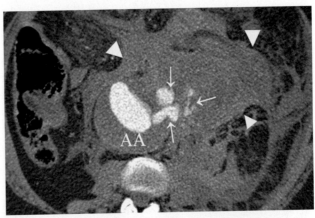

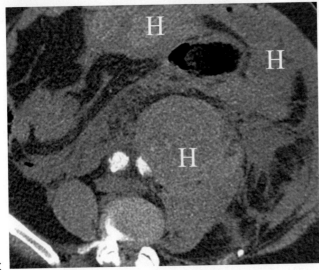

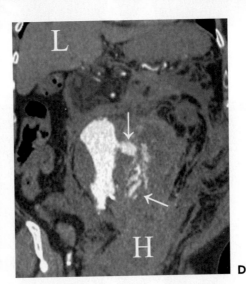

Figure 17-18   Ruptured abdominal aortic aneurysm. **A:** Contrast-enhanced axial computed tomography image shows normal aorta at renal artery (*arrow*) level. Retroperitoneal hematoma from ruptured infrarenal aortic aneurysm (*arrowheads*). K, kidneys. **B:** Ruptured infrarenal aortic aneurysm with active extravasation (*arrows*) of contrast into the retroperitoneum. Large retroperitoneal hematoma is on the left side (*arrowheads*). AA, aortic aneurysm. **C:** Extension of retroperitoneal hematoma (H) in the pelvis. **D:** Coronal image shows ruptured aortic aneurysm with active extravasation (*arrows*). Retroperitoneal hematoma (H) extends into the left pelvis. L, liver.

Several CT signs of contained or impending rupture have also been described. The "draped aorta" sign occurs when the posterior aortic wall is not definable and the posterior margin of the aorta is closely applied to and follows the contour of the vertebral body (106). The presence of a crescent-shaped area of high attenuation within the wall or mural thrombus of the aneurysm has been associated with an intramural hematoma and is predictive of free or contained rupture of an AAA (10,296). In one study, the "crescent sign" had a 77% sensitivity and 93% specificity for rupture or intramural hematoma (208) (Fig. 17-21). The presence of either of these signs should raise the suspicion of impending or contained rupture particularly in patients with abdominal or back pain (208,296). The

amount of thrombus present and the circumference of the AAA involved by thrombus have not been shown to be different in patients with ruptured and nonruptured AAAs (79).

Because of its relatively long imaging time and the difficulty in monitoring critically ill patients, MRI has not been used to evaluate patients with suspected rupture of AAAs. Furthermore, MRI cannot distinguish acute hematoma from other fluid collections because of their similar signal intensities.

Chronic Pseudoaneurysm

In comparison with acute rupture, a chronic pseudoaneurysm (false aneurysm) appears as a well-defined,

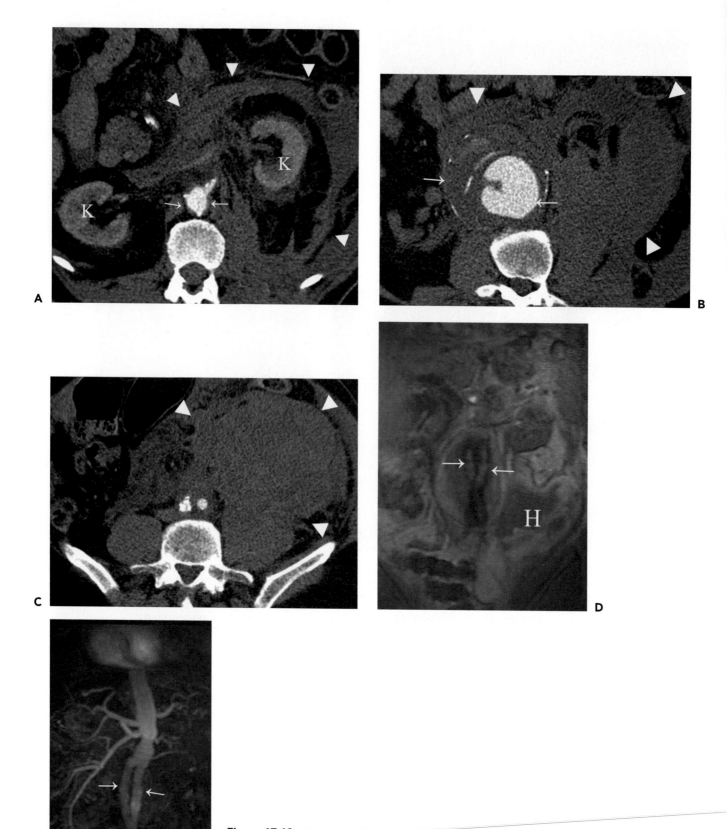

Figure 17-19 Ruptured abdominal aortic aneurysm treated with endovascular stenting. **A:** Contrast-enhanced computed tomography shows normal aorta (*arrows*) at renal arterial level. Note retroperitoneal hematoma secondary to ruptured infrarenal aneurysm (*arrowheads*). K, kidney. **B:** Ruptured aortic aneurysm (*arrows*) with retroperitoneal hematoma (*arrowheads*). **C:** Large retroperitoneal hematoma extending into pelvis from a ruptured aneurysm (*arrowheads*). **D:** Postendograft precontrast coronal T1-weighted magnetic resonance image (MRI) shows stent (*arrows*) in place. H, residual pelvic hematoma from recent aneurysm rupture. **E:** Postcontrast coronal MRI shows stent (*arrows*) in place.

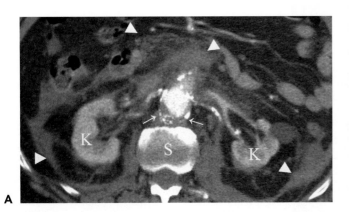

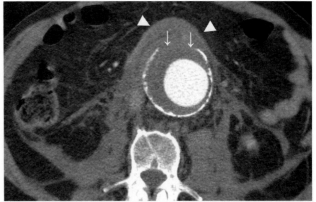

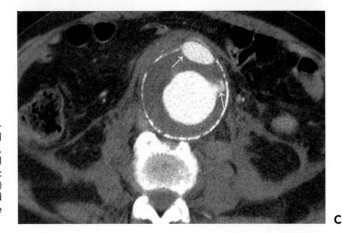

Figure 17-20 Ruptured abdominal aortic aneurysm. **A:** Contrast-enhanced axial computed tomography image at renal arterial level shows atherosclerotic changes in normal caliber aorta (*arrows*). Retroperitoneal hematoma anterior to aorta from ruptured infrarenal aortic aneurysm (*arrowhead*). K, kidneys; *S*, spine. **B:** Infrarenal aortic aneurysm with thrombus and break in calcification anteriorly (*arrows*) and retroperitoneal hematoma (*arrowheads*) resulting from ruptured aneurysm. **C:** Aortic aneurysm with active extravasation in the aneurysm sac (*arrows*).

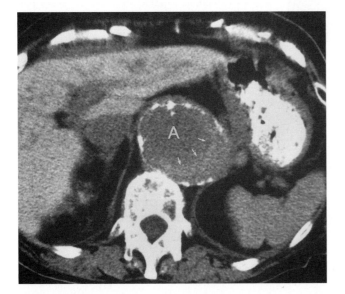

Figure 17-21 High-attenuating crescent in early rupture of an aortic aneurysm. Non–contrast-enhanced computed tomography scan shows an abdominal aortic aneurysm (A) with a high-attenuating crescent (*arrowheads*) posterolaterally. Emergent surgery in this 82-year-old woman with back pain disclosed very early aneurysm rupture at this site. (Courtesy of Jay Heiken, St. Louis, Missouri.)

usually round, mass with an attenuation value similar to or lower than that of the native aorta on noncontrast scans. On postcontrast scans, the lumen of the aneurysm as well as its communication with the aorta may enhance (Fig. 17-22).

Aortoenteric Fistula

Aortoenteric fistula (AEF) is most common in its secondary form in which communication between an aortic graft and adjacent bowel develops. Primary AEF, in which such communication occurs between native aorta and adjacent bowel, is rare. In over half of cases, the distal duodenum is the involved bowel segment, although involvement of the jejunum, ileum, and transverse colon has also been reported (40,195). Mechanical erosion of an aneurysm or graft into the adjacent bowel with secondary infection is the usual etiology (333). Preexisting septic aortitis, radiotherapy, or tumor are more unusual causes (36). Massive gastrointestinal hemorrhage is the most common symptom and is usually preceded by a smaller self-limited bleed. Fever, leukocytosis, and pain are also frequent symptoms (36). Diagnosis can be difficult and is frequently based on both endoscopy and CT. CT findings suspicious for AEF include perianeurysmal (or perigraft) soft tissue, fluid, and gas in the space between the aorta and duodenum (Figs. 17-23 and 17-24). Duode-

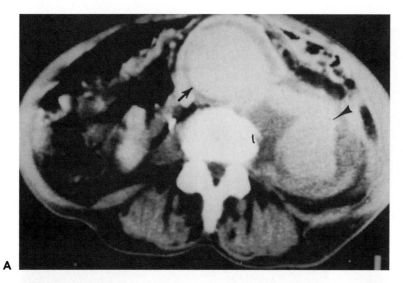

A

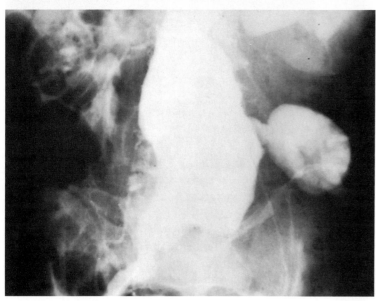

B

Figure 17-22 Aortic aneurysm and associated chronic pseudoaneurysm. **A:** Postcontrast computed tomography image demonstrates a large abdominal aortic aneurysm extending posterolaterally into the left paravertebral area. Note the centrally enhanced lumen in both the true (*arrow*) and the false (*arrowhead*) aneurysms. The lower density periphery represents either an atheroma or a thrombus. The left psoas muscle is obscured by the pseudoaneurysm. **B:** The abdominal arteriogram shows findings similar to those of the CT study.

nal fold thickening may also be noted (195). High-density clot or extravasated contrast may be visualized within the adjacent bowel in cases with intraluminal or intramural hemorrhage (255,370). For this reason, it is suggested that water be used instead of oral contrast in patients if AEF is a diagnostic consideration (255). On occasion, minimal or no CT findings are present; hence, a negative CT does not entirely preclude the possibility of AEF (195).

Aortocaval Fistula

Aortocaval fistulae are rare. The most common cause is rupture of an AAA into the adjacent IVC. Trauma, either iatrogenic or penetrating injury from a gunshot or stab wound, also causes fistulae. The most common symptom is an abdominal bruit with back pain and shock as common accompaniments. Severe leg swelling, scrotal edema, and renal insufficiency and hematuria are also noted from

the induced peripheral and pelvic venous hypertension (56). The CT findings that suggest this diagnosis include perivascular stranding around the IVC and fistulous tract and simultaneous enhancement of the aorta and IVC (Fig. 17-25). The IVC and iliac veins are noted to be distended. Retrograde opacification of the renal veins and perirenal stranding may also be observed (54,327). Similar findings have been reported on gadolinium-enhanced MRA (83). Although MRA takes longer to perform, its use may be indicated if renal insufficiency is present.

Aortic Dissection

Dissection of the aorta typically occurs when blood enters an intimal tear and progressively separates the intima from the underlying remainder of the wall. Alternatively, dissection may begin with an intramural bleed that ruptures through the intima to communicate with the lumen.

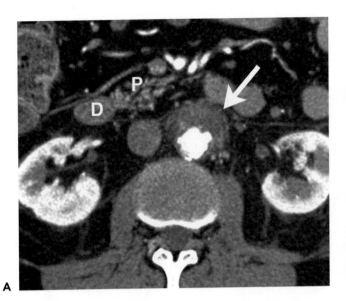

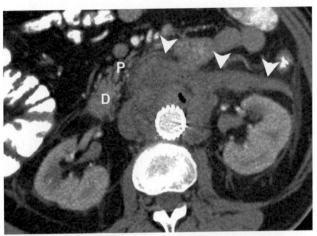

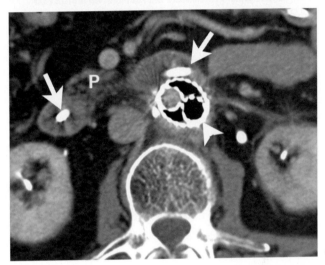

Figure 17-23 Aortitis with development of aortoenteric fistula. **A:** Initial contrast-enhanced computed tomography shows poorly circumscribed increased soft tissue around the anterior margin of the aorta (*arrow*). P, pancreas; D, duodenum. **B:** Two weeks later, following placement of an endograft, there is increased anterior soft tissue with air noted about the aorta and extending into the anterior pararenal space (*arrowheads*), indicative of aortic rupture with hematoma and infection. P, pancreas; D, duodenum. **C:** Seven weeks later, following placement of an additional endograft, there is air in the graft (*arrowhead*) with continuing pain, fevers, and gastrointestinal bleeding consistent with ongoing graft infection and aortoenteric fistula. Nasogastric tube (*arrows*) marks the location of the duodenum. P, pancreas.

In the vast majority of cases, dissection begins in the thoracic aorta. Isolated abdominal aortic involvement occurs in only 1% to 2% of dissection cases (73). Classification of dissection depends on the site of origin with Stanford type A lesions beginning proximal to the left subclavian artery and type B lesions starting distal to this vessel. Hypertension is the dominant predisposing factor, although diseases that affect wall integrity, such as Marfan syndrome, Turner syndrome, Ehlers-Danlos syndrome, and cystic medial necrosis also play a role. Other associations include bicuspid aortic valve, arteritis, and trauma (303). Dissection limited to the aorta presents classically with abrupt onset of sharp, severe midline pain. In lesions involving the ascending aorta, pain is frequently anterior, while with descending aortic involvement, pain is commonly posterior (104,303). If branch vessels within the abdomen are involved, ischemic damage to a variety of organs may occur and produce additional symptoms (291). Diagnosis can be difficult and in one series was missed in 38% of

patients on initial clinical evaluation and only established at autopsy in 11% (303).

The goal of imaging in aortic dissection is to verify the diagnosis, identify the type of dissection, identify the true and false lumen, and establish the extent of disease and presence of complications such as compromise of branch vessels (356). The diagnosis of an aortic dissection is based on demonstration of an intimal flap with enhancement of both the true and false lumina after intravenous administration of contrast medium. The true lumen can often be identified by its continuity with the undissected aortic lumen. When this observation is not available several other markers have been described to separate the true lumen from the false lumen. In general, the false lumen is larger than the true lumen and more likely to contain thrombus. The "beak" sign is a marker for the false lumen and occurs when there is an acute angle between the intimal flap and the outer wall (182). This angle may be enhanced or contain thrombus. Aortic "cobwebs," most likely representing

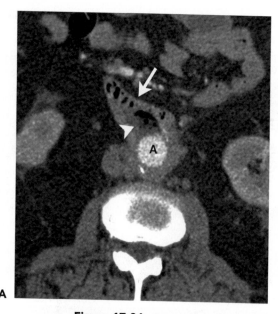

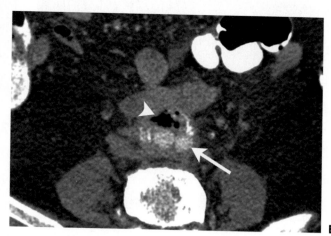

Figure 17-24   Aortoenteric fistula following open repair of an abdominal aortic aneurysm. **A:** Intravenous contrast–enhanced computed tomography scan shows an air and fluid collection (*arrowhead*) consistent with abscess sitting between aortic graft (A) and small bowel (*arrow*). **B:** Abscess (*arrowhead*) extends caudally in front of bilimbed portion of graft (*arrow*).

residual ribbons of media that have been incompletely sheared from the aortic wall during the dissection process, are occasionally seen, and serve as an anatomic marker of the false lumen (352). Markers of the true lumen include more rapid enhancement, outer wall calcification, and eccentric flap calcification. This latter occurs when there is calcification on one side of the intimal flap. The lumen facing that side is the true lumen (182,291).

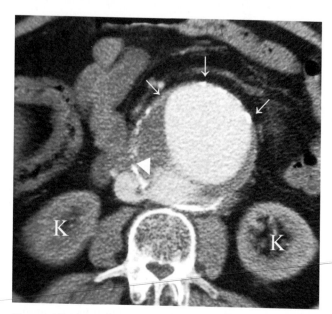

Figure 17-25   Aortocaval fistula. Contrast-enhanced computed tomography shows aortic aneurysm (*arrows*) with aortocaval fistula (*arrowhead*). K, kidneys.

When the false lumen does not fill with contrast medium, a diagnosis of aortic dissection still may be suggested if inward displacement of intimal calcification is present. However, it may not always be possible to distinguish thrombus calcification from displaced calcified intima because the two may appear similar (322). Although hyperdensity of the aortic wall at multiple levels has been reported to be specific for acute aortic dissection (118), 40% of patients without dissection in one series demonstrated this finding on noncontrast scans (174). Nevertheless, a hyperdense aortic wall tends to be uniformly thick throughout the vessel circumference in patients without dissection, whereas hyperdense thickening usually is eccentric in the uncommon form of dissection that occurs when intramural hematoma develops without intimal rupture (363).

When the dissection involves the abdominal aorta, the aortic branch vessels and the organs they supply should be carefully evaluated for possible ischemia. Two types of branch vessel obstruction have been described. Static obstruction occurs when the intimal flap intersects or enters the branch vessel and is treated with intravascular stenting. Dynamic obstruction occurs when the intimal flap is pressed against the branch vessel ostia like a curtain and is treated with fenestration (291,353). The number of abdominal organs with diminished enhancement on contrast-enhanced CTA had a strong correlation with postoperative death in one series of 48 patients with acute dissection extending into the abdomen (336).

Both CTA and MRA have a high sensitivity and specificity for the diagnosis of aortic dissection (302) (Figs. 17-26 to 17-28). Both work well for evaluation of extent of disease. Branch involvement may be better delineated with

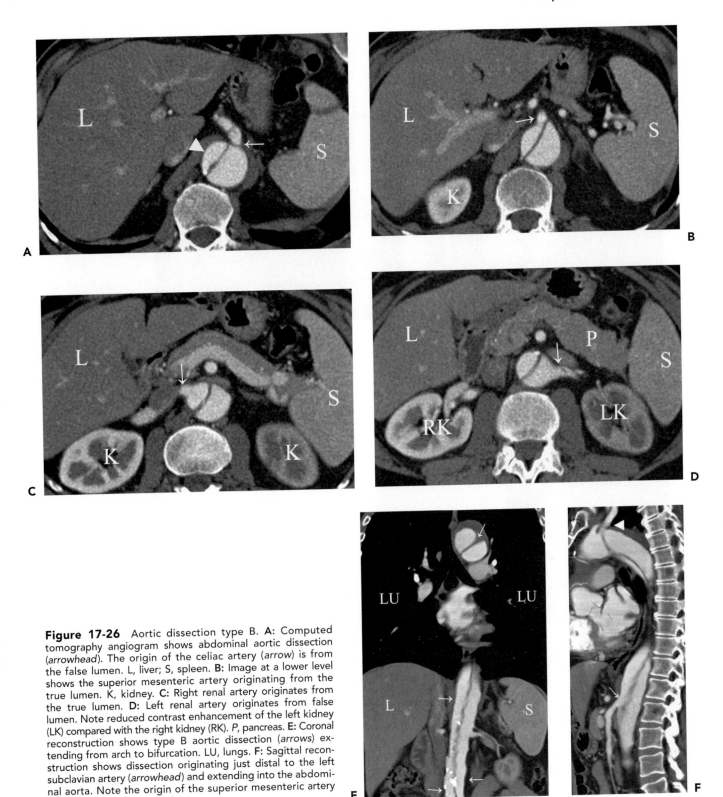

Figure 17-26 Aortic dissection type B. **A:** Computed tomography angiogram shows abdominal aortic dissection (*arrowhead*). The origin of the celiac artery (*arrow*) is from the false lumen. L, liver; S, spleen. **B:** Image at a lower level shows the superior mesenteric artery originating from the true lumen. K, kidney. **C:** Right renal artery originates from the true lumen. **D:** Left renal artery originates from false lumen. Note reduced contrast enhancement of the left kidney (LK) compared with the right kidney (RK). *P*, pancreas. **E:** Coronal reconstruction shows type B aortic dissection (*arrows*) extending from arch to bifurcation. LU, lungs. **F:** Sagittal reconstruction shows dissection originating just distal to the left subclavian artery (*arrowhead*) and extending into the abdominal aorta. Note the origin of the superior mesenteric artery from the true lumen (*arrow*).

MDCT CTA because of its improved spatial resolution (356). In general, because of its close proximity to the emergency department and short examination time, contrast-enhanced MDCT with multiplanar reconstructions has become the test of choice in the acute setting. In stable patients with a contraindication to iodinated contrast or in

follow-up of chronic dissection, MRI is a good alternative. The diagnosis of an aortic dissection can be made on unenhanced SE or GRE images (153,205). Flow-related signal void in both the true and false lumen outlines the thin intimal flap on unenhanced SE images. On occasion, intraluminal signal may appear in the false channel because of slow

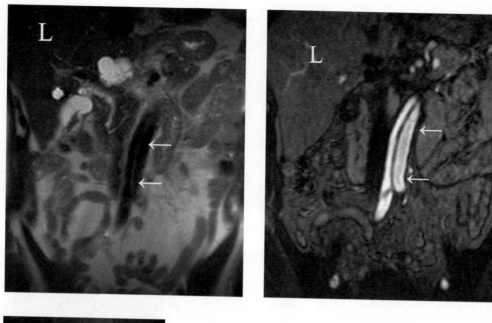

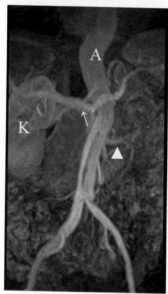

Figure 17-27 Aortic dissection. **A:** Coronal half Fourier snap shot turbo spin echo magnetic resonance (MR) image shows abdominal aortic dissection (*arrows*). L, liver. **B:** Coronal contrast-enhanced MRI shows dissection in abdominal aorta (*arrows*). L, liver. **C:** Coronal postcontrast maximum-intensity projection MRI shows aortic dissection with origin of the celiac axis (*arrow*) from true lumen and origin of left renal artery (*arrowhead*) from false lumen. A, aorta; K, kidney.

blood flow or thrombus (see Fig. 17-28). As stated previously, slow flow can be differentiated from a thrombus by comparing the signal intensity on the first and second echo image. They also can be differentiated on flow-sensitive gradient echo or phase images (205). Nonenhanced true fast imaging with steady-state precession (FISP) has also been used as a rapid (less than 4 minutes) evaluation for aortic dissection with good success (245). The use of contrast-enhanced 3D MRA provides a higher signal-to-noise ratio and superior visualization than noncontrast techniques and has become the technique of choice (113). In contradistinction to noncontrast imaging it also allows evaluation of organ perfusion. Imaging of the entire aorta and its branches can be completed within a breath-hold.

Contrast-enhanced 3D MRA provides accurate information regarding the entry and re-entry sites of the dissection, the length of the intimal flap, and the patency of branch vessels (340).

The inability of MRI to consistently demonstrate small calcifications is not of clinical significance in most patients. However, in the rare case of complete thrombosis of the false channel, the detection of an intimal flap by MRI may not be possible. In these patients, eccentric (or rarely concentric) aortic wall thickening may be the only sign of acute dissection (358). The wall thickening may be inhomogeneous with hyperintense foci and linear streaks or, less commonly, may be homogeneously isointense with muscle on the T1-weighted images (358).

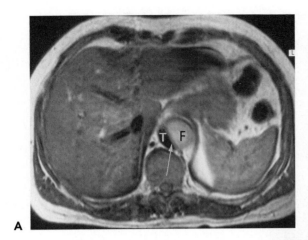

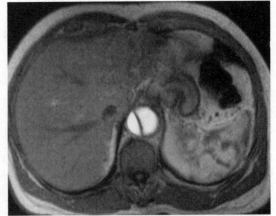

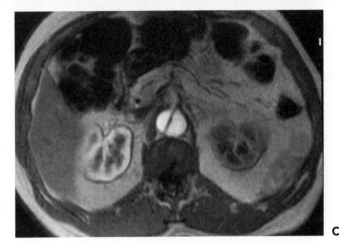

Figure 17-28 Aortic dissection. **A:** Transaxial gated T1-weighted spin echo image (repetition time, 1,219 milliseconds; echo time, 25 milliseconds) shows an intimal flap (*arrow*). Flow void in the true lumen (T) is a result of high-velocity flow, while signal in the false lumen (F) is a result of slow flow or thrombosis. **B:** Post-gadolinium T1-weighted fast low-angle shot image (repetition time, 140 milliseconds; echo time, 4 milliseconds; flip angle, 80 degrees) at the same level shows enhancement of both lumens with better delineation of the intimal flap. **C:** Image obtained at the level of the superior mesenteric artery takeoff demonstrates poor enhancement of the left kidney because of renal artery involvement.

Abdominal Aortic Aneurysm—Surgical and Endovascular Repair

Repair of an AAA can be performed with either a traditional open procedure or with more recently introduced endovascular techniques. In the former method, performed via either a transabdominal or retroperitoneal incision, the aneurysm sac is opened and a graft is inserted with its proximal end sewn to uninvolved aorta proximal to the aneurysm and its distal end either sewn to uninvolved aorta (tube graft) or to uninvolved common iliac or femoral vessels (bilimbed graft). The aneurysm sac is then closed over the graft and acts as a protective shell to decrease the incidence of postoperative AEFs. Endovascular repair involves the placement of an expandable stented graft that bridges the AAA either as a single-limbed or bifurcated graft (Figs. 17-29 and 17-30). The stent is placed via a femoral artery arteriotomy and guided fluoroscopically into position (233).

Although the first Western report of a successful repair of an AAA by endovascular approach was published in 1991 (242), results have been promising and demonstrate little difference in the mortality rates of endovascular

repair and conventional surgery (1,200,217). Advantages of endovascular repair include shorter hospital and/or intensive care stay, less blood loss, and fewer systemic complications (1,200). However, endovascular repair costs more than surgery and has a higher graft failure rate than conventional surgery (200).

Radiologic evaluation of an AAA is important before either open or endovascular repair. Prior to open repair it is important to note the size and extent of the AAA, involvement of the iliac vessels, and relationship of major vascular branches (renal arteries, superior mesenteric artery, celiac artery, inferior mesenteric artery). The presence of anomalous venous structures or horseshoe kidney should be noted, as well as the presence of inflammatory change about the aorta. Concomitant intraabdominal pathology, such as renal or colonic tumors or gallstones, should also be reported (148).

Careful patient selection is also of critical importance for a successful endovascular aneurysm repair (Fig. 17-31). Although precise criteria will differ depending on the device used, in general there should be at least 1.5 to 2 cm of normal caliber aorta proximal to the AAA and distal to the renal ostia. This "neck" should be cylindrical in shape,

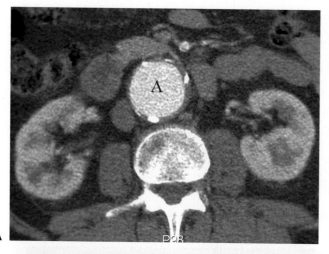

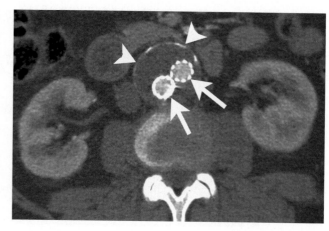

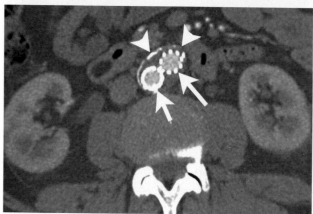

Figure 17-29 Abdominal aortic aneurysm treated with endograft repair. **A:** Contrast-enhanced axial computed tomography image of the abdominal aorta (A) with aneurysm and atherosclerotic changes. **B:** 2 months post–endograft repair of abdominal aortic aneurysm shows decrease in sac (*arrowhead*) size with endograft (*arrows*) in place. **C:** 8 months post–endograft repair of abdominal aortic aneurysm shows further decrease in sac (*arrowheads*) size with endograft (*arrows*) in place.

without significant flaring and should be free of thrombus. The angle between the neck and AAA should be less than 60 degrees. If the distal "landing" zone of the endovascular graft is in the aorta, it needs to be 2 to 2.5 cm in length, normal in caliber, and free of thrombus. In the more common situation, in which a bilimbed graft is used, the iliac vessels must be of normal caliber without significant tortuosity. If external iliac vessels are used, the internal iliac arteries must be embolized to prevent back filling of the aneurysm (233). The common and external iliac arteries must also be wide enough to accommodate the delivery device, although localized iliac stenosis is not itself a contraindication to endovascular repair since angioplasty can be performed at the time of the procedure. The presence of aberrant or accessory renal vessels or a patent inferior mesenteric artery or lumbar arteries should be noted. If they arise from the aneurysm sack, they may contribute to a persistent endoleak after the procedure or, if occluded by the graft, cause downstream ischemia if sufficient collaterals do not exist (233). Renal artery stenosis also may contribute to renal impairment and increases the risk of the procedure. The presence of perianeurysmal fibrosis or inflammatory change should also be noted, although its role in patient selection is controversial (329).

In conventional surgical repair, the size of the graft is determined by direct inspection of the vessels involved. In contradistinction, endovascular graft sizing is obtained noninvasively and typically involves either CTA or, less commonly, MRA (225,319,348). Measurements of diameter are best taken from planar images orthogonal to the long axis of the vessel and reflect the distance from wall to wall rather than lumen edge to lumen edge. Longitudinal measurements are typically taken from curved planar reconstructions along the centerline of the lumen. Commercially available software using CTA or MRA source data can expedite preoperative planning. Some versions allow the operator to place a 3D model of the proposed endograft within a 3D representation of the patient's aorta to preoperatively check fit (348).

Surgically Placed Aortic Grafts: Postoperative Complications and Evaluation

Aortic grafts are performed for replacing aneurysms and bypassing occlusive vascular disease. Their imaging appearance depends on the type of anastomoses performed and whether the graft is laid within the sac of the existing aneurysm (149).

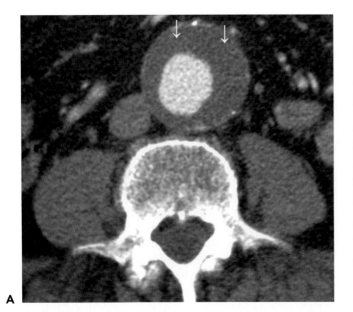

A

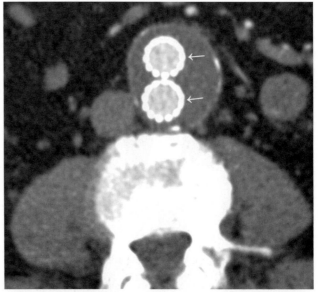

B

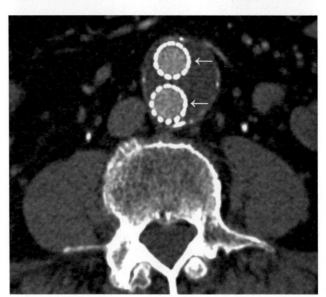

C

Figure 17-30 Abdominal aortic aneurysm treated with endograft repair. **A:** Contrast-enhanced axial computed tomography scan shows infrarenal aortic aneurysm with thrombus (*arrows*). **B:** 9 months following endograft (*arrows*) repair, the aneurysm sac has shrunk slightly in size. **C:** 16 months following endograft repair, there has been some further reduction in aneurysm sac size.

Postoperative aortas can be distinguished from native atherosclerotic aortas because the graft is of slightly higher attenuation than unenhanced blood on noncontrast CT scans and its lumen is perfectly round and smooth, whereas the patent lumen of an atherosclerosic aorta is usually slightly irregular. On MRI, the prosthetic graft itself does not produce any signal. In the case of an end-to-side anastomosis, the graft is seen ventral to the native aorta. The iliac branches of the graft are seen as two dense circular structures anterior to the calcified native iliac arteries, which are commonly thrombosed. The bifurcation of the graft is usually located 2 to 3 cm cephalad to the native aortic bifurcation.

The CT appearance of end-to-end anastomosis differs from that of end-to-side anastomosis in its complete interruption of the native aorta at the anastomotic site. Therefore, the distal native aorta is not opacified on postcontrast scans. In patients who have an end-to-end anastomosis

within the sac of an aneurysm (endoaneurysmorrhaphy), the aneurysm sac is wrapped around the graft to provide an additional layer between the graft and bowel to reduce the risk of AEF formation. A collection of serous fluid or soft tissue attenuation often can be identified between the synthetic graft and the native aortic wrap. This collection usually resolves by 2 to 4 months (257). Similarly, perigraft air may be seen in the immediate postoperative period (up to 38% of patients 6 to 9 days postsurgery) but usually resolves by three weeks (232,236,295). Larger aneurysms typically showed more periprosthetic air (232).

On MRI, a collection of fluid between the aneurysm sac and graft, which shows relatively low signal intensity on T1-weighted images and high signal intensity on T2-weighted images, is routinely seen on MRI studies obtained within several weeks of surgery and should be considered abnormal if present after 3 months (15). After

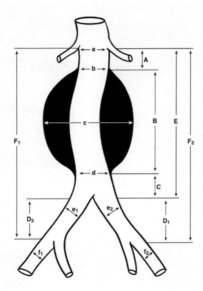

Figure 17-31 Measurements important for endovascular aneurysm repair. Diameter of: the aneurysm neck at the lowest renal artery (a), of the aorta 1.5 cm below the renal arteries (b), of the aneurysm sac (c), of the aorta 1.5 cm above the bifurcation (d), of the common iliac arteries (e1, e2), of the external iliac arteries (f1, f2). Length of the proximal aneurysm neck (A), of the abdominal aortic aneurysm (AAA) (B), of the distal aneurysm neck (C), of the common iliac arteries (D1, D2). Angle between the proximal neck and the AAA is also measured. (Adapted from Thurnher SA, Dorffner R, Thurnher MM, et al. Evaluation of abdominal aortic aneurysm for stent-graft placement: comparison of gadolinium-enhanced MR angiography versus helical CT angiography and digital subtraction angiography. *Radiology* 1997;205:341–352.)

7 to 10 weeks, a perigraft collar of low signal intensity is often seen on T1- and T2-weighted images and likely represents fibrosis or the wall of the native aorta adherent to the graft (graft incorporation) (15).

Postoperative complications of abdominal aortic graft surgery include hemorrhage and pseudoaneurysm formation, major vessel or graft limb occlusion, infection, and AEF (see Figs. 17-23 and 17-24). When acute hemorrhage is suspected, a noncontrast CT scan is often helpful for identification of the increased attenuation of fresh blood. Pseudoaneurysms typically occur at the anastomotic suture line and are more common in the femoral area than in the aortoiliac system (295). In one study of 69 patients with pseudoaneurysms, the time between graft insertion and pseudoaneurysm detection ranged from 1 to 238 months, with a median time of 92 months (331). Anastomotic pseudoaneurysms appear as paragraft collections containing thrombus. Portions of the pseudoaneurysm may communicate with the aortic lumen and enhance to the same degree on postcontrast scans. In other patients, the entire pseudoaneurysm may be filled with thrombus and appear as a diverticulum (101). The diagnosis of graft occlusion is based on the demonstration of a low-density lumen representing thrombus, with a lack of enhancement after administration of contrast medium.

Graft infection is the most serious complication of abdominal aortic graft surgery, with a mortality rate of 25% to 88% (39). Although diagnosis may be obvious, particularly if a femoral anastomoses is involved, it is often more subtle if the proximal aortic limb only is infected (39,236). Typically, when a graft becomes infected, an irregular collection of fluid and soft tissue attenuation is seen around the prosthesis, sometimes associated with multiple small bubbles of gas located posterior to or around the entire graft (195) (see Figs. 17-24). This is in contradistinction to a "normal" gas collection seen in the immediate postoperative period, which usually is solitary and anterior in location (103). Discontinuity of the enveloping aneurysm wrap and increased soft tissue/fluid (greater than 5 mm) between the wrap and graft have also been cited as signs of infection (195). Because gas and soft tissue/fluid may be a normal finding in the immediate postoperative period, needle aspiration of a suspicious perigraft collection is advised in any patient with suspected infection. Periprosthetic collections beyond three months after surgery, and periprosthetic gas beyond 4 to 7 weeks from surgery should be considered highly suspicious for infection (236). Although the overall sensitivity and specificity of CT for infection is high (195), nuclear medicine gallium scanning and labeled leukocyte scans may also be of value (144,295).

On MRI, perigraft abscesses appear as fluid collections that have low to medium signal intensity (iso- or hyperintense to muscle) on T1-weighted images and high intensity on T2-weighted images (iso- or hyperintense to fat) (146). Inflammation in surrounding tissues, characterized by a heterogeneous increased signal intensity of the psoas muscles adjacent to the graft, also can be seen (15). Gadolinium-enhanced T1-weighted fat-suppressed imaging accentuates the contrast difference between nonenhancing low signal abscess fluid and adjacent enhancing inflammatory tissue. However, the infected nature of the fluid cannot be ascertained on the basis of MR signal intensities alone. A significant limitation of MRI is its inability to detect small collections of gas. In addition, MRI cannot reliably differentiate between a collection of gas and a small cluster of calcifications (146).

Secondary AEF occurs between an aortic graft and adjacent bowel. CT features of secondary AEF are similar to those of graft infection and include perigraft soft tissue/fluid and extraluminal air (195). Although not specific, thickening of the small bowel, especially the third portion of the duodenum, adjacent to paragraft fluid, is highly suggestive of an AEF. Additional findings, such as extravasation of oral contrast material around the graft, intravasation of intravenous contrast material into unopacified small bowel, or small bowel hematomas, are rare.

Endografts: Postoperative Complications and Evaluation

Although endovascular stented grafts can be associated with many of the complications of surgically placed grafts, including

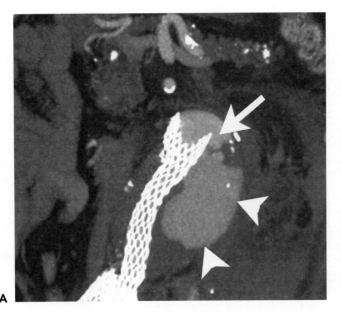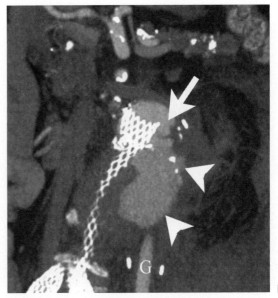

Figure 17-32 Type 1 endograft leak. **A, B:** Contrast-enhanced coronal computed tomography images demonstrate attempted endograft repair of an abdominal aortic aneurysm with a type 1 leak (*arrowheads*) originating at the neck of the graft (*arrow*). Infiltration of the fat in the left side of the retroperitoneum is sequela of recent iliac to left renal artery graft (G).

infection and rupture (243), they have unique problems that require long term follow-up and monitoring. These include, most prominently, endoleaks, continued aneurysm growth, endograft occlusion, and displacement or disruption of the stent itself (233,348). Endovascular stented graft leaks (endoleaks) are divided into four types (348,349):

Type 1 endoleak results from an incomplete seal at the proximal or distal end of the graft and the adjacent native aorta or iliac wall (Fig. 17-32).

Type 2 endoleak occurs when blood flows in a retrograde fashion into the aneurysm from patent aortic branch vessels (e.g., lumbar arteries, inferior mesenteric artery, accessory renal arteries) (Figs. 17-33 and 17-34).

Type 3 endoleak leaks occur from either a tear in the endograft fabric or other stent graft structural failure (Fig. 17-35).

Type 4 leaks are associated with porous graft material.

CT is the preferred modality for postoperative evaluation of endografts (11,193,263,) and may have a role in guiding percutaneous embolization of some endoleaks. The metallic stents are well visualized and allow direct evaluation of stent location and integrity. Intravenous contrast enhancement is necessary to evaluate endoleaks. These appear as collections of contrast within the aneurysmal sac. Biphasic scanning is suggested as some slow endoleaks are not apparent on the initial arterial phase images (92,281). Unenhanced scanning preceding the enhanced scans has also been suggested to be of benefit in distinguishing calcification from contrast leakage (281).

Reproducible evaluation of aneurysm size is crucial to ensure adequate exclusion of the aneurysm. Successful endograft placement will usually result in shrinkage of the aneurysm sac although this may depend on the type of graft employed (26,74). Any increase in aneurysm size is cause for concern, because progressive enlargement and rupture may occur even in the absence of demonstrable endoleak (323,350). The mechanism for this increase in aneurysm size is unclear but appears to result from increased pressure (termed endotension) within the aneurysm (66,350). Intravenous contrast–enhanced MRI has also been used successfully in the evaluation of endografts constructed with metals of low magnetic susceptibility, such as nickel–titanium alloys (nitinol) (76,133,193). Stainless steel–based stents cannot be adequately evaluated by MRI because of significant artifact (133,318). The use of MRI is favored in patients with impaired renal function or allergy to iodinated contrast and in younger patients in whom repeated examinations with ionizing radiation may be problematic (318).

INFERIOR VENA CAVA AND ITS TRIBUTARIES

Normal Anatomy

The IVC is formed by the confluence of the two common iliac veins at the level of the fifth lumbar vertebra. From this point, it ascends along the vertebral column to the

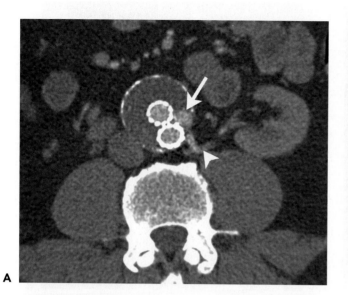

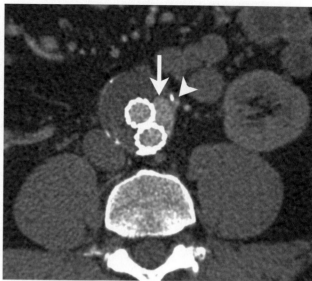

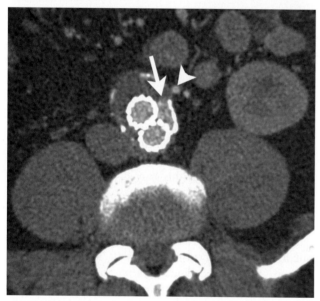

Figure 17-33 Type 2 endograft leaks. **A:** Contrast-enhanced axial computed tomography shows type 2 endograft leak (*arrow*) at site of entry of accessory left renal artery (*arrowhead*). **B:** Type 2 endograft leak (*arrow*) is also noted at the origin of the inferior mesenteric artery (*arrowhead*). **C:** Type 2 endograft leak (*arrow*). Inferior mesenteric artery (*arrowhead*).

right of the aorta to the level of the diaphragm and enters the chest terminating in the right atrium. Although it is in close proximity to the lumbar vertebral bodies in its most caudal position, it assumes a more ventral position at its cephalic end.

The shape, which may be round or flat, and the size of the IVC vary from patient to patient and even in the same patient at different levels. Performance of a Valsalva maneuver usually results in more distension of the IVC in normal subjects. In patients undergoing CT for abdominal trauma, a flat IVC at multiple levels may be a sign of hypovolemia resulting from major hemorrhage (139,299). In some cases, the demonstration of the collapsed IVC may precede the clinical detection of shock (139). It is important to note that a flattened IVC may also be seen in normotensive patients and may be related to respiratory variation as well as fluid status. In a study of 500 patients imaged for

nontraumatic indications, a flat IVC was noted at one or more level in 70 patients. Of these patients, only 30% had evidence of hypotension or hypovolemia (69). The renal veins, which are located ventral to the renal arteries, often can be seen in their entirety entering the vena cava. The left renal vein usually is longer than the right and passes across the midline between the abdominal aorta and the superior mesenteric artery. The main hepatic veins and their tributaries converge into the vena cava near the diaphragm. A small, oval collection of fat that lies medial to the IVC at or above the level of confluence of the hepatic veins and the IVC may be seen in approximately 0.5% of patients (214). It may occasionally mimic an intravascular lipoma or clot (123,262,285). This collection is contiguous with the fat around the subdiaphragmatic portion of the esophagus, and its presence or absence is not related to obesity (214).

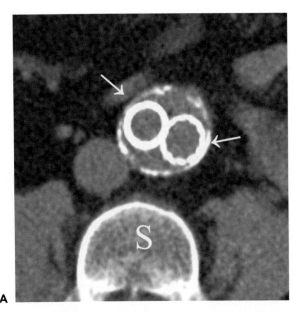

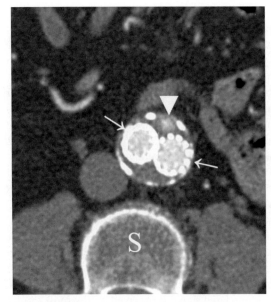

Figure 17-34 Type 2 endograft leak. **A:** Noncontrast axial computed tomography (CT) image obtained 1 month following endograft (*arrows*) repair of an abdominal aortic aneurysm. S, spine. **B:** Contrast-enhanced axial CT image obtained one month following endograft repair shows small leak (*arrowhead*) near origin of the inferior mesenteric artery that is consistent with a type 2 backflow leak.

The IVC, the iliac veins, and the renal veins can be easily seen even on noncontrast CT scans. The main hepatic veins and their tributaries also can be seen on noncontrast scans because they have a slightly lower attenuation than the normal hepatic parenchyma. At least a portion of normal caliber gonadal vein can be traced on consecutive contrast-enhanced scans in a majority of patients. Whereas the right gonadal vein drains directly into the IVC, approximately 4 cm below the junction of the right renal vein and the IVC (269), the left gonadal vein usually

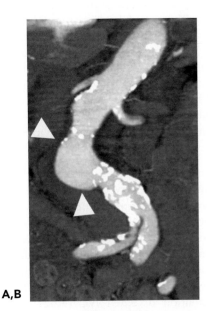

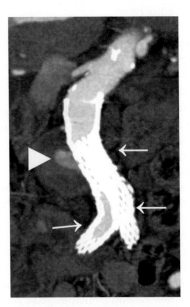

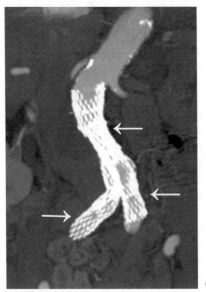

Figure 17-35 Type 3 endograft leak. **A:** Contrast-enhanced coronal maximum-intensity projection computed tomography image shows infrarenal aortic aneurysm (*arrowheads*). **B:** 1 month post–endograft placement, a type 3 leak is seen (*arrowhead*). *Arrows*, endograft. **C:** 4 months after endograft placement there has been resolution of the previously noted leak in the sac. The endograft (*arrows*) remains in place.

drains into the left renal vein. Below the left renal vein, the left gonadal vein is often seen posterior to the inferior mesenteric vein and anterior to the left psoas muscle. The gonadal veins may be enlarged in multiparous women and in men with varicoceles.

The attenuation value of the lumen of the IVC is similar to that of the abdominal aorta and thus varies with the hematocrit of the patient. However, in comparison to the aortic wall, the wall of the IVC is thin and rarely visible as a discrete structure, even in severely anemic patients.

The IVC and its tributaries are also well delineated by MRI because of the excellent contrast between vascular structures with flowing blood and adjacent soft tissue. The normal IVC demonstrates no intraluminal signal on SE images but appears as a high signal intensity structure on GRE sequences. As in the aorta, a flow-related enhancement effect (also called slice-entry phenomenon) can produce a signal in the IVC when transverse SE images are obtained. Unlike the aorta, the flow-related signal is observed on the most caudal slice of the imaged volume because of the opposite direction of the flow of blood.

Normal Variations (Congenital Anomalies)

Knowledge of the various developmental anomalies of the venous system and recognition of their CT/MRI appearances are critical for proper image interpretation and patient management. Venous anomalies may be mistaken for adenopathy or other pathology. Azygus continuation of the IVC may mimic aortic dissection (203). Preoperative identification of a venous anomaly may prevent iatrogenic injury particularly with abdominal aortic surgery (294). An association of IVC anomalies with other anomalies (e.g., asplenia, polysplenia, renal aplasia) as well as with deep venous thrombosis has also been noted (8,20,47,88,89,230).

The IVC is formed by the successive development and regression of three paired veins, the posterior cardinal, subcardinal, and supracardinal systems (23,81,207,213) (Fig. 17-36). The posterior cardinal system develops first at approximately six weeks but regresses without forming any of the normal IVC, although failure of complete regression of this segment is felt to be responsible for retrocaval ureter. The right subcardinal system, developing at 7 weeks, forms the IVC cephalad to the renal veins and anastomoses with the developing hepatic vessels to form the intrahepatic IVC. Anastomosis of the right and left subcardinal systems forms the normal left renal vein. The remainder of the subcardinal system regresses. The right supracardinal system, developing at approximately 8 weeks, forms the azygus system cephalad to the renal veins and the IVC caudal to the renal veins. The left supracardinal system gives rise to the hemiazygus system cephalad to the renal veins and normally regresses caudal to the renal vein.

Abnormal or absent regression of any of these venous structures results in different anomalies. For example, infrahepatic

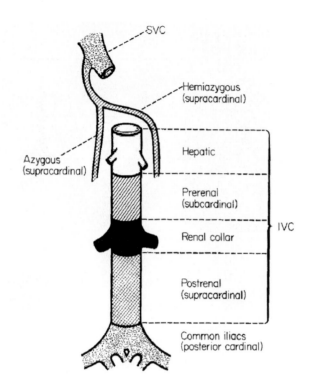

Figure 17-36 Schematic drawing showing the precursors of different segments of the inferior vena cava.

interruption of the IVC with azygus continuation occurs with failure of union of the right subcardinal system with the developing hepatic veins. Duplication of the IVC results from incomplete regression of the left supracardinal system. Schematic representations of these various anomalies are shown in Figure 17-37. Most of these venous anomalies can be confidently diagnosed on noncontrast CT or MRI scans by tracing their course on contiguous slices. If confusion persists, the vascular nature of these structures can be proven by intravenous contrast material administration. Whereas contiguous transverse CT or MR images are adequate for defining the anomalous venous anatomy, the entire system can be displayed more elegantly by 3D reconstructions of CTA or MRA data.

Interrupted Inferior Vena Cava with Azygos/Hemiazygos Continuation

When the right subcardinal vein fails to connect with the hepatic veins, blood returns to the heart through the azygos/hemiazygos system and the hepatic veins drain directly into the right atrium (Fig. 17-38). Rare variations include portal and hemiazygos continuation of the IVC (81) and hemiazygos continuation of a left IVC (32,223). This anomaly is seen with a prevalence of 0.6% and usually occurs as an isolated lesion (23). Occasionally, it can be associated with cardiac abnormalities, or other visceral anomalies such as the polysplenia syndromes (8,87).

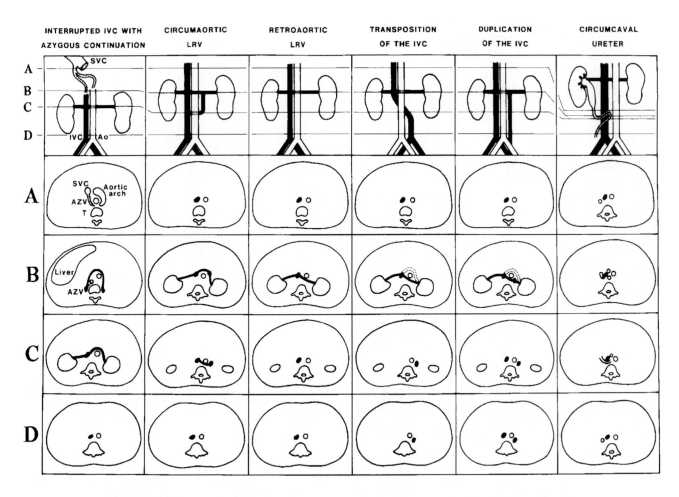

INTERRUPTED IVC WITH AZYGOUS CONTINUATION	CIRCUMAORTIC LRV	RETROAORTIC LRV	TRANSPOSITION OF THE IVC	DUPLICATION OF THE IVC	CIRCUMCAVAL URETER

Figure 17-37 Drawings showing relationships of aorta, inferior vena cava, and left renal vein in various congenital venous anomalies. (Adapted from Royal SA, Callen PW. CT evaluation of anomalies of the inferior vena cava and left renal vein. *J Comput Assist Tomogr* 1979;15:690–693.)

On transverse CT or MRI study, a normal IVC is seen from the confluence of the common iliac veins to the level of both kidneys. An intrahepatic segment of the IVC, which lies anterior to the right diaphragmatic crus and posterior to the caudate lobe of the liver, is absent. However, an enlarged azygos vein and often a hemiazygos vein as well can be seen in the retrocrural space on both sides of the aorta. The azygos vein can be further traced on more cephalic scans to the level where it arches anteriorly to join the superior vena cava just below the level of the aortic arch.

Circumaortic Left Renal Vein

There is a true vascular ring about the aorta in this anomaly. The preaortic left renal vein crosses from the left kidney to the IVC at the expected level of the renal veins. The additional retroaortic left renal vein(s) connects to the IVC by descending caudally and crossing the spine behind the aorta, usually one to two vertebrae below the level of the preaortic left renal vein (Fig. 17-39). Typically, the left gonadal vein drains into the aberrant retroaortic renal vein. This retroaortic renal vein is felt to represent a remnant of

the left supracardinal system and intrasupracardinal anastomosis and has a prevalence of 1.6% (3). On a CT or an MRI study, a normal, albeit somewhat diminutive, left renal vein can be seen in its preaortic position. The anomalous retroaortic left renal vein is identified in a more caudal position.

Retroaortic Left Renal Vein

In this anomaly, the anterior subcardinal veins regress completely and only the retroaortic left supracardinal vein and its anastomoses with the right supracardinal vein remain to drain the left kidney. The retroaortic left renal vein can be seen either at the same level as a normal left renal vein or in a more caudal position, sometimes as low as the confluence of iliac veins (Fig. 17-40). The prevalence of this anomaly is about 3% (3).

Left Inferior Vena Cava

Anomalous regression of the right supracardinal vein and persistence of the left supracardinal system result in transposition of the IVC. In this entity, a single IVC ascends on

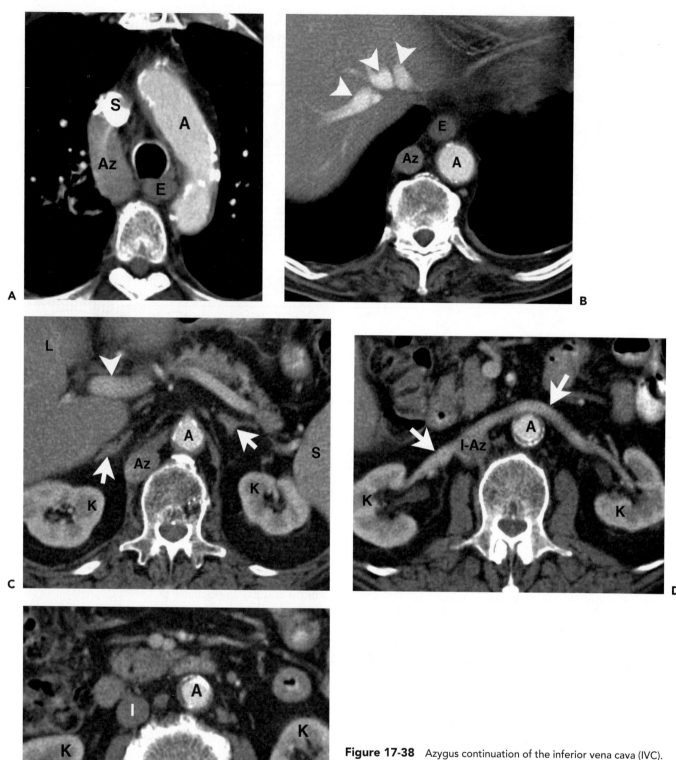

Figure 17-38 Azygus continuation of the inferior vena cava (IVC). **A:** Contrast-enhanced computed tomography scan shows prominent azygus arch (Az) emptying into superior vena cava (S). *A*, aorta; *E*, esophagus. **B:** At the level of the diaphragm, hepatic veins empty directly into the right atrium. Azygus vein is prominent. A, aorta; Az, azygus vein; E, esophagus. **C:** At level of porta vein (*arrowhead*), no intrahepatic IVC is present. Azygus vein (Az) is prominent. L, liver; S, spleen; K, kidney; *arrow*, adrenals. **D:** At the level of the renal veins (*arrows*), the azygus becomes the IVC (I-Az). K, kidney. **E:** A normal infrarenal IVC (I) is present. A, aorta; K, kidney.

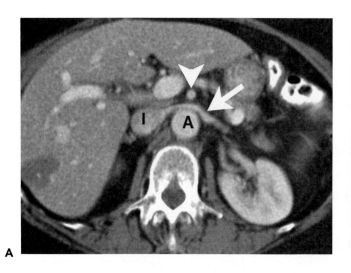

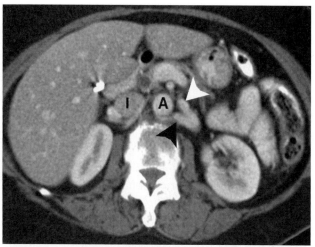

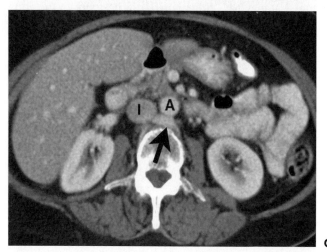

Figure 17-39 Circumaortic left renal vein. **A:** Contrast-enhanced computed tomography scan shows anterior portion of left renal vein (*arrow*) passing between the superior mesenteric artery (*arrowhead*) and aorta (A). I, inferior vena cava. **B:** The left renal vein divides into anterior and posterior branches (*arrowheads*). **C:** Retroaortic component of left renal vein is seen running posterior to aorta (A) to empty into inferior vena cava (I).

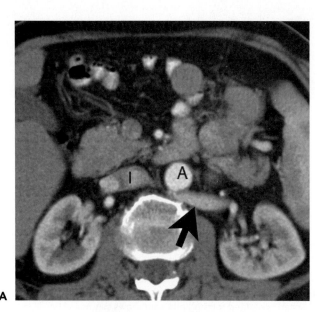

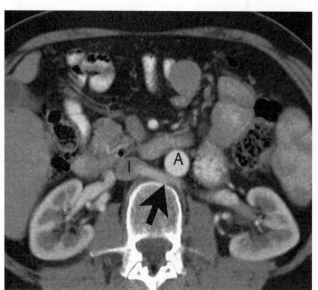

Figure 17-40 Retroaortic left renal vein. **A, B:** Contrast-enhanced computed tomography scan shows retroaortic left renal vein (*arrows*) extending behind the aorta (A) and emptying into the inferior vena cava (I).

the left side of the spine and crosses either anterior or posterior to the aorta at the level of the renal veins to ascend further to the right atrium on the right side of the spine. The characteristic appearance on CT or transverse MRI examination is a single IVC to the right of the aorta at levels above the renal vein, a vascular structure either crossing anterior or posterior to the aorta at the level of the renal veins, and a large single IVC to the left of the spine at levels below the renal veins (Fig. 17-41). The prevalence of this anomaly is 0.2% (3).

Duplication of the Inferior Vena Cava
In duplication of the IVC, there is an IVC, albeit smaller than usual in size, along the right side of the spine. In addition, a left-sided IVC ascends to the level of the renal veins to join the right-sided IVC through a vascular structure that may pass either anterior or posterior to the aorta at the level of the renal veins. Either vena cava can be the predominant vessel or they can be of equal size. This anomaly results from the persistence of both surpracardinal

veins and has a prevalence of 0.4% (3). On a CT or an MRI study, a single right-sided IVC is seen at levels above the renal veins. A vascular structure crossing either anterior or posterior to the aorta is seen at the level of the renal veins, and two vena cavae, one on each side of the aorta, are present below the level of the renal veins (Fig. 17-42). A duplicated left IVC can be differentiated from a dilated left gonadal vein by following its course on the more caudad scans. Whereas a duplicated left IVC joins the common iliac vein, a dilated left gonadal vein can be traced further inferiorly to the level of the inguinal canal.

Circumcaval Ureter (Synonym, Retrocaval Ureter)
Embryologically, a circumcaval ureter results from anomalous regression of the caudal segment of the right supracardinal vein and the persistence of the right posterior cardinal vein. Consequently, the ureter passes behind and around the medial aspect of the IVC as it courses to the bladder. Although more commonly described on the right, a left retrocaval ureter associated with a left IVC also has

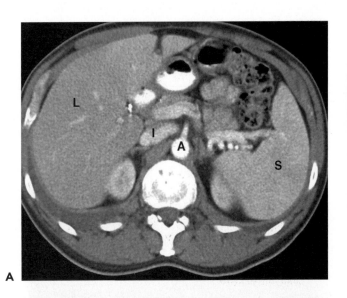

A

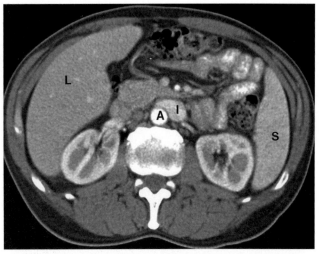

B

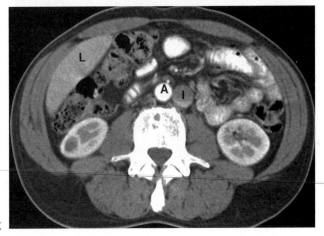

C

Figure 17-41 Left-sided inferior vena cava (IVC). **A:** Contrast-enhanced computed tomography scan shows suprarenal IVC (I) in the normal location. A, aorta; L, liver; S, spleen. **B:** IVC (I) crosses to left via left renal vein. **C:** IVC (I) remains to left of aorta (A). No normally positioned IVC is seen on the right.

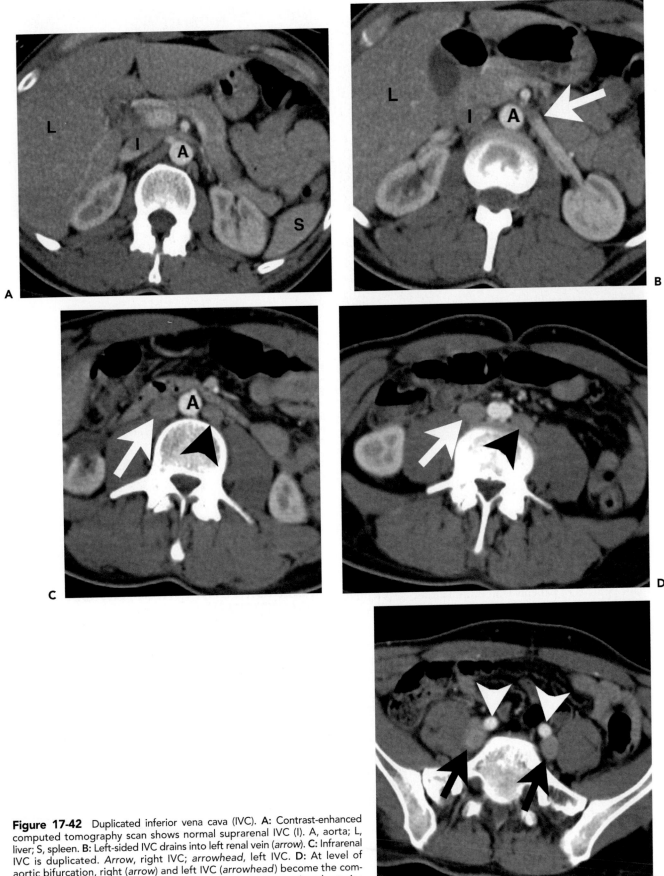

Figure 17-42 Duplicated inferior vena cava (IVC). **A:** Contrast-enhanced computed tomography scan shows normal suprarenal IVC (I). A, aorta; L, liver; S, spleen. **B:** Left-sided IVC drains into left renal vein (*arrow*). **C:** Infrarenal IVC is duplicated. *Arrow,* right IVC; *arrowhead,* left IVC. **D:** At level of aortic bifurcation, right (*arrow*) and left IVC (*arrowhead*) become the common iliac veins. **E:** Left and right common iliac veins (*arrows*) and arteries (*arrowheads*).

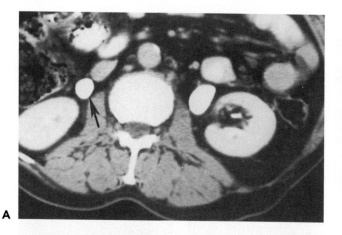

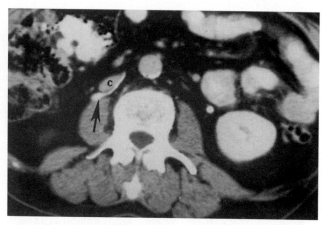

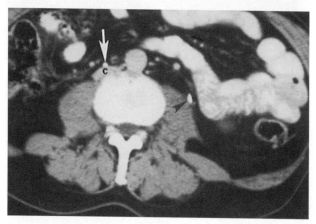

Figure 17-43 Circumcaval ureter. **A:** Postcontrast computed tomography image demonstrates a dilated proximal right ureter (*arrow*). **B:** At 1 cm caudal to (**A**), the right ureter (*arrow*) passes behind the inferior vena cava (c). **C:** At 1 cm caudal to (**B**), the right ureter (*arrow*) lies anterior to the inferior vena cava (c). This is in contrast to the normal left ureter (*arrowhead*), which lies along the anterolateral aspect of the psoas muscle.

been described (247). As in other types of vena caval anomalies, circumcaval ureter may be discovered as an incidental radiographic finding. However, patients with this condition sometimes present with signs and symptoms related to right ureteral obstruction. Whereas asymptomatic patients or patients with minimal caliectasis require only occasional follow-up, patients with significant renal obstruction often require surgical correction.

Circumcaval ureter has a characteristic appearance on excretory urography (medial deviation of the upper one third of the ureter with sharp turn toward the pedicle of the third or fourth lumbar vertebra producing a "reverse J" configuration). However, a definitive diagnosis by conventional imaging methods often requires concomitant opacification of the ureter and IVC. CT can simplify the diagnostic process. With CT, the proximal right ureter can be seen coursing medially behind and then anteriorly around the IVC so as to encircle it partially (Fig. 17-43). Three-dimensional rendering of images taken in the excretory phase has been reported to show the abnormality clearly (246).

Other Rare Anomalies

Other rare IVC anomalies have also been reported, including congenital portacaval shunts (18), absence of the

infrarenal IVC with preservation of the suprarenal segment (22), and combinations of previously described anomalies, such as duplicated IVC with azygus continuation (213).

INFERIOR VENA CAVA—PATHOLOGIC CONDITIONS

Aneurysm of the Inferior Vena Cava

IVC aneurysms are quite rare and can be classified as congenital (e.g., failure of regression or abnormal fusion of embryologic venous structures) or acquired (secondary to trauma, inflammation, increased flow, or pressure). Typically, these are true aneurysms containing all three layers of the normal wall, although the elastic and muscular layers may be attenuated (41). The lesions may be asymptomatic or present with symptoms secondary to thrombosis, obstruction, or embolism (192,309). The aneurysm may also mimic a solid tumor in appearance.

On contrast-enhanced CT or MRI, the aneurysm appears as a saccular or fusiform dilation of the IVC (Fig. 17-44) (292,367). Contrast enhancement may demonstrate the vascular nature of the lesion; however, mixing phenomenon or thrombosis may cause the lesion to mimic a solid

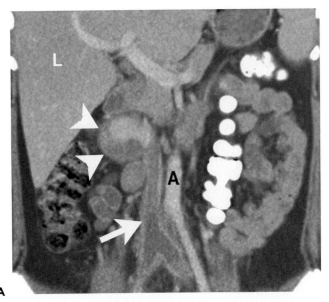

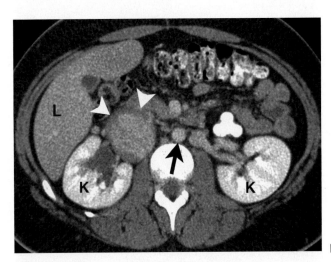

Figure 17-44 Inferior vena cava (IVC) aneurysm. **A:** Coronal reconstruction of intravenous contrast-enhanced computed tomography scan shows rounded structure with heterogeneous enhancement (*arrowheads*) coming off the right side of the IVC (*arrow*). Note extensive thrombosis within IVC. A, aorta; L, liver **B:** Axial image demonstrates IVC aneurysm (*arrowheads*), with mixing of contrast and unopacified blood. A, aorta; L, liver; K, kidney; *arrow*, aorta.

neoplasm (59). The "layered gadolinium" sign of normal hyperintense-enhanced blood sitting on top of a dark hypointense layer in the aneurysm has been described as a sign of an abdominal venous aneurysm (168).

Venous Thrombosis

Thrombosis in the IVC and other retroperitoneal veins may result from a variety of disorders. Surgical trauma,

inflammation, obstruction to outflow by retroperitoneal adenopathy or intravascular membrane, extension of thrombus from iliac or renal veins, and hypercoagulable states have all been reported to induce thrombosis (Figs. 17-45 and 17-46) (24). Similarly, intravascular tumor thrombus has been reported with a variety of neoplasms, including renal cell, transitional cell, adrenal cortical, and hepatocellular carcinoma, leiomyosarcoma, and malignant fibrohistiocytoma (Figs. 17-47 to 17-49) (48,72,147,215).

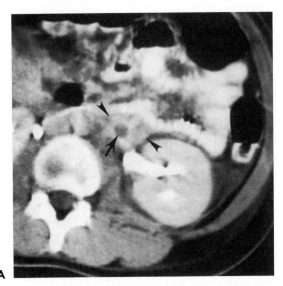

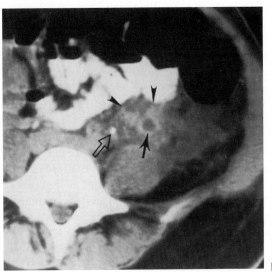

Figure 17-45 Postpartum septic thrombosis of the left ovarian vein. Sequential postcontrast computed tomography images demonstrate a thrombosed left ovarian vein (*arrow*) and its surrounding inflammatory changes (*arrowheads*) *Open arrow*, left ureter.

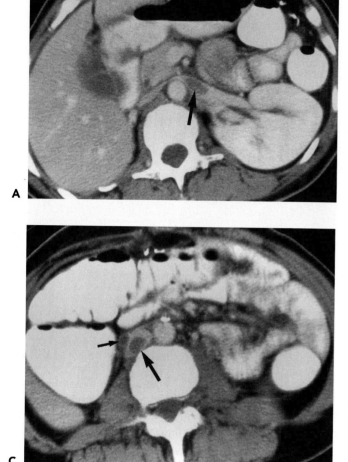

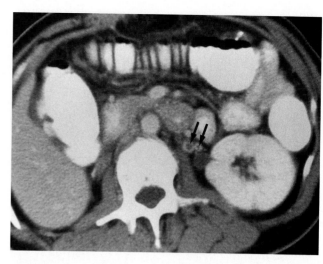

Figure 17-46 Thrombosis of multiple vessels in a patient with ovarian cancer: computed tomography (CT) appearance. Contrast-enhanced CT scan shows intraluminal hypodense filling defects representing thrombi within the opacified lumens of the left renal vein (*arrow*) (**A**), left gonadal veins (*arrows*) (**B**), and right gonadal vein (*small arrow*) and IVC (*large arrow*) (**C**).

The definitive diagnosis of venous thrombosis using CT depends on demonstration of an intraluminal thrombus (Fig. 17-50). Whereas a fresh thrombus has a density similar to or higher than that of circulating blood, an old thrombus is of lower density than the surrounding blood on non-contrast scans. In acute thrombosis, the vessel may appear larger than normal. This increased size is usually more focal than the generalized dilatation seen secondary to increased blood flow or increased vascular resistance at the level of the diaphragm/right atrium. However, in the case of chronic occlusion, the IVC may become atrophic and calcified. Following contrast administration, the thrombus will appear as either a low-density filling defect surrounded by contrast-enhanced blood, in the case of partial obstruction, or as a low-density mass obstructing the lumen. In acute thrombosis increased thickness and enhancement of the vessel wall may also be observed. Caution must be taken not to confuse true intraluminal defects with those caused by the laminar flow phenomenon in the dynamic stage of contrast administration. In this nonequilibrium

phase, slower flowing enhanced blood may stay closest to the vessel wall, with unopacified blood flowing centrally, suggesting a luminal thrombus. This "pseudothrombus" artifact is most noticeable in the suprarenal cava, where it is caused by poor mixing between the densely opacified renal venous effluent and the less densely opacified infrarenal caval blood (Fig. 17-51). This artifact can be differentiated from a true thrombus by its unsharp border, and the high attenuation of the pseudothrombus. The use of delayed equilibrium scans, in which adequate time has passed for homogeneous venous opacification, is recommended when venous thrombosis is suspected. Such delayed scans (beginning 3 minutes after the start of contrast administration) looking for the IVC and more proximal thrombus have been suggested as a useful adjunct in patients undergoing CT pulmonary angiography (194). In cases of complete caval obstruction, extensive venous collaterals may also be identified by CT (237). These include the paravertebral venous system and its communications with the ascending lumbar veins and the azygos/hemiazygos

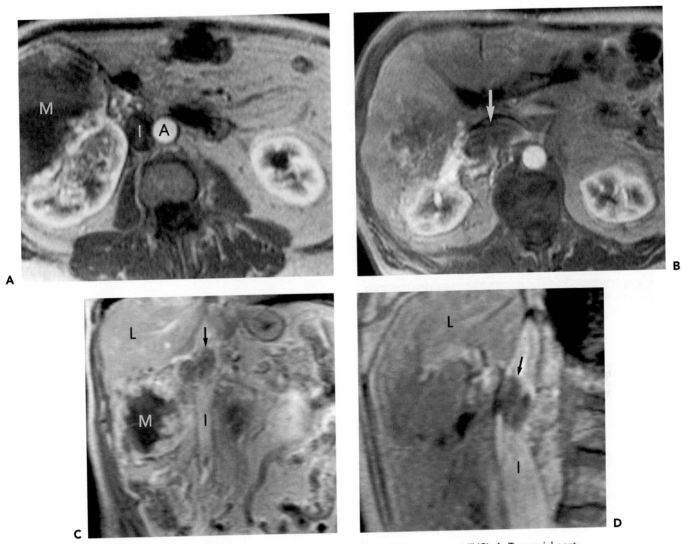

Figure 17-47   Renal cell carcinoma extending into the inferior vena cava (IVC). **A:** Transaxial post-gadolinium T1-weighted fast low-angle shot image (repetition time, 140 milliseconds; echo time, 4 milliseconds; flip angle, 80 degrees) shows a large necrotic right renal mass (M). A, aorta, I, IVC. **B:** Superiorly, enhancing tumor thrombus (*arrow*) is present within the dilated IVC. Coronal (**C**) and sagittal (**D**) images clearly demonstrate the cephalic extent of the tumor thrombus (*arrow*) within the infrahepatic IVC (I). *L*, liver.

system; gonadal, periureteric, and other retroperitoneal veins; abdominal wall veins; hemorrhoidal venous plexus; and the portal venous system.

On noncontrast MRI SE T1-weighted images, venous thrombus has a variable signal ranging from low to high and is seen against the signal void of flowing blood. Although slow flow may also produce intraluminal signal, it can be differentiated from thrombus by its showing an increase in signal intensity on the second echo image or by using a phase-sensitive imaging sequence (128,304). In contradistinction to SE images, venous thrombus appears as an area of lower signal on GRE images (13) and stands out against the bright signal of flowing blood. A homogeneous appearance of thrombus is seen with acute thrombus, while a heterogeneous pattern with hypointense dots

was seen in nonacute thrombus (301). Because GRE imaging takes less time than SE imaging, the former is the preferred noncontrast technique (304). MRA based on the GRE sequence is especially effective in demonstrating the entire venous system. However, false–positive diagnosis may occur at the confluence of vessels, where turbulent flow may reduce the signal of flowing blood, simulating a thrombus. Likewise, subacute thrombus, which is often hyperintense, may be confused with flowing blood and lead to a false–negative diagnosis. In one study (13), a combination of SE and GRE images significantly increased the accuracy of diagnosis of abdominal venous thrombosis. Alternatively, the potential problems with both noncontrast SE and GRE imaging can be resolved by using intravenous contrast (gadolinium chelate).

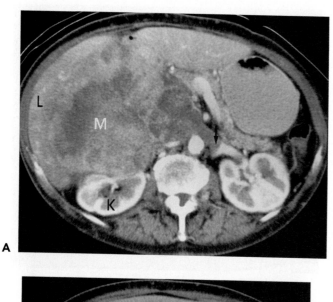

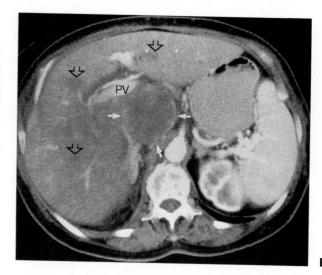

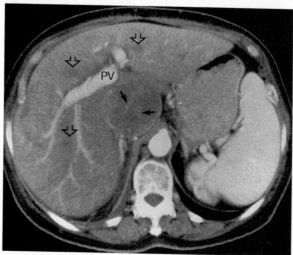

Figure 17-48   Leiomyosarcoma of the inferior vena cava (IVC). **A:** Contrast-enhanced computed tomography scan demonstrates a large, heterogeneously enhancing, soft tissue mass (M) abutting the right kidney (K) and liver (L). Tumor markedly expands the lumen of the IVC and extends into the left renal vein (*arrow*). **B, C:** Superiorly, note the thin rim of IVC wall enhancement (*white arrows*) and heterogeneous enhancement of the tumor thrombus (*black arrows*). PV, portal vein; *open arrows*, unopacified hepatic vein radicles.

In cases of catheter-induced septic thrombosis of the IVC, gas bubbles have been identified within the thrombi. In addition, inflammatory changes also can be observed surrounding the occluded vein (218).

Thrombosis of the renal and gonadal veins are also shown readily on CT and MRI. Because the right renal vein is shorter and more obliquely oriented than the longer, more horizontal left renal vein, direct demonstration of thrombus is achieved less frequently on the right than on the left. However, the use of thinner sections and the newer MDCT scanners improve visualization of both renal veins. The involved segment of the vein can be either normal in caliber or substantially enlarged. Thrombosis of ovarian vein, classically associated with postpartum (puerperal) endometritis, pelvic inflammatory disease, diverticulitis, appendicitis, and gynecologic surgery (137,288), also can occur in patients with malignant tumors, particularly those undergoing chemotherapy (136). Although puerperal ovarian vein thrombosis is associated with significant complications, including pulmonary embolism

and ureteral obstruction, patients with thrombosis associated with malignancy and chemotherapy are often asymptomatic and the need for therapy is uncertain (136). On CT, puerperal ovarian vein thrombosis appears as a well-defined tubular retroperitoneal mass extending from the pelvis to the infrarenal IVC (see Fig. 17-45). The mass corresponds to the dilated gonadal vein and usually contains a central low-attenuation region, representing thrombus (288). Other common CT findings include an inhomogeneously enhancing pelvic mass and fluid in an enlarged uterus. Inflammatory changes also may be seen around the occluded vein.

Tumoral and nontumoral thrombosis of the IVC can be identified but not differentiated from each other on CT scans unless hypervascularity is shown in the tumoral thrombus by contrast-enhanced CT (61). Expansion of the vein diameter is also indicative of tumor thrombus (see Fig. 17-48) (128). In some cases of tumor thrombus from renal cell carcinoma, hypervascularity is missing or difficult to demonstrate (369). Combined CT and

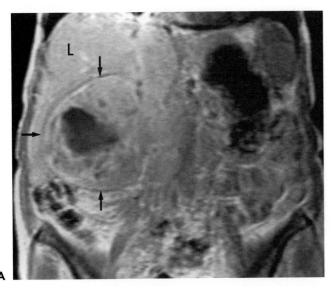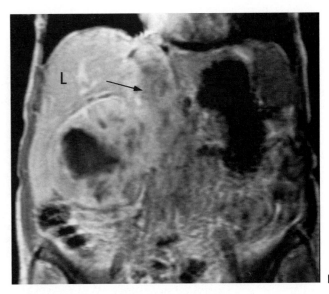

A **B**

Figure 17-49 Leiomyosarcoma of the inferior vena cava (IVC). Coronal pregadolinium **(A)** and post-gadolinium **(B)** T1-weighted fast low-angle shot images (repetition time, 140 milliseconds; echo time, 4 milliseconds; flip angle, 80 degrees) show a large retroperitoneal mass (*short arrows*) with peripheral enhancement. Central hypointensity is a result of tissue necrosis or cystic degeneration, commonly seen in leiomyosarcomas. Heterogeneously enhancing tumor extends into a dilated IVC (*long arrow*). L, liver.

fluorodeoxyglucose positron emission tomography (FDG-PET) scanning has been recently reported to be useful in distinguishing bland from tumor thrombus, with tumor thrombus showing abnormal FDG uptake (286). MRI may distinguish some tumor thrombus from bland thrombus on the basis of their signal characteristics. High signal intensity on the first and second echo images is indicative of a bland thrombus. Thrombi of intermediate signal intensity, however, can be seen in both bland and tumor thrombi (128). Enhancement after intravenous adminis-

tration of gadolinium favors tumor thrombus as does isointensity with the primary neoplasm (see Fig. 17-49). The reliability of MRI in differentiating between bland and tumor thrombi is yet to be determined in a large group of patients.

Transverse views are often sufficient for the diagnosis of caval thrombosis; however, sagittal and coronal sections from either MDCT or MRI more directly display the cephalocaudal extent of the thrombus. The latter information is particularly important for the planning of resection of the tumor thrombus.

US is a well-established technique for evaluating the IVC. It can detect caval thrombus from the level of the renal veins to the right atrium in most patients; however, US has limited ability to clearly demonstrate the rest of the IVC because of overlying bowel gas (147). Although gray scale sonography cannot distinguish bland thrombus from tumor thrombus, color Doppler US has been reported to be able to identify the neovascularity useful in making this distinction (129).

Intracaval Filters

Vena cava filters are used in patients when systemic anticoagulation is contraindicated or when recurrent pulmonary emboli have occurred despite systemic anticoagulation. Free-floating IVC or iliac thrombus alone has also been considered an indication for IVC filters. A variety of devices are available for percutaneous placement (158). CT has proved useful for evaluating the position of the IVC

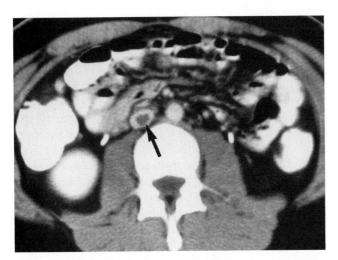

Figure 17-50 Thrombus within the inferior vena cava (IVC). Contrast-enhanced computed tomography scan shows a hypodense filling defect within the opacified lumen of the IVC (*arrow*).

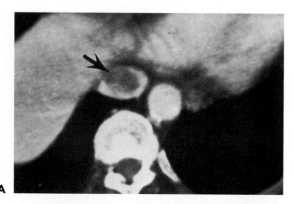
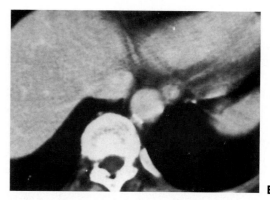

Figure 17-51   Pseudothrombus in the inferior vena cava (IVC). **A:** Computed tomography image at the level of the diaphragm obtained 1 minute after the bolus intravenous injection of contrast material into an arm vein shows a central hypodense defect within the IVC (*arrow*). **B:** Repeat image at the same level several minutes later demonstrates uniform enhancement of the IVC without evidence of a thrombus.

filters and their relation to the renal veins. It is also helpful in revealing complications including malposition, filter perforation, retroperitoneal hematoma, and recurrent thrombosis and pulmonary emboli (210,268). Filter leg perforations are a fairly common occurrence but are usually asymptomatic unless erosion into adjacent structures such as the duodenum or aorta occurs (143). MRI may also be used for evaluating patients with certain low-artifact caval filters. In general, titanium tantalum and low iron–based alloys create less artifact than those using stainless steel (313,314). SE and GRE images play complementary roles in such an evaluation.

Obliterative Hepatocavopathy (Synonym, Membranous Obstruction of the Inferior Vena Cava)

Obliterative hepatocavopathy or membranous or segmental obstruction of the IVC is a common cause of chronic Budd-Chiari syndrome in Asia and South Africa. The pathogenesis of the disorder had been thought to be congenital; however, many now suggest that it is the sequelae of previous bouts of IVC thrombosis (234,235). In obliterative hepatocavopathy, the hepatic segment of the IVC is obstructed by a fibrous membrane or replaced by cordlike fibrous tissue. In the former, the IVC usually ends abruptly at a thick membrane. In the latter, the IVC shows a more conical appearance tapering to an obliterated or narrowed segment ranging from 1 to 17 cm in length in one study (157). Calcification is seen in the obliterated segment in 34% of cases (157).

Sonography has been most useful in this disorder (188). Although CT will also usually demonstrate a narrowed or obliterated segment, simple axial images frequently miss membranous obstruction unless the membrane is calcified (162,188). In both situations (188), CT may show obliteration of hepatic veins, systemic collaterals such as

enlarged azygos and subcutaneous veins, and evidence of cirrhosis, portal hypertension, hepatic neoplasm, or ascites. The liver frequently demonstrates hypertrophy of the caudate and left lobe and atrophy of the right lobe. Linear, irregular, reticulate or wedge-shaped areas of hypoattenuation are noted in the periphery of the liver (157).

Iliocaval Compression Syndrome (Synonym, May-Thurner Syndrome)

Compression and partial obstruction of the left common iliac vein by the crossing right common iliac artery may result in chronic venous stasis or deep venous thrombosis in the left lower extremity. Although the diagnostic findings of external compression of the iliac vein, prestenotic enlargement of the proximal iliac vein, and prominent venous collaterals are most easily recognized using contrast venography, they have also been described using CT (50).

Primary Inferior Vena Cava Neoplasm

Leiomyosarcoma originating from the wall of the IVC is a rare retroperitoneal neoplasm. It occurs more commonly in women than men, with a mean age of 54 years in one large series (212). Typical presenting symptoms include abdominal pain, palpable mass, and lower limb edema. Tumors are most frequently located in the middle or lower section of the IVC below the hepatic veins (170,212). Typically, the tumors are large, averaging 10 to 11 cm in maximum diameter (124,212). Although an extraluminal growth pattern is most common, an intraluminal or dumbbell pattern (both intra- and extraluminal) is not infrequent (170,212). CT or MRI often shows a heterogeneously enhancing, well-circumscribed, lobulated right-sided retroperitoneal mass inseparable from the IVC, with displacement of adjacent organs such as the right kidney, pancreas, duodenum, and aorta (see Figs. 17-48 and 17-49) (334). The IVC is usually dilated in cases with primarily intraluminal growth. Calcification is uncommon (111). On MR images, leiomyosarcomas with extraluminal extent have homogeneous hypointensity to intermediate signal intensity on T1-weighted sequences and more heterogeneous intermediate to high signal intensity on T2-weighted sequences. Intraluminal tumor growth can be distinguished from blood thrombus on MRI. Blood thrombus has a signal intensity that is higher than that of tumor on both T1- and T2-weighted imaging (29,119). In upper IVC leiomyosarcomas, differentiation from a primary right adrenal carcinoma with venous extension may be difficult.

LYMPH NODES

Normal Anatomy

In the retroperitoneum, lymph nodes can be found surrounding the IVC and aorta (Fig. 17-52). Lymph nodes also can be seen in the root of the mesentery and along the course of the major venous structures draining to the IVC and portal vein. In the pelvis, lymph nodes can be identified in close proximity to the iliac vessels. Although less commonly seen, lymph nodes also can be found anterior to the psoas muscle and adjacent to the posterior iliac crest (44,351).

Normal lymph nodes in the abdomen and pelvis are routinely seen on CT or MR scans as small, oblong, soft tissue densities ranging from 3 to 10 mm in size (99,337). Short axis measurements should be used to minimize errors resulting from node orientation. The internal architecture of a lymph node generally is not discernible on CT or MRI, and distinguishing inflammatory adenopathy from neoplastic infiltration is usually not possible. Normal nodes typically show little enhancement with intravenous contrast—a fact that is useful in distinguishing small nodes from vascular structures, particularly in the mesentery and in the pelvis. The density of normal lymph nodes is similar to that of muscle on both contrast-enhanced and unenhanced CT scans. On MRI, the signal intensity of lymph nodes on T1-weighted images is slightly higher than that of muscle and diaphragmatic crura and is much lower than the signal intensity of fat. On rare occasions, however, lymph nodes may be nearly isointense to fat on T1-weighted images because of hemorrhage or melanin (Fig. 17-53). On T2-weighted images, the signal intensity of nodes increases, and hence, the contrast between lymph nodes and muscle increases and that between nodes and fat decreases. Thus, on T2-weighted images, lymph nodes are easily distinguished from muscle and diaphragmatic crura but may be difficult to differentiate from surrounding retroperitoneal fat because of their similar signal intensity.

In general, MRI is comparable to CT in the detection of retroperitoneal lymph nodes in adults (99,179,365). CT is generally performed with 5-mm sections and intravenous contrast. With MRI, T1-weighted images are most useful. Fat suppression techniques may aid visualization particularly with T2-weighted sequences or with gadolinium-enhanced T1-weighted sequences, because suppression of the retroperitoneal fat will render the higher signal intensity lymph nodes more conspicuous. Lymph nodes are also easily separated from blood vessels on either SE or GRE images without the use of intravenous contrast medium or following the use of gadolinium. As a result, displacement or encasement of blood vessels by lymphadenopathy is well demonstrated by MRI.

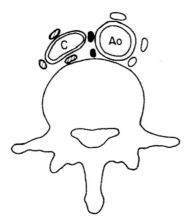

0 PERIAORTIC CHAIN
▮ INTERAORTO-CAVAL CHAIN
0 PERICAVAL CHAIN

A

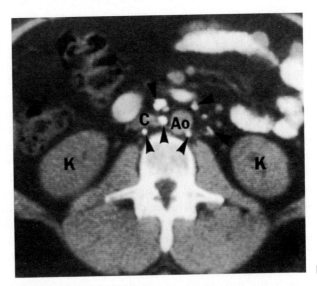

B

Figure 17-52 A: Schematic drawing denoting distribution of periaortic and pericaval lymph nodes. B: Computed tomography image in a patient after lymphangiography, showing normal distribution of retroperitoneal lymph nodes (*arrowheads*). Ao, aorta; C, inferior vena cava; K, kidney.

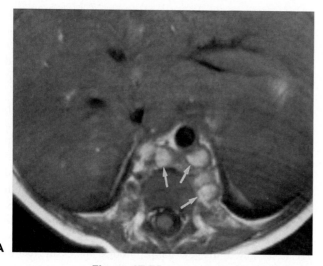
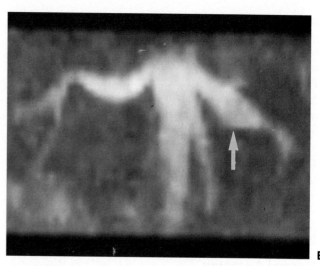

Figure 17-53 Hemorrhagic adenopathy in a patient with Kawasaki disease. **A:** Transaxial gated T1-weighted spin echo image (repetition time, 729 milliseconds; echo time, 15 milliseconds) shows multiple hyperintense enlarged retrocrural nodes (*arrows*) reflecting hemorrhagic contents. **B:** Maximum-intensity projection image of a magnetic resonance angiogram (three-dimensional fast imaging with steady-state precession; repetition time, 30 milliseconds; echo time, 7 milliseconds; flip angle, 25 degrees) shows a fusiform left renal artery aneurysm (*arrow*).

In general, multiplanar views either directly acquired, as with MRI, or reconstructed, as with CT, add little to the detection of normal or enlarged nodes. Axial views are generally preferred and sufficient.

LYMPH NODES—PATHOLOGIC CONDITIONS

Lymphadenopathy—General Considerations

The diagnosis of retroperitoneal lymphadenopathy by CT or MRI is based on recognition of nodal enlargement, sometimes concomitant with displacement or obscuration of normal structures in advanced disease (Figs. 17-54 to 17-56). For example, massive enlargement of retroaortic and retrocaval nodes may cause anterior displacement of these vessels. Except in unusually lean or cachetic patients, enlarged lymph nodes generally are well profiled by surrounding fat. Retrocrural and portahepatis nodes should not exceed 6 mm, whereas the upper limit of normal for gastrohepatic ligament nodes is 8 mm (38,65). Retroperitoneal, celiac axis, mesenteric, and pelvic nodes greater than 10 mm in size are considered abnormal, but multiple, slightly smaller (8 to 10 mm) nodes in these regions should be viewed with suspicion (65,99,337).

The presentation of lymphadenopathy may vary from (a) one or several discrete enlarged lymph nodes to (b) a more conglomerate group of contiguous enlarged nodes similar in size to the aorta or IVC to (c) a large homogeneous mass, in which individual nodes are no longer recognizable, obscuring the contours of normal surrounding

structures. Lymph node enlargement secondary to viral or granulomatous disease cannot be differentiated from lymphoma or metastases based on imaging findings alone, although the massive type of conglomeration is almost never seen with the benign conditions (Fig. 17-57).

Although most nodes have soft tissue density on CT, hypodense adenopathy may be seen with both malignant and benign disease. Testicular neoplasms, particularly teratocarcinoma and epidermoid carcinoma of the genitourinary tract often have low-density lymphadenopathy (Fig. 17-58). This may occur following therapy and represent areas of necrosis or liquefaction, or it may be present initially and correspond to epithelial-lined cystic areas (289). Low-density nodes are rarely noted in patients with lymphoma (252). Mycobacterium infection (more commonly *M. tuberculosis* than *M. avium intracellulare*) and histoplasmosis may also be associated with hypodense nodes (Fig. 17-59) (258,259). Whipple disease can demonstrate low-density adenopathy (Fig. 17-60). In this disease, the attenuation value of the enlarged lymph nodes often is quite low, ranging from +10 HU to 30 HU (186), and is most likely caused by the deposition of fat and fatty acids in the lymph nodes. Lymphangioleiomyomatosis has been associated with low-attenuation retroperitoneal masses and lymphadenopathy (16,360). Enlarged, low-density lymph nodes may also be seen in the cavitary lymph node syndrome associated with celiac sprue. This rare complication has a poor prognosis and may be associated with poorly controlled and long-standing disease (120,127). On CT, enlarged cavitary mesenteric nodes with fat–fluid levels have been reported (120).

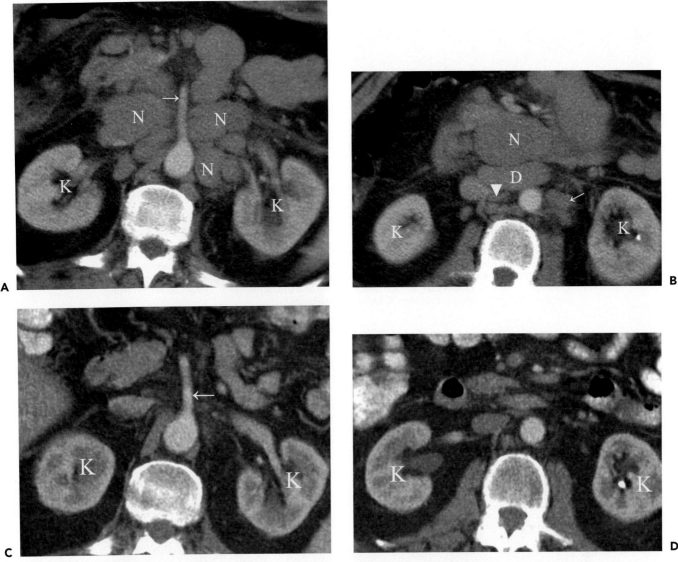

Figure 17-54 Burkitt lymphoma pre- and posttherapy. **A:** Contrast-enhanced axial computed tomography at the level of the celiac axis (*arrow*) shows bulky lymphadenopathy (N). K, kidney. **B:** Bulky mesenteric lymphadenopathy (N). *Arrow*, paraaortic lymph node; *arrowhead*, aortocaval node; K, kidney; D, duodenum. **C:** Following treatment, there has been almost complete resolution of the bulky adenopathy adjacent to the celiac axis (*arrow*). K, kidney. **D:** Mesenteric, paraaortic, and aortocaval lymphadenopathy has also almost completely resolved.

Both benign and malignant lymphadenopathy may exhibit mild to pronounced enhancement after intravenous administration of iodinated contrast material (Fig. 17-61) (131,251,252). Contrast enhancement may be homogeneous, inhomogeneous, or peripheral. Although the majority of lymphomas show only mild to moderate enhancement (199,252), hyperenhancing adenopathy has been reported in a number of disorders including metastasis from renal cell (Fig. 17-62) and bladder carcinoma, carcinoid, and Kaposi sarcoma (121,131), and in angioimmunoblastic lymphadenopathy (199) and Castleman disease (Fig. 17-63) (150). Pronounced enhancement may also be seen occasionally in mycobacterial infection. This is most commonly

peripheral, although homogeneous enhancement has also been noted (251).

Nodal calcification can occur in patients after granulomatous infection. It is also associated with a variety of malignancies including mucinous carcinoma, sarcomas, and treated (and rarely untreated) lymphomas (Fig. 17-64) (9,169).

Although *in vitro* study has shown that lymph nodes containing metastases have a significantly longer T2 than normal and hyperplastic nodes (345), *in vivo* tissue characterization based on relaxation times or signal intensities has not been possible (64,179). Enlarged lymph nodes resulting from malignant disease cannot be reliably distinguished

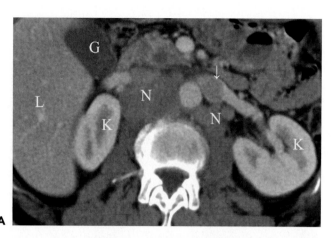
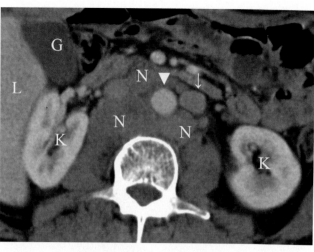

Figure 17-55 Prostate cancer metastases with left inferior vena cava (IVC). **A:** Contrast-enhanced axial computed tomography image at left renal vein level shows left IVC draining into left renal vein (*arrow*). Multiple matted retroperitoneal lymph nodes (N) are seen in this patient with lymphoma. K, kidney; L, liver; G, gallbladder. **B:** IVC (*arrow*) lies left of aorta (*arrowhead*). Lymph nodes (N) lifting aorta and IVC from the spine. L, liver; K, kidney; G, gallbladder.

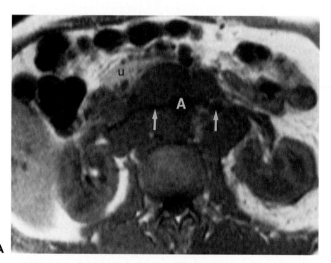
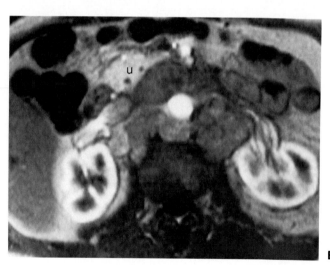

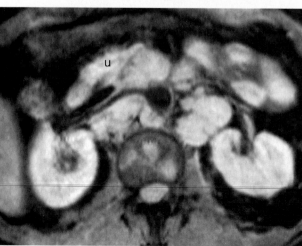

Figure 17-56 Extensive adenopathy resulting from metastatic prostate adenocarcinoma. **A:** Transaxial T1-weighted fast low-angle shot (FLASH) image (repetition time, 140 milliseconds; echo time, 4 milliseconds; flip angle, 80 degrees) shows lobulated circumaortic (A) tissue encasing the renal arteries (*arrows*). **B:** Transaxial postgadolinium T1-weighted FLASH image (repetition time, 140 milliseconds; echo time, 4 milliseconds; flip angle, 80 degrees) shows significant nodal enhancement. Note the anterior displacement of the aorta, a feature commonly seen with lymphadenopathy but not in retroperitoneal fibrosis. **C:** Transaxial postgadolinium, fat-saturated proton density–weighted, spin echo image (repetition time, 2,400 milliseconds; echo time, 15 milliseconds) shows the increased sensitivity to contrast enhancement using this sequence. *U*, uncinate process.

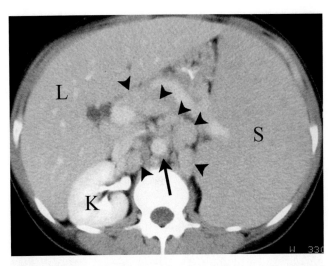

Figure 17-57 Sarcoidosis with adenopathy (*arrowheads*) and splenomegaly (S). L, liver; K, kidney; *arrow*, aorta.

by CT or routine MRI from those resulting from benign processes. Furthermore, lymph nodes that are of normal size but are partially or totally replaced with a neoplasm will not be identified as abnormal by routine MRI or CT.

Both MRI and CT can be used for evaluation of lymphadenopathy. MRI has several advantages over CT. One advantage is its ability to distinguish vascular structures from soft tissue structures without the use of iodinated contrast material. In particular, mildly enlarged pelvic lymph nodes may be difficult to detect by CT because of the great variability in location, diameter, and orientation of the pelvic arteries and veins. This is especially true in

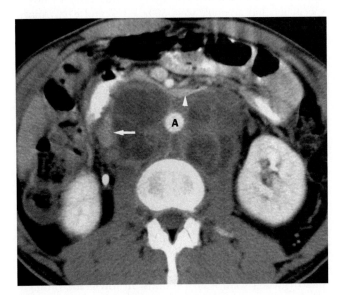

Figure 17-58 Low-density lymph nodes in a patient with metastatic seminoma. Contrast-enhanced computed tomography scan shows hypodense adenopathy surrounding the aorta. Note the elevation of the aorta (A), lateral displacement of the inferior vena cava (*arrow*), and anterior displacement of the left renal vein (*arrowhead*).

patients in whom adequate opacification of both the arteries and veins is not achieved because of technical reasons. Even with the administration of intravenous contrast material, mildly enlarged pelvic nodes still may be confused with pelvic vessels because both will enhance (131). In these instances, pelvic lymphadenopathy is more easily demonstrated by MRI. Venous anomalies, prominent gonadal veins, and collateral vessels all may mimic retroperitoneal lymphadenopathy on noncontrast CT studies, but are easily shown to be vascular structures by MRI. CT similarly has several advantages over MRI. Although a survey MRI examination of the abdomen and pelvis can be completed by T1-weighted GRE sequence in less than a minute, a thorough MR examination that consists of both T1- and T2-weighted sequences still takes more time than a comparable CT study. Furthermore, CT is less expensive and is more available than MRI. With optimal opacification of bowel loops, CT can also more easily detect lymphadenopathy in patients who have little retroperitoneal fat and in patients in whom the retroperitoneal tissue planes have been altered by surgery. Because of the poorer spatial resolution of MRI, a cluster of normal-size lymph nodes could appear as a single enlarged node on the MRI study. Finally, MRI is unable to detect small calcifications in lymph nodes, a limitation that is of greater significance in the evaluation of the mediastinum than in the retroperitoneum and pelvis.

In most institutions, CT remains the imaging procedure of choice for screening the retroperitoneum for evidence of lymphadenopathy. If the CT findings are equivocal, an MRI study could be performed. MRI should be considered as the primary imaging technique in those patients in whom exposure to ionizing radiation should be limited. This includes pediatric patients, especially if multiple follow-up examinations are anticipated, and pregnant patients in their second and third trimesters.

Other Modalities for Evaluating Lymphadenopathy

Bipedal lymphangiography (LAG) has been used in the past to evaluate neoplastic nodal involvement. In this procedure, methylene blue is initially injected into the dorsal aspect of the foot between the toes. This is picked up by the lymphatics, one of which is then exposed and cannulated. A small amount of an iodinated oil-based contrast agent is then slowly injected intralymphatically. Plain films of the abdomen are obtained over the next 24 hours and demonstrate lymphatic filling and nodal architecture. Neoplastic involvement is shown by alteration of the normal nodal architecture (100).

Although bipedal LAG was the mainstay of lymphatic imaging before the advent of CT and MRI, it has fallen out of favor for several reasons (338). The procedure itself is time-consuming, difficult to perform, and uncomfortable for the patient. In patients with severe cardiopulmonary

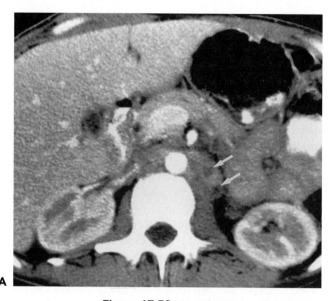
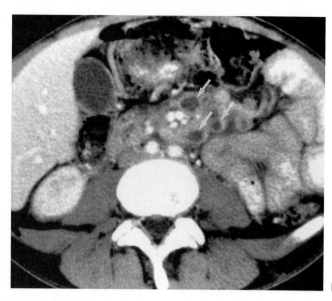

A   B

Figure 17-59 Low-density lymph nodes in an AIDS patient with *Mycobacterium avium intracellulare* (MAI) infection. Contrast-enhanced computed tomography scans show hypodense, enlarged nodes (*arrows*) in the (**A**) paraaortic region and (**B**) small bowel mesentery from culture-proved MAI.

disease, it may be medically contraindicated. False–positive lymphangiograms are not uncommon and can be produced by benign reactive hyperplasia (191). CT and MRI will also demonstrate nodal groups not routinely opacified during LAG (e.g. periportal, peripancreatic, retrocrural, and mesenteric nodes) as well as nodes completely replaced by tumor, which would not show up on LAG (163). And last, CT and MRI can evaluate both the local tumor and other abdominal viscera.

MR lymphangiography uses ferumoxtran-10, a contrast agent consisting of ultrasmall superparamagnetic iron

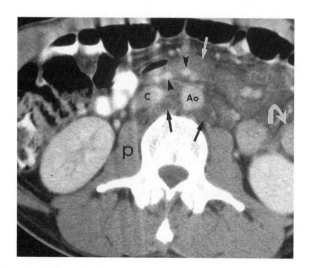

Figure 17-60 Whipple disease. Enlarged retroperitoneal (*black arrows*) and mesenteric (*white arrow*) lymph nodes are present. Note that the attenuation value of the lymph nodes is lower than that of psoas muscle (P). Ao, aorta; c, inferior vena cava; *black arrowhead*, superior mesenteric vessels; *curved white arrow*, thickened jejunum.

oxide particles (USPIO). When given intravenously, the particles accumulate in normal nodal tissue throughout the body, where they are then phagocytosed by macrophages. The susceptibility effect induced by the iron causes signal dropout in normal nodes on T2- or T2*-weighted images. In nodes wholly or partly replaced by tumor, this signal dropout is not noted. The usual analysis of images depends on comparison of pre- and post-USPIO contrast images (108,321). Initial studies using USPIO in the abdomen and pelvis have proved promising (108,109,321). In phase III clinical trial with abdominal and pelvic malignancy, sensitivity, specificity, and accuracy were 80%, 83%, and 81%, respectively, representing an improvement over noncontrast MRI in specificity and accuracy (7).

PET has shown utility in identifying metastatic adenopathy (165,321). The most common agent in current use is an 18-flourine labeled glucose analog (FDG) that is taken up by metabolically active cells, phosphorylated, and trapped. Many tumors, including lymphoma and lung, breast, esophageal, and colon carcinoma show increased activity on FDG-PET, and in these neoplasms, FDG-PET has proved useful in identifying nodal metastasis in both enlarged and normal-size nodes as well as extranodal disease (Fig. 17-65) (165,229,321). FDG-PET has been less successful in other tumors, including pulmonary carcinoid and prostate cancer (71,138,321). In the latter, other analogs (e.g., ^{11}C-acetate and ^{11}C-methione) have shown some value. False–negative FDG-PET results are noted with small (greater than 1 cm) lesions, in low-grade indolent tumors, and in areas adjacent to normal physiologic activity (e.g., ureters, bladder) (19). False–positive results can be seen with nodal inflammation, in granulation tissue, and where normal physiologic uptake is unusual or focal

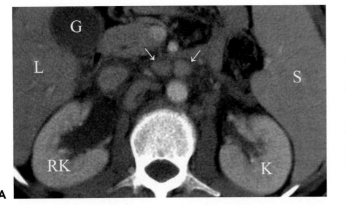

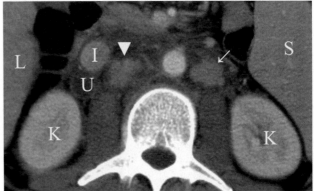

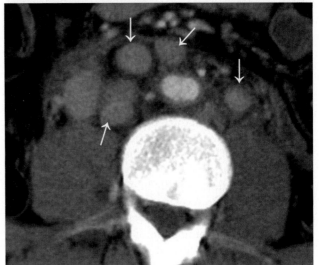

Figure 17-61 High-density cryptococcal lymphadenopathy in a patient with human immunodeficiency virus infection. **A:** Postcontrast computed tomography shows high-density lymph nodes in paraaortic region (*arrows*), hydronephrosis in right kidney (RK) resulting from ureteric obstruction by lymph nodes. K, left kidney; L, liver; G, gallbladder; S, spleen. **B:** High-density paraaortic (*arrow*) and aortocaval (*arrowhead*) lymph node displacing inferior vena cava (I). U, dilated right ureter; S, spleen; K, kidney; L, liver. **C:** Lower abdominal level shows high-density lymph nodes in paraaortic, aortocaval, and retroperitoneal regions (*arrows*).

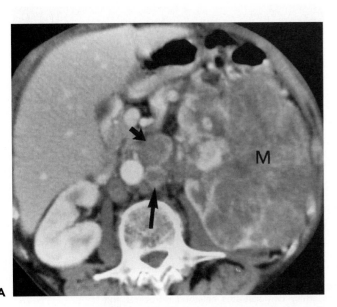

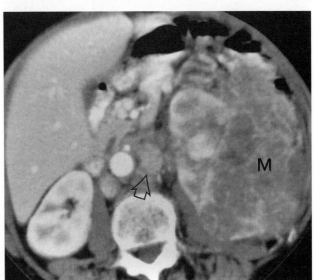

Figure 17-62 Enhancing adenopathy resulting from metastatic renal cell carcinoma. Contrast-enhanced computed tomography scans show paraaortic adenopathy demonstrating heterogeneous (*short arrow*) rim (*long arrow*) enhancement **(A)** and homogeneous (*open arrow*) enhancement **(B)**. Note the large renal mass (M). A, aorta; I, inferior vena cava.

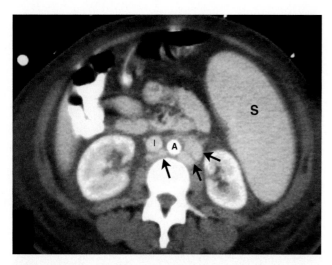

Figure 17-63 Castleman disease. Contrast-enhanced computed tomography scan shows brightly enhancing paraaortic and retrocaval adenopathy (*black arrows*). Splenomegaly (S) is also noted. I, inferior vena cava; A, aorta.

and mimics tumor. Although the inherent poor spatial resolution with PET was an early problem the development of combined PET/CT units and fusion imaging has overcome this to some degree.

US has been quite accurate in detecting retroperitoneal adenopathy (55); however, it is often difficult to obtain adequate scans of the lower abdomen because of bowel gas. In obese patients, examination of the retroperitoneal area by ultrasound also is difficult due to marked attenuation of the sound beam by the abundant subcutaneous and mesenteric fat

Differential Diagnosis

Other entities, such as retroperitoneal fibrosis, perianeurysmal fibrosis, saccular aortic aneurysm, and unopacified bowel may exhibit findings on CT or MRI resembling malignant lymphadenopathy. However, the soft tissue mass seen in idiopathic retroperitoneal fibrosis or perianeurysmal fibrosis usually has a more regular border than that seen with malignant lymphadenopathy (see Fig. 17-13). Aortic aneurysms usually can be distinguished from lymphadenopathy on postcontrast scans. Bowel loops can typically be followed along their course and identified. Although the inferior extent of the diaphragmatic crura, dilated lumbar lymphatics, or vascular abnormalities and anomalies such as an enlarged gonadal vein, a duplicated IVC, and a dilated azygos or hemiazygos vein could conceivably be confused with an enlarged lymph node, careful examination of multiple contiguous scans and concomitant use of intravenous iodinated contrast medium can separate these entities from lymphadenopathy (354).

Posttherapy Evaluation

An important application of imaging is in the evaluation of patients who have undergone radiation therapy or chemotherapy and have a residual retroperitoneal mass. CT is frequently unable to distinguish residual fibrotic changes from viable neoplasm (184,187). Several investigators have shown that MRI may be able to distinguish posttreatment fibrosis from residual or recurrent tumor (67,90,261). Demonstration of uniform low signal intensity (similar to that of muscle) on T1- and T2-weighted images suggests that the soft tissue mass represents mature fibrosis.

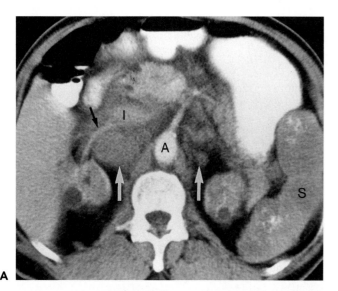

A

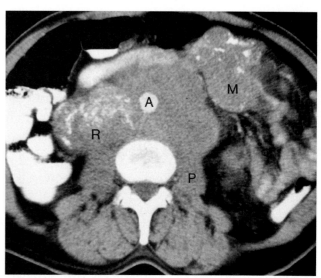

B

Figure 17-64 Calcified lymphoma before treatment. **A:** Contrast-enhanced computed tomography scan through the origin of the superior mesenteric artery demonstrates enlarged retrocaval and paraaortic nodes (*arrows*). Amorphous calcifications are noted in focal splenic lesions. Small renal cysts are present in both kidneys. S, spleen; *black arrow*, encased right renal artery. **B:** Computed tomography scan obtained 7 cm caudad shows calcified mesenteric (M) and retrocaval lymphadenopathy (R), an extremely atypical feature for untreated lymphoma. The rest of the retroperitoneal adenopathy is of soft tissue density. Note anterior displacement of the aorta (A) and obscuration of the psoas (P) margin.

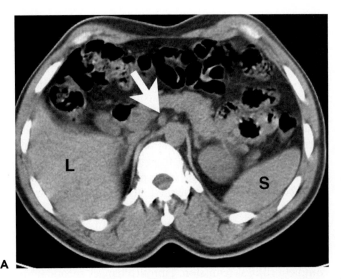
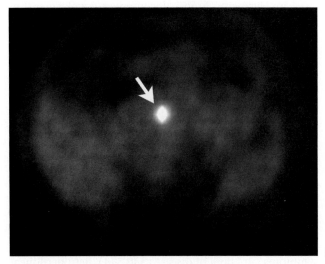

Figure 17-65 Normal-size node containing malignant cells and showing higher FDG-PET signal. **A:** Axial contrast-enhanced computed tomography (CT) scan shows a small right paraaortic node (*arrow*). L, liver; S, spleen. **B:** FDG-PET CT shows increased activity corresponding to normal-size node, consistent with a small metastatic deposit.

However, regions of intermediate to high signal intensity on T2-weighted images may represent not only viable tumor but benign processes such as necrosis, inflammation, or early fibrosis. This is especially true in the first six months after initiation of therapy (261). Caution is necessary because MR signal intensities reflect only gross histologic characteristics and cannot exclude microscopic foci of residual disease. Serial MRI studies may be of greater value than any one isolated examination in monitoring patients with suspected recurrent disease (261). FDG-PET has also been shown to have an important role in the evaluation of residual tumor posttherapy, with increased uptake seen in masses with residual tumor and lower uptake in fibrotic masses (165,272).

Lymphoceles are caused by the interruption of efferent lymphatics and the resulting accumulation of lymphatic fluid in the retroperitoneum. They are typically seen following lymphadenectomy. Spontaneous regression occurs in the majority of cases, however, a few may persist. Although usually asymptomatic when small, lymphoceles may cause symptoms, including venous obstruction and abdominal distension, and may become secondarily infected. They appear on CT or MRI as simple nonenhancing fluid collections with a thin wall and should not be mistaken for necrotic lymph nodes. Occasionally, negative attenuation values (HU) are seen in the fluid and, when present, are thought to be strongly suggestive of lymphocele. Mural calcification is uncommon (300,335,364).

Lymphoma

Lymphomas are a common cause of retroperitoneal lymphadenopathy. As a group, they span a wide variety of conditions ranging from indolent slow-growing malignancies to aggressive rapidly fatal disease. Lymphoma can be classified into two major categories: Hodgkin lymphoma,

which makes up 20% to 30% of cases in the United States and western Europe, and non-Hodgkin lymphoma (NHL) (277). Subclassification beyond this point has been a source of some confusion.

The 2001 World Health Organization Classification of Tumors of the Hematopoietic and Lymphomoid Tissues is the most recent effort at consensus and attempts to define subgroups based on a combination of morphology, immunophenotype, and genetic and clinical features. In this formulation, there are five subgroups of Hodgkin lymphoma: a nodular lymphocyte predominant form and the four classic subtypes—nodular sclerosis, lymphocyte rich, mixed cellularity, and lymphocyte depleted. Prognosis is best with the nodular lymphocyte predominant and nodular sclerosis forms and worse for the lymphocyte-depleted subgroup (277). The classification of NHL is considerably more complex, and the reader is referred to the pathology literature for more details (277).

Along with histologic classification and clinical presentation, staging is important in determining therapy. The Ann Arbor Staging Classification System is used in both Hodgkin lymphoma and NHL and is shown below (277,344):

Stage I: Involvement of a single lymph node region (I) or a single extralymphatic organ or site (IE).

Stage 2: Involvement of two or more nodal regions on the same side of the diaphragm (II) or localized involvement of an extralymphatic organ or site and one or more nodal regions on the same side of the diaphragm (IIE).

Stage III: Involvement of nodes on both sides of the diaphragm (III), which may be accompanied by localized involvement of an extralymphatic organ or site (IIIE) or spleen (IIIS) or both (IIISE).

Stage IV: Diffuse or disseminated involvement of one or more extralymphatic organs with or without node involvement. Biopsy-documented involvement of stage IV sites is denoted by letter suffixes: M = marrow, L = lung, H = liver, P = pleura, O = bone, D = skin and subcutaneous tissue.

- "A" is applied to asymptomatic patients; "B" to those with fever, sweats, and weight loss; and "X" to those with bulk disease (greater than 10 cm for nodes).

This schema is more helpful in therapy and prognosis in Hodgkin lymphoma than in NHL. Given the contiguous nature of spread via lymphatics in Hodgkin lymphoma, the extent of disease directly influences therapy. In contrast, NHL may spread hematogenously and commonly presents with discontiguous extensive nodal disease with more frequent involvement of extranodal sites (Fig. 17-66). Therefore, in NHL, therapy is governed more by histologic subtype, symptoms, and bulk of disease (338,344). Retroperitoneal nodal involvement is noted at the time of presentation in up to 55% of patients with NHL but in only 25% to 35% of Hodgkin lymphoma patients (338).

CT and MRI are both relatively accurate methods for detecting intraabdominal and pelvic lymphadenopathy in patients with lymphoma (see Fig. 17-66) (145). False–positive cases are largely a result of confusion with unopacified bowel loops or normal vascular structures, a problem that is easily resolved by rigorous attention to technique. False–positive diagnoses may also be a result of misinter-

pretation of lymphadenopathy secondary to benign inflammatory disease as malignant. False–negative interpretations almost always are secondary to the inability to recognize replaced but normal-sized or minimally enlarged lymph nodes as abnormal (338). Even with increasing experience in scan interpretation coupled with meticulous scanning techniques, this limitation remains a problem for CT and MRI. PET-CT scanning has been shown to be useful in this setting as well as for monitoring response to therapy (229). It should be noted, though, that low-grade lymphomas and some specific types of lymphoma (e.g., mucosa-associated lymphoid tissue lesions) may not accumulate FDG (125,141,229).

It should be emphasized that, in patients with massive lymphadenopathy on the initial study, the follow-up scans may not always revert to normal even when patients are in complete clinical remission. Fibrotic changes secondary to prior radiation or chemotherapy may appear either as discrete, albeit smaller, soft tissue masses or as a thin sheath causing obscuration of the discrete outlines of the aorta and IVC. Unfortunately, CT is incapable of differentiating between viable residual neoplasm and such fibrotic changes caused by chemotherapy or radiotherapy (264). T2-weighted MR images singly or sequentially, as well as PET-CT scanning, may help in distinguishing tumor from fibrosis, as discussed above (229). In difficult cases, surgical or percutaneous biopsy may be necessary for definitive proof.

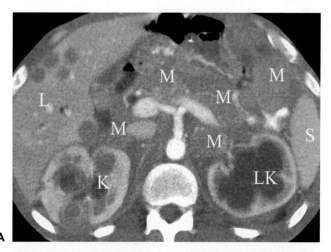

A

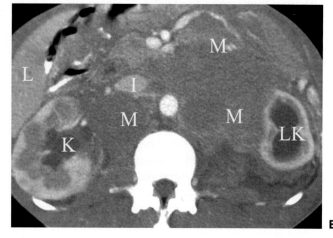

B

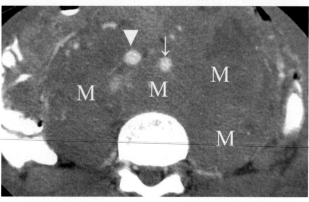

C

Figure 17-66 Burkitt lymphoma in a patient with AIDS. **A:** Axial contrast-enhanced computed tomography shows a large nodal mass (M) filling much of the retroperitoneum with hypodense lesions seen involving the liver (L) and right kidney (K). The left kidney (LK) is hydronephrotic as a result of ureteral compression. S, spleen. **B:** At a lower level, the large nodal mass (M) is seen displacing the inferior vena cava (IVC) (I) anteriorly and the left kidney (LK) laterally. Both kidneys are hydronephrotic. K, right kidney; L, liver. **C:** Further inferiorly, the large retroperitoneal nodal mass (M) displaces the aorta (*arrow*) and IVC (*arrowhead*) anteriorly.

Lymphomatous adenopathy is most commonly of soft tissue attenuation (40 to 50 HU) on noncontrast scans, although rarely lower attenuation (30 HU) values are seen (252). Maximal enhancement after intravenous contrast injection typically occurred at 1 to 2 minutes. In one study of 25 patients, a small (mean 16 HU) or moderate (31 HU) enhancement increment was seen in 9 and 12 patients, respectively (252). Pronounced enhancement (60 HU) was noted in 4 patients (252). Inhomogeneous enhancement is more common in patients with high-grade lymphoma, whereas homogeneous enhancement is seen more commonly in patients with low-grade disease (275). Calcification in lymphomatous nodes may occur following therapy; however, it may rarely be seen in untreated disease (9).

Abnormal lymph nodes usually have a homogeneous MRI appearance but may appear inhomogeneous as a result of calcification or necrosis. In one study, more than 60% of high-grade NHL nodes had an inhomogeneous MR appearance (corresponding to necrosis) on T2-weighted images, in contrast to low-grade NHL nodes, which were mostly homogeneous. Furthermore, patients with high-grade NHL and a homogeneous signal intensity pattern had a better survival rate than those with an inhomogeneous pattern (270). The administration of intravenous gadolinium contrast has been reported to improve the detectability of the inhomogeneities (271).

Testicular Neoplasms

Testicular neoplasms are the most common solid tumor in men 15 to 34 years old (30). Histologically, the germ cell testicular tumors are composed of different cell types but are grouped most commonly into seminomatous and nonseminomatous categories (30,279). Painless testicular enlargement is the classic presentation, although painful swelling is also noted and may mimic orchitis or epididymitis (30). Retroperitoneal, mediastinal, or pulmonary metastases may occur with only a small testicular mass, particularly in the nonseminomatous tumors (279). Treatment for both seminomatous and nonseminomatous tumors begins with radical inguinal orchiectomy. Radiation therapy directed at the ipsilateral pelvic and retroperitoneal nodes is then given in cases of seminoma, with adjuvant chemotherapy used in cases with more extensive disease (nodes greater than 5 cm or supradiaphragmatic nodes or visceral metastases) or relapse. In the nonseminomatous tumors, therapeutic options are less certain. In general, retroperitoneal lymph node dissection is used with or without adjuvant chemotherapy for local disease or disease limited to the retroperitoneum (stages 1 and 2) (30). Accurate determination of tumor extent helps in the design of radiation ports for seminomas and in the choice of initial mode of treatment in the nonseminomatous group.

Testicular tumors tend to metastasize via the lymphatic system. In general, the testicular lymphatics, which follow the course of the testicular arteries/veins, drain directly

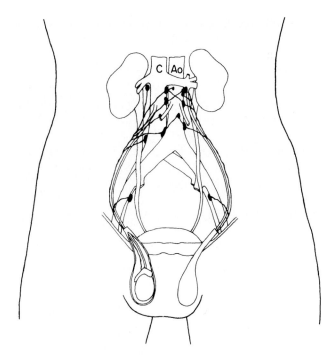

Figure 17-67 Schematic diagram showing lymphatic drainage from the testis and epididymis. The testis drains primarily into lymph nodes at or below the level of the renal hilum, whereas the epididymis drains into the distal aortic or proximal iliac nodal group.

into the lymph nodes in or near the renal hilus (Fig. 17-67). After involvement of these sentinel nodes, the lumbar paraaortic nodes become involved (unilaterally or bilaterally), followed by spread to the mediastinal and supraclavicular nodes or hematogenous dissemination to the lungs, liver, and brain (30).

Data from a large surgical series showed that nodal metastases from the right testis tend to be midline, with primary zones of involvement being the interaortocaval, precaval, and preaortic lymph node groups (Fig. 17-68).

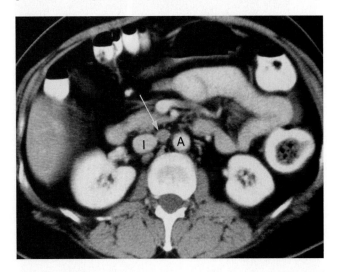

Figure 17-68 Interaortocaval adenopathy. This nodal region (*arrow*), between the aorta (A) and inferior vena cava (I), can be the first site of nodal metastasis from ovarian and testicular neoplasms, typically right-sided primaries.

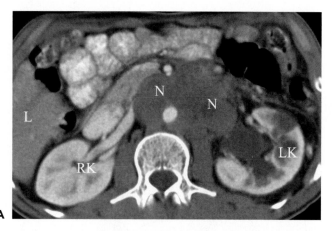

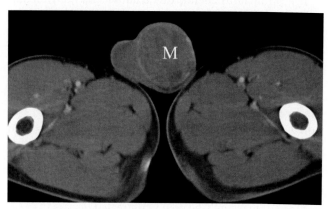

Figure 17-69 Metastatic seminoma. **A:** Contrast-enhanced axial computed tomography image at the level of the renal hila shows low-density retroperitoneal lymph nodes (N) causing hydronephrosis of the left kidney (LK). RK, right kidney; L, liver. **B:** Large mixed density mass is seen in the left testis.

Nodal metastases from the left testis show a predilection for preaortic followed by left paraaortic and interaortocaval nodal groups (63,267). In general, the presence of contralateral disease is unusual in the absence of ipsilateral or midline involvement. Similarly, suprahilar disease in the absence of infrahilar involvement is rare (Fig. 17-69) (63,267). Nodal involvement is also noted to be more likely in nodes anterior to a line bisecting the aorta than in posteriorly located nodes (122).

Involvement of inguinal lymph nodes is unusual unless there has been skin invasion, inadequate orchiectomy, or previous operation (e.g., herniorrhaphy) in the area (160).

CT and MRI may be used for evaluation of retroperitoneal involvement in testicular cancer (Fig. 17-70). Their sensitivity, however, suffer from an inability to recognize tumor in normal-size nodes (less than 1 cm). CT using a size criteria of greater than or equal to 10 mm shows a sensitivity of 40% and a specificity approaching 100% (35,122). Although lowering the size criteria for a normal lymph node from 10 mm to 4 mm increased the sensitivity of CT to 97% in one study, it was associated with a concomitant decrease in the specificity of the examination (from 100% to 58%) (122,306).

CT and MRI also play a role in the posttherapy follow-up of patients with testicular cancer. However, as with substantial lymphomatous lymph node involvement, residual retroperitoneal masses may remain on CT scans even after metastatic testicular carcinoma has been eradicated. Such

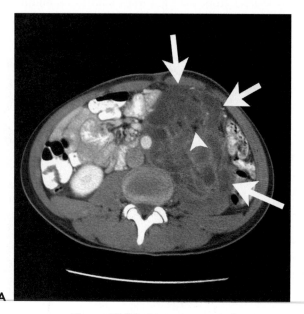

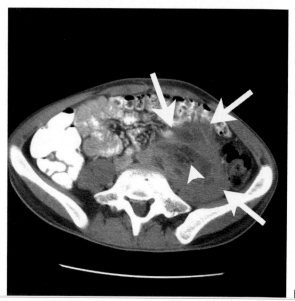

Figure 17-70 Metastatic testicular teatoma. **A and B:** Contrast-enhanced axial computed tomography images demonstrate a heterogeneous multilocular hypodense mass in the left paraaortic region (*arrows*). Note that the mass contains a small amount of fat (*arrowheads*). (Case courtesy of J. Kevin Smith, MD, PhD, Birmingham, AL.)

masses may represent posttreatment fibrosis or teratoma (usually in nonseminomatous germ cell tumor); they cannot be distinguished reliably from residual viable neoplasm by CT (307). In some cases, tumor masses may enlarge despite chemotherapy. Although these may represent a lack of response to chemotherapy (particularly if tumor markers [e.g., alpha fetoprotein (AFP) or human chorionic gonadotropin (HCG)] are increasing), it may also represent conversion of tumor to mature or immature teratoma. In the latter case, tumor markers are normal (238).

Other Retroperitoneal Metastasis

Retroperitoneal lymph nodes are frequently involved in a variety of malignancies from the gastrointestinal and genitourinary tract. The most common carcinomas associated with retroperitoneal lymphadenopathy are testicular, prostatic, cervical, endometrial, and renal (278). Because of the ability of CT and MRI to evaluate the liver, adrenals, and abdominal and pelvic lymph nodes simultaneously, they have been used as part of an abdominal oncologic survey in patients with known malignancy both in primary evaluation and in follow-up.

In contradistinction to lymphoma, nodal metastases from primary epithelial cancer of the genitourinary tract frequently cause replacement without enlarging the lymph node, a condition not discernible on routine CT or MRI scans (178). Identifying viable tumor in residual nodal masses is also problematic for many of these lesions. In these cases, PET using FDG or another agent may have a significant role in identifying otherwise occult disease. MR lymphangiography may also play a future role. A more complete discussion of the role of CT and MRI in pelvic malignancies is covered in Chapter 20.

RETROPERITONEAL HEMORRHAGE

Retroperitoneal hemorrhage has a number of etiologies. As previously described, it can occur secondary to rupture of an aortic aneurysm or atherosclerotic aorta. It can be seen following trauma, with injury to a retroperitoneal vessel or organ, or in patients who have undergone percutaneous renal biopsy or translumbar aortography. It may occur spontaneously in patients on anticoagulation therapy or with a bleeding diatheses or vasculitis. Several retroperitoneal tumors, including renal cell carcinoma and angiomyolipoma and adrenal pheochromocytoma and myelolipoma, as well as retroperitoneal metastasis may present with retroperitoneal bleeding (5,80,250,278,362).

Although acute onset of abdominal pain and development of an abdominal mass in association with a decreasing hematocrit are highly suggestive of retroperitoneal hemorrhage, clinical signs and symptoms may be ambiguous, delayed, or misleading (250). The diagnosis of retroperitoneal hemorrhage by plain abdominal radiographs lacks both sensitivity and specificity.

CT and MRI are both accurate noninvasive imaging methods for detecting retroperitoneal hemorrhage. On CT scans, it appears as an abnormal soft tissue density, either well localized or diffusely infiltrating the retroperitoneum (Fig. 17-71). Its location and attenuation characteristics depend on the source and duration of the hemorrhage (Figs. 17-72 to 17-74). Hemorrhage resulting from renal

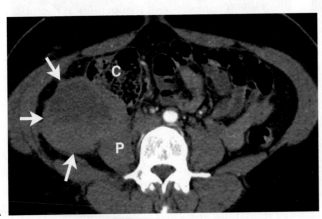

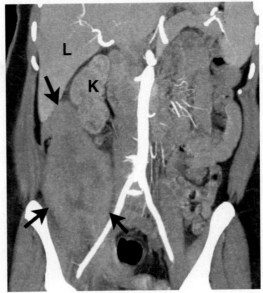

Figure 17-71 Retroperitoneal hematoma. **A:** Contrast-enhanced axial computed tomography image shows mixed attenuation mass (*arrows*) in the retroperitoneum displacing the ascending colon (C) anteriorly. P, psoas, **B:** Coronal reconstruction shows extent of retroperitoneal bleed (*arrows*). L, liver; K, kidney.

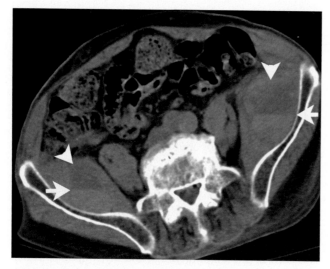

Figure 17-72 Bilateral iliacus hematomas in a patient on antico-agulant therapy. Non–contrast axial computed tomography image shows enlargement of both iliacus muscles by masses (*arrowheads*) containing fluid–fluid levels (*arrows*). The dependent portion is slightly hyperdense relative to muscle and represents settled blood products, with the lower density serum seen anteriorly.

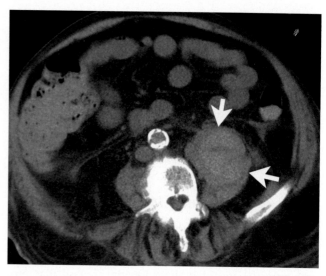

Figure 17-74 Psoas hematoma in a patient on anticoagulation for atrial fibrillation. Noncontrast axial computed tomography image shows a slightly hyperdense mass expanding the left psoas muscle (*arrows*).

biopsy or from renal tumor is centered around the kidney, whereas that associated with a leaking AAA or translumbar aortography generally surrounds the aorta before extending into the adjacent retroperitoneum. An acute hematoma (+70 to +90 HU) has a higher attenuation value than circulating blood because clot formation and retraction cause greater concentration of red blood cells (310,359). Contrast-enhanced CT may document active arterial extravasation either as a focal high-density area surrounded by a large

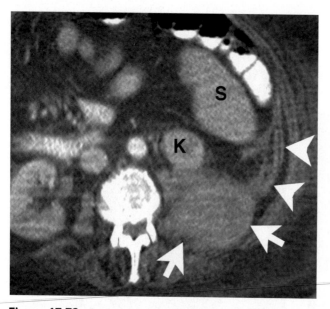

Figure 17-73 Psoas hematoma. Contrast-enhanced axial computed tomography image shows a mixed attenuation mass (*arrows*) expanding the psoas muscle. Extension into the posterior pararenal space and lateral conal fascia (*arrowheads*) is seen with displacement of the left kidney (*K*) anteriorly. *S*, spleen.

hematoma or as a diffuse area of high density (140). A subacute hematoma often has a lucent halo and a soft tissue density center. A chronic hematoma typically appears as a low-density mass (+20 to +40 HU) with a thick, dense rim (310). Peripheral calcification also may be present. Although hyperdensity is quite specific for acute hematoma, the appearance of retroperitoneal hemorrhage on CT is by no means pathognomonic. A subacute hematoma can be confused with a retroperitoneal tumor, and a chronic hematoma may have a similar appearance to an abscess, lymphocele, cyst, or urinoma. Differentiation among these entities often requires correlation with the patient's clinical history. The use of serial scanning, with decreasing size and attenuation value of the retroperitoneal mass, are reassuring signs that a the diagnosis of hematoma is correct in cases in which the clinical features are equivocal.

The MRI appearance of retroperitoneal hemorrhage depends on not only the age of the hematoma but also the magnetic field strength. The signal intensity of an acute hematoma imaged at low magnetic field (0.15 to 0.5 T) is less than or equal to that of muscle on T1-weighted images and higher than that of muscle on T2-weighted images (311). This is in contradistinction to the findings of acute hematoma when examined at high magnetic field (1.5 T). In that setting, acute hematoma has a similar signal intensity to that of muscle on T1-weighted images and marked hypointensity on T2-weighted images (94). Marked hypointensity on T2-weighted images is attributed to the presence of intracellular deoxyhemoglobin, which causes T2 shortening. This effect is more pronounced on GRE images than on SE images. A fluid–fluid level with greater signal in the dependent layer on T1-weighted images also has been described in large, acute hematomas (105).

As the hematoma ages, it assumes a more characteristic MRI appearance. On T1-weighted images, a subacute hematoma often has three distinct layers of signal: a thin, low-intensity rim corresponding to the hemosiderin-laden fibrous capsule, a slightly thicker, high-intensity (similar to fat) peripheral zone, and a medium intensity central core (slightly greater than muscle) (105,284,326). A similar three-ring appearance is noted on T2-weighted images, although the signal intensity of the central core is greater relative to the peripheral zone, whereas the rim remains low in intensity. With further maturation of the hematoma, the central core, which represents the retracted clot, continues to diminish in size, and the entire hematoma eventually becomes a homogeneous high signal intensity mass surrounded by a low-intensity rim on both T1- and T2-weighted images (Fig. 17-75). A progressive increase in signal intensity of a hematoma parallels the formation of methemoglobin (31,284)

Although hematoma may have a characteristic MRI appearance, it is important to note that hemorrhage into a tumor may be indistinguishable from a bland hematoma. Furthermore, fluid containing high protein content may have an appearance similar to that of a resolving hematoma. Fluid–fluid levels resulting from the settling of debris within an abscess may also simulate the appearance of sedimented blood.

Because of the ease with which the diagnosis of acute hematoma can be made on CT, CT will remain the procedure of choice in imaging patients with suspected acute retroperitoneal hemorrhage (less than 2 weeks duration). However, MRI may provide a more specific diagnosis than CT in less acute cases in which CT findings are nonspecific.

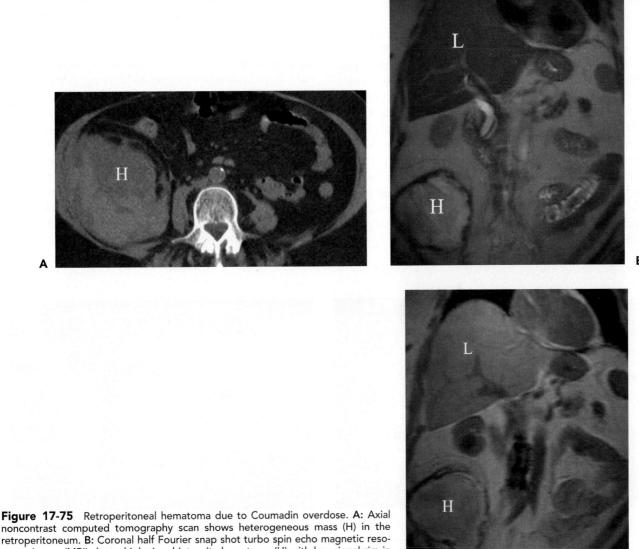

Figure 17-75 Retroperitoneal hematoma due to Coumadin overdose. **A:** Axial noncontrast computed tomography scan shows heterogeneous mass (H) in the retroperitoneum. **B:** Coronal half Fourier snap shot turbo spin echo magnetic resonance image (MRI) shows high signal intensity hematoma (H) with low signal rim in right retroperitoneal compartment. L, liver. **C:** Coronal T1-weighted MRI shows intermediate signal hematoma with low signal rim in right retroperitoneum. L, liver.

RETROPERITONEAL FIBROSIS

Retroperitoneal fibrosis is characterized by fibrous tissue proliferation along the posterior aspect of the retroperitoneum. Although the process can occur from the chest into the pelvis, the most commonly involved area lies between the renal hila and the pelvic brim. Extension anteriorly into the mesentery and posteriorly into the epidural space have also been reported (166). Vascular, ureteral, and even colonic encasement and obstruction can occur (130,274). The process is more common in men than in women and typically presents from 40 to 60 years of age. Symptoms are usually vague and poorly localized. Dull back or flank pain is most common, although weight loss, nausea, vomiting, and malaise are also reported. An elevated erythrocyte sedimentation rate is frequently seen. Azotemia may occur with ureteral obstruction (166).

Histologically, fibroblastic proliferation and collagen deposition are seen with varying amounts of inflammatory infiltrate. Early stages tend to be highly vascular and inflammatory, whereas late-stage disease often has become more fibrous and avascular (166,278). Although two thirds of cases are idiopathic (Ormond disease), certain drugs (e.g., methysergide), as well as primary or metastatic tumors (e.g., lymphoma and signet ring carcinoma), have all been associated with similar pathologic alterations in the retroperitoneum (6,278). The association of fibrosis and inflammation with some aortic aneurysms was discussed under the section on IAAAs. A similar idiopathic fibrosing disorder has been reported in the chest (fibrosing mediastinitis), thyroid (Reidel thyroiditis), orbit (pseudotumor), and biliary tree (sclerosing cholangitis). When these occur in combination, the process is referred to as multifocal fibrosclerosis (278). Each disease is thought to be a regional variation of a common immunologic hypersensitivity disorder .

Retroperitoneal fibrosis shows a variable appearance on CT and MRI (Fig. 17-76) Most patients present with a well-defined sheath of periaortic soft tissue density that surrounds the anterior and lateral surfaces of the aorta and IVC between the renal hila and sacral promontory. Loss of the normal fat planes surrounding these structures and the psoas musculature is common. On rare occasion, retroperitoneal fibrosis may show very asymmetric involvement or involvement of the retrocrural, mesenteric, peripancreatic, perirenal, or presacral regions (17,37,96,241,324,343). It may even present as single or multiple soft tissue masses with irregular borders, an appearance quite similar to that of primary retroperitoneal tumor or malignant lymphadenopathy (312,339). Unlike retroperitoneal tumors, the mass typically does not cause anterior displacement of the aorta or lateral displacement of the ureters or result in bony destruction (33,60).

On noncontrast CT scans, retroperitoneal fibrosis usually has an attenuation value similar to that of muscle although focal or uniform hyperdensity has also been reported (282, 339). With MRI, retroperitoneal fibrosis typically has a homogeneous low signal intensity similar to that of psoas muscle on T1-weighted images. The T2-weighted appearance varies depending on stage and activity of disease, with early-stage inflammatory lesions showing a hyperintense signal and late-stage lesions showing a hypointense signal (Fig. 17-77) (222). Variable contrast enhancement is noted on postcontrast scans, similarly reflecting the stage and activity of disease (282,339). Early-stage inflammatory fibrosis may show exuberant enhancement, whereas late stage disease hypoenhances (Fig. 17-78) (282,339).

Malignant retroperitoneal fibrosis tends to have a heterogeneous increased T2-weighted signal and enhancement following intravenous contrast administration) (Figs. 17-79 and 17-80). However, because of the variable appearance of

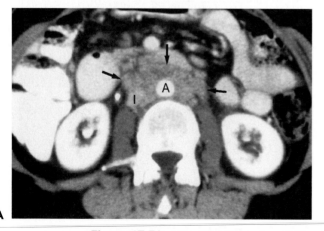
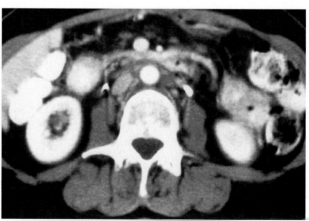

A   **B**

Figure 17-76   Idiopathic retroperitoneal fibrosis. **A:** Contrast-enhanced computed tomography scan shows mildly enhancing circumferential paraaortic soft tissue (*arrows*) encasing the inferior vena cava (I) and left ureter. Enhancement suggests an acute process or a malignant etiology. **B:** A follow-up study shows reduction of the paraaortic soft tissue after treatment with tamoxifen. Lack of enhancement is now consistent with chronic fibrosis.

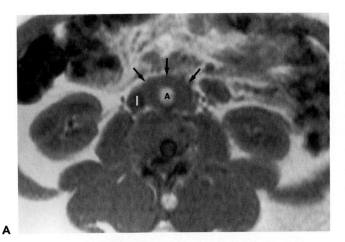
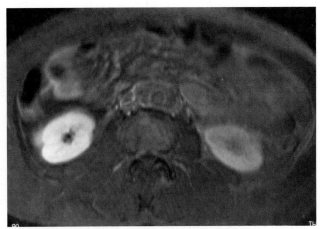

A   B

Figure 17-77 Chronic retroperitoneal fibrosis. **A:** Transaxial T1-weighted fast low-angle shot image (repetition time, 140 milliseconds; echo time, 4 milliseconds; flip angle, 80 degrees) shows sharply defined hypointense tissue (*arrows*) encasing the aorta (A). *I,* inferior vena cava. **B:** Post-gadolinium fat-saturated T1-weighted spin echo image (repetition time 600 milliseconds; echo time, 15 milliseconds) shows no enhancement of circumaortic tissue.

idiopathic retroperitoneal fibrosis, malignant causes of retroperitoneal fibrosis cannot be differentiated from non-malignant causes based on CT or MRI findings alone (166,282,339). If malignant retroperitoneal fibrosis is suspected and definitive proof is needed, biopsy is indicated. In these situations, it is recommended that multiple deep tissue samples be acquired, because relatively few malignant cells may be admixed with inflammatory cells of the collagen network (6,166).

Although US can demonstrate retroperitoneal fibrosis as a hypoechoic mass, CT or MRI are the modalities of choice for demonstrating the full extent of disease and associated organ compromise (282). In patients who are azotemic from ureteral obstruction, MRI is preferred because of the lack of nephrotoxicity of gadolinium-based contrast.

PRIMARY RETROPERITONEAL TUMORS

Primary retroperitoneal neoplasms comprise a rare and diverse group of tumors that arise in the retroperitoneum but are unassociated with retroperitoneal viscera (e.g., adrenals, kidneys, pancreas, lymph nodes). Lesions may be characterized pathologically as arising from either mesenchymal tissue (connective tissue, fat, muscle, blood vessels) or neurogenic tissue (nerve or nerve sheath, sympathetic ganglia, ectopic adrenal) or from embryonic or notochord remnants (240). Most tumors are malignant. Most tend to occur in middle age, although teratomas and neuroblastomas occur in children. Most tumors do not show a strong sex predilection; however, teratomas, ganglioneuromas, and leiomyosarcomas are more common in women, with liposarcomas, malignant fibrous histiocytomas, and chordomas more common in men. Patients are generally

asymptomatic until the tumors are large. Symptoms, which are often vague or nonspecific, are usually produced by compression of adjacent structures. Abdominal or back pain is common and may be produced by pressure or encroachment on nerve roots. Lower extremity swelling may be produced by venous compression. Compression or distortion of the gastrointestinal tract may produce anorexia, nausea, or weight loss with compression of genitourinary structures causing obstruction, frequency or hematuria (240). The primary treatment for retroperitoneal sarcomas is surgery. Five-year survival rates are poor because of difficulty in achieving a complete surgical excision in these often large lesions (75,185).

The diagnosis of tumors arising from the retroperitoneal tissues is readily accomplished with CT or MRI, even when the tumors are relatively small. Such neoplasms appear on CT or MRI generally as soft tissue masses that displace, compress, or obscure the normal retroperitoneal structures. Although it may sometimes be difficult to distinguish a true retroperitoneal neoplasm from a tumor arising from retroperitoneal viscera, the beak sign, phantom organ sign, embedded organ sign and prominent feeding artery sign may be useful (227). These signs, when present, suggest that the tumor is arising from a specific organ rather than the retroperitoneal soft tissue. For example, the beak sign occurs when a mass deforms its organ of origin into a beak shape at its margin. The phantom organ sign occurs when a mass originating in an organ has become so large that the organ is no longer discernable. The embedded organ sign occurs when the organ of origin appears embedded in a mass rather than deformed by it. The prominent feeding artery sign is seen when a mass originating in a specific viscera causes enlargement of the normal arterial supply to that organ (227).

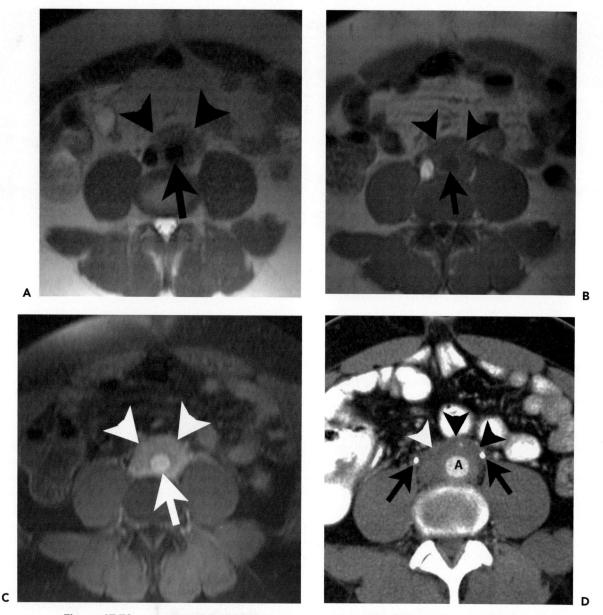

Figure 17-78 Acute retroperitoneal fibrosis. T2-weighted half Fourier snap shot turbo spin echo image **(A)** and T1-weighted fast low-angle shot image **(B)** show a hypointense rind of tissue (*arrowheads*) surrounding the aorta (*arrow*). **C:** Axial postgadolinium fat-saturated T1-weighted image shows significant tissue enhancement (*arrowheads*), reflecting the extensive capillary network present before fibrosis becomes chronic. *Arrow,* aorta. **D:** Contrast-enhanced computed tomography scan obtained following ureteral stent placement (*arrows*) shows soft tissue mass (*arrowheads*) surrounding the aorta (*A*).

Provided that some perivisceral fat is present, CT or MRI can accurately define the size, extent, and, to some degree, composition of the tumors as well as their effect on neighboring structures. Although sagittal and coronal images may be particularly useful in this regard, it should be noted that contiguity does not imply invasion because clear planes of separation between tumor and organ may be absent even when no invasion has occurred. Predictions as to definite invasion of normal structures, with implications toward surgical resectability, should be offered with caution.

CT and MRI can usually differentiate primary retroperitoneal neoplasms from retroperitoneal lymphomas. While the former tend to be heterogeneous on CT scans, lymphomas are usually homogeneous (52). Although most solid retroperitoneal tumors have an appearance similar to that of muscle tissue, it is occasionally possible to suggest a more limited differential diagnosis based on specific CT or MRI appearance (227). For example, the presence of fat is characteristic of lipomas and liposarcomas (Figs. 17-81 to 17-83). Although teratomas may also contain fat, they

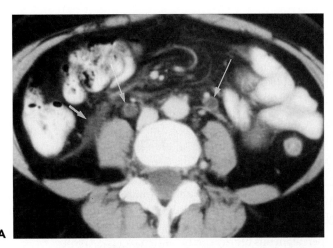

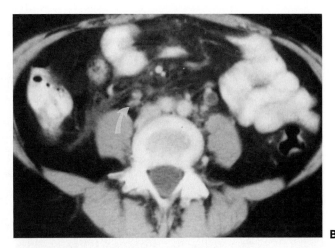

A

B

Figure 17-79 Malignant retroperitoneal fibrosis resulting from metastatic breast cancer. **A:** Contrast-enhanced computed tomography scan shows bilateral obstructive hydroureter (*long white arrows*) with a sheet of abnormal retroperitoneal soft tissue (*short white arrow*). **B:** Inferiorly, tissue extends to the right ureter with abnormal enhancement (*curved white arrow*) at the site of obstruction.

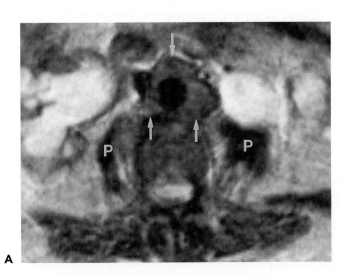

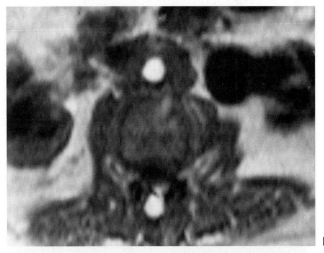

A

B

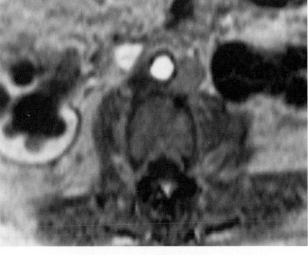

C

Figure 17-80 Malignant retroperitoneal fibrosis resulting from metastatic cervical carcinoma. **A:** Transaxial T2-weighted fast spin echo image (repetition time, 3,500 milliseconds; echo time, 93 milliseconds) shows circumaortic tissue (*arrows*) that is slightly hyperintense to psoas muscle (P). Note the bilateral obstructive hydronephrosis from disease in the pelvis. **B:** On a transaxial T1-weighted fast low-angle shot image (repetition time, 140 milliseconds; echo time, 4 milliseconds; flip angle 80 degrees), the tissue is isointense to the psoas muscle. **C:** Transaxial postgadolinium T1-weighted fast low-angle shot image (repetition time, 140 milliseconds; echo time, 4 milliseconds; flip angle, 80 degrees) shows mild enhancement of the tissue.

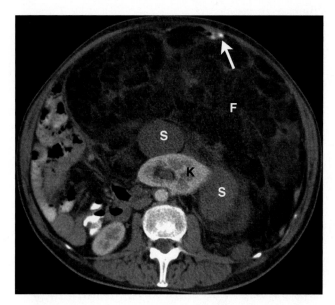

Figure 17-81 Retroperitoneal liposarcoma. Contrast-enhanced computed tomography scan shows a large retroperitoneal mass of mixed fat (F) and soft tissue (S) attenuation. The descending colon (*arrow*) and kidney (K) are displaced anteromedially indicating the retroperitoneal location of the tumor.

usually also show fat–fluid levels or calcification. A myxoid stoma with the resultant high signal appearance on T2-weighted imaging can be seen with some liposarcomas, malignant fibrous histiocytomas, and neurogenic tumors (371). Large areas of necrosis can be seen in any high-grade neoplasm but are typical of leiomyosarcoma (Figs. 17-84 and 17-85). Lymphangiomas, mucinous cystic lesions, and neurogenic tumors may show partially or completely cystic

regions. Vascularity also differs among tumor types, with lymphomas and low-grade liposarcomas being relatively hypovascular (227). Marked hypervascularity is noted in paragangliomas and hemangiopericytomas. Moderate hypervascularity characterizes leiomyosarcoma, malignant fibrous histiocytoma (MFH), and many of the other sarcomas. Growth pattern may offer a clue to the differential diagnosis. For example, neurogenic tumors involving the sympathetic ganglia often have an elongated shape as they grow along the sympathetic chain. Lymphangiomas, ganglioneuromas, and lymphomas tend to insinuate themselves between structures rather than compressing or displacing them (227,260). When more precise preoperative characterization is desired than imaging features allow, CT-guided percutaneous biopsy can be undertaken.

CT and or MRI also have an important role in following patients after tumor resection. In a study of 33 patients with recurrent retroperitoneal sarcoma, 85% had local or regional recurrence, with almost three fourths of recurrences being detected within 2 years of initial resection. As with the primary lesions, the majority of recurrent tumors showed a heterogeneous appearance on CT scans (102).

Lipoma and Liposarcoma

Lipomas and their malignant counterpart, liposarcomas, are the most common retroperitoneal soft tissue tumors (75,185,278). They are usually quite large at presentation and can be multiple. Liposarcomas can be categorized by the relative amount of intracellular fat and mucinous matrix they contain into lipogenic, myxoid, and pleomorphic types depending on the dominant component. Most lipogenic

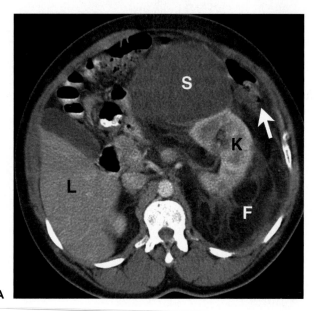

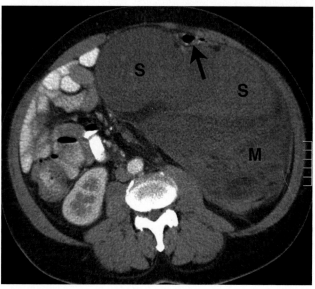

A   **B**

Figure 17-82 Dedifferentiated liposarcoma. A and B: Contrast-enhanced computed tomography scans at two levels of the midabdomen show a large retroperitoneal mass of fat (F), soft tissue (S), and mixed (M) attenuation displacing the descending colon (*arrow*) and kidney (K) anteromedially. In contrast to Figure 17-66, the mass shows more solid components, corresponding to dedifferentiated tumor. L, liver.

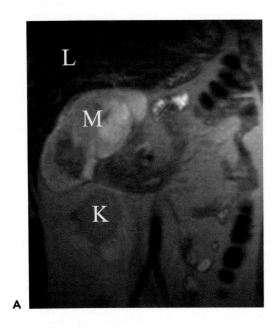

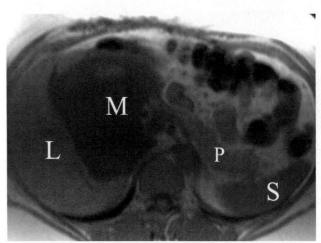

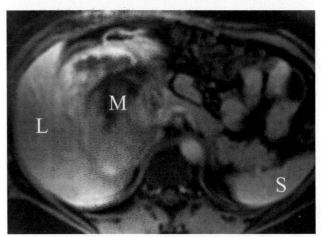

Figure 17-83 Dedifferentiated liposarcoma. **A:** Coronal half Fourier snap shot turbo spin echo magnetic resonance image (MRI) shows mixed signal retroperitoneal mass (M) displacing right kidney (K) inferiorly. L, liver. **B:** Axial T1-weighted MRI shows hypointense retroperitoneal mass (M) medial to the liver (L). P, pancreas; S, spleen. **C:** Contrast-enhanced T1-weighted MRI shows heterogeneous enhancement in the right retroperitoneal mass (M). L, liver; S, spleen.

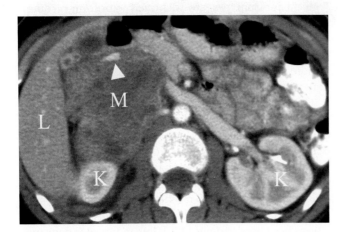

Figure 17-84 Leiomyosarcoma. Contrast-enhanced computed tomography shows a large heterogeneous mass (M) in right retroperitoneal compartment. The mass displaces inferior vena cava (*arrowhead*) anteriorly. L, liver; K, kidneys.

tumors are low-grade, well-differentiated lesions, with pleomorphic tumors being high-grade, poorly differentiated tumors. Myxoid tumors are the most common type and are typically of intermediate grade (341).

On CT or MRI, lipomas appear as sharply marginated, homogeneous masses with CT densities equal to that of normal fat and MR appearance consistent with that of simple fat on T1- and T2-weighted and fat-saturated sequences. Fine linear streaky densities may be present along with a thin border of denser tissue that defines the capsule. No significant soft tissue component is observed (82,341). In contradistinction, liposarcomas are poorly marginated infiltrative lesions that typically contain an admixture of fat and soft tissue density components (see Figs. 17-81 to 17-83). Although well-differentiated liposarcoma (lipogenic liposarcoma) may be virtually indistinguishable from benign lipoma, it more commonly contains some solid or infiltrative components that tend to be thicker, more

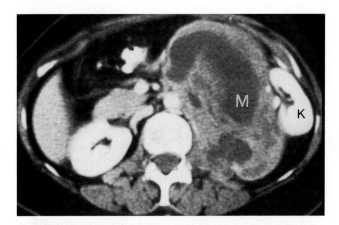

Figure 17-85 Retroperitoneal leiomyosarcoma. Contrast-enhanced computed tomography scan demonstrates a large, heterogeneously enhancing mass (M) displacing the left kidney (K) laterally. Irregular hypodense regions represent tissue necrosis and cystic degeneration commonly seen in leiomyosarcoma.

numerous, and less well defined than those seen with lipomas. They typically do not have a visible capsule and tend to blend into the adjacent fat. Myxoid liposarcomas have densities less than that of muscle and closer to that of water on CT. On MRI myxoid components have signal intensity similar to that of water. Following intravenous contrast, myxoid regions show gradual reticular enhancement. Although these lesions resemble complex cysts prior to contrast, following contrast they appear more solid. They may have sharp margins or calcification and most commonly do not contain demonstrable fat. Pleomorphic and round cell liposarcomas show a soft tissue density similar to that of muscle on CT. On T1-weighted MRI, they show a signal intensity similar to that of muscle, but have increased signal intensity on T2-weighted images, similar to that of fat. It has been suggested that MRI may be able to distinguish between the low-grade sclerotic soft tissue component sometimes seen in lipogenic and myxoid liposarcomas and the high-grade soft tissue component seen in pleomorphic and round cell liposarcomas. In the former, the signal intensity on T2-weighted images approximates that of muscle, whereas the signal intensity of the pleomorphic components is significantly higher, approximating that seen with fat (156,341).

Lesions other than lipoma and liposarcoma may also contain fat. A mature teratoma of the retroperitoneum may contain foci of mature fat. It typically can be differentiated from a lipoma or liposarcoma by the common presence of a fat–fluid level and calcifications, although these findings have, on rare occasions, been reported with lipoma or liposarcoma (57,171). Adrenal myelolipomas and renal angiomyolipomas may mimic liposarcomas; however, their usual origin from the adrenal or kidney should clarify the diagnosis. Enlarged vessels are also commonly visible in angiomyolipomas but unusual in liposarcomas (134). Rarely, an angiomyolipoma may originate in the perirenal fat and

be indistinguishable from a perirenal liposarcoma (325). Similarly, myelolipomas have been reported in the retroperitoneum and presacral region independent of the adrenal (152). A lymphangioma with a high lipid content can also simulate a lipoma on CT scans (58,82). A diffuse increase in retroperitoneal and or pelvic fat may also be seen in Cushing disease, with pelvic lipomatosis, with lipoplastic lymphadenopathy, and idiopathically (82). The symmetric nature of the fat and absence of encapsulation is helpful in distinguishing these lesions from lipomas.

Leiomyosarcoma

Leiomyosarcomas are the second most common type of retroperitoneal sarcoma (75,112,185) and are more common in women than men. They may demonstrate intravascular or extravascular growth or a combination of the two (112,172). As with the other retroperitoneal tumors, leiomyosarcomas can be huge, with measurements as great as 35 cm reported (320).

On CT scans, they typically present as a well-circumscribed, large muscle-density mass with areas of lower attenuation corresponding to necrosis (see Figs. 17-84 and 17-85). In general, the areas of necrosis are more extensive than that noted with other retroperitoneal malignancies (112,175). Intraluminal growth is most commonly seen involving the IVC between the diaphragm and renal veins. It typically expands the IVC and may extend into the heart (112). The MRI appearance is also quite heterogeneous. Lesions typically have low to intermediate signal on T1-weighted sequences and intermediate to high signal on T2-weighted sequences, reflecting the amount of cystic necrosis present (112,172).

Malignant Fibrous Histiocytoma

MFH is the third most common retroperitoneal sarcoma and has a broad range of histologic appearances (75,185). Four major subtypes are identified: storiform-pleomorphic, myxoid, giant cell, and inflammatory (161,224). Although most cases occur in the extremities, almost any site or organ can be involved. The tumor typically occurs in middle age or older patients. It is more common in men than women and usually presents with a mass or pain.

On CT or MRI, the lesions have a varied appearance, reflecting the underlying histologic pleomorphism. Tumors are usually quite large and may have circumscribed or ill-defined margins (161). Heterogeneous attenuation or signal intensity may be seen, particularly centrally, consistent with necrosis, hemorrhage, or myxoid material. Fluid levels are occasionally seen reflecting spontaneous hemorrhage. Fat is not seen, which may help to distinguish these lesions from liposarcomas (276). Enhancement is quite variable. Calcification is seen in only a minority of lesions (161). On MRI, the tumors usually display low or intermediate signal on T1-weighted sequences with high signal intensity seen on T2-weighted sequences. Myxoid material, if present, is typically hyperintense on T2-weighted sequences (224).

Neurogenic Tumors

Neurogenic tumors in the retroperitoneum can be categorized into those originating from ganglion cells (ganglioneuromas, ganglioneuroblastomas, and neuroblastoma), those arising from the paraganglionic system (pheochromocytomas, paragangliomas), and those arising from nerve sheath cells (neurilemomas, neurofibromas, and malignant nerve sheath tumors) (273). Lesions are typically seen from the adrenal to the organ of Zuckerkandl in a paraspinal location that mirrors the distribution of the sympathetic ganglia. Although neuroblastoma and ganglioneuroblastoma occur in infancy and childhood, the remainder of the neurogenic tumors occur in adults (273). Most lesions present with mass or pain; however, they may secrete substances, including catecholamines, vasoactive peptides, or androgenic hormones, that produce a variety of systemic symptoms.

Most neurogenic tumors appear as well-defined, simple or lobulated masses. They may be elongated in shape as they follow the course of the sympathetic nerves (227) (Figs. 17-86 and 17-87). Unlike other retroperitoneal tumors, they tend to insinuate themselves between vascular structures without causing vascular compromise or displacement (260). Calcification is common and can be seen in approximately 85% of cases of neuroblastoma and to a lesser degree in other neurogenic tumors. Most lesions are fairly homogeneous on CT, with attenuation similar to or less than that of muscle (21,117,260,273). Cystlike

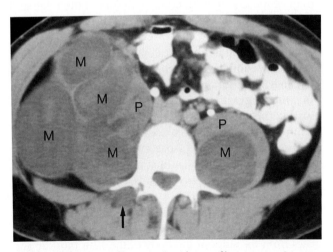

Figure 17-86 Neurofibromatosis with neurofibrosarcoma. Contrast-enhanced computed tomography scan demonstrates bilateral slightly enhancing, hypodense masses (M) extending along the course of the lumbar nerves and displacing the psoas muscles (P) anteriorly. The location is typical for a neurogenic tumor, and the gross asymmetry should raise suspicion for sarcomatous degeneration. A smaller neurofibroma lies posterior to the right transverse process (*arrow*).

spaces may be noted from areas of necrosis or myxoid degeneration (155). MRI demonstrates a low T1-weighted signal with moderate to markedly high T2-weighted signal intensity depending on the amount of myxoid matrix (114,273,371). A whorled appearance has been seen on T2-weighted images with ganglioneuroma (371). Variable enhancement is noted, with delayed enhancement described in tumors with myxoid stroma as contrast slowly diffuses into the myxoid regions (371). Paraganglionic tumors are typically hypervascular with marked enhancement, whereas ganglioneuromas show little early enhancement (Figs. 17-88 and 17-89). Ganglioneuromas also show a thin capsule, whereas neurofibromas are not encapsulated. The cystic degeneration seen in schwannomas is also not seen in ganglioneuromas (371). Although concern has been raised about inducing catecholamine release from pheochromocytoma with intravenous contrast use, a study of 10 patients with pheochromocytomas showed no increase in circulating epinephrine or norepinephrine following use of nonionic contrast (220).

Primary Germ Cell Tumors

Extragonadal germ cell tumors are thought to either arise from abnormal migration of primordial germ cells during embryogenesis or represent metastasis from occult gonadal primaries. Most extragonadal germ cell tumors occur in the midline. The mediastinum is the most common site, followed by the retroperitoneum (226). In children, there is no strong sex predilection in either benign or malignant germ cell tumors. Although in adults, benign tumors have similar sex parity, over 90% of malignant extragonadal germ cell tumors occur in men (226). Seminomatous and nonseminomatous germ cell tumors and teratomas all may occur in the retroperitoneum. Most patients present with back pain or an abdominal mass. Edema secondary to lymphatic obstruction is also noted. Elevation in serum biomarkers such as human chorionic gonadotropin (HCG) and alpha-fetoprotein (AFP) should be evaluated (226).

On CT or MRI, mature teratoma typically appear as a well-defined mass with cystic and solid components containing fat, fluid, and calcium. Fat may occur in several forms—solid fat, sebum, and admixed with hair—and show variation in density on CT and signal intensity on MRI (49). Fat–fluid levels may be noted and are strongly suggestive of teratoma (86). Malignant germ cell tumors appear as large, lobulated masses with mixed density components. The low-density regions presumably correspond to areas of necrosis or old hemorrhage (28).

Other Retroperitoneal Tumors

A variety of other neoplasms may involve the retroperitoneum. Most are quite rare, but several have distinctive imaging characteristics. Lymphangioma typically appears as a well-circumscribed, elongated, unicameral or septated

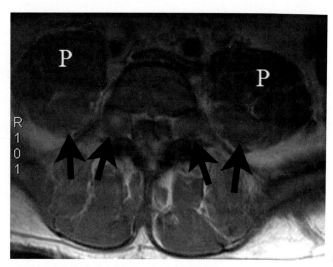

Figure 17-87 Neurofibromatosis with neurofibromas. **A:** T2-weighted magnetic resonance image demonstrates hyperintense lobulated masses (*arrows*) extending from the neural foramina bilaterally and displacing the psoas (P) anterolaterally. **B:** T1-weighted image shows the masses (*arrows*) to be similar to muscle in signal intensity.

fluid-filled mass. Septae are usually smooth and thin although approximately 20% showed thicker irregular walls. Calcification is unusual. Fluid is usually homogeneous and near water density, although a lesion containing chyle with fat density has been reported. High signal intensity on T2-weighted imaging is typical. T1-weighted signal is usually low unless hemorrhage has occurred (135). Layering debris may also be noted (58,183). Other rare cystic lesions of the retroperitoneum include primary mucinous cystadenoma, cystic teratoma, cystic mesothelioma, and a variety of congenital lesions (epidermoid, tailgut, bronchogenic cysts), as well as cystic change in solid neoplasms

(e.g., paraganglioma) (364). Hemangiopericytomas are large, complex masses showing multiple areas of irregular low density corresponding to regions of necrosis or hemorrhage. Hypervascularity in solid areas is characteristic but can also be found in leiomyosarcoma and MFH (4,91).

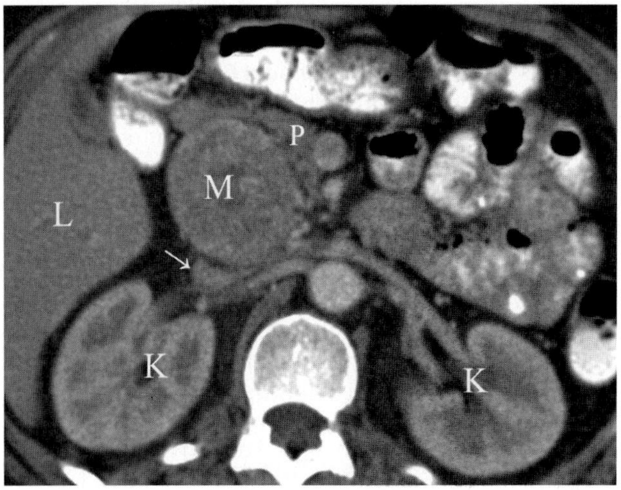

PSOAS

Normal Anatomy

The psoas major, psoas minor, and iliacus muscles are a group of muscles that function as flexors of the thigh and trunk. The psoas major muscle originates from fibers arising from the transverse processes of the 12th thoracic vertebra as well as all lumbar vertebrae. The muscle fibers fuse and pass inferiorly in a paraspinal location. As it exits from the pelvis, the psoas major assumes a more anterior location, merging with the iliacus to become the iliopsoas muscle. The iliopsoas passes beneath the inguinal ligament to insert on the lesser trochanter of the femur. At its superior attachment, the psoas muscle passes beneath the arcuate ligament of the diaphragm. The psoas muscle is in a fascial plane that directly extends from the mediastinum to the thigh.

The psoas minor is a long, slender muscle, located immediately anterior to the psoas major. When present, it arises from the sides of the body of the 12th thoracic and first lumbar vertebrae and from the fibrocartilage between them. It ends in a long, flat tendon that inserts on the iliopectineal eminence of the innominate bone.

On CT or MRI scans, the normal psoas major muscles are delineated clearly in almost every patient as paired paraspinal structures. The proximal portion of the psoas

Figure 17-88 Retroperitoneal paraganglioma. Contrast-enhanced computed tomography image shows a heterogeneously enhancing mass (M) in the region of the second part of the duodenum. Mass displaces the inferior vena cava (*arrow*) posteriorly and pancreatic head (P) anteromedially. K, kidney; L, liver.

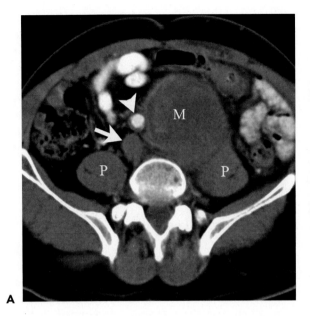

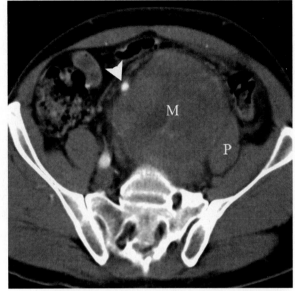

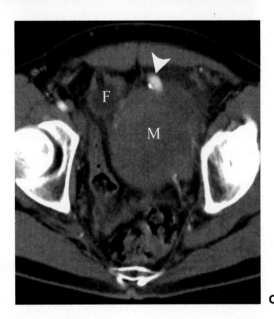

Figure 17-89 Retroperitoneal schwannoma. **A:** Contrast-enhanced computed tomography image shows a large paraaortic mass (M) displacing the aorta (*arrowhead*) and inferior vena cava (*arrow*) to the right. P, psoas. **B:** Mass (M) extends along the left common iliac artery (*arrowhead*), displacing it to the right. **C:** Mass is seen in the lower pelvis displacing left femoral artery anteromedially and the bladder, with contained Foley catheter (F), to the left.

muscle is triangular in shape, whereas the distal end has a more rounded appearance. The size of the psoas major muscle increases in a cephalocaudad direction. When visible, especially in young, muscular individuals, the psoas minor appears as a small, rounded, soft tissue mass anterior to the psoas major (Fig. 17-90). Caution must be taken not to confuse this muscle with an enlarged lymph node. The sympathetic trunk as well as the lumbar veins and arteries are sometimes seen as small soft tissue densities located just medial to the psoas muscles and lateral to the lumbar spine. However, differentiation between an artery, a vein, and a nerve in this location is not possible on non-contrast scans.

The psoas muscle has low signal intensity on both T1- and T2-weighted images. A T1-weighted pulse sequence provides the best contrast between the muscle and adjacent retroperitoneal fat; both T2-weighted and postgadolinium,

T1-weighted, fat-suppressed sequences can clearly differentiate normal muscle from most pathologic conditions (180,346).

To evaluate the psoas muscle, images in the transaxial plane should be obtained. If an abnormality is noted in the muscle, additional coronal or sagittal views may help delineate the extent of disease and determine if there is involvement of the spine (346).

Pathology

Neoplasm

A pathologic process can involve the psoas muscle by one of three mechanisms: (a) replacement, (b) medial displacement, and (c) lateral displacement (180). Lymphoma, other malignant

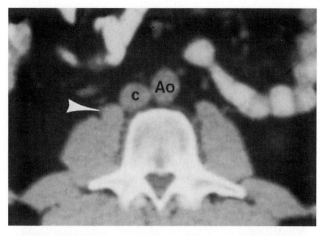

Figure 17-90 The psoas minor muscle (*arrowhead*), prominent in some muscular individuals, should not be confused with an enlarged lymph node. Ao, aorta; c, inferior vena cava.

retroperitoneal neoplasms, and metastasis may exhibit each of these appearances and result in a focal lesion, enlargement, or obscuration of the psoas muscle. The involved muscle most often has a CT attenuation value similar to the normal one, although areas of low attenuation also may be present (76). On MRI, the abnormal muscle has signal intensity higher than that of normal psoas on both T1- and T2-weighted images. On T1-weighted images, the signal intensity of the diseased muscle is less than that of fat unless

hemorrhage has occurred, in which case a high intensity signal may be observed in the abnormal region. Because of its superior contrast sensitivity, MRI is superior to CT in separating normal from abnormal psoas muscle. We have encountered cases in which the CT study showed apparent enlargement of the psoas muscle and subsequent MRI examination demonstrated that the psoas muscle was compressed and displaced laterally by a mass (180) (Fig. 17-91). However, neither examination can reliably differentiate mere contiguity from superficial invasion.

Inflammatory Lesions

Infection within the psoas muscle may occur either from direct extension from contiguous structures (secondary psoas abscess), such as the spine, kidney, bowel, and pancreas, or without a definite source (primary psoas abscess), in which case the infection is presumed to have arisen from hematogenous seeding (76,287,372). With the decreasing incidence in tuberculous involvement of the spine, the majority of psoas abscesses now encountered are of a pyogenic origin (76,372). On CT scans, the involved psoas muscle is often enlarged, with an abscess appearing as a focal low density area (0 HU to 30 HU) (Figs. 17-92 and 17-93) (76). The size and extent of the abscess usually can easily be delineated; visualization of the abscess is improved by intravenous administration of iodinated contrast material. Gas is noted in approximately

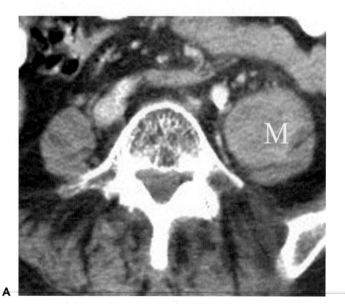

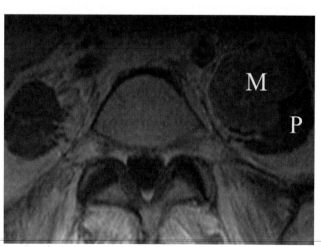

A   B

Figure 17-91 Non-Hodgkin lymphoma abutting left psoas muscle. **A:** Contrast-enhanced computed tomography (CT) shows enlargement of left psoas muscle by mass (M). Mass is not well delineated from muscle on CT. **B:** T1-weighted magnetic resonance image demonstrates mass (M) displacing psoas muscle (P) posterolaterally. Mass is slightly hyperintense relative to muscle.

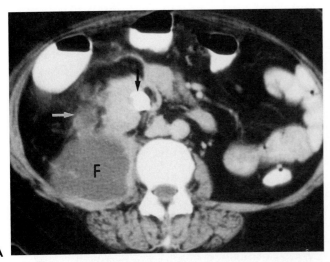
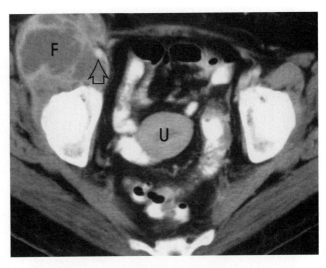

Figure 17-92 Psoas abscess from an infected urinoma. **A:** Contrast-enhanced computed tomography (CT) scan shows a fluid collection (F) tracking within the right psoas muscle. Note the obstructing renal calculus (*black arrow*) and the communication of the psoas collection with the right perinephric space (*white arrow*). **B:** CT scan at the level of the acetabulum demonstrates the inferior extent of this fluid collection to be located at the site of the right psoas muscle attachment. Note the enhancement of its wall and septations. Culture grew *Escherichia coli*. U, uterus; *open arrow*, external iliac artery.

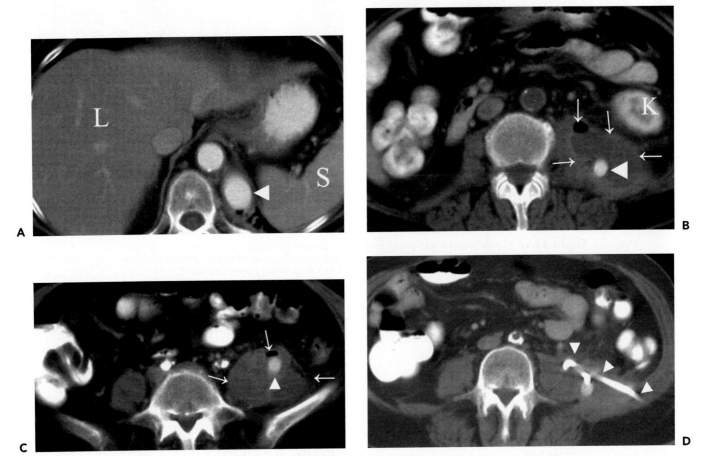

Figure 17-93 Abscess around aortofemoral graft: **A:** Contrast-enhanced computed tomography scan shows the proximal end of the aortofemoral graft (*arrowhead*). L, liver; S, spleen. **B:** At a lower level, a rim-enhancing low-density collection containing air (*arrows*) is seen surrounding the graft (*arrowhead*). K, kidney. The medial limb of the graft is patent; the lateral limb is thrombosed. **C:** At the level of the iliac crest, the low-density collection with air (*arrows*) is seen extending around the graft (*arrowhead*). **D:** Percutaneous placement of a drainage catheter (*arrowheads*) allows resolution of the abscess.

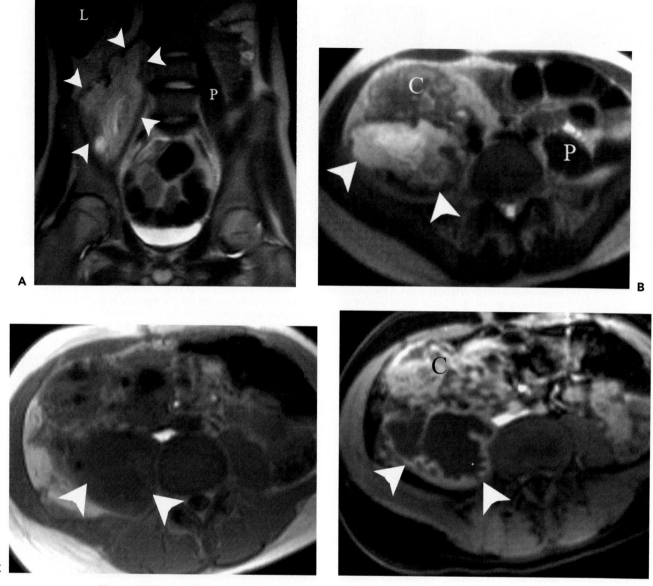

Figure 17-94   Crohn disease with psoas abscess. **A:** Coronal T2-weighted half Fourier snap shot turbo spin echo (HASTE) magnetic resonance (MR) image shows high signal intensity fluid collection (*arrowheads*) in right psoas muscle. L, liver; P, normal left psoas. **B:** Axial T2-weighted HASTE MRI shows inferior portion of high signal intensity abscess extending into right iliopsoas muscle (*arrowheads*). Note phlegmonous change around the cecum (C). P, left psoas. **C:** Axial T1-weighted MRI shows intermediate signal collection (*arrowheads*) virtually replacing the right psoas muscle. **D:** Axial T1-weighted contrast-enhanced fat-saturated MRI shows intense rim enhancement (*arrowheads*) around psoas abscess. Abnormal enhancement is also seen in the phlegmonous change about the cecum (C).

40% to 50% of cases (76,372). Psoas abscess can likewise be detected by MRI (Fig. 17-94). Abscesses have a signal intensity equal to or greater than that of normal muscle on T1-weighted images and a high signal intensity on T2-weighted images (180,346). A major limitation of MRI is its inability to consistently detect small collections of air that may be present within the abscess. If detected, a collection of air would appear as a focal region of signal void on both T1- and T2-weighted images. However, a focal

calcification in the muscle could have a similar appearance. Myositis without frank abscess formation has also been described and appears as muscle enlargement with increased T2-weighted signal corresponding to edema (95,361). In many cases, CT or MRI can help elucidate a source of infection such as appendicitis, Crohn disease, perirenal abscess, discitis, or sacroiliitis (372).

Enlargement of a psoas muscle with areas of lower density is not specific for an inflammatory process. In a study

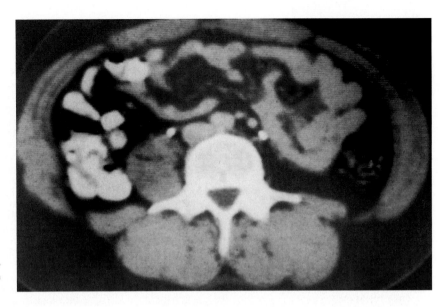

Figure 17-95 Psoas atrophy. Note absence of left psoas muscle in this patient with a history of polio. The right psoas is normal.

of 44 patients with iliopsoas abscess, tumor or hematoma, a correct diagnosis was made in only 48% of patients when clinical data were withheld (181). Irregular margins were seen in 67% of tumors but also 52% of abscesses. Low attenuation was noted in 100% of abscesses but also 67% of tumors. Diffuse involvement of the muscle was seen in 88% of hematomas but only 19% of abscesses. Although gas is usually significantly more common in abscess than tumor (76), in this series, gas was noted in three neoplasms and two abscesses (181). Gas has also been reported in the psoas muscle secondary to an intravertebral vacuum cleft (330). In cases in which the CT findings are nonspecific, CT can be used to guide percutaneous needle aspiration of the observed abnormality to obtain tissue for histologic examination and bacteriologic culture. In cases in which the diagnosis of psoas abscess is certain, CT can be used to guide percutaneous drainage (42,372).

Other Conditions

Although the psoas may undergo spontaneous hemorrhage due to overanticoagulation, a hematoma involving this muscle also can result from a leaking aortic aneurysm. As mentioned previously, the CT attenuation value of a hematoma varies from about +20 HU to +90 HU, depending upon its age (see Fig. 17-73). Hematoma, abscess, and neoplasm, with or without central necrosis, all can have a similar CT appearance (181). MRI may be helpful in cases of hemorrhage by demonstrating the characteristic increased signal on T1- and T2-weighted images of subacute blood (346).

Atrophy of the psoas muscle secondary to neuromuscular disorders is similarly easily identified and appears as a uniform decrease in the size of the muscle bulk on the involved side (Fig. 17-95). On occasion, the involved muscles have low density on CT because of partial fatty replacement.

REFERENCES

1. Adriaensen ME, Bosch JL, Halpern EF, et al. Elective endovascular versus open surgical repair of abdominal aortic aneurysms: systematic review of short-term results. *Radiology* 2002; 224:739–747.
2. Akkersdijk GJ, van Bockel JH. Ruptured abdominal aortic aneurysm: initial misdiagnosis and the effect on treatment. *Eur J Surg* 1998;164:29–34.
3. Aljabri B, MacDonald PS, Satin R, et al. Incidence of major venous and renal anomalies relevant to aortoiliac surgery as demonstrated by computed tomography. *Ann Vasc Surg* 2001; 15:615–618.
4. Alpern MB, Thorsen MK, Kellman GM, et al. CT appearance of hemangiopericytoma. *J Comput Assist Tomogr* 1986;10:264–267.
5. Amano T, Takemae K, Niikura S, et al. Retroperitoneal hemorrhage due to spontaneous rupture of adrenal myelolipoma. *Int J Urol* 1999;6:585–588.
6. Amis ES. Retroperitoneal fibrosis. *AJR Am J Roentgenol* 1991; 157: 321–329.
7. Anzai Y, Piccoli CW, Outwater EK, et al. Evaluation of neck and body metastases to nodes with ferumoxtran 10-enhanced MR imaging: phase III safety and efficacy study. *Radiology* 2003;228:777–788.
8. Applegate KE, Goske MJ, Pierce G, et al. Situs revisited: imaging of the heterotaxy syndrome. *Radiographics* 1999;19:837–852; discussion 853–854.
9. Apter S, Avigdor A, Gayer G, et al. Calcification in lymphoma occurring before therapy: CT features and clinical correlation. *AJR Am J Roentgenol* 2002;178:935–938.
10. Arita T, Matsunaga N, Takano K. Abdominal aortic aneurysm: rupture associated with the high-attenuating crescent sign. *Radiology* 1997;204:765–768.
11. Armerding MD, Rubin GD, Beaulieu CF, et al. Aortic aneurysmal disease: assessment of stent-graft treatment-CT versus conventional angiography. *Radiology* 2000;215:138–146.
12. Arrive L, Hricak H, Tavares NJ, et al. Malignant versus nonmalignant retroperitoneal fibrosis: differentiation with MR imaging. *Radiology* 1989;172:139–143.
13. Arrive L, Menu Y, Dessarts I, et al. Diagnosis of abdominal venous thrombosis by means of spin-echo and gradient-echo MR imaging: analysis with receiver operating characteristic curves. *Radiology* 1991;181:661–668.
14. Arrive L, Correas JM, Leseche G, et al. Inflammatory aneurysms of the abdominal aorta: CT findings. *AJR Am J Roentgenol* 1995;165:1481–1484.
15. Auffermann W, Olofsson PA, Rabahie GN, et al. Incorporation versus infection of retroperitoneal aortic grafts: MR imaging features. *Radiology* 1989;172:359–362.

16. Avila NA, Kelly JA, Chu SC, et al. Lymphangioleiomyomatosis: abdominopelvic CT and US findings. *Radiology* 2000;216:147–153.

17. Ayuso JR, Garcia-Criado A, Caralt TM, et al. Atypical retroperitoneal fibrosis: MRI findings. *Eur Radiol* 1999;9:937–939.

18. Badler R, Price AP, Moy L, et al. Congenital portacaval shunt: CT demonstration. *Pediatr Radiol* 2002;32:28–30.

19. Barrington SF, O'Doherty MJ. Limitations of PET for imaging lymphoma. *Eur J Nucl Med Mol Imaging* 2003;30[suppl 1]:S117–S127.

20. Basile A, Certo A, Ascenti G, et al. Embryologic and acquired anomalies of the inferior vena cava with recurrent deep vein thrombosis. *Abdom Imaging* 2003;28:400–403.

21. Bass JC, Korobkin M, Francis IR, et al. Retroperitoneal plexiform neurofibromas: CT findings. *AJR Am J Roentgenol* 1994;163:617–620.

22. Bass JE, Redwine MD, Kramer LA, et al. Absence of the infrarenal inferior vena cava with preservation of the suprarenal segment as revealed by CT and MR venography. *AJR Am J Roentgenol* 1999;172:1610–1612.

23. Bass JE, Redwine MD, Kramer LA, et al. Spectrum of congenital anomalies of the inferior vena cava: cross-sectional imaging findings. *Radiographics* 2000;20:639–652.

24. Bassilios N, Tassart M, Restoux A, et al. Inferior vena cava thrombosis due to acute pyelonephritis. *Nephrol Dial Transplant* 2004;19:981–983.

25. Bechtold RE, Dyer RB, Zagoria RJ, et al. The perirenal space: relationship of pathologic processes to normal retroperitoneal anatomy. *Radiographics* 1996;16:841–854.

26. Bertges DJ, Chow K, Wyers MC, et al. Abdominal aortic aneurysm size regression after endovascular repair is endograft dependent. *J Vasc Surg* 2003;37:716–723.

27. Bhalla S, Menias CO, Heiken JP. CT of acute abdominal aortic disorders. *Radiol Clin North Am* 2003;41:1153–1169.

28. Blomlie V, Lien HH, Fossa SD, et al. CT in primary malignant germ cell tumors of the retroperitoneum. *Acta Radiol* 1991;32:155–158.

29. Blum U, Wildanger G, Windfuhr M, et al. Preoperative CT and MR imaging of inferior vena cava leiomyosarcoma. *Eur J Radiol* 1995;20:23–27.

30. Bosl GJ, Motzer RJ. Testicular germ-cell cancer. *N Engl J Med* 1997;337:242–253.

31. Bradley WGJ, Schmidt PG. Effect of methemoglobin formation on the MR appearance of subarachnoid hemorrhage. *Radiology* 1985;156:99–103.

32. Brochert A, Reynolds T. Unusual duplication anomaly of the inferior vena cava with normal drainage of the right IVC and hemiazygous continuation of the left IVC. *J Vasc Interv Radiol* 2001;12:1453–1455.

33. Brooks AP, Reznek RH, Webb JAW. Aortic displacement on computed tomography of idiopathic retroperitoneal fibrosis. *Clin Radiol* 1989;40:51–52.

34. Brown PM, Pattenden R, Gutelius JR. The selective management of small abdominal aortic aneurysms: the Kingston study. *J Vasc Surg* 1992;125:21–27.

35. Bussar-Maatz R, Weissbach L. Retroperitoneal lymph node staging of testicular tumours: TNM study group. *Br J Urol* 1993;72:234–240.

36. Busuttil SJ, Goldstone J. Diagnosis and management of aortoenteric fistulas. *Semin Vasc Surg* 2001;14:302–311.

37. Buyl L, Oosterlinck W, Verstraete K, et al. An unusual case of unilateral periureteral retroperitoneal fibrosis. *Clin Radiol* 2003;58:492–494.

38. Callen PW, Korobkin M, Isherwood I. Computed tomographic evaluation of the retrocrural prevertebral space. *AJR Am J Roentgenol* 1977;129:907–910.

39. Calligaro KD, Veith FJ. Diagnosis and management of infected prosthetic aortic grafts. *Surgery* 1991;110:805–813.

40. Calligaro KD, Bergen WS, Savarese RP, et al. Primary aortoduodenal fistula due to septic aortitis. *J Cardiovasc Surg (Torino)* 1992;33:192–198.

41. Calligaro KD, Ahmad S, Dandora R, et al. Venous aneurysms: surgical indications and review of the literature. *Surgery* 1995;117:1–6.

42. Cantasdemir M, Kara B, Cebi D, et al. Computed tomography-guided percutaneous catheter drainage of primary and secondary iliopsoas abscesses. *Clin Radiol* 2003;58:811–815.

43. Carriero A, Iezzi A, Margarelli N, et al. Magnetic resonance angiography and colour-Doppler sonography in the evaluation of abdominal aortic aneurysms. *Eur Radiol* 1997;7:1495–1500.

44. Castellino RA. Lymph nodes of the posterior iliac crest: CT and lymphographic observations. *Radiology* 1990;175:687–689.

45. Castrucci M, Mellone R, Vanzulli A, et al. Mural thrombi in abdominal aortic aneurysms: MR imaging characterization—useful before endovascular treatment? *Radiology* 1995;197:135–139.

46. Catasca JV, Mirowitz SA. T2-weighted MR imaging of the abdomen: fast spin-echo vs conventional spin-echo sequences. *AJR Am J Roentgenol* 1994;162:61–67.

47. Chee YL, Culligan DJ, Watson HG. Inferior vena cava malformation as a risk factor for deep venous thrombosis in the young. *Br J Haematol* 2001;114:878–880.

48. Chesson JP, Theodorescu D. Adrenal tumor with caval extension—case report and review of the literature. *Scand J Urol Nephrol* 2002;36:71–73.

49. Choi BI, Chia JG, Kim SH, et al. MR imaging of retroperitoneal teratoma: correlation with CT and pathology. *J Comput Assist Tomogr* 1989;13:1083–1086.

50. Cil BE, Akpinar E, Karcaaltincaba M, et al. Case 76: May-Thurner syndrome. *Radiology* 2004;233:361–365.

51. Coady MA, Rizzo JA, Hammond GL, et al. Penetrating ulcer of the thoracic aorta: what is it? How do we recognize it? How do we manage it? *J Vasc Surg* 1998;27:1006–1016.

52. Cohan RH, Baker ME, Cooper C, et al. Computed tomography of primary retroperitoneal malignancies. *J Comput Assist Tomogr* 1988;12:804–810.

53. Coulam CH, Rubin GD. Acute aortic abnormalities. *Semin Roentgenol* 2001;36:148–164.

54. Cura M, Cura A, Bugnone A. Early enhancement of the inferior vena cava on helical CT. *Clin Imaging* 2003;27:236–238.

55. Damgaard-Pedersen K, von der Masse H. Ultrasound and ultrasound guided biopsy, CT and lymphography in the diagnosis of retroperitoneal metastases in testicular cancer. *Scand J Urol Nephrol* 1991;137:139–144.

56. Davidovic LB, Kostic DM, Cvetkovic SD, et al. Aorto-caval fistulas. *Cardiovasc Surg* 2002;10:555–560.

57. Davidson AJ, Hartman DS, Goldman SM. Mature teratoma of the retroperitoneum: radiologic, pathologic, and clinical correlation. *Radiology* 1989;172:421–425.

58. Davidson AJ, Hartman DS. Lymphangioma of the retroperitoneum: CT and sonographic characteristics. *Radiology* 1990;175:507–510.

59. de Bree E, Klaase JM, Schultze Kool LJ, et al. Aneurysm of the inferior vena cava complicated by thrombosis mimicking a retroperitoneal neoplasm. *Eur J Vasc Endovasc Surg* 2000;20:305–307.

60. Degesys GE, Dunnick NR, Silverman PM, et al. Retroperitoneal fibrosis: use of CT in distinguishing among possible causes. *AJR Am J Roentgenol* 1986;146:57–60.

61. Didier D, Racle A, Etievent JP, et al. Tumor thrombus of the inferior vena cava secondary to malignant abdominal neoplasms: US and CT evaluation. *Radiology* 1987;162:83–89.

62. Dobrin PB. Pathophysiology and pathogenesis of aortic aneurysms: current concepts. *Surg Clin North Am* 1989;69:687–703.

63. Donohue JP, Zachary JM, Maynard B. Distribution of nodal metastases in nonseminomatous testis cancer. *J Urol* 1982;128:315–330.

64. Dooms GC, Hricak H, Moseley ME, et al. Characterization of lymphadenopathy by magnetic resonance relaxation times: preliminary results. *Radiology* 1985;155:691–697.

65. Dorfman RE, Alpern MB, Gross BH, et al. Upper abdominal lymph nodes: criteria for normal size determined with CT. *Radiology* 1991;180:319–322.

66. Dubenec SR, White GH, Pasenau J, et al. Endotension. A review of current views on pathophysiology and treatment. *J Cardiovasc Surg (Torino)* 2003;44:553–557.

67. Ebner F, Kressel HY, Mintz MC, et al. Tumor recurrence versus fibrosis in the female pelvis: differentiation with MR at 1.5 T. *Radiology* 1988;166:333–340.

68. Edelman RR. MR angiography: present and future. *AJR Am J Roentgenol* 1993;161:1–11.

69. Eisenstat RS, Whitford AC, Lane MJ, et al. The "flat cava" sign revisited: what is its significance in patients without trauma? *AJR Am J Roentgenol* 2002;178:21–25.

70. Engellau L, Olsrud J, Brockstedt S, et al. MR evaluation ex vivo and in vivo of a covered stent-graft for abdominal aortic aneurysms: ferromagnetism, heating, artifacts, and velocity mapping. *J Magn Reson Imaging* 2000;12:112–121.

71. Erasmus JJ, McAdams HP, Patz EF Jr, et al. Evaluation of primary pulmonary carcinoid tumors using FDG-PET. *AJR Am J Roentgenol* 1998;170:1369–1373.

72. Espiritu JD, Creer MH, Miklos AZ, et al. Fatal tumor thrombosis due to an inferior vena cava leiomyosarcoma in a patient with antiphospholipid antibody syndrome. *Mayo Clin Proc* 2002;77:595–599.

73. Farber A, Wagner WH, Cossman DV, et al. Isolated dissection of the abdominal aorta: clinical presentation and therapeutic options. *J Vasc Surg* 2002;36:205–210.

74. Farner MC, Carpenter JP, Baum RA, et al. Early changes in abdominal aortic aneurysm diameter after endovascular repair. *J Vasc Interv Radiol* 2003;14:205–210.

75. Feig BW. Retroperitoneal sarcomas. *Surg Oncol Clin N Am* 2003;12:369–377.

76. Feldberg MAM, Koehler PR, van Waes PFGM. Psoas compartment disease studied by computed tomography. *Radiology* 1983;148:505–512.

77. Fillinger MF, Raghavan ML, Marra SP, et al. In vivo analysis of mechanical wall stress and abdominal aortic aneurysm rupture risk. *J Vasc Surg* 2002;36:589–597.

78. Fillinger MF, Marra SP, Raghavan ML, et al. Prediction of rupture risk in abdominal aortic aneurysm during observation: wall stress versus diameter. *J Vasc Surg* 2003;37:724–732.

79. Fillinger MF, Racusin J, Baker RK, et al. Anatomic characteristics of ruptured abdominal aortic aneurysm on conventional CT scans: implications for rupture risk. *J Vasc Surg* 2004;39:1243–1252.

80. Frauenfelder T, Wildermuth S, Marincek B, et al. Nontraumatic emergent abdominal vascular conditions: advantages of multidetector row CT and three-dimensional imaging. *Radiographics* 2004;24:481–496.

81. Friedland GW, deVries PA, Nino-Murcia M, et al. Congenital anomalies of the inferior vena cava: embryogenesis and MR features. *Urol Radiol* 1992;13:237–248.

82. Friedman AC, Hartman DS, Sherman J, et al. Computed tomography of abdominal fatty masses. *Radiology* 1981;139:415–429.

83. Gaa J, Bohm C, Richter A, et al. Aortocaval fistula complicating abdominal aortic aneurysm: diagnosis with gadolinium-enhanced three-dimensional MR angiography. *Eur Radiol* 1999;9:1438–1440.

84. Gale ME, Johnson WC, Gerzof SG, et al. Problems in CT diagnosis of ruptured abdominal aortic aneurysms. *J Comput Assist Tomogr* 1986;10:637–641.

85. Ganaha F, Miller DC, Sugimoto K, et al. Prognosis of aortic intramural hematoma with and without penetrating atherosclerotic ulcer. A clinical and radiological analysis. *Circulation* 2002;106:342–348.

86. Gatcombe HG, Assikis V, Kooby D, et al. Primary retroperitoneal teratomas: a review of the literature. *J Surg Oncol* 2004;86:107–113.

87. Gayer G, Apter S, Jonas T, et al. Polysplenia syndrome detected in adulthood: report of eight cases and review of the literature. *Abdom Imaging* 1999;24:178–184.

88. Gayer G, Luboshitz J, Hertz M, et al. Congenital anomalies of the inferior vena cava revealed on CT in patients with deep vein thrombosis. *AJR Am J Roentgenol* 2003;180:729–732.

89. Gayer G, Zissin R, Strauss S, et al. IVC anomalies and right renal aplasia detected on CT: a possible link? *Abdom Imaging* 2003;28:395–399.

90. Glazer HS, Lee JKT, Levitt RG, et al. Radiation fibrosis: differentiation from recurrent tumor by MR imaging. *Radiology* 1985;156:721–726.

91. Goldman SM, Davidson AJ, Neal J. Retroperitoneal and pelvic hemangiopericytomas: clinical, radiologic, and pathologic correlation. *Radiology* 1988;168:13–17.

92. Golzarian J, Dussaussois L, Abada HT, et al. Helical CT of aorta after endoluminal stent-graft therapy: value of biphasic acquisition. *AJR Am J Roentgenol* 1998;171:329–331.

93. Golzarian J, Murgo S, Dussaussois L, et al. Evaluation of abdominal aortic aneurysm after endoluminal treatment: comparison of color Doppler sonography with biphasic helical CT. *AJR Am J Roentgenol* 2002;178:623–628.

94. Gomori JM, Grossman RI, Goldberg HI, et al. Intracranial hematomas: imaging by high field MR. *Radiology* 1985;157:87–93.

95. Gordon BA, Martinez S, Collins AJ. Pyomyositis: characteristics at CT and MR imaging. *Radiology* 1995;197:279–286.

96. Gossios K, Argyropoulou M, Akritidis N. Uncommon manifestations of retroperitoneal fibrosis. *Clin Radiol* 2003;58:331–333.

97. Goyen M, Ruehm SG, Debatin JF. MR-angiography: the role of contrast agents. *Eur J Radiol* 2000;34:247–256.

98. Greatorex RA, Dixon AK, Flower CDR, et al. Limitations of computed tomography in leaking abdominal aortic aneurysms. *BMJ* 1988;23:284–285.

99. Grubnic S, Vinnicombe SJ, Norman AR, et al. MR evaluation of normal retroperitoneal and pelvic lymph nodes. *Clin Radiol* 2002;57:193–200; discussion 201–194.

100. Guermazi A, Brice P, Hennequin C, et al. Lymphography: an old technique retains its usefulness. *Radiographics* 2003;23:1541–1558; discussion 1559–1560.

101. Guinet C, Buy JN, Ghossain MA, et al. Aortic anastomotic pseudoaneurysms: US, CT, MR, and angiography. *J Comput Assist Tomogr* 1992;16:182–188.

102. Gupta AK, Cohan RH, Francis IR. Patterns of recurrent retroperitoneal sarcomas. *AJR Am J Roentgenol* 2000;174:1025–1030.

103. Haaga JR, Baldwin N, Reich NE, et al. CT detection of infected synthetic grafts: preliminary report of a new sign. *AJR Am J Roentgenol* 1978;131:317–320.

104. Hagan PG, Nienaber CA, Isselbacher EM, et al. The international registry of acute aortic dissection (IRAD). New insights into an old disease. *JAMA* 2000;283:897–903.

105. Hahn PF, Saini S, Stark DD, et al. Intraabdominal hematoma: the concentric-ring sign in MR imaging. *AJR Am J Roentgenol* 1987;148:115–119.

106. Halliday KE, Al-Kutoubi A. Draped aorta: CT sign of contained leak of aortic aneurysms. *Radiology* 1996;199:41–43.

107. Hany TF, Debatin JF, Leung DA, et al. Evaluation of the aortoiliac and renal arteries: comparison of breath-hold, contrast-enhanced, three-dimensional MR angiography with conventional catheter angiography. *Radiology* 1997;204:357–362.

108. Harisinghani MG, Saini S, Weissleder R, et al. MR lymphangiography using ultrasmall superparamagnetic iron oxide in patients with primary abdominal and pelvic malignancies: radiographic-pathologic correlation. *AJR Am J Roentgenol* 1999;172:1347–1351.

109. Harisinghani MG, Barentsz J, Hahn PF, et al. Noninvasive detection of clinically occult lymph-node metastases in prostate cancer. *N Engl J Med* 2003;348:2491–2499.

110. Harris JA, Bis KG, Glover JL, et al. Penetrating atherosclerotic ulcers of the aorta. *J Vasc Surg* 1994;19:90–99.

111. Hartman DS. Retroperitoneal tumors and lymphadenopathy. *Urol Radiol* 1990;12:132–134.

112. Hartman DS, Hayes WS, Choyke PL, et al. Leiomyosarcoma of the retroperitoneum and inferior vena cava: radiologic-pathologic correlation. *Radiographics* 1992;12:1203–1220.

113. Hartnell GG. Imaging of aortic aneurysms and dissection: CT and MRI. *J Thorac Imaging* 2001;16:35–46.

114. Hayasaka K, Tanaka Y, Soeda S, et al. MR findings in primary retroperitoneal schwannoma. *Acta Radiol* 1999;40:78–82.

115. Hayashi H, Kumazaki T. Case report: inflammatory abdominal aortic aneurysm—dynamic Gd-DTPA enhanced magnetic resonance imaging features. *Br J Radiol* 1995;68:321–323.

116. Hayashi H, Matsuoka Y, Sakamoto I, et al. Penetrating atherosclerotic ulcer of the aorta: imaging features and disease concept. *Radiographics* 2000;20:995–1005.

117. Hayes WS, Davidson AJ, Grimley PM, et al. Extraadrenal retroperitoneal paraganglioma: clinical, pathologic, and CT findings. *AJR Am J Roentgenol* 1990;155:1247–1250.

118. Heiberg E, Wolverson MK, Saundaram M, et al. CT characteristics of aortic atherosclerotic aneurysm versus aortic dissection. *J Comput Assist Tomogr* 1985;9:78–83.

119. Hemant D, Krantikumar R, Amita J, et al. Primary leiomyosarcoma of inferior vena cava, a rare entity: imaging features. *Australas Radiol* 2001;45:448–451.

120. Herlinger H, Metz DC. Malabsorption states. In: Herlinger H, Maglinte DDT, Birnbaum BA, eds. *Clinical imaging of the small intestine*. New York: Springer, 1999:344–345.

121. Herts BR, Megibow AJ, Birnbaum BA, et al. High attenuation lymphadenopathy in AIDS patients: significance of findings at CT. *Radiology* 1992;185:777–781.

122. Hilton S, Herr HW, Teitcher JB, et al. CT detection of retroperitoneal lymph node metastases in patients with clinical stage I testicular nonseminomatous germ cell cancer: assessment of size and distribution criteria. *AJR Am J Roentgenol* 1997;169:521–525.

123. Hines J, Katz DS, Goffner L, et al. Fat collection related to the intrahepatic inferior vena cava on CT. *AJR Am J Roentgenol* 1999;172:409–411.

124. Hines OJ, Nelson S, Quinones-Baldrich WJ, et al. Leiomyosarcoma of the inferior vena cava: prognosis and comparison with leiomyosarcoma of other anatomic sites. *Cancer* 1999;85:1077–1083.

125. Hoffman M, Kletter K, Diemling M, et al. Positron emission tomography with fluorine-18-2-fluoro-2-deoxy-D-glucose (F18-FDG) does not visualize extranodal B-cell lymphoma of the mucosa associated lymphoid tissue (MALT)-type. *Ann Oncol* 1999;10:1185–1189.

126. Horejs D, Gilbert PM, Burstein S, et al. Normal aortoiliac diameters by CT. *J Comput Assist Tomogr* 1988;12:602–603.

127. Howat AJ, McPhie JL, Smith DA, et al. Cavitation of mesenteric lymph nodes: a rare complication of coeliac disease, associated with a poor outcome. *Histopathology* 1995;27:349–354.

128. Hricak H, Amparo E, Fisher MR, et al. Abdominal venous system: assessment using MR. *Radiology* 1985;156:415–422.

129. Hubsch P, Schurawitzki H, Susani M, et al. Color Doppler imaging of inferior vena cava: identification of tumor thrombus. *J Ultrasound Med* 1992;11:639–645.

130. Hulnick DH, Chatson GP, Megibow AJ, et al. Retroperitoneal fibrosis presenting as colonic dysfunction: CT diagnosis. *J Comput Assist Tomogr* 1988;12:159–161.

131. Husband JE, Robinson L, Thomas G. Contrast enhancing lymph nodes in bladder cancer: a potential pitfall on CT. *Clin Radiol* 1992;45:395–398.

132. Iino M, Kuribayashi S, Imakita S, et al. Sensitivity and specificity of CT in the diagnosis of inflammatory abdominal aortic aneurysms. *J Comput Assist Tomogr* 2002;26:1006–1012.

133. Insko EK, Kulzer LM, Fairman RM, et al. MR imaging for the detection of endoleaks in recipients of abdominal aortic stent-grafts with low magnetic susceptibility. *Acad Radiol* 2003;10:509–513.

134. Israel GM, Bosniak MA, Slywotzky CM, et al. CT differentiation of large exophytic renal angiomyolipomas and perirenal liposarcomas. *AJR Am J Roentgenol* 2002;179:769–773.

135. Iyer R, Eftekhari F, Varma D, et al. Cystic retroperitoneal lymphangioma: CT, ultrasound and MR findings. *Pediatr Radiol* 1993;23:305–306.

136. Jacoby WT, Cohan RH, Baker ME, et al. Ovarian vein thrombosis in oncology patients: CT detection and clinical significance. *AJR Am J Roentgenol* 1990;155:291–294.

137. Jain KA, Jeffrey RB. Gonadal vein thrombosis in patients with acute gastrointestinal inflammation. *Radiology* 1991;180:111–113.

138. Janzen NK, Laifer-Narin S, Han KR, et al. Emerging technologies in uroradiologic imaging. *Urol Oncol* 2003;21:317–326.

139. Jeffrey RBJ, Federle MP. The collapsed inferior vena cava: CT evidence of hypovolemia. *AJR Am J Roentgenol* 1988;150:431–432.

140. Jeffrey RBJ, Cardoza JD, Olcott EW. Detection of active intraabdominal arterial hemorrhage: value of dynamic contrast-enhanced CT. *AJR Am J Roentgenol* 1991;156:725–729.

141. Jerusalem G, Beguin Y, Najjar F, et al. Positron emission tomography (PET) with 18F-fluorodeoxyglucose (18F-FDG) for the staging of low-grade non-Hodgkin's lymphoma. *Ann Oncol* 2001;12:825–830.

142. Joarder R, Gedroyc WM. Magnetic resonance angiography: the state of the art. *Eur Radiol* 2001;11:446–453.

143. Joels CS, Sing RF, Heniford BT. Complications of inferior vena cava filters. *Am Surg* 2003;69:654–659.

144. Johnson KK, Russ PD, Bair JH, et al. Diagnosis of synthetic vascular graft infection: comparison of CT and gallium scans. *AJR Am J Roentgenol* 1990;154:405–409.

145. Jung G, Heindel W, von Bergwelt-Baildon M, et al. Abdominal lymphoma staging: is MR imaging with T2-weighted turbo-spin-echo sequence a diagnostic alternative to contrast-enhanced spiral CT? *J Comput Assist Tomogr* 2000;24:783–787.

146. Justich E, Amparo EG, Hricak H, et al. Infected aortoiliofemoral grafts: magnetic resonance imaging. *Radiology* 1985;154:133–136.

147. Kallman DA, King BF, Hattery RR, et al. Renal vein and inferior vena cava tumor thrombus in renal cell carcinoma: CT, US, MRI and venacavography. *J Comput Assist Tomogr* 1992;16:240–247.

148. Kalman PG, Johnston KW. Abdominal aortic aneurysms. In: Hobson RW 2nd, Wilson SE, Veith FJ, eds. *Vascular surgery principles and practice*, 3rd ed., revised and expanded. New York: Marcel Dekker, 2004:631–640.

149. Kam J, Patel S, Ward RE. Computed tomography of aortic and aortoiliofemoral grafts. *J Comput Assist Tomogr* 1982;6:298–303.

150. Kaneko T, Takahashi S, Takeuchi T, et al. Castleman's disease in the retroperitoneal space. *J Urol* 2003;169:265–266.

151. Kazerooni EA, Bree RL, Williams DM. Penetrating atherosclerotic ulcers of the descending thoracic aorta: evaluation with CT and distinction from aortic dissection. *Radiology* 1992;183:759–765.

152. Kenney PJ, Wagner BJ, Rao P, et al. Myelolipoma: CT and pathologic features. *Radiology* 1998;208:87–95.

153. Kersting-Sommerhoff BA, Higgins DB, White RD, et al. Aortic dissection: sensitivity and specificity of MR imaging. *Radiology* 1988;174:727–731.

154. Kim D, Edelman RR, Kent KC, et al. Abdominal aorta and renal artery stenosis: evaluation with MR angiography. *Radiology* 1990;174:727–731.

155. Kim SH, Choi BI, Han MC, et al. Retroperitoneal neurilemoma: CT and MR findings. *AJR Am J Roentgenol* 1992;159:1023–1026.

156. Kim T, Murakami T, Oi H, et al. CT and MR imaging of abdominal liposarcoma. *AJR Am J Roentgenol* 1996;166:829–833.

157. Kim TK, Chung JW, Han JK, et al. Hepatic changes in benign obstruction of the hepatic inferior vena cava: CT findings. *AJR Am J Roentgenol* 1999;173:1235–1242.

158. Kinney TB. Update on inferior vena cava filters. *J Vasc Interv Radiol* 2003;14:425–440.

159. Kissin EY, Merkel PA. Diagnostic imaging in Takayasu arteritis. *Curr Opin Rheumatol* 2004;16:31–37.

160. Klein FA, Whitmore WF Jr, Sogani PC, et al. Inguinal lymph node metastasis from germ cell testicular tumors. *J Urol* 1984;131:497–500.

161. Ko SF, Wan YL, Lee TY, et al. CT features of calcifications in abdominal malignant fibrous histiocytoma. *Clin Imaging* 1998;22:408–413.

162. Kobayashi A, Matsui O, Takashima T, et al. Calcification in caval membrane causing primary Budd-Chiari syndrome: CT demonstration. *J Comput Assist Tomogr* 1988;12:401–404.

163. Korobkin M, Callen PW, Fisch AE. Computed tomography of the pelvis and retroperitoneum. *Radiol Clin North Am* 1979;17:301–318.

164. Korobkin M, Silverman PM, Quint LE, et al. CT of the extraperitoneal space: normal anatomy and fluid collections. *AJR Am J Roentgenol* 1992;159:933–942.

165. Kostakoglu L, Agress H Jr, Goldsmith SJ. Clinical role of FDG-PET in evaluation of cancer patients. *Radiographics* 2003;23:315–340.

166. Kottra JJ, Dunnick NR. Retroperitoneal fibrosis. *Radiol Clin North Am* 1996;34:1259–1275.

167. Kramer CM, Cerilli LA, Hagspiel K, et al. Magnetic resonance imaging identifies the fibrous cap in atherosclerotic abdominal aortic aneurysm. *Circulation* 2004;109:1016–1021.

168. Krinsky G, Johnson G, Rofsky N, et al. Venous aneurysms: MR diagnosis with the "layered gadolinium" sign. *J Comput Assist Tomogr* 1997;21:623–627.

169. Kroepil P, Coakley FV, Graser A, et al. Appearance and distinguishing features of retroperitoneal calcifications at computed tomography. *J Comput Assist Tomogr* 2003;27:860–863.

170. Kulaylat MN, Karakousis CP, Doerr RJ, et al. Leiomyosarcoma of the inferior vena cava: a clinicopathologic review and report of three cases. *J Surg Oncol* 1997;65:205–217.

171. Kurosaki Y, Tanaka YO, Itai Y. Well-differentiated liposarcoma of the retroperitoneum with a fat-fluid level: US, CT, and MR appearance. *Eur Radiol* 1998;8:474–475.

172. Kurugoglu S, Ogut G, Mihmanli I, et al. Abdominal leiomyosarcomas: radiologic appearances at various locations. *Eur Radiol* 2002;12:2933–2942.

173. Kvilekval KHV, Best IM, Mason RA, et al. The value of computed tomography in the management of symptomatic abdominal aortic aneurysms. *J Vasc Surg* 1990;12:28–33.

174. Landay MJ, Virolainen H. "Hyperdense" aortic wall: potential pitfall in CT screening for aortic dissection. *J Comput Assist Tomogr* 1991;15:561–564.

175. Lane RH, Stephens DH, Reiman HM. Primary retroperitoneal neoplasms: CT findings in 90 cases with clinical and pathologic correlation. *AJR Am J Roentgenol* 1989;152:83–89.

176. Latifi HR, Heiken JP. CT of inflammatory abdominal aortic aneurysm: development from an uncomplicated atherosclerotic aneurysm. *J Comput Assist Tomogr* 1992;16:484–486.

177. Lederle FA, Johnson GR, Wilson SE, et al. Prevalence and associations of abdominal aortic aneurysm detected through screening. *Ann Intern Med* 1997;126:441–449.

178. Lee JKT, Stanley RJ, Sagel SS, et al. Accuracy of CT in detecting intraabdominal and pelvic lymph node metastases from pelvic cancers. *AJR Am J Roentgenol* 1978;131:675–679.

179. Lee JKT, Heiken JP, Ling D, et al. Magnetic resonance imaging of abdominal and pelvic lymphadenopathy. *Radiology* 1984;153:181–188.

180. Lee JKT, Glazer HS. Psoas muscle disorders: MR imaging. *Radiology* 1986;160:683–687.

181. Lenchik L, Dovgan DJ, Kier R. CT of the iliopsoas compartment: value in differentiating tumor, abscess, and hematoma. *AJR Am J Roentgenol* 1994;162:83–86.

182. LePage MA, Quint LE, Sonnad SS, et al. Aortic dissection: CT features that distinguish true lumen from false lumen. *AJR Am J Roentgenol* 2001;177:207–211.

183. Levy AD, Cantisani V, Miettinen M. Abdominal lymphangiomas: imaging features with pathologic correlation. *AJR Am J Roentgenol* 2004;182:1485–1491.

184. Lewis E, Bernardino ME, Salvador PG, et al. Post- therapy CT detected mass in lymphoma patients: is it viable tissue? *J Comput Assist Tomogr* 1982;6:792–795.

185. Lewis JJ, Leung D, Woodruff JM, et al. Retroperitoneal soft-tissue sarcoma: analysis of 500 patients treated and followed at a single institution. *Ann Surg* 1998;228:355–365.

186. Li DKB, Rennie CS. Abdominal computed tomography in Whipple's disease. *J Comput Assist Tomogr* 1981;5:249–252.

187. Libshitz HI, Jing BS, Wallace S, et al. Sterilized metastases: a diagnostic and therapeutic dilemma. *AJR Am J Roentgenol* 1983;140:15–19.

188. Lim JH, Park JH, Auh YH. Membranous obstruction of the inferior vena cava: comparison of findings at sonography, CT, and venography. *AJR Am J Roentgenol* 1992;159:515–520.

189. Lim JH, Kim B, Auh YH. Anatomical communications of the perirenal space. *Br J Radiol* 1998;71:450–456.

190. Limet R, Sakalihassan N, Albert A. Determination of the expansion rate and incidence of rupture of abdominal aortic aneurysm. *J Vasc Surg* 1991;14:540–548.

191. Lipson E, Polliak A, Bloom RA. Value of lymphangiography in the staging of Hodgkin lymphoma. *Radiology* 1994;193:757–759.

192. Lochbuehler H, Weber H, Mehlig U, et al. Aneurysm of the inferior vena cava in a 5-year-old boy. *J Pediatr Surg* 2002;37:E10.

193. Lookstein RA, Goldman J, Pukin L, et al. Time-resolved magnetic resonance angiography as a noninvasive method to characterize endoleaks: initial results compared with conventional angiography. *J Vasc Surg* 2004;39:27–33.

194. Loud PA, Grossman ZD, Klippenstein DL, et al. Combined CT venography and pulmonary angiography: a new diagnostic technique for suspected thromboembolic disease. *AJR Am J Roentgenol* 1998;170:951–954.

195. Low RN, Wall SD, Jeffrey RB, et al. Aortoenteric fistula and perigraft infection: evaluation with CT. *Radiology* 1990;175:157–162.

196. Macedo TA, Stanson AW, Oderich GS, et al. Infected aortic aneurysms: imaging findings. *Radiology* 2004;231:250–257.

197. Macura KJ, Corl FM, Fishman EK, et al. Pathogenesis in acute aortic syndromes: aortic dissection, intramural hematoma, and penetrating atherosclerotic aortic ulcer. *AJR Am J Roentgenol* 2003;181:309–316.

198. Macura KJ, Szarf G, Fishman EK, et al. Role of computed tomography and magnetic resonance imaging in assessment of acute aortic syndromes. *Semin Ultrasound CT MR* 2003;24:232–254.

199. Magnusson A, Andersson T, Larsson B, et al. Contrast enhancement of pathologic lymph nodes demonstrated by computed tomography. *Acta Radiol* 1989;30:307–310.

200. Maher MM, McNamara AM, MacEneaney PM, et al. Abdominal aortic aneurysms: elective endovascular repair versus conventional surgery—evaluation with evidence-based medicine techniques. *Radiology* 2003;228:647–658.

201. Mantello MT, Panaccione JL, Moriarty PE, et al. Impending rupture of nonaneurysmal bacterial aortitis: CT diagnosis. *J Comput Assist Tomogr* 1990;14:950–953.

202. Marston WA, Ahlquist R, Johnson G, et al. Misdiagnosis of ruptured abdominal aortic aneurysms. *J Vasc Surg* 1992;152:133–136.

203. Mathews R, Smith PA, Fishman EK, et al. Anomalies of the inferior vena cava and renal veins: embryologic and surgical considerations. *Urology* 1999;53:873–880.

204. Matsunaga N, Hayashi K, Sakamoto I, et al. Takayasu arteritis: protean radiologic manifestations and diagnosis. *Radiographics* 1997;17:579–594.

205. Matsunaga N, Hayashi K, Okada M, et al. Magnetic resonance imaging features of aortic diseases. *Top Magn Reson Imaging* 2003;14:253–266.

206. Mauro M. The query corner. Inflammatory aortic aneurysms. *Abdom Imaging* 1997;22:357–358.

207. Mayo J, Gray R, St. Louis E, et al. Anomalies of the inferior vena cava. *AJR Am J Roentgenol* 1983;140:339–345.

208. Mehard WB, Heiken JP, Sicard GA. High-attenuation crescent in abdominal aortic aneurysm wall at CT: sign of acute or impending rupture. *Radiology* 1994;192:359–362a(abst).

209. Meyers MA. The extraperitoneal spaces: normal and pathologic anatomy. In: Meyers MA, ed. *Dynamic radiology of the abdomen*, 5th ed. New York: Springer, 2000:333–477.

210. Miller CL, Wechsler RJ. CT evaluation of Kimray-Greenfield filter complications. *AJR Am J Roentgenol* 1986;147:45–50.

211. Mindell HJ, Mastromatteo JF, Dickey KW, et al. Anatomic communications between the three retroperitoneal spaces: determination by CT-guided injections of contrast material in cadavers. *AJR Am J Roentgenol* 1995;164:1173–1178.

212. Mingoli A, Cavallaro A, Sapienza P, et al. International registry of inferior vena cava leiomyosarcoma: analysis of a world series on 218 patients. *Anticancer Res* 1996;16:3201–3206.

213. Minniti S, Visentini S, Procacci C. Congenital anomalies of the venae cavae: embryological origin, imaging features and report of three new variants. *Eur Radiol* 2002;12:2040–2055.

214. Miyake H, Suzuki K, Ueda S, et al. Localized fat collection adjacent to the intrahepatic portion of the inferior vena cava: a normal variant on CT. *AJR Am J Roentgenol* 1992;158:423–425.

215. Miyazato M, Yonou H, Sugaya K, et al. Transitional cell carcinoma of the renal pelvis forming tumor thrombus in the vena cava. *Int J Urol* 2001;8:575–577.

216. Molmenti EP, Balfe DM, Kanterman RY, et al. Anatomy of the retroperitoneum: observations of the distribution of pathologic fluid collections. *Radiology* 1996;200:95–103.

217. Moore WS, Kashyap VS, Vescera CL, et al. Abdominal aortic aneurysm: a 6-year comparison of endovascular versus transabdominal repair. *Ann Surg* 1999;230:298–308.

218. Mori H, Fukuda T, Isomoto I, et al. CT diagnosis of catheter-induced septic thrombus of vena cava. *J Comput Assist Tomogr* 1990;14:236–238.

219. Moriyama Y, Yamamoto H, Hisatomi K, et al. Penetrating atherosclerotic ulcers in an abdominal aortic aneurysm: report of a case. *Surg Today* 1998;28:105–107.

220. Mukherjee JJ, Peppercorn PD, Reznek RH, et al. Pheochromocytoma: effect of nonionic contrast medium in CT on circulating catecholamine levels. *Radiology* 1997;202:227–231.

221. Muller BT, Wegener OR, Grabitz K, et al. Mycotic aneurysms of the thoracic and abdominal aorta and iliac arteries: experience with anatomic and extra-anatomic repair in 33 cases. *J Vasc Surg* 2001;33:106–113.

222. Mulligan SA, Holley HC, Koehler RE, et al. CT and MR imaging in the evaluation of retroperitoneal fibrosis. *J Comput Assist Tomogr* 1989;13:277–281.

223. Munechika H, Cohan RH, Baker ME, et al. Hemiazygos continuation of a left inferior vena cava: CT appearance. *J Comput Assist Tomogr* 1988;12:328–330.

224. Munk PL, Sallomi DF, Janzen DL, et al. Malignant fibrous histiocytoma of soft tissue imaging with emphasis on MRI. *J Comput Assist Tomogr* 1998;22:819–826.

225. Neschis DG, Velazquez OC, Baum RA, et al. The role of magnetic resonance angiography for endoprosthetic design. *J Vasc Surg* 2001;33:488–494.

226. Nichols CR, Fox EP. Extragonadal and pediatric germ cell tumors. *Hematol Oncol Clin North Am* 1991;5:1189–1209.

227. Nishino M, Hayakawa K, Minami M, et al. Primary retroperitoneal neoplasms: CT and MR imaging findings with anatomic and pathologic diagnostic clues. *Radiographics* 2003;23:45–57.

228. Nitecki SS, Hallet JW Jr, Stanson AW, et al. Inflammatory abdominal aortic aneurysms: a case-control study. *J Vasc Surg* 1996;23:860–869.

229. O'Doherty MJ, Macdonald EA, Barrington SF, et al. Positron emission tomography in the management of lymphomas. *Clin Oncol (R Coll Radiol)* 2002;14:415–426.

230. Obernosterer A, Aschauer M, Schnedl W, et al. Anomalies of the inferior vena cava in patients with iliac venous thrombosis. *Ann Intern Med* 2002;136:37–41.

231. Oderich GS, Panneton JM, Bower TC, et al. Infected aortic aneurysms: aggressive presentation, complicated early outcome, but durable results. *J Vasc Surg* 2001;34:900–908.

232. Ohara PJ, Borkowski GP, Hertzer NR, et al. Natural history of periprosthetic air on computerized axial tomographic examination of the abdomen following abdominal aortic aneurysm repair. *J Vasc Surg* 1984;1:429–433.

233. Ohki T, Lipsitz EC, Veith FJ. Endovascular grafts for aneurysms, occlusive disease, and vascular injuries. In: Hobson RW 2nd, Wilson SE, Veith FJ, eds. *Vascular surgery principles and practice*, 3rd ed., revised and expanded. New York: Marcel Dekker, 2004:363–393.

234. Okuda K. Membranous obstruction of the inferior vena cava (obliterative hepatocavopathy, Okuda). *J Gastroenterol Hepatol* 2001;16:1179–1183.

235. Okuda K. Inferior vena cava thrombosis at its hepatic portion (obliterative hepatocavopathy). *Semin Liver Dis* 2002;22:15–26.

236. Orton DF, LeVeen RF, Saigh JA, et al. Aortic prosthetic graft infections: radiologic manifestations and implications for management. *Radiographics* 2000;20:977–993.

237. Pagani JJ, Thomas JL, Bernardino ME. Computed tomographic manifestations of abdominal and pelvic venous collaterals. *Radiology* 1982;142:415–419.

238. Panicek DM, Tonger GC, Heelan RT, et al. Nonseminomatous germ cell tumors: enlarging masses despite chemotherapy. *Radiology* 1990;175:499–502.

239. Papanicolaou N, Wittenberg J, Ferrucci JTJ, et al. Preoperative evaluation of abdominal aortic aneurysms by computed tomography. *AJR Am J Roentgenol* 1986;146:711–715.

240. Papanicolaou N, Yoder IC, Lee MJ. Primary retroperitoneal neoplasms: how close can we come in making the correct diagnosis? *Urol Radiol* 1992;14:221–228.

241. Park BK, Kim SH, Moon MH. Idiopathic presacral retroperitoneal fibrosis: report of two cases. *Br J Radiol* 2003;76:570–573.

242. Parodi JC, Palmaz JC, Barone HD. Transfemoral intraluminal graft implantation for abdominal aortic aneurysms. *Ann Vasc Surg* 1991;5:491–499.

243. Parra JR, Lee C, Hodgson KJ, et al. Endograft infection leading to rupture of aortic aneurysm. *J Vasc Surg* 2004;39:676–678.

244. Participants TUKSAT. Long-term outcomes of immediate repair compared with surveillance of small abdominal aortic aneurysms. *N Engl J Med* 2002;346:1445–1452.

245. Pereles FS, McCarthy RM, Baskaran V, et al. Thoracic aortic dissection and aneurysm: evaluation with nonenhanced true FISP MR angiography in less than 4 minutes. *Radiology* 2002;223:270–274.

246. Pienkny AJ, Herts B, Streem SB. Contemporary diagnosis of retrocaval ureter. *J Endourol* 1999;13:721–722.

247. Pierro JA, Soleimanpour M, Bory JL. Left retrocaval ureter associated with left inferior vena cava. *AJR Am J Roentgenol* 1990;155:545–546.

248. Pistolese GR, Ippoliti A, Mauriello A, et al. Postoperative regression of retroperitoneal fibrosis in patients with inflammatory abdominal aortic aneurysms: evaluation with spiral computed tomography. *Ann Vasc Surg* 2002;16:201–209.

249. Platt JF, Ellis JH, Korobkin M, et al. Potential renal donors: comparison of conventional imaging with helical CT. *Radiology* 1996;198:419–423.

250. Pode D, Caine M. Spontaneous retroperitoneal hemorrhage. *J Urol* 1992;147:311–318.

251. Pombo F, Rodriquez E, Mato J, et al. Patterns of contrast enhancement of tuberculous lymph nodes demonstrated by computed tomography. *Clin Radiol* 1992;46:13–17.

252. Pombo F, Rodriquez E, Caruncho MV, et al. CT attenuation values and enhancing characteristics of thoracoabdominal lymphomatous adenopathies. *J Comput Assist Tomogr* 1994;18:59–62.

253. Powell JT, Greenhalgh RM. Small abdominal aortic aneurysms. *N Engl J Med* 2003;348:1895–1901.

254. Prince MR, Narasimham DL, Stanley JC, et al. Breath-hold gadolinium-enhanced MR angiography of the abdominal aorta and its major branches. *Radiology* 1995;197:785–792.

255. Puvaneswary M, Cuganesan R. Detection of aortoenteric fistula with helical CT. *Australas Radiol* 2003;47:67–69.

256. Quanadli SD, Mesurolle B, Coggia M, et al. Abdominal aortic aneurysm: pretherapy assessment with dual-slice helical CT angiography. *AJR Am J Roentgenol* 2000;174:181–187.

257. Qvarfordt PG, Reilly LM, Mark AS, et al. Computerized tomographic assessment of graft incorporation after aortic reconstruction. *Am J Surg* 1985;150:227–231.

258. Radin DR. Disseminated histoplasmosis: abdominal CT findings in 16 patients. *AJR Am J Roentgenol* 1991;157:955–958.

259. Radin DR. Intraabdominal *Mycobacterium tuberculosis* vs *Mycobacterium avium-intracellulare* infections in patients with AIDS: distinction based on CT findings. *AJR Am J Roentgenol* 1991;156:487–491.

260. Radin R, David CL, Goldfarb H, et al. Adrenal and extra-adrenal retroperitoneal ganglioneuroma: imaging findings in 13 adults. *Radiology* 1997;202:703–707.

261. Rahmouni A, Tempany C, Jones R, et al. Lymphoma: monitoring tumor size and signal intensity with MR imaging. *Radiology* 1993;188:445–451.

262. Raju NL, Austin JH. Case 37: juxtacaval fat collection—mimic of lipoma in the subdiaphragmatic inferior vena cava. *Radiology* 2001;220:471–474.

263. Raman KG, Missig-Carroll N, Richardson T, et al. Color-flow duplex ultrasound scan versus computed tomographic scan in the surveillance of endovascular aneurysm repair. *J Vasc Surg* 2003;38:645–651.

264. Rankin SC. Assessment of response to therapy using conventional imaging. *Eur J Nucl Med Mol Imaging* 2003;30[suppl 1]:S56–S64.

265. Raptopolous V, Touliopoulos P, Lei QF, et al. Medial border of the perirenal space: CT and anatomic correlation. *Radiology* 1997;205:777–784.

266. Rasmussen TE, Hallett JW Jr. Inflammatory aortic aneurysms: a clinical review with new perspectives in pathogenesis. *Ann Surg* 1997;225:155–164.

267. Ray B, Hajdu SI, Whitmore WF. Distribution of retroperitoneal lymph node metastases in testicular germinal tumors. *Cancer* 1974;33:340–348.

268. Ray CE Jr, Kaufman JA. Complications of inferior vena cava filters. *Abdom Imaging* 1996;21:368–374.

269. Rebner M, Gross BH, Korobkin M, et al. CT appearance of right gonadal vein. *J Comput Assist Tomogr* 1989;13:460–462.

270. Rehn SM, Nyman RS, Glimelius BLG, et al. Non-Hodgkin lymphoma: predicting prognostic grade with MR imaging. *Radiology* 1990;176:249–253.

271. Rehn SM, Sperber GO, Nyman RS, et al. Quantification of inhomogeneities in malignancy grading of non-Hodgkin lymphoma with MR imaging. *Acta Radiol* 1993;34:3–9.

272. Reske SN. PET and restaging of malignant lymphoma including residual masses and relapse. *Eur J Nucl Med Mol Imaging* 2003;30[suppl 1]:S82–S88.

273. Rha SE, Byun JY, Jung SE, et al. Neurogenic tumors in the abdomen: tumor types and imaging characteristics. *Radiographics* 2003;23:29–43.

274. Rhee RY, Gloviczki P, Luthra HS, et al. Iliocaval complications of retroperitoneal fibrosis. *Am J Surg* 1994;168:179–183.

275. Rodriguez M. Computed tomography, magnetic resonance imaging, and positron emission tomography in non Hodgkin's lymphoma. *Acta Radiol* 1998;417:1–36.

276. Ros PR, Viamonte M Jr, Rywlin AM. Malignant fibrous histiocytoma: mesenchymal tumor of ubiquitous origin. *AJR Am J Roentgenol* 1984;142:753–759.

277. Rosai J. Lymph nodes. In: Rosai J, ed. *Rosai and Ackerman's surgical pathology*. New York: Mosby, 2004:1917–1961.

278. Rosai J. Peritoneum, retroperitoneum and related structures. In: Rosai J, ed. *Rosai and Ackerman's surgical pathology*. New York: Mosby, 2004:2373–2415.

279. Rosai J. Male reproductive system: testis. In: Rosai J, ed. *Rosai and Ackerman's surgical pathology*. New York: Mosby, 2004:1412–1456.

280. Royal SA, Callen PW. CT evaluation of anomalies of the inferior vena cava and left renal vein. *J Comput Assist Tomogr* 1979;15: 690–693.

281. Rozenblit AM, Patlas M, Rosenbaum AT, et al. Detection of endoleaks after endovascular repair of abdominal aortic aneurysm: value of unenhanced and delayed helical CT acquisitions. *Radiology* 2003;227:426–433.

282. Rubenstein WA, Gray G, Auh YH, et al. CT of fibrous tissues and tumors with sonographic correlation. *AJR Am J Roentgenol* 1986; 147:1067–1074.

283. Rubin GD, Drake MD, Napel S, et al. Spiral CT of renal artery stenosis: comparison of three-dimensional rendering techniques. *Radiology* 1994;190:181–189.

284. Rubin JI, Gomori JM, Grossman RI, et al. High-field MR imaging of extacranial hematomas. *AJR Am J Roentgenol* 1987;148:813–817.

285. Ryan MF, Atri M. Fat collection related to the intrahepatic portion of the inferior vena cava. *AJR Am J Roentgenol* 2001;177: 251–252.

286. Rydberg JN, Sudakoff GS, Hellman RS, et al. Positron emission tomography-computed tomography imaging characteristics of an inferior vena cava tumor thrombus with magnetic resonance imaging correlation. *J Comput Assist Tomogr* 2004; 28:517–519.

287. Santaella RO, Fishman EK, Lipsett PA. Primary vs secondary iliopsoas abscess. Presentation, microbiology, and treatment. *Arch Surg* 1995;130:1309–1313.

288. Savader SJ, Otero RR, Savader BL. Puerperal ovarian vein thrombosis: evaluation with CT, US, and MR imaging. *Radiology* 1988;167:637–639.

289. Scatarige JC, Fishman EK, Kuhajda FP, et al. Low attenuation nodal metastasis in testicular carcinoma. *J Comput Assist Tomogr* 1983;9:463–465.

290. Schoellnast H, Tillich M, Deutschmann HA, et al. Abdominal multidetector row computed tomography: reduction of cost and contrast material dose using saline flush. *J Comput Assist Tomogr* 2003;27:847–853.

291. Sebastia C, Pallisa E, Quiroga S, et al. Aortic dissection: diagnosis and follow-up with helical CT. *Radiographics* 1999;19:45–60.

292. Sheth R, Hanchate V, Rathod K, et al. Aneurysms of the inferior vena cava. *Australas Radiol* 2003;47:94–96.

293. Shin MS, Berland LL, Ho KJ. Small aorta: CT detection and clinical significance. *J Comput Assist Tomogr* 1990;14:102–103.

294. Shindo S, Kubota K, Kojima A, et al. Anomalies of inferior vena cava and left renal vein: risks in aortic surgery. *Ann Vasc Surg* 2000;14:393–396.

295. Siegel CL, Cohan RH. CT of abdominal aortic aneurysms. *AJR Am J Roentgenol* 1994;163:17–29.

296. Siegel CL, Cohan RH, Korobkin M. Abdominal aortic aneurysm morphology: CT features in patients with ruptured and nonruptured aneurysms. *AJR Am J Roentgenol* 1994;163:1123–1129.

297. Singh K, Bonaa KH, Jacobsen BK, et al. Prevalence of and risk factors for abdominal aortic aneurysms in a population-based study: the Tromso study. *Am J Epidemiol* 2001;154::236–244.

298. Singh K, Jacobsen BK, Solberg S, et al. Intra- and interobserver variability in the measurements of abdominal aortic and common iliac artery diameter with computed tomography. The Tromso study. *Eur J Vasc Endovasc Surg* 2003;25:399–407.

299. Sivit CJ, Taylor GA, Bulas DI, et al. Posttraumatic shock in children: CT findings associated with hemodynamic instability. *Radiology* 1992;182:723–726.

300. Solberg A, Angelsen A, Bergan U, et al. Frequency of lymphoceles after open and laparoscopic pelvic lymph node dissection in patients with prostate cancer. *Scand J Urol Nephrol* 2003;37: 218–221.

301. Soler R, Rodriguez E, Lopez MF, et al. MR imaging in inferior vena cava thrombosis. *Eur J Radiol* 1995;19:101–107.

302. Sommer T, Fehske W, Holzknecht N, et al. Aortic dissection: a comparative study of diagnosis with spiral CT, multiplanar transesophageal echocardiography, and MR imaging. *Radiology* 1996;199:347–352.

303. Spittell PC, Spittell JA, Joyce JW, et al. Clinical features and differential diagnosis of aortic dissection: experience with 236 cases (1980-1990). *Mayo Clin Proc* 1993;68:642–651.

304. Spritzer CE, Norconk JJ Jr, Sostman HD, et al. Detection of deep venous thrombosis by magnetic resonance imaging. *Chest* 1993;104:54–60.

305. Stella A, Gargiulo M, Faggioli GL, et al. Postoperative course of inflammatory abdominal aortic aneurysms. *Ann Vasc Surg* 1993; 7:229–238.

306. Stomper PC, Fung CY, Socinski MA, et al. Detection of retroperitoneal metastases in early-stage nonseminomatous testicular cancer: analysis of different CT criteria. *AJR Am J Roentgenol* 1987;149:1187–1190.

307. Stomper PC, Kalish LA, Garnick MB, et al. CT and pathologic predictive features of residual mass histologic findings after chemotherapy for nonseminomatous germ cell tumors: can residual malignancy or teratoma be excluded? *Radiology* 1991;180: 711–714.

308. Sueyoshi E, Sakamoto I, Matsuoka Y, et al. Aortoiliac and lower extremity arteries: comparison of three-dimensional dynamic contrast-enhanced subtraction MR angiography and conventional angiography. *Radiology* 1999;210:683–688.

309. Sullivan VV, Voris TK, Borlaza GS, et al. Incidental discovery of an inferior vena cava aneurysm. *Ann Vasc Surg* 2002;16:513–515.

310. Swensen SJ, McLeod RA, Stephens DH. CT of extracranial hemorrhage and hematomas. *AJR Am J Roentgenol* 1984;143:907–912.

311. Swensen SJ, Keller PL, Berquist TH, et al. Magnetic resonance imaging of hemorrhage. *AJR Am J Roentgenol* 1985;145:921–927.

312. Takashima T, Onoda N, Ishikawa T, et al. Tumor-forming idiopathic retroperitoneal fibrosis: report of a case. *Surg Today* 2004;34: 374–378.

313. Teitelbaum GP, Bradley WGJ, Klein BD. MR imaging artifacts, ferromagnetism and magnetic torque of intravascular filters, stents, and coils. *Radiology* 1988;16:657–664.

314. Teitelbaum GP, Ortega HV, Vinitski S, et al. Low-artifact intravascular devices: MR imaging evaluation. *Radiology* 1988;168: 713–719.

315. Tennant WG, Hartnell GG, Baird RN, et al. Inflammatory aortic aneurysms: characteristic appearances on magnetic resonance imaging. *Eur J Vasc Surg* 1992;6:399–402.

316. Tennant WG, Hartnell GG, Baird RN, et al. Radiologic investigation of abdominal aortic aneurysm disease: comparison of three modalities in staging and the detection of inflammatory change. *J Vasc Surg* 1993;17:703–709.

317. Thornton FJ, Kandiah SS, Monkhouse WS, et al. Helical CT evaluation of the perirenal space and its boundaries: a cadaveric study. *Radiology* 2001;218:659–663.

318. Thurnher S, Cejna M. Imaging of aortic stent-grafts and endoleaks. *Radiol Clin North Am* 2002;40:799–833.

319. Thurnher SA, Dorffner R, Thurnher MM, et al. Evaluation of abdominal aortic aneurysm for stent-graft placement: comparison of gadolinium-enhanced MR angiography versus helical CT angiography and digital subtraction angiography. *Radiology* 1997;205:341–352.

320. Todd CS, Michael H, Sutton G. Retroperitoneal leiomyosaroma: eight cases and a literature review. *Gynecol Oncol* 1995;59:333–337.

321. Torabi M, Aquino SL, Harisinghani MG. Current concepts in lymph node imaging. *J Nucl Med* 2004;45:1509–1518.

322. Torres WE, Maurer DE, Steinberg HV, et al. CT of aortic aneurysms: the distinction between mural and thrombus calcification. *AJR Am J Roentgenol* 1988;150:1317–1319.

323. Torsello GB, Klenk E, Kasprzak B. Rupture of abdominal aortic aneurysm previously treated by endovascular stentgraft. *J Vasc Surg* 1998;28:184–187.

324. Triantopoulou C, Rizos S, Bourli A, et al. Localized unilateral perirenal fibrosis: CT and MRI appearances. *Eur Radiol* 2002; 12:2743–2746.

325. Tseng CA, Pan YS, Su YC, et al. Extrarenal retroperitoneal angiomyolipoma: case report and review of the literature. *Abdom Imaging* 2004;29:721–723.

326. Unger EC, Glazer HS, Lee JKT, et al. MRI of extracranial hematomas: preliminary observations. *AJR Am J Roentgenol* 1986; 146:403–407.

327. Unterweger M, Wiesner W, Pretre R, et al. Spiral CT in an acute spontaneous aorto-caval fistula. *Eur Radiol* 2000;10:733–735.

328. Vaccari G, Caciolli S, Calamai G, et al. Intramural hematoma of the aorta: diagnosis and treatment. *Eur J Cardiothorac Surg* 2001; 19:170–173.

329. Vallabhaneni SR, McWilliams RG, Anbarasu A, et al. Perianeurysmal fibrosis: a relative contra-indication to endovascular repair. *Eur J Vasc Endovasc Surg* 2001;22:535–541.

330. Van Bockel SR, Mindelzun RE. Gas in the psoas muscle secondary to an intravertebral vacuum cleft: CT characteristics. *J Comput Assist Tomogr* 1987;11:913–915.

331. van den Akker PJ, Brand R, van Schilfgaarde R, et al. False aneurysms from prosthetic reconstructions for aortoiliac obstructive disease. *Ann Surg* 1989;210:658–666.

332. Van Hoe L, Baert AL, Gryspeerdt S, et al. Supra- and juxtarenal aneurysms of aorta: preoperative assessment with thin-section spiral CT. *Radiology* 1996;198:443–448.

333. van Olffen TB, Knippenberg LH, van der Vliet JA, et al. Primary aortoenteric fistula: report of six new cases. *Cardiovasc Surg* 2002;10:551–554.

334. van Rooij WJJ, Martens F, Verbeeten BJ, et al. CT and MR imaging of leiomyosarcoma of the inferior vena cava. *J Comput Assist Tomogr* 1988;12:415–419.

335. vanSonnenberg E, Wittich GR, Casola G, et al. Lymphoceles: imaging characteristics and percutaneous management. *Radiology* 1986;161:593–596.

336. Vernhet H, Serfaty JM, Serhal M, et al. Abdominal CT angiography before surgery as a predictor of postoperative death in acute aortic dissection. *AJR Am J Roentgenol* 2004;182:875–879.

337. Vinnicombe SJ, Norman AR, Nicholson V, et al. Normal pelvic lymph nodes: evaluation with CT after bipedal lymphangiography. *Radiology* 1995;194:349–355.

338. Vinnicombe SJ, Reznek RH. Computerised tomography in the staging of Hodgkin's disease and non-Hodgkin's lymphoma. *Eur J Nucl Med Mol Imaging* 2003;30[suppl 1]:S42–S55.

339. Vivas I, Nicolas AI, Velazquez P, et al. Retroperitoneal fibrosis: typical and atypical manifestations. *Br J Radiol* 2000;73:214–222.

340. Vosshenrich R, Fischer U. Contrast-enhanced MR angiography of abdominal vessels: is there still a role for angiography? *Eur Radiol* 2002;12:218–230.

341. Waligore MP, Stephens DH, Soule EH, et al. Lipomatous tumors of the abdominal cavity: CT appearance and pathologic conditions. *AJR Am J Roentgenol* 1981;137:539–545.

342. Wallis F, Roditi GH, Redpath TW, et al. Inflammatory abdominal aortic aneurysms: diagnosis with gadolinium enhanced T1-weighted imaging. *Clin Radiol* 2000;55:136–139.

343. Warakaulle DR, Prematilleke I, Moore NR. Retroperitoneal fibrosis mimicking retrocrural lymphadenopathy. *Clin Radiol* 2004;59:292–293.

344. Warnke RA, Weiss LM, Chan JKC, et al. *Tumors of the lymph nodes and spleen*, Series 3 ed. Washington, DC: Armed Forces Institute of Pathology, 1994:53–62.

345. Weiner JI, Chako AC, Merten CW, et al. Breast and axillary tissue MR imaging: correlation of signal intensities and relaxation times with pathologic findings. *Radiology* 1986;160:299–305.

346. Weinreb JC, Cohen JM, Maravilla KR. Iliopsoas muscles: MR study of normal anatomy and disease. *Radiology* 1985;156:435–440.

347. Welch TJ, Stanson AW, Sheedy II PF, et al. Radiologic evaluation of penetrating aortic atherosclerotic ulcer. *Radiographics* 1990;10: 675–685.

348. Whitaker SC. Imaging of abdominal aortic aneurysm before and after endoluminal stent-graft repair. *Eur J Radiol* 2001;39:3–15.

349. White GH, May J, Waugh RC, et al. Type III and type IV endoleak: toward a complete definition of blood flow in the sac after endoluminal AAA repair. *J Endovasc Surg* 1998;5:305–309.

350. White GH, May J, Petrasek P, et al. Endotension: an explanation for continued AAA growth after successful endoluminal repair. *J Endovasc Surg* 1999;6:308–315.

351. William MP, Cook JV, Duchesne GM. Psoas nodes—an overlooked site of metastasis from testicular tumours. *Clin Radiol* 1989;40:607–609.

352. Williams DM, Joshi A, Drake MD, et al. Aortic cobwebs: an anatomic marker identifying the false lumen in aortic dissection—imaging and pathologic correlation. *Radiology* 1994;190: 167–174.

353. Williams DM, Lee DY, Hamilton BH, et al. The dissected aorta: part III. Anatomy and radiologic diagnosis of branch-vessel compromise. *Radiology* 1997;203:37–44.

354. Williams MP, Olliff JFC. Case report: computed tomography and magnetic resonance imaging of dilated lumbar lymphatic trunks. *Clin Radiol* 1989;40:321–322.

355. Willmann JK, Wildermuth S, Pfammatter T, et al. Aortoiliac and renal arteries: prospective intraindividual comparison of contrast-enhanced three-dimensional MR angiography and multidetector row CT angiography. *Radiology* 2003;226:798–811.

356. Willoteaux S, Lions C, Gaxotte V, et al. Imaging of aortic dissection by helical computed tomography. *Eur Radiol* 2004;14:1999–2008.

357. Wilmink AB, Forshaw M, Quick CR, et al. Accuracy of serial screening for abdominal aortic aneurysms by ultrasound. *J Med Screen* 2002;9:125–127.

358. Wolff KA, Herold CJ, Tempany CM, et al. Aortic dissection: atypical patterns seen at MR imaging. *Radiology* 1991;181:489–495.

359. Wolverson MK, Crepps LF, Sundaram M, et al. Hyperdensity of recent hemorrhage at body computed tomography: incidence and morphologic variation. *Radiology* 1983;148:779–784.

360. Woodring JH, Howard RS 2nd, Johnson MV. Massive low-attenuation mediastinal, retroperitoneal, and pelvic lymphadenopathy on CT from lymphangioleiomyomatosis. Case report. *Clin Imaging* 1994;18:7–11.

361. Wysoki MG, Angeid-Backman E, Izes BA. Iliopsoas myositis mimicking appendicitis: MRI diagnosis. *Skeletal Radiol* 1997;26: 316–318.

362. Yamada AH, Sherrod AE, Boswell W, et al. Massive retroperitoneal hemorrhage from adrenal gland metastasis. *Urology* 1992; 40:59–62.

363. Yamada T, Tada S, Harada J. Aortic dissection without intimal rupture: diagnosis with MR imaging and CT. *Radiology* 1988;168: 347–352.

364. Yang DM, Jung DH, Kim H, et al. Retroperitoneal cystic masses: CT, clinical and pathologic findings and literature review. *Radiographics* 2004;24:1353–1365.

365. Yang WT, Lam WWM, Yu MY, et al. Comparison of dynamic helical CT and dynamic MR imaging in the evaluation of pelvic lymph nodes in cervical cancer. *AJR Am J Roentgenol* 2000;175: 759–766.

366. Yasuhara H, Muto T. Infected abdominal aortic aneurysm presenting with sudden appearance: diagnostic importance of serial computed tomography. *Ann Vasc Surg* 2001;15:582–585.

367. Yekeler E, Genchellac H, Emiroglu H, et al. MDCT Appearance of idiopathic saccular aneurysm of the inferior vena cava. *AJR Am J Roentgenol* 2004;183:863–864.

368. Yucel EK, Silver MS, Carter AP. MR angiography of normal pelvic arteries: comparison of signal intensity and contrast-to-noise ratio for three different inflow techniques. *AJR Am J Roentgenol* 1994;163:197–201.

369. Zeman RK, Cronan JJ, Rosenfield AT, et al. Renal cell carcinoma: dynamic thin-section CT assessment of vascular invasion and tumor vascularity. *Radiology* 1988;167:393–396.

370. Zeppa MA, Forrest JV. Aortoenteric fistula manifested as an intramural duodenal hematoma. *AJR Am J Roentgenol* 1991;157: 47–48.

371. Zhang Y, Nishimura H, Kato S, et al. MRI of ganglioneuroma: histologic correlation study. *J Comput Assist Tomogr* 2001;25: 617–623.

372. Zissin R, Gayer G, Kots E, et al. Iliopsoas abscess: a report of 24 patients diagnosed by CT. *Abdom Imaging* 2001;26:533–539.

The Kidney and Ureter

18

Mark E. Lockhart   *J. Kevin Smith*   *Philip J. Kenney*

Renal imaging can be performed using any of a wide selection of radiologic modalities, including computed tomography (CT), magnetic resonance imaging (MRI), ultrasound, nuclear medicine, intravenous urography, or even conventional radiography. CT is especially useful in genitourinary imaging, because more protocols have been created to evaluate renal lesions, renal vasculature, and the urothelial structures. The last 5 to 10 years have seen dramatic changes in the ability of CT scanners to image faster with greater resolution. Using this new technology, CT has aided in the evaluation of urinary lithiasis, renal masses, and adrenal lesions. CT or MRI urography has potential to replace intravenous urography in the evaluation for transitional cell carcinoma. While the benefit of other imaging modalities cannot be forgotten, CT has become the workhorse of renal imaging in many institutions.

NORMAL ANATOMY

Anatomy

In the typical patient, there are two kidneys, each of which consists of a peripheral cortex, central medulla, renal sinus fat, vessels, and urothelial structures. The kidneys are located within the retroperitoneal space to each side of the vertebral bodies at the level of T10-L2 (Fig. 18-1). The left kidney is often located slightly more cranial than the right kidney. The kidneys are generally symmetric in size and appearance, but the left kidney may also be slightly longer than the right kidney. The kidneys are usually larger in male patients and should reach full size by the late teens. The normal range of the kidney size is variable based on patient height with median length 11 cm, and most are within a range of 9.8 to 12.3 cm. The cortical thickness of the kidneys is usually symmetric. The mean thickness of

the cortex is approximately 10 mm, based on sonographic studies (130).

The kidney margins are generally smooth, but there may be small indentations of the normal renal margin (Fig. 18-2). A thin capsule surrounds the kidney, but the capsule is not typically visualized by imaging in normal patients. It should be noted that in patients with renal artery occlusion the capsular region could be visible, as capsular arteries creating a thin rim of enhancement at the periphery of the kidney may supply it (187).

Beyond the renal capsule is the perinephric space, which contains fat and thin fibrous septations. The perinephric fat is contained within Gerota's fascia. Gerota's fascia also surrounds the adrenal, which is separated from the kidney by a transverse septum. The anterior and posterior renal fascias separate the kidney and adrenal from other adjacent spaces. If the fascia becomes thickened due to fluid or other causes, it may be visible (413).

Each kidney is supplied by one or more renal arteries, which originate from the aorta below the level of the superior mesenteric artery or rarely from the iliac arteries. Single bilateral renal arteries are the most common configuration and the renal arteries course anterior and medial to the kidney (see Fig. 18-2). However, in approximately 24% to 30% of kidneys, there will be multiple renal arteries (90,253). The right main renal artery typically passes posterior to the IVC, but precaval arteries are present in 5% of patients (562). The main renal artery typically divides at the renal hilum to form a dorsal and ventral branch. The dorsal and ventral branches subsequently divide into segmental renal arteries. In approximately one fifth of renal arteries, there may be early branching of the renal arteries within 2 cm of the origin of the main renal arteries (253). The renal arteries may also be in close association with the collecting system or proximal ureter. This may become

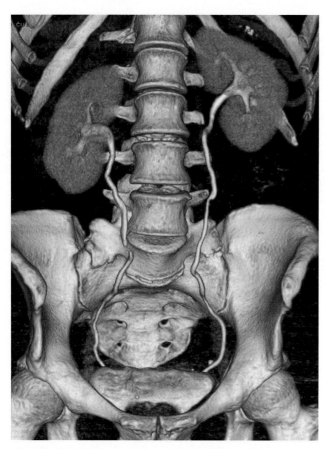

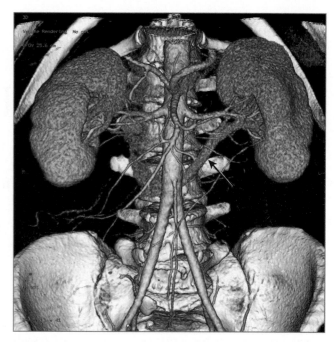

Figure 18-2 Normal renal CT angiogram. Volume rendered image from a CT angiogram on a potential renal donor. There are single renal arteries bilaterally with a slightly prehilar branch on the right. Note the somewhat lobular contour of the kidneys, the slight lateral tilt of the lower poles and the slight anterior rotation of the renal hila. There is also a retro-aortic left renal vein (*arrows*).

Figure 18-1 Normal CT urography. Abdominal CT with thin slices and excretory phase imaging demonstrates normal opacification of the collecting systems and ureters to the urinary bladder. Coronal volume rendered images present information in a format similar to intravenous urography.

GENERAL PRINCIPLES OF RENAL IMAGING

Computed Tomography: Normal Appearance and Technique

Normal Computed Tomography

Multiplanar imaging of the kidneys can provide exquisite anatomic detail. The normal smooth contours, craniocaudal orientations, and internal structures can be demonstrated easily and mimic gross pathological specimens. The densities of the renal medulla and renal cortex on non-enhanced CT are very similar, and they are similar to the attenuation of the liver. The renal parenchyma typically ranges from 27 to 47 Hounsfield units on non-enhanced CT (499). The renal sinus is most commonly anterior and medial to the parenchymal tissue, and it is easily differentiated from the parenchyma by its fat attenuation, even without intravenous contrast. The central renal sinus has fat attenuation with linear fluid-attenuation renal vessels coursing from the aorta and toward the inferior vena cava. The urothelial tract also originates in the renal sinus fat at the anteromedial aspect of the kidney, and in this region it includes the renal calyces and renal pelvis. The collecting system is usually collapsed, but there may be a small amount of calyceal fluid present.

The appearance of the kidneys varies with the timing of delay until image acquisition after the injection of intravenous iodinated contrast. On non-enhanced CT, the

important when there is obstruction because a crossing vessel may be associated with a ureteropelvic junction obstruction and may result in periureteral hemorrhage if the stenosis is treated endoscopically (444,487). The presence of a crossing vessel also significantly decreases the success rate of endopyelotomy for UPJ obstruction (345).

The renal venous drainage is extremely variable in number and location of the veins. The renal vein of the right kidney drains directly into the IVC. The renal vein of the left kidney is typically longer and courses anterior to the aorta until it reaches the IVC. Anomalous renal veins occur in approximately 11% of left kidneys (253). In the most common variant, two tributaries of a left renal vein may encircle the aorta (a circumaortic left renal vein) (Fig. 18-3). In the second most common variant, the left renal vein may course behind the aorta to the IVC (a retroaortic left renal vein) (see Fig. 18-2). The posterior component of a circumaortic or retroaortic renal vein is often located caudal to the level of the kidneys in its course to the IVC. The normal left adrenal vein and left gonadal vein drain into the left renal vein (Fig. 18-4).

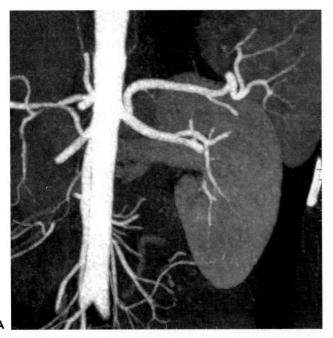
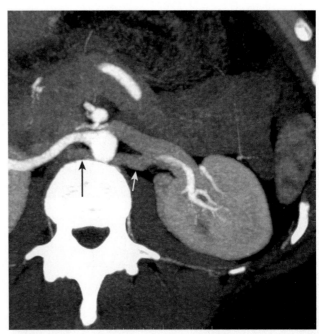

A   B

Figure 18-3 Circumaortic left renal vein. Coronal-obliqued maximum intensity projection (MIP) image **A:** axial-obliqued image **B:** from a CT angiogram on a potential renal donor shows the normally located anterior left renal vein and a smaller posterior branch (*arrows*). Note that the MIP reconstruction may artifactually appear as if the aorta is anterior to the vein.

central medullary portion of the parenchyma is not differentiated from the cortex in normal kidneys. Within 15 to 25 seconds of injection of intravenous contrast, the aorta and renal arteries opacify with contrast, as may be seen in CT an-

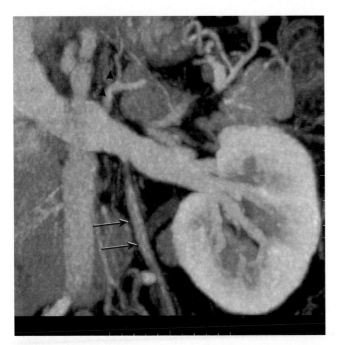

Figure 18-4 Normal left renal vein. Slab MIP image from a CT angogram on a potential renal donor show the left gonadal vein (*arrows*) and left adrenal vein (*arrowheads*) joining the left renal vein to the left of the aorta. Localizing these tributaries is critical during laparoscopic nephrectomy.

giography. During arterial phase of contrast enhancement, the cortex and medulla enhance at different rates with bright cortex juxtaposed to the less enhanced medulla (Fig. 18-5A). With standard injection rates, the cortex enhances to 70 HU during arterial phase and doubles to 145 HU within 40 seconds after injection. The medulla only enhances to less than 60 HU by 50 seconds (499). At approximately 100 to 120 seconds after contrast injection, during the nephrographic phase (Fig. 18-5B), the enhancement of the cortex and medulla equilibrates measuring at least 120 HU (499). The renal parenchyma of a normal kidney is homogeneous in the nephrographic phase with sharp delineation of the non-enhancing central renal sinus fat. After at least 3 minutes after injection, excretion from the renal tubules begins to fill the renal calyces and renal pelvis, known as the excretory phase (Fig. 18-5C). At this time, the renal medulla may be slightly more enhanced than the cortex as contrast is excreted from the renal tubules. During the excretory phase, dense contrast fills the collecting systems, the ureters, and eventually the urinary bladder.

Computed Tomography Technique

The CT technique that is chosen varies with the indication for the study. A decision must be made whether to use intravenous contrast. There are numerous indications, such as retroperitoneal hematoma or nephrolithiasis, that do not necessarily require intravenous contrast. Even in these situations, specific questions may arise which necessitate intravenous iodinated contrast administration. Often, the distal

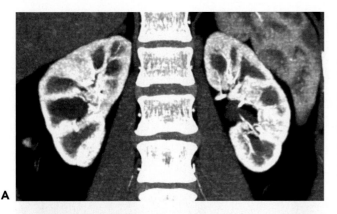

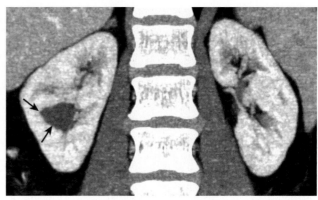

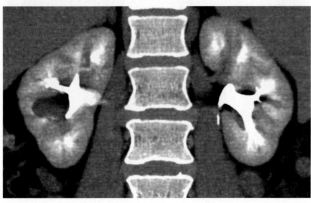

Figure 18-5 Different phases of normal renal contrast enhancement. Coronal thin slab reformatted images from a CT with contrast show the cortico-medullary phase (**A**), when the cortex has enhanced but the medulla is nearly unenhanced, the nephrographic phase (**B**), when the cortex and medulla are more similarly enhanced, and the urographic or excretory phase (**C**), when the cortex has started to wash out and the pyramids and collecting systems are intensely opacified. It is helpful to overhydrate patients or administer diuretic to dilute the urinary contrast to prevent CT artifacts. Note also single parapelvic cyst on the right (*arrows*).

ureters are difficult to visualize in the clinical question of nephrolithiasis, and intravenous contrast may enable the ureters to be separately visualized from any calcified pelvic phleboliths. Intravenous contrast should be judiciously administered since there is always a risk of anaphylactic reaction or even death. In patients with renal dysfunction, there is also the risk of contrast-induced nephrotoxicity, which may result in temporary renal insufficiency, permanent renal failure, or even death (330,512). The clinical benefit of intravenous contrast usually favors its administration despite the possible complications. Contrast enhancement significantly improves the visualization of the abdominal and pelvic structures and enables vascular characterization. After a delay, the urothelial system may be evaluated with thin slice CT, known as CT urography.

The selection of intravenous contrast also has several considerations. For many years, high-osmolar contrast was the standard of care. Research demonstrated reduced nephrotoxicity of low-osmolar contrast compared with high-osmolar agents (171). Because of a large difference in the cost of low-osmolar over high-osmolar contrast, universal administration of low-osmolar contrast was not immediately chosen. As the cost of low-osmolar contrast decreased and the difference in cost became less severe, universal administration of low-osmolar CT contrast became the standard in many hospitals. A similar situation is currently in consideration as new dimeric isosmolar nonionic contrast agents have been shown to have less nephrotoxicity than standard low-osmolar agents (13). These contrast

agents have a significantly higher cost than the standard low-osmolar agents, and based on institutional guidelines, they may be given in selected situations rather than as a universal policy.

Patients with mildly or moderately elevated creatinine are generally hydrated prior to intravenous contrast administration. A bicarbonate solution may be used to reduce the amount of contrast-induced nephrotoxicity when the creatinine is elevated (338). In these patients, we typically use the newer iso-osmolar contrast agents in an additional attempt to prevent nephrotoxicity. Usefulness of oral N-acetylcysteine has not been demonstrated in a recent large randomized trial (543). In cases of acute renal failure, severe renal failure not on dialysis, or severe prior allergic reaction, it may be thought that no iodinated contrast can be safely given. A premedication protocol for allergic reactions may be used, but patients may still have life-threatening allergic reactions in the face of standard premedication if the prior reaction was severe (313). In these cases, a combination of noncontrast CT and MRI or ultrasound may answer many clinical questions. MRI still has a very useful role in patients with renal insufficiency because intravenous gadolinium at routine dosage does not affect renal function. Intravenous gadolinium also does not have the similar high number of anaphylactic reactions as iodinated CT contrast, and contrast MRI is often chosen in patients with an allergic history (265).

In addition to the consideration of intravenous contrast, the administration of oral contrast may also pose a clinical dilemma. The standard of care for abdominal CT includes oral administration of 2 to 3 cups of diluted iodinated contrast. If possible, oral contrast is given time to pass into the small bowel to allow better characterization of the bowel and to improve detection of any free abdominal fluid. However, there are certain situations in which oral contrast may not be preferred. In the evaluation of nephrolithiasis, oral contrast may hinder the detection of ureteral calculi if dense contrast in bowel is adjacent to the ureter. In CT angiography, dense oral contrast will limit multiplanar and 3D reconstructions of the vascular system. Water may be used as a negative contrast agent to allow better characterization of the bowel in these patients. In an obtunded trauma patient with maxillofacial or cranial trauma, the trauma surgeons may prefer to rapidly perform the emergent trauma CT without oral contrast.

CT of renal disease often requires multiple series of images at different timings relative to intravenous contrast administration. Thin slices, 1 to 2 mm, are often performed on newer multidetector-row machines. The newest CT scanners have built-in dose reduction algorithms, but multiple series with thin slices will still administer a large dose of radiation to the patient. Each full sequence of images should be carefully considered as to whether it would provide significant additional information. At our institution, we will typically review noncontrast stone CT images to determine if the clinical question is answered before we decide whether repeated images with intravenous contrast should be performed. This is especially important with young patients who have nephrolithiasis and may often require numerous CT studies during their young adult years. Reduction of radiation dosage in these patients is important to limit potential carcinogenic effects at a later age. In patients with a known malignancy, the dosage issue is less of a clinical concern since the critical importance is accurate diagnosis and staging of tumor or tumor recurrence. In many of these cases, the expected life span of the patient will be significantly reduced if inadequate images do not detect recurrent disease.

Our multiphase renal mass protocol includes precontrast 3- to 5-mm images of the kidneys followed by 3- to 5-mm images of the abdomen and pelvis after intravenous contrast. If there is question of urothelial abnormality, 1-mm excretory phase images are obtained through the kidneys to the pelvis to allow CT urography reconstruction images. Images are performed after a 4- to 10-minute delay after intravenous contrast administration. At our institution, 4 cups of water are given prior to CT to help distend the ureters. Alternatively, a 250-mL normal saline infusion can be given immediately after the contrast injection to improve the distention of the renal pelvis and ureters for this evaluation (65,335). Some institutions also favor furosamide administration to improve ureteral distention. Thin slices, maximum intensity projection, and volumetric techniques of the CT data in a coronal plane (Fig. 18-6) are used to simulate the appearance of conventional intravenous urography.

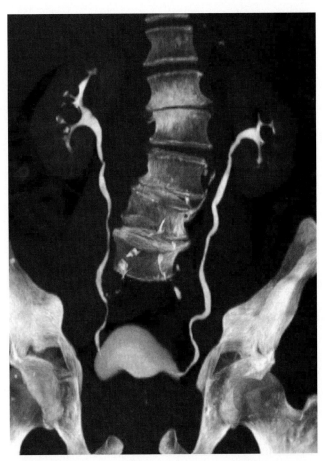

Figure 18-6 CT urogram. Coronal thick slab MIP projection from a CT urogram on a patient with hematuria simulates IVU, but with removal of overlapping structures such as the bowel and the sacrum. Adequate hydration or diuretic administration is important to achieve ureteral distension. An enlarged prostate causes elevation of the bladder floor.

MRI: NORMAL APPEARANCE AND TECHNIQUE

Normal Magnetic Resonance Imaging

On nonenhanced T1-weighted sequences, the signal intensity of the normal kidney on MRI is similar to the appearance of other abdominal organs, such as the liver. The renal cortical tissue has moderate T1 signal characteristics. In the absence of fat suppression, the renal sinus has typical fat intensity, consisting of high T1 (Fig. 18-7) and moderate T2 signals. However, T1 weighted images generally employ fat suppression. Fat saturation reduces the high signal from surrounding fat to allow improved visualization of the kidney (449). Moderately high T-2 signal characteristics are present in the renal medulla and cortex.

After gadolinium passes through the renal arteries to the kidneys, the cortex and medulla can be sharply differentiated if there is an imaging delay of less than 70 seconds after injection. The nephrographic phase, approximately 100 seconds after injection, will create a homogeneous

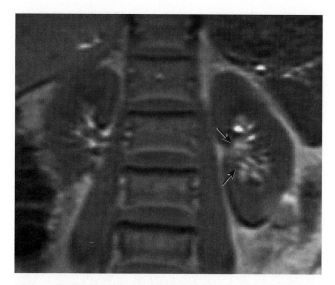

Figure 18-7 Normal T1-weighted MRI appearance of the kidney. The renal parenchyma is similar to other soft tissues and there is T1 bright fat in the renal hilum (arrows).

enhancement of the renal parenchyma, similar to CT. The perinephric fat will be similar to other areas of fat on all sequences. In later imaging during excretory phase, at least 3 to 5 minutes after contrast injection, the contrast in the renal collecting system is concentrated, and the concentrated contrast creates a signal void due to magnetic susceptibility (85,450).

MRI Technique

MRI has become a valuable tool in the evaluation of urinary tract disorders. Numerous techniques have been developed to provide rapid imaging with good spatial and contrast resolution. Respiratory gating techniques help to reduce motion artifact. T2-weighted imaging typically uses a fast spin-echo technique and may take approximately 3 to 5 minutes per series on standard machines. Axial, coronal, or sagittal source imaging is possible. For imaging of the entire urinary tract, coronal orientation may be useful, because axial imaging may be unable to include the entire system adequately in one series. Ultrafast half-Fourier transform techniques also allow T2-weighted imaging, but the spatial resolution is somewhat less than seen on FSE techniques; this limitation is partially offset by less motion or chemical shift artifacts (561). Standard spin-echo techniques are typically no longer performed, and have been replaced with gradient recalled echo images such as fast multiplanar spoiled gradient T1-weighted imaging. Newer three-dimensional volumetric T1 acquisition sequences also provide high resolution T1-weighted imaging of the kidneys.

MR angiography has evolved from previous noncontrast time-of-flight images based on flow of unenhanced blood to gadolinium enhanced breath-hold spoiled gradient evaluations, which have overcome previous in-plane

flow artifacts. Intravenous gadolinium contrast (0.1 to 0.3 mmol/kg) is used to shorten the T1 relaxation time of vascularized tissues and increase T1-weighted signal in enhanced structures. For arterial evaluation, MR angiographic images should use automated bolus-timing technique or test bolus to select the optimal time for imaging since a standardized 25-second delay may occasionally yield suboptimal contrast opacification. Coronal 3-mm or thinner images with no gap are performed. A phased-array surface coil can improve spatial resolution if it will cover the region of interest.

Standard MRI imaging of the kidney includes T1- and T2-weighted images. Either an axial or a coronal plane of imaging may be chosen. If a focal lesion is identified, a second plane of imaging may be helpful for further characterization and localization. Precontrast and postcontrast T1-weighted images are performed to evaluate the enhancement of the kidney and to quantitate enhancement of any focal lesions that are detected on the study. Fat-suppression techniques may assist in the detection of enhancement since there is improved signal difference between the renal parenchyma and the surrounding structures. T2-weighted images are not as useful in renal masses as T1-weighted images because of the nonspecific characteristic of most renal lesions on T2 sequences. One benefit of T2-weighted imaging is its ability to detect osseous metastases and assist in the detection of liver lesions.

Certain techniques may be useful in the evaluation of specific urologic questions. In the staging of a renal cell carcinoma, coronal T2-weighted and postcontrast T1-weighted images to the level of the heart may be helpful to characterize possible vena caval thrombus. Heavily T2-weighted coronal images of the urothelial system, MRI urography, can provide useful information regarding ureteral tumors, strictures, or obstruction based on signal obtained from the urine without intravenous contrast. For MRI urography, furosamide or saline bolus may be helpful to distend the ureters (372).

Limitations of Computed Tomography and Magnetic Resonance Imaging

CT and MRI are each excellent modalities for evaluation of the kidneys and ureters. Although both techniques have technical limitations, CT tends to be less expensive and more robust and is used as one of the first imaging studies alongside ultrasound. CT has excellent spatial and contrast resolution, which is improved by the use of intravenous contrast. Ultrafast acquisitions are possible with multidetector-row scanners so that motion artifact is reduced. CT is limited in patients who cannot receive intravenous iodinated contrast due to acute renal failure or history of anaphylactic reaction to iodinated contrast agents. In these patients, MRI is useful because intravenous gadolinium may still be given in the setting of renal insufficiency, and allergy to MRI contrast is extremely rare (356). However,

MRI has more susceptibility to motion artifacts, which are common in very sick patients. Ultrafast 3D MRI sequences are making progress to reduce these motion artifacts. Patients may have other contraindications to MRI that would not prevent performance of a CT examination (i.e., pacemaker or brain aneurysm clips).

In both CT and MRI, determination of whether true enhancement of a renal lesion is present may be difficult. MRI is more sensitive to vascularity within a lesion, but only relative enhancement can be generally described. CT allows absolute enhancement measurement, but the threshold may be changing in the setting of newer multidetector-row scanners. There may be significant pseudoenhancement of a lesion resulting from increased attenuation of the enhancing adjacent parenchyma. This is especially problematic in small lesions on multidetector-row CT (202). Radiation dosage and population radiation exposure by medical imaging is a concern specific to CT, but not ultrasound or MRI.

CONGENITAL ABNORMALITIES OF THE KIDNEYS

Abnormal Location or Fusion

Renal ectopia, or abnormal location of the kidney, occurs in approximately 1/500 to 900 persons (169). Renal ectopia occurs when the ureteral bud and metanephric blastema fail to migrate normally. The most common renal ectopia without fusion is a pelvic kidney (302). Often a pelvic kidney will be malrotated, and the renal hilum may be abnormally shaped with an everted appearance (Fig. 18-8).

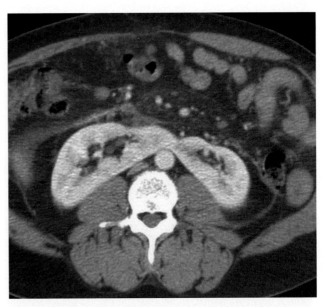

Figure 18-9 Horseshoe kidney. Axial image from a contrasted CT shows fusion of the lower poles anterior to the aorta.

Horseshoe kidney (Fig. 18-9) is a common type of renal ectopia that represents the most common renal fusion anomaly. It occurs in approximately 1/400 to 800 persons (339). A horseshoe kidney occurs when the poles of the kidneys (usually lower poles) are fused with an isthmus. The normal ascent of the kidney is halted at the level of the inferior mesenteric artery and the kidney remains located in the midline abdomen anterior to the aorta and spine. The lower poles, medially located relative to the upper poles, are located below the level of L3 vertebral body, a finding not common in normal kidneys. On CT, the two kidneys are medially located and are connected by a focal isthmus of tissue. The kidneys and isthmus typically enhance after intravenous contrast. The renal vasculature of a horseshoe kidney is usually abnormal with numerous vessels supplying the kidneys through a central hilum (443).

A horseshoe kidney is at risk for several complications. Because of the splaying of the vasculature and the shape of the kidney, there is increased risk of stasis in the collecting system. The stasis of urine in the collecting system may lead to urinary calculi or increased chance of urinary infection. Urinary calculi occur in 20% to 60% of cases (275,395), and most are calcium stones (411). In most patients, metabolic abnormalities contribute to stone formation (135). Ureteropelvic junction (UPJ) obstruction occurs in as many as 15% to 33% of patients (28,259), and there is association of crossing vessels in these patients. Vesicoureteral reflux is common in children with horseshoe kidney (448). There is increased risk of injury during trauma (255). The presence of a horseshoe kidney may also have an association with cryptorchiditism, hypospadias, polycystic kidneys, bladder extrophy, and ureteral anomalies (40).

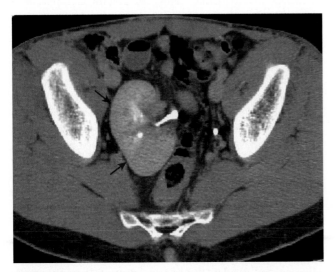

Figure 18-8 Pelvic kidney. Axial image from a CT with contrast shows the somewhat distorted, malrotated right pelvic kidney (arrows).

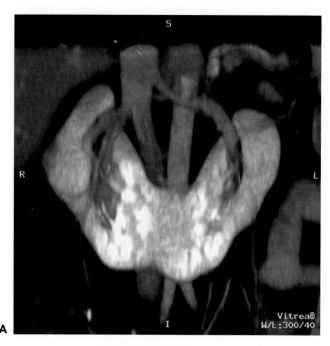 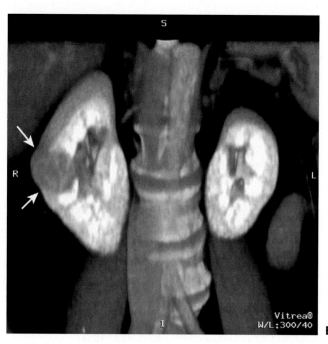

Figure 18-10 Renal carcinoma in a horseshoe kidney. Coronally oriented slap volume rendered images demonstrate the fusion of the lower renal poles and the renal arterial and venous anatomy (**A**) and the relationship of the vasculature to the right mid-renal tumor (arrows) (**B**).

In the horseshoe kidney, several neoplasms may occur; renal cell carcinoma (Fig. 18-10) is most common (436) but not at significantly increased risk over the general population (216). There is an increased incidence of transitional cell carcinoma (216,355), possibly resulting from stasis of urine in the collecting system. A rare tumor that occurs twice as often in a horseshoe kidney than in the general population is a Wilms tumor (339,367). Wilms tumor can be associated with a number of urologic abnormalities, including horseshoe kidney, cryptorchidism, hypospadias, pseudohermaphroditism, renal ectopia, or renal hypoplasia (339). In a horseshoe kidney, the location of Wilms tumor is evenly distributed among the right kidney, left kidney, and the small isthmus region (226,367). It presents with abdominal mass, hematuria, tumoral hemorrhage, or hypotension at a median age of 3 years (226). Surgical excision may be complicated by the abnormal vasculature supply that is common in horseshoe kidneys.

An extremely rare tumor that has a very high association with horseshoe kidney is known as a renal carcinoid tumor. Although only a small number of cases have been described, approximately 15% were discovered in horseshoe kidneys (272). These patients present with abdominal or flank pain (25). On ultrasound, the mass may be hyperechoic relative to the rest of the kidney, unlike many other renal lesions (234). On CT, the mass may be solid or appear as a nonenhancing hyperdense renal cystic lesion (234).

Another form of renal ectopia is termed *crossed ectopia*, which occurs in 1/1,000 persons (1) and is more common in males (144). This renal configuration occurs when one kidney crosses the midline and is attached to the lower pole

of the normally placed kidney. Most crossed kidneys are associated with renal parenchymal fusion (331). Rarely, there may be a solitary kidney with a single crossed ureter, or there may be two kidneys with crossing of the two ureters (331). In crossed fused ectopia, arterial and venous vasculature is usually atypical and may be complex (435). The malpositioned kidney is often malrotated. Crossed fused ectopia usually occurs with both kidneys on the right side of the abdomen (331). The ureter of the ectopic kidney inserts into the normal expected position at the left ureteral orifice of the bladder (331). There is increased risk for complications, and these may necessitate therapy. Complications may include urinary obstruction, renal calculi, urethral valves, hypospadias, and cryptorchidism (144).

CTA or MRI may provide useful information for preoperative assessment of fused kidneys (401,443). When necessary, renal surgery in these cases is often complex. Preoperative assessment of the vascular supply can be shown in great detail with CT angiography, thereby avoiding the added risk of catheter angiography prior to surgery. CT or MRI may demonstrate a point of fused parenchyma even if there is nonfunctional tissue in this region, unlike intravenous urography.

Rarely, an ectopic kidney may migrate cranially into the thorax with or without an associated diaphragmatic hernia (465). A thoracic kidney occurs in less than 1/10,000 persons (126). The abnormality is more common in males and usually occurs in the left hemithorax (126). It is usually detected incidentally because most are asymptomatic without the associated complications that occur in other ectopic kidneys (465). The kidney may be mistaken as a mass on radiography, but the diagnosis should be easily clarified on IVU, CT, or MRI. In one case, Stanley et al. (316) showed that the blood supply to the intrathoracic kidney came from the usual location.

Renal agenesis is extremely rare, and bilateral renal agenesis is lethal. The prevalence of bilateral renal agenesis and unilateral renal agenesis varies by population, but each occurs in less than 5 cases per 10,000 births (100,484). The left kidney is slightly more often absent (127). Other genitourinary abnormalities that may be associated with unilateral renal agenesis involve absence of the seminal vesicles, vas deferens, or epididymis in males and uterine, tubal, or vaginal anomalies in females (127). In patients who have renal agenesis or loss of the kidney during childhood, the remaining kidney will often enlarge; this process is known as compensatory renal hypertrophy. After nephrectomy, the remaining kidney volume can enlarge to a relative volume of approximately 120% within 3 years (491) (Fig. 18-11). The hypertrophied kidney usually will retain a normal location and orientation.

Abnormal Cortical Appearance

In a normally located kidney, another type of renal variant is visualized as an anomalous thickened appearance of the renal cortex, termed column of Bertin (Fig. 18-12). This prominent area of renal cortex may simulate a tumor, but it is often associated with a single central pyramid, which may suggest the diagnosis. Although the structure may appear hypoechoic on ultrasound and require additional imaging, the lesion usually has attenuation and enhancement patterns similar to the rest of the renal parenchyma on CT and MRI. A clue to the diagnosis is the external margin of the kidney should be smooth, and any distortion of the cortical margin should suggest an alternative diagnosis.

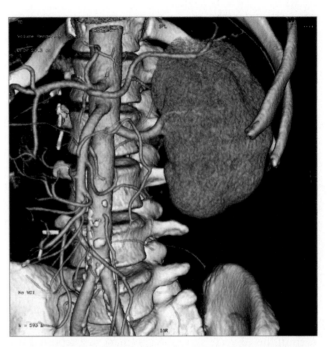

Figure 18-11 Compensatory hypertrophy of the left kidney after nephrectomy. Oblique coronal volume rendered image from a CT angiogram shows an enlarged left kidney and absent right kidney.

A junctional cortical defect is a common variant identified on ultrasound that has been suggested to represent an embryonic fusion defect (518). This variant is demonstrated as a focal area of cortical thinning at the anterosuperior or posterior inferior margin of the kidney. It is usually located between the lower pole and mid-portion at the junctions of renunculi (68). A linear cortical structure, known as an intermediate septum, is commonly associated with a junctional cortical defect (518). The enhancement pattern on CT and MRI differentiate this normal variant from a tumor. However, the appearance of a junctional defect may simulate cortical scarring.

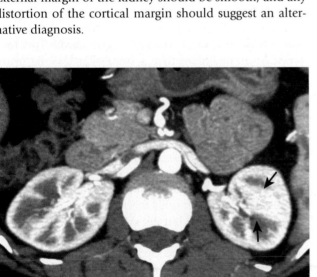
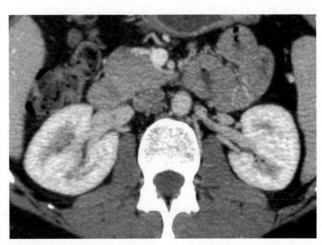

Figure 18-12 Prominent column of Bertin. Axial images of the left kidney from a multiphase renal CT reveals a prominent region of renal cortex (*arrows*) extending into the renal hilum on corticomedullary phase (**A**) and nephrographic phase (**B**).

A renal pseudotumor may also occur at the anterior aspect of the renal cortex. This has been termed as a hilar lip. This thickened region of cortex may be prominent on ultrasound, and it may even appear slightly hypoechoic to the adjacent parenchyma. However on CT or MRI, the characteristics are similar to the rest of the parenchyma on all sequences.

RENAL CALCIFIC DISEASE

Renal Stones

Whereas evaluation of suspected urinary lithiasis has relied on radiologic imaging for many years, the imaging done traditionally was conventional x-ray radiographs whether without or with intravenous iodinated contrast. For most of the 20th century, even for many years after CT was commonly available, the intravenous urogram (IVU) was considered the standard for such evaluations. However, in the 10 years since the landmark first reported use of noncontrast CT for detection of urinary calculi (472), CT has become the standard in the United States, virtually replacing the IVU.

With its currently recognized advantages of rapid, accurate diagnosis with minimal risk, one may wonder why it took so long after availability of CT for this transition to occur. The answers largely are, first, tradition, the acceptance of the usefulness of the IVU; second, the major cost differential especially in earlier days; and third, the greater limitation of CT before the advent of rapid spiral CT technology as well as wider penetration of CT in the medical care environment.

From the initial reports (472,473), confirmed by numerous independent investigators (78,150,368), unsurpassed accuracy was demonstrated for noncontrast CT, with a sensitivity 97% to 100% and specificity 92% to 100%. To emphasize the usefulness of CT, it has been shown that although nearly all calculi can be detected with CT, only about 60% are recognizable on conventional radiographs (298). CT has been shown to be more rapid and accurate than either the IVU or sonography (US). A number of studies have compared CT with US alone or in combination with plain radiographs (73,156,454,519). The sensitivity of US ranged from 24% to 77% versus 92% to 96% for CT, which also provided much more rapid results.

A considerable advantage of CT is the ability to detect noncalcific genitourinary (GU) pathology as well as non-GU abnormalities, which may be the cause of symptoms. The capability of the IVU for this is extremely limited, and although sonography may demonstrate gynecologic pathology, it is less capable of demonstrating gastrointestinal pathology such as diverticulitis, appendicitis, mesenteric adenitis, and pancreatitis, etc. In the 210 patients Smith studied (474), 30 were found with alternate diagnoses other than stones. Non-stone GU pathology in 14% and nongenitourinary lesions in

11% were reported by Fielding (150). Some have reported "indication creep" over the years (79,147), and decrease in positive rate (obstructing stone in ureter) from 49% to 28% with corresponding increase in alternate diagnosis rate from 16% to 49% has been considered a result of poor patient selection (79). However, one could argue that this is of little consequence if the patient presenting with pain, of whatever etiology, comes to rapid accurate diagnosis by CT and prompt treatment.

Although some argued that the IVU or other tests were necessary to look for evidence of the degree of obstruction, this argument has fallen out of favor. Many of the secondary signs on CT are in fact a result of the physiology of obstruction. More important, the presence or degree of obstruction does not significantly influence outcome or management. The size of the stone and the patient's symptoms are most critical, and it has been demonstrated that CT measurement of stone size is accurate (378).

Technique

No contrast is administered, thus no preparation is needed. After a scout view, scanning should include from at least just above the upper pole of kidneys (if not lung base) to perineum, and should be done in a single acquisition such that scrolling is continuous without pause or a gap. Typical parameters include 120- to 140-kilovolt (peak) (kV(p)) with 5-mm collimation and pitch 1.5:1. It may be possible that detection of tiny stones is better with pitch 1:1 or 2.5 mm collimation, or both, but this is not routinely necessary. If there is any question about the clinical suspicion, it is a good practice for a radiologist to assess the images before releasing the patient. If there are unsuspected findings, or a question as to whether a density lies in the ureter or not, or especially if the referring clinician has indicated concern about other diagnoses if no stone is detected, the radiologist can then make the decision whether to proceed with a contrasted study. The radiologist may also ask for a prone series to differentiate a stone that may lie in the bladder (usually lying at midline) but possibly in ureteral orifice (more lateral) (Fig. 18-13). In the experience at the author's institution, approximately 12% of studies proceed to contrast, although the actual frequency varies with the experience of the radiologist and the astuteness of the referring clinician. If contrast is given merely to opacify the ureter, the dose can be limited to 50 mL, and an appropriate delay (4 to 5 minutes) before scanning should be allowed. If a stone is identified in the ureter on the CT and is over 4 mm or 300 HU but not visible on the scout view, it may be helpful to obtain a conventional abdominal radiograph to follow the stone (565).

Interpretation

Interpretation is best done "soft copy" by scrolling sequentially through the images on a workstation. This improves

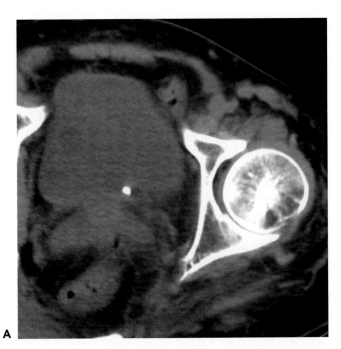
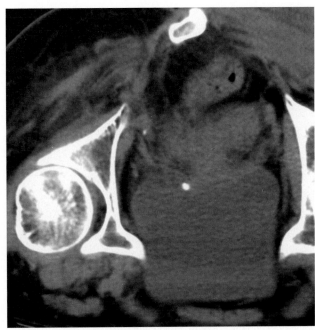

A   B

Figure 18-13 Stone lodged at the ureterovesicle junction (UVJ). Supine (**A**) and prone (**B**) images from a noncontrasted CT with a ureteral calculus at the UVJ apparently in the bladder. Prone image with the stone in a nondependent position confirms the stone has not yet passed.

the ability to follow the ureter even if it is nondilated as it courses caudally anterior to the psoas muscle, initially lateral to the ipsilateral gonadal vein, crossing medial to gonadal vein in the lower abdomen, through middle of the pelvis, and then anteriorly to the trigone (Fig. 18-14). This is most important because the key finding is that of a high attenuation structure within the ureter. A common (50% to 77%) (29,30) confirmatory finding is the soft tissue rim 1- to 2-mm thickening around the stone results from edema of the ureteral wall (Fig. 18-15), with a specificity of 92% (201).

Distinguishing a stone from a phlebolith is a common challenge, especially in the low pelvis if the ureter is nondilated. Several features may help in this distinction: phleboliths are always smooth and round; stones often are angular and may have fuzzy edges. Phleboliths rarely (0% to 20%) demonstrate a soft tissue rim sign (27,201,254). A soft tissue extension from a phlebolith is seen occasionally (21%) looking somewhat like a comet tail (Fig. 18-16) and representing the residual vein; this is not seen with a stone in the ureter (45). A central lucency is commonly (but not invariably) seen with phleboliths (sometimes requiring bone window settings) but is rare in stones. Comparison with previous studies can be illuminating—phleboliths remain in the same positions; if a prior study showed no density in a location of a current calcification, it probably is not a phlebolith. Phleboliths in the gonadal vein can be mistaken for stones if one is unfamiliar with their occurrence and the course of the gonadal vein. Although giving contrast too frequently is to be avoided, it may be necessary.

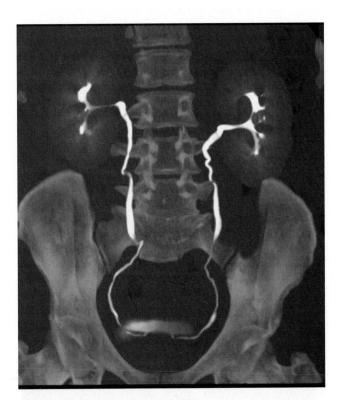

Figure 18-14 Normal course of the ureters. Coronal reconstructions of excretory phase CTU shows the proximal ureters coursing from the medial aspects of the kidneys into the pelvis. Note that there is mild elevation of the bladder with horizontal path of the distal ureters likely due to prostate enlargement.

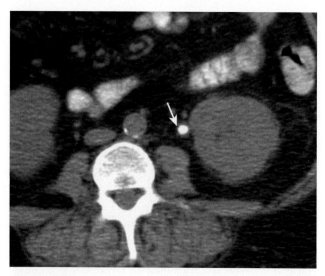

Figure 18-15 Soft tissue rim surrounding calculus. Noncontrast CT demonstrates a focal calcification (arrow) in the proximal ureter with a concentric rim of soft tissue density, indicating an impacted ureteral calculus. Note that there is also mild perinephric stranding, suggesting mild urinary obstruction.

Giving contrast to have absolute certainty is better than leaving the clinician unsure whether the patient has a stone or not, leading to unnecessary follow-up.

The obstruction resulting from a stone lodged in the ureter causes secondary signs (473). These include: hydronephrosis (69%) ureteral dilatation (67%), perinephric stranding (65%) periureteral stranding (65%) and swelling of the kidney (251). Detection of the secondary signs alone makes presence of a ureteral calculus as likely as 99% (473). Secondary signs, however, have their limitations because they are rather subjective. Absence of secondary signs does not by any means exclude a stone. Hydronephrosis

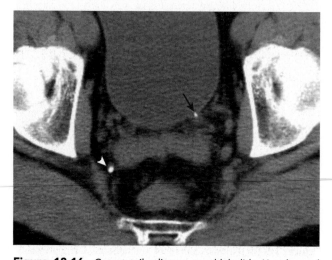

Figure 18-16 Comet tail adjacent to phlebolith. Unenhanced CT of the pelvis shows a phlebolith on the right with asymmetric "comet tail" soft tissue density (*arrowhead*). A stone in the distal left ureter (*arrow*) is also present.

can be overcalled due to extrarenal pelvis; assessment of the calyces at the poles is more reliable than the pelvis. Ureters can be dilated because of diureses, reflux, or prior obstruction. Perinephric stranding can be seen for many reasons; if bilaterally symmetric it is likely unimportant. When there is obstruction, increased lymphatic flow from the kidney, redirected to the capsular lymphatics due to the peripelvic pressure, produces this stranding (528). Frank perinephric fluid can be seen; at least some of the time this is actual calyceal rupture, and administration of contrast will show extravasation (Fig. 18-17). The renal edema also causes the loss of the hyperdense pyramid commonly seen in slightly dehydrated kidneys. It has been shown that obstructed kidney parenchyma measures 5-14 HU less than normal (172). It has been reported that the presence and severity of secondary signs correlates with degree of obstruction on IVU (44). It makes intuitive sense that the duration of symptoms correlates also with severity of secondary signs (528). In any case, these signs have not reliably been shown to correlate with outcome and thus cannot direct management. Stone size and position have consistently been shown to be the most reliable predictors of outcome. Approximately 90% of 1-mm stones will pass, proximal stones 5 mm or larger rarely pass; only 50% of stones larger than 7 mm pass, but some sizable distal stones may pass spontaneously (95,403). Most ureteral stones larger than 6 mm undergo intervention (149).

When conservative management is instituted, follow-up of the stone must be done. If a stone is clearly visible on scout view, it should be visible on conventional radiograph. However, less than 50% of stones are visible on scout view, but up to 60% can be seen on conventional radiograph. Nearly all calculi larger than 5 mm or greater than 300 HU will be radiographically visible, but those less than 2 mm or less than 200 HU may need to be followed with CT (565).

Pitfalls

Stones comprised of concretions of protease inhibitor crystals are not readily demonstrated as high attenuation lesions on CT. However, presumed diagnosis may be made in patients on this medication with symptoms of colic and secondary signs on CT. Several potentially significant non-stone GU diseases can cause pain but require contrast for diagnosis, including pyelonephritis, renal infarction, trauma, and renal tumors. Furthermore, diseases that do not relate to the genitourinary system are often undetected without intravenous or oral contrast. There has been some controversy regarding radiation exposure from CT for stones. There is comparable radiation dose to the patient for single-series CT compared with IVU (147), but the relative risk depends on the technique of each examination. However, frequent repeat examinations and follow-up with CT can increase the patient dose dramatically.

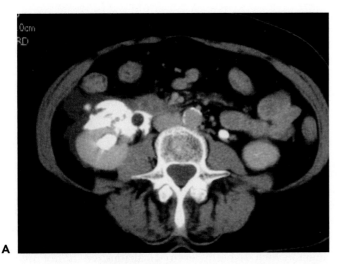
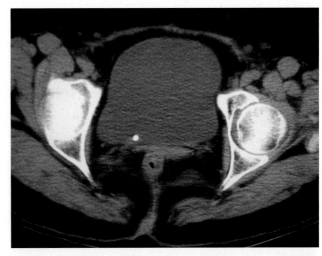

A

B

Figure 18-17 Pyelosinus rupture. Delayed CT images after intravenous contrast show extravasation of dense contrast-containing urine (**A**) due to backflow secondary to obstruction from distal ureteral stone (**B**).

Which method is best for diagnosis of urinary lithiasis in pregnant women is controversial. At the authors' institution, if sonography is not definitive and the patient's symptoms are strongly suspicious, noncontrast CT is performed. The radiation dose is controlled by initially performing a single test slice at the thickest part of the upper abdomen with dose reduced to the lowest level providing adequate image quality (usually 80 to 100mA maintaining kV at 120 to 140) and then proceeding with the study with those parameters to ensure rapid and accurate diagnosis on one study. Increasing the pitch to 2 also reduces the dose.

Because of its high contrast sensitivity, CT allows differentiation of tissues with much less attenuation difference than can be identified with radiography; thus, there is greater sensitivity for detection of small or faint calcifications than is possible with radiography. Although there is little published data, it is our experience that CT demonstrates more calculi in stone formers than does sonography (unpublished data), and CT is also much more sensitive than MRI. In the hands of a radiologist who is familiar with patterns of calcification, this sensitivity, combined with the precise localization and appearance of the calcification as well as other imaging features on CT, commonly allows correct diagnosis.

The normal kidney contains no calcification; thus, presence of calcification is always an indication of disease, but a wide range of disorders may result in renal calcification. Optimal evaluation of renal calcifications requires both unenhanced and contrast-enhanced images, because collecting system calculi may be obscured by contrast and because diagnosis of calcified renal tumors rests more on presence or absence of lesional enhancement than presence or absence of calcification (235).

Nephrolithiasis, that is, formation of stones in the collecting system, is one of the most common causes of calcifications in the urinary tract. Although the CT attenuation is

higher in stones with a significant calcium component, all commonly seen urinary stones, including urate and cysteine stones (with the exception of protease inhibitor concretions) (36), are "white" on CT images with usual soft tissue window and level settings. A critical factor in discriminating nephrolithiasis from other conditions is recognizing that the calculi lie only within the collecting system. Nephrocalcinosis most commonly results in calcifications within the medullary regions or within cortex depending on cause. In some patients, and particularly in patients with medullary sponge kidney, multiple fine medullary calcifications may be present in addition to collecting system stones. With very high resolution (1.25 mm or less) multidetector CT it may be possible to demonstrate also the "paint brush" appearance of the dilated medullary tubules of MSK after contrast (241), similar to IVU. With medullary nephrocalcinosis, the typical appearance is that of multiple small calcifications in numerous pyramids in both kidneys (Figs. 18-18 and 18-19). Cortical nephrocalcinosis may be seen as amorphous calcification limited to the cortex with sparing of medulla, calcification in both cortex and medulla, or with chronic cortical necrosis "tram-line" calcification on the periphery and corticomedullary junction (305).

Milk of calcium is well demonstrated on CT as a layer of high-attenuation material usually within a cystic structure (most commonly a calyceal diverticulum), sometimes in a hydronephrotic pelvis or ureterocele. Images delayed several minutes after contrast injection may be necessary to demonstrate communication of the calyceal diverticulum with the collecting system (Fig. 18-20). This can be particularly valuable when only a small amount of calcification is present, because the lesion may mistakenly be described as a complex cyst, raising concern for potential malignancy, whereas calyceal diverticula even with stones of milk of calcium have not been reported to have increased risk of malignancy.

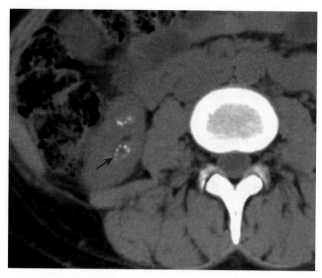

Figure 18-18 Medullary sponge kidney. Unenhanced CT of the kidney shows multiple punctate calcifications (*arrow*) within the renal pyramids.

CALCIFIED RENAL MASSES

Calcifications may occur in either benign or malignant renal masses (310)(549)(113). Approximately 25% to 30% of RCCs contain calcification on CT (34,566); less than 1% of cysts are calcified on radiography. The likelihood of calcification in RCC increases with size: only 3% of a series of RCCs less than 3 cm in diameter were calcified (560), whereas in another study 33% of RCCs larger than 3 cm contained calcification on CT (34). The exact location of the calcification and other features of the mass can be shown by CT, so that in many cases a definitive diagnosis can be made (264,549). Whereas MRI may help to evaluate such masses, it cannot demonstrate calcification well, showing only large calcifications as a relative signal void because of the low number of water protons.

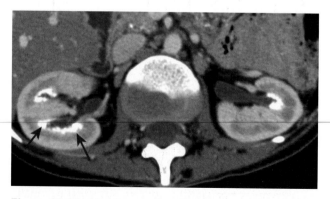

Figure 18-19 Medullary nephrocalcinosis. Contrasted CT of the kidneys demonstrates a line of calcifications (*arrows*) within the medullary regions of both kidneys. No contrast excretion has occurred on this corticomedullary phase study.

Calcified renal masses fall into three groups: (a) soft tissue masses containing calcification; (b) predominantly cystic masses with focal, mural, or septal calcification; and (c) indeterminate masses. Although the presence of calcification in a mass has for many years been considered a sign raising the concern for malignancy (RCC being the most common calcified renal mass) (113), it is probably not an independent risk factor (235). More important than the presence of calcification is the presence or absence of enhancing tissue within the lesion, whether or not there is significant calcification. CT is preeminent not only in detecting and displaying the location and appearance of the calcification, but also for detecting enhancement. As an alternative for patients who cannot receive iodinated contrast, MRI is effective in detecting or excluding enhancement, which is useful even if calcification is not well shown. Sonography is rarely useful for evaluating calcified renal masses, and dense cyst wall calcification prevents the sonographic interrogation of the lesional contents.

If CT shows calcification to be limited to the wall or septa of a cystic mass, and the mass otherwise fulfills criteria for a cyst (homogeneous water-attenuation contents, with no enhancing solid component or thick walls), a benign calcified cyst can be diagnosed with confidence. If the calcification is very dense or thick, follow-up is suggested. Diagnosis of a calcified tumor can be made in two situations—when the calcification is within the substance of an enhancing mass, or when there is peripheral calcification but also an enhancing area of soft tissue within the mass. A variety of patterns of calcification are found in RCC, including punctate, amorphous, linear, and curvilinear, peripheral calcification. Indeterminate calcified lesions are those in which there is some other disturbing feature in addition to calcification, such as high attenuation or heterogeneous contents, thick walls or septations, or questionable enhancement. Fine septal or mural calcification, without other disturbing features, in a cyst is most likely benign (Bosniak 2 category). Extensive, dense mural or septal calcification with no enhancement should probably be followed, although their likelihood of malignancy is probably less than 50% (thus, more properly Bosniak 2F than Bosniak 3). Calcifications with cysts are particularly common in autosomal dominant polycystic kidney disease (ADPKD), but when found in this entity should not be considered worrisome for malignancy, because there is no malignant predilection in this disease and the calcifications are usually the result of prior intracystic hemorrhage. Calcification can be seen in multicystic dysplastic kidney (MCDK), particularly in adults, but is not seen in multilocular cystic nephroma (MLCN).

RCC is the most common calcified enhancing mass, but other renal tumors may rarely contain calcifications, including Wilms tumor, TCC, squamous cell carcinoma, and metastases (16,196,274). About 10% of renal sarcomas may calcify, but calcification is virtually never seen in renal lymphoma. Although rare, calcification has been reported in both angiomyolipoma and oncocytoma.

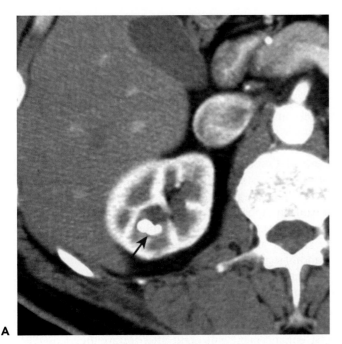
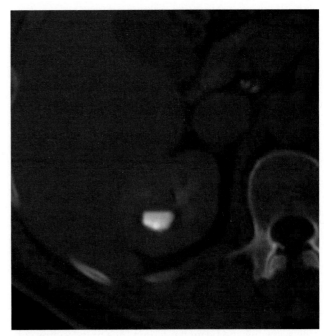

A   B

Figure 18-20   Stones in a calyceal diverticulum. Corticomedullary phase CT shows dense calculi (*arrow*) in the kidney prior to excretion. On delayed images, the stones are difficult to discern from the contrast within the calyceal diverticulum.

OTHER RENAL CALCIFICATIONS

Inflammatory masses and hematomas also may calcify. Staghorn calculi can be well shown on CT (sometimes correlation with scanned radiograph may be helpful to be certain of the contiguous branched configuration, indicative of a staghorn). CT can also distinguish the features of xanthogranulomatous pyelonephritis (XGP) from those cases with staghorn in a hydronephrotic or atrophic kidney. Hydatid cysts of the kidney often are calcified, and these may raise suspicion of RCC because hydatid disease is uncommon in the United States. Detection of daughter cysts suggests the diagnosis, because calcified RCC rarely is multilocular (111). Calcification is one feature that may be seen in renal tuberculosis (TB), most often as calcification within a parenchymal mass (tuberculoma). Although this may raise worry about renal carcinoma, usually other findings of TB are also present. Less commonly, calcification of urothelium (pelvis, ureter, or bladder) may result from TB. In immunocompromised patients, particularly those with AIDS, tiny multifocal renal calcifications can result from atypical mycobacteria (mycobacterium avium intracellulare) or pneumocystis (343).

A variety of vascular diseases can cause renal calcification. The most common is atherosclerosis, which causes calcified arterial plaques, usually at renal artery origins; there may be extensive calcification extending into intrarenal branches especially with chronic renal failure. Renal artery aneurysms and arteriovenous malformations may calcify. The relationship of the round, calcified aneurysm with the renal vasculature is usually well shown with CT, and contrast enhanced CT, especially with CT angiography techniques, can show the vascular nature (as well as other features such as engorgement and early filling of renal vein with arteriovenous malformation (AVM)) to allow correct diagnosis. Old hematomas may calcify; most commonly seen is a lenticular subcapsular calcified lesion owing to a remote subcapsular hematoma; there may be associated residual distortion of the kidney.

CYSTIC RENAL DISEASE

The most common renal mass in the adult is a cyst. Simple renal cysts arise from the cortex. If a lesion fulfills all the strict criteria for a cyst on sonography or CT, no further imaging evaluation is needed. Diagnostic features of simple cysts on CT are (a) smooth, round shape; (b) homogeneous water-attenuation fluid content; (c) smooth, sharp interface with adjacent renal parenchyma; and (d) imperceptible cyst wall (Fig. 18-21). Sometimes on CT, a thin rim of renal parenchyma may surround the cyst (especially polar cysts); also, two adjacent cysts may compress renal parenchyma between them (Fig. 18-22). Occasionally, a beak of renal parenchyma may be produced at the margin between cyst and kidney (446). If such masses otherwise fulfill CT criteria for a cyst, they should not be pursued aggressively. Although a variety of technical factors affect CT attenuation numbers, the latter can nevertheless be most useful in the diagnosis of renal masses. Simple cysts have homogeneous attenuation similar to that of water and should not have a attenuation over 20 HU. There should be

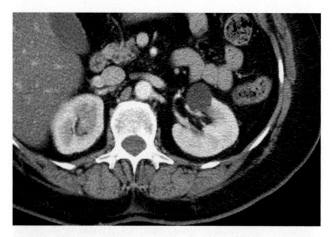

Figure 18-21 Simple cyst. Contrasted CT shows an exophytic cyst with lower attenuation than the adjacent renal parenchyma with no complexity or perceptible wall.

no significant increase in the attenuation after intravenous contrast. However, because of various factors, including volume averaging and beam hardening (due to the iodine concentrated in the adjacent renal parenchyma on enhanced scans), an increase of less than 10 HU should not be considered diagnostic of enhancement (46). Recent studies have shown that an increase of 15 to 20 HU may be more accurate in patients with bright enhancement of the renal cortex (314). This pseudoenhancement is more pronounced on multidetector CT than on single slice CT (202). The cyst contents should also remain homogeneous after contrast. Accurate assessment of enhancement requires appropriate section thickness—the slice thickness should be no more than half the diameter of the mass. Volume averaging may result in spurious "enhancement" when the slice includes part of the cyst and part of the renal parenchyma, because the CT attenuation value is an average of marked increase in attenuation of a small portion of renal parenchyma and the non-enhancing cyst contents.

Cysts may be solitary or multiple, and they can arise anywhere in the kidney. They tend to increase in size and number with age (112). Although cyst growth is slow, increase in size will be seen when followed for years. Cysts are usually asymptomatic. However, they may cause hematuria, and, if large, they may cause compressive mass effect, which can lead to hypertension or obstruction of the collecting system. In such circumstances, cyst aspiration and sclerosis, which can be done with CT or US guidance, is justified. Cyst aspiration currently has no role in diagnosis of complex cysts.

Although in general unnecessary, MRI demonstrates a distinctive appearance of simple renal cysts (250,320). Simple cysts have the same morphologic features on MRI as on CT: they are round and homogeneous, with a smooth, sharp interface with renal parenchyma and an imperceptible wall. Their signal intensity mirrors that of water (or cerebral spinal fluid); they are very hypointense on T1-weighted images, and they are very hyperintense (brighter than fat) on T2-weighted images (Fig. 18-23). No cyst enhancement will occur after intravenous Gd-DTPA (although volume averaging also occurs with MRI, and signal intensity numbers are not standardized, so no absolute numerical criteria can be used).

Calyceal diverticula may be discovered on CT as incidental findings, and on occasion they are imaged for further characterization after sonography, because these lesions may appear complicated, with calculi, debris, or milk of calcium within the diverticulum. These cystic spaces are lined by transitional epithelium and communicate with the collecting system through a narrow opening. They are commonly small and intrarenal, but they may be large and extend to the surface of the kidney (Fig. 18-24). They measure water attenuation on precontrast images unless calculi or milk of calcium is present. The latter is seen as a layered high attenuation, which will shift with change in patient position (495). On arterial phase, or routine

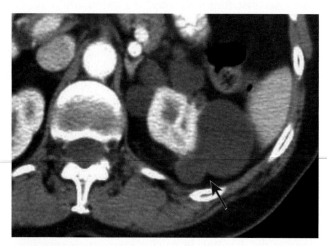

Figure 18-22 Pseudoseptation. Contrasted CT shows multiple adjacent simple cysts. The thin interface between two adjacent cysts (*arrow*) may simulate septation.

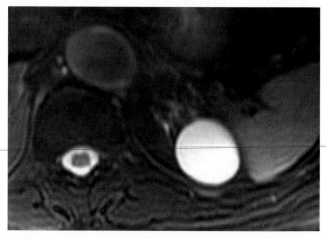

Figure 18-23 Simple cyst. Axial T2-weighted MRI image demonstrates homogenous high signal, consistent with fluid, in a simple left renal cyst.

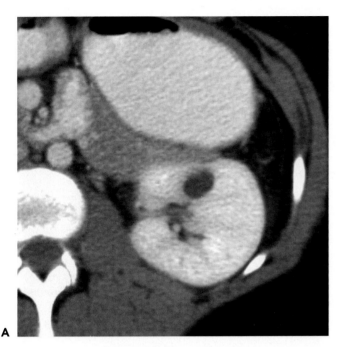
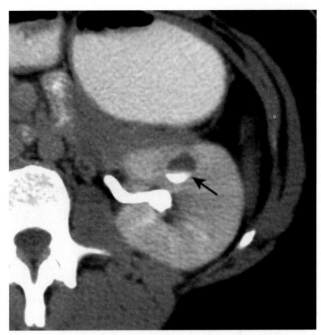

Figure 18-24 Layering contrast in calyceal diverticulum. **A:** Nephrographic phase CT shows a cortical hypodensity that is nonspecific. **B:** On delayed image, there is layer of excreted contrast (arrow), confirming a calyceal diverticulum.

early nephrographic CT images, a calyceal diverticulum will usually show water attenuation and may be misdiagnosed as complicated cyst if calcification is present. Excretory phase images (4 to 8 minutes after contrast administration) will show some filling with contrast in most cases, allowing correct diagnosis (Fig. 18-24B).

A variety of complex or complicated cystic masses occur, most of which are benign and of no clinical consequence. Nonetheless, they must be distinguished from renal malignancy (104,105). CT and MRI are very useful for this purpose, with CT playing the primary imaging role. A simple cyst may become complicated as a result of hemorrhage, infection, or other processes that thicken some or the entire wall and may increase the attenuation of the contents (46,194,425). Calcification within the wall or a septum may occur (105) (Fig. 18-25). Acute bleeding into a cyst may present with pain, and a fluid level may be seen within an acutely hemorrhagic cyst. The cyst may show increase in size on serial studies.

Hyperdense cysts have an attenuation value greater than renal parenchyma on precontrast CT images, commonly measuring 40 to 90 HU (46,93,101,197,569) (Fig, 18-26). This may be a result of bleeding into the cyst, with concentration of the protein components of blood. Some of these cysts contain a material as thick and dark as crankcase oil, and others contain inspissated white material (similar to milk of calcium), but some have clear amber fluid with a high protein content (152,493). Most hyperdense cysts are solitary, but they may be multiple; they are quite common in autosomal dominant polycystic disease (292). Hyperdense cysts may appear sonolucent, but in many cases

sonography shows internal echoes because of the thick nature of the contents. If the lesion is small (most are less than 3 cm), homogeneous, and shows no enhancement on postcontrast images, and if it has no other complicating factor (such as calcification), diagnosis of benign hyperdense cyst can be made. If CT first detects a hyperdense lesion, sonography may be helpful, because it may confirm the cystic nature. Follow-up of hyperdense cysts (with the exception of those in polycystic disease) is prudent to confirm their benign nature, because, rarely, renal carcinoma may have the appearance of a hyperdense cyst (129,197).

Several other findings may occur in cystic lesions that raise the level of suspicion for carcinoma. Thickening or irregularity of the wall, heterogeneity of the contents, calcification in the wall, and multilocularity or septation are all findings that may be seen in benign cystic lesions but also can be found in cystic renal neoplasms, including renal cell carcinoma, Wilms tumor, and others (104,195,194, 425). Bosniak has described a classification of renal cystic masses that is useful in clarifying the risk of malignancy and aids in the management of complicated cystic lesions (46). This classification is largely based on CT findings, but it includes information from sonography, MRI, and follow-up. This will be discussed further in the malignancy section.

Magnetic resonance imaging can be useful in evaluating complicated renal masses. The same morphologic criteria (e.g., homogeneity, sharp margination, thickness of wall and septa) can be used, as with CT. In addition, the great sensitivity of MRI to tissue characteristics can be useful because hemorrhage or other alteration of the cyst contents

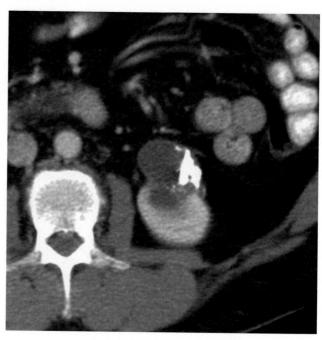

A   **B**

Figure 18-25   Benign cysts with thin (**A**) and thick (**B**) mural calcifications. Two images of a patient with multiple complex renal cysts show varying degrees of wall calcification. Stability over time confirmed benignity.

will be reflected by heterogeneity and change in the signal characteristics. Complicated cysts have higher signal intensity than water on T1-weighted images, and they demonstrate variable intensity on T2-weighted images (Fig. 18-27). If MRI shows a typical simple cyst (homogeneous low signal on T1 and high signal on T2), neoplasm is effectively excluded (320). However, when using only unenhanced T1- and T2-weighted images, complicated cysts cannot be reliably distinguished from renal neoplasms (224,320). The availability of MRI contrast agents provides the

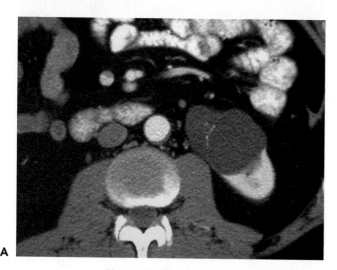

Figure 18-26   Hyperdense cysts. Contrasted CT shows a mildly hyperdense exophytic right renal cyst (*arrow*) without perceptible wall or solid component. There was no change in size over a three-year period.

opportunity to determine enhancement. As with CT, cysts do not enhance, but both benign and malignant neoplasms exhibit enhancement on postgandolinium studies. MRI is equivalent to CT for distinction of cysts from neoplasms (423,452), and currently it is the preferred procedure to evaluate complicated cysts in patients who cannot tolerate iodinated contrast. To clearly recognize enhancement, however, careful comparison of the appearance of the mass on the same type of sequence before and after Gd-DTPA is needed, because complicated cysts are typically hyperintense on T1-weighted images. Otherwise, such hyperintensity may be misconstrued as enhancement (449). As stated previously, it is easier to appreciate subtle contrast enhancement on fat-suppressed images than on non–fat-suppressed images.

PARAPELVIC CYSTS

Noncortical cysts occur adjacent to the renal parenchyma. Most cysts seen in the renal hilar region are believed to be of lymphatic origin and are usually called parapelvic cysts because of their location. These may be solitary but frequently are multiple. Etiology of this type of cyst is obscure, but no hereditary pattern is known. Such cysts typically replace the renal sinus fat and displace or compress adjacent structures, including renal parenchyma, pelvis, and hilar vessels. When solitary, these cysts are larger, often several centimeters in size, and appear round or oval. When multiple, they are usually smaller, and they may be ovoid or lobulated (Fig. 18-28). Parapelvic cysts are most

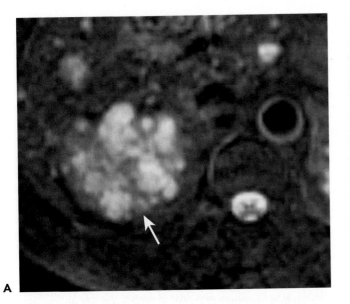

A

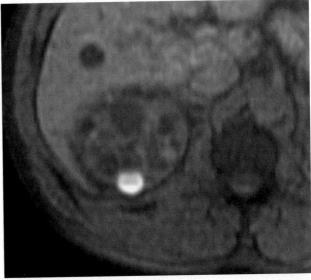

B

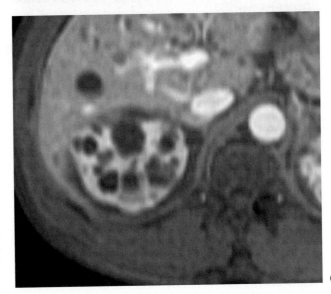

C

Figure 18-27 Complex renal cyst. **A:** Coronal Axial T2-weighted MRI shows complex renal cysts (*arrow*) among with subtle intermediate intensity among numerous simple other renal cysts in a patient with PCKD. **B:** On unenhanced T1-weighted images, the complex cysts havecyst has high signal relative to other cysts. **C:** On contrasted T2-weighted images, the complex cyst does not enhance (curved arrow)s have low signal intensity, possibly due to hemoglobin from prior hemorrhage.

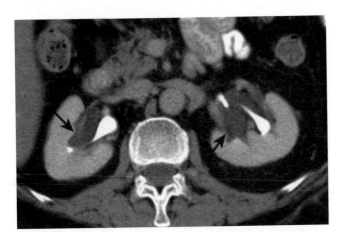

Figure 18-28 Parapelvic cysts. Excretory phase CT shows multiple fluid density cysts (*arrows*) within the renal pelvis. There is no communication with the mildly stretched collecting systems, which contain dense excreted contrast.

often of water attenuation but may be somewhat higher attenuation. There is neither enhancement nor communication with the collecting system after contrast medium administration (although increase in attenuation after retrograde pyelography has been reported, presumably due to extravasation and communication) (325). On unenhanced CT, MRI, or sonography, they may simulate hydronephrosis. However, their true nature is obvious on contrast-enhanced CT, as the contrast-filled infundibula are seen, effaced or compressed by the parapelvic cyst(s) (see Fig. 18-28). These lesions are of no clinical significance unless they enlarge enough to cause obstructive uropathy. Some of these cysts are thought to develop as a result of prior obstruction with resultant urine extravasation, the so-called parapelvic uriniferous pseudocysts (199,348).

CYSTIC DISEASES

Autosomal Dominant Polycystic Kidney Disease

Autosomal dominant polycystic kidney disease (ADPCKD) is a hereditary disorder that affects multiple organ systems; it has 100% penetrance but variable expressivity. In most patients (PKD1), the disease results from a genetic lesion on the short arm of chromosome 16 (383). Another slightly milder form of the disease has been shown to have a related but distinct genetic locus on chromosome 4 (PKD2). Renal disease is the predominant clinical feature, with between 5% and 10% of all end-stage renal disease resulting from ADPCKD, but the process affects many other organ systems. Hypertension is very common even before the onset of renal failure (157). Cerebral aneurysms occur in 5% to 10% (with cerebral hemorrhage occurring in about 8%), but the severity may be less than previously considered (442). These are usually small and involve the anterior circulation (164). Aortic aneurysm, aortic dissection, and valvular heart disease are much more common than in the general population (212). Cysts are found not only in the kidneys but also in the liver in approximately 60% to 80% of patients (352). They are present in the pancreas in about 7% of patients and in the spleen in less than 5% (212). Hepatic function is not usually impaired, however, even when the liver is diffusely involved.

Autosomal dominant polycystic kidney disease presents in several ways. The average age of onset of renal failure is in the sixth to seventh decade (157,212,383). Often the diagnosis is made because of screening, usually by sonography, of the offspring of an affected individual. Virtually all patients with the disease have sonographically detectable cysts by the age of 30 years (383). Patients may present with a palpable mass, because the kidneys become enlarged with increasing number and size of cysts. Not infrequently, patients present with complications of the renal disease, including flank pain, hematuria, or urinary tract infection. Nephrolithiasis (usually uric acid calculi) has been reported in up to 36% of cases (291).

Although CT and MRI are not usually indicated for screening of suspected subjects, they can be useful for evaluation of complications, and they both show typical patterns that are virtually diagnostic of the disorder. Multiple macroscopic cysts ranging from a few millimeters to several centimeters are seen throughout the full thickness of the renal parenchyma (Fig. 18-29) (281). Early in life, or in poorly penetrant forms, only a few cysts may be seen in the kidneys, overlapping with the appearance of multiple sporadic simple cysts. Detection of cysts in other organs are a useful clue to the diagnosis. With progression, the kidneys gradually enlarge as the cysts become more numerous, become larger, and replace the renal parenchyma (see Fig. 18-29). Bilateral involvement is usual, but sometimes the disease is quite asymmetric, and, rarely, only one

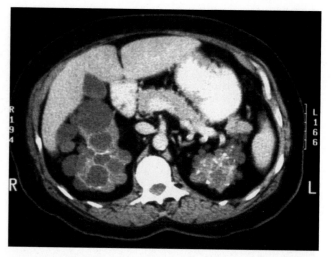

Figure 18-29 Autosomal dominant polycystic kidney disease. Contrasted CT image of the kidneys demonstrates diffuse cystic change in both kidneys with cysts of varying size and attenuation.

kidney shows significant disease (102,281,284,295). Although the cysts may have the typical appearance of simple cysts on CT, high-attenuation cysts are common, resulting from the frequency of hemorrhage into the cysts (292). Only 31% of patients in one study had no hyperdense cysts (292). Calcification of the cyst wall is also common, again most likely resulting from old hemorrhage. About 50% of ADPCKD patients have calcifications on CT, including calcified cysts and renal calculi (291). Calcification in these cysts does not carry the same degree of concern for renal carcinoma as it does in the general population. Although there is some controversy, no publications have convincingly established an increased incidence of renal cell carcinoma (RCC) in ADPCKD. Nevertheless, RCC does occur in these patients, and the same diagnostic criteria are used on CT as are used in general. Thus, it is very important to assess enhancement with pre- and postcontrast scans. Magnetic resonance imaging may be used as an alternative if there is a concern over the nephrotoxicity of iodinated contrast. CT is very useful in evaluating hematuria in patients with ADPCKD because it can detect cyst hemorrhage, can distinguish calculi from cyst calcification, and can diagnose renal neoplasms with higher accuracy than sonography can.

Magnetic resonance imaging may reveal a characteristic pattern in patients with ADPCKD. In addition to enlargement of the kidneys and the presence of multiple cysts scattered throughout the parenchyma, almost invariably cysts of varying signal intensity appear on both T1- and T2-weighted images (Fig. 18-30) (213). This is a result of hemorrhage of varying age within the cysts, so that some cysts are low signal on T1-weighted images and high on T2-weighted images, whereas others have high signal on T1-weighted images but remain low signal on T2-weighted images. The effect of hemorrhage into cysts is complex, but it may produce shortening of both T1 and T2 values, so

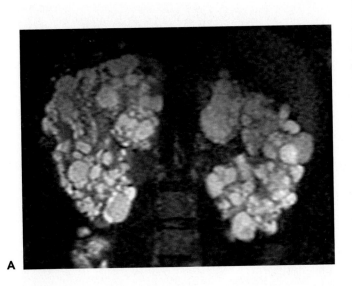

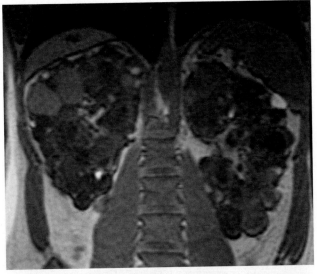

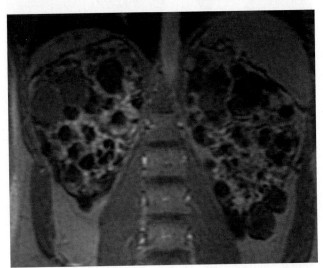

Figure 18-30 Autosomal dominant polycystic kidney disease on MRI. **A:** T2-weighted coronal image shows diffuse innumerable bright signal from innumerable cysts involving both kidneys. **B:** On uncontrasted T1-weighted image, the lesions have low-to-intermediate T1-weighted signal. **C:** There is no enhancement of the cysts on contrasted T1-weighted images, indicating lack of enhancement.

there may be increased signal on T1 but decreased on T2, unlike in simple cysts (213). Heterogeneity and layering may be seen, even in some cysts that are homogeneous on CT. Hemorrhagic cysts often show layering, with the dependent layer hyperintense on T1-weighted images but hypointense on T2-weighted images, and with the nondependent layer showing the reverse pattern (428). Renal carcinoma can be detected on MRI in these patients, as the tumor enhances with intravenous Gd-DTPA.

Sonography is commonly used and effective for both screening and initial diagnosis. Although currently primarily a research interest, volumetric evaluation of ADPKD may be of value in assessing progression of disease, as renal functional parameters (such as serum creatinine, glomerular filtration rate) do not worsen until relatively late in the disease process. Both CT (467) and MRI have been shown to be useful in such evaluation (76). The accuracy of volume measurements of total kidney volume, total cyst volume and changes over time has been well established (17).

MRI has particular advantages because of the lack of ionizing radiation and contrast with low renal toxicity, but it requires careful evaluation with multiple series (T1, T2, and gadolinium-enhanced T1) for complete assessment because of the variability in cyst signal intensity.

Acquired Cystic Disease of the Kidney

Nonhereditary cystic disease of the kidney (ACKD) is common in any form of end-stage renal disease, but it is particularly common in patients on chronic hemodialysis or peritoneal dialysis (323). The incidence of ACKD ranges from 47% to 87% (81,232,293), depending on the duration of dialysis, with an 80% likelihood reported after the third year (232). The exact etiology is not certain; ischemia, fibrosis, unknown metabolites, and inadequate control of renal disease have been postulated as causes. Hyperplasia of tubular epithelium occurs, which results in blockage and dilatation of nephrons, leading to cyst

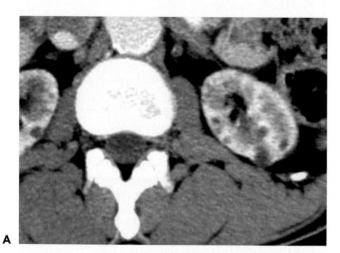

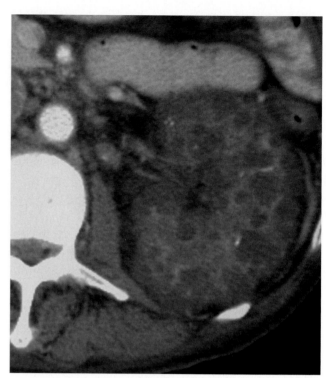

Figure 18-31   Acquired cystic renal disease. **A:** Contrast enhanced CT shows multiple small cysts in patient with end-stage renal disease. **B:** Contrasted CT in another patient shows marked enlargement of the end-stage kidney by countless cysts.

formation. There is a definite increase in renal carcinoma, with incidences between 5% and 19% reported (81,161,230, 232,293). Thus, routine evaluation of patients on dialysis longer than 3 years may be indicated.

Early in the disease process, the kidneys are small with only a few cysts (Fig. 18-31). The renal contour often is preserved, with most of the cysts small (less than 0.5 cm) and completely intrarenal. Although renal size may continue to decrease the first few years on dialysis, eventually the renal size begins to increase, as the cysts become more numerous and larger (2 to 3 cm). In a longitudinal CT study, 57% of patients had some cysts at the beginning of dialysis, whereas 87% did after 7 years. During this time, the kidney volume increased from 79 to 150 cc (297). Hemorrhage can occur either into the cyst or into the subcapsular or perinephric space. This can cause increased attenuation, heterogeneity, thickening, and calcification of the cyst walls. Eventually, after many years of dialysis, the kidneys may achieve an appearance nearly indistinguishable from that of ADPCKD (Fig. 18-32), even with calcifications (18). However, cysts do not occur in other organs in acquired disease.

As with ADPCKD, CT is superior to sonography for detection of complications, particularly RCC (509). Prevalence of renal carcinoma in hemodialysis patients has been reported to be as much as 40 times greater than in the general population (502). Intravenous contrast medium

can usually be used, if the patients already are on dialysis, but MRI is also an effective method for diagnosis of RCC. Detection of an enhancing lesion on either CT or MRI is presumptive evidence of RCC (Fig. 18-33). Although a renal adenoma may be suggested if the lesion is less than 3 cm,

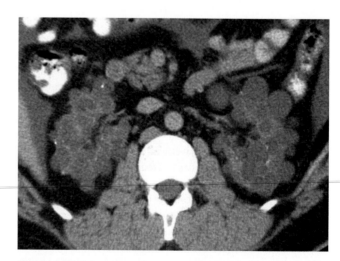

Figure 18-32   Acquired cystic renal disease (ACRD) mimics polycystic kidney disease (PCKD). A patient with severe acquired cystic renal disease has cystic enlargement of the kidneys simulating PCKD. ACRD is isolated to the kidneys, while the presence of cysts in the liver and pancreas would suggest PCKD.

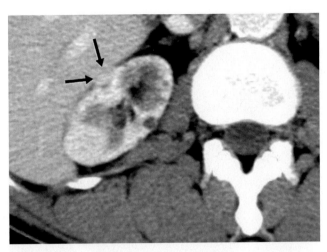

Figure 18-33 Small RCC in ACRD. Contrasted CT of the right kidney in patient with ACRD demonstrates a small focal enhancing mass (*arrows*) with disruption of the cortical margin. Patients with ACRD are at elevated risk for development of RCC.

size is not a reliable criterion. However, follow-up studies have shown that a significant proportion of RCC in ACKD patients are relatively indolent, 65% in one study having over 1 year doubling time. If the patient is not a good candidate for nephrectomy, or if the lesion is less than 2 cm, serial CT or MRI to determine biologic aggressiveness may be considered.

Although ACKD has been reported to regress after successful renal transplantation (232), it has also been reported that renal carcinoma may occur in native kidneys after transplantation (299). The premalignant potential of the cyst may remain for some time, and investigation of the native kidneys may be indicated in transplant patients with hematuria.

Autosomal Recessive Polycystic Kidney Disease

Autosomal recessive polycystic kidney disease, predominantly involving renal tubular ectasia and hepatic fibrosis, represents only 10% of PCKD patients and presents in infancy or childhood. It occurs in only 1 in 20,000 live births (568). The disease may present before birth, and infants with the disease do not typically survive. Children who present with the disease at a later age may survive into their teens or early adulthood. The most common method of detection is by ultrasound because of the risks of radiation associated with CT studies in children.

On ultrasound, the kidneys are usually symmetrically enlarged and may have cysts or a diffusely echogenic appearance (39,57). Discrete cysts are not usually identified on antenatal screening ultrasound, detected in only 4 of 27 patients in one study (57). On CT, the kidneys are large and hypodense. They demonstrate a striated appearance of

contrast enhancement (307). In a limited number of cases, MRI can detect early cystic lesions in these patients as well. Biliary fibrosis and manifestations of portal hypertension also occur. MRI is also more sensitive for biliary dilatation related to the hepatic manifestations of autosomal recessive PCKD than is ultrasound or CT (245).

Tuberous Sclerosis

Tuberous sclerosis (TS) is an autosomal dominant hereditary disorder resulting from a defect on chromosome 9 (61). It has somewhat variable presentation. Although the usual clinical features are seizure disorder, mental retardation, and cutaneous lesions, patients may not be recognized to have the disease until adulthood. Several renal lesions have been associated with TS, although the association with angiomyolipomas is best known (179,437). Cysts are seen in about 15% to 45% of patients, and cysts may be present in the first few months of life in some patients (69). Occasionally, numerous cysts are present in a pattern similar to that in AD-PCKD (see Fig. 18-27) (61)(344). Renal failure may occur, but it is uncommon. These cysts have a hyperplastic epithelial lining, as in acquired cystic disease. There may in fact be an increased incidence of RCC in TS patients, with an incidence of 1% reported (179,504).

Angiomyolipomas (AMLs) occur in 40% to 80% of patients with TS (526,399). Commonly, these are numerous, bilateral, and small (Fig. 18-34). However, they may be solitary or there may be only a few. Longitudinal studies have also shown that there is a propensity for AMLs in TS to grow and to hemorrhage, requiring angioembolization or surgery (69,526). The diagnosis of AML can be made if CT or MRI documents the presence of macroscopic fat (high T1, low T2 signal on MRI). Decreased signal on fat-saturated MRI sequences can help confirm the diagnosis if only small areas of fat are visible. Sonographic hyperechogenicity is not adequate, because small RCCs may also be hyperechoic (154). Fluid attenuation from hemorrhage may complicate the appearance. As AMLs increase in size, the risk of spontaneous hemorrhage increases, and therapy is recommended for lesions larger than 4 cm (376). All lesions greater than 10 cm should be evaluated for embolization, even if they are asymptomatic (188). For these large AMLs, selective arterial embolization may reduce the size of AMLs and their risk of bleeding (188,353).

The least common renal manifestation of TS is lymphangioleiomyomatosis. The process, most commonly seen in the chest, apparently results from smooth muscle proliferation that obstructs lymphatic channels, resulting in development of cystic lesions. Fluid-attenuation masses may be seen in the perinephric space in such cases (237).

Von Hippel-Lindau Disease

Another autosomal dominant hereditary disorder that may affect the kidney is von Hippel-Lindau (VHL) disease (84).

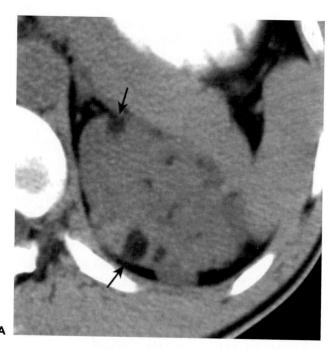

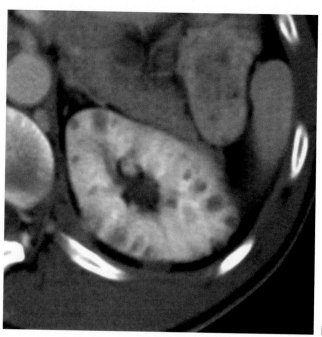

Figure 18-34   Tuberous Sclerosis (TS). Unenhanced (**A**) and contrasted (**B**) CT of the left kidney shows multiple round cortical lesions with fat attenuation values (*arrows*). The fat density of the lesions is consistent with angiomyolipomas, a common finding in TS.

The causative defect has been localized to the short arm of chromosome 3 (86,290,296). Several phenotypes exist. The most common includes presentation with retinal and CNS hemangioblastomas, renal cysts and cancers, and pancreatic cysts but not with pheochromocytoma. The next most common pattern includes hemangioblastomas, pheochromocytoma, and islet cell tumors of the pancreas but not pancreatic or renal cysts or renal cancers. In the least common form, hemangioblastomas, pheochromocytoma, and renal and pancreatic disease are found (86).

Renal cysts are found in 60% of patients; they are usually bilateral and may mimic ADPCKD, especially because pancreatic cysts may be seen (Fig. 18-35) (290). Of renal masses in VHL patients, 74% are cystic (87). Although it is uncommon for a cyst to degenerate into a tumor (87), many of the RCCs in VHL are partly cystic (Fig. 18-36). The presentation of RCC is in much younger patients in the setting of VHL than in the general population (210), and as many as 10% of patients with bilateral RCC are associated with VHL (238). RCC in patients with VHL has a slower growth rate and higher survival than patients with sporadic RCC (365). Still, RCC can be expected to develop in up to 45% of patients, and, historically, one third of the deaths have been caused by RCC (86).

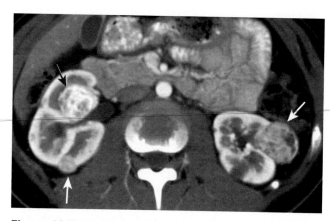

Figure 18-35 Von Hippel-Lindau (VHL). Multiple renal cysts present on contrasted CT are the most common renal lesions in this syndrome. The presence of pancreatic cysts (*arrows*) is also common in VHL.

Figure 18-36   Von Hippel-Lindau. On contrasted CT, the presence of multiple enhancing renal masses (*arrows*) is highly suspicious for multifocal RCC in this setting.

Angiography has been shown to have a sensitivity of only 35% for diagnosing RCC in VHL (342). Because the RCCs in these patients are commonly small when initially detected, CT is probably preferable to MRI, but no comparative study has yet been reported. Small tumors may be missed on initial CT, but with careful follow-up, enlarging lesions should be detected. In a patient with previous renal nephron-sparing surgeries or solitary kidney, MRI T1-weighted images may evaluate for lesional enhancement without the nephrotoxicity that is often associated with CT contrast agents. T2-weighted MRI is more sensitive than CT for detection of the renal mass pseudocapsule (500). This is best demonstrated as a thin low-T2-signal rim around the renal mass (500).

Removal of lesions that reach 3 cm in diameter is recommended, with an attempt at renal-conserving surgery rather than radical nephrectomy, because it is likely RCC will eventually develop in the contralateral kidney (86). For small tumors, enucleation, partial nephrectomy, and percutaneous ablation are possible therapies (459,539). A large series of VHL patients showed no cases of metastatic disease development when 3 cm was selected as the threshold for surgery. Furthermore, local resection was more often possible below this size, and fewer patients required dialysis or transplantation (128). On the other hand, tumors larger than 3 cm developed metastases in 27% of patients (128). If a new mass is detected on follow-up after previous normal studies, it is similarly followed until 3 cm large; then nephron-sparing surgery is performed because of the high likelihood of development of another RCC (86,204).

Other Cystic Diseases

Multilocular cystic nephroma is a localized cystic disease of the kidney believed by many to represent a benign neoplasm (20,194,312,385). It is uncommon and of unknown etiology and has no hereditary pattern. It is seen most often in two groups: young boys (3 months to 4 years of age) and adult women (over 30 years of age) (194,385). The pathologic characteristics are: (a) it is unilateral and solitary, (b) it consists of multiple noncommunicating epithelial-lined cysts separated by fibrous septa that contain no renal parenchyma, (c) a well-defined capsule is common, (d) the uninvolved kidney tissue is normal, and (e) the cysts do not communicate with the collecting system, but, not uncommonly, a portion of the mass may herniate into the renal pelvis. The usual multilocular cystic nephroma has no malignant potential and is often an incidental finding, but it may cause symptoms when large.

On CT, a multiloculated cystic mass ranging from a few centimeters to over 10 cm is shown. The cysts have water-attenuation value or slightly higher. The septa are usually thin with no enhancement (111) (Fig. 18-37). Usually the lesion has a thick capsule (5). Septal calcification is seen in about 10% of cases, and often it is curvilinear (312). High attenuation or other signs of hemorrhage are rarely seen in

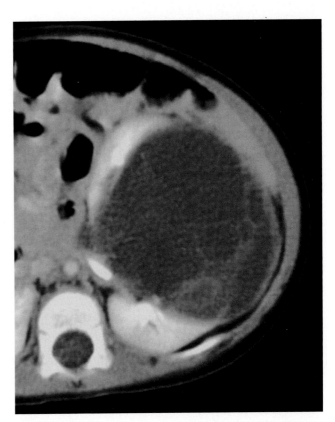

Figure 18-37 Multilocular cystic nephroma. Excretory phase CT of the left kidney demonstrates a large cystic mass with multiple thin septations. No solid or enhancing component was present.

multilocular cystic nephroma. In general, these lesions are in the Bosniak type 3 category, and they can be difficult to discriminate from cystic renal carcinoma (143,194–196, 385,386,425,553). On MRI, the cysts have low T1, high T2 signal intensity. The capsule is hypointense on T1 and T2 sequences. Intravenous gadolinium may demonstrate enhancement of the capsule (5). If CT or MRI shows thick or nodular enhancing septa, the mass must be considered renal carcinoma until proved otherwise, usually by resection. If there are no enhancing components, benign multiloculated cyst is likely, and the lesion may be followed if it is not so large as to cause symptoms (111).

Multicystic dysplastic kidney is usually encountered in neonates or infants, either as a finding on prenatal sonogram or as a palpable mass after birth. These can persist into adult life, but they are small masses in adults because they do not grow from childhood, and they often regress completely (488,533). The CT appearance is characteristic: a small- to moderate-sized cystic mass with peripheral calcification, occupying the expected location of a kidney (Fig.18-38) (501). The lesion may be uni- or multiloculated, and no contrast excretion occurs. The contralateral kidney often is hypertrophied, and may have ureteropelvic junction disproportion or partial obstruction.

Localized cystic disease, also known as segmental cystic disease, is a benign cystic condition that affects all or part

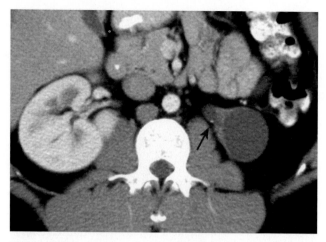

Figure 18-38 Multicystic dysplastic kidney. An atrophic left kidney (*arrow*) is visible with limited enhancement on contrasted CT.

of one kidney (see Fig. 18-22). It is not associated with PCKD or renal failure. On CT, a cluster of nonenhancing cysts without a capsule occurs in only one kidney. Calcifications may be present in cyst septations. Hyperdense cysts are uncommon. Findings are limited to one kidney, and the contralateral kidney is normal. On MRI, the findings are similar to those seen with CT (469).

RENAL MALIGNANCY

The most common symptoms and signs of renal malignancy are hematuria, weight loss, and flank pain. Tomography findings of transitional cell carcinoma include a small isodense filling defect within the collecting system. The lesion may be slightly hyperdense to the surrounding tissues on precontrast images. The tumor is much less dense than commonly is seen with stones. There is very little enhancement of the tumor after intravenous contrast. However, this small amount of contrast enhancement may help differentiate a transitional cell carcinoma from clot or hypodense calculus. Thin CT slices are required for evaluation. Recent development of CT urography has allowed generation of images that are equivalent to intravenous urography for demonstration of the collecting system and ureter. CT urography uses thin coronal slices with multiplanar reconstruction of images to form intravenous pyelogram-like images. The technique involves thin slices with overlap of the slices for reconstruction. Contrast is given, and standard CT images are obtained during arterial or portal phase. For detection of a renal mass, nephrographic phase images are superior to corticomedullary phase images (91). However, thin-slice CT images are repeated approximately 5 to 10 minutes after contrast injection (64,335). These images are reconstructed to show the pictures that resemble intravenous urography.

Renal Cell Carcinoma

Renal cell carcinoma, pathologically adenocarcinoma, is the most common primary renal malignancy in adults and occurs more commonly in males. Although most RCCs are sporadic, some may be associated with syndromes such as Von Hippel-Lindau. Renal cell carcinoma is associated with tobacco smoking (117). Other risk factors include exposure to petroleum products or asbestos (317). RCC is most commonly an incidentally discovered solid renal mass (438), but it may present with symptoms such as pain, hematuria, weight loss, or abdominal distension.

CT is very sensitive for focal lesions and is the most sensitive technique for characterizing renal enhancement. The typical amount of enhancement that is needed on CT is 10 HU, using single-slice scanner. However, with multidetector or multislice CT, more pseudoenhancement must be considered. Therefore, in these situations a threshold of 15 to 20 HU may be better for small renal masses (314). Lesions that do not enhance are typically considered benign, but the complexity of the lesion dictates further follow-up. In the cases of enhancing renal mass, the lesion is usually surgically resected if there is a high suspicion for malignancy. If the lesion is incidentally discovered, follow-up may be useful to document the benign or malignant nature of the lesion. Many radiologists prefer to have the follow-up in 3 to 6 months to allow adequate time for lesion growth.

The imaging appearance of renal cell carcinoma usually involves a focal renal mass centered in the renal cortex. The mass distorts the margins (Fig. 18-39) of the kidney in up to 94% of cases, regardless of tumor size (566). The prevalence of calcifications in a renal cell carcinoma is approximately 25% (566). Larger renal masses tend to have more calcifications than small renal lesions. CT is much more sensitive for calcifications than are conventional radiographs, ultrasound, or MRI. On CT, the calcifications of RCC may be punctate, amorphous, linear, or peripheral (260). There

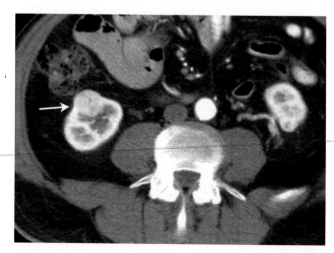

Figure 18-39 Small renal cell carcinoma. On corticomedullary phase CT, a small enhancing cortical mass is present. Even a small lesion such as this will usually disrupt the cortical margin (*arrow*).

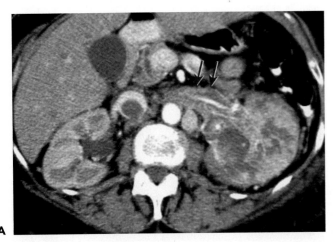
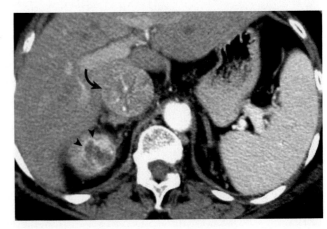

A   **B**

Figure 18-40 Large RCC with enhancing tumor thrombus. Two images of contrasted CT (**A, B**) show a large heterogenous left renal mass with extension of tumor into the left renal vein (arrows) and IVC. On the slightly more cranial image, the IVC (*curved arrow*) is expanded with enhancing tumor thrombus. Note is made of a synchronous enhancing lesion in the right kidney (*arrowheads*).

often is renal vein invasion, and the thrombus may extend into the inferior vena cava. The thrombus often is vascular and may show arterial enhancement (Fig. 18-40).

Renal cell carcinoma does not usually metastasize when less than 3 cm diameter, but exceptional cases do occur (105). RCC often metastasizes to the liver, bone, lungs, and nodes. One study suggests that more than two thirds of patients with stage IV disease have lung metastases (50). Liver metastases are often hypervascular (Fig. 18-41), and a metastasis may be visible only on arterial phase CT. The lesions, if small, are often invisible on portal phase imaging. When visualized on CT, the lesions on arterial phase are often bright. There may be a small peripheral rim, known as a pseudocapsule (392).

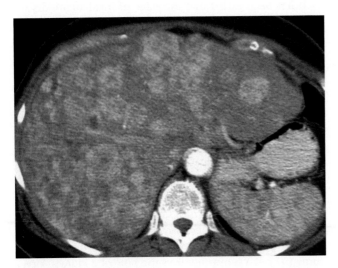

Figure 18-41 Hyperenhancing hepatic metastases. Numerous brightly enhancing liver lesions, consistent with metastases, are present on arterial phase CT in patient with known renal cell carcinoma. RCC metastases are commonly hypervascular.

Incidental renal lesions have a significantly lower likelihood of malignant potential and metastatic disease, as compared with lesions that present with symptoms. A greater percentage of incidental lesions are cystic than seen in symptomatic RCCs (33). Less than 15% of RCCs have cystic changes (195). Simple hypodense lesions are considered simple cysts, and do not need follow-up. However, if there is any complexity of the lesion, such as calcifications, septations, or a central location of the lesion, follow-up by CT is often recommended. Cystic RCC is usually asymptomatic and detected incidentally (96). When necrotic RCC is excluded and cystic lesions with less than 25% of the lesion appearing solid is considered, the malignant potential of these multilocular cystic RCCs is very low (361). If thick septations, enhancement, calcifications, or a significant amount of complexity with a solid component is present within a cystic lesion, the risk of malignancy is greater (195). Obviously, the presence of metastatic disease or venous invasion suggests malignant potential. In cystic RCC, MRI may also be more sensitive than CT for enhancement (361).

MRI is another modality for the characterization of a focal renal mass. RCC is typically mildly hypointense to the renal cortex on T1-weighted imaging (Fig. 18-42). On T2-weighted images, the lesion is mildly high T2 signal intensity (225) MRI is very sensitive to enhancement because of gadolinium contrast, and most renal carcinomas will show enhancement (see Fig. 18-42C). However, MRI is unable to provide exact enhancement measurements, unlike CT Hounsfield units. The enhancement of renal tumors on MRI is measured without units. Based on T1-weighted images, a 15% to 20% enhancement is considered diagnostic. Enhancement of septations or solid component is also consistent with neoplasm. However, as in CT, renal adenoma may also enhance. Most RCCs have a hypointense pseudocapsule at the periphery of the tumor (559).

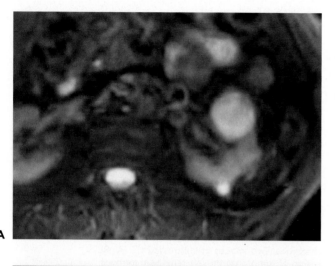

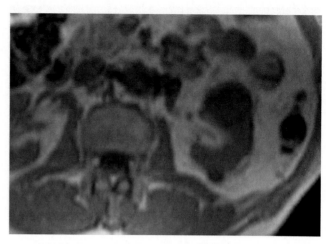

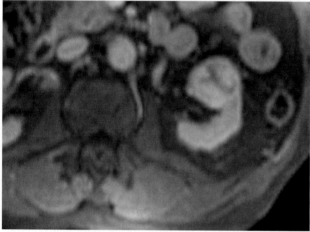

Figure 18-42 RCC on MRI. A small cortical lesion in the left kidney has high T2 signal (**A**), and mildly low T1 signal intensity (**B**). On T1-weighted image after intravenous gadolinium (**C**), there is bright enhancement of the lesion with small central scar or necrosis. Note that the appearance is very similar to an oncocytoma.

Fat-saturated images are recommended because gross fat may be detected with an angiomyolipoma. Therefore, if there is a signal dropout on fat-saturated images, the diagnosis of angiomyolipoma can be made. It is extremely rare for renal cell carcinoma to contain microscopic fat. MRI is less sensitive than CT for detection of calcifications.

Staging of Renal Cell Carcinoma

Staging of renal cell carcinoma is a critical part of the evaluation of a patient with renal mass. The staging affects the survival of the patient (515) and often the therapeutic approach. The main classifications schemes are Robson's classification (422) and TNM classification scheme (7). The staging depends on the lesion size, extension beyond the kidney margins, and invasion of the perinephric fat. Involvement beyond Gerota's fascia is a negative clinical indicator. Local spread to regional nodes or vascular invasion are classification factors. Previous studies have shown that CT is very accurate in the staging of RCC (419). A recent study of 3D MRI showed very high (97%) accuracy for staging of renal masses. In this study there was 100% sen-

sitivity for collecting system invasion (227). However, another recent study of combined staging of RCC by CT and MRI was only 67% accurate (538).

It has been noted that the stage of incidentally discovered RCCs is generally lower than that in symptomatic patients. Furthermore, stage-for-stage survival is higher in patients with incidental RCCs (270) Most incidental enhancing renal masses are renal cell carcinomas, but approximately 82% are stage I lesions as opposed to 37% stage I tumors in suspected cases (379).

Stage I and II RCCs are limited by the renal capsule and Gerota's fascia, respectively (422). By TNM classification, stage T1a tumors are less than 4 cm, stage T1b measure 4 to 7 cm, and stage II tumors are larger than 7 cm (7). These tumors may be treated with local resection for cure. Surgery may involve radical nephrectomy for large tumors or masses in the midportion or collecting system regions. However, the use of partial nephrectomy has increased in recent years with complication rates similar to those of radical nephrectomy (97). If a tumor involves the pole of a kidney, then a partial nephrectomy may be possible. Small tumors may be resected or enucleated laparoscopically, but higher complication rates have been reported (412). The size of the mass as well as the presence of adenopathy influences the choice of resection technique. For small isolated tumors, the cancer-specific 5-year survival rate is 89% after nephron-sparing surgery compared with a 91% 5-year survival rate after radical nephrectomy (133,183,289). Therefore, in these cases, nephron-sparing surgery is preferable. Radiofrequency ablation is a safe and effective therapy for localized tumors, especially when they are smaller than 3 cm and exophytic. In tumors between 3 and 5 cm, as many as 44% may require a second ablation procedure (162).

For stages I and II lesions, CT may have limitations in discerning whether there is extension beyond Gerota's capsule (243). Thickening of structures in the perinephric space may suggest stage III disease, but the finding is not specific because it may result from edema or hyperemia (271). Although CT is limited in its ability to detect local extension into the capsule, this finding does not significantly affect management and outcome because both stages are resectable with good prognosis. MRI is similar to CT in its limited accuracy for assessing extension of tumor through Gerota's fascia (142,359), but again, this distinction does not affect treatment if radical nephrectomy is performed. However, the differentiation is more important if nephron-sparing surgery is considered.

Stage III tumor classification includes invasion of the renal vein, IVC, adrenal involvement, or regional adenopathy (7,422). In as many as 30% of patients with renal cell carcinoma, there is tumor thrombus in the renal vein or IVC (see Fig. 18-40) that will need to be removed at the time of surgery (122,177,211,422,496). IVC involvement is rare in small tumors (248). A determinant of the complexity of surgery is whether the tumor thrombus extends into

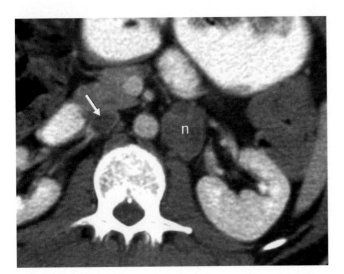

Figure 18-43 RCC nodal metastasis. A large left para-aortic nodal mass (n) lies adjacent to the left renal hilum. This is a common location for nodal metastases. Note the thrombus (*arrow*) in the IVC.

the right atrium. In this case, a combined surgery by urology and cardiothoracic surgery is often necessary. Metastatic adenopathy in the retroperitoneal space (Fig. 18-43) also has poor prognostic significance (327). In these cases, nodal dissection may be performed. CT can detect local adenopathy, and criteria have generally used a 1-cm threshold (489). However, this criterion has been unsuccessful in differentiating reactive nodes from metastatic adenopathy. A significant proportion of nodes with minimum diameter measuring at least 1 cm do not contain malignancy on pathologic examination (458). For this reason, surgery is still pursued in patients with isolated retroperitoneal adenopathy. On the other hand, nodes less than 1 cm in diameter may contain microscopic metastases. The presence of an adrenal mass should prompt concurrent adrenalectomy at the time of surgery, unless it fits attenuation criteria for a benign adenoma. Adrenal metastatic involvement occurs in less than 10% of RCC patients (166).

CT is very specific for renal vein invasion by tumor thrombus with 98% specificity (548). A hypodense filling defect outlined by contrast in the renal vein on a CT using corticomedullary or nephrographic phase timing is diagnostic for thrombus (319). Heterogeneous enhancement of the thrombus on nephrographic phase can confirm tumor thrombus. The inflow of unenhanced blood from the pelvis may be mistaken for IVC thrombus (482), and in certain cases delayed images may be needed to determine whether an IVC defect is inflow or thrombus. Tumor thrombus often enlarges the caliber of the IVC, and it may be heterogeneous and invade the IVC wall (see Fig. 18-40). There may be bland thrombus inferior to tumor thrombus in the IVC as a result of occlusion of the lumen.

In stage III disease, MRI is more sensitive for IVC thrombosis, and the diagnosis is aided by multiplanar ability of MRI to image the IVC in a coronal plane. MRI is more sensitive for IVC wall invasion to confirm tumor thrombus (357). It has a similar accuracy to CT for characterization of stage III disease. However, magnetic resonance imaging is more accurate than CT for the venous vascular invasion or tumor thrombus within the IVC (222,247,248,410). Gradient echo images may detect a low signal defect within the high signal lumen of the IVC (429) or high signal in the low signal flow void (Fig. 18-44). Contrast-enhanced MRI has the ability to perform coronal source images during contrast injection to evaluate for thrombus as a filling defect. Furthermore, T2-weighted images in the axial or coronal planes may be useful to evaluate for vascular invasion.

The ability of MRI to detect nodes is similar to that of CT, but it is similarly limited in its ability to differentiate reactive and malignant nodes. Based on nodal size criteria alone, MRI and CT are similar in sensitivity and specificity for metastatic adenopathy. More than 50% of abnormally enlarged nodes (greater than 1 cm) in the setting of RCC are a result of inflamed, nonmetastatic nodes (489).

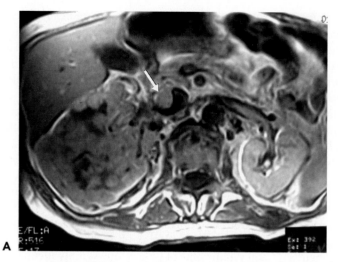 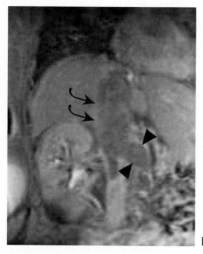

Figure 18-44   RCC with caval invasion. **A:** On axial T1 weighted MRI, a high signal intensity lesion (arrow) is present within the normal flow void in the IVC, consistent with thrombus formation. **B:** In another patient, contrasted coronal T1-weighted image shows an intermediate intensity thrombus expanding the IVC (*curved arrows*) and left renal vein (*arrowheads*).

However, recent ultrasmall supramagnetic iron oxide particle MRI contrast agents have shown promise for differentiating reactive nodes from metastatic nodes on delayed MRI imaging, even when traditional diagnostic criteria such as size are normal. A normal node will take up this agent, and the particles create a drop in T2* signal. Metastatic nodes do not take up the particles and demonstrate no drop in signal (189).

Stage IV cancer involves distant metastases or spread to adjacent organs (see Figs. 18-41 and 18-45), other than the adrenal (422). Metastatic disease to distant organs commonly involves the lung, liver, bone, or brain. RCC rarely metastasizes when it is less than 3 cm in diameter (105). However, once organs are invaded by the tumor, the prognosis is extremely poor. In stage IV disease, the therapy is palliative because a surgical cure is not possible. However, an isolated metastasis may be treated with local resection or percutaneous therapy. Radiofrequency ablation of a solitary hepatic metastasis may prolong survival. CT is very accurate in staging renal masses with distant metastases (243).

Direct invasion of adjacent organs, like distant metastases, is a specific indicator of poor prognosis. Large tumors may directly invade the adjacent muscles, liver, pancreas, colon, or spleen. Invasion of adjacent organs may limit surgical resection or increase the amount of time at surgery. Occasionally a renal mass may appear to invade the liver or spleen, when it actually is only distorting the margin of the organ without direct invasion (243). Multiplanar CT reconstructions or MRI acquisitions may be beneficial to help differentiate invasion of the organ from extension adjacent to the organ, but there are no specific signs of minimal invasion. MRI may underestimate T4 stage dis-

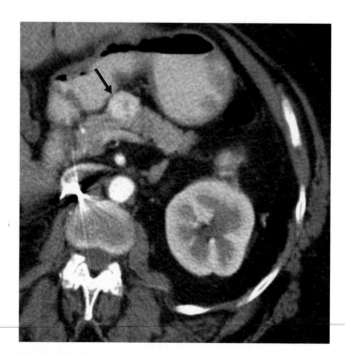

Figure 18-45   RCC with metastasis to pancreas. On contrasted CT in a patient with prior right nephrectomy (surgical clip visible), a brightly enhancing mass (*arrow*) is present in the pancreatic body. RCC metastases are often hypervascular.

ease by underestimating direct organ invasion (132). MRI may differentiate high T2 signal of tumor from the low T2 signal of normal structures such as the psoas muscle (247).

Treatment and Follow-up Imaging

The treatment of RCC depends on the staging of the tumor. For small RCCs, especially those that are incidentally discovered, the metastatic rate is low when lesions measure less than 3 cm in diameter. For minimally complex lesions, follow-up is usually chosen unless there are other considerations or risk factors. In patients who choose surgery for a Bosniak I or II lesion, postsurgical follow-up is based on clinical risk factors. For cystic lesions that are at least Bosniak III category, surgery is most commonly preferred if clinically possible, and closer postsurgical follow-up is warranted because of the increased risk of recurrence. Baseline CT and follow-up CT at 6-month intervals for 2 years is generally recommended. The most likely sites for recurrence of tumor are in the nephrectomy site or the adjacent structures. Solid organ recurrence may also occur in the liver, contralateral kidney, or adrenal.

Partial nephrectomy or nephron sparing surgery is more commonly performed for small lesions and have shown a similar tumor recurrence rate to nephrectomy (133,183, 289). Low-grade lesions measuring less than 4 cm are candidates for nephron-sparing surgery (289). Partial nephrectomy has become especially useful in the treatment of the incidentally discovered renal mass, which are often small and of lower stage (517). This procedure is often performed laparoscopically. Partial nephrectomy should be especially considered in a patient with abnormal contralateral kidney. After partial nephrectomy, it is important to follow all patients with RCC treated by nephron-sparing surgery, because there may be synchronous lesions in the remaining kidneys (371); however, the timing of follow-up may vary based on the underlying tumor (374). For small and exophytic lesions, percutaneous radiofrequency ablation is a safe, effective therapy (162).

Cystic Lesions and Rare Tumor Types

Whereas most renal cell carcinomas are solid enhancing lesions, some are cystic. The classification system developed by Bosniak has been used to stratify cystic renal lesions into risk of malignancy (47). A simple cyst is classified as a Bosniak type I lesion (see Figs. 18-21, 18-22, and 18-23), with no significant risk of malignancy. This appearance includes an imperceptible wall, without septations, calcifications, or enhancement. The lesion should include at least 25% of the margin of the kidney so that the wall can be evaluated. A type II cyst (see Fig. 18-25A) has characteristics that are minimally worrisome but do not fit strict criteria for a simple cyst. Thin septations, calcifications, or a central location fulfills a Bosniak II criterion. Hyperdense cysts that do not demonstrate enhancement also fit into this cate-

gory. The risk of malignancy in these patients is usually less than 14% (103). A Bosniak type III cyst (see Fig. 18-25B) has more worrisome features than a Bosniak II cyst. These characteristics may include thicker calcifications or thicker septations. A small amount of enhancement may be visualized in the periphery of the lesion (47). With the exception of a single small series of four cases with a high rate, Bosniak III lesions have a 25% to 59% likelihood of malignancy (103). A Bosniak IV cyst (Fig. 18-46) has characteristics consistent with cystic renal malignancy. This includes enhancement of the lesion. Thick septations and calcifications are often present. Usually there is more than one worrisome finding of malignancy in these cysts. The likelihood of renal cell carcinoma in these patients is approximately 95%. If clinically possible, surgery is recommended in Bosniak III or Bosniak IV cyst. There has been follow-up of Bosniak III cysts in patients who were higher risk for surgery. The Bosniak classification system was developed for CT evaluation of cystic renal lesions. The criteria do not exactly hold for ultrasound or MRI imaging. Because of the increased ability of ultrasound to detect septations, it is possible that ultrasound would overestimate the risk of malignancy based on septations. However, CT is more sensitive for calcifications.

MRI is more sensitive for contrast enhancement but less sensitive for calcifications. The characteristics of a simple cyst on MRI are a homogeneous, bright T2-weighted signal without visible septations or wall thickening. After intra-

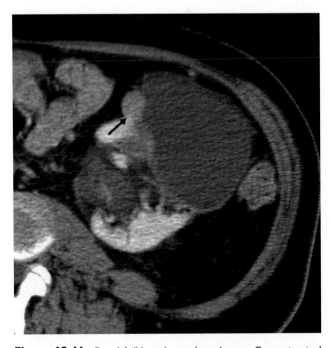

Figure 18-46 Bosniak IV cystic renal carcinoma. On contrasted CT, cystic left renal mass has thickened wall and a focal enhancing nodule (*arrow*) within the cyst wall. This finding suggests a high likelihood of malignancy, necessitating surgical management.

venous gadolinium contrast, there is no enhancement of the lesion on T1-weighted images (320). The presence of high T1-weighted signal on precontrast images is useful to help detect heme products. This helps improve the diagnosis of hemorrhagic renal cyst in the absence of intravenous contrast enhancement.

Subsequent to the initial research by Bosniak, a modification of the classification system was made. A Bosniak II F category was created. Lesions in this category have Bosniak II characteristics, but they have more worrisome features such that a follow-up study is recommended to confirm stability of size. Stability of size over a 2-year period is considered necessary to document stability. However, even slow-growing renal malignancies may have minimal change over 2 years. The presence of two simple cysts adjacent to one another is a potential pitfall of the Bosniak classification system. In these cases, the two cysts may resemble a single cyst with a septation. However, if there are no other worrisome findings, the appearance is consistent with a very low likelihood of malignancy.

Acquired cystic renal disease (see Fig. 18-31) is a risk factor for RCC. Acquired cystic disease develops after approximately 3 to 10 years of hemodialysis (323). There is increased incidence of RCC in these patients (323). The detection of RCC in these patients is best on early phase at approximately 40 seconds after injection of contrast, because of the relative paucity of normal cortical enhancement relative to tumors. Furthermore, this timing allows detection of papillary RCC, the most common RCC type in acquired cystic disease, which has less enhancement during later phases (503).

Chromophobe RCC is a recently classified subtype of RCC. It occurs in males or females (358). The tumor is typically large at presentation and homogenous in appearance without necrosis or hemorrhage. The mass is generally hypovascular on contrast-enhanced CT relative to clear cell RCC (358).

Transitional Cell Carcinoma

Urothelial tumors are less common in the upper urinary tract than renal cell carcinoma (283). However, transitional cell carcinoma (TCC) is the second most common renal neoplasm in adults and represents the vast majority of urothelial tumors. It is most common in the urinary bladder, followed in frequency by the ureter and renal pelvis. Only approximately 10% of urothelial tumors are of other etiologies (160). The next most common etiology is squamous cell carcinoma, associated with inflammation, nephrolithiasis, and leukoplakia (35,206,363). Squamous cell carcinoma is aggressive and may present as an infiltrating mass, a thickening of the renal pelvic wall, or as a filling defect in the collecting system (360). Adenocarcinomas represent less than 1% of urothelial malignancies (160), and they are associated with ureteritis glandularis and chronic inflammation (268).

Risk factors for TCC include nonsterioidal anti-inflammatory drug (NSAID) abuse, tobacco use, and some occupational exposures (11). TCC is more common in males (328). The incidence of TCC may be increased in horseshoe kidney (355). Patients with TCC most commonly present with hematuria (407) or, less commonly, with pain or weight loss. Initial detection of an urothelial lesion in a symptomatic patient has been most often made by intravenous urography. The findings on IVU include a filling defect outlined by excreted contrast. There may be obstruction of the kidney with non-opacification of the collecting system or ureter. The collecting system may be distorted by mass. In small tumors, only a small polypoid defect may be visible. Occasionally, sonography may detect a collecting system lesion in the calyces or renal pelvis. Prior to CT urography and MR urography techniques, initial detection of collecting system lesions was limited in cross-sectional imaging. For CT or MRI evaluation, it is important to include images in the excretory phase (3 to 5 minutes after injection) to show low-attenuation mass margins involving the collecting system or ureter, as outlined by concentrated dense contrast.

There are three general CT imaging appearances of a small transitional cell carcinoma. On CT, the most common appearance of TCC is a small, hypodense lesion in the renal collecting system (Fig. 18-47) (534). The lesion will have soft tissue attenuation (less than 40 HU) that is less attenuating than is common for urinary calculi, excluding indinivir stones. The attenuation of TCC is also slightly lower than a blood clot within the collecting system but higher than the attenuation of urine (160). TCC will enhance 10 to 50 HU after intravenous contrast (160,364,384). The amount of enhancement is less than

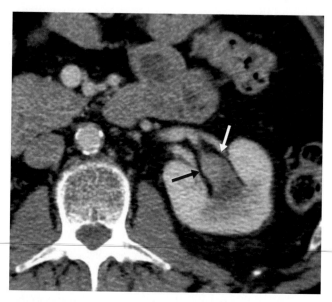

Figure 18-47 TCC filling defect in renal pelvis. On nephrographic phase CT, a hypodense filling defect expands the left renal pelvis (*arrows*).

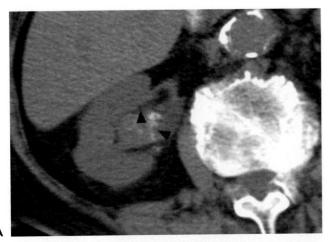

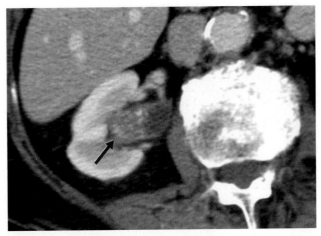

A

B

Figure 18-48 Renal pelvis TCC with stippled calcification. **A:** On precontrast image, a focal soft tissue density lesion fills the right renal pelvis. The mass has multiple stippled calcifications (*arrowheads*), which are the most common appearance of calcifications in TCC. **B:** After intravenous contrast, mild enhancement (*arrow*) of the mass is present.

the surrounding renal parenchyma, and therefore the lesion appears hypodense relative to the kidney (21). Still, this mild enhancement of TCC differentiates this cause from other nontumorous diagnoses, such as stone or clot. In the kidney, TCC is usually more central than RCC owing to its origin in the urothelium. Transitional cell carcinomas may contain stippled calcification (124) (Fig. 18-48). Necrosis within a larger mass is not uncommon (53). TCC is bilateral in less than 2% of patients (218). Unlike renal cell carcinoma, a transitional cell carcinoma does not commonly involve the renal vein, although even cases involving the inferior vena cava have been reported (288). Renal pelvis transitional cell carcinoma does occasionally arise within the proximal ureter (Fig.18-49).

TCC may present as a locally aggressive infiltrative renal mass (Fig. 18-50) (193). The tumor may be large and necrotic (53). The margins of the mass may be ill defined. Involvement of the renal parenchyma can be detected by finding a hypoenhancing mass involving the parenchyma or a heterogeneous abnormal hypoenhancement disrupting the normal enhancing parenchyma on nephrographic phase (523). The mass originates from the central region of the kidney and expands the kidney symmetrically (21,53,283). The renal contours are usually not disrupted, unlike in RCC, but this may rarely occur with TCC (53) (Fig. 18-51).

A third appearance of TCC is thickening of the collecting system urothelium or ureteral wall (21) (Fig. 18-52).

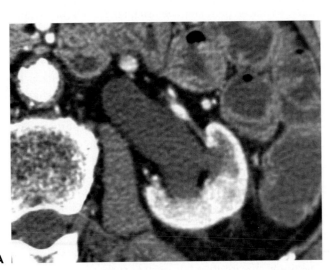

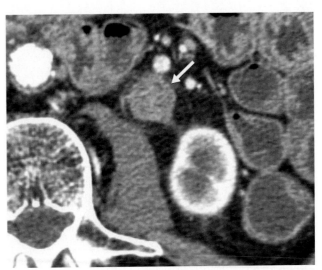

A

B

Figure 18-49 TCC in proximal ureter with obstruction. **A:** Contrast enhanced CT at the level of the renal hilum shows moderate hydronephrosis. **B:** Image of the proximal ureter on same series has a focal mass (*arrow*) causing the obstruction, consistent with TCC.

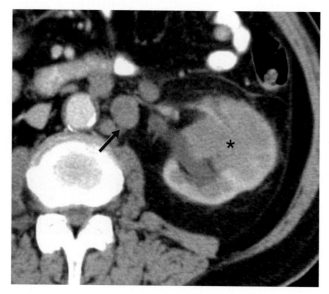

Figure 18-50 Infiltrative TCC. Contrast enhanced CT shows a poorly marginated central renal mass (*) invading the renal hilum. Hilar adenopathy is also present (arrow).

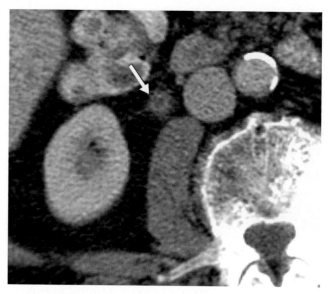

Figure 18-52 TCC thickening of the ureter. Contrasted CT shows concentric thickening (*arrow*) of the right ureter with periureteral stranding.

The thickening may be symmetric or eccentric, and there may be expansion of the collecting system above the area of thickening (160,375). In some cases, the mass may extend from the collecting system into the ureter. There may be thickening of the ureter wall. The thickening usually involves a focal portion of the ureter and may cause obstruction. In acute urinary obstruction, there may be delayed uptake and excretion of contrast by the kidney.

For upper tract transitional cell carcinoma, the likelihood of development of another TCC in the kidneys, ureters, or urinary bladder is 40% (242). However, after

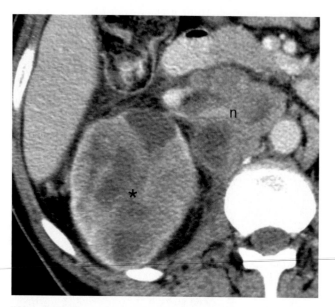

Figure 18-51 TCC expanding kidney. Infiltrative tumor diffusely expands the kidney with minimal disruption of the cortical margin. This mass exhibits areas of necrosis (*arrow*) and massive retroperitoneal adenopathy (n).

radical cystectomy for urinary bladder transitional cell carcinoma, the likelihood of upper track metastases is only 2% (497).

Staging of transitional cell carcinomas of the upper urinary tract has different prognostic indicators than renal cell. Overall accuracy of CT staging for upper tract TCC is 43% to 60% (60,396,445). Carcinoma *in situ* and tumors limited to the submucosa have the best prognosis. Tumors invading beyond the subepithelial tissue (stage II) and muscularis (stage III) have worsened prognostic outcomes, and determination of muscle invasion is important in therapeutic planning (8). Unfortunately, IVU and CT are not accurate for differentiating whether there is muscular invasion by a small tumor (21,283). Other indicators of stage III disease are tumor invasion of the renal parenchyma or peripelvic/periureteral fat. CT has shown variable accuracy in the detection of nodal involvement (stage IV). One study has shown sensitivity and specificity for nodal metastases as high as 87% and 98%, respectively. Other studies have shown less promising accuracy for characterization of the presence or absence of malignant nodal disease (329,445).

For stage I and stage II tumors, surgical nephroureterectomy is generally recommended, but some patients may now be amenable to localized surgical resection (522). Indicators of worse prognosis are invasion of the parenchyma or periureteral tissue (stage III) for which CT has shown mixed results in detecting (14,523). Another finding consistent with stage III disease is soft tissue infiltration of the peripelvic fat (523). Stage IV disease is characterized by invasion of adjacent organs, lymph node metastases, or metastatic disease to other organs, such as bone or lung (523). Generally, if there are distant metastases, surgery is not performed and systemic therapy is used.

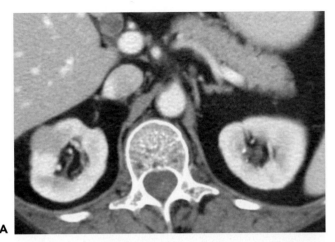
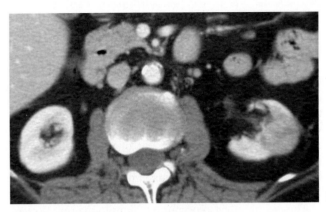

Figure 18-53 Lymphoma as bilateral focal renal masses. Contrast enhanced CT show homogenous, mildly enhancing renal masses in the right (**A**) and left (**B**) kidney. This is the most common appearance of renal involvement by systemic lymphoma.

MR appearance of a small TCC usually appears as a focal lesion involving the renal pelvis or calyceal system. The lesion may demonstrate low signal intensity on precontrast T1-weighted images. After intravenous gadolinium contrast, the lesions can demonstrate enhancement on similar T1-weighted sequences. In the ureters, both MRI and CT have shown good sensitivity and specificity for staging in a small series (14). For the urinary bladder, contrast enhancement with gadolinium agents may allow differentiation of mucularis mucosal invasion, which is limited on CT (508). The role and accuracy of MR urography is still undetermined for detection of upper tract urothelial tumors.

Lymphoma

Renal lymphoma is usually a part of a systemic disease and is associated with adenopathy or involvement of other organs such as the liver and gastrointestinal tract (418). Systemic lymphoma often involves the kidneys on pathologic review at autopsy (426). Renal involvement by lymphoma is often asymptomatic (146). The detection of renal involvement usually occurs at imaging study, such as CT or MRI, detected in less than 6% of cases (441). Non-Hodgkin's lymphoma is much more common than Hodgkin's lymphoma in renal involvement (418).

CT is more sensitive than ultrasound in detection of renal lymphoma (547). There are four common presentations of renal lymphoma. The most common type is involvement of the kidneys by multiple focal renal lesions occurring in approximately one third of cases (418) (Fig. 18-53). Focal solitary renal parenchymal mass is a common CT appearance, but renal lymphoma is more often multiple and commonly bilateral (6,418). On CT, focal renal masses have attenuation similar to or slightly different from the renal parenchyma on nonenhanced images. After intravenous contrast, the enhancement of the lesions is less

than that of the surrounding renal parenchyma. Small lesions are generally homogeneous. In larger lesions, there may be necrosis and heterogeneity. Calcifications are rare unless there has been therapy.

Invasion of the kidney by a renal hilum mass is also possible (Fig. 18-54). Renal lymphoma does not usually involve the renal vein or IVC, although it may rarely occur (537). In cases of renal involvement, there is a perinephric involvement of the lymphoma in approximately one third of patients, most of which also have parenchymal involvement (334,418).

A third appearance of renal involvement by lymphoma is a perinephric rind of soft tissue (Fig. 18-55) around the kidney without a focal parenchymal lesion. The soft tissue has

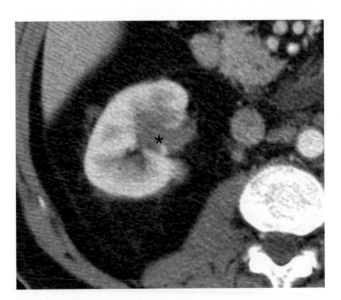

Figure 18-54 Lymphoma infiltrating the renal hilum. Infiltrative lymphoma (*) on contrasted CT is usually less enhanced than the renal parenchyma and may closely resemble TCC.

a low attenuation, and commonly directly invades the renal parenchyma. The perinephric adenopathy may compress adjacent renal hilar structures. The kidney parenchyma may appear affected through direct involvement by perirenal tumor or renal hilar mass (433).

Another less common appearance is diffuse infiltrative involvement of the kidney (Fig. 18-56) (192). In this case, there may be diffuse renal enlargement by a low-attenuation infiltrative mass. The mass uniformly expands the kidney, with or without a focal exophytic lesion (418). There is usually predominant involvement of the renal medulla, with relative sparing of the cortical margins. The mass usually involves the renal hilum, and encasement of the renal vessels may result in decreased renal enhancement (451).

The morphologic appearance of lymphoma on MRI has many similar characteristics to CT. The various patterns of lymphomatous renal involvement can be well demonstrated on MRI in a patient with a contraindication to CT. Renal lymphoma is generally slightly hypointense to the renal parenchyma on non-enhanced T1-weighted imaging. On T2-weighted images, the lesions are mildly hyperintense relative to the renal parenchyma. There is mild heterogeneous enhancement of the tumors, but the amount of enhancement is much less than that of the surrounding parenchyma on T1-weighted images after intravenous gadolinium contrast (451).

Primary renal lymphoma is a form of NHL that arises directly from the renal parenchyma. Primary renal lymphoma is extremely rare because the normal kidney is free of lymphatic tissue (83,481). It presents with acute renal failure or possibly abdominal pain (80). The tumor is aggressive with rapid progression (108,440). However, renal function may return after systemic therapy. CT of primary renal NHL demonstrates enlargement of the kidney. Of the few reported cases, 43% demonstrated bilateral renal involvement (108). Another extremely rare hematologic malignancy of the kidney is chronic lymphocytic leukemia. However, there is renal involvement in as many as 90% of

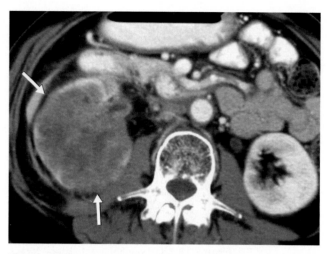

Figure 18-56 Lymphoma diffusely infiltrating and expanding the kidney. On contrasted CT, the infiltrative, hypodense central renal mass (*arrows*) enlarges the kidney with only minimal cortical margin disruption, similar in appearance to infiltrative TCC.

cases of this rare malignancy. This renal disease may be associated with membranous glomerulonephitis and occasionally with renal failure (108).

Metastases

Metastases to the kidney most commonly are seen in the setting of other metastatic disease (380). Renal metastases are present in approximately 10% to 20% of patients, depending on tumor type (2,388). Excluding lymphoma and leukemia, the most common primary sites for renal metastases include lung, colon, and breast carcinoma; melanoma; and reproductive organ malignancies such as testicular or ovarian carcinoma. Melanoma, when present, frequently metastasizes to the kidneys, but it is less common than the other types of primary malignancies (58,145).

Metastases to the kidney are usually asymptomatic and are discovered on imaging studies (88,380). Rarely, patients with renal metastases may have hematuria (88). Metastatic disease to the kidney usually represents hematogenous spread of disease, but it rarely may be the only site of metastasis (32,88).

CT is very sensitive for renal metastases (88). The most common appearance of renal metastatic disease is usually multifocal small renal masses (Fig. 18-57), and they may involve both kidneys (219). However, solitary renal metastases are not uncommon (88). Renal metastases are typically hypodense and do not commonly demonstrate hyperenhancement (219). The lesions measure 20 to 40 HU on nonenhanced CT images and have minimal enhancement after intravenous contrast of 5 to 15 HU (88). Large renal lesions may be associated with breast, lung, or colon carcinoma metastases, and those from colon carcinoma often disrupt the renal cortical margins (88). Invasion of

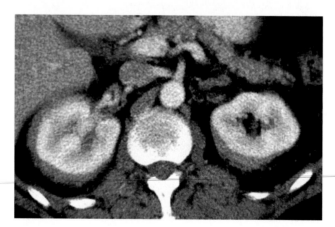

Figure 18-55 Perinephric lymphoma. Bilateral perinephric rinds of soft tissue density surround the cortex of both kidneys on contrasted CT.

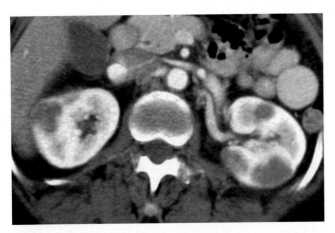

Figure 18-57 Metastases. Contrasted CT in a patient with lung carcinoma has multiple hypodense focal lesions that are consistent with metastatic disease.

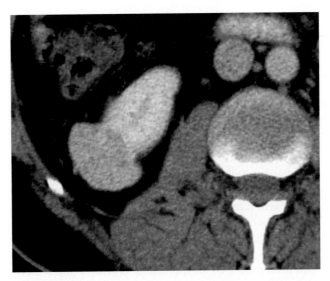

Figure 18-58 Primary renal sarcoma. Focal homogenous mass on contrasted CT is centered beyond the expected margin of the renal cortex. The exophytic nature of the mass should suggest the diagnosis of a capsular sarcoma.

the perinephric space by a renal metastasis is seen in metastases from melanoma or lung carcinoma (88,551). This type of perirenal metastatic disease usually represents lymphatic spread. Diffuse infiltrative metastases may also occur (32,388). Hemorrhagic renal metastases are most closely associated with melanoma primaries but may occur with other primaries, such as pheochromocytomas and leiomyosarcomas (145).

In the setting of a known malignancy, renal metastasis is much more common than RCC, but rarely there is a clinical question of RCC versus metastasis (88). Renal metastases are bilateral in more than 50% of patients (535). Solitary metastasis may resemble RCC, but RCC typically has more necrosis. Other findings, such as hyperenhancement and renal vein thrombosis, help suggest RCC over metastasis (32,145,380). In our experience, the margination of metastases is often less well-defined than is seen in RCC. However, in the setting of a single renal lesion in a patient with recent malignancy, the clinical question is important. This is because the therapy for renal cell carcinoma is often different from the therapy for metastatic disease. There has been increased use of radiofrequency ablation techniques for the treatment of an isolated renal mass. This is more commonly used to treat a small renal cell carcinoma or rarely an isolated metastasis (162). In the setting of renal metastases, the treatment would likely be palliative.

Renal Sarcoma

Renal sarcomas have several different cell types and may arise from the renal parenchyma or the capsule (Fig. 18-58). They are most common in patients more than 40 years of age, and they present with hematuria, abdominal distension, weight loss, or pain (461). Leiomyosarcoma is the most common type of renal sarcoma, composing as many as half of renal sarcomas (140). They are commonly located in the retroperitoneum and may be located in the

perinephric space (277). These tumors are treated with surgical resection but generally have a poor prognosis (321,478). On CT, these tumors are heterogeneous. Fibrous tissue components have delayed enhancement, and spindle cell components exhibit early enhancement. On MRI, the tumors have low T1 signal with mixed areas of high and low signal on T2-weighted sequences.

Liposarcoma of the kidney usually arises from the capsule and may present with mass, pain, or weight loss, without hematuria (62). On CT, liposarcomas appear as a retroperitoneal mass that contains areas of macroscopic fat. Perinephric tumors are usually large, averaging more than 10 cm in diameter. The tumors are generally hypovascular. A tumor capsule may be present, and the tumor may displace the kidney (236). Invasion of the renal parenchyma is not typical. Also, liposarcoma of the renal parenchyma is extremely rare (326); therefore, no renal cortical defect should exist. Unlike AMLs, liposarcomas are relatively avascular and without enlarged vessels (236). Diagnosis of perinephric liposarcoma on CT relies on differentiating it from AML by noting the absence of enlarged vessels emanating from the kidney as well as the absence of a low-attenuation renal cortical defect associated with AMLs (236).

Clear cell sarcoma of the kidney is a rare but aggressive neoplasm that is most common in neonates and young children. It presents with hematuria, abdominal distension, or weight loss/lethargy (167). This tumor metastasizes preferentially to bone, as compared with other renal neoplasms (24). It may also metastasize to the liver, nodes, and lung. Treatment usually requires a combination of surgery and systemic therapy. On CT, the tumors are large and heterogeneous and enhance less than the normal renal parenchyma (167). Multiple small foci are common. Necrosis, hemorrhage, and calcification may be present (167).

Sarcomatoid RCC is a tumor comprising RCC and TCC elements (140) and may be difficult to differentiate from sarcoma. The CT appearance is similar to the pattern of clear cell renal carcinoma (461).

Wilms Tumor

Wilms tumor is a common renal tumor in the pediatric population. The tumor most commonly occurs in children aged 3 to 4 years (77) and presents as a palpable abdominal mass. In some cases, Wilms tumor has been associated with WAGR syndrome (Wilms, aniridia, GU abnormalities, retardation), DRASH syndrome (Wilms, congenital nephropathy, pseudo-hermaphroditism), or Beckwith-Wiedemann syndrome (omphalocele, macroglossia, gigantism, macrosomia, hemi-hypertrophy) (311). On CT, Wilms tumor appears as a focal solid renal mass with an appearance similar to that of renal cell carcinoma. The mass typically enhances heterogeneously and may exhibit areas of cystic change or necrosis (416)(Fig. 18-59). There may be perinephric extension by the mass and metastatic adenopathy may be present (77)(151). Vascular invasion by the tumor has been frequently described (77). Unlike neuroblastomas, Wilms tumor does not usually encase the aorta (311). Calcifications are rare. Metastases most commonly involve the lungs (178).

On MRI, Wilms tumors demonstrate mildly low T1-signal and high T2-signal characteristics. Areas of necrosis may result in heterogeneous signal within the mass and heterogeneous enhancement. MRI is able to demonstrate renal vein and IVC involvement better than CT does, and coronal images may be useful (544).

Collecting Duct Carcinoma

Collecting duct carcinoma (CDC), also known as Bellini duct carcinoma or renal medullary carcinoma, is a rare tumor that arises from the cells lining the epithelium of the distal collecting tubules of the kidney (532). The tumor usually presents with hematuria, pain, or weight loss (390). It is more common in men than women (125) and commonly occurs at mean age range of 50 to 60 years, with a wide age range (393). It is an aggressive tumor with a poor prognosis that usually has metastatic disease at the time of diagnosis (116). Chao et al. noted that 83% of patients presented with stage IV disease (74). Nodal metastases and lung metastases occur in 78% and 27% of cases, respectively (390). Other common sites of metastases include the adrenal gland and liver (116). Therapy includes nephrectomy, but it is only curative in the few patients who have disease limited to the kidney (12,74). In patients with metastases, the median survival after surgery is 11 to 16 months (12,74).

On CT, the mass is a solid or complex solid and cystic mass in the central portion of the kidney. The tumor usually involves the renal pelvis, but it may also commonly grow into the cortex or even distort the renal margins. The tumor may be invasive and/or expansile (158,393). In one study, punctate or rim calcifications were present in 4 of 17 cases (393). On noncontrast CT, the tumor occasionally was mildly hyperdense to the rest of the cortex. After intravenous contrast, the tumor was hypodense to the normal parenchyma, with only mild to moderate enhancement. The right kidney was more commonly involved, in 82% of cases. Metastatic disease, usually adenopathy, was visible on CT in 41% of patients (393).

On MRI, CDC usually is a central renal mass with T1 signal that is isointense to normal renal parenchyma unless there are cystic components that are hypointense. On T2-weighted imaging, low T2 signal relative to the parenchyma is present. No pseudocapsule is visible (393). The low T2 signal is not typical of RCC and should suggest the diagnosis of CDC (393). On gallium-67 radioscintigraphy, the tumor may have uptake, and this should prompt consideration of the diagnosis (492).

Renal medullary carcinoma (RMC) is a rare, distinctive tumor with an aggressive nature similar to that of CDC. It occurs in young African-American children and adults, with a male predominance, and commonly has metastases present at the time of presentation (15,498). RMC occurs in higher association with sickle cell trait or, rarely, disease (498). The most common presentation is hematuria, pain, or mass (498). Like CDC, the mass is typically central and it also has a predilection for the right kidney (in 82% of patients) (566). It is a hypodense central renal mass and there may be associated adenopathy. Most patients do not respond to therapy, and survival is less than 16 months (498).

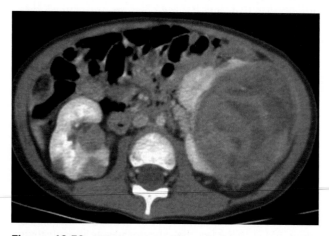

Figure 18-59 Wilm's tumor with nephroblastomatosis. Contrasted CT in a 3-year-old child demonstrates a markedly heterogeneous solid and cystic mass expanding the left kidney. Multiple small lesions are present in the right kidney. (Courtesy of Stuart A. Royal).

BENIGN RENAL LESIONS

Oncocytoma

Renal oncocytoma is a benign tumor (349,424). It is a solid tumor that has specific genetic differences from renal cell carcinoma (75). It appears as a solid, enhancing mass

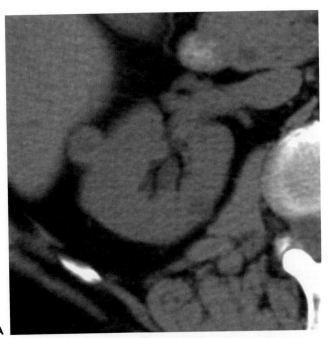
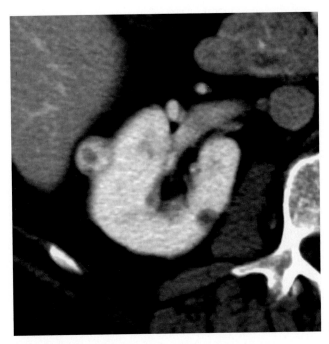

A   B

Figure 18-60 Small exophytic oncocytoma. Precontrast (**A**) and contrasted (**B**) CT show a small enhancing cortical mass distorting the renal margin, diagnosed as oncocytoma on pathology. The appearance is not distinguishable from RCC.

with many characteristics that are similar to those of RCC (Fig. 18-60). In fact, the appearance of renal oncocytoma, when typical, cannot be differentiated from that of RCC. These lesions vary in size and occur in a wide range of patient ages. Renal oncocytomas are more common in men (82,389,424). Most oncocytomas are asymptomatic (approximately 80%), but a few may present with hematuria, pain, or mass (424). They are uncommon, but the incidence of renal oncocytoma is higher in incidentally discovered renal masses, as compared with patients who have urinary symptoms (389).

Rarely, the tumors may be multiple and bilateral (9,531), but nephron-sparing surgery is possible even in these cases (398). Metachronous lesions may occur in 4% of patients (119). Bilateral renal oncocytomatosis (Fig. 18-61) is extremely rare (3).

On CT, oncocytomas are typically solid, well-marginated tumors that are slightly hypodense to the rest of the renal parenchyma on nonenhanced images (406,514). They typically show homogeneous enhancement after intravenous contrast. Although oncocytomas are more commonly homogeneous than renal cell carcinomas are, a significant number of renal cell carcinomas have a homogeneous appearance (115). A capsule may be present around the tumor (22). Some lesions may exhibit a central scar that is low attenuation with a branched appearance, regardless of lesion size (273). The scar is typically nonenhancing (294). Unfortunately, central necrosis associated with RCC may occasionally mimic the central scar of a renal oncocytoma (115,303). Renal capsular pathologic invasion into the perinephric fat occurs in 11% of cases (9).

Currently, there is no specific CT finding to differentiate oncocytoma from RCC (424). Therefore, in the absence of previously documented oncocytoma or known stability of the lesion, surgery is generally performed for these lesions. However, nephron-sparing surgery should be considered. An oncocytoma with atypical features does not have a significantly different outcome but should be closely followed (424). There should be no adenopathy or vascular invasion associated with the mass, because it is a benign neoplasm. The presence of a central scar with absence of calcification, necrosis, or hemorrhage should suggest the diagnosis, although there is some overlap with small RCCs (19).

The MRI appearance of renal oncocytoma is typically hypointense to normal renal parenchyma on nonenhanced T1-weighted images. However, approximately 27% may be isointense on T1 (190). The lesions enhance homogeneously after intravenous gadolinium contrast administration and may exhibit a spoke-wheel pattern of central enhancement (228). There is usually high signal intensity of the lesion on T2-weighted images (190). When the central scar is present, it is usually hypointense on T2-weighted sequences, as opposed to the high T2 signal of necrosis (190). The MRI characteristics of renal oncocytoma cannot be reliably differentiated from RCC (19,405).

Percutaneous biopsy of renal oncocytoma may be unable to differentiate it from RCC (54,75). Differentiation of oncocytoma and chromophobe RCC is especially difficult (75). Because the confirmation of the benign nature often cannot be obtained, surgical excision may be necessary. There is also an increased association of clear cell carcinoma in these patients in either kidney (301).

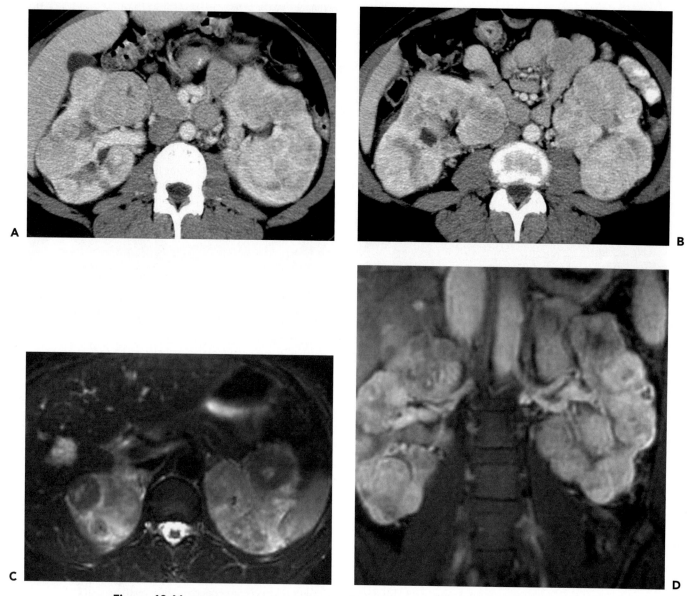

Figure 18-61 Multiple bilateral oncocytomas. On contrasted CT (**A**, **B**), numerous enhancing renal masses enlarge the kidneys without distant metastases. Axial T2-weighed (**C**) and coronal T1 contrasted (**D**) images of the kidneys have appearance that is indistinguishable from multifocal RCC.

Renal adenoma is a small solid renal tumor that is also indistinguishable from RCC. The lesions exhibit enhancement after intravenous contrast, similar to RCC or oncocytoma. Other solid enhancing renal masses, such as small solid renal fibromas, are less common. Renal leiomyoma is another rare lesion that may have a solid appearance and enhancement.

Angiomyolipoma

Angiomyolipomas are commonly isolated sporadic tumors or associated with tuberous sclerosis (TS) (286). Sporadic AMLs without TS are commonly detected in females during the fifth to seventh decade or later and are more often larger and solitary than those found associated with syndromes (286,506). Tuberous sclerosis is the most commonly associated syndrome and consists of mental retardation, seizures, and typical skin lesions. Multiple angiomyolipomas (Fig. 18-62) should suggest the diagnosis of TS, as described earlier in this chapter. Approximately 80% of patients with TS have angiomyolipomas (185). However, only 20% of cases of angiomyolipoma subsequently yield a diagnosis of TS. Angiomyolipomas may be rarely associated with neurofibromatosis-1, von Hippel-Lindau, or ADPKD.

Angiomyolipoma is a common benign renal mass and is detected as an incidental finding on imaging or resulting from symptoms in the setting of lesion hemorrhage. Patients without TS are more often symptomatic (483). Signs of hemorrhage include pain or evidence of shock (397).

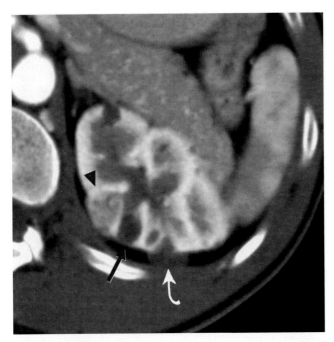

Figure 18-62 Angiomyolipoma. Contrast enhanced CT shows three types of AML in patient with tuberous sclerosis—fatty intrarenal (*arrow*), lipid poor (*arrowhead*), and "mushroom" (*curved arrow*).

On sonography, lesions are generally echogenic, because of the presence of fat.

CT is generally the most accurate imaging technique for detection and characterization of angiomyolipomas. The lesions are usually low attenuation with fat measurements (Fig. 18-63), and the presence of gross fat is characteristic

for these lesions. The ROIs of these lesions are typically less than −10 HU (48). Thin slices are necessary to demonstrate fat in small AMLs because of volume averaging. Higher specificity can be obtained using threshold measurements of −15 to −30 HU. On CT, the fat attenuation of an AML may be interposed with solid components. A subset of lesions will not meet fat attenuation criteria because of volume averaging or intratumoral hemorrhage (286). Other AMLs do not meet fat attenuation criteria because they are relatively fat-poor and appear denser than the surrounding renal cortex on nonenhanced CT images (240). In one series of dense AMLs, the fat content still ranged from 5% to 15% (381). If there are only small areas of fat within the lesion, the diagnosis of AML is made, but rarely a well-differentiated renal cell carcinoma could have this appearance (200).

The presence of other typical AMLs in the contralateral or ipsilateral kidney helps in the diagnosis of an atypical AML. AMLs are usually well marginated but do not have a true capsule (236) (see Fig. 18-62). The lesion is usually at the margin of the kidney, and the exophytic component may expand, or "mushroom," beyond a small hypodense wedge-shape defect in the renal parenchyma (Fig. 18-64). This wedge defect is diagnostic of angiomyolipoma (236). Large vessels may be identified (236). These lesions are often vascular and show moderate enhancement after intravenous contrast. Intratumoral aneurysms are commonly present, and aneurysms greater than 5 mm in diameter correlate with increased risk of hemorrhage (558).

Approximately 58% to 75% of these lesions will grow over time (287,483,526). However, growth of an isolated

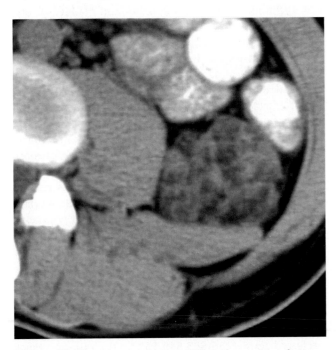

Figure 18-63 Angiomyolipoma. Diffuse fatty and soft tissue densities are present in this exophytic mass arising from the renal margin. Note that liposarcoma may also have this appearance.

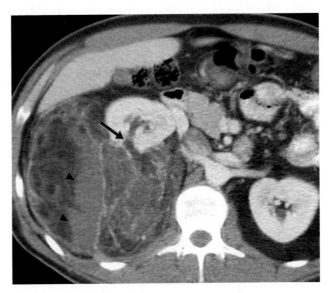

Figure 18-64 Angiomyolipoma with hemorrhage. The intermediate density fluid within the AML is consistent with hemorrhage (*arrowheads*), common in large lesions. A renal notch (*arrow*) with vessels entering tumor and spontaneous hemorrhage confirm the diagnosis of AML.

AML without TS is much less common than with TS or in the presence of multiple lesions (287). Annual follow-up of asymptomatic lesions is commonly performed, unless they are larger than 4 cm in diameter, with increased risk of hemorrhage necessitating semiannual evaluation (376). However, even small AMLs may rarely bleed (249). In small, isolated AMLs, less frequent follow-up examinations may be performed once initial size stability is confirmed. For large symptomatic lesions, embolization may reduce the size of the lesion and prevent subsequent hemorrhagic risk (353,536)(see Fig. 18-64).

MRI can also demonstrate the fat component of an angiomyolipoma. On MRI, AMLs have a characteristic high T1 signal intensity that is consistent with fat signal. Fat-saturated T1 images show a significant drop in signal intensity within the lesion, as compared with the adjacent renal parenchyma (228). Likewise, opposed-phase T1-weighted images show relatively low signal intensity compared with in-phase T1-weighted imaging. AMLs may display enhancement on T1-weighted images after gadolinium contrast but are usually hypointense to the surrounding parenchyma. T2-weighted images may show moderately high intensity (228).

Pathology may have difficulty differentiating a well-differentiated liposarcoma from angiomyolipoma. Occasional spindle cells may yield an incorrect diagnosis unless the radiologic appearance is considered, so that adequate specimen volume is obtained and evaluated (536). In patients with coexistent angiomyolipoma and oncocytoma, 36% were associated with tuberous sclerosis (394).

Non-neoplastic Benign Solid Renal Lesions

Multiple solid renal masses may be visualized in non-neoplastic situations. Sarcoidosis may occasionally have a pseudotumorous appearance with multiple hypodense lesions involving both kidneys (306) (Fig. 18-65). A solid renal lesion may be suspected on ultrasound if there are two areas of renal cortical scarring that are adjacent to an area that is spared from scarring. A prominent renal column of Bertin is a common clinical dilemma on ultrasound. Typically, this lesion may be separated from malignancy based on its similar enhancement to the rest of the kidney on CT or MRI. The lesion does not usually distort the renal margin. There is central extension of the column of Bertin in most patients. It is important to differentiate these lesions from renal malignancy.

RENAL INFECTIONS

Acute Infection

In most cases, clinical signs such as fever, chills, flank pain or tenderness, and laboratory results such as leukocytosis (80%), pyuria, and bacteriuria indicate the presence of acute urinary tract infection. Urine cultures are positive in

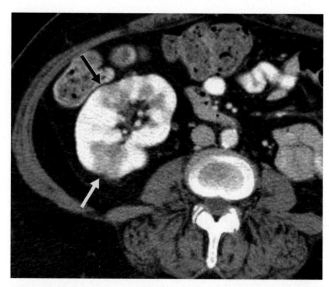

Figure 18-65 Renal sarcoidosis. Contrasted CT shows bilateral hypodense renal masses (*arrows*). This is described as the pseudotumorous form of renal sarcoid.

75% and blood cultures in 50% (49). In many cases, no imaging is needed if there is prompt clinical response to appropriate antibiotics. If clinical signs and symptoms are unclear, or if response to treatment is poor, imaging is often performed to detect potential complications. Urinary tract infection (UTI) is best considered as an interaction between host and pathogen with a variety of factors on both sides determining the likelihood of a significant infection. CT may be useful in the setting of recurrent UTIs for detection of anatomic factors such as stones, obstruction including congenital anomalies and bladder, or urethral diverticula.

It is less important to document acute pyelonephritis, which almost invariably responds to antibiotics, than to identify complicating factors such as hydronephrosis, calculi, and abscess. Intravenous urography is rarely used for serious infections, because it often fails to show any abnormality in cases of acute pyelonephritis or small renal abscesses; conversely, several different processes can result in nonvisualization of the kidney, such as severe pyelonephritis, or pyonephrosis (173,513). Although sonography can detect hydronephrosis, calculi, and some abscesses, it is much less revealing than CT (49,173,477). In many cases of acute pyelonephritis, sonography will appear normal although CT shows definite abnormalities (505). Although radionuclide scintigrams are very sensitive to renal changes resulting from infection, they do not distinguish the various pathologic processes in adults. CT is usually the most revealing imaging procedure for renal infections.

A variety of terms have been promulgated for acute bacterial infection of the kidney, but *acute pyelonephritis* is the preferred term (285,505,545,567). Others terms (such as *acute focal bacterial nephritis* and *lobar nephronia*) have enjoyed popular usage (505); however, neither pathology

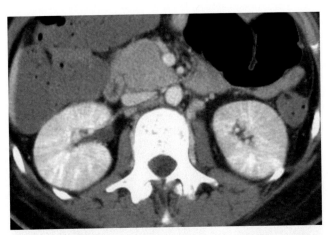

Figure 18-66 Pyelonephritis with striated nephrogram. Bilateral symmetric striated nephrograms are present on contrasted CT. The symmetric involvement and lack of perinephric stranding would be atypical for infection.

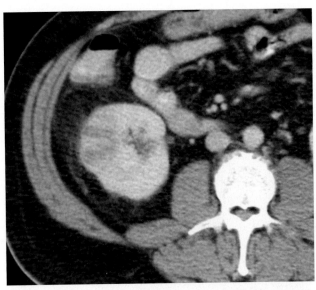

Figure 18-67 Focal pyelonephritis. Focal areas of diminished enhancement in the renal cortex after intravenous contrast are consistent with pyelonephritis. Although not shown here, focal areas of nonenhancement may be seen with early abscess formation.

nor treatment is different from what is classically called acute pyelonephritis. The CT features of acute pyelonephritis are: (a) renal swelling, producing enlargement of the affected kidney; (b) focal hypoattenuation; and (c) mass effect. There are round or wedge-shaped areas in the parenchyma whose attenuation is normal, decreased (because of edema or necrosis), or occasionally increased (because of hemorrhage) (421) on precontrast images. After contrast, these areas show diminished enhancement compared to normal parenchyma on early images (Fig. 18-66) (49,173,477). The wedge-shaped areas in fact do enhance, but much less than normal parenchyma, as a result of edema or vasospasm caused by the infection. On delayed images up to 24 hours, there may be increased attenuation within, or at the periphery of, these areas (233).

In some cases, one or more focal areas of the kidney are severely involved, with sparing of other regions (173,477). There may be a single mass-like region as a result of swelling resulting from edema (this is focal pyelonephritis, formerly called acute focal bacterial nephritis to distinguish it from neoplasm) (285) (Fig. 18-67). Patchy decreased enhancement may be limited to this focal mass. A frequent (77%) finding in acute infections is thickening of the renal fascia and thickening of the septa in the perinephric space, a result of hyperemia and inflammatory edema (477).

Despite treatment with adequate antibiotics, CT abnormalities may persist for several weeks to months (476). Persistence of a focal mass may increase the suspicion of tumor, but it must be recognized as a possible sequela of infection until followed for up to 6 months (476). With the severe parenchymal infection that causes focal CT abnormalities, scar formation is not uncommon, and polar or global atrophy may be seen (476).

Emphysematous pyelonephritis (EPN) is classically considered a potentially life-threatening, gas-forming infection of the kidney. Contributing factors to development of EPN are high tissue level of glucose, presence of glucose fermenting bacteria, poor vascular supply/poor tissue oxygen tension, impaired host immunity, and obstruction (although this last is not an absolute requirement). Because of these causative factors, this process is usually seen in diabetics (229,377,427,530). Patients may present with signs of acute infection, but often they are found comatose from diabetic ketoacidosis. In fact there are signs, symptoms or laboratory data that distinguish patients with EPN from those with other upper urinary tract infections (462). Imaging is necessary for diagnosis.

Although in the past diagnosis may have been made using IVU (mottled gas in nonfunctioning kidney), several studies have shown that CT is the best means for diagnosis and has also demonstrated some features not recognizable by either IVU or US (462,540,541,507). CT demonstrates not only the presence and location of gas, but also presence of perinephric fluid collections or renal or perirenal abscesses (Fig. 18-68). Wan differentiated two types of EPN. Type 1, "classic" EPN, is characterized by intraparenchymal gas (which may be streaky, mottled, bubbly, or loculated) but no perinephric fluid or focal abscess. In classic EPN, gas may extend to the subcapsular, perinephric, and pararenal spaces and may cross to the contralateral retroperitoneal spaces, even when the other kidney is not infected.

Type 2 EPN was characterized by "presence of renal or perirenal fluid in association with bubbly or loculated gas or by gas in collecting system" (Fig. 18-69). In a clinical series, Wan found 69% mortality in type 1 EPN, but only 18% in type 2 (540). Negative prognostic factors included type 1 EPN, severe thrombocytopenia, impaired renal function, and high levels of hematuria. Nephrectomy was required in 16 and drainage in 13; all but 1 were diabetic.

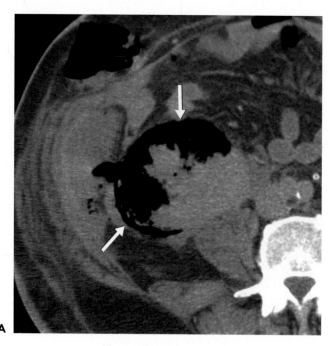

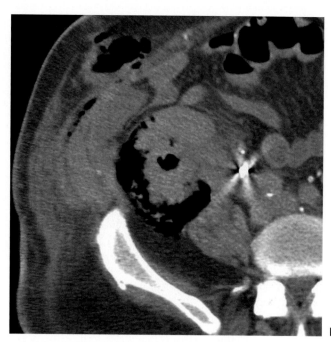

Figure 18-68 Emphysematous pyelonephritis in a transplant kidney. Two uncontrasted CT images of transplanted kidney (**A, B**) in the right lower quadrant show severe distortion and destruction of the kidney with large amounts of gas in the expected regions of renal cortex (*arrows*). Gas also tracks in the abdominal wall.

A series of 20 patients showed typical characteristics of EPN in the modern era (462). Diabetes was present in 80%, 75% were female, mean age was 55 years, and left kidney was slightly more common (60%). Only 50% had obstruction. Infectious agent was *Escherichia coli* in 70%, mortality was 20%, but nephrectomy was performed in all. While the definition of type 2 EPN includes what may be called "emphysematous pyelitis," this subset of gas-forming renal infections should be recognized as distinct. In a small series of 5 patients with gas in the collecting system but no perinephric fluid, there was no mortality. Furthermore, only 1 of the 5 had diabetes; 4 of the 5 had urinary lithiasis (431).

The importance of these recent studies is that overall mortality is not as high as in the past but that EPN remains life threatening. The presence or absence of fluid and its character may be as important as the presence and location of gas. Parenchymal gas in a nonfunctioning kidney with no associated fluid probably remains the most severe form. Gas in the collecting system with no fluid is the least severe and can be treated medically (with relief of obstruction if needed). However, gas in association with perinephric fluid or abscess is intermediate severity, and if treated conservatively should be followed closely with CT. Because carbon dioxide (CO_2) is rapidly absorbed, there should be rapid decrease in the gas if there is a good response to medical therapy, and persistent gas on follow-up CT indicates ongoing infection (340). If the gas and fluid do not improve with antibiotics and drainage, nephrectomy may still be required.

Pyonephrosis results from infection of a hydronephrotic kidney. This may present as either an acute or a chronic infection, with up to 15% of patients being afebrile (563). Thus, this entity must be distinguished from acute pyelonephritis, renal abscess, and XGP. Urography is of little use, because the kidney is usually nonfunctioning. Sonography is usually diagnostic and can guide percutaneous aspiration and nephrostomy placement. However, CT is often used in such

Figure 18-69 Emphysematous pyelonephritis—Gram negative rods, Enterobacter. Contrasted CT of the right kidney demonstrates gas within the collecting system of the left kidney. The nephrogram has a patchy appearance.

a setting. CT shows dilation of the collecting system and poor excretion. Thickening of the pelvic wall and of Gerota's fascia is common (159); increased attenuation or heterogeneity of the pelvic contents may be seen but is rare. CT also can show the cause of the obstruction.

The role of MRI in evaluation of acute renal infection is limited to patients who either cannot undergo a contrast-enhanced CT study or have equivocal CT examination results. Little experience exists with MRI in the diagnosis of urinary tract infections. It is more difficult with MRI than with CT to produce good images of very ill patients because of the susceptibility of MRI to motion. The changes resulting from pyelonephritis are not specific, with variable heterogeneous enhancement of parenchyma on breath-hold GRE T1-weighted images after Gd-DTPA. Renal abscesses may be demonstrated as low signal, nonenhancing regions on contrast-enhanced T1-weighted images, with variable surrounding enhancing wall and perinephric inflammatory stranding (55).

RENAL ABSCESS

Renal abscess is increasingly uncommon, largely because most acute infections are effectively treated. Most renal abscesses currently are a result of an ascending infection and are usually caused by gram-negative urinary pathogens, particularly *E. coli* (36%) (49,155). Less than 10% result from hematogenous seeding usually caused by *Staphylococcus* (49,155). Renal abscesses also may be a complication of trauma, surgery, contiguous spread from other organs, or lymphatic spread (49,278). In most cases today, a renal abscess results from breakdown and coalescence of microabscesses due to acute pyelonephritis that is inadequately treated. An abscess is a necrotic, devascularized cavity, often filled with pus. Although many patients present with acute infection, the diagnosis is sometimes obscure if the patient has only vague symptoms such as flank pain, weakness, and weight loss (49,155,455). Fever is absent in one third of patients, a normal urinalysis is found in one fourth, and positive urine cultures are present in only one third of patients (351). Thus, renal abscess (Fig. 18-70) must be distinguished both from acute pyelonephritis and from renal tumors. CT is the best procedure for this evaluation, identifying 96% of abscesses in two large series (155)(477). Although sonography will identify an abnormality, it is less sensitive than CT (155,477), and the appearance may not be distinguishable from a renal neoplasm. A rare type of abscess, secondary to actinomycosis, may also mimic a renal mass. It can have low signal intensity on T1- and T2-weighted MRI with a focal appearance (223).

In many cases of renal abscess (50%), the entire kidney is enlarged (477). In some, a focal mass bulges the renal contour. Inflammatory changes in the perinephric space and thickening of Gerota's fascia are common (77% and 42%, respectively) (477). A focal low-attenuation area

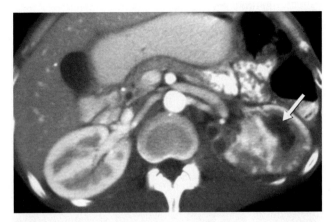

Figure 18-70 Pyelonephritis and renal abscess on CT. Patchy enhancement of the left kidney is present with liquifactive necrosis in the medullary portion of the kidney (*arrow*). The right kidney has a normal appearance.

(near water attenuation) is seen on precontrast images; there will be no enhancement in the center of the lesion. Commonly there is a thick, slightly irregular and ill-defined rind of enhancing tissue surrounding the abscess cavity (Fig. 18-71). There may be septations within the abscess (Fig. 18-72). The remainder of the kidney may be normal, or it may show changes of pyelonephritis. The presence of gas in the lesion is pathognomonic of abscess, but it is unusual.

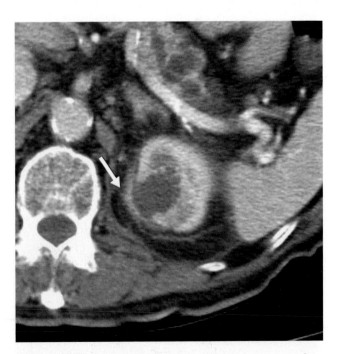

Figure 18-71 Renal abscess—Enterobacter Aerogenes. Contrasted CT of the left upper pole demonstrates poorly marginated collection with extension through the cortex and marked thickening of perinephric fascia (*arrow*). Changes of chronic pancreatitis are noted in the tail of the pancreas.

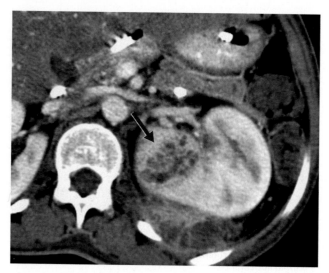

Figure 18-72 Multiple renal and perirenal abscesses with loculation/septations. On contrasted CT, parenchymal loculated collection (*arrow*) has a separate complex collection in the posterior perinephric space. Culture revealed Methycillin Resistant Staphylococcus aureus (MRSA).

Perinephric abscess has also declined in frequency in the modern era. It is now uncommon but still occurs, usually as extension of a renal infection into the perinephric space. It is characterized on CT as a discrete, loculated fluid collection in the perinephric space usually with a recognizable enhancing rim (Fig. 18-73). It may be adjacent to a renal parenchyma abscess and may contain gas. Although perinephric abscess carries a reputation of high mortality,

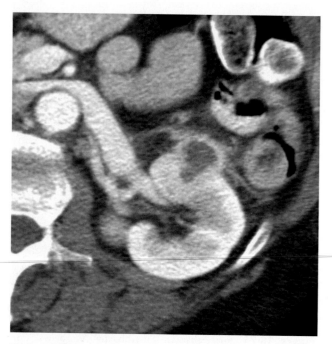

Figure 18-73 Perinephric abscess—*E. coli*. Thick walled complex collection on contrasted CT is secondary to extension of a renal abscess into the perinephric space. Renal abscess may commonly extend beyond the cortical margins.

based on prior experience of over 50% mortality (336), the rapid availability and accuracy of CT allows for earlier detection and correct diagnosis. In a series of 25 patients with perinephric abscess, only 4 required nephrectomy, and mortality was only 12% (336). The 10 patients with abscesses smaller than 1.8 cm were successfully treated with antibiotics alone; 11 had antibiotics and percutaneous drainage with successful outcome.

It is sometimes difficult to distinguish an indolent abscess from a necrotic renal tumor (106). In such a case, percutaneous needle biopsy may be required. In general, once an abscess is identified, needle aspiration should be done for definitive diagnosis, for culture, and for placement of drains, which has been shown to improve outcome (278). Despite therapy, CT will show sequelae of renal abscesses for weeks to months, especially if treated without drainage. Focal scarring often results (476).

CHRONIC RENAL INFECTIONS

The characteristic changes of chronic pyelonephritis on urography are also readily identified with CT. A focal parenchymal scar overlying a blunted calyx indicates the diagnosis, whether single or multiple areas are involved. This is distinct from scarring related to infarct, in which the calyx is not blunted.

Xanthogranulomatous pyelonephritis is an uncommon chronic infection that has a specific pathologic appearance, typically occurring in an obstructed kidney. There is accumulation of lipid-laden macrophages (xanthoma cells) and a granulomatous infiltrate because of the failure of local immune response (198). In 85% of cases, the entire kidney is involved, but the disease may be focal. CT is very useful, because the findings on sonography and urography are nonspecific (175,198,207,387,529). On CT, XGP is associated with (a) a large central calculus, often a staghorn; (b) enlargement of the kidney (or of a segment); (c) poor or no excretion of contrast into the collecting system; and (d) multiple focal low-attenuation (−10 to +30 HU) masses scattered throughout the involved portions of the kidney (Fig. 18-74). The low-attenuation collections represent dilated, debris-filled calyces and xanthoma collections. The collections themselves do not enhance, and there is no excretion of contrast, but there is bright enhancement of the rims of the collections because of inflammatory hypervascularity. Although XGP is usually found in the setting of chronic obstruction, often the renal pelvis is less dilated than might be expected for high-grade chronic obstruction. Also, the renal sinus fat is often obliterated by inflammation (387). Perinephric extension occurs in about 14% and is well shown on CT (89,175, 207,529), fistulae may develop (494), and gas rarely may be seen. Some variations occur: the kidney may be small, and calculi may be absent, making it difficult to distinguish XGP from other infections or neoplasm. Nephrectomy is

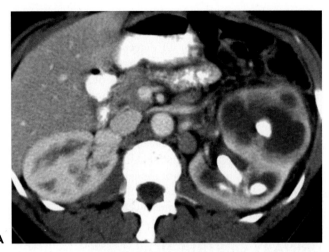

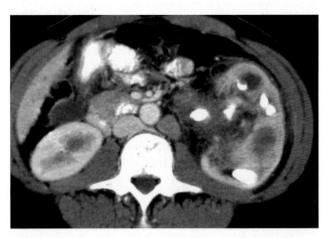

A

B

Figure 18-74   Xanthogranulomatous pyelonephritis (XGP). **A, B:** On contrasted CT, the left kidney is enlarged, very poorly enhancing, and contains a fragmented staghorn calculus. The collecting system is markedly dilated and distorted by xanthogranulomatous debris; perinephric stranding is present.

indicated in any case, but partial nephrectomy can be performed for the focal form.

Renal tuberculosis (TB) is uncommon, but its frequency has recently been increasing because of resistant organisms and the increase in patients with AIDS. A variety of findings may be shown, depending on the stage of involvement (110,137,174,404). CT is capable of demonstrating parenchymal masses and cavities, parenchymal scarring, calcifications, thickening of renal pelvis or ureter, hydronephrosis or hydrocalicosis, autonephrectomy, and extrarenal manifestations (Fig. 18-75). Detection of moth-eaten calyces and amputated infundibulum may be better shown by IVU, although experience with multidetector CTU is limited. Each individual finding of renal TB is nonspecific, but a

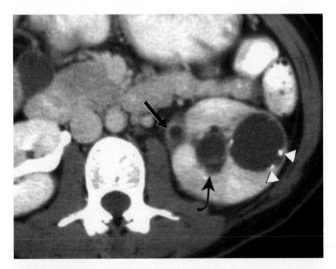

Figure 18-75   Renal tuberculosis. Contrasted CT shows a dilated infundibulum (*curved arrow*) proximal to a stricture, thickening of the proximal ureter wall (*arrow*) and renal abscess with peripheral calcifications (*arrowheads*).

combination of findings can be suggestive—in one study, cases with parenchymal masses showed at least one other finding; the most frequent combination on CT was hydronephrosis or hydrocalicoses with parenchymal scarring. The "autonephrectomy," a small nonfunctioning kidney with diffuse amorphous calcification, is easily recognized on CT. Demonstration of a small hydronephrotic kidney with a contracted and thick-walled renal pelvis is also suggestive of TB. Marked thickening of the wall of the ureter or pelvis may be seen on CT. CT also is excellent for demonstrating perirenal extension or fistulae to adjacent organs, such as the colon or duodenum.

The incidence of fungal infections in the kidney is also on the rise with the increasing population of immune-compromised patients, including transplant recipients, patients with malignancies, and AIDS patients (554). Fungi can cause pyelonephritis and renal abscess with the same CT appearance as bacterial infections (106,153). Fungal infection is suggested when multiple microabscesses are seen in the kidney, spleen, or liver (460). Slough of urothelium, inflammatory cells, and mycelia into the collecting system can form a fungus ball. Such patients often have poor renal function, and careful attention to the attenuation of the pelvic contents is required to recognize a fungus ball on noncontrast CT. In these patients, the pelvis is dilated and filled with material of soft tissue attenuation, rather than water attenuation.

Malacoplakia is a very uncommon chronic infection that can affect the kidney, although it is more commonly found in other organs, particularly the bladder. Renal malacoplakia is much more common in women than in men, and patients are usually debilitated or immune suppressed; it can occur in renal transplants. It results when a bacterial infection, most often *E. coli*, cannot be eradicated because of a local immune failure, and a chronic granulomatous inflammatory process develops. The process is often multi-focal, and it may be bilateral. Multiple soft tissue masses of varying size may be seen on CT (231). These lesions enhance less than normal renal parenchyma after intravenous contrast, but enhancement does occur because of the inflammatory vascularity. Hydronephrosis, nephrolithiasis, and lesional calcification are not seen. There may be perinephric involvement. If unifocal, the lesion can mimic RCC; when multifocal, metastases or lymphoma may be considered. Pathologic examination is often needed for diagnosis; large histiocytes (von Hanseman cells) and basophilic intracytoplasmic inclusions (Michaelis-Gutmann bodies) are pathognomonic (231).

Hydatid disease is very uncommon in North America, but it is endemic in parts of the world and may be seen in immigrants or travelers. The kidneys are involved in only about 2% to 3% of cases (4). The disease results from infestation by the larval form of *Echinococcus granulosus*. Signs and symptoms are nonspecific, including flank mass, hematuria, dysuria, fever, and hypertension. The cysts may rupture into the collecting system, and renal colic may be a presenting symptom due to hydatiduria (4). The CT appearance may be characteristic, usually showing a multilocular cystic mass with mural calcification. There may be enhancement of the thick walls. The presence of small daughter cysts within the main cyst is characteristic, and it is different from the usual appearance of a calcified RCC. However, occasionally there may be a noncalcified unilocular cyst, which may be difficult to distinguish from an infected simple cyst (4).

In patients with AIDS, a number of conditions can affect the kidneys, and CT may be useful in demonstrating these diseases. Kaposi sarcoma, lymphoma, or RCC may produce renal masses in AIDS patients (343). All types of renal infections, including pyelonephritis, abscess, fungal infections, and TB, are more common in AIDS patients. Opportunistic infectious agents, such as pneumocystis, *Mycobacterium avium-intracellulare,* and cytomegalovirus can involve the kidney; all of these can produce multiple, small calcifications scattered throughout the kidneys (343). Human immunodeficiency virus (HIV)-associated nephropathy is most often seen in HIV patients who are young, black men with a history of intravenous drug abuse. On CT, the kidneys are normal to large in size; there may be a striated nephrogram after intravenous contrast (343).

Renal replacement lipomatosis is a quite unusual process that produces a striking CT appearance (220,369). It is associated with chronic infection and calculi, commonly central and often obstructing (182,490,511). The kidney may be large or small but is usually nonfunctioning. Most of the renal parenchyma has been replaced by fat, in many cases leaving only a ghost of a kidney containing calculi. Pararenal fascia is thickened, and there may be fistulae. A fatty mass causing displacement of adjacent structures, suggestive of liposarcoma, can also be seen (369).

Papillary necrosis can result from a variety of causes and is associated with UTI and diabetes, although it may also be a result of vascular disease, hemoglobinopathies and others. Although usually diagnosed with IVU in the past, there may be potential for CT detection, although further investigation is needed. Use of extremely fine resolution MDCTU in excretory phase is capable of demonstrating blunted calyces and medullary cavities, but no large study has documented sensitivity and specificity of this technique. One study reported that early changes of papillary swelling and diminished enhancement could be seen early in the course, best demonstrated in the nephrographic phase. However, only some of these progressed on follow-up IVU to classic changes of papillary necrosis, perhaps because of successful intervention (280).

URINARY OBSTRUCTION

CT and sonography are useful imaging methods for the detection of obstruction. Each has the capacity to visualize kidneys with any degree of function, because the visualization is not dependent on excretion of contrast. More important, gas or bone does not impede CT visualization, unlike with sonography, so CT can demonstrate the full length of the ureters. CT can display the changes of acute obstruction—swelling, perirenal stranding, pyelocaliectasis, and delayed excretion (Fig. 18-76). The changes of chronic obstruction—renal parenchymal atrophy, hydronephrosis, poor excretion—are also well displayed. Detection of hydroureteronephrosis is not dependent on excretion of contrast, and the true strength of CT is its ability to show the entire course of the ureter, the point of change in caliber of an obstructed ureter, and intrinsic causes of obstruction such as high attenuation stones or ureteral tumors with soft tissue attenuation and postcontrast enhancement. Extrinsic causes of obstruction such as extrinsic tumors, retroperitoneal fibrosis, and retrocaval ureter or congenital anomalies such as ectopic ureterocoeles can be easily seen.

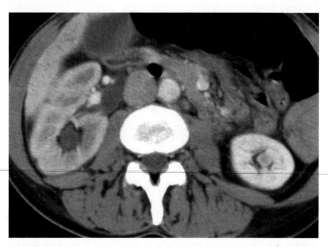

Figure 18-76 Obstruction of the right ureter. Delayed right renal enhancement is present on contrasted CT compared to left kidney. Note the right kidney is malrotated.

One hallmark of chronic obstruction is symmetric atrophy of the entire obstructed kidney (or one segment in ureteral duplication), in contrast to focal and irregular atrophy resulting from infarcts or chronic pyelonephritis. Careful analysis thus allows CT to distinguish true obstructive dilation from some potential pitfalls. The other hallmark is hydronephrosis, which is easily displayed on CT. Some potential pitfalls, such as extrarenal pelvis, multiple parapelvic cysts, postobstructive dilatation, diuretic state, bladder outlet obstruction, and others, may be avoided with enhanced scans, showing either a normal excretion pattern or the collecting system separate from cysts. Delayed images may be helpful to fill the collecting system and ureters. Although not emphasized as a significant finding in the literature, ureteral jets can often be seen on CT, documenting flow to the bladder as with sonography.

MRI is also useful in detecting or excluding obstruction, although with perhaps slightly less spatial resolution than CT. It is capable of demonstrating the anatomic changes as described previously of acute or chronic obstruction. With water-sensitive techniques (fat-suppressed T2, RARE type sequences), not only can the dilated collecting system and ureter be easily displayed, but the perirenal edema and stranding that occur with acute obstruction can also be seen. However, detection of small calculi on MRI is more difficult than on CT; larger stones may be indicated as a hypointense filling defect or meniscus at the bottom of a columned ureter. Magnetic resonance urography (MRU) techniques have been developed that have some potential for diagnosis of the presence and cause of obstructive uropathy. In the setting of chronic obstruction with significant dilatation, T2-sensitive techniques are very useful (and when gadolinium contrast-enhanced techniques limited by the poor excretion of the chronically obstructed kidney). In the setting of acute obstruction, T2 methods are less effective, and T1-weighted gadolinium-enhanced methods to opacify the collecting system and ureter may be more useful. However, the minimally dilated or normal system may be less well displayed unless some diuretic agents (e.g., intravenous fluid or furosamide) are used (37, 372). For complete analysis, however, particularly when obstruction is caused by a mass lesion, MRU methods may be used to identify the location of obstruction; axial MR imaging methods focused on this location then should be employed to diagnose the causative lesion.

RENAL FAILURE

Although more expensive than sonography and less quantitative than nuclear medicine techniques, CT can be useful in evaluation of nonobstructive renal failure in general. Although it is nonspecific for diagnosis of the wide variety of acute and chronic parenchymal disorders, CT or CTA can clearly demonstrate vascular compromise, particularly renal arterial occlusion or stenosis, as well as renal vein thrombosis. MRI or MRA is similarly effective for vascular

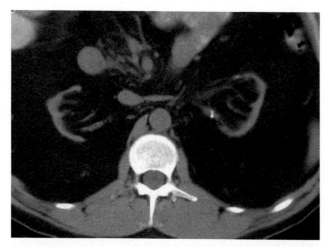

Figure 18-77 End-stage renal failure. Unenhanced CT shows bilaterally atrophied kidneys (*arrows*) with vascular calcification and absence of collecting system dilatation. Renal sinus fat fills the void.

evaluation, particularly in patients with contraindications to iodinated contrast. Although CT can often distinguish the features of acute nonobstructive renal failure (normal to swollen, nonhydronephrotic kidney with poor excretion) from chronic (small kidneys with diffuse atrophy but no hydronephrosis) (see Fig. 18-77), distinction of the exact cause (e.g., acute tubular necrosis versus drug-induced nephrotoxicity) usually is not possible. HIV-associated nephropathy may be suggested by nephromegaly and poor excretion in a setting of severe renal failure and nephrotic syndrome (343). In a patient with no history of preexisting renal failure but recent contrast exposure, CT demonstration of persistent high attenuation on unenhanced scans 24 to 48 hours later is suggestive of acute contrast nephrotoxicity, and additional contrast should be avoided (309) (Fig. 18-78). Contrast excretion into the gallbladder is often also seen in such cases.

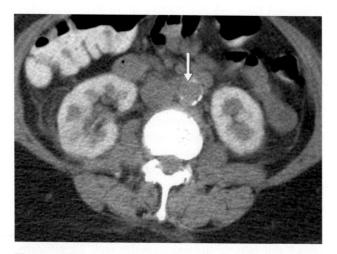

Figure 18-78 Acute tubular necrosis with abnormally persisting nephrogram. Unenhanced CT shows persistent contrast staining of the renal cortices one day after previous intravenous contrast administration. Note there is no contrast within the aorta (*arrow*).

RENAL TRAUMA

The kidney is the most commonly injured urinary tract organ, with renal injuries seen in 8% to 10% of victims of blunt or penetrating trauma, motor vehicle accident being the most frequent (23,362). CT has superseded the intravenous urogram and is the most useful imaging technique for renal trauma, as well as for trauma in general, not only because of its unsurpassed accuracy and detection of urinary injuries, but also its ability to evaluate multiple organ systems. Trauma commonly affects multiple systems, and treatment of the whole patient with early recognition of all the injuries is key. The current trend is toward non-operative management; the ability to accurately detect injuries as well as grade them with CT helps make this possible. CT is a most accurate imaging tool to provide a comprehensive evaluation of the total patient, to stage injuries, and to provide a baseline for follow-up. It can be most effective when installed as close to the trauma bay as possible.

Patient selection

Although most significant renal injuries (95%) are associated with hematuria, hematuria has limited usefulness as a selection criterion. It is nonspecific as to the source of bleeding. It may be absent even with significant injury, particularly renal infarction and ureteropelvic junction disruption (43,480). In addition, only about 1 to 5 in 1,000 patients with hematuria but no hypotension after trauma have a significant injury (71,205,370). CT may be selected for use specifically to detect GU trauma in patients with gross hematuria, microhematuria and shock, or findings associated with renal injury such as lumbar fractures. Patients with penetrating injury and any degree of hematuria should be imaged. However in practice, CT is commonly performed in patients with any abdominal symptoms, hypotension, depressed level of consciousness, and evidence of high-velocity trauma whether hematuria is present or not.

Imaging Methods

Although conventional radiography remains a standard segment of the trauma evaluation of skeletal injuries, it does not offer acceptable accuracy for detection of renal injuries. Likewise, CT has superseded intravenous urography (IVU). The IVU has less sensitivity and specificity than properly performed CT, can evaluate only the urinary tract, actually takes longer to perform and is difficult to perform well in the unprepped trauma patient.

Ultrasound evaluation of trauma in general is controversial and beyond the scope of this text. Nevertheless, solid organ injuries, including renal ones, are clearly more evident on CT than on US (332,333). Although US is sensitive to the presence of intraperitoneal fluid, up to 65% of renal injuries are not associated with intraperitoneal fluid, and US is not sensitive for retroperitoneal fluid. Whereas US may show abnormality of the kidney or perinephric space, CT has superior sensitivity as well as better ability to classify the severity of injury to allow for proper management.

The accuracy of CT, including its ability to show vascular injuries and active extravasation, has essentially eliminated the usefulness of catheter angiography in the acute setting, although angiographic techniques remain useful for treatment of complications such as traumatic pseudoaneurysm, persistent active bleeding, and hypertension. Retrograde pyelography has a very limited role, although it can be useful to document ureteral injury before placement of a stent. MRI at present plays no substantial role, largely because of the difficulty of its use in the emergency department setting and with unstable patients, although its role may expand in the future.

CT Technique

Rapid and accurate evaluation of trauma patients is necessary, and CT, especially multidetector helical CT, allows this. Accurate diagnoses can be made with axial CT or single detector helical CT, but MDCT affords more rapid imaging, thus reducing the artifact due to motion and breathing artifact. Detection of injuries such as arterial extravasation is optimized with the use of MDCT, and it also decreases the time the patient must remain in the scan room. The more efficient tube-heat capacity characteristic of MDCT also allows for quick performance of multiple consecutive CT examinations (e.g., head, chest-abdomen-pelvis, spine, and pelvic bone examinations).

Acceptable accuracy in abdominal trauma CT requires administration of intravenous contrast, because solid organ and urinary tract injuries may be unapparent on unenhanced studies. A useful protocol is 120 to 150 mL low osmolar iodinated contrast for adults (1.5 to 2.0 mL/kg for children) with power injector set preferably at 3 to 4 mL per second (although 2 mL per second is acceptable in the case of limited intravenous access). Oral contrast, although not necessary for urinary tract injuries, is routinely used in most trauma centers, even though delay for passage of contrast through the small bowel is not advisable (141). To avoid volume averaging artifacts, image thickness should be 5 mm or less. A pitch of 1.5:1 on single-slice helical CT is acceptable; with MDCT high speed (pitch greater than 1) increases image acquisition speed while maintaining excellent image quality. Retrospective reconstruction of thinner slices can be done (sometimes useful for subtle injuries) if scans are performed at less than maximum table speed. Kilovolt (peak) of 140 and milliampere seconds of 100 to 300 are adequate, depending on patient body size and scan mode. At present the authors use HS mode on a 4-slice GE scanner in the ED with 5 mm images, table speed 15 mm per second, 0.8-second scanning with delay of 45 seconds for chest, 75 seconds for abdomen and a pause of 180 seconds before scanning the pelvis. (The authors currently use 16 ∞ 1.5 mm detector collimation, pitch approximately 1:1, and scan delay of 45 seconds for chest, continuing straight through abdomen and pelvis in one scan.) This does not allow for bladder filling; if there are reasons to suspect a bladder injury, formal CT cystography should be performed (350). To detect or exclude collecting-system involvement, delayed scans through the kidneys may be necessary. These can be done routinely (4 to 8 minutes), but our practice is to check the images while patient is in the scan room and perform delayed images only when there is a renal parenchymal abnormality, perinephric fluid, or peripelvic fluid. Urethral injuries cannot be accurately assessed with CT.

Image review is best using a PACS workstation and scrolling through images multiple times with soft tissue, bone, and lung window settings. Although focus here is on renal injuries, the radiologist must evaluate all abdominal structures with thoroughness and attention to detail in trauma patients.

Classification of Renal Injuries

Although the scoring system devised by the American Association for the Surgery of Trauma (AAST) was developed initially for research purposes, it is often used for clinical management purposes, because it has been shown to correlate with general severity of injury and with perceived need for surgical treatment (347). Although it is not strictly based on imaging features and clusters different imaging patterns of injury, it behooves the radiologist to be familiar with the language and how it is used in triage. In this system, renal injuries are graded according to the depth of injury as well as involvement of vessels and collecting system:

Grade 1
    Hematuria with normal imaging studies
    Contusion
    Non-expanding subcapsular hematoma
Grade 2
    Non-expanding perinephric hematoma confined
        to retroperitoneum
    Superficial cortical laceration less than 1 cm in
        depth without collecting system injury
Grade 3
    Renal laceration greater than 1 cm in depth and
        does not involve the collecting system
Grade 4
    Renal laceration extending through the kidney into
        the collecting system
    Injuries involving the main renal artery or vein
        with contained hemorrhage
    Segmental infarction without associated hematoma
Grade 5
    Shattered kidney
    UPJ avulsion

Complete laceration, occlusion, or thrombosis of the main renal artery or vein

Grade 1 Injuries
Hematuria with normal imaging studies, renal contusion, and small subcapsular hematomas, each classified as grade 1 injuries, account for roughly 80% of kidney injuries. Contusions on CT are usually seen as poorly marginated areas of diminished enhancement and excretion. Unlike with segmental infarcts, there is some enhancement (Fig. 18-79). A high-attenuation fluid collection limited between the surface of the kidney and the true renal capsule, not extending through to the perinephric space, is a typical appearance of a subcapsular hematoma (Fig. 18-80). These usually form a crescentic shape around only a portion of the renal circumference. They are less common than perinephric hematomas and can develop significant pressure, resulting in deformation of the adjacent kidney; this pressure, if great enough, can result in hypertension.

Grades 2 and 3 Injuries
A perinephric hematoma may be an isolated finding but often is seen in conjunction with a renal parenchymal laceration. Thus, when a perinephric hematoma is identified, a careful search for an even subtler renal laceration should be made. On CT, perinephric hematoma appears as an ill-defined, somewhat high-attenuation collection of varying volume between the renal surface and Gerota's fascia (Fig. 18-81). Because the perinephric space is more expandable and the hematoma can track inferiorly into the retroperitoneal space, pressure rarely develops to deform the kidney.

An irregular or linear defect in the renal parenchyma on contrast-enhanced CT images is the hallmark of a renal laceration. These may be higher attenuation than water attenuation and do not enhance. If there is no extravasation from the collecting system and the depth is less than 1 cm, the

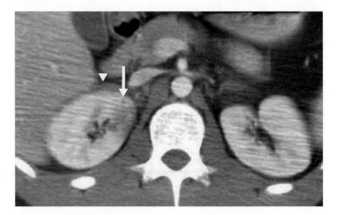

Figure 18-79 Renal contusion. In a patient with recent trauma, a focal region of decreased enhancement (*arrow*) is seen within the medial aspect of the right kidney, with a trace of perinephric hematoma (*arrowhead*).

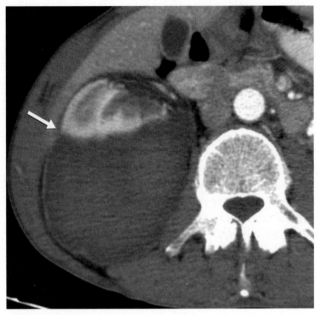

Figure 18-80 Subcapsular hematoma. CT image after intravenous contrast shows a crescent-shaped hematoma surround part of the left kidney. There is distortion of the renal cortex (*arrow*) at the posterior aspect of the renal margin.

laceration is AAST grade 2, and if deeper than 1 cm, AAST grade 3 (Fig. 18-82). These injuries are most often successfully managed non-operatively, unless there is active arterial extravasation, which can also be managed with vascular interventional techniques (52,98,123,267).

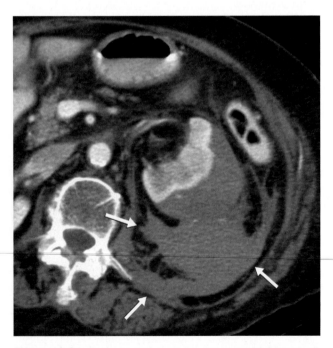

Figure 18-81 Subcapsular hematoma. On contrasted CT, a large left subcapsular hematoma compresses and distorts the left renal cortex. Perinephric and posterior pararenal space hematomas (*arrows*) are also present.

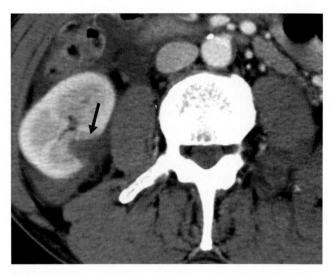

Figure 18-82 Grade 3 renal laceration. On a contrasted CT, a laceration (*arrow*) extends more than one centimeter centrally through the renal cortex, and a moderate perinephric hematoma is noted.

Grade 4 Injuries

Lacerations that extend not only through renal parenchyma but also into either the collecting system or major vessels are categorized as grade 4 and are more significant injuries. On CT vascular extravasation can be recognized if there is an abnormal collection of contrast during the early parenchyma phase before filling of the collecting system has occurred. Arterial extravasation is more common than venous extravasation. If there is any perinephric or peripelvic fluid, imaging in excretory phase is needed to evaluate for extravasation of opacified urine from the collecting system (Fig. 18-83). Even large amounts of urinary extravasation often resolve with nonoperative management, although stent placement is often performed for treatment of injuries with moderate and large urine extravasations. If vascular extravasation persists, embolization or surgery may be needed.

Thrombosis, dissection or laceration of a segmental artery can lead to a segmental infarction of parenchyma, also a grade 4 injury. The typical features on CT are a well-delineated, linear or wedge-shaped area of complete absence of enhancement. There should be neither bulging nor indentation of the renal contour. Segmental infarctions extend through the kidney in a radial pattern and may be associated with other injuries. They may be multifocal and may resolve on follow-up examinations (Fig. 18-84), probably as result of clot lysis before permanent ischemic damage, or lead to residual scarring (67,70). A possible long-term complication is hypertension (6% to 20%) (31,56).

Grade 5 Injuries

This class includes shattered or devascularized kidneys, UPJ avulsion, and complete laceration or thrombosis of the main renal artery or vein. Shattered kidney (Fig. 18-85)

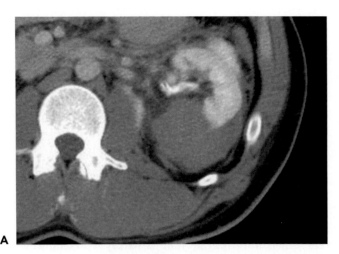

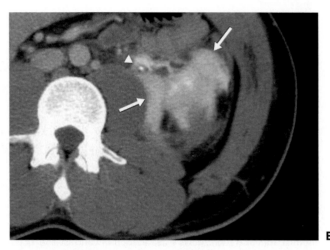

A   B

Figure 18-83   Grade 4 renal trauma. **A:** Excretory CT demonstrates renal laceration with associated hematoma. **B:** Delayed slightly more caudal image of the same CT shows urinary contrast extravasation (*arrows*) into the perinephric space and around the ureter (*arrowhead*). A fractured left
kidney with perinephric hematomas, nevertheless, shows some parenchymal enhancement.

lies at the extreme end of the spectrum of lacerations, with
multiple deep lacerations commonly, with collecting-
system extravasation, and often with some devascularized
regions. Rapid deceleration, such as occurs with high-
speed impact, results in a hyperextension that can cause
disruption of the ureteropelvic junction (Fig. 18-86), because the kidney moves forward with momentum, pulling
away from the more fixed ureter (and/or the artery and
vein). An avulsion of the UPJ can be partial, which is more
easily treated with a ureteral stent, or complete. Complete
avulsion may require early surgical repair to salvage an
otherwise uninjured kidney and avoid chronic urinoma.
Fluid medial to the pelvis or around proximal ureter suggests this injury, and delayed views may demonstrate
extravasation (191)(256)(261). The presence of contrast

in the distal ureter (which should always be searched
for in every trauma CT) indicates a partial disruption.
Although a serious injury, hematuria is often minimal or
absent (256, 261). Careful attention to detail with knowledge of the CT features can allow for correct diagnosis and
renal salvage; missed diagnosis can result in chronic urinoma and eventual nephrectomy.

The stretching of the elastic renal artery in deceleration injury can result in an incomplete vascular tear,
with resultant thrombosis of the main renal artery, and
devascularization of the kidney. Hematuria is often absent,
and because there is not active hemorrhage, there may not
be hypotension, unless the patient has other injuries (180).
This lesion is readily recognizable on contrasted CT, because the kidney is normal size but shows no enhancement;

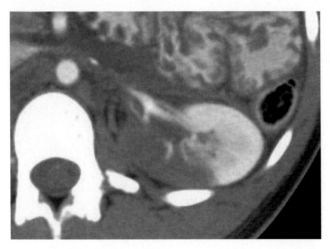

Figure 18-84   Renal Infarct. Contrasted CT shows absence of
enhancement in the dorsal aspect of the left kidney, in a vascular
distribution, consistent with occlusion/disruption of a dorsal branch
of the left renal artery.

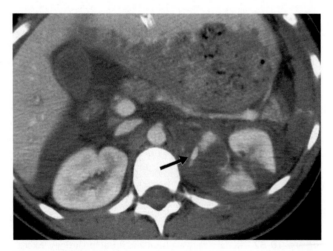

Figure 18-85   Renal laceration with arterial extravasation. Although no contrast excretion has yet occurred on this contrasted CT,
extravasation of densely contrasted blood (*arrow*) is present medial
to the renal cortex. Multiple renal lacerations are also present.

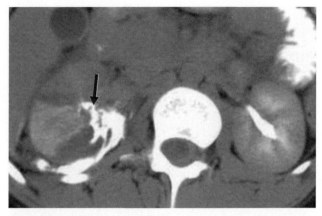

Figure 18-86 Post-traumatic urinoma. Delayed CT images after contrast administration shows extravasation of contrast-enhanced urine from the right collecting system (*arrow*), which tracks posterior to the kidney.

it may be possible to see cutoff of the enhancement in the renal artery, and absence of hematoma in retroperitoneum is typical (Fig. 18-87). There may be retrograde filling of the renal vein, and a cortical rim sign may be seen, although more often this is evident some time after the initial insult. It is possible to see active extravasation and massive retroperitoneal hematoma from complete laceration of the main renal artery, but patients with such injuries are unstable and are seen in the CT suite only with very rapid transit to hospital and scan room in the emergency department. Renal vascular injuries are the result of very-high-energy trauma and are often associated with other severe injuries. This, plus the poor outcome of attempted surgical repair, has led to the current practice at most centers of conservative management of arterial thrombosis. Late complication of hypertension occurs in 40% to 50% of patients managed conservatively; vascular

intervention to infarct the remaining underperfused renal tissue or nephrectomy may be needed (180,266).

A serious but much less common vascular injury is thrombosis or laceration of the main renal vein. A filling defect may be demonstrated on CT, or there may only be non-enhancement of the vein with a delayed or persistent nephrogram resulting from the occlusion (38,191). A medially located or circumrenal subcapsular or perinephric hematoma can result from a renal vein disruption.

Vascular Contrast Extravasation

In early-phase contrast-enhanced CT, images that show an area of enhancement of similar intensity to that of adjacent vessels in or near an injured kidney represent active bleeding, a finding that should be searched for and recognized on trauma CT. If contained, a well-circumscribed area of such bright enhancement within the renal parenchyma is likely a pseudoaneurysm. Such post-traumatic pseudoaneurysms may persist and enlarge and can cause delayed bleeding or hypertension. Renal lacerations can also cause arteriovenous fistulae, which also can enlarge and lead to bleeding, hypertension, or high-output cardiac failure.

Active free hemorrhage is more ill defined and may have a flame or waterfall shape, usually with associated fresh (high-attenuation) hematoma (Fig. 18-88). On delay images, the attenuation remains high but less than on early images (whereas leak of contrast-enhanced urine

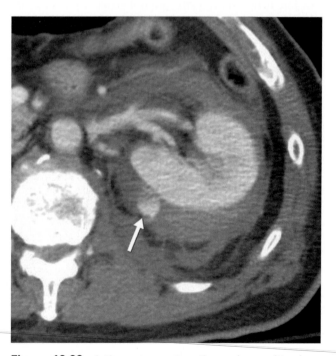

Figure 18-88 Active extravasation. On nephrographic phase CT, a large perinephric hematoma is present and focal arterial extravasation of contrasted blood is visible (*arrow*) in a patient with a motor vehicle trauma patient.

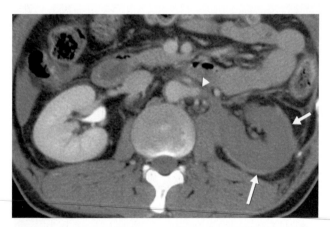

Figure 18-87 Renal artery avulsion and infracted kidney. Excretory phase CT shows non-enhancement of the left kidney with a thin rim of capsular enhancement (*arrows*) secondary to intact capsular arteries. A focal injury is present in the proximal aspect of the main renal artery (*arrowhead*).

tends to continue to increase). As with such active bleeding in other areas of the body, active extravasation from renal parenchymal or vascular laceration may necessitate urgent surgery or transvascular intervention because exsanguination can result (239,276,453,552).

Properly performed trauma CT, especially with MDCT located in the emergency department close to the trauma bay, provides accurate diagnosis or exclusion of renal injuries, aiding optimal, rapid, and effective therapy. Although other imaging means have some potential role, the accuracy of CT and, in particular, its ability to stage the severity of the injury and detect life-threatening findings, such as active bleeding, give CT the predominant role. Accuracy in diagnosis and staging is key because of the trend toward non-operative management. This is particularly true with renal injuries; it has been shown that even with very severe renal injuries, conservative, non-operative management in the long run usually results in better preservation of functioning renal tissue compared with early operation, which often results in nephrectomy (52,267).

RENAL VASCULAR DISEASE

Arterial phase images may be useful to evaluate for vascular anatomy or pathology and for surgical planning. They can be obtained by using bolus tracking features of the CT scanner, sequential low-dose slices after a small test injection prior to the actual scan, or a standard delay of 20 to 30 seconds from the beginning of the contrast injection of 75 to 150 mL of intravenous contrast at 4 to 5 mL per second. Imaging at approximately 20 seconds helps decrease any renal vein opacification, which may obscure the arteries with standard maximum intensity projection (MIP) images. With volume rendering or targeted region of interest MIP, this is less of a problem; the better opacification of the renal veins obtained by scanning nearer 30 seconds delay may help in the detection of renal vein anomalies or tumor extension. Low-osmolar contrast may help decrease the chance of nausea and subsequent patient motion and reduce the risk of nephrotoxicity and of tissue injury if contrast extravasation occurs. Images should be obtained with 1- to 3-mm collimation, subsecond scan time, and pitch of up to 2:1 to allow coverage of the area of interest in a single breath-hold (coverage time is no longer a problem on 16+ slice scanners). Hyperventilation or oxygen by nasal cannula may be helpful to increase breath-holding time with single-slice scanners. To improve stenosis detection and characterization, as well as the quality of off-axis and 3D reconstructions, images should be reconstructed with 50% overlap.

Imaging the kidneys in the corticomedullary phase of enhancement is probably not essential for renal evaluation if images are obtained in the nephrographic phase. However, corticomedullary images are often obtained when scan timing in the upper abdomen is optimized for evaluation of the liver for metastases if renal tumor is present or suspected.

Image Review

Most diagnoses can be made from review of the axial image set, but multiplanar reformatting may be very useful for renal artery evaluation and surgical planning. Multiplanar reformatted images in the coronal or sagittal planes can be helpful to better show lesions at the upper and lower poles and within the collecting system. Commonly used 3D visualization techniques include MIP, volume rendering and occasionally shaded surface rendering. MIP images are obtained by projecting visual "rays" through the volume of data, keeping only the maximum value encountered. MIP images do not show complicated anatomic relationships as well because there is no depth information, and they do not typically show intrarenal pathology well. The MIP technique does provide a more accurate depiction of renal artery stenosis, however (148). Generation of MIP images may also require the editing out of unwanted high-density structures such as bones, and this can often be tedious on older workstations; therefore, sometimes limited volume or "slab" MIP images may be generated. Volume rendering has many of the advantages of both surface rendering and MIP. Volume rendering uses the entire volume of data and can provide life-like images including color, translucency or transparency of different density ranges, and lighting and shading. Measurement of degree of stenosis with volume rendering may be problematic, however, because of the variable opacity of objects and distortions often introduced to portray perspective. Curved planar reformatted images along the centerline of the renal arteries are most accurate for depicting the precise degree of stenosis, especially when the contrast column is partly obscured by calcium (148). As with all planar imaging, they should be constructed in two orthogonal orientations to accurately portray stenosis.

Even if only the axial images are viewed, it is still helpful to review a large number of images on a workstation or CT scanner to allow rapid paging through the images. Soft copy review may help to cope with "image overload," because a study with thin slices and three or more phases can easily occupy more view boxes than many reading rooms have. Reviewing the images at a workstation also avoids the delay of waiting for the images to be filmed, potentially speeding patient care. This paging, or "cine," review can facilitate detection of subtle lesions in the arteries, renal parenchyma, and collecting system, where the anatomic relations are complex or obliquely oriented. The intense enhancement of the arteries and renal parenchyma resulting from rapid injection for the arterial-phase scan may cause the kidneys and arteries to be too bright and "burnt out" for optimal viewing if filmed at standard window and level settings. Soft copy review eliminates this problem by allowing rapid review of optimized or multiple window and level settings.

CTA for Renal Artery Stenosis, Renal Artery Stents, and Renal Perfusion

Renal artery stenosis is a common cause of secondary hypertension and an important and growing cause of renal impairment. Renal artery stenosis is generally defined as greater than 50% diameter narrowing of at least one main renal artery. Up to 90% of renal artery stenosis is from atherosclerotic vascular disease and usually occurs in the ostial or proximal renal arteries (42). Medial fibroplasia accounts for almost all of the remaining 10% of renal artery stenosis and usually occurs in women, typically younger than 55 years of age, within the distal two thirds of the main renal artery or in branch renal arteries (42). Medial fibroplasia, often called fibromuscular dysplasia, is an inflammatory vasculitis that may result in multiple short stenoses and intervening areas of dilatation, producing a "beaded" appearance of the renal artery (42). Diagnosis of renal artery stenosis is important because treatment of the stenosis may result in improvement in hypertension and possible improvement or stabilization of renal function.

Imaging modalities for evaluation of renal artery stenosis include captopril nuclear renal scan, sonography with Doppler, CT angiography, MR angiography, and catheter angiography. Currently, the best screening modality is still controversial (42). Both captopril renal scan and Doppler ultrasound can provide assessment of the renal physiology and therefore may be important in predicting which patients will have benefit from revascularization (42,318,409). Captopril renal scan has been demonstrated to have a relatively high sensitivity and specificity, both about 90%, and is especially useful in predicting improvement after revascularization. Interpretation may be difficult, however, in patients with bilateral disease, those with impaired renal function, or those with only one kidney (42,318,409). Sonography is noninvasive and can also provide physiologic information but may be very operator-dependent. With color and spectral Doppler examination, sonography has been to shown to have sensitivity of up to 95% and specificity of 90% (42,486). Decreased diastolic flow, or elevated "resistive index," demonstrated by Doppler ultrasound is also highly predictive that hypertension will fail to improve with correction of the stenosis (486).

Both CT angiography and MR angiography complement the physiologic information provided by captopril nuclear scan and duplex Doppler ultrasound by providing noninvasive means to obtain anatomic information similar to catheter angiography (Fig. 18-89). They both provide more information about other renal and extrarenal abnormalities than does catheter angiography alone. Early imaging strategies have been shown to be more cost effective in the management of renal artery stenosis (66). MR angiography is especially helpful in evaluation of patients with poor renal function, but it is sensitive to motion artifacts and has lower spatial resolution than CT angiography (181,516).

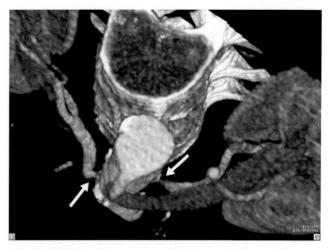

Figure 18-89 Bilateral renal artery stenosis. Bilateral renal artery origin narrowing (*arrows*) is well shown on obliqued reconstruction in a cephalocaudal orientation of arterial phase CT.

Sensitivity and specificity for significant renal artery stenosis with single-slice helical CT are in the range of 89% to 99% and 82% to 99%, respectively, compared with catheter angiography (148,246). Sensitivity with current x-ray tubes and techniques is likely at the high end of this range. The increasing availability of 16-row and higher MDCT should improve the results even further, because evaluation of renal arteries challenges the technical limits of slice thinness and coverage on single-slice helical CT and even some early multislice scanners. The measured specificity of CT may be falsely low due to some false–negative angiograms when a stenosis at the origin is obscured by the overlying aorta because of suboptimal obliquity of the images (246). One limitation of CT angiography is the limited resolution for peripheral stenoses and fibromuscular dysplasia (FMD) (246). However, the spatial resolution of modern multislice CT scanners with ample coverage length using 0.5- to 1-mm slices may be sufficient to consistently detect mild or peripheral FMD (Fig. 18-90) as demonstrated on conventional angiography (186,246). After endovascular stent placement for the treatment of renovascular disease, CT angiography may also be a useful noninvasive tool to evaluate for possible restenosis (26,59,315414).

Renal Artery Aneurysm

Renal artery aneurysms are uncommon and often not associated with atherosclerosis or aortic aneurysm disease. Most appear due to medial fibroplasia ("fibromuscular dysplasia"), and they are more common in women. There is also an association with hypertension and with multiple pregnancies (131,203). Other vasculitidies, connective tissue disorders such as neurofibromatosis and Ehlers-Danlos, and inflammatory processes such as septic emboli and mycotic aneurysms are other uncommon causes. Many are

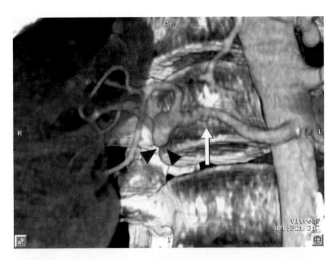

Figure 18-90 Fibromuscular dysplasia with renal artery aneurysm. Arterial phase CT with coronal oblique reconstruction shows irregular "beaded" appearance of distal main renal artery (*arrow*). Focal renal artery aneurysm is noted (*arrowheads*).

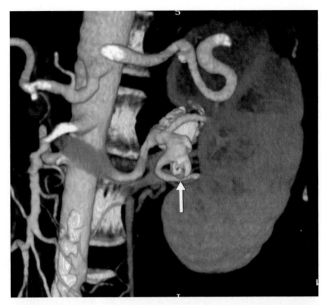

Figure 18-91 Saccular renal artery aneurysm. Coronal obliqued volume reconstruction image of CT angiography demonstrates a saccular left renal artery aneurysm (*arrow*) in a middle-aged woman.

now discovered incidentally during imaging for other reasons, and most patients are asymptomatic.

Indications for repair versus medical management are still not well defined. Renal artery aneurysms less than 1.5 cm may safely be followed in most patients (184). Increased risk of rupture during pregnancy is a known risk of renal artery aneurysm, so expectations for future pregnancy and increasing or large size of an aneurysm are fairly well established indications for surgical therapy (184). However, improvement in hypertension has more recently been documented in patients treated surgically compared with those treated medically, so surgery may also be indicated in patients with hypertension that is difficult to control (203,391,322,415). Renal artery aneurysms tend to occur at branch points where there may be discontinuities in the internal elastic lamina, even in normal people. Saccular aneurysms are the most common and usually occur at the first or second branching of the main renal artery in the renal hilum, but they may be within the renal parenchyma; they are mostly a result of medial fibroplasia or atherosclerosis (see Fig.18-90). Mural calcification and mural thrombus are common, especially in larger aneurysms (257,457,524) (Fig. 18-91). Fusiform aneurysms may occur at any point in the renal arterial system and are usually a result of medial fibroplasia (257). Intrarenal aneurysms may also be caused by polyarteritis nodosa and Wegener granulomatosis or may actually represent pseudoaneurysms.

Pseudoaneurysms also occur in the kidneys and may lead to exsanguinating hematuria or perinephric hematoma, or they may cause or be secondary to arteriovenous fistula. They may be secondary to penetrating or blunt trauma or iatrogenic injury during intravascular procedures or may occur following renal or renovascular surgery. Inflammatory processes and tumors also sometimes result in intrarenal pseudoaneurysms. Intrarenal location of aneurysm and clinical information should suggest the diagnosis of renal

pseudoaneurysm. Historically pseudoaneurysms have been evaluated with catheter angiography, but arterial or early venous-phase CT may also reveal them and allow for characterization of associated renal abnormalities (346).

Vasculitis

In addition to stenoses and aneurysms, small vessel vasculitis associated with diseases such as polyarteritis nodosa, Wegener granulomatosis, and systemic lupus erythematosis may cause abnormalities of renal perfusion at the subsegmental level, resulting in a striated nephrogram or frank infarctions leading to scars (Fig. 18-92). Polyarteritis nodosa and Wegener granulomatosis may also be a cause of

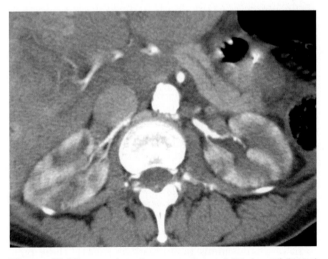

Figure 18-92 Vasculitis. Contrast enhanced CT shows bilateral striations involving the renal cortices. This appearance resembles pyelonephritis, but no perinephric stranding is present. The clinical presentation was not consistent with acute pyelonephritis.

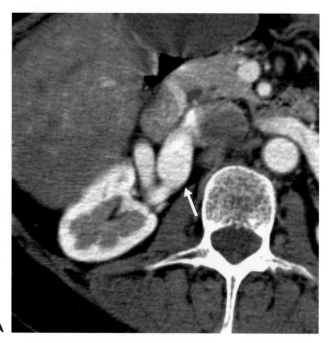 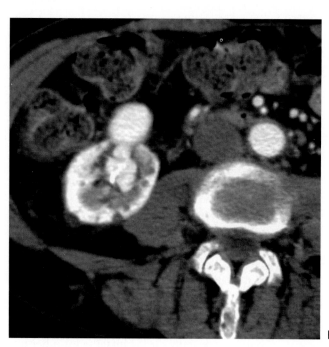

Figure 18-93   Arteriovenous malformation. **A:** Contrasted CT shows early filling of a dilated renal vein (*arrow*). **B:** On a slightly caudal image, a brightly enhancing central renal lesion is present.

spontaneous perinephric hemorrhage (114). Patients with systemic lupus erythematosis may have enlarged kidneys during the acute phase or diminished renal size later in the disease. They may have arterial findings similar to those of other small vessel vasculitidies but are also at very high risk for renal vein thrombosis, which may occur in up to one third of patients with SLE and nephrotic syndrome (51,464).

Arteriovenous Communications

Direct communication between arteries and veins may be visible on CT and MRI examinations of the kidneys. They are most commonly iatrogenic, such as from renal biopsy or blunt or penetrating trauma in the form of arteriovenous fistula (AVF), and are often asymptomatic and usually spontaneously resolve. They may sometimes present with congestive heart failure or a flank bruit if there is very high flow. AVFs may cause persistent or delayed hematuria and rarely may result in hypertension, thought to result from segmental ischemia peripheral to the AVF (99,176, 221,257). AVFs may also occur because of inflammatory processes, tumors, or adjacent aneurysms eroding into a vein. There is typically a single dilated feeding artery and a single very dilated draining vein. Direct communication between the renal arteries and veins without an intervening capillary bed may rarely occur spontaneously in the form of arteriovenous malformations (AVM). These typically involve multiple small connections between the artery and vein and may present with gross hematuria if located adjacent to the collecting system or with subcapsular or

perinephric hematoma if there is cortical involvement (99,221,257). CT and MRI during early phases of contrast can show the dilated vascular structures (Fig. 18-93) as well as early enhancement of the inferior vena cava and ipsilateral renal vein.

Renal Artery Dissection

Dissection of the renal artery and its branches may result in stenosis, aneurysmal dilatation, or both. Dissection may be secondary to blunt trauma, arterial catheterization, extension of aortic dissection or result from primary renal artery pathology such as atherosclerosis or intimal or perimedial fibroplasias (257,354,470). CT with thin sections may show the intimal flap or aneurysm and any associated perfusion abnormalities or infarctions. Dissection with impaired renal flow may cause impaired renal function or secondary hypertension, and these are generally considered indications for revascularization. Aneurysms secondary to dissection are generally considered unstable and are repaired (354,391,470).

Renal Vein Thrombosis

Renal vein thrombosis is an uncommon vascular pathology that may be a cause of renal dysfunction and may also present with flank pain and hematuria. Renal vein thrombosis is usually associated with hypercoagulable states, renal disease, or both (304,555). It most commonly occurs in patients with nephrotic syndrome, especially that caused by membranous glomerulonephritis (304), and in patients with lupus, who may have both nephritis and a hypercoagulable state (51,464). Renal cell carcinoma has a predilection for direct extension into the renal vein and vena cava and transitional cell carcinoma may also more rarely cause tumor thrombus (72,458,524). In children, renal vein thrombus occurs secondary to dehydration in infants and from extension of Wilms tumor (257). Trauma to the kidney or renal hilum may cause disruption or thrombosis of the renal vein and occurs in all age groups. Extension of IVC or left ovarian vein thrombus may rarely cause secondary thrombosis of the renal vein (257).

Ultrasound and MRI with MRV are preferred imaging techniques if there is renal dysfunction. CT with intravenous contrast may be used if there is not substantial renal dysfunction. Renal vein thrombus may be seen secondarily on CT performed primarily for evaluation of hematuria, hypercoagulable state, renal tumors, or trauma.

Renal vein thrombus involves the left renal vein slightly more often than the right, possibly because of the longer course of the left renal vein (257). Acute renal vein thrombus presents with an expanded, non-enhancing, or only peripherally enhancing, thick walled vein, typically with edema around the vein and kidney (168). Tumor thrombus may show enhancement, sometimes with early enhancement of tumor arteries within the renal vein tumor. There may be renal enlargement of and poor or no excretion (168). Ultrasound shows decreased or reversed diastolic arterial flow and absent or diminished venous flow. Chronic renal vein thrombosis demonstrates attenuation of the renal vein and enlarged collateral veins around the renal hilum and upper ureter (257,510).

Nutcracker Syndrome

In patients with "nutcracker syndrome" the left renal vein is compressed between the aorta and an abnormally steeply angled origination of the superior mesenteric artery. The resultant left renal vein hypertension leads to the development of varices around the renal hilum and proximal ureter (118,217). Severe pain or recurrent gross hematuria may require intervention, usually by renal vein transposition to lower on the inferior vena cava (215), or more recently renal vein stent placement (107,447,546).

In patients with nutcracker syndrome, severe narrowing of the renal vein crossing the aorta and dilatation of the vein proximal to this or obvious varices around the renal hilum or upper ureter may be demonstrated by CT, MRI, or ultrasound. Thin-section CT with sagittal and coronal reformated images or MR angiography with sagittal images may be helpful in demonstrating an abnormally steep origination of the superior mesenteric artery (463). Pressure gradient may need to be measured in the renal vein directly in equivocal cases, but there is overlap with normal range (up to 10 cm water) (217).

Computed Tomography Angiography for Surgical Planning for Tumors

CT is widely used in the detection and staging of renal masses. When a radical nephrectomy is planned for renal cell carcinoma, delineation of the detailed renal artery anatomy may not be necessary; however, segmental nephrectomy is an increasingly used option for small carcinomas or indeterminate tumors that may be benign and for localized renal tumors where there is a need for a nephron-sparing procedure. Radical and segmental nephrectomy can each be performed laparoscopically in appropriate patients (165). Indications for nephron-sparing surgery include tumors arising in a single kidney, renal dysfunction, multiple synchronous tumors, abnormality of the contralateral kidney, or hereditary conditions such as von Hippel-Lindau disease (373). In preoperative management, CT with CT angiography allows the surgical approach to be planned using information on the relationship of the kidney and lesion to the ribs, iliac crest and spine, renal vasculature, renal margins, and collecting system (94). Thin-slice CT with multidetector-row CT may also allow for better evaluation of even minimal invasion of the perirenal fat, an important sign indicating that nephron-sparing surgery may not be possible (72). Volume-rendering techniques are especially useful in presenting this complex data for surgical planning and can show the images in a "surgical orientation" (Fig. 18-94) and allow interactive or videotaped progressive removal of layers to depict the key anatomic relationships for surgical planning (94,458,564).

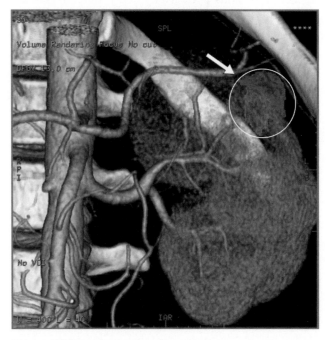

Figure 18-94 Assistance for surgical planning. Volume reconstruction of CT arteriogram is further annotated with color in the region of a focal cortical mass prior to nephron sparing surgery. The study shows the relation of the tumor (*arrow*) to the adjacent ribs.

UPJ Obstruction

CT with CT angiography is also useful for the identification of potential complications during the repair of UPJ obstruction. In the current treatment of UPJ obstruction, percutaneous or ureteroscopic therapy has become a standard option that avoids an open surgery. However, up to 40% of patients may have a crossing accessory artery that may be related to the UPJ obstruction and increase the likelihood of complication from hemorrhage as well as increase the failure rate of endoscopic therapy (527). Most of the crossing vessels are anterior to the UPJ, so the procedure involves a cut in the ureteropelvic junction in the posterior-lateral direction. Significant numbers of crossing vessels are posterior (345), however, and some surgeons advocate routine evaluation of patients for crossing vessels preoperatively with catheter or CT angiography. Especially if there is kinking at the UPJ, an open or laparoscopic procedure is performed for patients with crossing vessels (382,521). Renal CT with CT angiography allows depiction of any crossing vessels in the potential incision site prior to endoscopic surgery and shows the anterior or posterior relationship of the artery to the UPJ that is not shown with catheter angiography (Fig. 18-95), if patients are still considered for endoscopic surgery (262,345,408,430,466, 479,521).

Computed Tomography and Computed Tomographic Angiography for Renal Donors

Traditional evaluation of potential renal donors has included intravenous pyelography (IVP) and catheter angiography. CT with CT angiography is supplanting both the IVP and catheter angiogram in many institutions and allows for a single, noninvasive outpatient procedure.

Findings that affect the transplant procedure include accessory renal arteries, early renal artery branching, fibromuscular dysplasia, renal venous anomalies, and duplicated collecting systems. Although many of these variants may still allow transplantation, their presence may complicate the surgery or favor selection of the contralateral kidney for donation. Other findings such as nephrolithiasis, renal ectopia, renovascular disease, renal asymmetry, numerous renal arteries, renal tumor, or extrarenal abnormalities may even preclude donation (373,471).

Laparoscopy has more recently been used for harvesting transplant kidneys and reduces the risk, discomfort, and recovery time of donors when compared with open nephrectomy. However, the visualization of adjacent vascular structures at surgery may be more restricted during laparoscopic nephrectomy. Venous anatomic variants can have serious consequences and may result in hemorrhage or conversion to an open procedure (373,471).

Compared with catheter angiography, CT angiography has a sensitivity of 95% to 100% and specificity 99% to 100% for accessory renal artery detection and sensitivity 93% to 100% and specificity 99% to 100% for prehilar branches (120,148,253,258,263,400,471). Most studies also show at least some accessory arteries that are better seen with CT, and they suggest that venous and renal parenchymal abnormalities are better seen with CT (109,252,400, 434,471) (Figs. 18-96, 18-97, and 18-98). Even for centers that do not perform renal donor evaluation, this research demonstrates the ability of CT angiography to accurately depict renal arterial abnormalities and tiny accessory arteries.

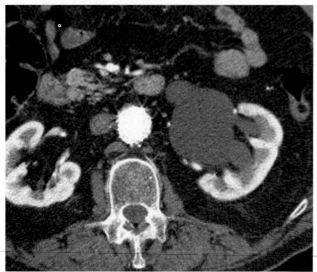 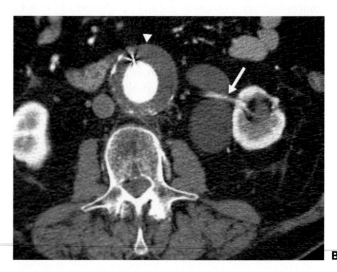

A **B**

Figure 18-95 Crossing vessel. **A:** CT arteriogram shows dilatation of the left renal pelvis and calyces. **B:** On slightly caudal image, a crossing vessel (*arrow*) is present. There is a high association of crossing vessel with ureteropelvic junction obstruction. Note the study was performed to evaluate the aortic aneurysm (*arrowhead*).

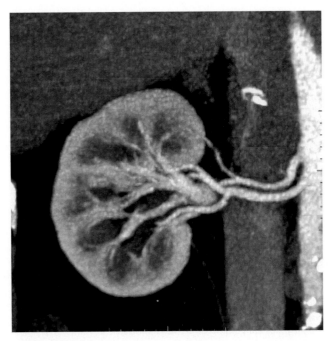

Figure 18-96 Renal donor CT arteriogram. Two right renal arteries are present in a patient being evaluated for renal donation.

RENAL SURGERY

Renal Biopsy

The use of minimally invasive techniques in radiology has increased in the urinary system. Although surgery is the current therapy for most primary renal neoplasms, biopsy

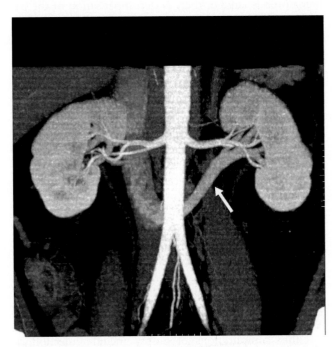

Figure 18-97 Retroaortic left renal vein. On CT angiography coronal reconstruction for evaluation of renal donor, a retroaortic left renal vein (*arrow*) courses caudally to the normal renal vein location. This is important in surgical planning.

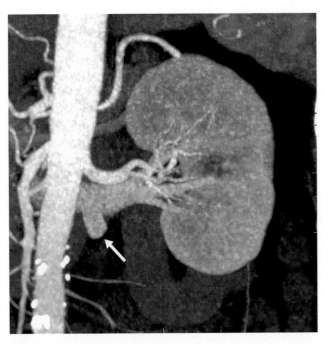

Figure 18-98 Venous variant. A large lumbar vein (*arrow*) drains into the left renal vein on this coronal reconstruction of a renal donor CT arteriogram. Although the image appears as if the vein is retroaortic, this is artifactual due to the maximum intensity projection technique.

of renal disease is a safe, accurate method that can help in certain clinical situations (550,557). Biopsy may be useful if the patient is a poor surgical candidate and localized percutaneous therapy is available. It may help to prevent surgery if metastasis is clinically suspected. Preoperative diagnosis of atypical renal histopathologies may guide nonsurgical therapy. Considerations during renal biopsy should include the potential to affect subsequent therapy, potential for inadequate specimen, and potential complications. Homogeneous multiple renal masses may raise the question of renal lymphoma. In renal lymphoma, surgery may not be the preferred method of treatment, and biopsy can be especially helpful. Percutaneous biopsy has sensitivity of 90% and negative predictive value of 64%. However, in small or very large masses, the negative predictive value is low (439). Insufficient tissue is the most common cause for false–negative results (557). For CT-guided biopsies, the accuracy was similar in all lesions, regardless of size (134). The accuracy of CT-guided core biopsy for tumor type is 90%, but it was less accurate for grading of tumors (282,366). For the diagnosis of malignancy, ultrasound-guided core biopsy is extremely accurate (63). In indeterminate cystic renal lesions, there is increased likelihood of an incorrect diagnosis by imaging-guided biopsy with sensitivity for malignancy 71% (279). CT-guided biopsy may also be helpful to evaluate borderline enlarged lymph nodes in the retroperitoneum before nephrectomy (Fig. 18-99).

As the number of incidental renal masses continues to increase, efforts are being made to reduce the occurrence of

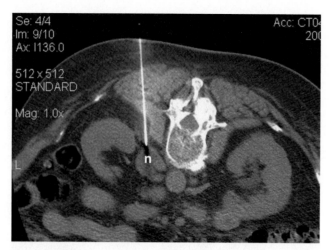

Figure 18-99 Percutaneous biopsy. Prone CT guided biopsy is performed with visualization of the needle tip in a hilar nodal mass (n) in a patient with renal cell carcinoma.

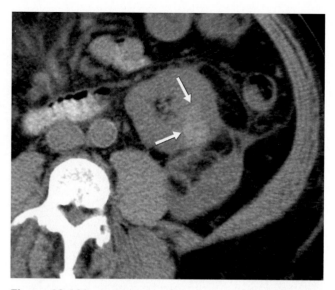

Figure 18-100 Complication of renal biopsy. Uncontrasted CT after renal biopsy demonstrates dense hematoma in the left renal parenchyma (*arrows*) with associated perinephric hematoma. Hematomas are common after renal biopsy.

nephrectomy for benign lesion. Percutaneous biopsy of a renal mass is more commonly being performed in these cases. The diagnosis can be determined in 72% of these patients, but many are insufficient for definitive diagnosis (420). The incidence of seeding from a low potential tumor is very low, but has been documented (121,468, 566). However, the risk may be reduced with the use of cutting needles (282). The likelihood of tract seeding is higher for biopsy of TCC, and biopsy should be avoided in these patients (209,468).

Biopsy for differentiation of metastatic disease from a concurrent RCC in a patient with a malignancy may also help guide therapy. In one series with known extrarenal malignancies, biopsy of solid renal masses found synchronous RCC more often than metastasis (439). If RCC is confirmed, surgical therapy or radiofrequency ablation may be performed. However, if the lesion is diagnosed as a metastatic lesion, systemic therapy may be indicated rather than surgery. Patients referred for renal biopsy should be evaluated for bleeding risk factors or coagulation dysfunction. At our institution, we typically prefer an INR of 1.3 or less for core biopsy. The level of platelets should be at least 60,000, but 100,000 is preferred. Hemoglobin and hematocrit levels should be known before the procedure so that the patient may be followed if hemorrhage is suspected. Commonly, two to five biopsies are performed with guidance (63).

CT appearance after biopsy may commonly demonstrate moderate attenuation subcapsular hematoma (Fig. 18-100) or hemorrhage in the perinephric space (282). Postbiopsy imaging does not usually include intravenous contrast unless there is high suspicion of active extravasation. However, if there is significant hematocrit drop in the hours after biopsy, repeat CT is performed and contrast can be used if active extravasation is suspected.

MRI is sensitive for hemorrhage after biopsy. The heme products are usually detectable by a combination of T1

and T2 sequences. The signal characteristics will depend on the time of imaging relative to the hemorrhage.

Renal biopsy is associated with several potential complications (170). The most common complication after biopsy is localized hemorrhage in the retroperitoneal space, as high as 17% using a 14-gauge biopsy gun needle (402). Small perinephric hematoma is common after a biopsy but does not require further therapy unless the hematoma is large or there is decompensation of the patient because of blood loss. The incidence of severe hemorrhage is less than 3% for 18-gauge biopsy and less than 4% for 14-gauge biopsy (475). The risk of major complication is lower in biopsy of a transplanted kidney allograft, approximately 1% (41). Even for large retroperitoneal hemorrhage, active bleeding usually subsides owing to tamponade effect by the hematoma in the confined space. However, if there is intraperitoneal extension of the hemorrhage, surgery is indicated because the hemorrhage will not likely tamponade.

Another possible complication of renal biopsy is arterial venous fistula formation. The complication is not typically visible at the time of biopsy or on immediate follow-up. However, on subsequent examinations, an arterial venous communication is often visible after prior renal biopsy. The findings on CT include an abnormal early enhancement of the renal vein, which appears dilated relative to the other renal vein. There may be early contrast opacification of the IVC. The renal artery may be dilated. Rarely, an AVM may be exophytic to the renal parenchyma.

Other complications of biopsy include infection or nontarget organ injury. The rate of infection is low because of the high vascularity of the kidney, but it may occur. Renal abscess or pyelonephritis can usually be treated with medical therapy using antibiotics. The most severe of complications in the adjacent organs for CT-guided renal biopsy is perforation of the colon. Whereas small bowel perforation typically heals, there is repeated distention of the colon in the physiologic state and the patient may require surgical correction if there is colonic perforation. Other organs adjacent to the kidneys that may be injured during biopsy are the liver, spleen, pancreas, and aorta as well as the inferior vena cava. However, the rate of nontarget complication is low.

Renal Transplant Preoperative Evaluation: Recipient

Patients with chronic renal failure are commonly evaluated for renal transplantation. Renal transplantation has been shown to be the most effective treatment of chronic renal failure with the greatest success in the long term. Because of the high cost and complexity of the surgery, as well as the shortage of adequate donor kidneys, a rigorous evaluation is performed in the potential transplant recipient prior to surgery. The recipient will be chronically treated with immunosuppression; therefore, the presence of a tumor must be excluded before the surgery, because immunosuppression may allow a low-grade tumor to worsen or metastasize. In patients with polycystic kidney disease, the native kidneys may be especially large and may limit the amount of space in the peritoneum. In some cases, a native kidney may be surgically removed at the time of transplantation surgery. There may be some residual impact of the polycystic kidneys on creatinine clearance and fluid balance, so bilateral nephrectomy is not performed without consideration.

At our institution, there is a large hemodialysis population. As patients remain on hemodialysis for longer times, there is increased vascular calcification of the arterial system (456). There have been several cases in which the iliac arteries were severely calcified to the extent that the ability of the surgeon to place a transplant kidney was severely limited. There have been cases where the transplant allograft was lost because of this problem (10). In one series from Spain, approximately 29% of chronic dialysis patients had severe iliac calcifications that would limit transplant anastomosis formation (10). Patients evaluated to possibly receive a transplant kidney are routinely evaluated with abdominal radiography for pelvis calcifications. In patients with minimal or no calcifications, no further evaluations are performed of the arteries. However, if there are moderate or severe iliac calcifications, a CT examination is performed to characterize the extent of calcifications. Our surgeons require a 3-cm region of the external iliac arteries that is essentially free of calcifications for placement of the allograft. In some situations, the transplant may be performed despite the presence of small calcifications in this region. To closely evaluate these patients with moderate to severe calcifications, pelvis CT is performed with contiguous 5-mm-thick slices without intravenous or oral contrast. The radiology report should detail the extent of pelvis calcifications as well as describe any incidental findings.

Renal Transplant Preoperative Evaluation: Donor

The renal donor is evaluated especially closely before donation of a kidney. Comprehensive testing is performed to minimize the risk that a patient with intrinsic renal disease or potential for future renal failure donates a kidney. The traditional method of evaluation of these patients has included IVU, nuclear renal scan, and conventional angiography. More recently, multiphase CT with CT urography has been performed in lieu of IVU and angiography. Precontrast images are initially obtained to exclude urinary calculus. The precontrast images also allow for localization of the kidneys before CT and CT angiography. Using rapid intravenous contrast bolus, CT angiography with thin slices is performed and 3D volumetric reconstruction images are obtained to simulate the findings of conventional angiography. Portal venous phase images are subsequently performed to detect any small renal tumors or urinary abnormalities prior to surgery. At our institution, a CT urogram is immediately obtained after the CT to characterize the appearance and number of ureters.

The sensitivity of CT for renal calculus is higher than has been previously detectable on IVP. CT is also more specific for characterizing a focal renal abnormality. In fact, most abnormal IVP findings in renal donors are not malignant, but require further study. These patients are typically evaluated with CT before further consideration for transplantation. Early detection of calculi in the evaluation process may prevent the potential donor from undergoing further, more invasive testing. The purpose of CT angiography is to characterize the location and number of renal arteries. Approximately 30% of patients have multiple renal arteries in at least one kidney (90). The left kidney is generally preferred for transplantation, if all else is equal, because of the longer left renal vein. However, if there are multiple left renal arteries and a solitary right renal artery, the right kidney may be taken. The presence of multiple ureters on the left is also a potential indication for donation of the right kidney. If there is a focal cyst or potential renal lesion in the right kidney, the abnormal kidney will be resected and evaluated, and if the lesion is benign, the kidney will be placed in the transplant recipient. An overriding principle in renal transplant donation is that the renal donor retains the kidney that has the best potential for function if the kidneys are possible to resect.

MRI may be used to evaluate patients in a similar way to CT. The sensitivity for calcifications is less than that of CT, and MRI is more sensitive to motion artifact degrading the study. MR angiography is performed during the arterial phase. T2-weighted images, precontrast T1-weighted images, and multiphase contrasted T1-weighted images should be used with intravenous injection of gadolinium contrast.

Renal Transplant Postoperative Evaluation and Acute Complications

A patient receiving a transplant kidney undergoes a complex procedure in which the renal artery and renal vein are anastomosed to their respective vessels in the iliac region. The transplant ureter is anastomosed to the urinary bladder for drainage of urine. The surgical procedure may take several hours, and there is potential for several complications. In living related donor donation, complications occur in approximately 16% of patients, and many of these can be detected by CT (269).

Transplant renal artery stenosis (Fig. 18-101), a common problem in renal transplants (136), may result in severe impairment of renal perfusion, causing allograft dysfunction. The most severe of all complications is renal artery thrombosis with loss of the transplant kidney. This is extremely rare, but it is devastating and is best imaged by ultrasound in the emergent setting (525). In renal arterial thrombosis, the kidney may demonstrate a complete or segmental lack of enhancement on contrasted CT.

Renal vein thrombosis (Fig. 18-102) is also a severe complication in the transplanted kidney. Postsurgical arteriovenous fistula is another potential complication, occurring in 10% to 15% of biopsy follow-up studies (337,341). In fact,

fistulae in the transplant kidneys are much more common than fistulae in the native kidneys. Other complications of renal transplantation include acute tubular necrosis or acute rejection. In these cases, the transplant kidneys may be patchy in appearance and may show reduced concentration of intravenous contrast. Typically an elevated creatinine in these patients will preclude contrast CT until the creatinine has been reduced. In these patients, ultrasound or MRI is usually preferred as the initial form of imaging.

Transplant Postoperative Chronic Complications

In a patient with a renal transplant, monitoring for other long-term complications should be performed. Hydronephrosis, hydroureter, renal arterial disease, and chronic rejection may all occur in a transplanted kidney. Hydronephrosis resulting from urinary obstruction (Fig. 18-103) occurs in approximately 8% of renal transplant allografts (485). CT is very sensitive and specific for transplant hydronephrosis. MRI is also very accurate in the diagnosis of renal transplant complications, such as hydronephrosis (92).

Lymphoceles or peritransplant seromas may require treatment in approximately 7% of transplant patients, according to one large series (269) and infection of a collection is consistent with abscess (Fig. 18-104). These may extrinsically compress the adjacent vessels. Post-transplant lymphoproliferative disorder (PTLD) (Fig. 18-105) may occur and cause renal artery stenosis or hydronephrosis (308).

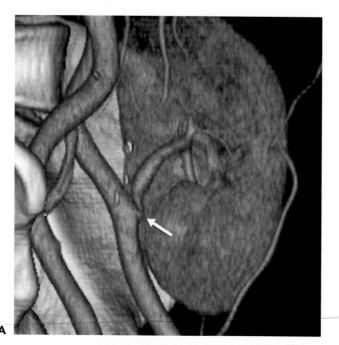

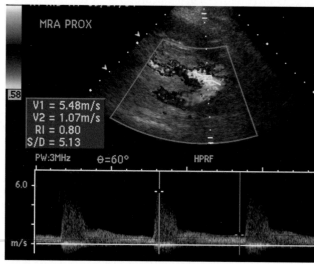

A   B

Figure 18-101 Transplant renal artery stenosis. **A:** In a patient with transplant dysfunction, volume reconstruction of the transplanted kidney shows transplant renal artery narrowing (*arrow*). **B:** Spectral Doppler ultrasound has elevated peak systolic velocity, also consistent with the diagnosis.

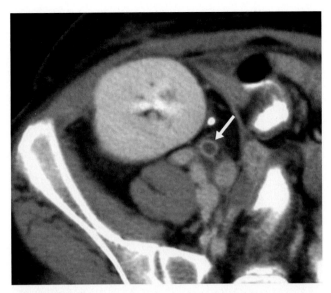

Figure 18-102 Transplant renal vein thrombosis. The transplant renal vein shows absence of normal contrast opacification (*arrow*) during excretory phase images in a patient with transplant dysfunction.

Radiofrequency Ablation of Renal Mass

In a small number of hospitals, radiofrequency ablation (RFA) has increased in use as alternative to nephrectomy for selected renal masses (162) (Fig. 18-106). Even in these institutions, laparoscopic or open surgery is usually the standard of care. In certain situations, as patients with a

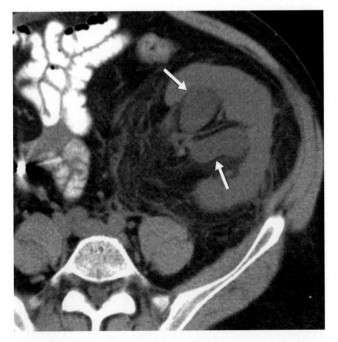

Figure 18-103 Transplant hydronephrosis. On pelvic CT of transplanted kidney, moderate hydronephrosis is present (*arrows*). The transplant ureter was obstructed within a hernia (*not shown*).

previous partial or total nephrectomy, a contraindication preventing nephrectomy such as high surgical risk patients, or in patients who refuse open surgery, RFA may be indicated as an alternative to expectant management (138). It may be useful in patients who need nephron sparing due to multiple lesions in diseases such as VHL.

The RFA procedure begins with proper screening of the patient for risk factors that would preclude a large needle placement, such as coagulopathy. Imaging evaluation should be completed to prevent localized therapy in a patient with diffuse systemic metastases. Although general anesthesia and conscious sedation have been described in the literature, adequate sedation is crucial because of the discomfort associated with the procedure (138,163). Biopsy should be considered before ablation, because a large percentage of renal lesions referred for RFA are not actually RCCs (520). Ultrasound, CT, or rarely MRI may be used to guide needle placement. Ultrasound can provide real-time guidance for needle placement, but often the ablation site becomes nonvisible owing to gas generated during the procedure (300). CT does not suffer from this limitation in case additional portions of the tumor require additional needle placements for ablation. The RFA may be performed percutaneously or in conjunction with localized surgical access by the urologist. A variety of probes are commercially available, and there is some variability in the methods of needle cooling and prevention of unintended charring. The size of the ablation defect also varies with the type of probe. After the procedure, in-patient monitoring and laboratory evaluation is needed because of the possibility of complication or need for vascular intervention. A competing technology is cryoablation, which uses extreme cold to destroy tumor cells in the same way that RFA use radiofrequency and impedance.

In the periprocedure period, fluid and gas may be associated with the ablated tissue at the RFA site. The gas and stranding eventually resolve, leaving a nonenhancing defect in the parenchyma of the kidney. Unlike open surgery, RFA requires frequent follow-up imaging by multiphase CT or MRI to detect residual enhancing tumor that might require re-ablation. Multiple studies are performed in the first 6 months, when risk of recurrence is highest. Subsequent imaging studies may be performed on a semiannual basis (138,163). For tumors larger than 4 cm, there is a significant rate of need for reablation (162). On contrasted CT, the radiographic features and evolution of radiofrequency ablation of renal tumors varies based on the location of the tumor within the kidney. Central renal tumors appear after ablation as a hypodense, wedge-shaped defect without enhancement. There may be fat attenuation located between the ablated lesion and normal kidney. Exophytic masses also show absence of enhancement after ablation but retain their original shape (Fig. 18-106C). Residual tumor after ablation demonstrates focal contrast enhancement within the ablated region (324). On MRI, a 15% increase in ROI

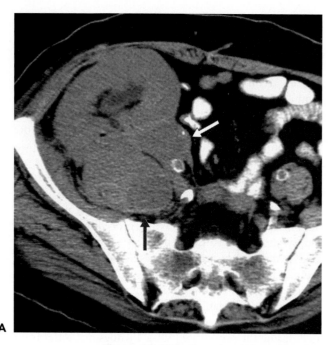
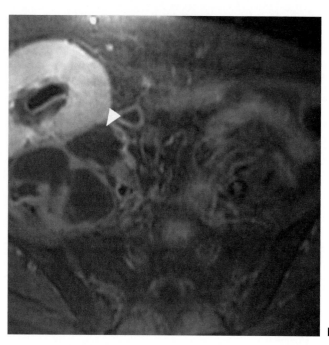

A **B**

Figure 18-104 Transplant kidney abscess. **A:** On CT, a complex lesion (*arrows*) is present in the transplant renal hilar region. **B:** Contrast enhanced T1-weighted MRI shows complexity of the lesion with peripheral enhancement and areas of central necrosis (*arrowheads*). Post-transplant lymphoproliferative disease could have this appearance.

using the same T1-weighted parameters suggests residual tumor (214). However, small areas of viable tumor may persist in regions that do not enhance (417).

The most common complications of ablation procedures are hematoma, pain, and paraesthesia at the skin where the needle is placed. Complications occur in 11% of patients, but major complications and death are rare (244). Hematomas may occur, but rarely require transfusion (162). Overall, RFA is a safe procedure that is well tolerated by patients and has a low complication rate (432).

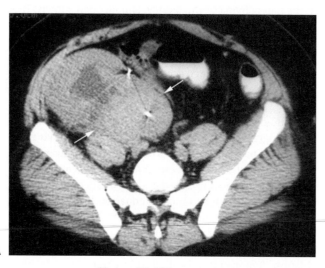
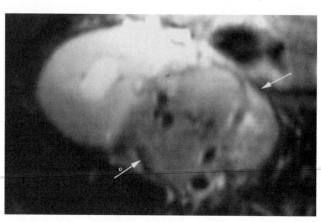

A **B**

Figure 18-105 Post-transplant lymphoproliferative disease. **A:** Uncontrasted CT demonstrates a large mass in the transplant kidney hilum (arrows). **B:** Contrasted MRI shows mild heterogeneous enhancement of the mass (*arrows*). (Courtesy of Robert Lopez-Ben).

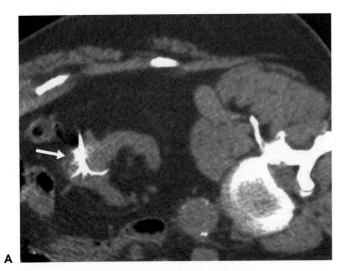

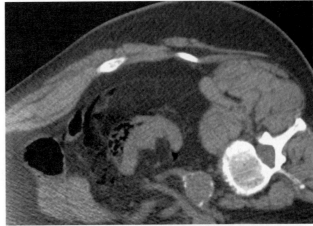

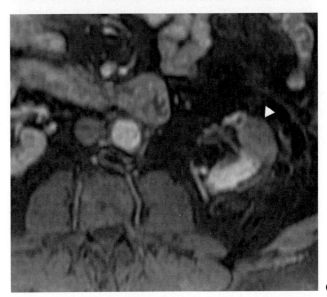

Figure 18-106 Radiofrequency ablation of renal tumor. **A:** CT during ablation shows metallic tynes (*arrow*) of the ablation needle within a renal mass. **B:** Image obtained immediately after the ablation demonstrates gas in the ablation site. **C:** Follow-up contrasted CT shows lack of abnormal enhancement (*arrowhead*) confirming the ablation of the mass.

REFERENCES

1. Abeshouse BS, Bhisitkul I. Crossed renal ectopia with and without fusion. *Urologia Internationalis* 1959; 9:63–91.
2. Abrams HL, Spiro R, Goldstein N. Metastases in carcinoma; analysis of 1000 autopsied cases. *Cancer* 1950:3(1):74–85.
3. Ac'h S, Chapuis H, Mottet N. Metachronous renal oncocytomatosis. *Urologia Internationalis* 2003;70(3):241–243.
4. Afsar H, Yagci F, Meto S, et al. Hydatid disease of the kidney: evaluation and features of diagnostic procedures. *J Urol* 1994;151(3):567–570.
5. Agrons GA, Wagner BJ, Davidson AJ, et al. Multilocular cystic renal tumor in children: radiologic-pathologic correlation. *Radiographics* 1995;15(3):653–669.
6. Ambos MA, Bosniak MA, Madayag MA, et al. Infiltrating neoplasms of the kidney. *Am J Roentgenol* 1977;129(5):859–864.
7. American Joint Committee on Cancer. Kidney. In: Greene FL, Page DL, Fleming ID, et al., ed. *AJCC cancer staging manual*, 6th ed. New York: Springer;2002:323–328.
8. American Joint Committee on Cancer. Renal pelvis and ureter. In: Greene FL, Page DL, Fleming ID, et al., ed. *AJCC cancer staging manual*, 6th ed. New York: Springer;2002:329–334.
9. Amin MB, Crotty TB, Tickoo SK, et al. Renal oncocytoma: a reappraisal of morphologic features with clinicopathologic findings in 80 cases. *Am J Surg Pathol* 1997;21(1):1–12.
10. Andres A, Revilla Y, Ramos A, et al. Helical computed tomography angiography is the most efficient test to assess vascular calcifications in the iliac arterial sector in renal transplant candidates. *Transplant Proc* 2003;35(5):1682–1683.
11. Anton-Culver H, Lee-Feldstein A, Taylor TH. Occupation and bladder cancer risk. *Am J Epidemiol* 1992;136(1):89–94.
12. Antonelli A, Portesi E, Cozzoli A, et al. The collecting duct carcinoma of the kidney: a cytogenetical study. *Eur Urol* 2003;43(6):680–685.
13. Aspelin P, Aubry P, Fransson SG, et al. Nephrotoxic effects in high-risk patients undergoing angiography. *N Engl J Med* 2003;348(6):491–499.
14. Atasoy C, Yagci C, Fitoz S, et al. Cross-sectional imaging in ureter tumors: findings and staging accuracy of various modalities. *Clin Imaging* 2001;25(3):197–202.
15. Avery RA, Harris JE, Davis CJ Jr, et al. Renal medullary carcinoma: clinical and therapeutic aspects of a newly described tumor. *Cancer* 1996;78(1):128–132.
16. Ayres R, Curry NS, Gordon L, et al. Renal metastases from osteogenic sarcoma. *Urologic Radiology* 1985;7(1):39–41.
17. Bae KT, Commean PK, Lee J. Volumetric measurement of renal cysts and parenchyma using MRI: phantoms and patients with polycystic kidney disease. *J Comput Assist Tomog* 2000;24(4):614–619.
18. Bakir AA, Hasnain M, Young S, et al. Dialysis-associated renal cystic disease resembling autosomal dominant polycystic kidney

disease: a report of two cases. *Am J Nephrol* 1999;19(4), 519–522.

19. Ball DS, Friedman AC, Hartman DS, et al. Scar sign of renal oncocytoma: magnetic resonance imaging appearance and lack of specificity. *Urol Radiol* 1986;8(1):46–48.

20. Banner MP, Pollack HM, Chatten J, et al. Multilocular renal cysts: radiologic-pathologic correlation. *Am J Roentgenol* 1981;136(2):239–247.

21. Baron RL, McClennan BL, Lee JK, et al. Computed tomography of transitional-cell carcinoma of the renal pelvis and ureter. *Radiology* 1982;144(1):125–130.

22. Barth KH, Menon M. Renal oncocytoma. Further diagnostic observations. *Diagnostic Imaging* 1980;49(5):259–265.

23. Baverstock R, Simons R, McLoughlin M. Severe blunt renal trauma: a 7-year retrospective review from a provincial trauma centre. *Can J Urol* 2001;8(5):1372–1376.

24. Beckwith JB, Palmer NF. Histopathology and prognosis of Wilms tumors: results from the First National Wilms Tumor Study. *Cancer* 1978;41(5):1937–1948.

25. Begin LR, Guy L, Jacobson SA, et al. Renal carcinoid and horseshoe kidney: a frequent association of two rare entities—a case report and review of the literature. *J Surg Oncol* 1998;68(2):113–119.

26. Behar JV, Nelson RC, Zidar JP, et al. Thin-section multidetector CT angiography of renal artery stents. *Am J Roentgenol* 2002;178(5):1155–1159.

27. Bell TV, Fenlon HM, Davison BD, et al. Unenhanced helical CT criteria to differentiate distal ureteral calculi from pelvic phleboliths. *Radiology* 1998;207(2):363–367.

28. Bellman GC, Yamaguchi R. Special considerations in endopyelotomy in a horseshoe kidney. I 1996, 47(4):582–585.

29. Belville JS, Morgentaler A, Loughlin KR, et al. Spontaneous perinephric and subcapsular renal hemorrhage: evaluation with CT, US, and angiography. *Radiology* 1989;172(3):733–738.

30. Bernardino ME, deSantos LA, Johnson DE, et al. Computed tomography in the evaluation of post-nephrectomy patients. *Radiology* 1979;130(1):183–187.

31. Bertini JE Jr, Flechner SM, Miller P, et al. The natural history of traumatic branch renal artery injury. *J Urol* 1986, 135(2):228–230.

32. Bhatt GM, Bernardino ME, Graham SD Jr. CT diagnosis of renal metastases. *J Comput Assist Tomog* 1983;7(6):1032–1034.

33. Bielsa O, Lloreta J, Gelabert-Mas A. Cystic renal cell carcinoma: pathological features, survival and implications for treatment. *Br J Urol* 1998;82(1):16–20.

34. Birnbaum BA, Bosniak MA, Krinsky GA, et al. Renal cell carcinoma: correlation of CT findings with nuclear morphologic grading in 100 tumors. *Abdom Imaging* 1994;19(3):262–266.

35. Blacher EJ, Johnson DE, Abdul-Karim FW, et al. Squamous cell carcinoma of renal pelvis. *Urology* 1985;25(2):124–126.

36. Blake SP, McNicholas MM, Raptopoulos V. Nonopaque crystal deposition causing ureteric obstruction in patients with HIV undergoing indinavir therapy. *Am J Roentgenol* 1998;171(3):717–720.

37. Blandino A, Gaeta M, Minutoli F, et al. MR urography of the ureter. *Am J Roentgenol* 2002;179(5):1307–1314.

38. Blankenship B, Earls JP, Talner LB. Renal vein thrombosis after vascular pedicle injury. *Am J Roentgenol* 1997;168(6):1574.

39. Blickman JG, Bramson RT, Herrin JT. Autosomal recessive polycystic kidney disease: long–term sonographic findings in patients surviving the neonatal period. *Am J Roentgenol* 1995;164(5):1247–1250.

40. Boatman DL, Kolln CP, Flocks RH. Congenital anomalies associated with horseshoe kidney. *J Urol* 1972;107(2):205–207.

41. Bogan ML, Kopecky KK, Kraft JL, et al. Needle biopsy of renal allografts: comparison of two techniques. *Radiology* 1990;174(1):273–275.

42. Bokhari SW, Faxon DP. Current advances in the diagnosis and treatment of renal artery stenosis. *Rev Cardiovasc Med* 2004;5(4):204–215.

43. Boone TB, Gilling PJ, Husmann DA. Ureteropelvic junction disruption following blunt abdominal trauma. *J Urol* 1993;150(1):33–36.

44. Boridy IC, Kawashima A, Goldman SM, et al. Acute ureterolithiasis: nonenhanced helical CT findings of perinephric edema for prediction of degree of ureteral obstruction. *Radiology* 1999;213(3):663–667.

45. Boridy IC, Nikolaidis P, Kawashima A, et al. Ureterolithiasis: value of the tail sign in differentiating phleboliths from ureteral calculi at nonenhanced helical CT. *Radiology* 1999;211(3):619–621.

46. Bosniak MA. The current radiological approach to renal cysts. *Radiology* 1986;158(1):1–10.

47. Bosniak MA. The small (less than or equal to 3.0 cm) renal parenchymal tumor: detection, diagnosis, and controversies. *Radiology* 1991;179(2):307–317.

48. Bosniak MA, Megibow AJ, Hulnick DH, et al. CT diagnosis of renal angiomyolipoma: the importance of detecting small amounts of fat. *Am J Roentgenol* 1988;151(3):497–501.

49. Bova JG, Potter JL, Arevalos E, et al. Renal and perirenal infection: the role of computerized tomography. *J Urol* 1985;133(3):375–378.

50. Bracken RB. Renal carcinoma: clinical aspects and therapy. *Semin Roentgenol* 1987;22(4):241–247.

51. Bradley WG Jr, Jacobs RP, Trew PA, et al. Renal vein thrombosis: occurrence in membranous glomerulonephropathy and lupus nephritis. *Radiology* 1981;139(3):571–576.

52. Brandes SB, McAninch JW. Reconstructive surgery for trauma of the upper urinary tract. *Urol Clin North Am* 1999;26(1):183–199.

53. Bree RL, Schultz SR, Hayes R. Large infiltrating renal transitional cell carcinomas: CT and ultrasound features. *J Comput Assist Tomogr* 1990;14(3):381–385.

54. Brierly RD, Thomas PJ, Harrison NW, et al. Evaluation of fine-needle aspiration cytology for renal masses. *Br J Urol Int* 2000;85(1):14–18.

55. Brown ED, Brown JJ, Kettritz U, et al. Renal abscesses: appearance on gadolinium-enhanced magnetic resonance images. *Abdom Imaging* 1996;21(2):172–176.

56. Bruce LM, Croce MA, Santaniello JM, et al. Blunt renal artery injury: incidence, diagnosis, and management. *Am Surg* 2001;67(6):550–554.

57. Brun M, Maugey-Laulom B, Eurin D, et al. Prenatal sonographic patterns in autosomal dominant polycystic kidney disease: a multicenter study. *Ultrasound Obstet Gynecol* 2004;24(1):55–61.

58. Bruneton JN, Drouillard J, Laurent F, et al. Imaging of renal metastases. *J Radiol* 1988;69(11):639–643.

59. Bucek RA, Puchner S, Reiter M, et al. Multidetector CT angiography with perfusion analysis in the surveillance of renal artery stents. *J Endovasc Ther* 2004;11(2):139–143.

60. Buckley JA, Urban BA, Soyer P, et al. Transitional cell carcinoma of the renal pelvis: a retrospective look at CT staging with pathologic correlation. *Radiology* 1996;201(1):94–198.

61. Campos A, Figueroa ET, Gunasekaran S, et al. Early presentation of tuberous sclerosis as bilateral renal cysts. *J Urol* 1993;149(5):1077–1079.

62. Cano JY, D'Altorio RA. Renal liposarcoma: case report. *J Urol* 1976;115(6),:47–49.

63. Caoili EM, Bude RO, Higgins EJ, et al. Evaluation of sonographically guided percutaneous core biopsy of renal masses. *Am J Roentgenol* 2002;179:373–378.

64. Caoili EM, Cohan RH, Korobkin M, et al. Urinary tract abnormalities: initial experience with multi-detector row CT urography. *Radiology* 2002;222:353–360.

65. Caoili EM, Inampudi P, Cohan RH, et al. Optimization of multidetector row CT urography: effect of compression, saline administration, and prolongation of acquisition delay. *Radiology* 2005;235(1):116–123.

66. Carlos RC, Axelrod DA, Ellis JH, et al. Incorporating patient-centered outcomes in the analysis of cost-effectiveness: imaging strategies for renovascular hypertension. *Am J Roentgenol* 2003;181(6):1653–1661.

67. Carroll PR, McAninch JW, Klosterman P, et al. Renovascular trauma: risk assessment, surgical management, and outcome. *J Trauma* 1990;30(5):547–552.

68. Carter AR, Horgan JG, Jennings TA, et al. The junctional parenchymal defect: a sonographic variant of renal anatomy. *Radiology* 1985;154(2):499–502.

69. Casper KA, Donnelly LF, Chen B, et al. Tuberous sclerosis complex: renal imaging findings. *Radiology* 2002;225(2):451–456.

70. Cass AS, Luxenberg M. Traumatic thrombosis of a segmental branch of the renal artery. *J Urol* 1987;137(6):1115–1116.

71. Cass AS, Luxenberg M, Gleich P, et al. Clinical indications for radiographic evaluation of blunt renal trauma. *J Urol* 1986; 136(2):370–371.

72. Catalano C, Fraioli F, Laghi A, et al. High-resolution multidetector CT in the preoperative evaluation of patients with renal cell carcinoma. *Am J Roentgenol* 2003;180(5):1271–1277.

73. Catalano O, Nunziata A, Altei F, et al. Suspected ureteral colic: primary helical CT versus selective helical CT after unenhanced radiography and sonography. *Am J Roentgenol* 2002;178(2): 379–387.

74. Chao D, Zisman A, Pantuck AJ, et al. Collecting duct renal cell carcinoma: clinical study of a rare tumor. *J Urol* 2002;167(1): 71–74.

75. Chao DH, Zisman A, Pantuck AJ, et al. Changing concepts in the management of renal oncocytoma. *Urology* 2002;59(5):635–642.

76. Chapman AB, Guay-Woodford LM, Grantham JJ, et al. Renal structure in early autosomal-dominant polycystic kidney disease (ADPKD): The Consortium for Radiologic Imaging Studies of Polycystic Kidney Disease (CRISP) cohort. *Kidney Int* 2003; 64(3):1035–1045.

77. Charles AK, Vujanic GM, Berry PJ. Renal tumours of childhood. *Histopathology* 1998;32(4):293–309.

78. Chen MY, Zagoria RJ. Can noncontrast helical computed tomography replace intravenous urography for evaluation of patients with acute urinary tract colic? *J Emerg Med* 1999;17(2):299–303.

79. Chen MY, Zagoria RJ, Saunders HS, et al. Trends in the use of unenhanced helical CT for acute urinary colic. *Am J Roentgenol* 1999;173(6):1447–1450.

80. Chin KC, Perry GJ, Dowling JP, et al. Primary T-cell-rich B-cell lymphoma in the kidney presenting with acute renal failure and a second malignancy. *Pathology* 1999;31(4):325–327.

81. Cho C, Friedland GW, Swenson RS. Acquired renal cystic disease and renal neoplasms in hemodialysis patients. *Urologic Radiology* 1984, 6(3–4), 153–157.

82. Choi H, Almagro UA, McManus JT, et al. Renal oncocytoma. A clinicopathologic study. *Cancer* 1983;51(10):1887–1896.

83. Choi JH, Choi GB, Shim KN, et al. Bilateral primary renal non-Hodgkin's lymphoma presenting with acute renal failure: successful treatment with systemic chemotherapy. *Acta Haematologica* 1997;97(4):231–235.

84. Choyke PL, Filling-Katz MR, Shawker TH, et al. Von Hippel-Lindau disease: radiologic screening for visceral manifestations. *Radiology* 1990;174(3 Pt 1):815–820.

85. Choyke PL, Frank JA, Girton ME, et al. Dynamic Gd-DTPA-enhanced MR imaging of the kidney: experimental results. *Radiology* 1989;170(3 Pt 1):713–720.

86. Choyke PL, Glenn GM, Walther MM, et al. Von Hippel-Lindau disease: genetic, clinical, and imaging features. *Radiology* 1995; 194(3):629–642.

87. Choyke PL, Glenn GM, Walther MM, et al. The natural history of renal lesions in von Hippel-Lindau disease: a serial CT study in 28 patients. *Am J Roentgenol* 1992;159(6):1229–1234.

88. Choyke PL, White EM, Zeman RK, et al. Renal metastases: clinicopathologic and radiologic correlation. *Radiology* 1987;162(2): 359-363.

89. Chuang CK, Lai MK, Chang PL, et al. Xanthogranulomatous pyelonephritis: experience in 36 cases. *J Urol* 1992;147(2):333–336.

90. Cochran ST, Krasny RM, Danovitch GM, et al. Helical CT angiography for examination of living renal donors. *Am J Roentgenol* 1997;168:1569–1573.

91. Cohan RH, Sherman LS, Korobkin M, et al. Renal masses: assessment of corticomedullary-phase and nephrographic-phase CT scans. *Radiology* 1995;196(2):445–451.

92. Cohnen M, Brause M, May P, et al. Contrast-enhanced MR urography in the evaluation of renal transplants with urological complications. *Clin Nephrol* 2002;58(2):111–117.

93. Coleman BG, Arger PH, Mintz MC, et al. Hyperdense renal masses: a computed tomographic dilemma. *Am J Roentgenol* 1984;143(2):291–294.

94. Coll DM, Herts BR, Davros WJ, et al. Preoperative use of 3D volume rendering to demonstrate renal tumors and renal anatomy. *Radiographics* 2000;20(2):431–438.

95. Coll DM, Varanelli MJ, Smith RC. Relationship of spontaneous passage of ureteral calculi to stone size and location as revealed by unenhanced helical CT. *Am J Roentgenol* 2002;178(1): 101–103.

96. Corica FA, Iczkowski KA, Cheng L, et al. Cystic renal cell carcinoma is cured by resection: a study of 24 cases with long-term followup. *J Urol* 1999;161(2):408–411.

97. Corman JM, Penson DF, Hur K, et al. Comparison of complications after radical and partial nephrectomy: results from the National Veterans Administration Surgical Quality Improvement Program. *Br J Urol Int* 2000;86(7):782–789.

98. Corr P, Hacking G. Embolization in traumatic intrarenal vascular injuries. *Clin Radiol* 1991;43(4):262–264.

99. Crotty KL, Orihuela E, Warren MM. Recent advances in the diagnosis and treatment of renal arteriovenous malformations and fistulas. *J Urol* 1993;150(5 Pt 1):1355–1359.

100. Cunniff C, Kirby RS, Senner JW, et al. Deaths associated with renal agenesis: a population-based study of birth prevalence, case ascertainment, and etiologic heterogeneity. *Teratology* 1994;50(3):200–204.

101. Curry NS, Brock G, Metcalf JS, et al. Hyperdense renal mass: unusual CT appearance of a benign renal cyst. *Urologic Radiology* 1982;4(1):33–35.

102. Curry NS, Chung CJ, Gordon B. Unilateral renal cystic disease in an adult. *Abdom Imaging* 1994;19(4):366–368.

103. Curry NS, Cochran ST, Bissada NK. Cystic renal masses: accurate Bosniak classification requires adequate renal CT. *Am J Roentgenol* 2000;175(2):339–342.

104. Curry NS, Reinig J, Schabel SI, et al. An evaluation of the effectiveness of CT vs. other imaging modalities in the diagnosis of atypical renal masses. *Invest Radiol* 1984;19(5):447–454.

105. Curry NS, Schabel SI, Betsill WL Jr. Small renal neoplasms: Diagnostic Imaging, pathologic features, and clinical course. *Radiology* 1986;158(1):113–117.

106. Cyran KM, Kenney PJ. Asymptomatic renal abscess: evaluation with gadolinium DTPA-enhanced MRI. *Abdom Imaging* 1994; 19(3):267–269.

107. d'Archambeau O, Maes M, De Schepper AM. The pelvic congestion syndrome: role of the "nutcracker phenomenon" and results of endovascular treatment. *JBR-BTR* 2004;87(1):1–8.

108. Da'as N, Polliack A, Cohen Y, et al. Kidney involvement and renal manifestations in non-Hodgkin's lymphoma and lymphocytic leukemia: a retrospective study in 700 patients. *Eur J Haematol* 2001;67(3):158–164.

109. Dachman AH, Newmark GM, Mitchell MT, et al. Helical CT examination of potential kidney donors. *Am J Roentgenol* 1998; 171(1):193–200.

110. Dahlene DH Jr, Stanley RJ, Koehler RE, et al. Abdominal tuberculosis: CT findings. *J Comput Assist Tomogr* 1984;8(3):443–445.

111. Dalla-Palma L, Pozzi-Mucelli F, di Donna A, et al. Cystic renal tumors: US and CT findings. *Urologic Radiology* 1990;12(2):67–73.

112. Dalton D, Neiman H, Grayhack JT. The natural history of simple renal cysts: a preliminary study. *J Urol* 1986;135(5):905–908.

113. Daniel WW Jr, Hartman GW, Witten DM, et al. Calcified renal masses. A review of ten years experience at the Mayo Clinic. *Radiology* 1972;103(3):503–508.

114. Daskalopoulos G, Karyotis I, Heretis I, et al. Spontaneous perirenal hemorrhage: a 10-year experience at our institution. *Int Urol Nephrol* 2004;36(1):15–19.

115. Davidson AJ, Hayes WS, Hartman DS, et al. Renal oncocytoma and carcinoma: failure of differentiation with CT. *Radiology* 1993;186:693–696.

116. Davis CJ Jr, Mostofi FK, Sesterhenn IA. Renal medullary carcinoma. The seventh sickle cell nephropathy. *Am J Surg Pathol* 1995;19(1):1–11.

117. Dayal H, Kinman J. Epidemiology of kidney cancer. *Semin Oncol* 1983;10(4):366–377.

118. de Schepper A. "Nutcracker" phenomenon of the renal vein and venous pathology of the left kidney. *Journal Belge de Radiologie* 1972;55(1):507–511.

119. Dechet CB, Bostwick DG, Blute ML, et al. Renal oncocytoma: multifocality, bilateralism, metachronous tumor development and coexistent renal cell carcinoma. *J Urol* 1999;162(1):40–42.

120. Del Pizzo JJ, Sklar GN, You-Cheong JW, et al. Helical computerized tomography arteriography for evaluation of live renal donors undergoing laparoscopic nephrectomy. *Urology* 1999;162(1): 31–34.

121. Denton KJ, Cotton DW, Nakielny RA, et al. Secondary tumour deposits in needle biopsy tracks: an underestimated risk? *J Clin Pathol* 1990;43(1):83.

122. Didier D, Racle A, Etievent JP, et al. Tumor thrombus of the inferior vena cava secondary to malignant abdominal neoplasms: US and CT evaluation. *Radiology* 1987;162(1 Pt 1):83–89.

123. Dinkel HP, Danuser H, Triller J. Blunt renal trauma: minimally invasive management with microcatheter embolization experience in nine patients. *Radiology* 2002;223(3):723–730.

124. Dinsmore BJ, Pollack HM, Banner MP. Calcified transitional cell carcinoma of the renal pelvis. *Radiology* 1988;167(2):401–404.

125. Dobronski P, Czaplicki M, Kozminska E, et al. Collecting (Bellini) duct carcinoma of the kidney—clinical, radiologic and immunohistochemical findings. *Int Urol Nephrol* 1999;31(5):601–609.

126. Donat SM, Donat PE. Intrathoracic kidney: a case report with a review of the world literature. *J Urol* 1988;140(1):131–133.

127. Doroshow LW, Abeshouse BS. Congenital unilateral solitary kidney: report of 37 cases and a review of the literature. *Urologic Survey* 1961;11:219–249.

128. Duffey BG, Choyke PL, Glenn G, et al. The relationship between renal tumor size and metastases in patients with von Hippel-Lindau disease. *J Urol* 2004;172(1):63–65.

129. Dunnick NR, Korobkin M, Clark WM. CT demonstration of hyperdense renal carcinoma. *J Comput Assist Tomogr* 1984;8(5):1023–1024.

130. Emamian SA, Nielsen MB, Pedersen JF, et al. Kidney dimensions at sonography: correlation with age, sex, and habitus in 665 adult volunteers. *Am J Roentgenol* 1993;160:83–86.

131. English WP, Pearce JD, Craven TE, et al. Surgical management of renal artery aneurysms. *J Vascular Surg* 2004;40(1):53–60.

132. Ergen FB, Hussain HK, Caoili EM, et al. MRI for preoperative staging of renal cell carcinoma using the 1997 TNM classification: comparison with surgical and pathologic staging. *Am J Roentgenol* 2004;182(1):217–225.

133. Eschwege P, Saussine C, Steichen G, et al. Radical nephrectomy for renal cell carcinoma 30 mm. or less: long-term follow results. *J Urol* 1996;155(4):1196–1199.

134. Eshed I, Elias S, Sidi AA. Diagnostic value of CT-guided biopsy of indeterminate renal masses. *Clin Radiol* 2004;59(3):262–267.

135. Evans WP, Resnick MI. Horseshoe kidney and urolithiasis. *J Urol* 1981;125(5):620–621.

136. Faenza A, Spolaore R, Poggioli G, et al. Renal artery stenosis after renal transplantation. *Kidney Int* 1983;23(suppl. 14):S54–S59.

137. Fan ZM, Zeng QY, Huo JW, et al. Macronodular multi-organs tuberculoma: CT and MR appearances. *J Gastroenterol* 1998;33(2):285–288.

138. Farrell MA, Charboneau WJ, DiMarco DS, et al. Imaging-guided radiofrequency ablation of solid renal tumors. *Am J Roentgenol* 2003;180(6):1509–1513.

139. Farres MT, Pedron P, Gattegno B, et al. Helical CT and 3D reconstruction of ureteropelvic junction obstruction: accuracy in detection of crossing vessels. *J Comput Assist Tomogr* 1998;22(2):300–303.

140. Farrow GM, Harrison EG Jr, Utz DC. Sarcomas and sarcomatoid and mixed malignant tumors of the kidney in adults. III. *Cancer* 1968;22(3):556–563.

141. Federle MP, Yagan N, Peitzman AB, et al. Abdominal trauma: use of oral contrast material for CT is safe. *Radiology* 1997;205(1):91–93.

142. Fein AB, Lee JK, Balfe DM, et al. Diagnosis and staging of renal cell carcinoma: a comparison of MR imaging and CT. *Am J Roentgenol* 1987;148(4):749–753.

143. Feldberg MA, van Waes PF. Multilocular cystic renal cell carcinoma. *Am J Roentgenol* 1982;138(5):953–955.

144. Felzenberg J, Nasrallah PF. Crossed renal ectopia without fusion associated with hydronephrosis in an infant. *Urology* 1991;38(5):450–452.

145. Ferrozzi F, Bova D, Campodonico F. Computed tomography of renal metastases. *Semin Ultrasound CT MR* 1997;18(2):115–121.

146. Ferry JA, Harris NL, Papanicolaou N, et al. Lymphoma of the kidney. A report of 11 cases. *Am J Surg Pathol* 1995;19(2):134–144.

147. Fielding JR, Fox LA, Heller H, et al. Spiral CT in the evaluation of flank pain: overall accuracy and feature analysis. *J Comput Assist Tomogr* 1997:21(4):635–638.

148. Fielding JR, Silverman SG, Rubin GD. Helical CT of the urinary tract. *Am J Roentgenol* 1999;172(5):1199–1206.

149. Fielding JR, Silverman SG, Samuel S, et al. Unenhanced helical CT of ureteral stones: a replacement for excretory urography in planning treatment. *Am J Roentgenol* 1998;171(4):1051–1053.

150. Fielding JR, Steele G, Fox LA, et al. Spiral computerized tomography in the evaluation of acute flank pain: a replacement for excretory urography. *J Urol* 1997;157(6):2071–2073.

151. Fishman EK, Hartman DS, Goldman SM, et al. The CT appearance of Wilms tumor. *J Comput Assist Tomogr* 1983;7(4):659–665.

152. Fishman MC, Pollack HM, Arger PH, et al. High protein content: another cause of CT hyperdense benign renal cyst. *J Comput Assist Tomogr* 1983;7(6):1103–1106.

153. Flechner SM, McAninch JW. Aspergillosis of the urinary tract: ascending route of infection and evolving patterns of disease. *J Urol* 1981;125(4):598–601.

154. Forman HP, Middleton WD, Melson GL, et al. Hyperechoic renal cell carcinomas: increase in detection at US. *Radiology* 1993;188(2):431–434.

155. Fowler JE Jr, Perkins T. Presentation, diagnosis and treatment of renal abscesses: 1972–1988. *J Urol* 1994;151(4):847–851.

156. Fowler KA, Locken JA, Duchesne JH, et al. US for detecting renal calculi with nonenhanced CT as a reference standard. *Radiology* 2002;222(1):109–113.

157. Freedman BI, Soucie JM, Chapman A, et al. Racial variation in autosomal dominant polycystic kidney disease. *Am J Kidney Dis* 2000;35(1):35–39.

158. Fukuya T, Honda H, Goto K, et al. Computed tomographic findings of Bellini duct carcinoma of the kidney. *J Comput Assist Tomog* 1996;20(3):399–403.

159. Fultz PJ, Hampton WR, Totterman SM. Computed tomography of pyonephrosis. *Abdom Imaging* 1993;18(1):82–87.

160. Gatewood OM, Goldman SM, Marshall FF, et al. Computerized tomography in the diagnosis of transitional cell carcinoma of the kidney. *J Urol* 1982;127(5):876–887.

161. Gehrig JJ Jr, Gottheiner TI, Swenson RS. Acquired cystic disease of the end-stage kidney. *Am J Med* 1985;79(5):609–620.

162. Gervais DA, McGovern FJ, Arellano RS, et al. Radiofrequency ablation of renal cell carcinoma. Part 1: Indications, results, and role in patient management over a 6-year period and ablation of 100 tumors. *Am J Roentgenol* 2005;185(1):64–71.

163. Gervais DA, McGovern FJ, Arellano RS, et al. Renal cell carcinoma: clinical experience and technical success with radio-frequency ablation of 42 tumors. *Radiology* 2003;226(2):417–424.

164. Gibbs GF, Huston J 3rd, Qian Q, et al. Follow-up of intracranial aneurysms in autosomal-dominant polycystic kidney disease. *Kidney Int* 2004;65(5):1621–1627.

165. Gill IS, Matin SF, Desai MM, et al. Comparative analysis of laparoscopic versus open partial nephrectomy for renal tumors in 200 patients. *J Urol* 2003;170(1):64–68.

166. Gill IS, McClennan BL, Kerbl K, et al. Adrenal involvement from renal cell carcinoma: predictive value of computerized tomography. *J Urol* 1994;152(4):1082–1085.

167. Glass RB, Davidson AJ, Fernbach SK. Clear cell sarcoma of the kidney: CT, sonographic, and pathologic correlation. *Radiology* 1991;180(3):715–717.

168. Glazer GM, Francis IR, Gross BH, et al. Computed tomography of renal vein thrombosis. *J Comput Assist Tomogr* 1984;8(2):288–293.

169. Gleason PE, Kelalis PP, Husmann DA, et al. Hydronephrosis in renal ectopia: incidence, etiology and significance. *J Urol* 1994;151(6):1660–1661.

170. Goethuys H, Van Poppel H, Oyen R, et al. The case against fine-needle aspiration cytology for small solid kidney tumors. *Eur Urol* 1996;29(3):284–287.

171. Goldfarb S, Spinler S, Berns JS, et al. Low-osmolality contrast media and the risk of contrast-associated nephrotoxicity. *Invest Radiol* 1993;28 (suppl 5):S7–S10.

172. Goldman SM, Faintuch S, Ajzen SA, et al. Diagnostic value of attenuation measurements of the kidney on unenhanced helical

CT of obstructive ureterolithiasis. *Am J Roentgenol* 2004;182(5): 1251–1254.

173. Goldman SM, Fishman EK. Upper urinary tract infection: the current role of CT, ultrasound, and MRI. *Semin Ultrasound CT MRI* 1991;12(4):335–360.

174. Goldman SM, Fishman EK, Hartman DS, et al. Computed tomography of renal tuberculosis and its pathological correlates. *J Comput Assist Tomogr* 1985;9(4):771–776.

175. Goldman SM, Hartman DS, Fishman EK, et al. CT of xanthogranulomatous pyelonephritis: radiologic-pathologic correlation. *Am J Roentgenol* 1984;142(5):963–969.

176. Goldman SM, Sandler CM. Urogenital trauma: imaging upper GU trauma. *Eur J Radiol* 2004;50(1):84–95.

177. Goncharenko V, Gerlock AJ Jr, Kadir S, et al. Incidence and distribution of venous extension in 70 hypernephromas. *Am J Roentgenol* 1979;133(2):263–265.

178. Grundy P, Breslow N, Green DM, et al. Prognostic factors for children with recurrent Wilms tumor: results from the Second and Third National Wilms Tumor Study. *J Clin Oncol* 1989;7(5): 638–647.

179. Gutierrez OH, Burgener FA, Schwartz S. Coincident renal cell carcinoma and renal angiomyolipoma in tuberous sclerosis. *Am J Roentgenol* 1979;132(5):848–850.

180. Haas CA, Dinchman KH, Nasrallah PF, et al. Traumatic renal artery occlusion: a 15-year review. *J Trauma* 1998;45(3):557–561.

181. Hacklander T, Mertens H, Stattaus J, et al. Evaluation of renovascular hypertension: comparison of functional MRI and contrast-enhanced MRA with a routinely performed renal scintigraphy and DSA. *J Comput Assist Tomogr* 2004;28(6):823–831.

182. Hadar H, Meiraz D. Renal sinus lipomatosis: differentiation from space-occupying lesion with aid of computed tomography. *Urology* 1980;15(1):86–90.

183. Hafez KS, Fergany AF, Novick AC. Nephron sparing surgery for localized renal cell carcinoma: impact of tumor size on patient survival, tumor recurrence and TNM staging. *J Urol* 1999;162(6): 1930–1933.

184. Hageman JH, Smith RF, Szilagyi E, et al. Aneurysms of the renal artery: problems of prognosis and surgical management. *Surgery* 1978;84(4):563–572.

185. Hajdu SI, Foote FW Jr. Angiomyolipoma of the kidney: report of 27 cases and review of the literature. *J Urol* 1969;102(4): 396–401.

186. Hallscheidt PJ, Thorn M, Radeleff BA, et al. Comparison of spatial resolution in high-resolution multislice computed tomography and digital subtraction angiography using renal specimens. *J Comput Assist Tomogr* 2003;27(6):864–868.

187. Hann L, Pfister RC. Renal subcapsular rim sign: new etiologies and pathogenesis. *Am J Roentgenol* 1982;138(1):51–54.

188. Harabayashi T, Shinohara N, Katano H, et al. Management of renal angiomyolipomas associated with tuberous sclerosis complex. *J Urol* 2004;171(1):102–105.

189. Harisinghani MG, Saini S, Weissleder R, et al. MR lymphangiography using ultrasmall superparamagnetic iron oxide in patients with primary abdominal and pelvic malignancies: radiographic-pathologic correlation. *Am J Roentgenol* 1999;172(5): 1347–1351.

190. Harmon WJ, King BF, Lieber MM. Renal oncocytoma: magnetic resonance imaging characteristics. *J Urol* 1996;155(3):863–867.

191. Harris AC, Zwirewich CV, Lyburn ID, et al. CT findings in blunt renal trauma. *Radiographics* 2001;21 Spec:S201–S214.

192. Hartman DS, David CJ Jr, Goldman SM, et al. Renal lymphoma: radiologic-pathologic correlation of 21 cases. *Radiology* 1982; 144(4):759–766.

193. Hartman DS, Davidson AJ, Davis CJ Jr, et al. Infiltrative renal lesions: CT-sonographic-pathologic correlation. *Am J Roentgenol* 1988;150(5):1061–1064.

194. Hartman DS, Davis CJ, Sanders RC, et al. The multiloculated renal mass: considerations and differential features. *Radiographics* 1987;7(1):29–52.

195. Hartman DS, Davis CJ Jr, Johns T, et al. Cystic renal cell carcinoma. *Urology* 1986;28(2):145–153.

196. Hartman DS, Davis CJ Jr, Madewell JE, et al. Primarymalignant renal tumors in the second decade of life: Wilms tumor versus renal cell carcinoma. *J Urol* 1982;127(5):888–891.

197. Hartman DS, Weatherby E 3rd, Laskin WB, et al. Cystic renal cell carcinoma: CT findings simulating a benign hyperdense cyst. *Am J Roentgenol* 1992;159(6):1235–1237.

198. Hayes WS, Hartman DS, Sesterbenn IA. From the archives of the AFIP. Xanthogranulomatous pyelonephritis. *Radiographics* 1991;11(3):485–498.

199. Healy ME, Teng SS, Moss AA. Uriniferous pseudocyst: computed tomographic findings. *Radiology* 1984;153(3):757–762.

200. Hélénon O, Chrétien Y, Paraf F, et al. Renal cell carcinoma containing fat: demonstration with CT. *Radiology* 1993;188: 429–430.

201. Heneghan JP, Dalrymple NC, Verga M, et al. Soft-tissue "rim" sign in the diagnosis of ureteral calculi with use of unenhanced helical CT. *Radiology* 1997;202(3):709–711.

202. Heneghan JP, Spielmann AL, Sheafor DH, et al. Pseudoenhancement of simple renal cysts: a comparison of single and multidetector helical CT. *J Comput Assist Tomogr* 2002;26(1):90–94.

203. Henke PK, Cardneau JD, Welling TH 3rd, et al. Renal artery aneurysms: a 35-year clinical experience with 252 aneurysms in 168 patients. *Ann Surg* 2001;234(4):454–462; discussion 462–463.

204. Herring JC, Enquist EG, Chernoff A, et al. Parenchymal sparing surgery in patients with hereditary renal cell carcinoma: 10-year experience. *J Urol* 2001;165(3):777–781.

205. Herschorn S, Radomski SB, Shoskes DA, et al. Evaluation and treatment of blunt renal trauma. *J Urol* 1991;146(2):274–276.

206. Hertle L, Androulakakis P. Keratinizing desquamative squamous metaplasia of the upper urinary tract: leukoplakia—cholesteatoma. *J Urol* 1982;127(4):631–635.

207. Hertle L, Becht E, Klose K, et al. Computed tomography in xanthogranulomatous pyelonephritis. *Eur Urol* 1984;10(6):385–388.

208. Herts BR. Helical CT and CT angiography for the identification of crossing vessels at the ureteropelvic junction. *Urol Clin North Am* 1998;25(2):259–269.

209. Herts BR, Baker ME. The current role of percutaneous biopsy in the evaluation of renal masses. *Semin Urol Oncol* 1995;13(4): 254–261.

210. Hes FJ, Feldberg MA. Von Hippel-Lindau disease: strategies in early detection (renal-, adrenal-, pancreatic masses). *Eur Radiol* 1999;9(4):598–610.

211. Hietala SO, Ekelund L, Ljungberg B. Venous invasion in renal cell carcinoma: a correlative clinical and radiologic study. *Urol Radiol* 1988;9(4):210–216.

212. Higashihara E, Aso Y, Shimazaki J, et al. Clinical aspects of polycystic kidney disease. *J Urol* 1992;147(2):329–332.

213. Hilpert PL, Friedman AC, Radecki PD, et al. MRI of hemorrhagic renal cysts in polycystic kidney disease. *Am J Roentgenol* 1986;146(6):1167–1172.

214. Ho VB, Allen SF, Hood MN, et al. Renal masses: quantitative assessment of enhancement with dynamic MR imaging. *Radiology* 2002;224(3):695–700.

215. Hohenfellner M, D'Elia G, Hampel C, et al. Transposition of the left renal vein for treatment of the nutcracker phenomenon: long-term follow-up. *Urology* 2002;59(3):354–357.

216. Hohenfellner M, Schultz-Lampel D, Lampel A, et al. Tumor in the horseshoe kidney: clinical implications and review of embryogenesis. *J Urol* 1992;147(4):1098–1102.

217. Hohenfellner M, Steinbach F, Schultz-Lampel D, et al. The nutcracker syndrome: new aspects of pathophysiology, diagnosis and treatment. *J Urol* 1991;146(3):685–688.

218. Holmang S, Johansson SL. Synchronous bilateral ureteral and renal pelvic carcinomas: incidence, etiology, treatment and outcome. *Cancer* 2004;101(4):741–747.

219. Honda H, Coffman CE, Berbaum KS, et al. CT analysis of metastatic neoplasms of the kidney. Comparison with primary renal cell carcinoma. *Acta Radiologica* 1992;33(1):39–44.

220. Honda H, McGuire CW, Barloon TJ, et al. Replacement lipomatosis of the kidney: CT features. *J Comput Assist Tomogr* 1990;14(2):229–231.

221. Honda H, Onitsuka H, Naitou S, et al. Renal arteriovenous malformations: CT features. *J Comput Assist Tomogr* 1991;15(2): 261–264.

222. Horan JJ, Robertson CN, Choyke PL, et al. The detection of renal carcinoma extension into the renal vein and inferior vena cava: a

prospective comparison of venacavography and magnetic resonance imaging. *J Urol* 1989;142(4):943–947.

223. Horino T, Yamamoto M, Morita M, et al. Renal actinomycosis mimicking renal tumor: case report. *South Med J* 2004;97(3):316–318.

224. Hovsepian DM, Levy H, Amis ES Jr, et al. MR evaluation of renal space-occupying lesions: diagnostic criteria. *Urologic Radiology* 1990;12(2):74–79.

225. Hricak H, Thoeni RF, Carroll PR, et al. Detection and staging of renal neoplasms: a reassessment of MR imaging. *Radiology* 1988;166(3):643–649.

226. Huang EY, Mascarenhas L, GH. M. Wilms tumor and horseshoe kidneys: a case report and review of the literature. *J Pediatr Surg* 2004;39(2):207–212.

227. Huang GJ, Israel G, Berman A, et al. Preoperative renal tumor evaluation by three-dimensional magnetic resonance imaging: staging and detection of multifocality. *Urology* 2004;64(3):453–457.

228. Huch Boni RA, Debatin JF, Krestin GP. Contrast-enhanced MR imaging of the kidneys and adrenal glands. *Magn Res Imaging Clin N Am* 1996;4(1):101–131.

229. Hudson MA, Weyman PJ, van der Vliet AH, et al. Emphysematous pyelonephritis: successful management by percutaneous drainage. *J Urol* 1986;136(4):884–886.

230. Hughson MD, Hennigar GR, McManus JF. Atypical cysts, acquired renal cystic disease, and renal cell tumors in end stage dialysis kidneys. *Lab Invest* 1980;42(4):475–480.

231. Hurwitz G, Reimund E, Moparty KR, et al. Bilateral renal parenchymal malacoplakia: a case report. *J Urol* 1992;147(1):115–117.

232. Ishikawa I. Uremic acquired cystic disease of kidney. *Urology* 1985;26(2):101–108.

233. Ishikawa I, Tateishi K, Onouchi Z, et al. Persistent wedge-shaped contrast enhancement of the kidney. *Urol Radiol* 1985;7(1):45–47.

234. Isobe H, Takashima H, Higashi N, et al. Primary carcinoid tumor in a horseshoe kidney. *Int J Urol* 2000;7(5):184–188.

235. Israel GM, Bosniak MA. Calcification in cystic renal masses: is it important in diagnosis? *Radiology* 2003;226(1):47–52.

236. Israel GM, Bosniak MA, Slywotzky CM, et al. CT differentiation of large exophytic renal angiomyolipomas and perirenal liposarcomas. *Am J Roentgenol* 2002;179(3):769–773.

237. Jacobs JE, Sussman SK, Glickstein MF. Renal lymphangiomyoma—-a rare cause of a multiloculated renal mass. *Am J Roentgenol* 1989;152(2):307–308.

238. Jacobs SC, Berg SI, Lawson RK. Synchronous bilateral renal cell carcinoma: total surgical excision. *Cancer* 1980;46(11):2341–2345.

239. Jeffrey RB, Cardoza JD, Olcott EW. Detection of active intraabdominal arterial hemorrhage: value of dynamic contrast-enhanced CT. *Am J Roentgenol* 1991;156(4):725–729.

240. Jinzaki M, Tanimoto A, Narimatsu Y, et al. Angiomyolipoma: imaging findings in lesions with minimal fat. *Radiology* 1997;205(2):497–502.

241. Joffe SA, Servaes S, Okon S, et al. Multi-detector row CT urography in the evaluation of hematuria. *Radiographics* 2003;23(6):1441–1455.

242. Johansson S, Angervall L, Bengtsson U, et al. Uroepithelial tumors of the renal pelvis associated with abuse of phenacetin-containing analgesics. *Cancer* 1974;33(3):743–753.

243. Johnson CD, Dunnick NR, Cohan RH, et al. Renal adenocarcinoma: CT staging of 100 tumors. *Am J Roentgenol* 1987;148(1):59–63.

244. Johnson DB, Solomon SB, Su LM, et al. Defining the complications of cryoablation and radio frequency ablation of small renal tumors: a multi-institutional review. *J Urol* 2004;172(3):874–877.

245. Jung G, Benz-Bohm G, Kugel H, et al. MR cholangiography in children with autosomal recessive polycystic kidney disease. *Pediatr Radiol* 1999;29(6):463–466.

246. Kaatee R, Beek FJ, de Lange EE, et al. Renal artery stenosis: detection and quantification with spiral CT angiography versus optimized digital subtraction angiography. *Radiology* 1997;205(1):121–127.

247. Kabala JE, Gillatt DA, Persad RA, et al. Magnetic resonance imaging in the staging of renal cell carcinoma. *Br J Radiol* 1991;64(764):683–689.

248. Kallman DA, King BF, Hattery RR, et al. Renal vein and inferior vena cava tumor thrombus in renal cell carcinoma: CT, US, MRI and venacavography. *J Comput Assist Tomogr* 1992;16(2):240–247.

249. Kaneti J, Krugliak L, Hirsch M, et al. Rupture of renal angiomyolipoma: conservative surgery. *J Urol* 1983;129(4):810–811.

250. Karstaedt N, McCullough DL, Wolfman NT, et al. Magnetic resonance imaging of the renal mass. *J Urol* 1986;136(3):566–570.

251. Katz DS, Lane MJ, Sommer FG. Unenhanced helical CT of ureteral stones: incidence of associated urinary tract findings. *Am J Roentgenol* 1996;166(6):1319–1322.

252. Kawamoto S, Lawler LP, Fishman EK. Evaluation of the renal venous system on late arterial and venous phase images with MDCT angiography in potential living laparoscopic renal donors. *Am J Roentgenol* 2005;184(2):539–545.

253. Kawamoto S, Montgomery RA, Lawler LP, et al. Multidetector CT angiography for preoperative evaluation of living laparoscopic kidney donors. *Am J Roentgenol* 2003;180(6):1633–1638.

254. Kawashima A, Sandler CM, Boridy IC, et al. Unenhanced helical CT of ureterolithiasis: value of the tissue rim sign. *Am J Roentgenol* 1997;168(4):997–1000.

255. Kawashima A, Sandler CM, Corl FM, et al. Imaging of renal trauma: a comprehensive review. *Radiographics* 2001;21(3):557–574.

256. Kawashima A, Sandler CM, Corriere JN Jr, et al. Ureteropelvic junction injuries secondary to blunt abdominal trauma. *Radiology* 1997;205(2):487–492.

257. Kawashima A, Sandler CM, Ernst RD, et al. CT evaluation of renovascular disease. *Radiographics* 2000;20(5):1321–1340.

258. Kaynan AM, Rozenblit AM, Figueroa KI, et al. Use of spiral computerized tomography in lieu of angiography for preoperative assessment of living renal donors. *J Urol* 1999;161(6):1769–1775.

259. Keeley FX Jr, Bagley DH, Kulp-Hugues D, et al. Laparoscopic division of crossing vessels at the ureteropelvic junction. *J Endourol* 1996;10(2):163–168.

260. Kenney PJ, McClennan BL. The kidney. In: Lee J, Sagel S, Stanley RJ, Heiken JP, eds. *Computed body tomography with MRI correlation*, vol. 2, 3rd ed. Philadelphia: Lippincott-Raven Publishers; 1998:1087–1170.

261. Kenney PJ, Panicek DM, Witanowski LS. Computed tomography of ureteral disruption. *J Comput Assist Tomogr* 1987;11(3):480–484.

262. Khaira HS, Platt JF, Cohan RH, et al. Helical computed tomography for identification of crossing vessels in ureteropelvic junction obstruction-comparison with operative findings. *Urology* 2003;62(1):35–39.

263. Kim TS, Chung JW, Park JH, et al. Renal artery evaluation: comparison of spiral CT angiography to intra-arterial DSA. *Journal of Vascular and Interventional Radiology* 1998;9(4):553–559.

264. Kim WS, Goldman SM, Gatewood OM, et al. Computed tomography in calcified renal masses. *J Comput Assist Tomogr* 1981;5(6):855–860.

265. Kirchin MA, Runge VM. Contrast agents for magnetic resonance imaging: safety update. *Top Magn Reson Imaging* 2003;14(5):426–435.

266. Knudson MM, Harrison PB, Hoyt DB, et al. Outcome after major renovascular injuries: a Western trauma association multicenter report. *J Trauma* 2000;49(6):1116–1122.

267. Knudson MM, Maull KI. Nonoperative management of solid organ injuries. Past, present, and future. *Surg Clin North Am* 1999;79(6):1357–1371.

268. Kobayashi S, Ohmori M, Akaeda T, et al. Primary adenocarcinoma of the renal pelvis. Report of two cases and brief review of literature. *Acta Pathologica Japonica* 1983;33(3):589–597.

269. Kocak T, Nane I, Ander H, et al. Urological and surgical complications in 362 consecutive living related donor kidney transplantations. *Urologia Internationalis* 2004;72(3):252–256.

270. Konnak JW, Grossman HB. Renal cell carcinoma as an incidental finding. *J Urol* 1985;134(6):1094–1096.

271. Kopka L, Fischer U, Zoeller G, et al. Dual-phase helical CT of the kidney: value of the corticomedullary and nephrographic phase

for evaluation of renal lesions and preoperative staging of renal cell carcinoma. *Am J Roentgenol* 1997;169(6):1573–1578.

272. Krishnan B, Truong LD, Saleh G, et al. Horseshoe kidney is associated with an increased relative risk of primary renal carcinoid tumor. *J Urol* 1997;157(6):2059–2066.

273. Krizanac S, Vranesic D, Oberman B. Oncocytomas of the kidney. *Br J Urol* 1987;60(3):189–192.

274. Kumar R, Amparo EG, David R, et al. Adult Wilms' tumor: clinical and radiographic features. *Urol Radiol* 1984;6(3–4):164–169.

275. Lampel A, Hohenfellner M, Schultz-Lampel D, et al. Urolithiasis in horseshoe kidneys: therapeutic management. *Urology* 1996; 47(2):182–186.

276. Lane MJ, Katz DS, Shah RA, et al. Active arterial contrast extravasation on helical CT of the abdomen, pelvis, and chest. *Am J Roentgenol* 1998;171(3):679–685.

277. Lane RH, Stephens DH R, Reiman HM. Primary retroperitoneal neoplasms: CT findings in 90 cases with clinical and pathologic correlation. *Am J Roentgenol* 1989;152(1):83–89.

278. Lang EK. Renal, perirenal, and pararenal abscesses: percutaneous drainage. *Radiology* 1990;174(1):109–113.

279. Lang EK, Macchia RJ, Gayle B, et al. CT-guided biopsy of indeterminate renal cystic masses (Bosniak 3 and 2F): accuracy and impact on clinical management. *Eur Radiol* 2002;12(10):2518–2524.

280. Lang EK, Macchia RJ, Thomas R, et al. Detection of medullary and papillary necrosis at an early stage by multiphasic helical computerized tomography. *J Urol* 2003;170(1):94–98.

281. Lawson TL, McClennan BL, Shirkhoda A. Adult polycystic kidney disease: ultrasonographic and computed tomographic appearance. *J Clin Ultrasound* 1978;6(5):297–302.

282. Lechevallier E, Andre M, Barriol D, et al. Fine-needle percutaneous biopsy of renal masses with helical CT guidance. *Radiology* 2000;216(2):506–510.

283. Leder RA, Dunnick NR. Transitional cell carcinoma of the pelvicalices and ureter. *Am J Roentgenol* 1990;155(4):713–722.

284. Lee JK, McClennan BL, Kissane JM. Unilateral polycystic kidney disease. *Am J Roentgenol* 1978;130(6):1165–1167.

285. Lee JK, McClennan BL, Melson GL, et al. Acute focal bacterial nephritis: emphasis on gray scale sonography and computed tomography. *Am J Roentgenol* 1980;135(1):87–92.

286. Lemaitre L, Claudon M, Dubrulle F, et al. Imaging of angiomyolipomas. *Semin Ultrasound CT MRI* 1997;18(2):100–114.

287. Lemaitre L, Robert Y, Dubrulle F, et al. Renal angiomyolipoma: growth followed up with CT and/or US. *Radiology* 1995;197(3): 598–602.

288. Leo ME, Petrou SP, Barrett DM. Transitional cell carcinoma of the kidney with vena caval involvement: report of 3 cases and a review of the literature. *J Urol* 1992;148(2 Pt 1):398–400.

289. Lerner SE, Blute ML, Bergstralh EJ, et al. Analysis of risk factors for progression in patients with pathologically confined prostate cancers after radical retropubic prostatectomy. *J Urol* 1996; 156(1):137–143.

290. Levine E, Collins DL, Horton WA, et al. CT screening of the abdomen in von Hippel-Lindau disease. *Am J Roentgenol* 1982; 139(3):505–510.

291. Levine E, Grantham JJ. Calcified renal stones and cyst calcifications in autosomal dominant polycystic kidney disease: clinical and CT study in 84 patients. *Am J Roentgenol* 1992;159(1):77–81.

292. Levine E, Grantham JJ. High-density renal cysts in autosomal dominant polycystic kidney disease demonstrated by CT. *Radiology* 1985;154(2):477–482.

293. Levine E, Grantham JJ, Slusher SL, et al. CT of acquired cystic kidney disease and renal tumors in long-term dialysis patients. *Am J Roentgenol* 1984;142(1):125–131.

294. Levine E, Huntrakoon M. Computed tomography of renal oncocytoma. *Am J Roentgenol* 1983;141(4):741–746.

295. Levine E, Huntrakoon M. Unilateral renal cystic disease: CT findings. *J Comput Assist Tomogr* 1989;13(2):273–276.

296. Levine E, Lee KR, Weigel JW, et al. Computed tomography in the diagnosis of renal carcinoma complicating Hippel-Lindau syndrome. *Radiology* 1979;130(3):703–706.

297. Levine E, Slusher SL, Grantham JJ, et al. Natural history of acquired renal cystic disease in dialysis patients: a prospective longitudinal CT study. *Am J Roentgenol* 1991;156(3):501–506.

298. Levine JA, Neitlich J, Verga M, et al. Ureteral calculi in patients with flank pain: correlation of plain radiography with unenhanced helical CT. *Radiology* 1997;204(1):27–31.

299. Levine LA, Gburek BM. Acquired cystic disease and renal adenocarcinoma following renal transplantation. *J Urol* 1994;151(1): 129–132.

300. Leyendecker JR, Dodd GD 3rd, Halff GA, et al. Sonographically observed echogenic response during intraoperative radiofrequency ablation of cirrhotic livers: pathologic correlation. *Am J Roentgenol* 2002;178(5):1147–1151.

301. Licht MR, Novick AC, Tubbs RR, et al. Renal oncocytoma: clinical and biological correlates. *J Urol* 1993;150(5 Pt 1):1380–1383.

302. Lingeman JE, Lifshitz DA, Evan AP. Surgical management of urinary lithiasis. In: Walsh PC, Vaughan ED, ed. *Campbell's urology*, Vol 4. Philadelphia: Elsevier Science; 2002:3361–3451.

303. Liu J, Fanning CV. Can renal oncocytomas be distinguished from renal cell carcinoma on fine-needle aspiration specimens? A study of conventional smears in conjunction with ancillary studies. *Cancer* 2001;93(6):390–397.

304. Llach F, Papper S, Massry SG. The clinical spectrum of renal vein thrombosis: acute and chronic. *Am J Med* 1980;69(6):819–827.

305. Lloyd-Thomas HG, Balme RH, Key JJ. Tram-line calcification in renal cortical necrosis. *Br Med J* 1962;5282: 909–911.

306. Lockhart ME, Smith JK, Kenney PJ, et al. Pseudotumorous renal involvement of sarcoidosis. *J Urol* 2001;165(3):895.

307. Lonergan GJ, Rice RR, Suarez ES. Autosomal recessive polycystic kidney disease: radiologic-pathologic correlation. *Radiographics* 2000;20(3):837–855.

308. Lopez-Ben R, Smith JK, Kew CE II, et al. Focal posttransplantation lymphoproliferative disorder at the renal allograft hilum. *Am J Roentgenol* 2000;175(5):1417–1422.

309. Love L, Lind JA Jr, Olson MC. Persistent CT nephrogram: significance in the diagnosis of contrast nephropathy. *Radiology* 1989; 172(1):125–129.

310. Love L, Yedlicka J. Computed tomography of internally calcified renal cysts. *Am J Roentgenol* 1985;145(6):1225–1227.

311. Lowe LH, Isuani BH, Heller RM, et al. Pediatric renal masses: Wilms tumor and beyond. *Radiographics* 2000;20(6):1585–1603.

312. Madewell JE, Goldman SM, Davis CJ Jr, et al. Multilocular cystic nephroma: a radiographic-pathologic correlation of 58 patients. *Radiology* 1983;146(2):309–321.

313. Madowitz JS, Schweiger MJ. Severe anaphylactoid reaction to radiographic contrast media. Recurrences despites premedication with diphenhydramine and prednisone,. JAMA 1979;241(26): 2813–2815.

314. Maki DD, Birnbaum BA, Chakraborty DP, et al. Renal cyst pseudoenhancement: beam-hardening effects on CT numbers. *Radiology* 1999;213(2):468–472.

315. Mallouhi A, Rieger M, Czermak B, et al. Volume-rendered multidetector CT angiography: noninvasive follow-up of patients treated with renal artery stents. *Am J Roentgenol* 2003;180(1): 233–239.

316. Malter IJ, Stanley RJ. The intrathoracic kidney: with a review of the literature. *J Urol* 1972;107(4):538–541.

317. Mandel JS, McLaughlin JK, Schlehofer B, et al. International renal-cell cancer study. IV. Occupation. *IntJ Cancer* 1995;61(5): 601–605.

318. Mann SJ. Captopril renal scans for detecting renal artery stenosis. *Arch Intern Med* 2003;163(5):630; author reply 630–631.

319. Marks WM, Korobkin M, Callen PW, et al. CT diagnosis of tumor thrombosis of the renal vein and inferior vena cava. *Am J Roentgenol* 1978;131(5):843–846.

320. Marotti M, Hricak H, Fritzsche P, et al. Complex and simple renal cysts: comparative evaluation with MR imaging. *Radiology* 1987;162(3):679–684.

321. Martin J, Garcia M, Duran A, et al. Renal vein leiomyosarcoma: a case report and literature review. *Urol Radiol* 1989;11(1):25–29.

322. Martin RS 3rd, Meacham PW, Ditesheim JA, et al. Renal artery aneurysm: selective treatment for hypertension and prevention of rupture. *J Vasc Surg* 1989;9(1):26–34.

323. Matson MA, Cohen EP. Acquired cystic kidney disease: occurrence, prevalence, and renal cancers. *Medicine* (Baltimore) 1990;69(4):217–226.

324. Matsumoto ED, Watumull L, Johnson DB, et al. The radiographic evolution of radio frequency ablated renal tumors. *J Urol* 2004;172(1):45–48.

325. Mayer DP, Baron RL, Pollack HM. Increase in CT attenuation values of parapelvic renal cysts after retrograde pyelography. *Am J Roentgenol* 1982;139(5):991–993.

326. Mayes DC, Fechner RE, Gillenwater JY. Renal liposarcoma. *Am J SurgPathol* 1990;14(3):268–273.

327. McClennan BL. Computed tomography in the diagnosis and staging of renal cell carcinoma. *Semin Urol* 1985;3(2):111–131.

328. McClennan BL, Balfe DM. Oncologic imaging: kidney and ureter. *International Journal of Radiation Oncology, Biology, Physics* 1983;9(11):1683–1704.

329. McCoy JG, Honda H, Reznicek M, et al. Computerized tomography for detection and staging of localized and pathologically defined upper tract urothelial tumors. *J Urol* 1991;146(6):1500–1503.

330. McCullough PA, Wolyn R, Rocher LL, et al. Acute renal failure after coronary intervention: incidence, risk factors, and relationship to mortality. *Am J Med* 1997;103(5):368–375.

331. McDonald JH, McClellan DS. Crossed renal ectopia. *Am J Surg* 1957;93(6):995–1002.

332. McGahan JP, Richards JR, Jones CD, et al. Use of ultrasonography in the patient with acute renal trauma. *J Ultrasound Med* 1999;18(3):207–213.

333. McGahan JP, Rose J, Coates TL, et al. Use of ultrasonography in the patient with acute abdominal trauma. *J Ultrasound Med* 1997;16(10):653–662.

334. McMillin KI, Gross BH. CT demonstration of peripelvic and periureteral non-Hodgkin lymphoma. *Am J Roentgenol* 1985;144(5):945–946.

335. McTavish JD, Jinzaki M, Zou KH, et al. Multi-detector row CT Urography: comparison of strategies for depicting the normal urinary collecting system. *Radiology* 2002;225(3):783–790.

336. Meng MV, Mario LA, McAninch JW. Current treatment and outcomes of perinephric abscesses. *J Urol* 2002;168(4 Pt 1):1337–1340.

337. Merkus JWS, Zeebregts CJAM, Hoitsma AJ, et al. High incidence of arteriovenous fistula after biopsy of kidney allografts. *Br J Surg* 1993;80(3):310–312.

338. Merten GJ, Burgess WP, Gray LV, et al. Prevention of contrast-induced nephropathy with sodium bicarbonate: a randomized controlled trial. *JAMA* 2004;291(19):2328–2334.

339. Mesrobian HG, Kelalis PP, Hrabovsky E, et al. Wilms tumor in horseshoe kidneys: a report from the National Wilms Tumor Study. *J Urol* 1985;133(6):1002–1003.

340. Michaeli J, Mogle P, Perlberg S, et al. Emphysematous pyelonephritis. *J Urol* 1984;131(2):203–208.

341. Middleton WD, Picus Daniel D, Marx MV, et al. Color Doppler sonography of hemodialysis vascular access: comparison with angiography. *Am J Roentgenol* 1989;152:633–639.

342. Miller DL, Choyke PL, Walther MM, et al. Von Hippel-Lindau disease: inadequacy of angiography for identification of renal cancers. *Radiology* 1991;179(3):833–836.

343. Miller FH, Parikh S, Gore RM, et al. Renal manifestations of AIDS. *Radiographics* 1993;13(3):587–596.

344. Mitnick JS, Bosniak MA, Hilton S, et al. Cystic renal disease in tuberous sclerosis. *Radiology* 1983;147(1):85–87.

345. Mitsumori A, Yasui K, Akaki S, et al. Evaluation of crossing vessels in patients with ureteropelvic junction obstruction by means of helical CT. *Radiographics* 2000;20(5):1383–1393.

346. Mizodata Y, Yokota J, Fujimura I, et al. Successful evaluation of pseudoaneurysm formation after blunt renal injury with dual-phase contrast-enhanced helical CT. *Am J Roentgenol* 2001;177(1):136–138.

347. Moore EE, Shackford SR, Pachter HL, et al. Organ injury scaling: spleen, liver, and kidney. *J Trauma* 1989;29(12):1664–1666.

348. Morag B, Rubinstein ZJ, Hertz M, et al. Computed tomography in the diagnosis of renal parapelvic cysts. *J Comput Assist Tomogr* 1983;7(5):833–836.

349. Morales A, Wasan S, Bryniak S. Renal oncocytomas: clinical, radiological and histological features. *J Urol* 1980;123(2):261–264.

350. Morgan DE, Nallamala LK, Kenney PJ, et al. CT cystography: radiographic and clinical predictors of bladder rupture. *Am J Roentgenol* 2000;174(1):89–95.

351. Morgan WR, Nyberg LM Jr. Perinephric and intrarenal abscesses. *Urology* 1985;26(6):529–536.

352. Mosetti MA, Leonardou P, Motohara T, et al. Autosomal dominant polycystic kidney disease: MR imaging evaluation using current techniques. *J Magn Reson Imaging* 2003;18(2):210–215.

353. Mourikis D, Chatziioannou A, Antoniou A, et al. Selective arterial embolization in the management of symptomatic renal angiomyolipomas. *Eur J Radiol* 1999;32(3):153–159.

354. Muller BT, Reiher L, Pfeiffer T, et al. Surgical treatment of renal artery dissection in 25 patients: indications and results. *J Vasc Surg* 2003;37(4):761–768.

355. Murphy DM, Zincke H. Transitional cell carcinoma in the horseshoe kidney: report of 3 cases and review of the literature. *Br J Urol* 1982;54(5):484–485.

356. Murphy KP, Szopinski KT, Cohan RH, et al. Occurrence of adverse reactions to gadolinium-based contrast material and management of patients at increased risk: a survey of the American Society of Neuroradiology Fellowship Directors. *Acad Radiol* 1999;6(11):656–664.

357. Myneni L, Hricak H, Carroll PR. Magnetic resonance imaging of renal carcinoma with extension into the vena cava: staging accuracy and recent advances. *Br J Urol* 1991;68(6):571–578.

358. Nagashima Y, Inayama Y, Kato Y, et al. Pathological and molecular biological aspects of the renal epithelial neoplasms, up-to-date. *Pathol Int* 2004;.54(6):377–386.

359. Narumi Y, Hricak H, Presti JC Jr, et al. MR imaging evaluation of renal cell carcinoma. *Abdom Imaging* 1997;22(2):216–225.

360. Narumi Y, Sato T, Hori S, et al. Squamous cell carcinoma of the uroepithelium: CT evaluation. *Radiology* 1989;173(3)853–856.

361. Nassir A, Jollimore J, Gupta R, et al. Multilocular cystic renal cell carcinoma: a series of 12 cases and review of the literature. *Urology* 2002;60(3):421–427.

362. National Center for Injury Prevention and Control. *Injury fact book 2001–2002*. Atlanta, GA: Centers for Disease Control and Prevention; 2001.

363. Nativ O, Reiman HM, Lieber MM, et al. Treatment of primary squamous cell carcinoma of the upper urinary tract. *Cancer* 1991;68(12):2575–2578.

364. Negru D, Ghiorghiu DC, Reut R, et al. Role of computerized tomography in the diagnosis of transitional cell carcinoma of the upper urinary tract. *Revista medico-chirurgicala a Societatii de Medici si Naturalisti din Iasi* 2003;107(3):613–617.

365. Neumann HP, Bender BU, Berger DP, et al. Prevalence, morphology and biology of renal cell carcinoma in von Hippel-Lindau disease compared to sporadic renal cell carcinoma. *J Urol* 1998;160(4):1248–1254.

366. Neuzillet Y, Lechevallier E, Andre M, et al. Accuracy and clinical role of fine needle percutaneous biopsy with computerized tomography guidance of small (less than 4.0 cm) renal masses. *J Urol* 2004;171(5):1802–1805.

367. Neville H, Ritchey ML, Shamberger RC, et al. The occurrence of Wilms tumor in horseshoe kidneys: a report from the National Wilms Tumor Study Group (NWTSG). *J Pediatr Surg* 2002;37(8):1134–1137.

368. Niall O, Russell J, MacGregor R, et al. A comparison of noncontrast computerized tomography with excretory urography in the assessment of acute flank pain. *J Urol* 1999;161(2):534–537.

369. Nicholson DA. Case report: replacement lipomatosis of the kidney—unusual CT features. *Clin Radiol* 1992;45(1):42–43.

370. Nicolaisen GS, McAninch JW, Marshall GA, et al. Renal trauma: re-evaluation of the indications for radiographic assessment. *J Urol* 1985;133(2):183–187.

371. Nissenkorn I, Bernheim J. Multicentricity in renal cell carcinoma. *J Urol* 1995;153(3 Pt 1):620–622.

372. Nolte-Ernsting CC, Bucker A, Adam GB, et al. Gadolinium-enhanced excretory MR urography after low-dose diuretic injection: comparison with conventional excretory urography. *Radiology* 1998;209(1):147–157.

373. Novick AC. Laparoscopic and partial nephrectomy. *Clin Cancer Res* 2004;10(18 Pt 2):6322S–6327S.

374. Novick AC. Nephron-sparing surgery for renal cell carcinoma. *Annu Rev Med* 2002;53:393–407.

375. Nyman U, Oldbring J, Aspelin P. CT of carcinoma of the renal pelvis. *Acta Radiol* 1992;33(1):31–38.

376. Oesterling JE, Fishman EK, Goldman SM, et al. The management of renal angiomyolipoma. I 1986;135(6):1121–1124.

377. Olazabal A, Velasco M, Martinez A, et al. Emphysematous pyelonephritis. *Urology* 1987;29(1):95–98.

378. Olcott EW, Sommer FG, Napel S. Accuracy of detection and measurement of renal calculi: in vitro comparison of three-dimensional spiral CT, radiography, and nephrotomography. *Radiology* 1997;204(1):19–25.

379. Ozen H, Colowick A, Freiha FS. Incidentally discovered solid renal masses: what are they? *Br J Urol* 1993;72(3):274–276.

380. Pagani JJ. Solid renal mass in the cancer patient: second primary renal cell carcinoma versus renal metastasis. *J Comput Assist Tomogr* 1983;7(3):444–448.

381. Paivansalo M, Lahde S, Hyvarinen S, et al. Renal angiomyolipoma. Ultrasonographic, CT, angiographic, and histologic correlation. *Acta Radiol* 1991;32(3):239–243.

382. Pardalidis NP, Papatsoris AG, Kosmaoglou EV. Endoscopic and laparoscopic treatment of ureteropelvic junction obstruction. *J Urol* 2002;168(5):1937–1940.

383. Parfrey PS, Bear JC, Morgan J, et al. The diagnosis and prognosis of autosomal dominant polycystic kidney disease. *N Engl J Med* 1990;323(16):1085–1090.

384. Parienty RA, Ducellier R, Pradel J, et al. Diagnostic value of CT numbers in pelvocalyceal filling defects. *Radiology* 1982;145(3):743–747.

385. Parienty RA, Pradel J, Imbert MC, et al. Computed tomography of multilocular cystic nephroma. *Radiology* 1981;140(1):135–139.

386. Parienty RA, Pradel J, Parienty I. Cystic renal cancers: CT characteristics. *Radiology* 1985;157(3):741–744.

387. Parker MD, Clark RL. Evolving concepts in the diagnosis of xanthogranulomatous pyelonephritis. *Urol Radiol* 1989;11(1):7–15.

388. Pascal RR. Renal manifestations of extrarenal neoplasms. *Hum Pathol* 1980;11(1):7–17.

389. Perez-Ordonez B, Hamed G, Campbell S, et al. Renal oncocytoma: a clinicopathologic study of 70 cases. *Am J Surg Pathol* 1997;21(8):871–883.

390. Peyromaure M, Thiounn N, Scotte F, et al. Collecting duct carcinoma of the kidney: a clinicopathological study of 9 cases. *J Urol* 2003;170(4 Pt 1):1138–1140.

391. Pfeiffer T, Reiher L, Grabitz K, et al. Reconstruction for renal artery aneurysm: operative techniques and long-term results. *J Vasc Surg* 2003;37(2):293–300.

392. Pickhardt PJ, Lonergan GJ, Davis CJ Jr, et al. From the archives of the AFIP. Infiltrative renal lesions: radiologic-pathologic correlation. Armed Forces Institute of Pathology. *Radiographics* 2000;20(1):215–243.

393. Pickhardt PJ, Siegel CL, McLarney JK. Collecting duct carcinoma of the kidney: are imaging findings suggestive of the diagnosis. *Am J Roentgenol* 2001;176(3):627–633.

394. Pillay K, Lazarus J, Wainwright HC. Association of angiomyolipoma and oncocytoma of the kidney: a case report and review of the literature. *J Clin Pathol* 2003;56(7):544–547.

395. Pitts WR Jr, Muecke EC. Horseshoe kidneys: a 40-year experience. *J Urol* 1975;113(6)743–746.

396. Planz B, George R, Adam G, et al. Computed tomography for detection and staging of transitional cell carcinoma of the upper urinary tract. *Eur Urol* 1995;27(2):146–150.

397. Pode D, Meretik S, Shapiro A, et al. Diagnosis and management of renal angiomyolipoma. *Urology* 1985;25(5):461–467.

398. Ponholzer A, Reiter WJ, Maier U. Organ sparing surgery for giant bilateral renal oncocytoma. *J Urol* 2002;168(6):2531–2532.

399. Povey S, Burley MW, Attwood J, et al. Two loci for tuberous sclerosis: one on 9q34 and one on 16p13. **Ann Hum Genet** 1994;58 (Pt 2):107–127.

400. Pozniak MA, Balison DJ, Lee FT Jr, et al. CT angiography of potential renal transplant donors. *Radiographics* 1998;18(3):565–587.

401. Pozniak MA, Nakada SY. Three-dimensional computed tomographic angiography of a horseshoe kidney with ureteropelvic junction obstruction. *Urology* 1997;49(2):267–268.

402. Preda A, Van Dijk LC, Van Oostaijen JA, et al. Complication rate and diagnostic yield of 515 consecutive ultrasound-guided biopsies of renal allografts and native kidneys using a 14-gauge Biopty gun. *Eur Radiol* 2003;13(3):527–530.

403. Preminger GM, Vieweg J, Leder RA, et al. Urolithiasis: detection and management with unenhanced spiral CT—a urologic perspective. *Radiology* 1998;207(2):308–309.

404. Premkumar A, Lattimer J, Newhouse JH. CT and sonography of advanced urinary tract tuberculosis. *Am J Roentgenol* 1987;148(1):65–69.

405. Pretorius ES, Siegelman ES, Ramchandani P, et al. Renal neoplasms amenable to partial nephrectomy: MR imaging. *Radiology* 1999;212(1):28–34.

406. Quinn MJ, Hartman DS, Friedman AC, et al. Renal oncocytoma: new observations. *Radiology* 1984;153(1):49–53.

407. Raabe NK, Fossa SD, Bjerkehagen B. Carcinoma of the renal pelvis. Experience of 80 cases. *Scand J Urol Nephrol* 1992;26(4):357–361.

408. Rabah D, Soderdahl DW, McAdams PD, et al. Ureteropelvic junction obstruction: does CT angiography allow better selection of therapeutic modalities and better patient outcome? *J Endourol* 2004;18(5):427–430.

409. Radermacher J, Chavan A, Bleck J, et al. Use of Doppler ultrasonography to predict the outcome of therapy for renal-artery stenosis. *N Engl J Med* 2001;344(6):410–417.

410. Rahmouni A, Mathieu D, Berger JF, et al. Fast magnetic resonance imaging in the evaluation of tumoral obstructions of the inferior vena cava. *J Urol* 1992;148(1):14–17.

411. Raj GV, Auge BK, Weizer AZ, et al. Percutaneous management of calculi within horseshoe kidneys. *J Urol* 2003;170(1):48–51.

412. Ramani AP, Desai MM, Steinberg AP, et al. Complications of laparoscopic partial nephrectomy in 200 cases. *J Urol* 2005;173(1):42–47.

413. Raptopoulos V, Kleinman PK, Marks S Jr, et al. Renal fascial pathway: posterior extension of pancreatic effusions within the anterior pararenal space. *Radiology* 1986;158(2):367–374.

414. Raza SA, Chughtai AR, Wahba M, et al. Multislice CT angiography in renal artery stent evaluation: prospective comparison with intra-arterial digital subtraction angiography. *Cardiovasc Intervent Radiol* 2004;27(1):9–15.

415. Reiher L, Grabitz K, Sandmann W. Reconstruction for renal artery aneurysm and its effect on hypertension. *Eur J Vasc Endovasc Surg* 2000;20(5):454–456.

416. Reiman TA, Siegel MJ, Shackelford GD. Wilms tumor in children: abdominal CT and US evaluation. *Radiology* 1986;160(2):501–505.

417. Rendon RA, Kachura JR, Sweet JM, et al. The uncertainty of radio frequency treatment of renal cell carcinoma: findings at immediate and delayed nephrectomy. *J Urol* 2002;167(4):1587–1592.

418. Reznek RH, Mootoosamy I, Webb JA, et al. CT in renal and perirenal lymphoma: a further look. *Clin Radiol* 1990;42(4):233–238.

419. Richie JP, Garnick MB, Seltzer S, et al. Computerized tomography scan for diagnosis and staging of renal cell carcinoma. *J Urol* 1983;129(6):1114–1116.

420. Richter F, Kasabian NG, Irwin RJ Jr, et al. Accuracy of diagnosis by guided biopsy of renal mass lesions classified indeterminate by imaging studies. *Urology* 2000;55(3):348–352.

421. Rigsby CM, Rosenfield AT, Glickman MG, et al. Hemorrhagic focal bacterial nephritis: findings on gray-scale sonography and CT. *Am J Roentgenol* 1986;146(6):1173–1177.

422. Robson CJ, Churchill BM, Anderson W. The results of radical nephrectomy for renal cell carcinoma. *J Urol* 1969;101(3):297–301.

423. Rominger MB, Kenney PJ, Morgan DE, et al. Gadolinium-enhanced MR imaging of renal masses. *Radiographics* 1992:12(6):1097–1116.

424. Romis L, Cindolo L, Patard JJ, et al. Frequency, clinical presentation and evolution of renal oncocytomas: multicentric experience from a European database. *Eur Radiol* 2004;45(1):53–57.

425. Rosenberg ER, Korobkin M, Foster W, et al. The significance of septations in a renal cyst. *Am J Roentgenol* 1985;144(3):593–595.

426. Rosenberg SA, Diamond HD, Jaslowitz B, et al. Lymphosarcoma: a review of 1269 cases. *Medicine* 1961;40:31–84.

427. Rosi P, Selli C, Carini M, et al. Xanthogranulomatous pyelonephritis: clinical experience with 62 cases. *Eur Urol* 1986;12(2):96–100.

428. Roubidoux MA. MR imaging of hemorrhage and iron deposition in the kidney. *Radiographics* 1994;14(5):1033–1044.

429. Roubidoux MA, Dunnick NR, Sostman HD, et al. Renal carcinoma: detection of venous extension with gradient-echo MR imaging. *Radiology* 1992;182(1):269–272.

430. Rouviere O, Lyonnet D, Berger P, et al. Ureteropelvic junction obstruction: use of helical CT for preoperative assessment—comparison with intraarterial angiography. *Radiology* 1999;213(3):668–673.

431. Roy C, Pfleger DD, Tuchmann CM, et al. Emphysematous pyelitis: findings in five patients. *Radiology* 2001;218(3):647–650.

432. Roy-Choudhury SH, Cast JE, Cooksey G, et al. Early experience with percutaneous radiofrequency ablation of small solid renal masses. *Am J Roentgenol* 2003;180(4):1055–1061.

433. Rubin BE. Computed tomography in the evaluation of renal lymphoma. *J Comput Assist Tomogr* 1979;3(6):759–764.

434. Rubin GD. Helical CT of potential living renal donors: toward a greater understanding. *Radiographics* 1998;18(3):601–604.

435. Rubinstein ZJ, Hertz M, Shahin N, et al. Crossed renal ectopia: angiographic findings in six cases. *Am J Roentgenol* 1976;126(5):1035–1038.

436. Rubio Briones J, Regalado Pareja R, Sanchez Martin F, et al. Incidence of tumoural pathology in horseshoe kidneys. *Eur Radiol* 1998;33(2):175–179.

437. Rumancik WM, Bosniak MA, Rosen RJ, et al. Atypical renal and pararenal hamartomas associated with lymphangiomyomatosis. *Am J Roentgenol* 1984;142(5):971–972.

438. Russo P. Renal cell carcinoma: presentation, staging, and surgical treatment. *Semin Oncol* 2000;27(2):160–176.

439. Rybicki FJ, Shu KM, Cibas ES, et al. Percutaneous biopsy of renal masses: sensitivity and negative predictive value stratified by clinical setting and size of masses. *Am J Roentgenol* 2003;180(5):1281–1287.

440. Saito S. Primary renal lymphoma. Case report and review of the literature. *Urol Int* 1996;56(3):192–195.

441. Salem YH, Miller HC. Lymphoma of genitourinary tract. *J Urol* 1994;151(5):1162–1170.

442. Schrier RW, Belz MM, Johnson AM, et al. Repeat imaging for intracranial aneurysms in patients with autosomal dominant polycystic kidney disease with initially negative studies: a prospective ten-year follow-up. *J Am Soc Nephrol* 2004;15(4):1023–1028.

443. Schubert RA, Soldner J, Steiner T, et al. Bilateral renal cell carcinoma in a horseshoe kidney: preoperative assessment with MRI and digital subtraction angiography. *Eur Radiol* 1998;8(9):1694–1697.

444. Schwartz BF, Stoller ML. Complications of retrograde balloon cautery endopyelotomy. *J Urol* 1999;162(5):1594–1598.

445. Scolieri MJ, Paik ML, Brown SL, et al. Limitations of computed tomography in the preoperative staging of upper tract urothelial carcinoma. *Urology* 2000;56(6):930–934.

446. Segal AJ, Spitzer RM. Pseudo thick-walled renal cyst by CT. *Am J Roentgenol* 1979;132(5):827–428.

447. Segawa N, Azuma H, Iwamoto Y, et al. Expandable metallic stent placement for nutcracker phenomenon. *Urology* 1999;53(3):631–633.

448. Segura JW, Kelalis PP, Burke EC. Horseshoe kidney in children. *J Urol* 1972;108(2):333–336.

449. Semelka RC, Hricak H, Stevens SK, et al. Combined gadolinium-enhanced and fat-saturation MR imaging of renal masses. *Radiology* 1991;178(3):803–809.

450. Semelka RC, Hricak H, Tomei E, et al. Obstructive nephropathy: evaluation with dynamic Gd-DTPA-enhanced MR imaging. *Radiology* 1990;175(3):797–803.

451. Semelka RC, Kelekis NL, Burdeny DA, et al. Renal lymphoma: demonstration by MR imaging. *Am J Roentgenol* 1996;166(4):823–827.

452. Semelka RC, Shoenut JP, Kroeker MA, et al. Renal lesions: controlled comparison between CT and 1.5-T MR imaging with nonenhanced and gadolinium-enhanced fat-suppressed spin-echo and breath-hold FLASH techniques. *Radiology* 1992;182(2):425–430.

453. Shanmuganathan K, Mirvis SE, Sover ER. Value of contrast-enhanced CT in detecting active hemorrhage in patients with blunt abdominal or pelvic trauma. *Am J Roentgenol* 1993;161(1):65–69.

454. Sheafor DH, Hertzberg BS, Freed KS, et al. Nonenhanced helical CT and US in the emergency evaluation of patients with renal colic: prospective comparison. *Radiology* 2000;217(3):792–797.

455. Sheinfeld J, Erturk E, Spataro RF, et al. Perinephric abscess: current concepts. *J Urol* 1987;137(2)(February):191–194.

456. Shemesh J, Koren-Morag N, Apter S, et al. Accelerated progression of coronary calcification: four-year follow-up in patients with stable coronary artery disease. *Radiology* 2004;233(1):201–209.

457. Sheth S, Fishman EK. Multi-detector row CT of the kidneys and urinary tract: techniques and applications in the diagnosis of benign diseases. *Radiographics* 2004;24(2):e20.

458. Sheth S, Scatarige JC, Horton KM, et al. Current concepts in the diagnosis and management of renal cell carcinoma: role of multidetector CT and three-dimensional CT. *Radiographics* 2001;21:S237–S254.

459. Shingleton WB, Sewell PE Jr. Percutaneous renal cryoablation of renal tumors in patients with von Hippel-Lindau disease. *J Urol* 2002;167(3):1268–1270.

460. Shirkhoda A. CT findings in hepatosplenic and renal candidiasis. *J Comput Assist Tomogr* 1987;11(5):795–798.

461. Shirkhoda A, Lewis E. Renal sarcoma and sarcomatoid renal cell carcinoma: CT and angiographic features. *Radiology* 1987;162(2):353–357.

462. Shokeir AA, El-Azab M, Mohsen T, et al. Emphysematous pyelonephritis: a 15-year experience with 20 cases. *Urology* 1997;49(3):343–346.

463. Shokeir AA, el-Diasty TA, Ghoneim MA. The nutcracker syndrome: new methods of diagnosis and treatment. *Br J Urol* 1994;74(2):139–143.

464. Si-Hoe CK, Thng CH, Chee SG, et al. Abdominal computed tomography in systemic lupus erythematosus. *Clin Radiol* 1997;52(4):284–289.

465. Sidhu R, Gupta R, Dabra A, et al. Intrathoracic kidney in an adult. *Urol Int* 2001;66(3):174–175.

466. Siegel CL, McDougall EM, Middleton WD, et al. Preoperative assessment of ureteropelvic junction obstruction with endoluminal sonography and helical CT. *Am J Roentgenol* 1997;168(3):623–626.

467. Sise C, Kusaka M, Wetzel LH, et al. Volumetric determination of progression in autosomal dominant polycystic kidney disease by computed tomography. *Kidney Int* 2000;58(6):2492–2501.

468. Slywotzky C, Maya M. Needle tract seeding of transitional cell carcinoma following fine-needle aspiration of a renal mass. *Abdom Imaging* 1994;19(2):174–176.

469. Slywotzky CM, Bosniak MA. Localized cystic disease of the kidney. *Am J Roentgenol* 2001;176(4):843–849.

470. Smith BM, Holcomb GW 3rd, Richie RE, et al. Renal artery dissection. *Ann Surg* 1984;200(2):134–146.

471. Smith PA, Ratner LE, Lynch FC, et al. Role of CT angiography in the preoperative evaluation for laparoscopic nephrectomy. *Radiographics* 1998;18(3):589–601.

472. Smith RC, Rosenfield AT, Choe KA, et al. Acute flank pain: comparison of non-contrast-enhanced CT and intravenous urography. *Radiology* 1995;194(3):789–794.

473. Smith RC, Verga M, Dalrymple N, et al. Acute ureteral obstruction: value of secondary signs of helical unenhanced CT. *Am J Roentgenol* 1996;167(5):1109–1113.

474. Smith RC, Verga M, McCarthy S, et al. Diagnosis of acute flank pain: value of unenhanced helical CT. *Am J Roentgenol* 1996;166(1):97–101.

475. Song JH, Cronan JJ. Percutaneous biopsy in diffuse renal disease: comparison of 18- and 14-gauge automated biopsy devices. *J Vasc Intervent Radiol* 1998;9(4):651–655.

476. Soulen MC, Fishman EK, Goldman SM. Sequelae of acute renal infections: CT evaluation. *Radiology* 1989;173(2):423–426.

477. Soulen MC, Fishman EK, Goldman SM, et al. Bacterial renal infection: role of CT. *Radiology* 1989;171(3):703–707.

478. Srinivas V, Sogani PC, Hajdu SI, et al. Sarcomas of the kidney. *J Urol* 1984;132(1):13–16.

479. Stabile Ianora AA, Scardapane A, Chiumarullo L, et al. Congenital stenosis of ureteropelvic junction: assessment with multislice CT. *Radiol Med* (Torino) 2003;105(4):315–325.

480. Stables DP, Fouche RF, de Villiers van Niekerk JP, et al. Traumatic renal artery occlusion: 21 cases. I 1976;115(3):229–233.

481. Stallone G, Infante B, Manno C, et al. Primary renal lymphoma does exist: case report and review of the literature. *J Nephrol* 2000;13(5):367–372.

482. Steele JR, Sones PJ, Heffner LT Jr. The detection of inferior vena caval thrombosis with computed tomography. *Radiology* 1978; 128(2):385–386.

483. Steiner MS, Goldman SM, Fishman EK, et al. The natural history of renal angiomyolipoma. *J Urol* 1993;150(6):1782–1786.

484. Stoll C, Alembik Y, Dott B, et al. Prenatal detection of internal urinary system's anomalies. A registry-based study. *Eur J Epidemiol* 1995;11(3):283–290.

485. Straiton JA, McMillan A, Morley P. Ultrasound in suspected obstruction complicating renal transplantation. *Br J Radiol* 1989; 62(741):803–806.

486. Strandness DE Jr. Duplex imaging for the detection of renal artery stenosis. *Am J Kidney Dis* 1994;24(4):674–678.

487. Streem SB, Geisinger MA. Prevention and management of hemorrhage associated with cautery wire balloon incision of ureteropelvic junction obstruction. *J Urol* 1995;153:1904–1906.

488. Strife JL, Souza AS, Kirks DR, et al. Multicystic dysplastic kidney in children: US follow-up. *Radiology* 1993,;186(3):785–788.

489. Studer UE, Scherz S, Scheidegger J, et al. Enlargement of regional lymph nodes in renal cell carcinoma is often not due to metastases. *J Urol* 1990;144(2 Pt 1):243–245.

490. Subramanyam BR, Bosniak MA, Horii SC, et al. Replacement lipomatosis of the kidney: diagnosis by computed tomography and sonography. *Radiology* 1983;148(3):791–792.

491. Sugaya K, Ogawa Y, Hatano T, et al. Compensatory renal hypertrophy and changes of renal function following nephrectomy. *Hinyokika Kiyo* 2000;46(4):235–240.

492. Sumi Y, Ozaki Y, Shindoh N, et al. Gallium-67 uptake in Bellini duct carcinoma of the kidney. *Ann Nucl Med* 1999;13(2): 117–120.

493. Sussman S, Cochran ST, Pagani JJ, et al. Hyperdense renal masses: a CT manifestation of hemorrhagic renal cysts. *Radiology* 1984;150(1):207–211.

494. Sussman SK, Gallmann WH, Cohan RH, et al. CT findings in xanthogranulomatous pyelonephritis with coexistent renocolic fistula. *J Comput Assist Tomogr* 1987;11(6):1088–1090.

495. Sussman SK, Goldberg RP, Griscom NT. Milk-of-calcium hydronephrosis in patients with paraplegia and urinary-enteric diversion: CT demonstration. *J Comput Assist Tomogr* 1986;10(2): 257–259.

496. Svane S. Tumor thrombus of the inferior vena cava resulting from renal carcinoma. A report on 12 autopsied cases. *Scand J Urol Nephrol* 1969;3(3):245–256.

497. Sved PD, Gomez P, Nieder AM, et al. Upper tract tumour after radical cystectomy for transitional cell carcinoma of the bladder: incidence and risk factors. *BJU International* 2004;94(6): 785–789.

498. Swartz MA, Karth J, Schneider DT, et al. Renal medullary carcinoma: clinical, pathologic, immunohistochemical, and genetic analysis with pathogenetic implications. *Urology* 2002;60(6): 1083–1089.

499. Szolar DH, Kammerhuber F, Altziebler S, et al. Multiphasic helical CT of the kidney: increased conspicuity for detection and characterization of small (<3-cm) renal masses. *Radiology* 1997;202(1):211–217.

500. Takahashi S, Ueda J, Furukawa T, et al. Renal cell carcinoma: preoperative assessment for enucleative surgery with angiography, CT, and MRI. *J Comput Assist Tomogr* 1996;20(6):863–870.

501. Takao R, Amamoto Y, Matsunaga N, et al. Computed tomography of multicystic kidney. *J Comput Assist Tomogr* 1980;4(4): 548–549.

502. Takebayashi S, Hidai H, Chiba T, et al. Renal cell carcinoma in acquired cystic kidney disease: volume growth rate determined by helical computed tomography. *Am J Kidney Dis* 2000;36(4): 759–766.

503. Takebayashi S, Hidai H, Chiba T, et al. Using helical CT to evaluate renal cell carcinoma in patients undergoing hemodialysis: value of early enhanced images. *Am J Roentgenol* 1999;172(2): 429–433.

504. Takeyama M, Arima M, Sagawa S, et al. Preoperative diagnosis of coincident renal cell carcinoma and renal angiomyolipoma in nontuberous sclerosis. *J Urol* 1982;128(3):579–581.

505. Talner LB, Davidson AJ, Lebowitz RL, et al. Acute pyelonephritis: can we agree on terminology? *Radiology* 1994;192(2):297–305.

506. Tamboli P, Ro JY, Amin MB, et al. Benign tumors and tumor-like lesions of the adult kidney. Part II: benign mesenchymal and mixed neoplasms, and tumor-like lesions. *Adv Anat Pathol* 2000;7(1):47–66.

507. Tang HJ, Li CM, Yen MY, et al. Clinical characteristics of emphysematous pyelonephritis. *J Microbiol Immunol Infect* 2001;34(2): 125–130.

508. Tanimoto A, Yuasa Y, Imai Y, et al. Bladder tumor staging: comparison of conventional and gadolinium-enhanced dynamic MR imaging and CT. *Radiology* 1992;185(3):741–747.

509. Taylor AJ, Cohen EP, Erickson SJ, et al. Renal imaging in long-term dialysis patients: a comparison of CT and sonography. *Am J Roentgenol* 1989;153(4):765–767.

510. Theodorescu D, Witchell S, Connolly J. Chronic adult renal vein thrombosis: two unusual cases and a review of the literature. *Int Urol Nephrol* 1991;23(5):429–435.

511. Thierman D, Haaga JR, Anton P, et al. Renal replacement lipomatosis. *J Comput Assist Tomogr* 1983;7(2):341–343.

512. Thomsen HS. Contrast-medium-induced nephrotoxicity: are all answers in for acetylcysteine? *Eur J Radiol* 2001;11(12):2351–2353.

513. Thornbury JR. Acute renal infections. *Urol Radiol* 1991;12(4): 209–213.

514. Tikkakoski T, Paivansalo M, Alanen A, et al. Radiologic findings in renal oncocytoma. *Acta Radiol* 1991;32(5):363–367.

515. Tomaszewski JE. The pathology of renal tumors. *Semin Roentgenol* 1995;30(2):116–127.

516. Tsuda K, Murakami T, Kim T, et al. Helical CT angiography of living renal donors: comparison with 3D Fourier transformation phase contrast MRA. *J Comput Assist Tomogr* 1998;22(2):186–193.

517. Tsui KH, Shvarts O, Smith RB, et al. Renal cell carcinoma: prognostic significance of incidentally detected tumors. *J Urol* 2000;163(2):426–430.

518. Tsushima Y, Sato N, Ishizaka H, et al. US findings of junctional parenchymal defect of the kidney. *Nippon Igaku Hoshasen Gakkai Zasshi* 1992;52(4):436–442.

519. Tublin ME, Dodd GD 3rd, Verdile VP. Acute renal colic: diagnosis with duplex Doppler US. *Radiology* 1994;193(3):697–701.

520. Tuncali K, vanSonnenberg E, Shankar S, et al. Evaluation of patients referred for percutaneous ablation of renal tumors: importance of a preprocedural diagnosis. *Am J Roentgenol* 2004; 183(3):575–582.

521. Turk IA, Davis JW, Winkelmann B, et al. Laparoscopic dismembered pyeloplasty—-the method of choice in the presence of an enlarged renal pelvis and crossing vessels. *Eur Urol* 2002;42(3): 268–275.

522. Urban BA, Buckley J, Soyer P, et al. CT appearance of transitional cell carcinoma of the renal pelvis: Part 1. Early-stage disease. *Am J Roentgenol* 1997;169(1):157–161.

523. Urban BA, Buckley J, Soyer P, et al. CT appearance of transitional cell carcinoma of the renal pelvis: Part 2. Advanced-stage disease. *Am J Roentgenol* 1997;169(1):163–168.

524. Urban BA, Ratner LE, Fishman EK. Three-dimensional volume-rendered CT angiography of the renal arteries and veins: normal anatomy, variants, and clinical applications. *Radiographics* 2001;21(2):373–386.

525. Urbancic A, Buturovic-Panikvar J. Emergency intra- and perioperative Doppler after kidney transplantation—-a guide for immediate surgical intervention. *Transplant Proc* 2001;33:3320–3321.

526. van Baal JG, Smits NJ, Keeman JN, et al. The evolution of renal angiomyolipomas in patients with tuberous sclerosis. *J Urol* 1994;152(1):35–38.

527. Van Cangh PJ, Wilmart JF, Opsomer RJ, et al. Long-term results and late recurrence after endoureteropyelotomy: a critical analysis of prognostic factors. *J Urol* 1994;151(4):934–937.

528. Varanelli MJ, Coll DM, Levine JA, et al. Relationship between duration of pain and secondary signs of obstruction of the urinary tract on unenhanced helical CT. *Am J Roentgenol* 2001;177(2):325–330.

529. Varma DG, Rojo JR, Thomas R, et al. Computed tomography of xanthogranulomatous pyelonephritis. *J Comput Assist Tomogr* 1985;9(3):241–247.

530. Vas W, Carlin B, Salimi Z, et al. CT diagnosis of emphysematous pyelonephritis. *Comput Radiol* 1985;9(1):37–39.

531. Velasquez G, Glass TA, D'Souza VJ, et al. Multiple oncocytomas and renal carcinoma. *Am J Roentgenol* 1984;142(1):123–124.

532. Verdorfer I, Culig Z, Hobisch A, et al. Characterisation of a collecting duct carcinoma by cytogenetic analysis and comparative genomic hybridisation. *Int J Oncol* 1998;13(3):461–464.

533. Wacksman J, Phipps L. Report of the Multicystic Kidney Registry: preliminary findings. *J Urol* 1993;150(6):1870–1872.

534. Wadsworth DE, McClennan BL, Stanley RJ. CT of the renal mass. *Urol Radiol* 1982;4(2–3):85–94.

535. Wagle DG, Moore RH, Murphy GP. Secondary carcinomas of the kidney. *J Urol* 1975;114(1):30–32.

536. Wagner BJ, Wong-You-Cheong JJ, Davis CJ Jr. Adult renal hamartomas. *Radiographics* 1997;17(1):155–169.

537. Wagner JR, Honig SC, Siroky MB. Non-Hodgkin's lymphoma can mimic renal adenocarcinoma with inferior vena caval involvement. *Urology* 1993;42(6):720–723.

538. Walter C, Kruessell M, Gindele A, et al. Imaging of renal lesions: evaluation of fast MRI and helical CT. *Br J Radiol* 2003;76(910):696–703.

539. Walther MM, Choyke PL, Weiss G, et al. Parenchymal sparing surgery in patients with hereditary renal cell carcinoma. *J Urol* 1995;153(3 Pt 2):913–916.

540. Wan YL, Lee TY, Bullard MJ, et al. Acute gas-producing bacterial renal infection: correlation between imaging findings and clinical outcome. *Radiology* 1996;198(2):433–438.

541. Wan YL, Lo SK, Bullard MJ, et al. Predictors of outcome in emphysematous pyelonephritis. *J Urol* 1998;159(2):369–373.

542. Waters WB, Richie JP. Aggressive surgical approach to renal cell carcinoma: review of 130 cases. *J Urol* 1979;122(3):306–309.

543. Webb JG, Pate GE, Humphries KH, et al. A randomized controlled trial of intravenous N-acetylcysteine for the prevention of contrast-induced nephropathy after cardiac catheterization: lack of effect. *Am Heart J* 2004;148(3):422–429.

544. Weese DL, Applebaum H, Taber P. Mapping intravascular extension of Wilms' tumor with magnetic resonance imaging. *J Pediatr Surg* 1991;26(1):64–67.

545. Wegenke JD, Malek GH, Alter AJ, et al. Acute lobular nephronia. *J Urol* 1986;135(2):343–345.

546. Wei SM, Chen ZD, Zhou M. Intravenous stent placement for treatment of the nutcracker syndrome. *J Urol* 2003;170(5):1934–1935.

547. Weinberger E, Rosenbaum DM, Pendergrass TW. Renal involvement in children with lymphoma: comparison of CT with sonography. *Am J Roentgenol* 1990;155(2):347–349.

548. Welch TJ, LeRoy AJ. Helical and electron beam CT scanning in the evaluation of renal vein involvement in patients with renal cell carcinoma. *J Comput Assist Tomogr* 1997;21(3):467–471.

549. Weyman PJ, McClennan BL, Lee JK, et al. CT of calcified renal masses. *Am J Roentgenol* 1982;138(6):1095–1099.

550. Whittier WL, Korbet SM. Timing of complications in percutaneous renal biopsy. *J Am Soc Nephrol* 2004;15(1):142–147.

551. Wilbur AC, Turk JN, Capek V. Perirenal metastases from lung cancer: CT diagnosis. *J Comput Assist Tomogr* 1992;16(4):589–591.

552. Willmann JK, Roos JE, Platz A, et al. Multidetector CT: detection of active hemorrhage in patients with blunt abdominal trauma. *Am J Roentgenol* 2002;179(2):437–444.

553. Wills JS. Cystic adenocarcinoma of the kidney mimicking multilocular renal cyst. *Urol Radiol* 1983;5(1):51–53.

554. Wise GJ, Silver DA. Fungal infections of the genitourinary system. *J Urol* 1993;149(6):1377–1388.

555. Witz M, Kantarovsky A, Morag B, et al. Renal vein occlusion: a review. *J Urol* 1996;155(4):1173–1179.

556. Wolf JS Jr. Evaluation and management of solid and cystic renal masses. *J Urol* 1998;159(4):1120–1133.

557. Wood BJ, Khan MA, McGovern F, et al. Imaging guided biopsy of renal masses: indications, accuracy and impact on clinical management. *J Urol* 1999;161(5):1470–1474.

558. Yamakado K, Tanaka N, Nakagawa T, et al. Renal angiomyolipoma: relationships between tumor size, aneurysm formation, and rupture. *Radiology* 2002;225(1):78–82.

559. Yamashita Y, Honda S, Nishiharu T, et al. Detection of pseudocapsule of renal cell carcinoma with MR imaging and CT. *Am J Roentgenol* 1996;166(5):1151–1155.

560. Yamashita Y, Takahashi M, Watanabe O, et al. Small renal cell carcinoma: pathologic and radiologic correlation. *Radiology* 1992;184(2):493–498.

561. Yamashita Y, Tang Y, Abe Y, et al. Comparison of ultrafast half-Fourier single-shot turbo spin-echo sequence with turbo spin-echo sequences for T2-weighted imaging of the female pelvis. *J Magn Reson Imaging* 1998;8(6):1207–1212.

562. Yeh BM, Coakley FV, Meng MV, et al. Precaval right renal arteries: prevalence and morphologic associations at spiral CT. *Radiology* 2004;230(2):429–433.

563. Yoder IC, Pfister RC, Lindfors KK, et al. Pyonephrosis: imaging and intervention. *Am J Roentgenol* 1983;141(4):735–740.

564. Young GS, Silverman SG, Kettenbach J, et al. Three-dimensional computed tomography for planning urologic surgery. *Urol Clin North Am* 1998;25(1):103–111.

565. Zagoria RJ, Khatod EG, Chen MY. Abdominal radiography after CT reveals urinary calculi: a method to predict usefulness of abdominal radiography on the basis of size and CT attenuation of calculi. *Am J Roentgenol* 2001;176(5):1117–1122.

566. Zagoria RJ, Wolfman NT, Karstaedt N, et al. CT features of renal cell carcinoma with emphasis on relation to tumor size. *Invest Radiol* 1990;25(3):261–266.

567. Zaontz MR, Pahira JJ, Wolfman M, et al. Acute focal bacterial nephritis: a systematic approach to diagnosis and treatment. *J Urol* 1985;133(5):752–757.

568. Zerres K, Mucher G, Becker J, et al. Prenatal diagnosis of autosomal recessive polycystic kidney disease (ARPKD): molecular genetics, clinical experience, and fetal morphology. *Am J Med Genet* 1998;76(2):137–144.

569. Zirinsky K, Auh YH, Rubenstein WA, et al. CT of the hyperdense renal cyst: sonographic correlation. *Am J Roentgenol* 1984;143(1):151–156.

The Adrenal Glands

19

Suzan M. Goldman   *Philip J. Kenney*

Computed tomography (CT) is the primary diagnostic imaging method for evaluation of adrenal disorders. When optimal CT scanning technique is used, the normal or pathologic adrenal glands can be well visualized in virtually 100% of patients.(2,76,110,176) Large and small masses and hyperplasia can be readily detected when present. With modern CT scanners, imaging of the adrenals can be achieved even in the most emaciated patients, and in patients who are unable to suspend respiration.

The adrenals can be well imaged with axial slices. Most large adrenal masses can be detected with rapid scanning with the 5-mm contiguous slice technique. However, thinner slices (2.5 to 3 mm contiguous) should be made if small lesions are suspected or if initial screening is negative in a patient strongly suspected of having adrenal disease (Fig. 19-1).

The development of helical and multislice CT scanners has allowed even greater reduction in slice thickness without compromising the examination quality or time span. There has been no scientific study of the most appropriate technique for helical CT based on pathologic series, but in clinical practice normal adrenals and adrenal lesions are well demonstrated with the following technique: Slice thickness 2.5 to 3 mm with 1.5- to 3-mm interval through adrenal region, following oral contrast, performed before and after intravenous injection of 100 to 150 mL of low osmolar iodinated contrast. Slices thinner than 2 mm tend to have more noise and have not been shown to be necessary to detect even small lesions. No study has documented an optimal timing of imaging after contrast; lesions can usually be well seen in "routine" or "portal venous phase" images 90 to 120 seconds postinjection, with no diagnostic advantage yet demonstrated for "arterial phase" images at 25 seconds. With a four-slice multislice CT scanner, lesions can be seen using HS mode (pitch 1.5 or "6") with 1.25 mm detectors, 2.5-mm slice thickness with table speed at 7.5 mm/rotation

(1.5 pitch × 1.25 mm detector × four row) or in HQ mode (pitch 0.75 or "3"), 2.5 mm detectors, slice thickness of 2.5 mm with table speed 7.5 mm/rotation (0.75 pitch × 2.5 mm detector × four row). Multislice CT scanners with 16 detectors offer more options, but for adrenal imaging neither the finest resolution nor lowest pitch is necessary, and using less than maximum table speed avoids unacceptable slice profile broadening. Excellent images of the adrenals are obtained with 16-slice multidetector CT with 1.25-mm detectors with pitch 0.938, table speed 18.76 mm/rotation, or 1.375 pitch, table speed 27.5 mm/rotation, or 1.75 and 35 mm/rotation.

Both helical and multislice CT thin slices allow better reformatted images (in sagittal or coronal plane), which sometimes can be useful in determining whether a mass arises from the adrenal, liver, or kidney. Helical and multislice CT also will avoid the potential problem of slice misregistration resulting from erratic breathing by the patient. Although helical CT images have slightly less edge sharpness, daily practice shows no effects on diagnostic accuracy in detecting small lesions.

The normal adrenal glands and most masses can usually be detected without the use of intravenous iodinated contrast material. However, intravenous contrast is useful to characterize the enhancement pattern of masses, improving the ability to make a specific diagnosis. Whereas general screening can be adequately done with postcontrast scans only, performance of pre- and postcontrast scans can be useful for the most accurate differential diagnosis of a mass (e.g., for distinguishing adenoma, myelolipoma, and malignancy). Rapid sequential imaging of the adrenal region after bolus injection of contrast is also helpful in distinguishing adrenal masses from adjacent vascular structures and other organs, such as the kidney, liver, and pancreas (10,14,108). Oral contrast should be used routinely because it helps delineate the gastrointestinal structures of the upper abdomen and it

1311

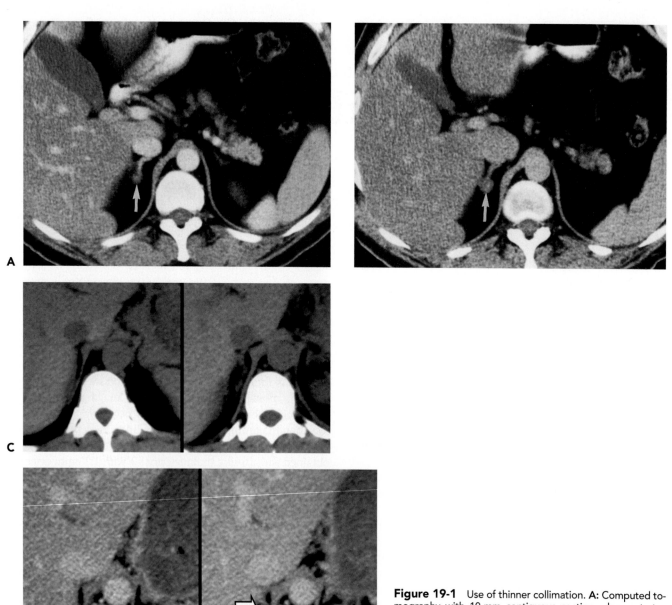

Figure 19-1 Use of thinner collimation. **A:** Computed tomography with 10-mm contiguous sections demonstrates an equivocal right adrenal nodule (*arrow*). **B:** Repeat with contiguous 3-mm sections clearly shows a small nodule (*arrow*). **C:** In another patient with hyperaldosteronism, initial image with 7-mm helical slice technique shows no abnormality. **D:** In the same patient, 3-mm slice technique reveals a small (3-mm) nodule of the medial limb of the right adrenal (*arrow*).

helps avoid mistaking a bowel structure for an adrenal mass (10,147,148).

Great strides have been made in magnetic resonance imaging (MRI) of the abdomen; and with current techniques, the adrenals also can be delineated in nearly all patients with MRI (23,44,111,114,146). Patients who are claustrophobic, are unstable or erratic breathers, exceed the size limits, or have pacemakers cannot be evaluated with MRI. State-of-the-art MRI scanners now produce thin sections (3 to 5 mm) with good spatial resolution and signal-to-noise ratio. The use of respiratory compensation

techniques, or rapid imaging sequences that can be performed during suspended respiration, produce images without significant motion artifacts. Fat-suppression methods allow avoidance of chemical shift artifact that can obscure fine detail on transverse relaxation time (T2)-weighted images. Fat suppression also makes normal adrenals very conspicuous on T2-weighted images: they are bright, in contrast to surrounding retroperitoneal fat. Intravenous contrast agents now available for MRI provide information about enhancement patterns of masses that is similar to that obtained with contrast-enhanced CT. Techniques sensitive to the presence of lipid (such as in phase, out of phase, and fat suppression) are most useful in differentiating between subacute hemorrhage and fat-containing adrenal masses, both of which can appear as high signal lesions on longitudinal relaxation time (T1)-weighted spin echo images.

An MRI evaluation of the adrenals should usually consist of both T1- and T2-weighted images. Either spin echo or gradient refocused echo (GRE) T1-weighted images are acceptable, with rapid GRE T1-weighted images during a breath-hold preferred because they take less time and provide sharper images. T2-weighted images done with fat suppression also provide better margination of the adrenals and masses.

Equipment with higher field strength and stronger gradients allow the acquisition of images with excellent space and time resolution, apart from the ability to achieve thinner and thinner slices with no harm to image quality. The appropriate MRI study protocol of adrenal glands should include: T1-weighted gradient echo sequences in and out of phase in the axial and coronal planes, slice thickness of 3 to 5 mm; T2-weighted TSE sequences with lipid saturation in the axial plane, slice thickness of 3 to 5 mm; and T2-weighted HASTE sequences of the coronal plane, slice thickness of 5 mm. The use of intravenous contrast agents should be limited to cases for which there rests a doubt, (to differentiate solid lesions from hemorrhages), and in cases of pheochromocytoma. The use of such contrast media is not yet established in the diagnosis of adenomas.

T1-weighted GRE images performed with an echo time at which lipid and water protons are in opposed phases are useful, because loss of signal documents the presence of lipid (106). Dynamic serial T1-weighted images obtained after intravenous administration of gadolinium diethylenetriamine penta-acetic acid (DTPA) are used to show enhancement patterns of adrenal masses (94). Whereas axial images are standard, coronal and sagittal images may be useful for displaying anatomic relationships of large adrenal masses, and for detecting the organ of origin of a large mass. Despite the many improvements in MRI that allow more rapid data acquisition, an MRI examination of the adrenals is still a relatively lengthy procedure compared with CT, because several different imaging sequences must be performed.

MRI imaging of the adrenal glands is most useful as an alternative to CT in patients who cannot tolerate intravenous iodinated contrast, in cases of suspected pheochromocytoma and when confirming a diagnosis of hemorrhage.

NORMAL ANATOMY

The adrenal glands are paired retroperitoneal organs that lie in a suprarenal location and are enclosed within the perinephric fascia. They are surrounded by a variable amount of retroperitoneal fat. The right adrenal is usually seen directly superior to the upper pole of the right kidney (Figs. 19-2 and 19-3), with its most caudal portion just anterior to the upper pole. The right adrenal is directly posterior to the inferior vena cava and insinuates between the right lobe of the liver and the right crus of the diaphragm. If there is a paucity of retroperitoneal fat, the right adrenal can be difficult to visualize, but with state-of-the-art CT it is usually recognizable (see Fig. 19-2). The left adrenal may be seen at the same level as the right, but often it is slightly more caudal. It is anteromedial to the upper pole of the left kidney and is usually seen on CT in the same slice as the left kidney. The left adrenal lies lateral to the aorta and the left diaphragmatic crus, and superior to the left renal vein. A portion of the pancreas or the splenic vessels may be immediately anterior to the left adrenal. When performing a dedicated (thin-section) CT of the adrenals, it is important to obtain a sufficient number of images because the adrenals each extend about 2 to 4 cm in the craniocaudal direction and because masses may protrude superiorly or inferiorly, with other slices showing apparently normal adrenal morphology.

The adrenals have a complex three-dimensional shape; this results in a variety of appearances on cross-sectional images. Both glands anatomically have a medial and a lateral limb extending posteriorly from a central ridge. The right adrenal may appear as a linear structure paralleling the diaphragmatic crus (see Fig. 19-2). This appearance is a result of visualization of the medial limb, without recognition of the lateral limb, which is often closely apposed to the liver. With excellent technique, both limbs of the right adrenal can be seen, resulting in an inverted tuning fork shape (see Fig. 19-2). Inverted V, Y, L, and other configurations may be seen (110,176). The left adrenal most often has an inverted V or Y shape, but it may be triangular or have other shapes (110,176) (see Fig. 19-2). Commonly, the adrenals in an individual have a slightly different configuration on each slice (see Fig. 19-3). The most caudal portions of both adrenals may appear as horizontal linear structures. The adrenals have the same shape on axial MRI as on CT (Figs. 19-4 and 19-5). On coronal views, the adrenals usually are seen as inverted V- or Y-shaped structures just superior to the upper poles of the kidneys (see Fig. 19-4).

On precontrast CT, the adrenals have a soft tissue density similar to that of the liver. If very early postcontrast scans are obtained, there is considerable enhancement, which fades quickly to moderate enhancement—slightly less than that of liver (Fig. 19-6). The adrenal cortex and medulla cannot be reliably distinguished by either CT or MRI. On T1-weighted MRI images, the adrenals have a medium signal intensity, similar to that of the liver, somewhat greater than the diaphragmatic crus but much less than the surrounding fat (26,28). On standard T2-weighted images, the adrenals are hypointense to fat and isointense to liver, but they are hyperintense to the crus (see Fig. 19-4). There is less difference between adrenal and fat signal intensities on T2-weighted images, and significant chemical shift artifact may obscure details of the normal adrenals (see Fig. 19-4B). On fat-suppressed T2-weighted images, however, the

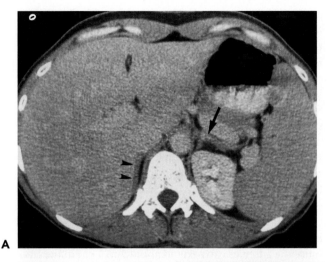

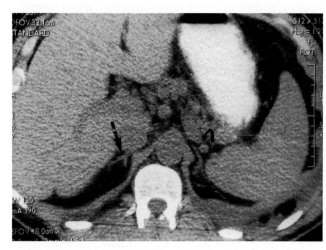

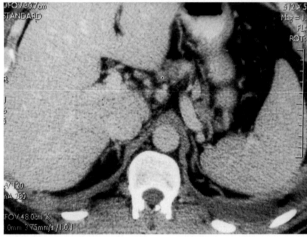

Figure 19-2 Normal adrenal glands on computed tomography. **A:** In this thin patient, the right adrenal (*arrowheads*) appears as a linear structure posterior to the inferior vena cava and the left as an inverted-Y-shaped structure (*arrow*) anterior to the left kidney. **B:** In another patient, a precontrast 3-mm image demonstrates the right adrenal as inverted V (*arrow*) and the left as an inverted Y (*curved arrow*). **C:** After contrast the adrenals can be seen as enhanced.

normal adrenals appear somewhat brighter than liver, and are much brighter than the suppressed fat (see Fig. 19-5). Thus, normal adrenals and small masses are best seen on T1-weighted or fat-suppressed T2-weighted images. The normal adrenals do not demonstrate marked enhancement after intravenous administration of gadolinium compounds. The adrenals can be clearly separated from adjacent vessels because of the signal void phenomenon on spin echo images or flow enhancement on GRE images.

There is considerable variability in the lengths of the limbs. The surface of the normal adrenal glands should be quite smooth, without protruding nodules, and the limbs should have uniform thickness. Although no strict measurements have been standardized, any area thicker than 10 mm is abnormal (76,110). A study of 55 normal patients with neither endocrine or other adrenal disease nor severe nonadrenal disease that might result in hyperplasia reported the mean maximum width of the central portion of the right adrenal on axial CT images to be 0.61 cm with 95th percentile 0.99 cm. The medial limb had mean of 0.28, 95th percentile 0.44, and lateral limb 0.28 and 0.39, respectively. The left adrenal, which sometimes is more triangular, may have slightly larger dimensions. In this study,

mean maximum width of the central portion of left adrenal was 0.79 cm, 95th percentile 1.22, medial limb 0.33 and 0.47, lateral limb 0.30 and 0.48 (169,170). A useful rough estimate of normal size is that the thickness of the gland's limbs should not exceed the thickness of the ipsilateral diaphragmatic crus at the same level. It must be recognized that in the face of stress (as may be seen in severely ill patients), the adrenals may become enlarged in response to physiologically high circulating adrenocorticotropic hormone (ACTH) levels (see Fig. 19-7).

Congenital absence of the adrenal glands is quite rare (130). The vast majority of patients with renal agenesis or ectopy do have an ipsilateral adrenal gland (79,130). However, in such patients the adrenal is in the shape of a flat disc parallel to the spine. On cross-sectional images with CT or MRI, these glands will be seen as linear structures (Fig. 19-8), either in the expected location or slightly more caudal. In contrast, in patients who have had simple nephrectomy, or who have undergone severe renal atrophy, the adrenals have a normal shape (79). There may be greater difficulty evaluating the adrenals in such patients, because removal of the perinephric fascia and the kidneys allows other organs to move adjacent to the adrenals—bowel loops on the right;

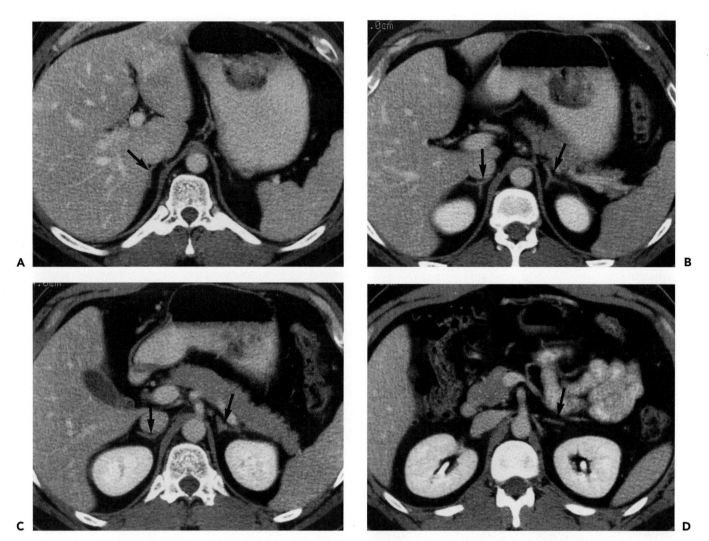

Figure 19-3 Normal adrenal glands on computed tomography. **A, B, C:** Note the different shape of the adrenals (*arrows*) on each sequential section. **D:** The left adrenal ends at the level of the left renal vein.

medial movement of the tail of the pancreas; and bowel loops, splenic vessels, or spleen on the left.

PSEUDOTUMORS

A variety of normal structures may simulate an adrenal mass if meticulous technique is not used (10). The routine use of oral contrast and rapid scanning after bolus intravenous contrast will usually allow these pseudotumors to be distinguished from true adrenal masses. Pseudotumors are less common on the right, because there are fewer adjacent organs. Rarely, the duodenum, stomach or colon may produce a mass-like appearance (148) (Fig. 19-9A). One should be careful when interpreting images of previously splenectomized patients, some of which develop splenosis and the small splenic tissue nodules may mimic tumors when near the adrenal space (Fig. 19-9).

Either an accessory spleen or the presence of the pancreatic tail in an unusual location may produce a rounded structure in the region of the left adrenal (Fig. 19-10). Most often, a splenic lobulation can be seen to connect with the spleen if contiguous slices are done, and both splenic lobulations and accessory spleens will have the same attenuation value as the spleen on pre- and postcontrast scans. Either tortuous or dilated splenic arteries or veins can simulate a left adrenal mass (10,14,108). This is particularly common when portal hypertension is present; the left inferior phrenic vein that passes immediately anterior to the left adrenal may dilate as a collateral pathway from the splenic vein to the left renal vein (14). These vascular pseudotumors can be identified by their tubular nature, which can be recognized on sequential contiguous slices as well as by their bright enhancement after intravenous administration of iodinated contrast medium. Adjacent bowel, particularly a gastric diverticulum (147,154) or redundant gastric fundus

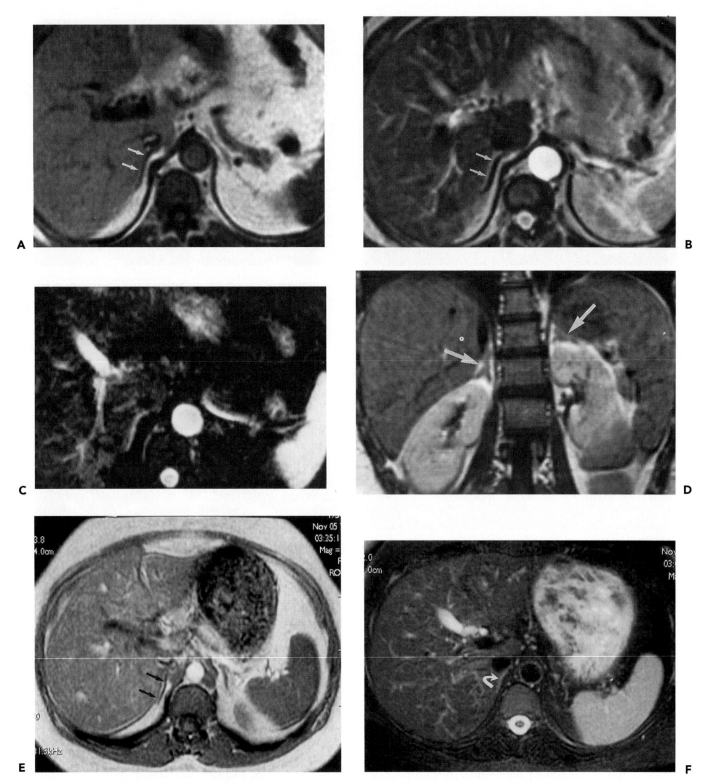

Figure 19-4 Normal adrenal glands on magnetic resonance imaging. **A:** The linear-appearing normal right adrenal *(arrows)* is clearly seen with lower signal than the liver on this longitudinal relaxation time (T1)-weighted gradient refocused echo (GRE) scan (two dimensional fast low-angle shot) (130/4/80 degrees) performed during suspended respiration without fat suppression. **B, C:** On heavily transverse relaxation time (T2)-weighted fat-suppressed, fast spin echo image (????2300/90), the right *(curved arrows)* and left adrenals *(arrow)* are seen free of chemical shift artifact, but the gland appears hyperintense to liver. **D:** Fat-suppressed T1-weighted GRE image (150/4.2/90) after gadolinium diethylene-triamine penta-acetic acid depicts the enhancing right adrenals *(arrow)*. **E:** In another patient, breath-hold GRE T1-weighted image clearly shows linear right adrenal *(arrows)*. **F:** Fat-suppressed T2-weighted image also shows the normal right adrenal *(curved arrow)* well, slightly higher signal than liver.

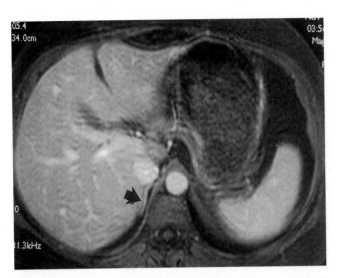

Figure 19-4 (*continued*) **G:** Gadolinium-enhanced breath-hold fat-suppressed T1-weighted GRE shows the enhancing right adrenal (*arrow*).

(Fig. 19-11), and occasionally a small bowel loop, may be misconstrued as a left adrenal mass if there is not adequate oral contrast.

Pseudotumors present less of a difficulty to MRI, partly because of the multiplanar imaging capability and partly because of the ease with which pathologic masses, which have moderate signal intensity, can be distinguished from vessels, which either have signal void on spin echo images or very bright signal on GRE sequences.

PATHOLOGY

A variety of pathologic processes can affect the adrenal glands. Some cause endocrine disorders (functional diseases), either hyperfunction or adrenal insufficiency, and some do not produce biochemical abnormalities. Although both CT and MRI provide accurate depiction of the adrenal morphology, both functional and nonfunctional disorders may produce similar appearances, so correlation of imaging findings with the endocrine status is usually necessary for diagnosis. In patients with biochemical evidence of adrenal hyperfunction, a CT examination is valuable because of its ability to differentiate between a focal mass, hyperplastic glands, and normal adrenals. A pathologic diagnosis can usually be made based on the imaging appearance of an adrenal mass and the clinical history, even when there is no adrenal dysfunction. Thus, other diagnostic studies can be avoided. MRI has diagnostic capabilities equivalent to those of CT. Detection of small masses and documentation of normal adrenal morphology can probably be better done with CT, because of its better spatial resolution. However, MRI has better tissue characterization capabilities, which may be useful in certain circumstances.

The accuracy of CT for diagnosis of adrenal masses has been reported as being better than 90% (2,41,92). With proper technique, masses smaller than 5 mm can be detected. A normal appearance of the adrenal effectively excludes the presence of an adrenal tumor. Because many small adrenal masses are isodense with adrenal tissue, they are detected as focal bulges on the otherwise smooth adrenal surface. Focal enlargement is a more important finding than any measurement. Some small masses have only a minimal attachment to the adrenal, whereas large masses may obliterate the adrenal glands. Inability to visualize a normal adrenal is suggestive of adrenal origin, but extra-adrenal malignant masses can engulf or invade the adrenal. If an adrenal mass becomes very large, its exact site of origin can be difficult to determine, especially on conventional axial and helical CT with thicker slices. Multislice CT allows the performance of thinner slices with isotropic reconstruction in any plane, without loss of image sharpness, becoming as advantageous as multiplanar MRI. Large

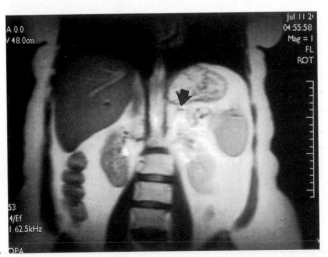

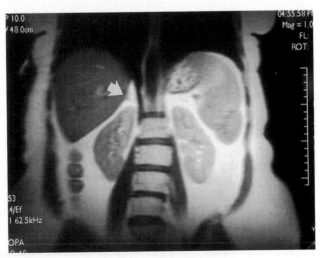

A   B

Figure 19-5 Normal adrenal glands on magnetic resonance imaging. **A:** Coronal breath-hold fast spin echo (1053/32) shows normal left adrenal (*arrow*). **B:** With same technique, normal right adrenal is barely visible (*arrow*). (*continued*)

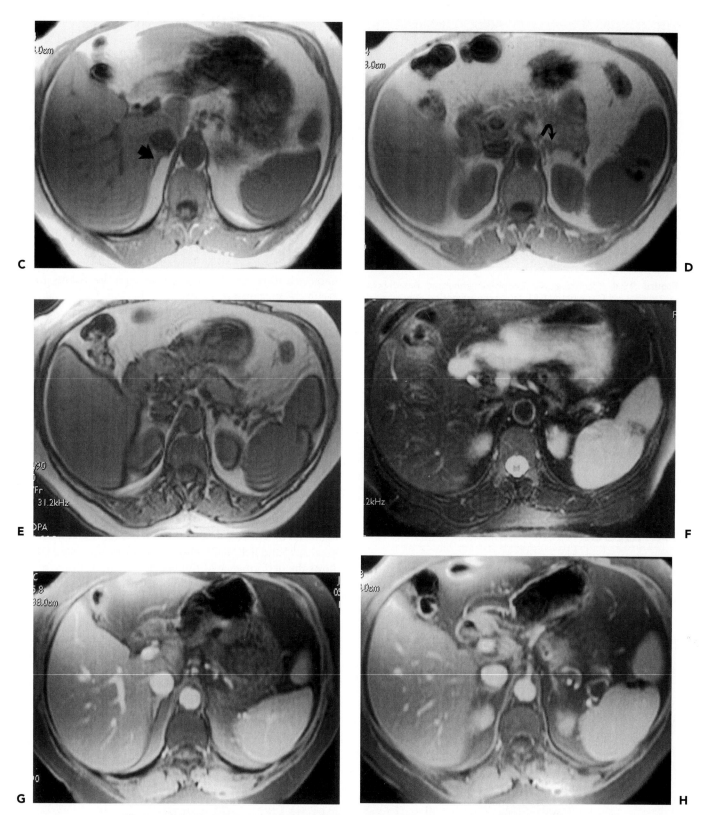

Figure 19-5 *(continued)* **C, D:** Right *(arrow)* and left *(curved arrow)* adrenals are well shown on breath-hold in phase T1-weighted image (150/4.2/90), somewhat less well on the opposed phase image (150/1.8/90) **E:** due to phase shift artifact. **F:** Fat-suppressed T2-weighted image (5217/85/90) also shows both normal adrenals well. **G, H:** Both adrenals are well seen with enhancement evident on fat-suppressed T1-weighted image (200/4.2/90) following intravenous gadolinium diethylene-tri-amine penta-acetic acid.

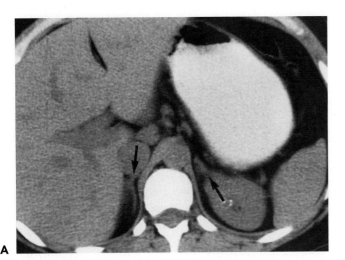

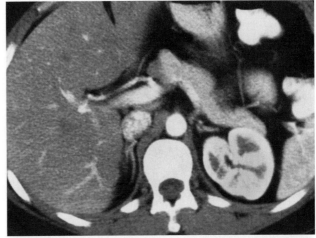

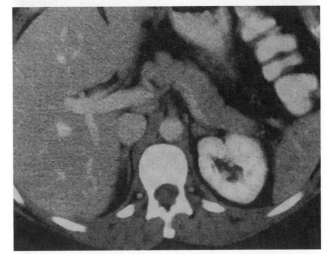

Figure 19-6 Normal adrenal glands: enhancement pattern on helical computed tomography. **A:** Precontrast computed tomography image shows both right and left adrenal glands (*arrows*) have attenuation similar to the diaphragmatic crura. **B:** Immediately following rapid bolus intravenous injection of 125 mL of nonionic iodinated contrast, both adrenals show bright enhancement, brighter than liver or crura. **C:** At 90 seconds after contrast, the enhancement is similar to that of the liver.

hepatic, renal, or retroperitoneal tumors may simulate an adrenal mass. In these cases, demonstration of a normal adrenal gland essentially excludes the possibility that the mass is adrenal in origin. Conversely, the presence of adrenal hyperfunction confirms an adrenal origin. The pattern of displacement of organs likewise may be helpful in determining the center of origin, because most tumors grow centrifugally. Right adrenal masses typically displace the kidney inferiorly, and the inferior vena cava anteriorly, whereas hepatic masses rarely displace the vena cava anteriorly. Computed reconstructions along other orthogonal planes may help in recognizing the origin of such a large mass. On MRI, with multiplanar imaging and better tissue contrast, it is often easier to determine the organ of origin of an upper abdominal mass. The distinction between an adrenal and a renal mass can be achieved by MRI if the upper pole renal cortex is shown to be intact.

Adrenal hyperplasia may result in diffuse thickening of the adrenal glands, but retention of the normal shape (Fig. 19-12). This enlargement is usually smooth, but there may be nodularity. However, bilateral enlargement, whether smooth or nodular, is indicative of hyperplasia. A significant number of patients with clinical and biochemical evidence

of hyperplasia will have normal adrenals with CT (66,128). In part, this is because there may be significant hyperfunction of the adrenal cortex before enough thickening has occurred to be recognizable. Thus, a normal appearance of the adrenals does not exclude hyperplasia. With current CT technique, focal nodules are frequently noted in hyperplastic glands. These are usually smaller than 5 mm, but they can be several centimeters in size (33,159). Adrenal hyperplasia can be diagnosed when there are bilateral nodules or when there is nodularity associated with bilateral adrenal thickening. With primary functional adrenal tumors, the ipsilateral remaining adrenal tissue and contralateral adrenal gland should be normal or atrophic. However, it is not always possible to distinguish an adenoma from a solitary hyperplastic nodule by CT.

Detection of hyperplasia is important in evaluation of patients with functional disorders. Although both MRI and CT can show markedly enlarged glands, CT is preferable because it is better able to detect subtle alterations of adrenal morphology. On MRI, hyperplastic adrenals can be seen to be enlarged, but the signal intensity of the tissue is similar to that of normal adrenal gland. On occasion, the

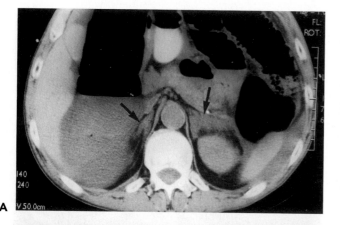

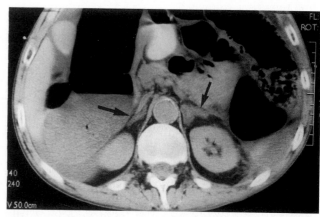

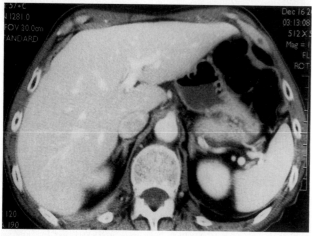

Figure 19-7 Stress-induced adrenal hyperplasia. **A, B:** Both adrenals (*arrows*) show diffuse thickening in this patient presenting with bowel ischemia. **C:** Follow-up study several weeks after successful treatment shows adrenals have returned to normal size.

adrenals are found to be enlarged in patients with no evidence of adrenal dysfunction. These findings are not clinically significant. A number of conditions have been associated with such nonspecific hyperplasia, including acromegaly (100%), hyperthyroidism (40%), aortic aneurysm and dissection (55%), hypertension with arteriosclerosis (16%), diabetes mellitus (3%), and a variety of malignancies (56b,159,170). In some cases, this adrenal enlargement is

a response to physiologic stress (see Fig. 19-7). On imaging, the appearance is indistinguishable from hyperplasia producing adrenal hyperfunction.

The advantages of MRI over axial CT have been questioned since the arrival of helical CT and now multislice CT. Still, MRI has advantages in the evaluation of adrenal pathologies such as pheochromocytoma and hemorrhage. Magnetic susceptibility effect of acute hemorrhage is best demonstrated

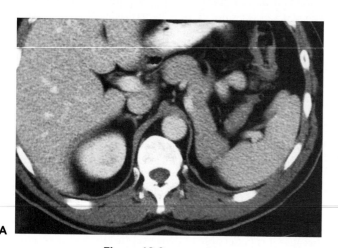

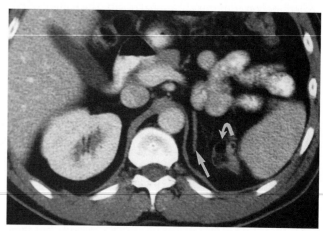

Figure 19-8 Anomalous adrenal in a patient with renal agenesis. **A:** Note the normal right adrenal, and the posteromedial placement of the tail of the pancreas. **B:** More inferiorly, the left adrenal (*arrow*) is seen with a linear configuration; note the medially placed splenic flexure of the colon (*curved arrow*).

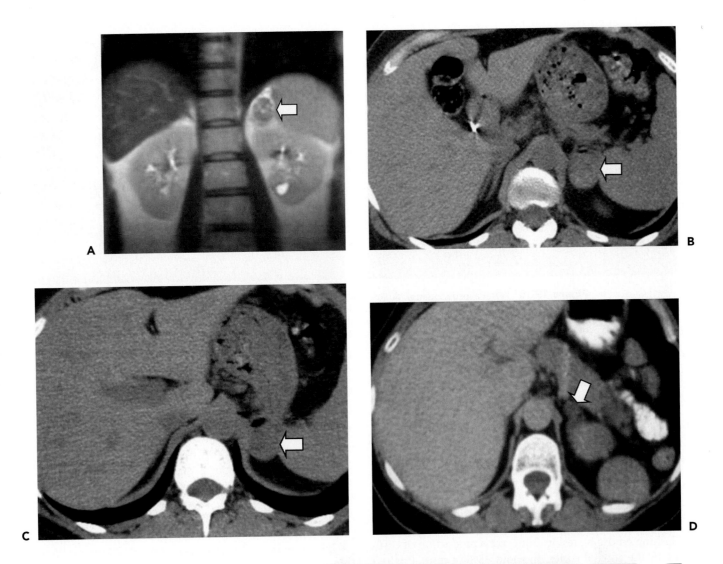

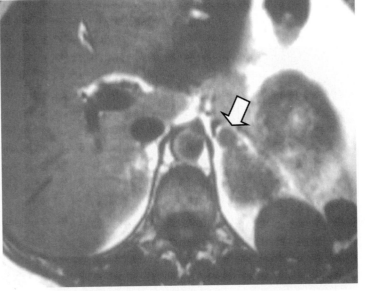

Figure 19-9 Adrenal pseudotumors. **A:** Coronal T2-weighted magnetic resonance imaging shows what appears to be a left suprarenal mass (*arrow*). **B:** On computed tomography (CT) there also appears to be an adrenal mass (*arrow*); note normal right adrenal. **C:** At a more cranial level, gas is seen within the suspicious structure, which is a gastric diverticulum. Splenosis: note on this splenectomized patient being evaluated for possible hyperaldosteronism, a small nodule (*arrow*) near the left adrenal is shown both on (**D**) computed tomography and (**E**) magnetic resonance imaging. This was a splenule.

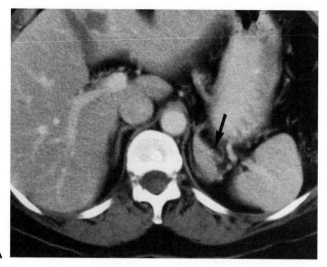
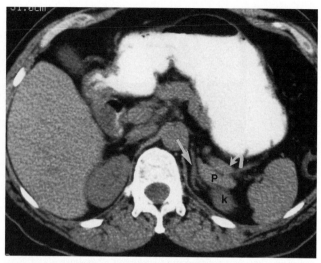

Figure 19-10 Adrenal pseudotumor. **A:** Routine computed tomography performed with 10-mm contiguous slice technique shows a possible left adrenal mass (*arrow*). **B:** Repeat computed tomography with contiguous 3-mm slices shows the normal left adrenal (*arrow*); volume averaging of the tail of the pancreas accounted for the adrenal pseudotumor. P, Pancreas; k, upper pole of left kidney; splenic vein (*curved arrow*).

on GRE images, subacute hematoma can be best seen on T1-weighted GRE or spin echo sequences. Although mature fat can be identified on T1-weighted or fat-suppressed images, other lipid-containing structures are discernible by using opposed phase imaging. MRI has been shown to be comparable with CT in detection of adrenal masses.

CUSHING SYNDROME

Cushing syndrome results from excess production of cortisol by the adrenal cortex. In about 85% of cases, this is a result of excess ACTH production (an ACTH-dependent

disorder) resulting from a pituitary adenoma or hyperplasia (80%), or coming from an ectopic source (74). The dexamethasone suppression test can aid in distinguishing pituitary from ectopic sources of elevated ACTH, because urinary cortisol secretion is not suppressed in cases of ectopic ACTH (74). About 15% of cases of Cushing syndrome are ACTH independent, usually due to a cortical adenoma or adrenal carcinoma, rarely secondary to primary nodular hyperplasia (74,127). Adrenal CT is performed in patients with Cushing syndrome to distinguish ACTH-dependent (hyperplasia) from ACTH-independent (focal mass) disorders, and to determine the location of the focal mass in the latter. In patients with an adenoma or

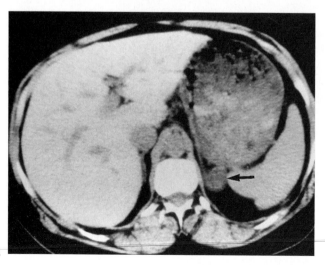
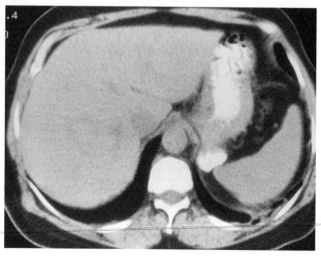

Figure 19-11 Adrenal pseudotumor. **A:** An apparent mass is seen in the region of the left adrenal (*arrow*) on this computed tomography done without oral contrast. **B:** Following oral contrast administration, computed tomography shows the apparent mass was a gastric diverticulum. The normal left adrenal was seen more inferiorly.

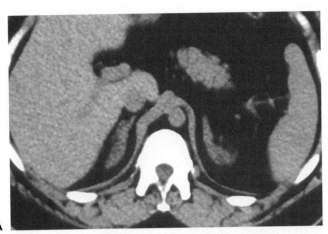
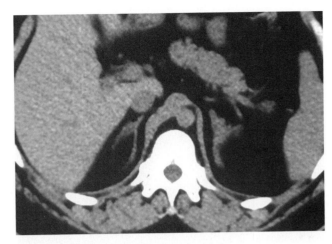

A   B

Figure 19-12 Congenital hyperplasia. **A, B:** Note the irregular, nodular thickening of both adrenal glands on unenhanced computed tomography.

a carcinoma, the remaining ipsilateral and the contralateral adrenals are normal or atrophic. Surgical removal of an adenoma (or of a resectable carcinoma) is curative. Biochemical testing can be extremely useful.

CT is virtually 100% accurate for detection of adrenal adenomas resulting in hypercortisolism (39,41,66). These adenomas are almost always larger than 2 cm at the time of presentation, are usually in the range 2 to 5 cm (36), and are readily seen on CT, especially because these patients have abundant retroperitoneal fat (Figs. 19-13, 19-14). The masses are smooth, round or oval, and relatively

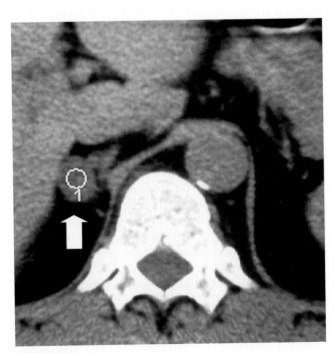

Figure 19-13 Cushing syndrome due to a cortical adenoma. **A:** A small (1.5-cm) round 18 HU attenuation mass is seen in the right adrenal (*arrow*). The left adrenal is atrophic. Surgery confirmed a cortical adenoma.

homogeneous, with little enhancement after intravenous contrast. Most often they have a soft tissue attenuation value, but they may have near water attenuation because of relatively high lipid content (109,144), in addition to the fact that most of them also demonstrate rapid washout at 15 minutes, in excess of 60% from baseline attenuation (87). Calcification can be found in adenomas, although it is rare (80) (Fig. 19-15).

The contralateral adrenal is commonly visibly thinner than normal, indicating atrophy from ACTH suppression (see Fig. 19-14). With these findings, and in the proper clinical setting, no further investigation is needed. It should be noted that no CT characteristic has been reported that distinguishes whether an adenoma produces excess cortisol or aldosterone or whether it is not hyperfunctioning (137).

MRI is equally accurate in patients with cortisol producing adenomas, because of their size (127). Typically, the signal intensity of the adenomas is similar to that of liver on T1-weighted images, and similar or only slightly greater on T2-weighted images (Fig. 19-16) (44,135). After intravenous administration of gadolinium compounds, enhancement is only moderate, it is relatively homogeneous, and it shows significant washout in 10 minutes in most cases (95). The presence of intracellular lipid can be documented by the phase-contrast method (106). Although adrenal adenomas and cysts may have similar attenuation values on CT, they are readily distinguished on MRI, because cysts are very hyperintense on T2-weighted images and do not enhance.

A normal CT or MRI appearance does not exclude hyperplasia (128). In fact, in the absence of a focal mass, a patient with biochemical evidence of hypercortisolism and normal adrenals can confidently be given the diagnosis of hyperplasia as long as exogenous steroid use is excluded. Most often, both adrenals become smoothly thickened due to excess ACTH. The thickening may become massive, especially with ectopic ACTH production (36) (Fig. 19-17).

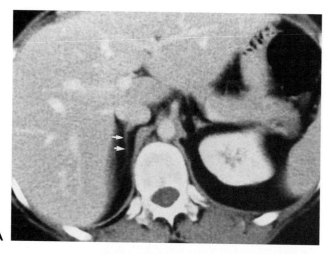
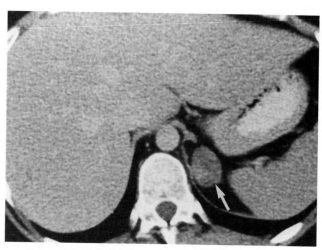

Figure 19-14 Cushing syndrome due to a cortical adenoma. **A:** The right adrenal (*arrows*) is atrophic in this patient with hypercortisolism. **B:** More superiorly, there is a 2.5 × 3 cm left adrenal mass (*arrow*).

Adrenal nodules ranging in size from 6 mm to 7 cm may be seen in 12% to 15% of patients with ACTH-dependent Cushing syndrome (36) (Figs. 19-18, 19-19). Although usually bilateral, such nodules may be unilateral (128). Careful examination usually shows some evidence of bilateral enlargement. Primary pigmented nodular adrenocortical disease is a rare disorder producing Cushing syndrome. It tends to present in younger patients more frequently than the other types of Cushing syndrome. Elevated cortisol is found, with very low ACTH levels. On CT,

multiple bilateral nodules up to 3 cm are typical. Unlike macronodular hyperplasia due to excess ACTH, the cortex between the nodules is atrophic (37,38). On MRI, the nodules are relatively low signal on both T1- and T2-weighted images.

PRIMARY ALDOSTERONISM

Primary aldosteronism (Conn syndrome) results from excess adrenal production of the mineralocorticoid aldosterone. It is characterized by reduced plasma renin levels, hypokalemia, and hypertension. Biochemical tests for the disorder indicate the inability to suppress aldosterone excretion with normal saline infusion, and the lack of change in serum aldosterone levels with postural change (15). As many as 95% of cases result from an autonomous cortical adenoma (aldosteronoma); most of the remaining cases result from primary idiopathic bilateral hyperplasia (132). A few rare cases have been reported to have resulted from bilateral adenomas, unilateral hyperplasia, and adrenal carcinoma (56,160). Correct diagnosis is important, because surgical removal of an aldosteronoma is curative (132), but partial and even bilateral total adrenalectomy commonly fails to cure hypertension in patients with hyperplasia (60).

On CT, aldosteronomas appear as round or oval lesions, similar to other adenomas, but typically smaller than cortisol-producing adenomas (40,51,132,175) (Fig. 19-20). They are rarely larger than 3 cm and are usually in the range 5 to 35 mm with a median size of 16 to 17 mm (Figure 19-21) (40,132). Because of a relatively high lipid content, they often (50%) have an attenuation value similar to that of water (−10 to +10) (Fig. 19-22) (40,109). This propensity for low attenuation should be recognized so that a low-attenuation mass discovered in a patient with documented hyperaldosteronism is not misdiagnosed as a cyst.

Figure 19-15 Atypical adenoma. **A:** Unenhanced computed tomography demonstrates a small right adrenal mass (*arrow*). The lesion is overall of low attenuation, but contains a focus of calcification (*curved arrow*). Calcification is rare in benign adenomas, but does occur.

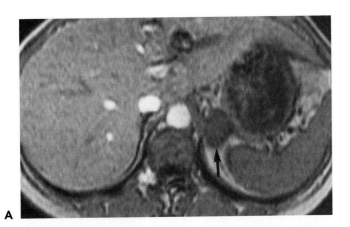

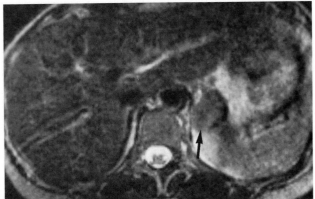

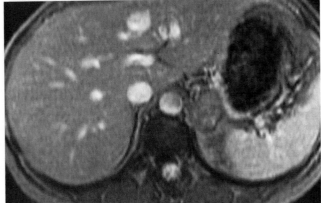

Figure 19-16 Cushing syndrome due to a cortical adenoma. **A:** Longitudinal relaxation time (T1)-weighted gradient refocused echo (144/6/75 degrees) image done during suspended respiration shows a homogeneous 2.2 × 3.2 cm mass in the left adrenal *(arrow)* with signal intensity slightly less than that of liver. **B:** On transverse relaxation time (T2)-weighted image (2000/90), the mass *(arrow)* is lower signal than fat, similar to liver. **C:** Following intravenous administration of gadolinium diethylene-triamine pentaacetic acid. T1-weighted gradient refocused echo scan (144/6/75 degrees) shows only mild enhancement, which rapidly washed out. Surgery confirmed the lesion was a cortical adenoma.

Because aldosteronomas are typically small, they present a greater challenge than cortisol-producing adenomas. Early publications reported a sensitivity of 70% with several false–negative CT images because of inability to detect small aldosteronomas (51,175). With better quality, thin-section CT, a sensitivity of 80% to 90% has been achieved (40,70). With the 5-mm-section technique, false

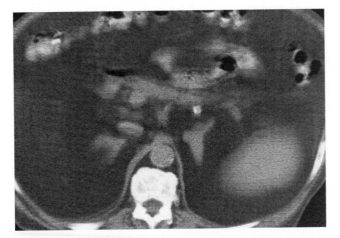

Figure 19-17 Adrenal hyperplasia due to ectopic adrenocorticotropic hormone. This patient with carcinoma of the lung developed hypercortisolism. Computed tomography shows increased retroperitoneal fat and marked, smooth thickening of both adrenals.

negatives are uncommon (12% to 14%) (40,56). No recent report using multislice helical CT has been published regarding accuracy of detection of aldosteronomas. Given the quality of superfine slices possible with this technology, even greater sensitivity may be predicted.

Primary adrenal hyperplasia causing aldosteronism may be micronodular or macronodular. The adrenals may appear normal or diffusely thickened on CT (Fig. 19-23). One or more discrete nodules ranging from 7 to 16 mm may be seen (Fig. 19-24) (132). Diagnostic errors may occur because of a unilateral nodule that simulates an adenoma on CT. Conversely, tiny bilateral nodules that are present in 25% of patients with aldosteronomas (34) may result in an erroneous diagnosis of hyperplasia. An accuracy of 80% for CT showing lack of lateralization (either both glands are normal, both are enlarged, or there are bilateral nodules) has been reported (56). Because of these potential difficulties, adrenal venous sampling still can be useful in certain patients. Some have advocated routine adrenal venous sampling if bilateral nodules are seen on CT (33). When properly performed, biochemical testing of adrenal vein samples can have a diagnostic accuracy of nearly 100% (16,51); however, technical failures are common in inexperienced hands. Misleading information can result if the data are not obtained and interpreted correctly (56). For example, an inadequate sample from the right adrenal vein would result in apparent lateralization to the

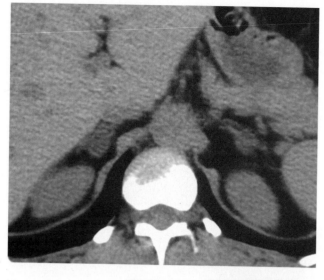

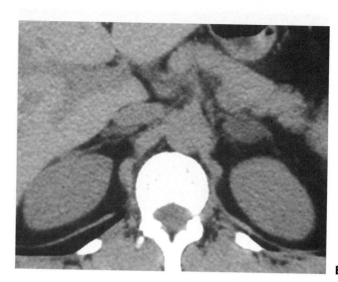

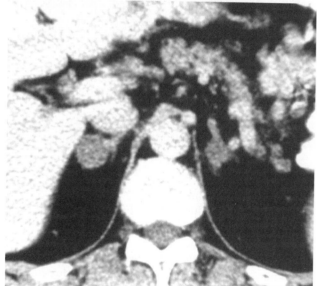

Figure 19-18   Nodular hyperplasia, Cushing disease. **A, B, C:** At several levels, both adrenal glands show multiple focal nodules resulting in bilateral enlargement. (**C** shows different patient from **A** and **B**.)

left adrenal in a case of bilateral hyperplasia. Obtaining both aldosterone and cortisol levels in all blood samples and correlation of venous sampling results with CT will help to avoid such errors.

Although aldosteronomas can be shown with MRI, there is no advantage of MRI over CT (see Fig. 19-21) (70). Because many aldosteronomas are small, the lesser spatial resolution of MRI is a theoretical disadvantage. Aldosteronomas are not distinguishable from other adenomas by any MRI feature. In fact, as with CT, no MRI feature has been described that indicates whether an adenoma is hyperfunctional or nonhyperfunctional (157).

Adrenal CT should be performed first to evaluate a patient with biochemical evidence of primary hyperaldosteronism. Certain biochemical features are strongly indicative of an aldosteronoma (15), and CT should be done to lo-

cate the tumor before surgical removal. If the imaging study is inconclusive, adrenal venous sampling should be done and all diagnostic studies correlated prior to surgery.

ADRENAL CARCINOMA

Adrenal carcinoma is a highly malignant neoplasm that arises in the adrenal cortex. It is rare, with an incidence estimated at two cases per million people (68). It can occur at any age, with a median age of about 40 years (47,69,129). Men and women are affected about equally, although there is a slightly greater propensity for women to have functioning neoplasms (69). About 50% of adrenal carcinomas will produce an endocrine disorder. Cushing syndrome is most common, seen in about 50% of adrenal carcinoma pa-

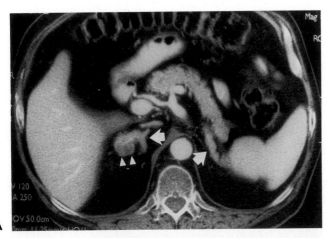
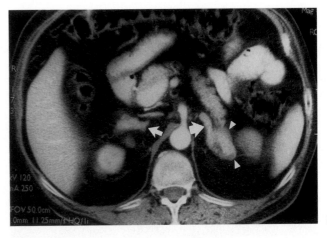

A   B

Figure 19-19 Cushing syndrome due to massive nodular hyperplasia. In this patient with pituitary adenoma, computed tomography reveals marked enlargement of both (**A**) right (*arrow*) and (**B**) left (*arrow*) adrenals consisting of diffuse thickened in addition to focal nodules (*arrowheads*), resulting in odd shapes.

tients, and it accounts for 65% of the functional disorders. Cushing syndrome may be seen alone or in combination with virilization. Virilization alone, feminization, and aldosteronism may be seen, in order of decreasing frequency (11,69,128,160).

Adrenal carcinomas often are very large when first detected. This is especially true of nonfunctioning tumors, which remain clinically silent until very advanced, when they may be discovered because of flank pain, fatigue, palpable mass, or evidence of metastases. Even functioning tumors are usually large when presenting, which may be a result of relatively inefficient production of hormone, so that a very large mass is needed to produce enough functioning hormone to result in a clinical disorder (101). Average size at presentation is 12 cm (range 3 to 30 cm)

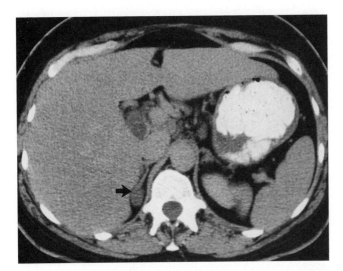

Figure 19-20 Aldosteronoma. Computed tomography image shows a 1-cm mass in the medial limb of the left adrenal (*arrow*). The mass has an attenuation value slightly lower than that of adjacent normal adrenal tissue.

(47,69). Today, however, with the widespread use of imaging, some of these neoplasms are discovered incidentally (69) and are smaller than previously reported. There is frequently concern with an incidentally discovered adrenal mass that the patient may have adrenal carcinoma. Adenomas typically are small, round, or ovoid; homogeneous with less than 10 HU attenuation on precontrast CT and signal drop on opposed phase images on MRI; and show very slow growth (88). Adrenal carcinoma typically shows rapid growth (Fig. 19-25). As a result, if there is concern, a single 6-month follow-up CT can readily distinguish these entities; lack of growth effectively excludes adrenal carcinoma

The histology of adrenocortical carcinoma is variable. It can be difficult to distinguish a well-differentiated carcinoma from an adenoma, even with a resected specimen. Needle biopsy may be nondiagnostic (Fig. 19-28). Correlation of histology with radiologic features, and sometimes biologic behavior, is needed for diagnosis (30). The overall prognosis is very poor, with 5-year survival of 20% to 25% (11,129). However, prognosis is better (42% to 57%) for localized (stage I) adrenal carcinomas if complete surgical resection can be accomplished (11,69,129). Effective chemotherapy is not available.

Adrenal carcinomas are readily detected by CT. Most often they are seen as large, irregularly shaped, heterogeneous masses in the adrenal region (Figs. 19-26 and 19-27). Both right and left are affected equally, with bilateral disease seen in less than 10% (11). At least some central areas of low attenuation are common (47) because of necrosis. Calcification is found in about 40% (80) (see Fig. 19-27). Heterogeneous enhancement after intravenous contrast is typical, with strong enhancement of the periphery and little enhancement centrally (47). The tumors may be poorly marginated, or they may show local invasion. Invasion of the inferior vena cava, liver metastases, and retroperitoneal

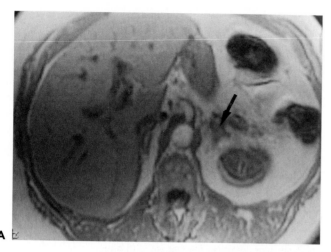

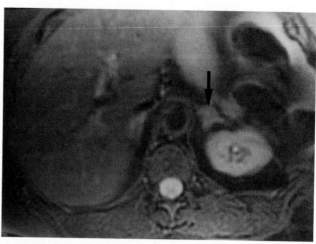

Figure 19-21 Aldosteronoma. **A:** Breath-hold gradient echo longitudinal relaxation time (T1) image in this patient with biochemical hyperaldosteronism shows normal right adrenal and small nodule on left (*arrow*). **B:** Fat-suppressed transverse relaxation time (T2) image shows nodule (*arrow*) is not markedly hyperintense. A 1.2-cm aldosteronoma was resected laparoscopically.

lymph adenopathy may be seen. In general, especially in functioning cases, adrenal carcinomas can be diagnosed by CT, as the features noted previously are clearly different from those of an adenoma or hyperplasia. If an incidental tumor is seen, however, it may be more difficult to discriminate from an adenoma on CT, as both may be less than 5 cm, well circumscribed, and homogeneous (47).

On MRI, adrenal carcinomas are easily seen as large heterogeneous masses in the adrenal bed, with areas isointense or hypointense to liver on T1-weighted images, and isointense or hyperintense to fat on T2-weighted images (23,135,156) (Fig. 19-29). Areas of hemorrhage may result in variable signal intensity dependent on the age of the hemorrhage. With multiplanar capability and the high tis-

sue contrast of T2-weighted images, MRI can be useful to define the adrenal origin and the extent of disease (see Figs. 19-27, 19-29). After injection of gadolinium, bright heterogeneous enhancement is seen (95) (see Fig. 19-29). The high sensitivity of MRI for venous involvement and liver disease make it helpful for staging; venous extension is a poor prognostic sign (135), and if metastases are present, surgery is not indicated. Although poorly differentiated malignant tissue does not contain lipid, more, well-differentiated areas in functioning tumors may show a slight decrease in signal on the opposed phase images, thereby simulating adenoma (145). However, a correct diagnosis can be made confidently when all imaging features are taken into account.

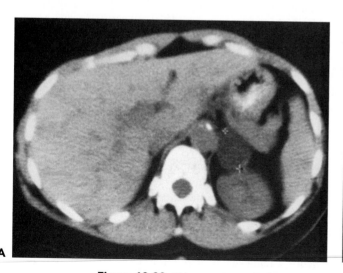

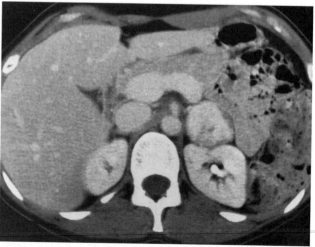

Figure 19-22 Aldosteronomas. **A:** Computed tomography without intravenous contrast in this patient with hyperaldosteronism shows a low-attenuation (−14 HU) mass arising in the left adrenal; although the homogeneous low attenuation simulates a cyst, a 3-cm solid aldosteronoma (with a large lipid component) was resected. **B:** A 4-cm left adrenal mass with marked heterogeneous enhancement is shown in this patient with hyperaldosteronism; surgical resection confirmed aldosteronoma.

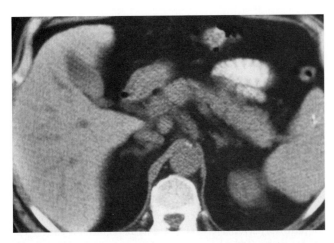

Figure 19-23 Conn syndrome due to adrenal hyperplasia. Computed tomography shows no focal mass; adrenal venous sampling revealed bilateral elevated aldosterone levels.

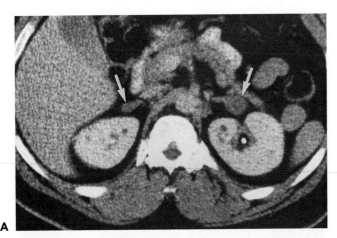

A

B

Figure 19-24 Conn syndrome due to adrenal hyperplasia. **A:** Bilateral nodular enlargement of the adrenals (*arrows*) is shown by computed tomography. **B:** Longitudinal relaxation time (T1)-weighted magnetic resonance image also shows bilateral nodularity (*arrows*). Adrenal venous sampling confirmed bilateral excess aldosterone levels.

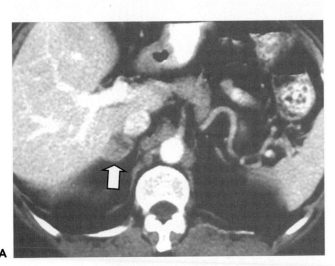

A

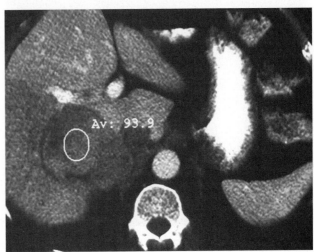

B

Figure 19-25 Adrenal carcinoma with rapid growth. **A:** Initial enhanced computed tomography demonstrated a small right adrenal mass (*arrow*) as an incidental finding. Despite its heterogeneity it was thought most likely an adenoma. **B:** Follow-up 9 months later shows marked increase in size, a feature most worrisome for adrenal carcinoma, which was confirmed pathologically.

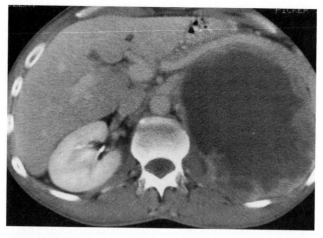

Figure 19-26 Adrenal carcinoma. Contrast-enhanced computed tomography reveals a large mass with low-attenuation center and irregular, nodular, enhancing wall, which displaced the left kidney inferiorly, the spleen superiorly, and the stomach and pancreas anteriorly.

PHEOCHROMOCYTOMA

A pheochromocytoma is a neoplasm of the adrenal medulla that contains chromaffin cells and causes excess catecholamine production. When such a tumor arises outside the adrenal, it is properly labeled a paraganglioma, because such lesions arise from paraganglia, neural crest cell derivatives that are in close proximity to the sympathetic chain. Most are benign, although about 10% are malignant. Sporadic cases are usually unilateral, affecting the right adrenal slightly more frequently; about 5% are bilateral (104) (Fig. 19-30). Most patients are hypertensive. Although paroxysmal hypertensive episodes, including symptomatic hypertensive crises are considered classic, 15% have sustained hypertension without paroxysms (104). Between paroxysmal episodes, some patients are normotensive and others have sustained hypertension (104). The increased catecholamine production is usually reflected by

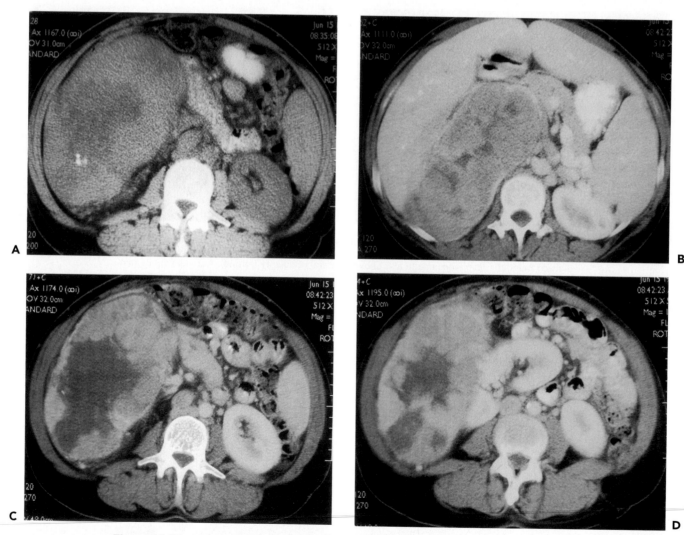

Figure 19-27 Adrenal carcinoma. **A:** Precontrast computed tomography shows a large heterogeneous right adrenal mass containing a small amount of calcification. **B, C:** The mass shows moderate, heterogeneous enhancement after contrast with central necrosis. **D:** The mass is intimately associated with the displaced kidney, unclear on computed tomography whether of renal or adrenal origin. (*continued*)

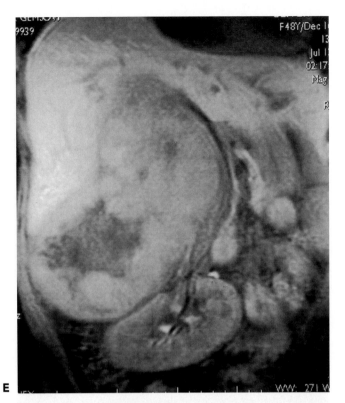

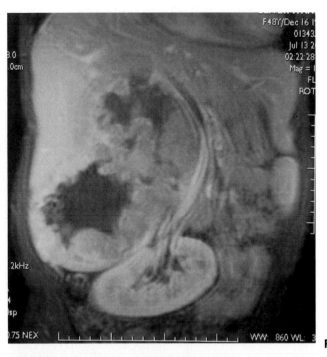

E

F

Figure 19-27 (*continued*) Magnetic resonance image also shows the mass to be heterogeneously enhancing, but (**E**) precontrast and (**F**) postcontrast magnetic resonance imaging coronal longitudinal relaxation time (T1)-weighted breath-hold gradient refocused echo images show the mass is separate from both liver and kidney thus most likely adrenal carcinoma, confirmed at surgery.

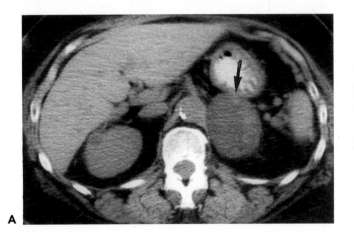

A

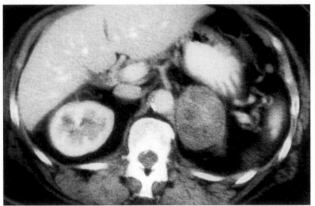

B

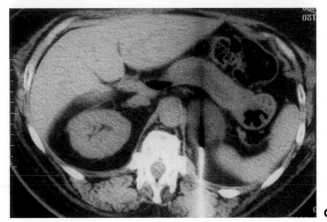

C

Figure 19-28 Adrenal carcinoma. **A:** This patient presented with abdominal pain but was found to be hypertensive. Unenhanced computed tomography reveals 5 (6 cm left adrenal mass [*arrow*], attenuation 21 HU. **B:** Enhanced scan shows moderate heterogeneous enhancement. **C:** Percutaneous biopsy was performed, but report was "Adrenal cortical neoplasm, nonspecific." The mass was resected with final pathology adrenal carcinoma.

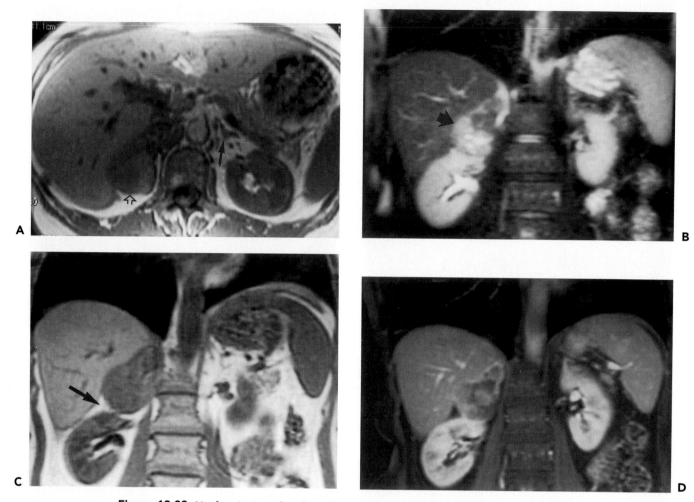

Figure 19-29 Nonfunctioning adrenal carcinoma. Patient was referred for what was thought on outside computed tomography to be a renal mass; she had no endocrine signs or symptoms. **A:** longitudinal relaxation time (T1)-weighted gradient refocused echo sequence shows an irregularly shaped slightly heterogeneous 4.5 × 5.0 cm right adrenal mass (*open arrow*); note the normal left adrenal (*arrow*). **B:** Coronal breath-hold transverse relaxation time (T2)-weighted (HASTE) image shows the heterogeneously hyperintense mass (*arrow*) indents but is separate from the right kidney. **C:** The suprarenal origin is very clear on coronal breathhold T1 (*arrow*). **D:** Following intravenous administration of gadolinium diethylene-triamine penta-acetic acid (150/6/70 degrees 7), there is heterogeneous enhancement.

elevated serum or urinary catecholamine levels, or by urine vanillylmandelic acid (VMA) or metanephrine levels. There are more false–negative results with VMA than metanephrines. In most cases, diagnosis of pheochromocytoma can be established with biochemical testing, especially if the plasma catecholamine levels are markedly elevated (>2,000 pg/mL) (16). However, biochemical tests are expensive, time consuming, and fraught with difficulty because such factors as episodic catecholamine production, concurrent medication, stress, inadequate urine collection for 24-hour samples, and other factors can contribute to both false–positive and false–negative results for every known test. Detection and localization are important because surgical resection is curative, and because there is no effective medical therapy. Unrecognized and untreated pheochromocytoma often results in untimely death resulting from complications of surgery or owing to long-term

complications such as myocardial infarction or cerebral and renal vascular disease (142). Thus, imaging can play an important role in evaluation of patients suspected of pheochromocytoma.

Pheochromocytoma is found in less than 1% of the hypertensive population and in 0.3% of autopsies (142). Clinical signs suggestive of the diagnosis include labile hypertension, including paroxysms of hypertension and tachycardia, headache, palpitation, diaphoresis, pallor, and weight loss (142). There is an increased likelihood of pheochromocytoma in patients with neurofibromatosis, von Hippel-Lindau disease, and multiple endocrine neoplasia (MEN) syndromes (50% in MEN 2 and 90% in MEN 2b). In such syndromes, and in children, multiple or bilateral cases are more likely. In MEN 2b, bilateral tumors are so common that bilateral adrenalectomy is recommended because lesions may recur after unilateral surgery (16,73) (Fig. 19-31).

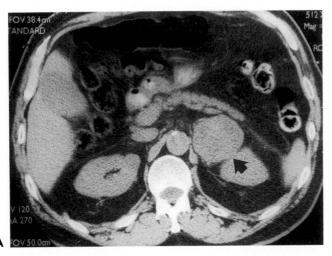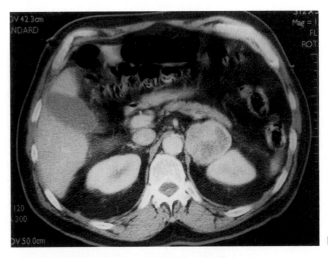

Figure 19-30 Pheochromocytoma. This patient developed malignant hypertension during a surgical procedure, stimulating evaluation. **A:** Precontrast computed tomography shows a 5 × 6 cm left adrenal mass (*arrow*), attenuation is that of soft tissue, 27 HU. **B:** The mass shows heterogeneous enhancement after intravenous contrast.

Although 90% of pheochromocytomas arise in the adrenal, up to 10% are extra-adrenal (Figs. 19-31 to 19-33), with many such lesions (7%) in the infrarenal portion of the retroperitoneum, arising in the organ of Zuckerkandl (63) (see Fig. 19-33). Paragangliomas can be single or multiple, and they may have greater malignant potential (63). Paragangliomas also can be found in the neck, the mediastinum, and the wall of the urinary bladder. The latter patients can present with a distinct clinical picture of headache, diaphoresis, and hypertension related to a distended bladder, or to urination.

Pheochromocytomas are usually larger than 3 cm at presentation and invariably should be identified by CT (173). If small, the tumors are round and have homogeneous soft tissue–attenuation values (see Figs. 19-30 and 19-34). Because pheochromocytomas are hypervascular neoplasms,

they have a propensity to undergo hemorrhagic necrosis even when benign, accounting for the central low attenuation seen in large neoplasms (Figs. 19-35 and 19-36). Central necrosis may be so extensive as to simulate a cyst (20,42). Calcification is uncommon; when present, it may have an eggshell pattern (32,59,78). After intravenous administration of iodinated contrast medium, pheochromocytomas exhibit heterogeneous enhancement, a pattern indistinguishable from that of a malignant adrenal neoplasm. Correlation with biochemical function is required to establish the correct diagnosis.

Because pheochromocytomas are large, they can be detected even with unenhanced CT (133). Some concern has been raised about the use of intravenous contrast in patients with pheochromocytoma. Plasma catecholamine levels can be raised by intravenous injection of iodinated

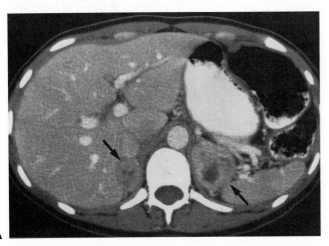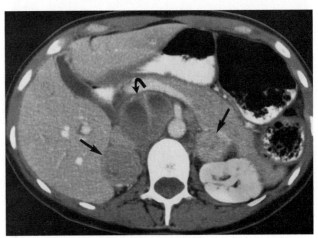

Figure 19-31 Multiple pheochromocytomas in multiple endocrine neoplasia 2b. **A:** Computed tomography shows bilateral heterogeneous adrenal tumors (*arrows*). **B:** At a more inferior level, additional bilateral adrenal tumors (*arrows*) are seen, as well as an extra-adrenal lesion (*curved arrow*).

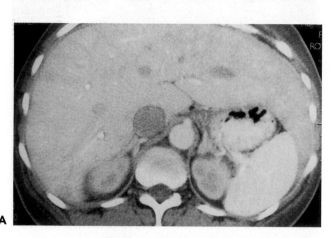

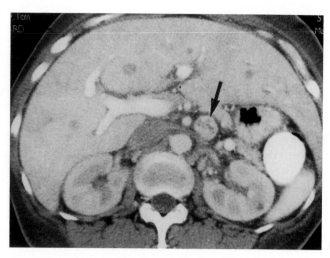

Figure 19-32 Paraganglioma. **A:** Note the adrenals are normal in this hypertensive woman with end stage renal disease. **B:** A 1.8-cm heterogeneous brightly enhancing retroperitoneal mass (*arrow*) is present. Paraganglioma was confirmed by surgical resection.

contrast medium, but symptomatic blood pressure elevations do not usually result (133). Only if a patient has known hypertensive episodes and has not had adequate pharmacologic adrenergic blockade is it necessary to avoid contrast. Contrast is especially useful for detection of extraadrenal lesions. Although paragangliomas can usually be identified on CT (see Fig. 19-32), they have a nonspecific appearance. The CT features of malignant paragangliomas in particular overlap with those of other retroperitoneal malignancies (63). Radionuclide metaiodobenzylguanidine (MIBG) scintigraphy can be useful to document whether a retroperitoneal mass is in fact a paraganglioma (63,131). Another method used in cases of a suspected

paraganglioma is dosage of catecholamines. The presence of high levels of norepinephrine alone indicates that the suspected mass is more likely a paraganglioma. However, the presence of both epinephrine and norepinephrine is highly suggestive of a pheochromocytoma in the adrenal.

Pheochromocytomas have a rather characteristic appearance on MRI (44,53,135). Because they are several centimeters in diameter, they are readily detected, with a sensitivity of 100% in one report (149). When small, they usually are homogeneous and isointense to muscle, hypointense to liver on T1-weighted images, and markedly hyperintense to fat on T2-weighted images (44,165) (Figs. 19-37 and 19-38). As pheochromocytomas grow and develop central necrosis,

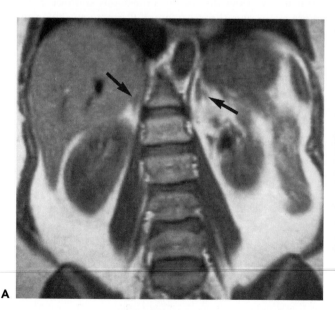

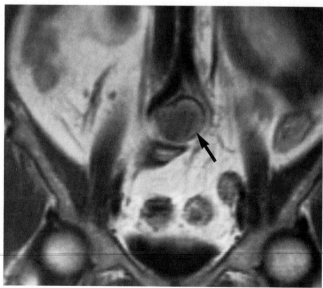

Figure 19-33 Organ of Zuckerkandl paraganglioma. **A:** Coronal longitudinal relaxation time (T1)-weighted image (500/20) shows the adrenals (*arrows*) are normal. **B:** A mass is present at the aortic bifurcation (*arrow*).

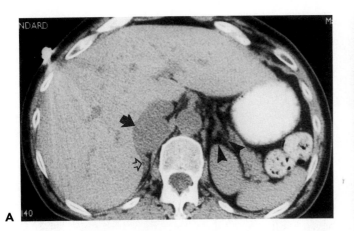

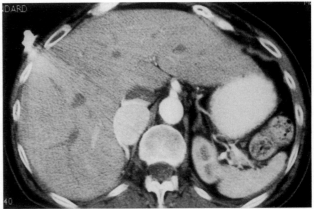

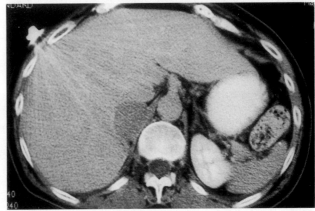

Figure 19-34 Pheochromocytoma. **A:** Unenhanced computed to-mography in this patient with episodic hypertension shows homogeneous 4-cm right adrenal mass (*arrow*); note remaining normal portion of right adrenal (*open arrow*), and normal left adrenal (*arrowheads*). Attenuation was 21 HU. **B:** Corticomedullary phase image after intravenous contrast show striking homogeneous enhancement of the mass, 150 HU. **C:** On 15-minute delay, the attenuation fell to 53 HU. A benign pheochromocytoma was resected after positive biochemical evaluation.

some central areas may be hyperintense on both T1- and T2-weighted images (138) (see Fig. 19-35). MR findings may enable characterization of pheochromocytomas because the signal intensity of these tumors is sometimes very high on T2-weighted images. Such a high signal intensity, which is probably caused by the presence of a cystic component, may be especially useful for extra-adrenal tumors. If present, it can also help distinguish a pheochromocytoma from an adrenal adenoma (27,93).

Exuberant, persistent enhancement after intravenous gadolinium is typical (95,165) (see Fig. 19-38). Because no lipid is found in pheochromocytoma, there is no decrease in signal on opposed phase images. Paragangliomas have similar distinctive imaging characteristics; as a result, MRI is superior to CT for diagnosis of paragangliomas (131), and nearly as sensitive as MIBG (165). Because most such tumors lie in the adrenal or retroperitoneum, sagittal or coronal MRI can quickly and effectively show the area of abnormality (138) (see Figs. 19-35, 19-37, 19-38).

Because the prevalence of pheochromocytoma/paraganglioma is low, no imaging should be performed unless there is some clinical or biochemical evidence of its existence. Either CT or MRI can effectively detect or exclude an adrenal pheochromocytoma. If adrenal CT or MRI is negative, no further imaging should be performed without strong biochemical findings. If there is strong clinical or

biochemical evidence, imaging of the entire retroperitoneum as well as the adrenals should be performed; either CT or MRI can be used, although MRI may be preferred because of greater specificity and less concern about contrast effects. Biopsy of a mass suspected to be a pheochromocytoma is not recommended, especially if adequate hypertensive control has not been achieved, because several episodes of severe hemorrhage and even death have resulted following percutaneous biopsy (21,102). MIBG has both high sensitivity and high specificity, and it can detect a paraganglioma in any part of the body (49). However, it is an expensive test that requires up to 72 hours to complete and is not widely available. Furthermore, it does not provide sufficient anatomic detail for surgical planning. It is most useful in evaluating patients with a strong clinical suspicion and in whom CT or MRI is normal or equivocal, or for follow-up of malignant lesions.

The follow-up for these patients should be very judicious, and information on clinical presentations and surgical data should be included and taken into account during analysis of examination results, whether from a CT or from an MR. The presence of hypertension in this group of patients is not always indicative of persistence or recurrence of the disease. Other causes of hypertension should be evaluated, such as renal changes resulting from chronic disease. Surgical materials such as Surgicell (Ethicon, Inc.,

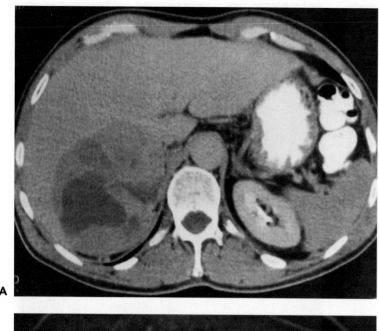

A

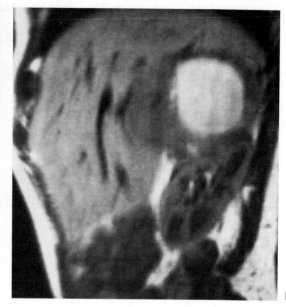

B

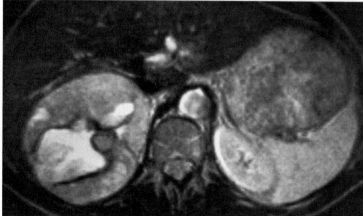

C

Figure 19-35 Pheochromocytoma. **A:** Contrast computed tomography shows a 10-cm right suprarenal mass with marked heterogeneity. **B:** Sagittal longitudinal relaxation time (T1)-weighted image (366/20) show the mass is clearly separate from the kidney, as the renal cortex is intact. Note the areas with signal as intense as fat that correspond to the low-attenuation areas on computed tomography, probably representing hemorrhage. **C:** Transverse relaxation time (T2)-weighted magnetic resonance imaging (1800/80) shows most of the mass is more intense than liver, similar to fat, but the hemorrhagic areas are more intense than fat.

Somerville, NJ) are frequently applied and may present as a "mass" occupying perhaps the space previously taken by the gland. This can lead to misinterpretations of exam results (Fig. 19-39).

NONHYPERFUNCTIONING NEOPLASMS

Nonhyperfunctioning adrenal neoplasms are clinically silent until they become very large, although they may present with pain if they hemorrhage. Currently, most such masses are found incidentally on studies performed for other reasons. About 30% of all adrenal masses are incidentally detected by CT (1). An adrenal mass is seen in about 4% of all abdominal CT scans, with one third being serendipitous findings; the remainder are either metastases in patients with known malignancies, or they are functioning lesions (1). Most incidental adrenal masses are benign and of no clinical significance, especially in patients with no known malignancy. In two large series, only 6.7% and

9% of serendipitous adrenal masses were subsequently proved malignant (3,50). Although historically size has been considered an important factor, with larger tumors having a greater likelihood of malignancy, size is an imperfect criterion. Although malignant neoplasms were all larger than 6.5 cm in one study (3) and although most benign masses are less than 5 cm (1,24), there is considerable overlap. Most incidental masses greater than 5 cm are still benign in patients with no history of malignancy (82), and lesions as small as 1 cm may be metastases (85). Thus, it is imperative to use imaging features other than size to make a diagnosis.

NONHYPERFUNCTIONING ADENOMAS

Adrenal adenomas that do not produce clinically significant excess hormones are not infrequent, being found in some 2% to 8% of autopsies (1,65) and in 1% to 2% of abdominal CT scans (1,7,55). They are commonly

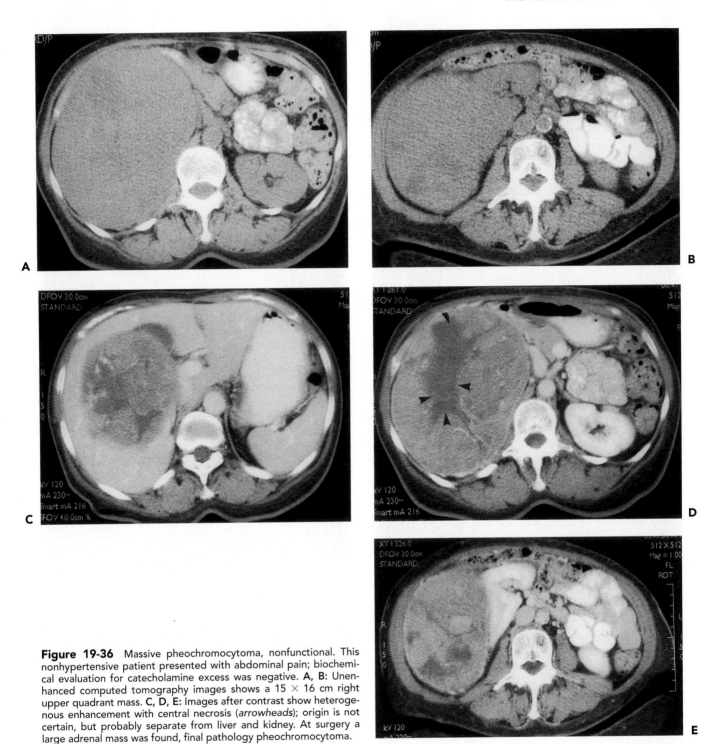

Figure 19-36 Massive pheochromocytoma, nonfunctional. This nonhypertensive patient presented with abdominal pain; biochemical evaluation for catecholamine excess was negative. **A, B:** Unenhanced computed tomography images shows a 15 × 16 cm right upper quadrant mass. **C, D, E:** Images after contrast show heterogenous enhancement with central necrosis (*arrowheads*); origin is not certain, but probably separate from liver and kidney. At surgery a large adrenal mass was found, final pathology pheochromocytoma.

unilateral, although, seldom, bilateral adenomas do occur (Fig. 19-40). Although nonhyperfunctioning adenomas may be 6 cm or larger (85), most are 3 cm or less, and only 5% exceed 5 cm (3). The incidence is slightly higher in diabetic (16%) and hypertensive patients (12%) (85). Because of the fact that they do function, they are "warm nodules" on adrenal scintigrams. Calcification may be present (80,107)

Nonhyperfunctioning adenomas have a CT appearance indistinguishable from other adenomas, except that contralateral atrophy is not present. They are smooth, round or oval, with a well-defined margin. These adenomas are usually homogeneous without a perceptible wall on noncontrast scans.

CT densitometry can be used to accurately differentiate benign from malignant adrenal masses. Lee et al. (97) reported the use of nonenhanced CT attenuation values for the characterization of adrenal masses where most adenomas had attenuation values lower than those of malignant

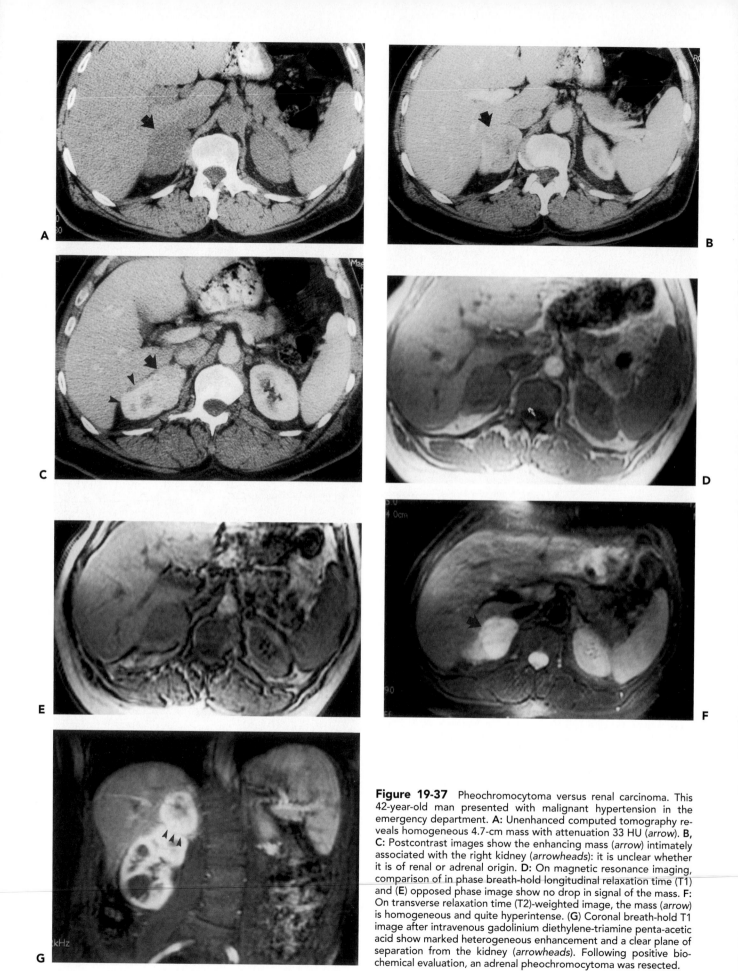

Figure 19-37 Pheochromocytoma versus renal carcinoma. This 42-year-old man presented with malignant hypertension in the emergency department. **A:** Unenhanced computed tomography reveals homogeneous 4.7-cm mass with attenuation 33 HU (*arrow*). **B, C:** Postcontrast images show the enhancing mass (*arrow*) intimately associated with the right kidney (*arrowheads*): it is unclear whether it is of renal or adrenal origin. **D:** On magnetic resonance imaging, comparison of in phase breath-hold longitudinal relaxation time (T1) and (**E**) opposed phase image show no drop in signal of the mass. **F:** On transverse relaxation time (T2)-weighted image, the mass (*arrow*) is homogeneous and quite hyperintense. (**G**) Coronal breath-hold T1 image after intravenous gadolinium diethylene-triamine penta-acetic acid show marked heterogeneous enhancement and a clear plane of separation from the kidney (*arrowheads*). Following positive biochemical evaluation, an adrenal pheochromocytoma was resected.

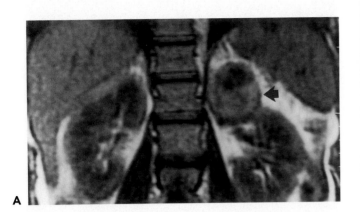

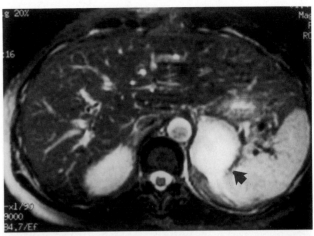

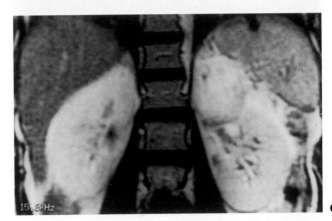

Figure 19-38 Pheochromocytoma. **A:** longitudinal relaxation time (T1)–weighted gradient refocused echo image during suspended respiration shows a 4-cm heterogeneous left adrenal mass (*arrow*). **B:** On fat-suppressed transverse relaxation time (T2)–weighted image, the mass (*arrow*) is markedly hyperintense. **C:** Following intravenous gadolinium diethylene-triamine penta-acetic acid, the mass shows marked heterogeneous enhancement, which persisted for several minutes.

masses. Korobkin et al. (12) and Boland et al. (90) confirmed these findings. Boland et al. pooled the data from 10 articles and showed that a sensitivity of 71% and a specificity of 98% result from choosing a threshold value of 10 HU for the diagnosis of adrenal adenoma (Figs. 19-41, 19-42) (12). Of homogeneous adrenal masses with a nonenhanced CT attenuation value of 10 HU or less, 98% will be benign (most will be adenomas), whereas 29% of adenomas will have an attenuation value of more than 10 HU and will be indistinguishable from most nonadenomas, including metastases.

Another approach to CT densitometry for characterization of adrenal masses makes use of the "histogram" function available on most scanners. The authors placed a circular region of interest covering the center two thirds (avoiding the periphery to limit volume averaging) of adrenal masses including 90 adenomas on unenhanced CT, 184 adenomas on enhanced CT, and 31 adrenal metastases on enhanced CT (4). The histogram is a plot of pixel attenuation along the x axis with the frequency of each attenuation value along the y axis, and also provides mean attenuation, number of pixels, and range of pixel attenuation. The authors showed that none of the adrenal metastases contained any negative pixels on enhanced CT,

whereas 52% of the adenomas did, 51% having more than 10% negative pixels. On unenhanced CT, 87 of the 90 adenomas had negative pixels, including 14 of the 16 that had mean attenuation above 10 HU (4). Thus use of this method may allow a quick option to diagnose adenoma even after contrast, although potential pitfalls could result from variance in scan technique (may be susceptible to artifact from high noise profile) and calibration.

Chemical shift MRI can be used to differentiate adrenal nodules. A relative loss in signal intensity in an adrenal mass, when opposed-phase and in-phase images are compared, can also be used to characterize many adrenal masses as benign adenomas (Figs. 19-42, 19-43). Adrenal adenomas, unlike most metastases and other nonadenomas, often contain large amounts of intracellular lipid (106). The sensitivity and specificity for the diagnosis of adrenal adenoma are similar for chemical shift MR imaging and nonenhanced CT densitometry (121). A histologic study of resected adenomas that had undergone presurgical CT or MR imaging showed a linear correlation between the percentage of lipid-rich cortical cells and both the nonenhanced CT attenuation value and the relative change in signal intensity on opposed-phase chemical shift MR images (91).

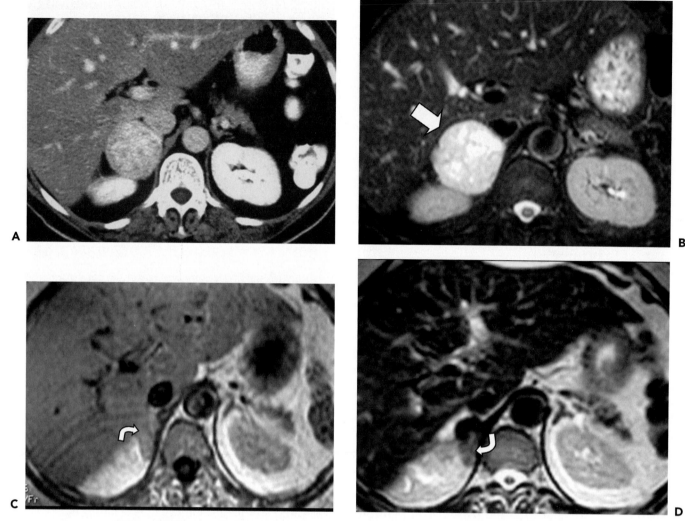

Figure 19-39 Pheochromocytoma; postoperative finding. **A:** Enhanced computed tomography in this hypertensive patient demonstrates a vigorously enhancing right adrenal mass. **B:** The mass (*arrow*) is markedly hyperintense on fat-suppressed transverse relaxation time (T2)-weighted image. Pheochromocytoma was confirmed by surgical resection. Post-adrenalectomy (**C**) longitudinal relaxation time (T1) and (**D**) T2-weighted magnetic resonance images show a small mass-like lesion in adrenalectomy bed (*curved arrow*). At surgery, the adrenal bed was packed with Surgicel for hemostasis.

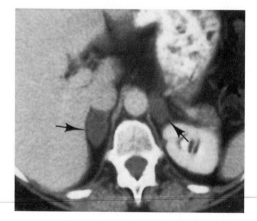

Figure 19-40 Biopsy-proved bilateral nonhyperfunctioning adenomas in a patient with bronchogenic carcinoma. Postcontrast computed tomography image demonstrates bilateral adrenal masses (*arrows*), each measuring 1.5 cm in diameter. Both masses have homogeneous near-water attenuation values. This computed tomography appearance is characteristic of a nonhyperfunctioning adenoma.

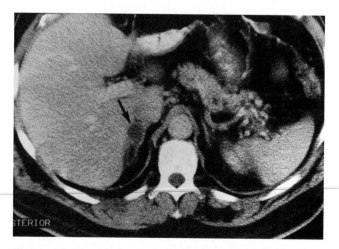

Figure 19-41 Adenoma. An 18-mm low-attenuation (−18 HU) right adrenal adenoma (*arrow*) was discovered incidentally in this asymptomatic man. The computed tomography finding of a mass with attenuation this low excludes malignancy.

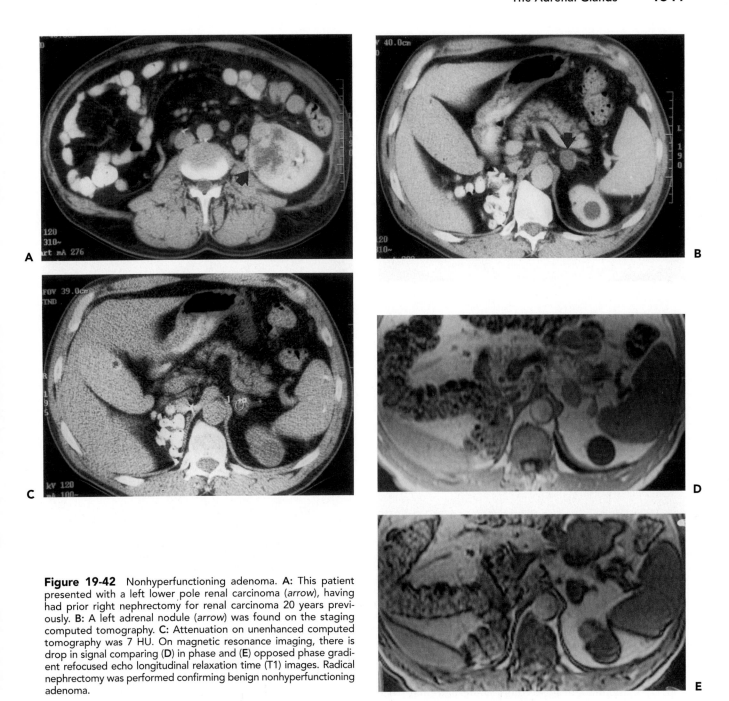

Figure 19-42 Nonhyperfunctioning adenoma. **A:** This patient presented with a left lower pole renal carcinoma (*arrow*), having had prior right nephrectomy for renal carcinoma 20 years previously. **B:** A left adrenal nodule (*arrow*) was found on the staging computed tomography. **C:** Attenuation on unenhanced computed tomography was 7 HU. On magnetic resonance imaging, there is drop in signal comparing (**D**) in phase and (**E**) opposed phase gradient refocused echo longitudinal relaxation time (T1) images. Radical nephrectomy was performed confirming benign nonhyperfunctioning adenoma.

A substantial minority of adrenal adenomas is lipid-poor and cannot be characterized by means of their nonenhanced CT attenuation (Figs. 19-44, 19-45). Korobkin (87), established washout curve values for adenomas. The adenomas, notwithstanding the presence and quantities of lipids in their composition, have the property of presenting rapid loss of enhancement and attenuation values at 15 minutes, which can be used to differentiate adenomas from other masses (Fig. 19-45).

The established formula for this calculation includes the density of the lesion during the precontrast, portal (60-second) and 15-minute delay phases. The examination should be performed with an appropriate technique with thin slices and density measurements with region of interest spanning one half to two thirds of the area of the lesion, always in the same position. Calcification and necrosis areas should be avoided when taking the measurements. Adrenal masses that contain substantial portions of inhomogeneously low attenuation, which indicate substantial components of necrosis or cystic change, cannot be characterized by means of delayed enhancement washout calculations. The abnormal or absent capillary beds in these excavated regions will probably show slow enhancement washout regardless of the original underlying histologic cause (15). In the equation % enhancement washout = (E-D/E-U) −100, where E = enhancement: attenuation at portal

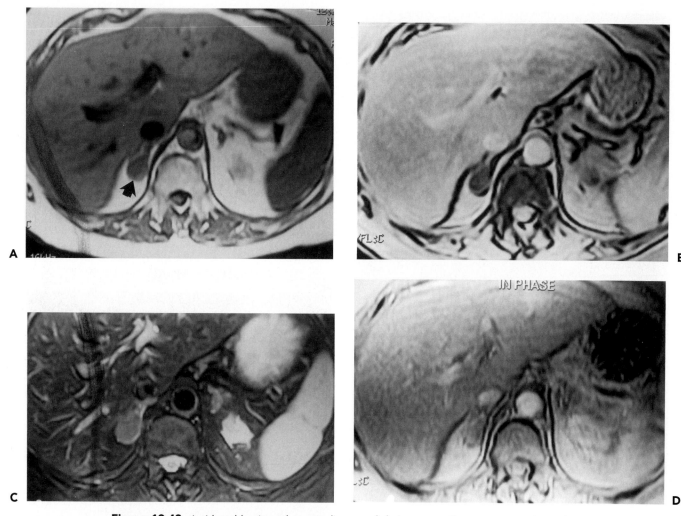

Figure 19-43 Incidental benign adenoma, discovered during magnetic resonance angiography for renal artery stenosis. **A:** In-phase longitudinal relaxation time (T1) gradient refocused echo (GRE) magnetic resonance imaging images shows small right adrenal nodule (*arrow*) near isointense with spleen. **B:** Opposed-phase GRE T1 image shows lesion is clearly much less intense than spleen, this signal drop indicating presence of intracellular lipid. **C:** On fat-suppressed transverse relaxation time (T2)-weighted image, the lesion is only slightly more intense than liver. **D:** T1 GRE image after intravenous gadolinium diethylene-triamine penta-acetic acid shows mild enhancement.

phase, D = delayed enhanced attenuation at 15 minutes, and U = attenuation at precontrast, the percentage enhancement washout represents the percentage of the initial wash in of enhancement that is washed out at the time of delayed scanning, as follows: percentage enhancement washout equals (enhancement washout divided by enhancement) multiplied by 100.

The relative enhancement washout can also be used and is an approximation of the true enhancement washout; it relates the enhancement washout to the enhanced attenuation value instead of the enhancement wash in, as follows: relative percentage enhancement washout equals (enhancement washout divided by enhanced attenuation) multiplied by 100 (87).

The relative enhancement washout of an adrenal mass was a concept introduced as an approximation to the true

enhancement washout that could be used when a delayed enhanced scan is obtained after an adrenal mass is depicted on a standard enhanced CT scan, without knowledge of the nonenhanced attenuation. It is not a physiologic construct, however, because it relates the amount of attenuation loss to only the enhanced attenuation value and not to the gain in attenuation value after the administration of a contrast material (88).

$$\text{Relative washout} = E/D \times 100$$

Most adrenal cortical carcinomas are larger than 6 cm at presentation and often have demonstrable metastases. Typically, these tumors also have large amounts of necrosis, which would invalidate attempts to assess enhancement washout. Despite this more common presentation of adrenal cortical carcinoma, the possibility of differentiating the

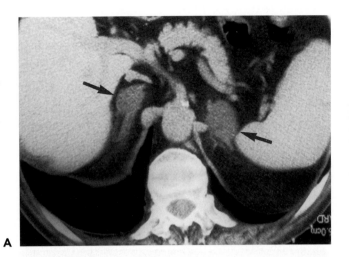

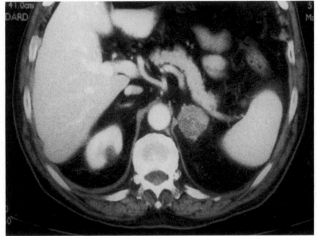

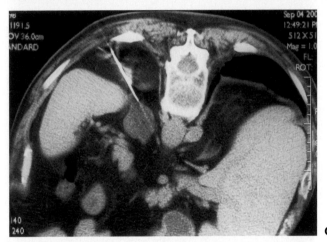

Figure 19-44 Atypical adrenal adenoma. **A:** Staging computed tomography in this patient presenting with lung cancer revealed bilateral adrenal masses (*arrows*), 2 cm on the right and 3.5 cm on left. Both measured −5 HU on unenhanced computed tomography. **B:** Note on this enhanced the left adrenal lesion is somewhat heterogeneous. **C:** Because of the size and heterogeneity, biopsy of the left adrenal mass was performed, revealing benign adenoma.

rare small adrenal cortical carcinoma from the more common adrenal adenoma between 3 and 6 cm in diameter by using enhancement washout calculations has not yet been systematically assessed (88).

The evaluation of a known adrenal mass starts by using nonenhanced CT. If the attenuation of the mass is 10 HU or less the diagnosis is, in most cases, a lipid-rich adrenal adenoma, and a small fraction of these will be cysts. In such a case, there is no need for further evaluation. If the attenuation is more than 10 HU, the mass is considered to be indeterminate and an enhanced and 15-minute-delayed enhanced CT scan should be performed. If the enhancement washout is more than 60%, the most likely diagnosis is of a lipid-poor adenoma. Again, there is no need for further evaluation. If the enhancement washout is less than 50%, the mass is considered indeterminate. Percutaneous adrenal biopsy is recommended if the patient has a primary neoplasm without other evidences of metastases. In a patient without cancer, surgery is recommended if the mass measures more than 4 to 5 cm. Follow-up CT, or adrenal scintigraphy with the use of radio-iodinated norcholesterol, can also be performed in this group of patients.

Nonhyperfunctioning adenomas also have characteristic MRI features. On MRI, the mass is homogeneous with signal intensity usually less than that of fat but greater than that of muscle on all sequences (23). In most cases, the signal intensity is similar to that of normal liver on both T1- and T2-weighted images (23,26,44,53,135) (Fig. 19-46). However, signal intensities are affected by many factors and can be variable, such that diagnosis based only on signal intensities may be indeterminate in as much as 21% to 31% (5,26,134). After intravenous administration of gadolinium compounds, adenomas show limited enhancement (<100% signal intensity increase over baseline) with rapid washout (<30% residual enhancement at 10 minutes) (94,95). Many adenomas contain a significant amount of intracellular lipid, which accounts for the relatively low attenuation value on CT (109). This can be achieved by showing a decrease in signal intensity comparing the same gradient echo sequence with echo time in or out of phase (106,163) (Fig. 19-47). However, some adenomas do not contain large amounts of lipid, so lack of signal drop does not prove malignancy. Using all these MRI features, correct diagnosis can be made in most cases.

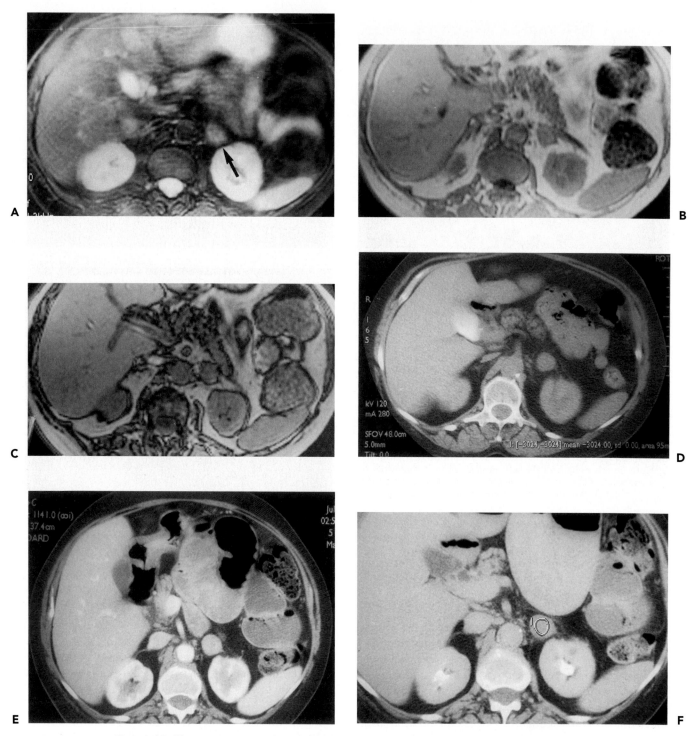

Figure 19-45 Lipid poor adrenal adenoma. **A:** Gadolinium-enhanced fat-suppressed longitudinal relaxation time (T1) magnetic resonance imaging demonstrates small left adrenal mass *(arrow),* and incidental finding on prior routine computed tomography. Comparison of in phase **(B)** and opposed phase **(C)** T1 gradient refocused echo images show no drop in signal. **D:** Attenuation unenhanced computed tomography is 34 HU. **E:** Initial enhanced attenuation 110 HU. **F:** On 15-minute delay, the attenuation fell to 50 HU, a washout consistent with lipid poor adenoma. The lesion has not changed on follow-up.

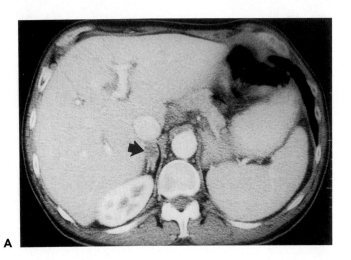

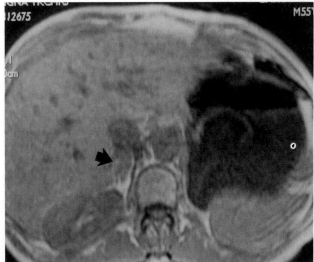

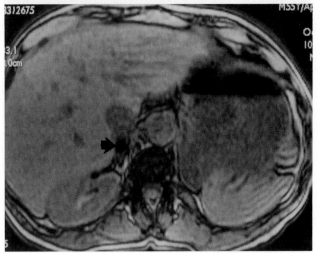

Figure 19-46 Nonhyperfunctioning adenoma. **A:** A right adrenal nodule (*arrow*) was an incidental finding on routine enhanced computed tomography in this asymptomatic patient. **B:** On longitudinal relaxation time (T1)-weighted breath-hold gradient refocused echo magnetic resonance imaging image, the nodule (*arrow*) is slightly less intense than the spleen. **C:** Striking drop in signal (*arrow*) is shown on opposed phase image.

METASTATIC DISEASE

Metastases to the adrenals are common from a variety of primary malignancies, including thyroid, renal, gastric, colon, pancreatic, and esophageal carcinomas, and melanoma. Lung and breast cancer, however, are the most common sources, with adrenal metastases found on CT in approximately 19% of lung cancer patients (150,166). Because adrenal metastases are so common in lung cancer, and because the adrenals may be the only site of metastasis (123,143), the adrenal glands should be included in the CT examination of all patients presenting with a lung cancer (52,115). Surgery is not indicated if adrenal metastases are present in non-small cell lung cancer; accurate staging can help determine the prognosis in patients with small cell cancer (166). Not all adrenal masses found in cancer patients, however, are metastases (see Fig. 19-40). Even in patients with lung cancer, about one third of adrenal masses are benign (52,119). Thus, the imaging features must be used to help make the correct diagnosis. If the

imaging findings are equivocal, a percutaneous CT-guided biopsy should be performed to establish a histologic diagnosis (Fig. 19-48). A baseline CT at the time of presentation of patients with lung cancer is a useful aid in follow-up. Detection of a new small adrenal mass on follow-up is clear evidence of metastasis if the baseline showed normal adrenals (Fig. 19-49).

Adrenal metastases can vary considerably on CT. A normal appearance does not absolutely exclude metastasis, especially with lung cancer (22,123), but most often careful examination will reveal some focal bulge of the adrenal contour. Size can range from less than a centimeter to extremely large; the size, however, overlaps with that of adenomas (Figs. 19-49–19-54) (85). Adrenal metastases may be unilateral or bilateral. When small (less than 5 cm), they commonly are fairly well circumscribed, round or oval, and of soft tissue density (see Fig. 19-49). They may have smooth or irregular, lobulated contours. They may show local invasion, a sign of malignancy. Calcification is rare (80), and they may hemorrhage (see Fig. 19-55) (152).

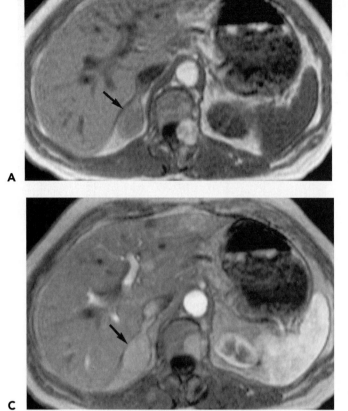

A

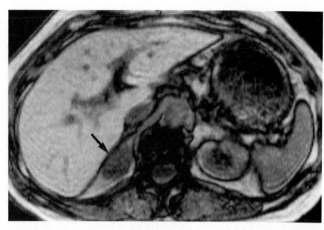

B

C

Figure 19-47 Nonhyperfunctioning adenoma. **A:** On longitudinal relaxation time (T1)-weighted gradient refocused echo magnetic resonance imaging image (two-dimensional FLASH), a right adrenal mass (*arrow*) isointense with liver is shown. **B:** Opposed-phase T1-weighted GRE image shows the mass (*arrow*) with signal intensity less than the liver. **C:** Following intravenous gadolinium diethylene-triamine penta-acetic acid, the mass (*arrow*) shows moderate homogeneous enhancement.

Small adrenal metastases are solid tumors and thus usually have homogeneous soft tissue attenuation values, similar to or higher than that of muscle on noncontrast scans (see Fig. 19-49). Larger metastases may develop cen-

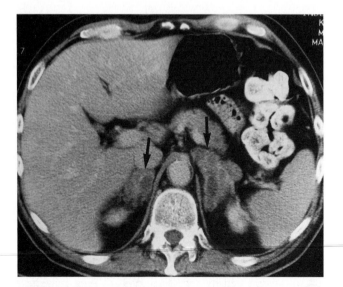

Figure 19-48 Adrenal metastases from primary non-small cell bronchogenic carcinoma. Bilateral adrenal masses (*arrows*) with focal low attenuation areas are noted on this contrast computed tomography. Percutaneous biopsy documented metastatic disease.

tral necrosis and thus are heterogeneous (Figs. 19-50 and 19-51); if hemorrhage has occurred, slightly high density areas may be seen on noncontrast scans. Even if there is central necrosis, however, the density is not lower than that of water, because malignant tumors do not produce lipid (97). Korobkin et al. (89,90), after studying a large series of adrenal nodules, including adenomas and metastases, showed that no metastases show attenuation values of less than 18UH precontrast. In studies from various authors, who evaluated the behavior of adenomas and metastases, no metastases showed a washout curve superior to 60%.

Following intravenous administration of iodinated contrast material, there may be homogeneous enhancement, but commonly enhancement is heterogeneous, especially with larger tumors. A thick, nodular enhancing rim also may be seen (9) (Figs. 19-52 and 19-50).

Adrenal metastases can vary in size and appearance on MRI. On T1-weighted images, metastases usually have signal intensity similar to or lower than that of normal liver tissue, not distinctly different from that of adenomas. They may be heterogeneous (23,44,53,135). On T2-weighted images, they are often heterogeneous, and they are usually hyperintense compared with normal liver, often similar to or of higher intensity than fat, unlike the typical adenoma (Figs. 19-56 and 19-57) (23,44,135). Numerous calculations

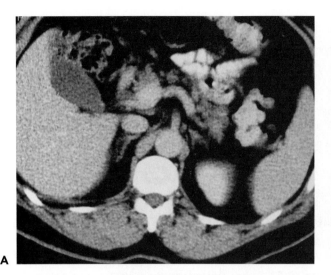
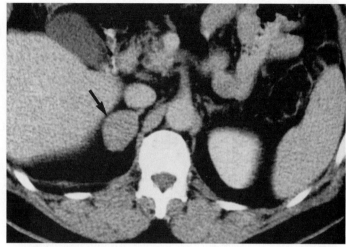

Figure 19-49 Adrenal metastasis. **A:** Baseline computed tomography in this patient presenting with lung cancer shows normal adrenals. **B:** Follow-up 8 months later shows a homogeneous 4-cm mass in the right adrenal (*arrow*). The appearance is not inconsistent with an adenoma, but, because it is new, it is clearly a metastasis.

based on signal intensity ratios, or calculated T2 values, have been investigated, but none have been found to be reliable in practice for distinguishing metastases from adenomas (23,26,53,83,135). Because metastases do not produce lipid, there is no decrease in signal on opposed phase images (106,162). This has been shown to be a more consistent finding than T2 values (167). After intravenous administration of gadolinium compounds,

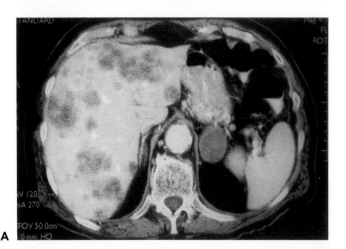
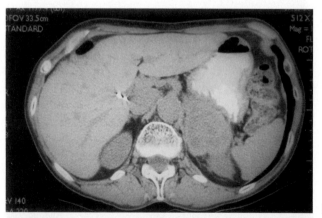
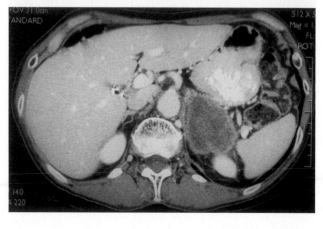

Figure 19-50 Adrenal metastases. **A:** Numerous liver metastases as well as left adrenal mass are shown on enhanced computed tomography (CT). Although the appearance of the adrenal mass not definitive, biopsy is not needed. **B:** In another patient, unenhanced CT shows somewhat irregularly shaped mildly heterogeneous left adrenal mass. **C:** On enhanced CT image, a thick enhancing rim is shown, a finding seen in metastases.

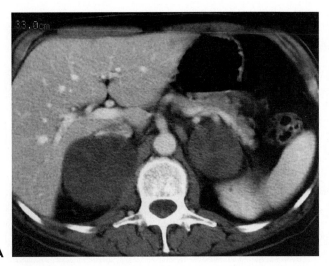

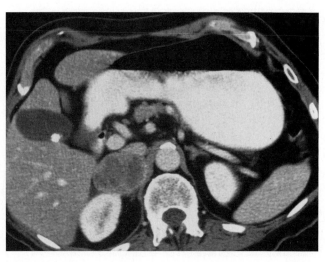

Figure 19-51 Adrenal metastases. Large heterogeneous adrenal masses are present bilaterally (right, 8 cm; left, 5 cm) in this man with bronchogenic carcinoma.

Figure 19-52 Adrenal metastasis. The ovoid 3- × 4-cm right adrenal mass in this patient with lung cancer shows an irregular enhancing rim on this computed tomography image performed with rapid scanning after bolus intravenous contrast.

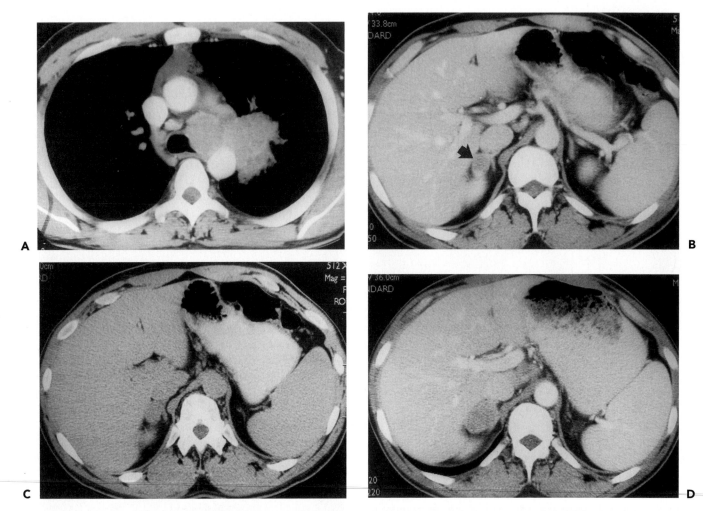

Figure 19-53 Adrenal metastasis. **A:** Staging computed tomography (CT) was done in this patient with lung cancer. **B:** A small (1.6 × 1.7 cm) right adrenal nodule (*arrow*) was detected on routine enhanced CT, attenuation 60 HU. **C:** On 15-minute delay, attenuation was 45 HU, not typical of adenoma. **D:** Follow-up CT 4 months later shows considerable increase in size of the metastasis, now 2.5 × 3.7 cm.

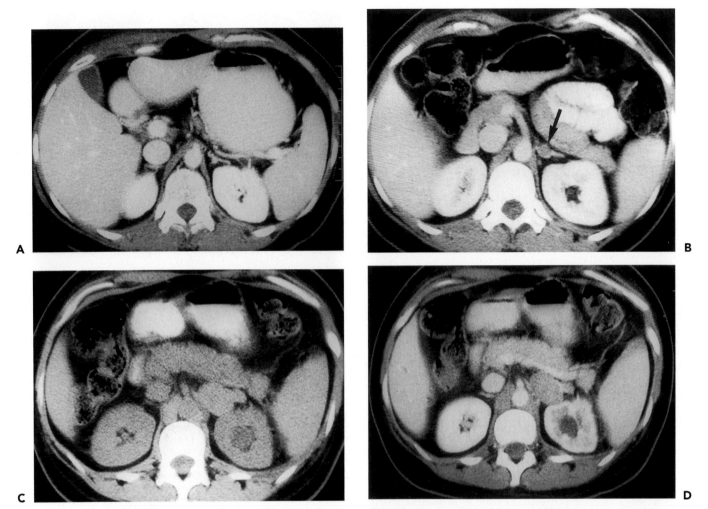

Figure 19-54 Adrenal metastasis. **A:** Baseline computed tomography (CT) in this patient with breast cancer shows both adrenal glands have normal appearance. **B:** Follow-up CT 1 year later reveals a tiny (7-mm) nodule has developed (*arrow*); although nonspecific, this must represent metastasis. **C:** Follow-up unenhanced CT 10 months later shows the mass is considerably larger, 2.1 × 2.5 cm, attenuation 37 HU. **D:** Enhanced CT shows moderate enhancement; note also retrocrural lesion.

metastases exhibit exuberant and heterogeneous enhancement that persists for several minutes, an enhancement pattern quite different from that of adenomas (see Fig. 19-57) (95). MRI is readily able to demonstrate or exclude local invasion because of the great contrast between neoplastic and normal tissue, especially on fat-suppressed T2-weighted images.

CT is the most cost-effective method for screening and following patients with malignancies. In most cases, adrenal metastases can be diagnosed or excluded by a well-performed CT. MRI can be valuable in cases in which CT could not be performed. Percutaneous biopsy under CT guidance can be very effective, with accuracy and negative predictive value of more than 90% (64,155,167). However, complications can occur (75,167), (Fig. 19-58) and biopsy is not needed if the imaging findings are diagnostic. Follow-up by CT can be diagnostic, because adenomas are very slow growing and do not change in size over a period of a few months, whereas metastases show growth.

Neoplastic patients frequently show a diffuse enlargement of the adrenal glands but with no masses or changes in contours. Biochemical studies carried out with this group of patients have demonstrated a number of changes in the gland function, which are shown to be consistent with hyperplasia. A definite association between malignant neoplasms and adrenal gland hyperplasia is observed; there is a higher prevalence of adrenal gland hyperplasia in tumors patients when compared to the general population (56a).

ADRENAL LYMPHOMA

Adrenal masses occasionally result from involvement by lymphoma, with diffuse non-Hodgkin disease the commonest type (54,72,124). This may be found at presentation or at follow-up, with adrenal lymphoma reported in 1% to 4% of patients being followed for lymphoma (54,72,124). Adrenal involvement is most commonly seen in conjunction

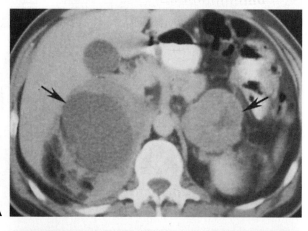

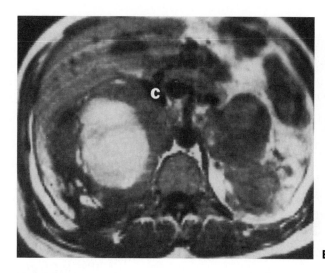

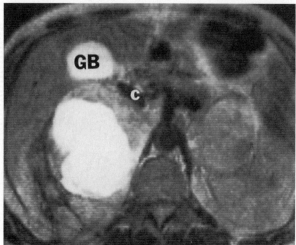

Figure 19-55 Hemorrhagic adrenal metastases due to melanoma. **A:** Postcontrast computed tomography (CT) image demonstrates bilateral, inhomogeneous adrenal masses (*arrows*), the right being more irregular than the left. **B:** Longitudinal relaxation time (T1)-weighted image (500/35) shows basically the same findings as CT. The extremely high signal intensity seen in the right adrenal mass is due to subacute hemorrhage. **C:** transverse relaxation time (T2)-weighted image (2100/90). With the exception of hemorrhage, both adrenal masses have signal intensities similar to that of fat. *C*, Inferior vena cava; *GB*, gallbladder.

with an extra-adrenal disease site (45). Primary adrenal lymphoma is rare and is believed to arise from hematopoietic cells in the adrenal (43). Lymphomatous adrenal masses are bilateral in one third of cases; when bilateral, the patient may develop Addison disease (67,105,124) (Figs. 19-59 and 19-60).

On CT, adrenal lymphomas usually are seen as large soft tissue masses (40 to 60 HU) replacing the adrenal. They usually alter the shape of the adrenal, but the adrenal may markedly expand while retaining a somewhat adreniform shape. Mild to moderate enhancement is seen after intravenous administration of iodinated contrast (see Figs. 19-59, 19-60 and 19-61). The lesions may be homogeneous, but they are often heterogeneous with low attenuation areas even before therapy (6,43). Sometimes the growth pattern can suggest lymphoma, as it is more likely to infiltrate or insinuate around the upper pole of the kidney than displace it, as would be typical of carcinoma (Fig. 19-62). There may be hemorrhage, and calcification can be found especially after chemotherapy (43). On MRI, adrenal lymphomas are indistinguishable from other malig-

nancies. They are usually heterogeneous, with low signal on T1-weighted images (less intense than normal liver, but more intense than muscle) and more intense than fat on T2-weighted images (23,53,96) (Fig. 19-63).

MYELOLIPOMA

Myelolipoma is an uncommon, benign, nonfunctioning neoplasm of the adrenal, found in less than 1% of autopsies (120). It is composed of variable amounts of fat and hematopoietic tissue, including myeloid and erythroid cells and megakaryocytes. The etiology is unclear, but myelolipoma may be a result of metaplasia of cells in the adrenal, possibly myeloid cells misplaced during embryogenesis (31). It affects men and women equally. Although this is a nonfunctioning tumor, in 10% it is associated with endocrine disorders, including Cushing syndrome (8,172), congenital adrenal hyperplasia (118), and Conn syndrome (174). Most myelolipomas (80%) are asymptomatic and are of no clinical significance. Some (10%) become large and cause vague symptoms or

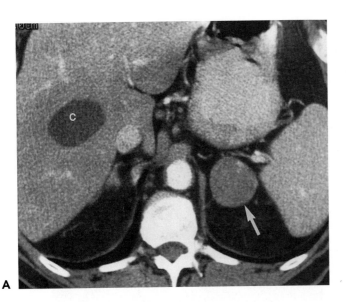

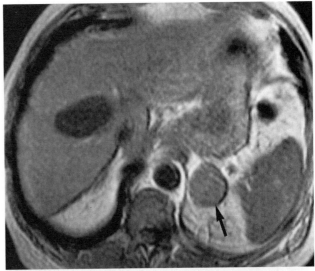

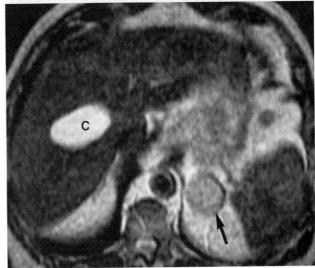

Figure 19-56 Adrenal metastasis from a primary esophageal carcinoma. **A:** A 4-cm left adrenal mass (*arrow*) is homogeneous except for a few tiny high-attenuation foci, a pattern that could represent a nonhyperfunctioning adenoma. *C*, Incidental liver cyst. **B:** The mass (*arrow*) is isointense with liver on longitudinal relaxation time (T1)-weighted gradient refocused echo image (50/5/35 degrees). **C:** On transverse relaxation time (T2)-weighted magnetic resonance imaging image (2000/80/), the mass (*arrow*) is more intense than liver, but not as intense as the cyst (*C*).

pain (46). Large myelolipomas may hemorrhage, which can be the cause of pain. Size ranges from 1 to 15 cm, with a mean of about 4 cm.

On CT, most myelolipomas are well-circumscribed masses, sometimes with a discrete thin apparent capsule (Fig. 19-64). Occasionally, the mass may appear to extend into the retroperitoneum (168). Nearly all contain some definite fat density (less than −20 HU). However, the amount of fat is widely variable, ranging from nearly all fat, to more than half fat (50%), to only a few tiny foci of fat in a soft tissue mass (10%) (81,113,136,140) (Figs. 19-64–19-69). Occasionally, the mass has an attenuation value between that of fat and water because the fat and myeloid elements are diffusely mixed. Calcification is seen in 30%, often punctate (81,140) (see Fig. 19-64). With hemorrhage, high-density areas can be seen (Fig. 19-67). Bilateral myelolipomas occur in about 10% (136).

The presence of fat in an adrenal mass also can be recognized on MRI, because fat is typically bright on both T1- and T2-weighted images (114) (Figs. 19-68 and 19-69). Decrease in signal with fat suppression or phase cancellation is confirmatory (106) (see Fig. 19-69). However, if the mass is nearly all mature fat, there will not be loss of signal with opposed phase images because the loss of signal occurs only with phase cancellation in areas with an admixture of fat and water protons (163). Overall, myelolipomas are often heterogeneous because the nonfatty areas will have signal intensity similar to that of hematopoietic bone marrow (112). The lesions enhance brightly after intravenous administration of gadolinium (Fig. 19-69).

The presence of fat in an adrenal mass is the key to the diagnosis of myelolipoma, because virtually no other adrenal lesion contains fat. Teratoma and liposarcoma of the adrenals are extraordinarily rare. An angiomyolipoma of the upper pole of a kidney may be mistaken to be an adrenal myelolipoma. However, this is of no clinical significance, because both these lesions are benign. If necessary, diagnosis can be confirmed by percutaneous needle biopsy

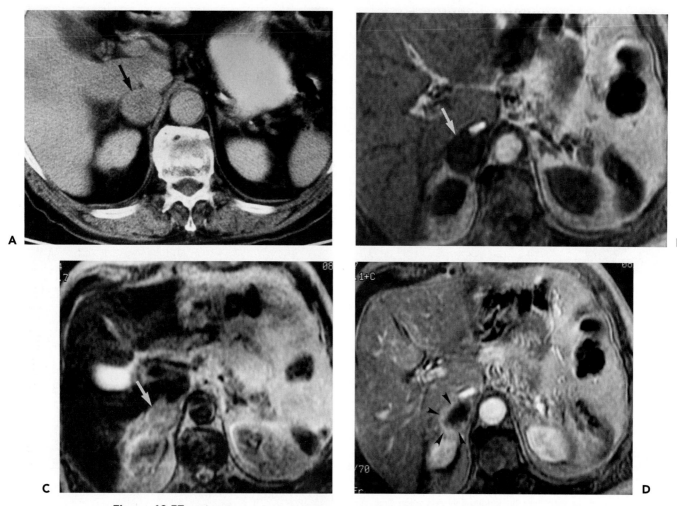

Figure 19-57 Adrenal metastasis. **A:** Contrast-enhanced computed tomography shows a fairly homogeneous right adrenal mass (*arrow*) in this patient with a history of bladder cancer; no other abnormality was found in the chest or abdomen. **B:** The mass (*arrow*) has lower signal than liver on longitudinal relaxation time (T1)-weighted gradient refocused echo image (114/4.2/70 degrees). **C:** The mass (*arrow*) is nearly isointense with fat on transverse relaxation time (T2)-weighted spin echo image. **D:** There is heterogeneous enhancement (*arrowheads*) after intravenous gadolinium diethylene-triamine penta-acetic acid (144/4.2/70 degrees).

(29,58). If the biopsy reveals bone marrow elements and the mass contains fat, the diagnosis is assured, because extramedullary hematopoiesis does not contain fat (84). The presence of megakaryocytes also is an important diagnostic histologic feature (29). A definite diagnosis is important because surgical resection is not indicated unless there has been significant hemorrhage. In nearly all cases, a diagnosis of adrenal myelolipoma can be made confidently based on CT or MRI findings alone.

ADRENAL CYSTS

Adrenal cysts are rare, found in only 1 of 1,400 autopsies (171). They are nonfunctional and usually found incidentally. The most common (45%) type is endothelial cyst (25).

These are predominantly lymphangiomatous cysts, typically small and asymptomatic (77). Thirty-nine percent are pseudocysts, which lack an endothelial lining and are most often a sequela of remote adrenal hemorrhage (48,77,125). These are the type most often detected by CT. These can be quite large and may produce symptoms because of their size. The remaining cystic lesions of the adrenals are parasitic cysts (7%), caused by *Echinococcus*, and true epithelial cysts (9%) (125).

On CT, adrenal cysts are large masses (5 to 20 cm) that are well circumscribed and round. They are suprarenal in location, but it may be difficult on CT to recognize that they arise in the adrenal rather than the kidney or liver. Sonography or MRI may better show their true origin. They usually are of near-water attenuation, but they can have higher or mixed attenuation values resulting from old

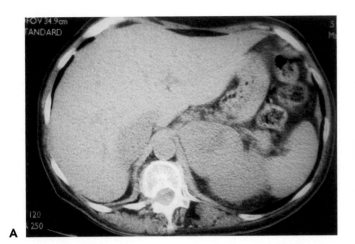

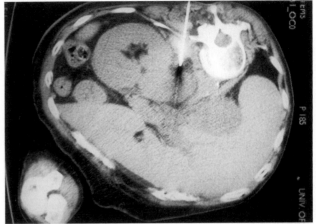

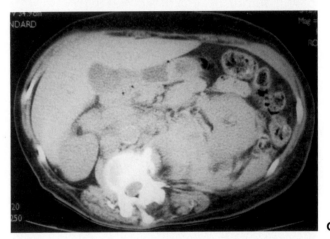

Figure 19-58 Adrenal metastases, complication of biopsy. **A:** Bilateral adrenal masses worrisome for metastases were found on investigation of failure to thrive in this nursing home patient. **B:** Percutaneous biopsy was done for diagnosis, revealing poorly differentiated malignancy, possibly a breast primary malignancy. **C:** Following the biopsy, the patient had pain and declining hematocrit. Unenhanced CT demonstrates large hemorrhage.

hemorrhage (Figs. 19-70 and 19-71). The wall may be thick and can show contrast enhancement. Calcification is common (75%) (80), being usually curvilinear in shape and often limited to the inferior aspect of the wall (80,164).

Although MRI may show typical cystic features, homogeneous low intensity on T1-weighted images and extreme hyperintensity on T2-weighted images, signal intensity can vary depending on the age of hemorrhage. There is no

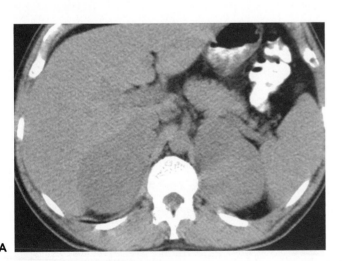

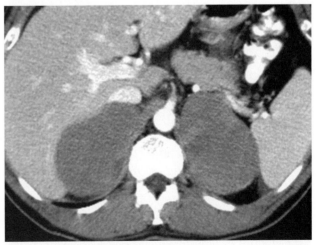

Figure 19-59 Bilateral adrenal lymphoma. **A:** Unenhanced computed tomography shows relatively homogeneous large bilateral adrenal masses. **B:** Computed tomography after intravenous contrast shows slight homogeneous enhancement, a pattern commonly seen in lymphoma.

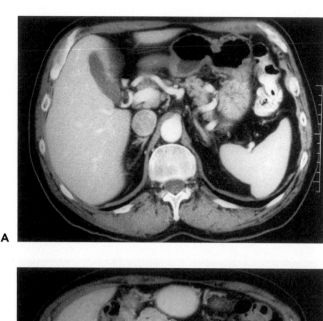

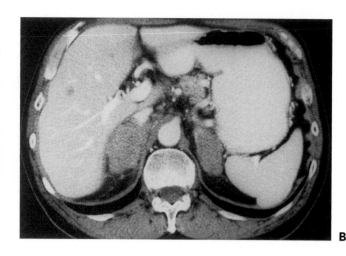

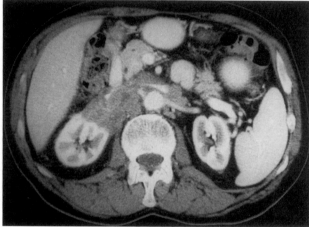

Figure 19-60 Adrenal lymphoma. **A:** Baseline computed tomography in this patient with lymphoma shows both adrenals appear normal. **B:** Follow-up enhanced computed tomography scan shows development of bilateral slightly lobular adrenal masses. **C:** New retroperitoneal adenopathy is also present.

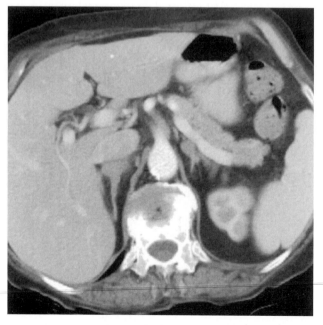

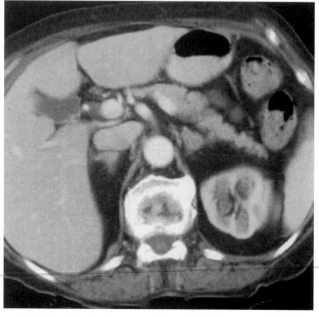

Figure 19-61 Nodular adrenal lymphoma. **A, B:** Note multiple focal nodules in both adrenal glands, with normal appearance of intervening uninvolved areas. Typically with nodular adrenal cortical hyperplasia, nodules are superimposed on thickened glands (see Fig. 19-19).

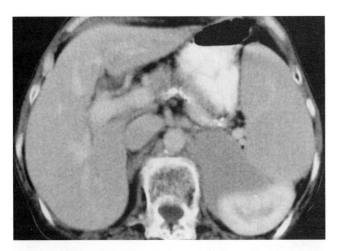

Figure 19-62 Adrenal lymphoma. A homogeneous mass arising in the region of the left adrenal insinuates itself around the left kidney without deforming it.

central enhancement on either CT or MRI. Adrenal cysts are of no clinical significance, and surgical removal is unnecessary if the diagnosis can be established by imaging. Concern about malignancy is reasonable only in complicated cysts, which may have high attenuation values, a thick enhancing wall, and septations. In such cases, percutaneous needle aspiration may be helpful for both diagnosis and treatment (164).

INFLAMMATORY DISEASE

Inflammatory processes in the adrenals are uncommon. Adrenal abscesses occur rarely; they sometimes represent adrenal hematomas that became infected (116). More often, adrenal inflammation is a result of chronic granulomatous disease, with tuberculosis (TB) and histoplasmosis being

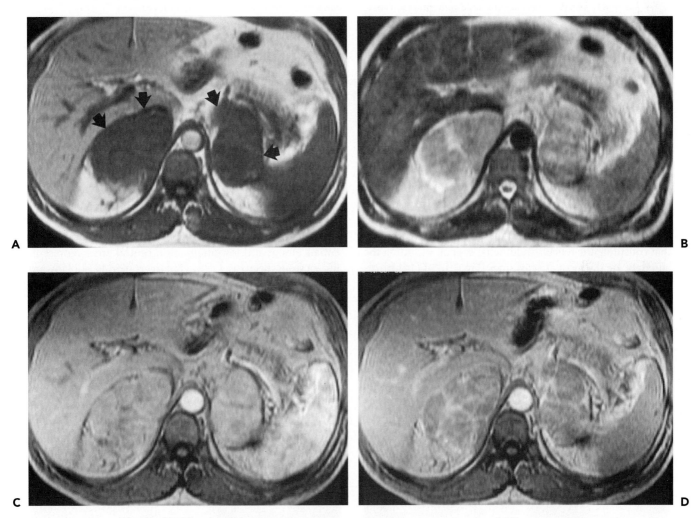

Figure 19-63 Primary adrenal lymphoma: magnetic resonance imaging (MRI) appearance. **A:** Longitudinal relaxation time (T1)-weighted image (500/35) shows two oblong-shaped adrenal masses (*M*). **B:** transverse relaxation time (T2)-weighted image (2100/90). The masses are slightly inhomogeneous and have a signal intensity similar to that of fat. Based on MRI signal characteristics, adrenal lymphoma cannot be distinguished from metastases. *K,* Kidney; *c,* inferior vena cava; *L,* liver; *S,* spleen. **C:** T1 gradient refocused echo image immediately after gadolinium diethylene-triamine penta-acetic acid (DTPA) injection shows bright heterogeneous enhancement of both masses. **D:** Thirteen minutes after gadolinium DTPA injection, the enhancement is not as bright.

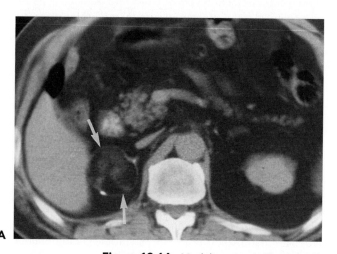
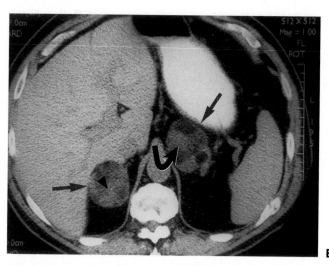

Figure 19-64 Myelolipomas. **A:** The right adrenal contains a partly fatty mass (*arrows*) with a capsule; note the calcification. **B:** In another patient, bilateral adrenal masses (*arrows*) are demonstrated on unenhanced computed tomography. These are of mixed attenuation with focal areas measuring 55 HU (*arrowhead*) and 58 HU (*curved arrow*).

most common, (Fig. 19-72) although North American blastomycosis has been reported to involve the adrenals (61).

Paracoccidioidomycosis, or South American blastomycosis, is the most common systemic mycosis in South America, with Brazil responsible for about 70% of total world cases. Its etiologic agent is *Paracoccidioides brasiliensis*. This disease chiefly involves the respiratory tract, and its presentation can vary from acute and self-limited to a progressive pulmonary disease or extrapulmonary dissemination. Hormonal or occupational factors (especially agricultural labor) can increase susceptibility. Diagnosis is made by lesion biopsy and fungal culture, serologic tests, and chest radiograph (61). The organs that constitute the reticuloendothelial system, including the adrenals, are the most affected ones (Fig. 19-73) (141).

Granulomatous disease of the adrenals can cause a variety of appearances depending on the stage of disease. In most cases, there is bilateral enlargement of the adrenals (35,62,103,179). Bilateral adrenal enlargement in a patient with a reactive tuberculin skin test or with chest radiographic changes of TB, paracoccidioidomycosis or histoplasmosis, should suggest the diagnosis, even if pulmonary cultures are nondiagnostic (179).

With active adrenal TB or paracoccidioidomycosis, both glands are usually enlarged to some degree for a disease course of less than 3 months (acute stage) (Fig. 19-73). The masses are frequently heterogeneous, with heterogeneous enhancement and low-attenuation central areas representing caseous necrosis (178). Enlarged glands and inward

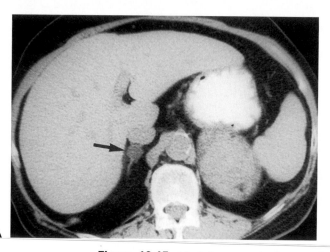
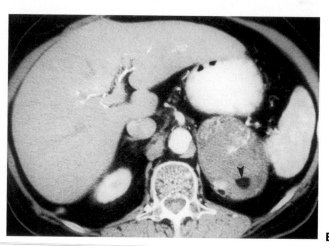

Figure 19-65 Myelolipoma and adenoma. **A:** On computed tomography (CT) performed for vague symptoms, bilateral adrenal masses were incidentally discovered in this normotensive patient. Unenhanced CT shows small right adrenal nodule (*arrow*); this measured 9 HU. **B:** Left adrenal mass is largely of soft tissue attenuation, with enhancement demonstrated on this enhanced CT, but a small focus (*arrowhead*) measures –67 HU, indicating myelolipoma.

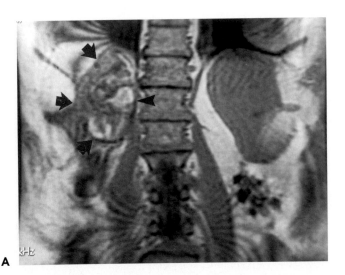

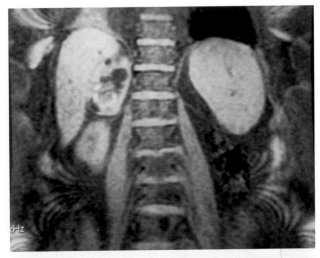

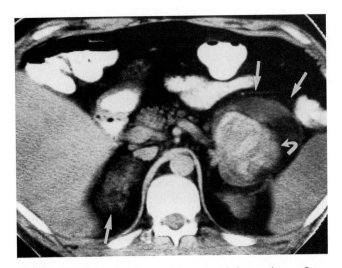

Figure 19-66 Myelolipoma. **A:** Right adrenal mass was discovered on magnetic resonance imaging performed for suspected renal artery stenosis. Coronal breath-hold gradient refocused echo longitudinal relaxation time (T1) shows heterogeneous suprarenal mass (*arrows*); note areas of high signal (*arrowhead*) on this nonfat-suppressed scan. **B:** The mass shows enhancement on the fat suppressed T1 image after intravenous gadolinium diethylene-triamine penta-acetic acid. However, note the loss of signal of central foci, indicative of fat. **C:** Unenhanced computed tomography confirms the presence of fat (*arrow*) and also shows small foci of calcification (*arrowhead*).

Figure 19-67 Bilateral myelolipomas with hemorrhage. Computed tomography, performed because of acute left flank pain, shows bilateral fat containing adrenal masses (*arrows*). The left mass contains a high-attenuation area (*curved arrow*), confirmed to be an acute hemorrhage at surgery.

atrophic areas are found in the subacute stage of the disease (disease course of 6 to 24 months) (57).

Calcification is present in nearly half of cases of adrenal TB or Pb (35,161). Atrophy is seen at the chronic stage, when the disease duration exceeded 24 months. In some cases, at a late stage of disease, dense calcification with no soft tissue mass may be seen (35). Active adrenal histoplasmosis most often presents with mild to marked symmetrical enlargement of both adrenals, which retain the normal shape (99,179). There is low attenuation in the center with higher peripheral density, because of caseous necrosis (99,179) (Fig. 19-74). Calcification is not usually seen in the acute phase, but it may be seen with healing (179).

With TB, paracoccidioidomycosis and histoplasmosis, there may be associated lymphadenopathy. Both may cause adrenal insufficiency. The diagnosis usually is suggested because of the CT appearance of the glands and the clinical presentation, especially when there is adrenal insufficiency. Percutaneous biopsy can be done to confirm the diagnosis (35,61,179).

The MRI signal intensity of inflammatory adrenal masses is nonspecific (Fig. 19-75). It has signal intensity similar to

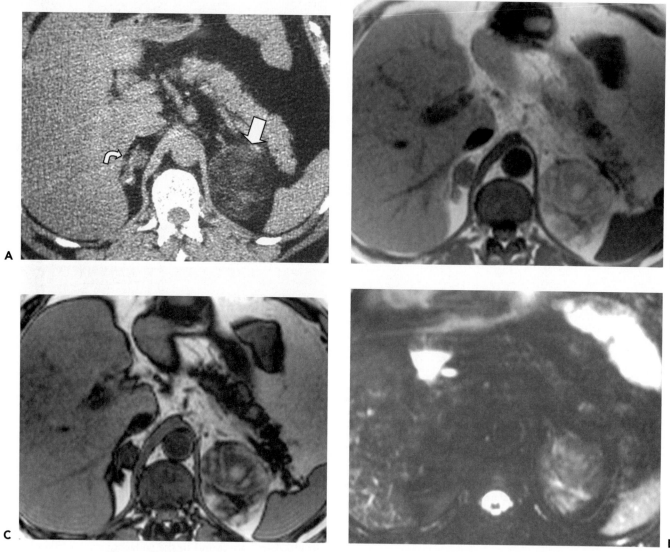

Figure 19-68 Myelolipoma and hyperplasia. **A:** Unenhanced computed tomography demonstrates nodularity of right adrenal gland (*curved arrow*), and a large fat-containing left adrenal mass (*arrow*). Comparison of **B:** in phase longitudinal relaxation time (T1)-weighted breath-hold gradient refocused echo image and **C:** opposed phase image shows drop in signal of right adrenal nodule. Note that fatty portions of left adrenal mass do not show drop in signal, due to the proponderance of fat. **D:** Fat-suppressed T2-weighted image does show loss of signal in the left adrenal myelolipoma.

spleen on T1-weighted images, and similar to or higher than fat on T2-weighted images (5). Enhancement patterns have not been described. Calcification is difficult to recognize.

ADRENAL HEMORRHAGE

Adrenal hemorrhage occurs in three distinct settings: neonatal hemorrhage, spontaneous (atraumatic) hemorrhage in the adult and severe trauma. Neonatal hemorrhage is the most common, resulting partly from the large fetal adrenal that is prone to injury during birth trauma. Because it is

primarily the regressing fetal adrenal tissue that is involved, such patients do not develop adrenal insufficiency, and in the adult the only sequela is calcification of the adrenal without an associated mass (80).

Adrenal hemorrhage in the adult may be seen in the setting of severe illness, such as sepsis, including but not limited to meningococcemia, burns, hypotension, and other life-threatening illnesses. In these circumstances, it is likely the stress-related hyperplasia makes the adrenal prone to spontaneous rupture. About one third of cases of adrenal hemorrhage are associated with anticoagulant therapy. Commonly, the bleeding occurs in the first 3 weeks of

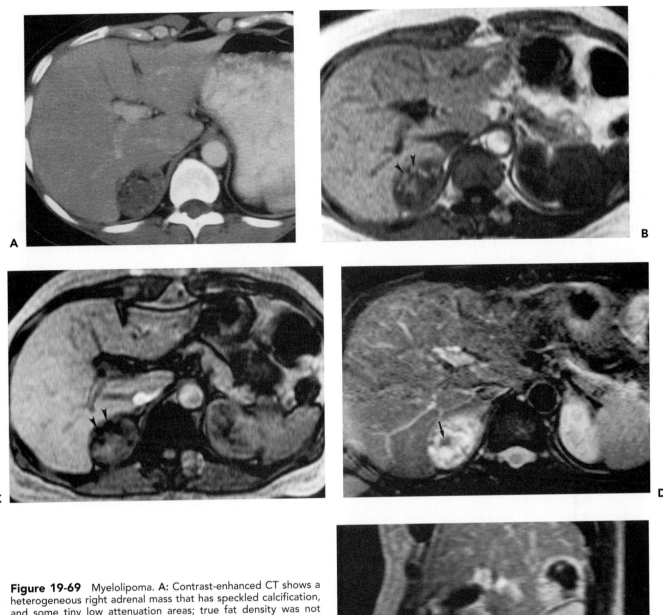

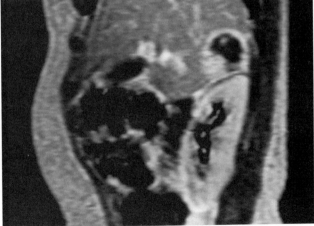

Figure 19-69 Myelolipoma. **A:** Contrast-enhanced CT shows a heterogeneous right adrenal mass that has speckled calcification, and some tiny low attenuation areas; true fat density was not measured. **B:** longitudinal relaxation time (T1)-weighted gradient refocused echo magnetic resonance imaging (154/4/70 degrees) shows several foci (*arrowheads*) isointense with fat in the mass that is mostly isointense with muscle. **C:** On the opposed-phase image (echo time 7 msec), the bright areas (*arrowheads*) have lost signal. **D:** On fat-suppressed transverse relaxation time (T2)-weighted image (3000/90), much of the mass is hyperintense, whereas the small fat foci are low signal (*arrow*). **E:** Sagittal T1-weighted gradient refocused echo image (154/4/70 degrees) after intravenous gadolinium diethylene-triamine penta-acetic acid shows bright peripheral enhancement, confirming that the lesion does not arise from the kidney.

anticoagulation (117,181). This is probably not caused by excessive anticoagulation but is partly a result of stress-related hyperplasia resulting from the illness that necessitated the anticoagulation (100). The boggy hyperplastic adrenals are more prone to disruption and hemorrhage.

On CT, adrenal hemorrhage results in unilateral or bilateral adrenal masses that are usually ovoid, about 3 cm in diameter, and of about muscle density or higher with poor enhancement, if any, after intravenous administration of iodinated contrast (Fig. 19-76). With larger hemorrhages,

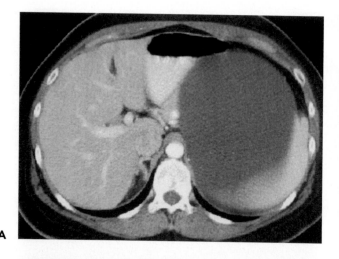

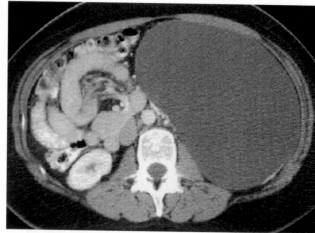

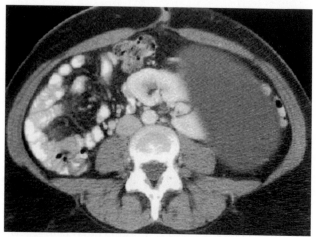

Figure 19-70 Giant adrenal cyst. **A:** A homogeneous water-density mass is seen originating high in the left upper quadrant, no normal adrenal visible. **B:** The cyst occupies most of the left abdomen. **C:** The left kidney is displaced inferomedially. A huge benign unilocular cyst of the left adrenal was removed at open surgery.

the masses may be heterogeneous and may have ill-defined margins (Fig. 19-77). The size and attenuation value decrease over time if followed with CT (101,180). Calcification may develop in several weeks to months. If the hemorrhage is bilateral, adrenal insufficiency may occur. It may be important to suggest this possibility so that an ACTH stimulation test can be done to confirm adrenal insufficiency because the clinical signs may be subtle. As mentioned previously, small metastases rarely cause adrenal insufficiency.

The adrenal glands are well protected in the retroperitoneum. Posttraumatic adrenal hemorrhage is not common, reported to be seen in 2% of patients undergoing CT for severe abdominal injury (Figs. 19-78 to 19-80) (19). Because of lack of specific clinical signs for acute traumatic adrenal hemorrhage, the condition usually is detected as an incidental finding in CT studies performed for evaluation of acute blunt trauma. It has long been recognized that the right adrenal is more prone to traumatic hemorrhage (19,149). Based on pathologic analysis at autopsies, Sevitt (151) postulated this may be a result of one of two mechanisms: direct trauma may more likely affect the right adrenal as it is in a confined space between liver and spine.

Alternatively, blunt force trauma produces a compressive force that results in an acute elevation of pressure in the abdomen, transmitted via the inferior vena cava directly to the right adrenal through the short right adrenal vein, while this compressive force is dissipated into the left renal vein with little change in pressure of the left adrenal vein. However bilateral and isolated left adrenal hematomas occur.

The largest study of adrenal hematomas detected on CT reported on 54 adrenal hematomas in 51 patients found in 2,692 (1.8%) patients who had abdominal CT for severe trauma over a 54-month period (133a). The total number of trauma patients seen during that period in that institution, including those who did not require CT on clinical grounds, was 6,808, for prevalence of 0.8%. Right adrenal hematomas were seen in 42 patients and left adrenal hematomas in 12, with 3 patients having bilateral adrenal hematomas. The hematomas had mean maximum diameter of 2.8 cm, mostly ovoid and some round, and 98% had stranding in adjacent fat. The mean attenuation on routine contrasted scans was 52 HU. There may be concern in the acute setting whether a patient has an adrenal hematoma or an incidental mass, and, because trauma scans usually are done only after contrast, the density readings are not specific.

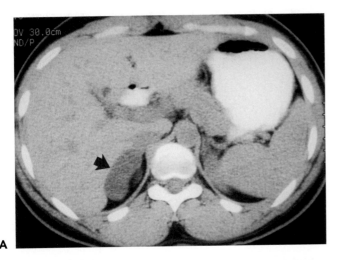

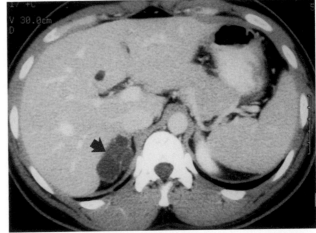

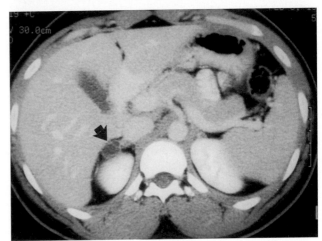

Figure 19-71 Multiloculated adrenal cyst. **A:** Lobular water attenuation mass (*arrow*) in the suprarenal region is shown on this unenhanced computed tomography. **B, C:** The mass shows septations but no enhancement of contents on the enhanced images. This may represent epithelial cyst and is stable on follow-up.

If the lesion is thought to probably represent an incidental adenoma (absence of stranding or other injury), a repeat CT without contrast can be performed because hematomas are typically more than 50 HU, whereas adenomas commonly are less than 10 HU. Alternatively, a delayed follow-up CT will show decreased attenuation and size in most hematomas and complete resolution in some, whereas incidental masses will remain similar size.

In this study, patients with adrenal hematomas had significantly more serious injury than the trauma patients without adrenal hematomas, most likely due to the requirement for severe force of trauma to injure the adrenal. The group with adrenal hematomas had a statistically higher Injury Severity Score, length of intensive care unit stay and hospital stay, and mortality rate (9.8% for those with adrenal hematoma versus 3.7% for those without). Mortality was particularly high when active extravasation was noted in the adrenal bed (two of the three patients with this finding died). Other injuries were common: of the 51 patients with adrenal hematoma, 26 had hepatic lacerations, 24 had splenic injuries, seven had right renal injuries, nine had left renal injuries, and 10 had right and

15 had left pneumothoraces; many had orthopedic injury as well. Only one patient with an adrenal hematoma had no other significant injury. The adrenal injury itself is usually less clinically significant than the other injuries. However, a potential risk of adrenal insufficiency exists if bilateral adrenal adenomas are present (19,180,181).

One distinctive type of surgical trauma may result in an adrenal hematoma. When orthotopic liver transplantation is performed, a segment of the recipient's inferior vena cava must be excised, requiring ligation and division of the right adrenal vein, which can result in infarction and sometimes in hemorrhage in the right adrenal region (13,158) (Fig. 19-81). This may be seen in 2% of patients who undergo such surgery and should be recognized as a surgical complication of no clinical significance as long as the contralateral adrenal is intact (13).

Metastases to the adrenal will hemorrhage, but only rarely. This usually can be distinguished from other adrenal hemorrhages because there is a large heterogeneous mass, with more extensive infiltrative retroperitoneal bleeding (152). Because these patients usually have advanced disease, neoplasm elsewhere is also usually evident.

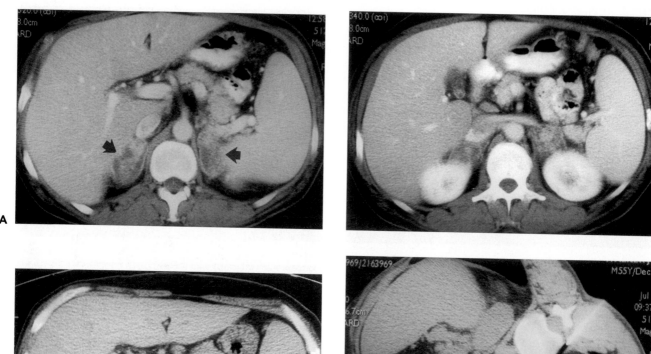

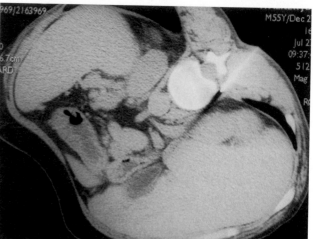

Figure 19-72 Histoplasmosis of adrenals. **A, B:** Heterogenous bilateral adrenal masses (*arrows*) were discovered in this patient with low grade fever, mediastinal adenopathy and pulmonary disease. **C:** Prior to biopsy, unenhanced images show the masses with attenuation 34 HU. **D:** Because of concern for metastases, percutaneous biopsy was performed revealing histoplasmosis.

On MRI, adrenal hemorrhage will produce a mass that can have varying signal intensities dependent on the age of the blood. They can be recognized because they usually have a pattern different from that of adenoma or malignancy. A subacute hematoma usually has high signal intensity on both T1- and T2-weighted images (86). In some cases of subacute hematoma, on T1-weighted images the center may be low intensity because of the presence of intracellular deoxyhemoglobin, and the periphery may have high signal because of free methemoglobin; because both substances are high signal on T2, the mass is all high signal on T2. In chronic adrenal hematoma, the center consists of methemoglobin and thus this is of high signal on T1- and T2-weighted images, whereas the periphery contains hemosiderin, which is low signal on both T1- and T2-weighted images. This ring pattern is distinctive and is suggestive of the diagnosis (71).

ADDISON DISEASE

Adrenal insufficiency may result from a variety of causes including bilateral hemorrhage, inflammatory disease, and idiopathic autoimmune primary Addison disease. Although metastases to the adrenals are common, they rarely lead to Addison disease. When it occurs, the disease is either in an advanced stage or is associated with spontaneous hemorrhage (150). Another rare cause is hemochromatosis, which can be recognized on CT because the adrenals are normal or small in size but have increased attenuation values (35).

CT is indicated in evaluation of patients with Addison disease. In one study, all cases of idiopathic Addison disease could be distinguished from other causes (161). CT can also determine the stage of the disease: acute, subacute and chronic, as discussed previously (Figs. 19-74 and 19-83) (57).

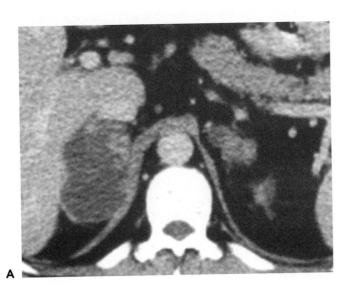

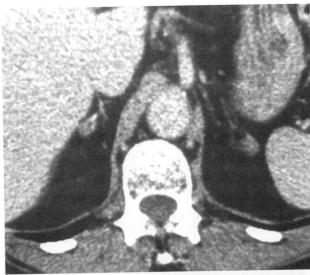

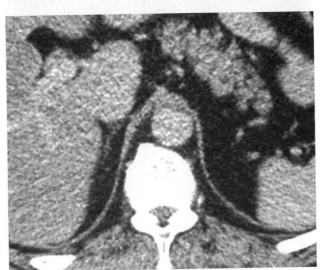

Figure 19-73 Paracoccidioidomycosis. **A:** Enhanced computed tomography in acute phase shows bilateral enlargement of adrenals with large low attenuation mass on right consistent with granulomatous inflammation. **B:** Follow-up demonstrates typical subacute phase, mild nodular enlargement bilaterally. **C:** With further delay, the adrenals have become atrophic in chronic phase.

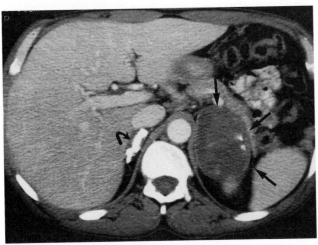

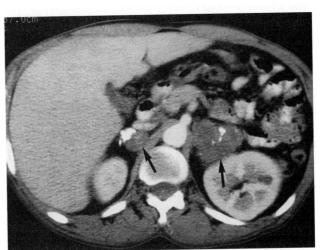

Figure 19-74 Adrenal tuberculosis. **A:** Computed tomography reveals a densely calcified right adrenal (*curved arrow*) and a heterogeneous left adrenal mass (*arrows*) in this patient with disseminated tuberculosis. **B:** More inferiorly, both adrenals show heterogeneous, somewhat low-attenuation small masses (*arrows*). The patient was addisonian.

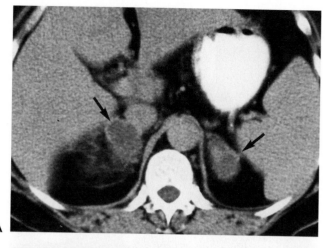

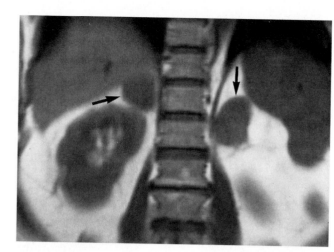

A

B

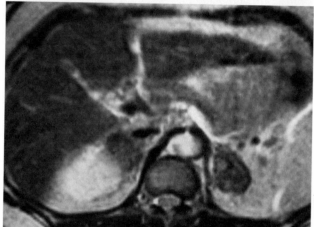

C

Figure 19-75   Bilateral adrenal enlargement due to histoplasmosis. **A:** Bilateral heterogeneous adrenal masses with low-attenuation centers and denser rims are seen on computed tomography (*arrows*). **B:** On longitudinal relaxation time (T1)-weighted coronal magnetic resonance image (416/2.0) the masses (*arrows*) are isointense with the spleen. **C:** The masses are of mixed signal on T2 (1600/80), with some central areas isointense with fat, presumably the areas of caseous necrosis.

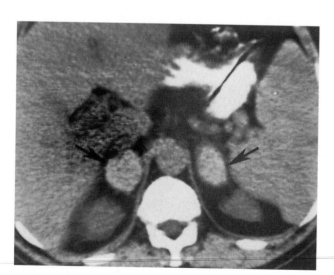

Figure 19-76   Acute adrenal hemorrhage. Noncontrast computed tomography image demonstrates bilateral adrenal masses (*arrows*), each measuring 3.5 cm in diameter. The attenuation value of both masses is uniformly higher than that of paraspinal muscle.

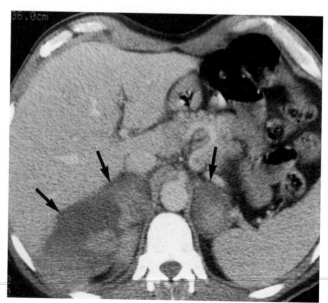

Figure 19-77   Spontaneous adrenal hemorrhage. Bilateral heterogeneous adrenal masses (*arrows*) with some high-attenuation areas were found in this patient with severe heart disease who was recently anticoagulated.

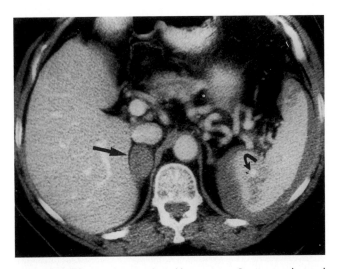

Figure 19-78 Traumatic adrenal hematoma. Contrast-enhanced computed tomography in a patient who was in a motor vehicle accident shows ovoid right adrenal mass (*arrow*) as well as splenic laceration with active extravasation (*curved arrow*).

Adrenal atrophy that results from autoimmune disease results in small glands without calcification (35,66,161) (Fig. 19-83). This must be distinguished from adrenal atrophy resulting from exogenous steroids, which has a similar appearance, by careful history. Conversely, adrenal hemorrhage, neoplasms, or inflammatory disease show either adrenal masses or calcification, as discussed previously (101,103,179) (see Figs. 19-59 and 19-74). Small adrenals that are partly or completely calcified suggest old granulomatous disease (particularly TB and Pb), whereas very dense calcifications with no soft tissue component suggest remote adrenal hemorrhage.

COMPUTED TOMOGRAPHY AND OTHER IMAGING TECHNIQUES

Except in a pediatric population, ultrasound is not used as a primary imaging method for adrenal disease, because it has both lower sensitivity and specificity than CT or MRI. The adrenals are often difficult to identify on sonography;

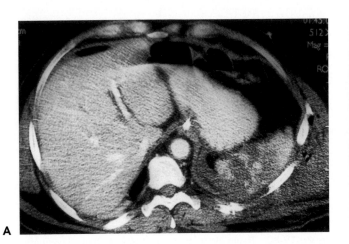

A

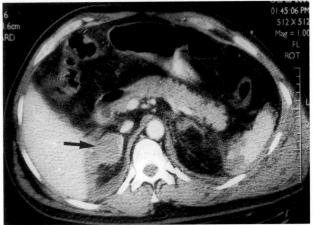

B

C

Figure 19-79 Traumatic adrenal hematoma. **A:** Trauma computed tomography (contrast enhanced) following motor vehicle collision demonstrates complex splenic laceration. **B:** More inferiorly, a 50-HU attenuation right adrenal mass is present (*arrow*). The patient also had renal injury. **C:** Follow-up computed tomography 2 weeks later shows the mass is lower in attenuation, now 30 HU; this evolution confirms this is a hematoma.

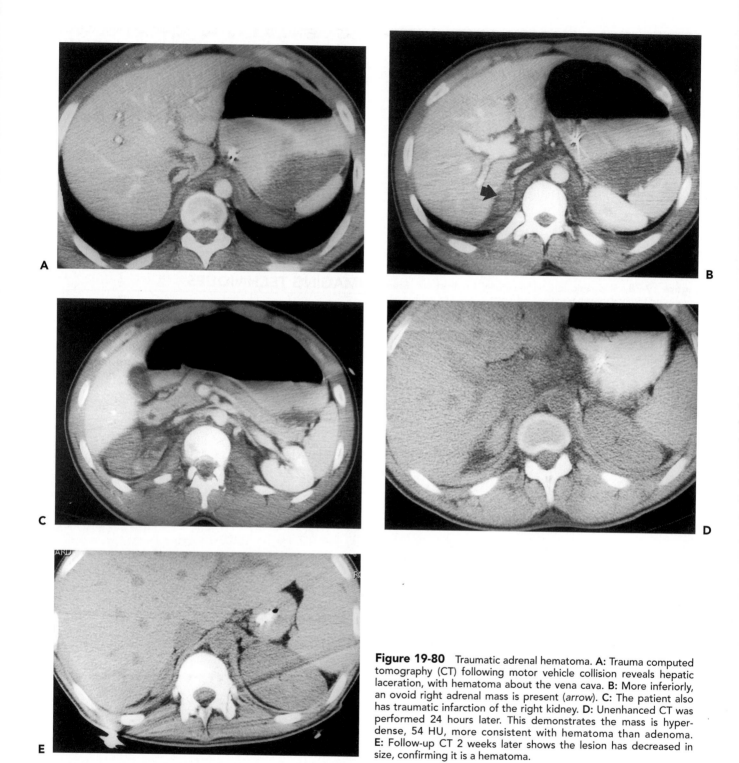

Figure 19-80   Traumatic adrenal hematoma. **A:** Trauma computed tomography (CT) following motor vehicle collision reveals hepatic laceration, with hematoma about the vena cava. **B:** More inferiorly, an ovoid right adrenal mass is present (*arrow*). **C:** The patient also has traumatic infarction of the right kidney. **D:** Unenhanced CT was performed 24 hours later. This demonstrates the mass is hyperdense, 54 HU, more consistent with hematoma than adenoma. **E:** Follow-up CT 2 weeks later shows the lesion has decreased in size, confirming it is a hematoma.

the left adrenal in particular is frequently obscured by bowel gas. Sonography can be useful in limited circumstances, such as to help determine the exact origin of a large upper abdominal mass or to determine whether a mass is cystic or solid.

CT and MRI have replaced adrenal angiography and venography. Adrenal venous sampling remains useful in certain cases. In patients with hyperaldosteronism and equivocal CT findings, adrenal venous sampling is helpful in distinguishing aldosteronoma from bilateral hyperplasia.

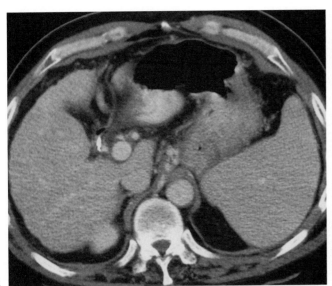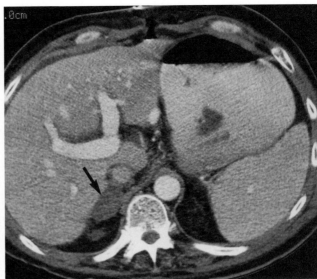

Figure 19-81 Iatrogenic adrenal hematoma. **A:** The right adrenal is normal in this preoperative computed tomography. **B:** After liver transplantation, a right adrenal mass (*arrow*) with slightly ill-defined margins has developed.

Venous sampling, however, is almost never necessary in evaluation of Cushing syndrome or suspected pheochromocytoma. Adrenal venography and venous sampling nevertheless do have potential for inadequate samples and complications, including hemorrhage and infarction of the adrenal (51).

Despite many years of investigation, adrenal scintigraphy remains little used. Compared with CT, it is expensive and requires several days before results are available. There is limited availability of the radiopharmaceutical agents, some of which are still investigational. Radioiodine-labeled MIBG does have some usefulness in certain clinical circumstances, although both CT and MRI are highly accurate and more widely available. One advantage of ^{131}I-MIBG is that images of the entire body can be produced in a patient suspected of having primary extra-adrenal or malignant metastatic pheochromocytomas. Although MIBG could be used to screen patients suspected of having pheochromocytoma, it is quicker and more cost effective to image the adrenals and retroperitoneum with CT or MRI because most pheochromocytomas are found there. MIBG can be done in patients with strong clinical and biochemical evidence of a catecholamine-producing neoplasm but negative CT or MRI. Nevertheless, MIBG does not provide enough anatomic detail to allow surgical planning, and some imaging study must be done even if MIBG is positive.

Although MRI is able to demonstrate both normal and abnormal adrenal glands accurately, it remains limited in utility because of its longer examination time, greater cost,

and more stringent patient requirements as compared with CT. However, MRI is extremely useful in selected cases. As stated previously, MRI can distinguish between nonhyperfunctioning adenoma and metastasis better than CT can. Regarding functional disorders, MRI is probably preferable to CT for evaluation of suspected pheochromocytoma, because it is as accurate for adrenal mass detection (and better for paraganglioma detection), but the findings are more specific. MRI is equivalent to CT in evaluation of Cushing syndrome. However, CT is preferred for evaluation of hyperaldosteronism and adrenal insufficiency. MRI can be useful to further characterize lesions detected on CT, including more clearly demonstrating the extent of a mass, its exact organ of origin, and detection of vascular or other local extension. MRI can be useful in evaluating an adrenalectomy bed for possible recurrence of a malignancy, because spin echo images show less degradation by clip artifact than CT shows. Last, pregnant patients suspected of having adrenal disease can be more safely studied with MRI than with CT.

A few studies have been reported on the potential role of positron emission tomography (PET) and PET/CT fusion for assessment of renal malignancies, mostly renal carcinoma. However, most studies are of relatively small numbers of patients without long-term follow-up. It is unlikely PET will replace CT (or alternatively MRI) for initial diagnosis of renal carcinoma. Sensitivity of PET for renal carcinoma has been reported to be between 77% and 94%, at best equivalent to the detection accuracy of CT (153). The real potential role for PET may lie in improving accu-

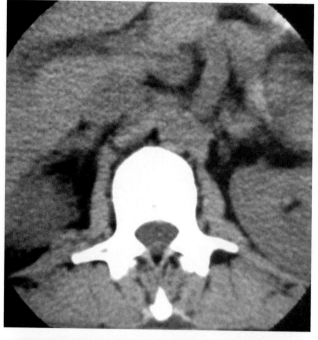

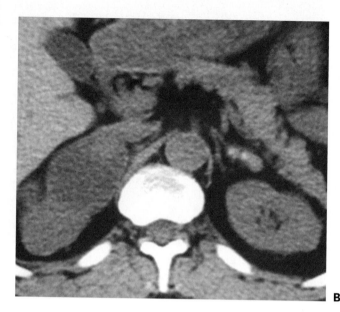

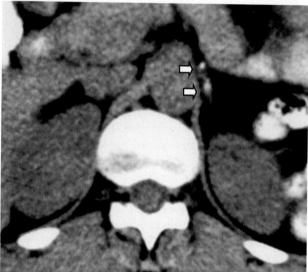

Figure 19-82 Addison disease. **A:** Initial computed tomography in acute phase of adrenal tuberculosis shows slightly thickened and slightly ill-defined adrenals. **B:** In subacute phase bilateral enlargement with large low attenuation mass on right has developed. **C:** With further delay, adrenals have become atrophic in chronic phase (*arrows, left adrenal*).

racy for initial staging and posttreatment monitoring, particularly as it is a whole-body method. Accuracy in detecting lymph node metastases has been reported to be increased from 83% for CT to near 100% and detection of postoperative recurrence increased from 70% with CT to 100% with PET (although only 10 patients followed) (153). Further study is needed to clearly define the role of PET for adrenal masses (Fig. 19-84).

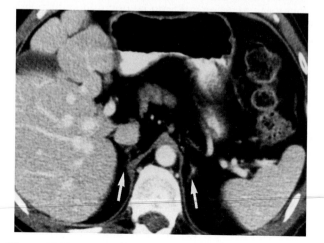

Figure 19-83 Idiopathic Addison disease. In this patient presenting with adrenal insufficiency, both adrenals (*arrows*) are markedly atrophic.

ACKNOWLEDGMENT

We thank Joseph K. T. Lee, co-author of this chapter in the previous edition, for his valuable assistance.

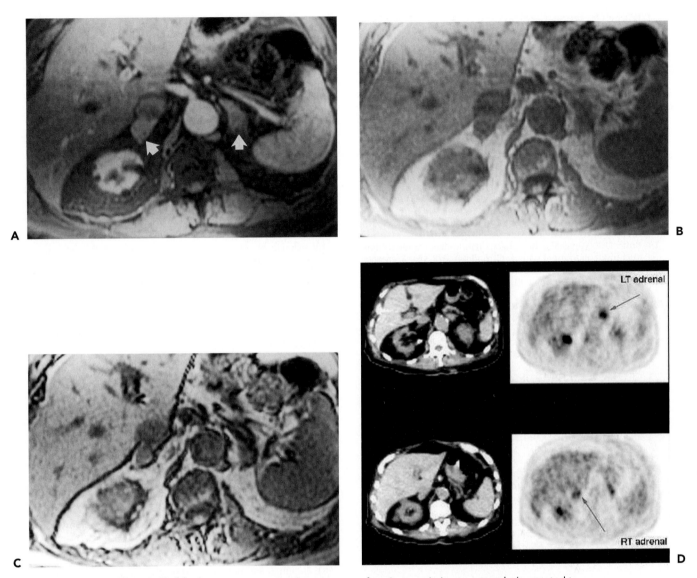

Figure 19-84 Metastases versus adenomas: use of positron emission tomography/computed tomography. **A:** Staging evaluation of this patient with lung cancer revealed bilateral nonspecific adrenal masses on computed tomography. The small lesions (*arrows*) are well demonstrated on fat suppressed longitudinal relaxation time (T1)-weighted magnetic resonance image after intravenous gadolinium diethylene-triamine penta-acetic acid. Comparison of (**B**) in phase and (**C**) opposed phase T1 gradient refocused echo images shows no drop in signal. **D:** positron emission tomography/computed tomography was performed showing abnormal metabolic activity in the adrenal nodules (*arrows*) indicating these are small metastases.

REFERENCES

1. Abecassis M, McLoughlin MJ, Langer B, et al. Serendipitous adrenal masses: prevalence, significance and management. *Am J Surg.* 1985;149:783–788.

2. Abrams HI, Siegelman SS, Adams DF. Computed tomography versus ultrasound of the adrenal gland: a prospective study. *Radiology* 1982;143:121–128.

3. Aso Y, Homma Y. A survey on incidental adrenal tumors in Japan. *J Urol.* 1992;147:1478–1481.

4. Bae KT, Fuangtharnthip P, Prasad SR, et al. Adrenal masses: CT characterization with histogram analysis Method 1. *Radiology* 2003;228:735–742

5. Baker ME, Spritzer C, Blinder R, et al. Benign adrenal lesions mimicking malignancy on MR imaging: report of two cases. *Radiology* 1987;163:669–671.

6. Baskal NN, Erdogan G, Kamel AN, et al. Localized non-Hodgkin's lymphoma of the adrenal and thyroid glands. *Endocrinol Jpn.* 1992;39:269–276.

7. Belldegrun A, Hussain S, Seltzer SE, et al. Incidentally discovered mass of the adrenal gland. *Surg Gynecol Obstet.* 1986;163: 203–208.

8. Bennett DB, McKenna TJ, Hough AJ, et al. Adrenal myelolipoma associated with Cushing's disease. *Am J Clin Pathol.* 1980;73: 443–447.

9. Berland LL, Koslin DB, Kenney PJ, et al. Differentiation between small benign and malignant adrenal masses with dynamic incremented CT. *AJR Am J Roentgenol.* 1988;151:95–101.

10. Berliner L, Bosniak MA, Megibow A. Adrenal pseudotumors on computed tomography. *J Comput Assist Tomogr.* 1982;6:281–285.

11. Bodie B, Novick AC, Pontes JE, et al. The Cleveland Clinic experience with adrenal cortical carcinoma. *J Urol.* 1989;141:257–260.

12. Boland GW, Lee MJ, Gazelle GS, et al. Characterization of adrenal masses using unenhanced CT: An analysis of the CT literature. *AJR Am J Roentgenol.* 1998;171:201–204

13. Bowen A, Keslar PJ, Newman B, et al. Adrenal hemorrhage after liver transplantation. *Radiology* 1990;176:85–88.

14. Brady TM, Gross BH, Glazer GM, et al. Adrenal pseudo masses due to varices: angiographic-CT-MRI-pathologic correlations. *AJR Am J Roentgenol.* 1985;145:301–304.

15. Bravo EL, Tarazi RC, Dustan HP, et al. The changing clinical spectrum of primary aldosteronism. *Am J Med.* 1983;74: 641–651.

16. Bravo EL. Adrenal medullary function. In: Moore WT, Eastman RC, eds. *Diagnostic endocrinology.* Philadelphia: BC Becker; 1990; 218–226.

17. Brink JA, Heiken JP, Balfe DM, et al. Spiral CT: decreased spatial resolution in vivo due to broadening of section-sensitivity profile. *Radiology* 1992;185:469–474.

18. Brunt LM, Wells SA Jr. The multiple endocrine neoplasia syndromes. *Invest Radiol.* 1985;20:916–927.

19. Burks DW, Mirvis SE, Shanmuganathan K. Acute adrenal injury after blunt abdominal trauma: CT findings. *AJR Am J Roentgenol.* 1992;158:503–507.

20. Bush WH, Elder JS, Crane RE, et al. Cystic pheochromocytoma. *Urology* 1985;25:332–334.

21. Casola G, Nicolet V, van Sonnenberg E, et al. Unsuspected pheochromocytoma: risk of blood-pressure alterations during percutaneous adrenal biopsy. *Radiology* 1986;159:733–735.

22. Cedermark BJ, Ohlsen H. Computed tomography in the diagnosis of metastases of the adrenal glands. *Surg Gynecol Obstet.* 1981;152:13–16.

23. Chang A, Glazer HS, Lee JKT, et al. Adrenal gland: MR imaging. *Radiology* 1987;163:123–128.

24. Chang SY, Lee S, Ma CP, et al. Non-functioning tumors of the adrenal cortex. *Br J Urol.* 1989;63:462–464.

25. Cheema P, Cartagena R, Staubitz W. Adrenal cysts: diagnosis and treatment. *J Urol.* 1981;120:396.

26. Chezmar JL, Robbins SM, Nelson RC, et al. Adrenal Masses: characterization with T1-weighted MR imaging. *Radiology* 1988; 166:357–359.

27. Cirillo RL Jr, Bennett WF, Vitellas KM, et al. Pathology of the adrenal gland: Imaging features. *AJR Am J Roentgenol.* 1998;18: 1425–1440.

28. Davis PL, Hricak H, Bradley WG Jr. Magnetic resonance imaging of the adrenal glands. *Radiol Clin North Am.* 1984;22:891–895.

29. DeBlois GG, DeMay RM. Adrenal myelolipoma diagnosis by computed-tomography-guided fine-needle aspiration. *Cancer* 1985;55:848–850.

30. Desai MB, Kapadia SN. Feminizing adrenocortical tumors in male patients: adenoma versus carcinoma. *J Urol.* 1988;139: 101–103.

31. Dieckmann KP, Hamm B, Pickartz H, et al. Adrenal myelolipoma: clinical, radiologic and histologic features. *Urology* 1987;29:1–8.

32. Disler DG, Chew FS. Adrenal pheochromocytoma. *AJR Am J Roentgenol.* 1992;158:1056.

33. Doppman JL. The dilemma of bilateral adrenocortical nodularity in Conn's and Cushing's syndromes. *Radiol Clin North Am.* 1993;31:1039–1050.

34. Doppman JL, Gill JR, Miller DL, et al. Distinction between hyperaldosteronism due to bilateral hyperplasia and unilateral aldosteronoma: reliability of CT. *Radiology* 1992;184:677–682.

35. Doppman JL, Gill JR Jr, Nienhuis AW, et al. CT findings in Addison's disease. *J Comput Assist Tomogr.* 1982;6:757–761.

36. Doppman JL, Miller DL, Dwyer AJ, et al. Macronodular adrenal hyperplasia in Cushing disease. *Radiology* 1988;166:347–352.

37. Doppman JL, Nieman LK. Travis WD, et al. CT and MR imaging of massive macronodular adrenocortical disease: a rare cause of autonomous primary adrenal hypercortisolism. *J Comput Assist Tomogr.* 1991;15:773–779.

38. Doppman JL, Travis WD, Nieman L, et al. Cushing syndrome due to primary pigmented nodular adrenocortical disease: findings at CT and MR imaging. *Radiology* 1989;172:415–420.

39. Dunnick NR, Doppman JL, Gill JR, et al. Localization of functional adrenal tumors by computed tomography and venous sampling. *Radiology* 1982;142:429–433.

40. Dunnick NR, Leight GS Jr, Roubidoux MA, et al. CT in the diagnosis of primary aldosteronism: sensitivity in 29 patients. *AJR Am J Roentgenol.* 1993;160:321–324.

41. Eghrari M, McLoughlin MJ, Rosen IE, et al. The role of computed tomography in assessment of tumoral pathology of the adrenal glands. *J Comput Assist Tomogr.* 1980;4:71–77.

42. Falappa P, Mirk P, Rossi M, et al. Case report. Bilateral pseudocystic pheochromocytoma. *J Comput Assist Tomogr.* 1980;4: 860–862.

43. Falchook FS, Allard JC. Case report. CT of primary adrenal lymphoma. *J Comput Assist Tomogr.* 1991;15:1048–1050.

44. Falke TH, te-Strake L, Shaff MI, et al. MR imaging of the adrenals: correlation with computed tomography. *J Comput Assist Tomogr.* 1986;10:242–253.

45. Feldberg MAM, Hendriks MJ, Klinkhamer AC. Massive bilateral non-Hodgkin's lymphomas of the adrenals. *Urol Radiol.* 1986;8: 85–88.

46. Fink DW, Wurtzebach LR. Symptomatic myelolipoma of the adrenal. *Radiology* 1980;134:451–452.

47. Fishman EK, Deutch BM, Hartman DS, et al. Primary adrenocortical carcinoma: CT evaluation with clinical correlation. *AJR Am J Roentgenol.* 1987;148:531–535.

48. Foster DG. Adrenal cysts. *Arch Surg.* 1966;92:131–143.

49. Francis IR, Glazer GM, Shapiro B, et al. Complementary roles of CT and ^{131}I-MIBG scintigraphy in diagnosing pheochromocytoma. *AJR Am J Roentgenol.* 1983;141:719–725.

50. Gajraj H, Young AE. Adrenal incidentaloma. *Br J Surg.* 1993;80: 422–426.

51. Geisinger MA, Zelch MG, Bravo EL, et al. Primary hyperaldosteronism: comparison of CT, adrenal venography, and venous sampling. *AJR Am J Roentgenol.* 1983;141:299–302.

52. Gillams A, Roberts CM, Shaw P, et al. The value of CT scanning and percutaneous fine needle aspiration of adrenal masses in biopsy-proven lung cancer. *Clin Radiol.* 1992;46:18–22.

53. Glazer GM, Woolsey EJ, Borrello J, et al. Adrenal tissue characterization using MR imaging. *Radiology* 1986;158:73–79.

54. Glazer HS, Lee JKT, Balfe DM, et al. Non-Hodgkin lymphoma: computed tomographic demonstration of unusual extranodal involvement. *Radiology* 1983;149:211–217.

55. Glazer HS, Weyman PJ, Sagel SS, et al. Nonfunctioning adrenal masses: incidental discovery on computed tomography. *AJR Am J Roentgenol.* 1982;139:81–85.

56. Gleason PE, Weinberger MH, Pratt JH, et al. Evaluation of diagnostic tests in the differential diagnosis of primary aldosteronism: unilateral adenoma versus bilateral micronodular hyperplasia. *J Urol.* 1993;150:1365–1368.

56a. Goldman SM, Borri M L, Abbehusen C, Faiçal S, Szenjnfeld J, Ajzen S. Prevalence of non-metastatic adrenal glands' enlargement in patients with malignant neoplasms evaluated by computed tomography (CT). Presented at SUR/SGR meeting 2000, Hawaii.

56b. Goldman SM, Palacio G, Borri ML, et al. Prevalence of adrenal gland enlargement in patients with aortic aneurysm or aortic dissection. Presented at SUR Annual Meeting, 2000.

57. Goldman SM, Palacios GG, Falcao MA. Determining phase of Addison's disease: value of computed tomography. *Eur Radiol.* 2002;12(P):D6.

58. Gould JD, Mitty HA, Pertsemlidis D, et al. Adrenal myelolipoma: diagnosis by fine needle aspiration. *AJR Am J Roentgenol.* 1987;148:921–922.

59. Grainger RG, Lloyd GAS, Williams JL. Eggshell calcification: a sign of pheochromocytoma. *Clin Radiol.* 1967;18:282–286.

60. Grant CS, Carpenter P, Van Heerden JA, et al. Primary aldosteronism. Clinical management. *Arch Surg.* 1984;119:585–590.

61. Halvorsen RA Jr, Heaston DK, Johnston WW, et al. Case report. CT guided thin needle aspiration of adrenal blastomycosis. *J Comput Assist Tomogr.* 1982;6:389–391.

62. Hauser H, Gurret JP. Miliary tuberculosis associated with adrenal enlargement: CT appearance. *J Comput Assist Tomogr.* 1986;10: 254–256.

63. Hayes WS, Davidson AJ, Grimley PM, et al. Extra adrenal retroperitoneal paraganglioma: clinical, pathologic, and CT findings. *AJR Am J Roentgenol.* 1990;155:1247–1250.

64. Heaston DK, Handel DB, Ashton PR, et al. Narrow gauge needle aspiration of solid adrenal masses. *AJR Am J Roentgenol.* 1982;138: 1143–1148.

65. Hedeland H, Östberg G, Hökfelt B. On the prevalence of adrenocortical adenomas in an autopsy material in relation to hypertension and diabetes. *Acta Med Scand.* 1968;184:211–214.

66. Huebener KH, Treugut H. Adrenal cortex dysfunction: CT findings. *Radiology* 1984;150:195–199.

67. Huminer D, Garty M, Lapidot M, et al. Lymphoma presenting with adrenal insufficiency. *Am J Med.* 1988;84:169–172.

68. Hutler AM, Kayhoe E. Adrenal cortical carcinoma: clinical features in 138 patients. *Am J Med.* 1966;41:572.

69. Icard P, Chapuis Y, Andreassian B, et al. Adrenocortical carcinoma in surgically treated patients: a retrospective study on 156 cases by the French Association of Endocrine Surgery. *Surgery* 1992;112:972–980.

70. Ikeda DM, Francis IR, Glazer GM, et al. The detection of adrenal tumors and hyperplasia in patients with primary aldosteronism: comparison of scintigraphy, CT and MR imaging. *AJR Am J Roentgenol.* 1989;153:301–306.

71. Itoh K, Yamashita K, Satoh Y, et al. Case report. MR imaging of bilateral adrenal hemorrhage. *J Comput Assist Tomogr.* 1988;12: 1054–1056.

72. Jafri SZ, Francis IR, Glazer GM, et al. CT detection of adrenal lymphoma. *J Comput Assist Tomogr.* 1983;7:254–256.

73. Jansson S, Tisell LE, Fjalling M, et al. Early diagnosis of and surgical strategy for adrenal medullary disease in MEN II gene carriers. *Surgery* 1988;103:11–18.

74. Kamilaris TC, Chrousos GP. Adrenal diseases. In: Moore WT, Eastman RC, eds. *Diagnostic Endocrinology.* Philadelphia: BC Becker; 1990:79–109.

75. Kane NM, Korobkin M, Francis IR, et al. Percutaneous biopsy of left adrenal masses: prevalence of pancreatitis after anterior approach. *AJR Am J Roentgenol.* 1991;157:777–780.

76. Karstaedt N, Sagel SS, Stanley RJ, et al. Computed tomography of the adrenal gland. *Radiology* 1978;129:723–730.

77. Kearny GP, Mahoney EM, Maher E, et al. Functioning and nonfunctioning cysts of the adrenal cortex and medulla. *Am J Surg.* 1977;134:363–368.

78. Kenney PJ. Letters to the editor. Adrenal pheochromocytoma. *AJR Am J Roentgenol.* 1993;160:209–210.

79. Kenney PJ, Robbins GL, Ellis DA, et al. Adrenal glands in patients with congenital renal anomalies: CT appearance. *Radiology* 1985;155:181–182.

80. Kenney PJ, Stanley RJ. Calcified adrenal masses. *zUrol Radiol.* 1987;9:9–15.

81. Kenney PJ, Wagner BJ, Rao P, et al. Myelolipoma: CT and pathologic features. *Radiology* 1998;208:87–95.

82. Khafagi FA, Gross MD, Shapiro B, et al. Clinical significance of the large adrenal mass. *Br J Surg.* 1991;78:828–833.

83. Kier R, McCarthy S. MR characterization of adrenal masses: field strength and pulse sequence considerations. *Radiology* 1989;171: 671–674.

84. King BF, Kopecky KK, Baker MK, et al. Extramedullary hematopoiesis in the adrenal glands: CT characteristics. *J Comput Assist Tomogr.* 1987;11:342–343.

85. Kobayshi S, Seki T, Nonomura K, et al. Clinical experience of incidentally discovered adrenal tumor with particular reference to cortical function. *J Urol.* 1993;150:8–12.

86. Koch KJ, Cory DA. Simultaneous renal vein thrombosis and bilateral adrenal hemorrhage: MR demonstration. *J Comput Assist Tomogr.* 1986;10:681–683.

87. Korobkin M. Combined unenhanced and delayed enhanced CT for characterization of adrenal masses. *Radiology* 2002;222: 629–633.

88. Korobkin M. CT characterization of adrenal masses: The time has come. *Radiology* 2000;217:629–632.

89. Korobkin M, Brodeur FJ, Francis IR, et al. CT time-attenuation washout curves of adrenal adenomas and nonadenomas. *AJR Am J Roentgenol.* 1998;170:747–752.

90. Korobkin M, Brodeur FJ, Yutzy GG, et al. Differentiation of adrenal adenomas from nonadenomas using CT attenuation values. *AJR Am J Roentgenol.* 1996;166:531–536.

91. Korobkin M, Giordano TJ, Brodeur FJ, et al. Adrenal adenomas: Relationship between histologic lipid and CT and MR findings. *Radiology* 1996;200:743–747.

92. Korobkin M, White EA, Kressel HY, et al. Computed tomography in the diagnosis of adrenal disease. *AJR* 1979;132:231–238.

93. Krebs TL, Wagner BJ. MR imaging of the adrenal gland: Radiologic–pathologic correlation. *Radiographics* 1998;18:1424–1440.

94. Krestin GP, Friedmann G, Fischbach R, et al. Evaluation of adrenal masses in oncologic patients: dynamic contrast-enhanced MR vs CT. *J Comput Assist Tomogr.* 1991;15:104–110.

95. Krestin GP, Stenbrich W, Friedman G. Adrenal masses: evaluation with fast gradient-echo MR imaging and Gd-DTPA-enhanced dynamic studies. *Radiology* 1989;171:675–680.

96. Lee FT, Thornbury JR, Grist TM, et al. MR imaging of adrenal lymphoma. *Abdom Imaging* 1993;18:95–96.

97. Lee MJ, Hahn PF, Papanicolaou N, et al. Benign and malignant adrenal masses: CT distinction with attenuation coefficients, size, and observer analysis. *Radiology* 1991;179:415–418.

98. Leroy-Willig A, Bittoun J, Luton JP, et al. In vivo MR spectroscopic imaging of the adrenal glands: distinction between adenomas and carcinomas larger than 15 mm based on lipid content. *AJR Am J Roentgenol.* 1989;153:771–773.

99. Levine E. CT evaluation of active adrenal histoplasmosis. *Urol Radiol.* 1991;13:103–106.

100. Ling D, Korobkin M, Silverman PM, et al. CT demonstration of bilateral adrenal hemorrhage. *AJR Am J Roentgenol.* 1983;141: 307–308.

101. Lipsell MB, Hertz R, Ross GT. Clinical and pathophysiologic aspects of adrenocortical carcinoma. *Am J Med.* 1963;35: 374–383.

102. McCorkell SJ, Niles NL. Fine-needle aspiration of catecholamine-producing adrenal masses: a possible fatal mistake. *AJR Am J Roentgenol.* 1985;145:113–114.

103. McMurray JF Jr, Long D, McClure R, et al. Addison's disease with adrenal enlargement on computed tomographic scanning. Report on two cases of tuberculosis and review of the literature. *Am J Med.* 1984;77:365–368.

104. Melicow MM. One hundred cases of pheochromocytoma (107 tumors) at the Columbia-Presbyterian Medical Center, 1926–1976: a clinicopathological analysis. *Cancer* 1977;40: 1987–2004.

105. Mersey JH, Bowers B, Jezic DV, et al. Adrenal insufficiency due to invasion by lymphoma: documentation by CT scan. *South Med J.* 1986;79:71–73.

106. Mitchell DG, Crovello M, Matteucci T, et al. Benign adrenocortical masses: diagnosis with chemical shift MR imaging. *Radiology* 1992;185:345–351.

107. Mitnick JS, Bosniak MA, Megibow AJ, et al. Non-functioning adrenal adenomas discovered incidentally on computed tomography. *Radiology* 1983;148:495–499.

108. Mitty HA, Cohen BA, Sprayregen S, et al. Adrenal pseudotumors on CT due to dilated portosystemic veins. *AJR Am J Roentgenol.* 1983;141:727–730.

109. Miyake H, Maeda H, Tashiro M, et al. CT of adrenal tumors: frequency and clinical significance of low-attenuation lesions. *AJR Am J Roentgenol.* 1989;152:1005–1007.

110. Montagne JP, Kressel HY, Korobkin M, et al. Computed tomography of the normal adrenal gland. *AJR Am J Roentgenol.* 1978;130:963–966.

111. Moon KL, Hricak H, Crooks LE, et al. Nuclear magnetic resonance imaging of the adrenal gland: a preliminary report. *Radiology* 1983;147:155–160.

112. Musante F, Derchi LE, Bazzocchi M, et al. MR imaging of adrenal myelolipomas. *J Comput Assist Tomogr.* 1991;15:111–114.

113. Musante F, Derchi LE, Zappasodi F, et al. Myelolipoma of the adrenal gland: sonographic and CT features. *AJR Am J Roentgenol.* 1988;151:961–964.

114. Newhouse JH. MRI of the adrenal gland. *Urol Radiol.* 1990; 12:1–6.

115. Nielsen ME Jr, Heaston DK, Dunnick NR, et al. Preoperative CT evaluation of adrenal glands in non-small-cell bronchogenic carcinoma. *AJR Am J Roentgenol.* 1982;139:317–320.

116. O'Brien WM, Choyke PL, Copeland J, et al. Computed tomography of adrenal abscess. *J Comput Assist Tomogr.* 1987;11:550–551.

117. O'Connell TX, Aston SJ. Acute adrenal hemorrhage complicating anticoagulant therapy. *Surg Gynecol Obstet.* 1974;139:355–357.

118. Oliva A, Duarte B, Hammadeh R, et al. Myelolipoma and endocrine dysfunction. *Surgery* 1988;103:711–715.

119. Oliver TW, Bernardino ME, Miller JI, et al. Isolated adrenal masses in non-small-cell bronchogenic carcinoma. *Radiology* 1984;153:217–218.

120. Olsson CA, Krane RJ, Klugo RC, et al. Adrenal myelolipoma. *Surgery* 1973;73:665–670.

121. Outwater EK, Siegelman ES, Huang AB, et al. Adrenal masses: correlation between CT attenuation value and chemical shift ratio at MR imaging with in-phase sequences. *Radiology* 1996;200: 743–747.

122. Pagani JJ. Non-small-cell lung carcinoma adrenal metastases. Computed tomography and percutaneous needle biopsy in their diagnosis. *Cancer* 1984;53:1058–1060.

123. Pagani JJ. Normal adrenal glands in small cell lung carcinoma: CT-guided biopsy. *AJR Am J Roentgenol.* 1983;140:949–951.

124. Paling MR, Williamson BRJ. Adrenal involvement in non-Hodgkin lymphoma. *AJR Am J Roentgenol.* 1983;141:303–305.

125. Pasciak RM, Cook WA. Case report. Massive retroperitoneal hemorrhage owing to a ruptured adrenal cyst. *J Urol.* 1988;130:98–100.

126. Pena CS, Boland GW, Hahn PF, et al. Characterization of indeterminate lipid-poor adrenal masses: Use of washout characteristics at contrast-enhanced CT. *Radiology* 2000;217:798–802.

127. Perry RR, Nieman LK, Cutler GB, et al. Primary adrenal causes of Cushing's syndrome: diagnosis and surgical management. *Ann Surg.* 1989;210:59–68.

128. Pojunas KW, Daniels DL, Williams AL, et al. Pituitary and adrenal CT of Cushing syndrome. *AJR Am J Roentgenol.* 1986;146: 1235–1238.

129. Pommier RF, Brennan MF. An eleven-year experience with adrenocortical carcinoma. *Surgery* 1992;112:963–971.

130. Potter EL. *Pathology of the fetus and newborn.* Chicago: Year Book Medical Publishers; 1952.

131. Quint LE, Glazer GM, Francis IR, et al. Pheochromocytoma and paraganglioma: comparison of MR imaging with CT and I-131 MIBG scintigraphy. *Radiology* 1987;165:89–93.

132. Radin DR, Manoogian C, Nadler JL. Diagnosis of primary hyperaldosteronism: importance of correlating CT findings with endocrinologic studies. *AJR Am J Roentgenol.* 1992;158:553–557.

133. Raisanen J, Shapiro B, Glazer GM, et al. Plasma catecholamines in pheochromocytoma: effect of urographic contrast media. *AJR Am J Roentgenol.* 1984;143:43–46.

133a.Rana AI, Kenney PJ, Lockhart ME, et al. Adrenal hematomas in trauma patients. Presented at ARRS, 2001.

134. Reinig JW, Doppman JL, Dwyer AJ, et al. MRI of indeterminate adrenal masses. *AJR Am J Roentgenol.* 1986;147:493–496.

135. Reinig JW, Doppman JL, Dwyer AJ, et al. Adrenal masses differentiated by MR. *Radiology* 1986;158:81–84.

136. Rao P, Kenney PJ, Wagner BJ, et al. Imaging and pathologic features of myelolipoma. *Radiographics* 1997;17:1373–1385.

137. Remer EM, Weinfeld RM, Glazer GM, et al. Hyperfunctioning and nonhyperfunctioning benign adrenal cortical lesions: characterization and comparison with MR imaging. *Radiology* 1989;171:681–685.

138. Rink IJ, Reinig JW, Dwyer AJ, et al. MR imaging of pheochromocytomas. *J Comput Assist Tomogr.* 1985;9:454–458.

139. Ritchey ML, Kinard R, Novicki DE. Adrenal tumors: involvement of the inferior vena cava. *J Urol.* 1987;138:1134–1136.

140. Rofsky NM, Bosniak MA, Megibow AJ, et al. Adrenal myelolipomas: CT appearance with tiny amounts of fat and punctate calcification. *Urol Radiol.* 1989;11:148–152.

141. Rosa S, Peterson RE, Roberts RB. Recovery of adrenal reserve following treatment of disseminated South American blastomycosis. *Am J Med.* 1981;71:298.

142. St. John Sutton MG, Sheps SG, Lie JT. Prevalence of clinically unsuspected pheochromocytoma: review of a 50-year autopsy series. *Mayo Clin Proc.* 1981;56:354–360.

143. Sandler MA, Perlberg JL, Madrazo BL, et al. Computed tomographic evaluation of the adrenal gland in the preoperative assessment of bronchogenic carcinoma. *Radiology* 1982;145:733–736.

144. Schaner EG, Dunnick NR, Doppman JL, et al. Adrenal cortical tumors with low attenuation coefficients: a pitfall in computed tomography diagnosis. *J Comput Assist Tomogr.* 1978;2:11–15.

145. Schulund JF, Kenney PJ, Brown ED, et al. Adrenal cortical carcinoma: MRI appearance using current technique. *J Magn Reson Imaging.* 1995;5:171–174.

146. Schultz CL, Haaga JR, Fletcher BD, et al. Magnetic resonance imaging of the adrenal glands: a comparison with computed tomography. *AJR Am J Roentgenol.* 1984;143:1235–1240.

147. Schwartz AN, Goiney RC, Graney DO. Gastric diverticulum simulating an adrenal mass: CT appearance and embryogenesis. *AJR Am J Roentgenol.* 1986;146:553–554.

148. Schwartz JM, Bosniak MA, Megibow AJ, et al. Case report. Right adrenal pseudotumor caused by colon: CT demonstration. *J Comput Assist Tomogr.* 1988;12:153–154.

149. Scully RE, Mark EJ, McNeely BU. Case 28, case records of the Massachusetts General Hospital: weekly clinicopathological exercises. *N Engl J Med.* 1984;311:783–790.

150. Seidenwurm DJ, Elmer EB, Kaplan LM, et al. Metastases to the adrenal glands and the development of Addison's disease. *Cancer* 1984;54:552–557.

151. Sevitt S. Post traumatic adrenal apoplexy. *J Clin Pathol.* 1955;8: 185–194.

152. Shah HR, Love L, Williamson MR, et al. Hemorrhagic adrenal metastases: CT findings. *J Comput Assist Tomogr.* 1989;13:77–81.

153. Shvarts O, Han K, Seltzer M, et al. Positron emission tomography in urologic oncology. *Cancer Control* 2002;9:335–342.

154. Silverman PM. Gastric diverticulum mimicking adrenal mass: CT demonstration. *J Comput Assist Tomogr.* 1986;10:709–710.

155. Silverman SG, Mueller PR, Pinkney LP, et al. Predictive value of image-guided adrenal biopsy: analysis of results of 101 biopsies. *Radiology* 1993;187:715–718.

156. Smith SM, Patel SK, Turner DA, et al. Magnetic resonance imaging of adrenal cortical carcinoma. *Urol Radiol.* 1989;11:1–6.

157. Sohaib SA, Peppercorn PD, Allan C, et al. Primary hyperaldosteronism (Conn syndrome): MR imaging findings. *Radiology* 2000;214:527–531

158. Solomon N, Sumkin J. Right adrenal gland hemorrhage as a complication of liver transplantation: CT appearance. *J Comput Assist Tomogr.* 1988;12:95–97.

159. Sommers SC. Adrenal glands. In: Anderson WAD, Kissane JM, eds. *Pathology,* vol 2. St. Louis: Mosby; 1977;1658–1679.

160. Stone NN, Janoski A, Muakkassa W, et al. Mineralocorticoid excess secondary to adrenal cortical carcinoma. *J Urol.* 1984;132: 962–965.

161. Sun ZH, Nomura K, Toraya S, et al. Clinical significance of adrenal computed tomography in Addison's disease. *Endocrinol Japan* 1992;39:563–569.

162. Tsushima Y, Ishizaka H, Matsumoto K, et al. Differential diagnosis of adrenal masses using out-of-phase flash imaging. A preliminary report. *Acta Radiologica* 1992;33:262–265.

163. Tsushima Y, Ishizaka H, Matsumoto M. Adrenal masses: differentiation with chemical shift, fast low-angle shot MR imaging. *Radiology* 1993;186:705–709.

164. Tung GA, Pfister RC, Papanicolaou N, et al. Adrenal cysts: imaging and percutaneous aspiration. *Radiology* 1989;173: 107–110.

165. van Gils APG, Falke THM, van Erkel AR, et al. MR imaging and MIBG scintigraphy of pheochromocytomas and extra-adrenal functioning paragangliomas. *Radiographics* 1991;11:37–57.

166. Vas W, Zylak CJ, Mather D, et al. The value of abdominal computed tomography in the pre-treatment assessment of small cell carcinoma of the lung. *Radiology* 1981;138:417–418.

167. Vassiliades VG, Bernardino ME. Percutaneous renal and adrenal biopsies. *Cardiovasc Intervent Radiol.* 1991;14:50–54.

168. Vick CW, Zeman RK, Mannes E, et al. Adrenal myelolipoma: CT and ultrasound findings. *Urol Radiol.* 1984;6:7–13.

169. Vincent JM, Morrison ID, Armstrong P, et al. The size of normal adrenal glands on computed tomography. *Clin Radiol.* 1994;49: 453–455.

170. Vincent JM, Morison ID, Armstrong P, et al. Computer tomography of diffuse, non-metastatic enlargement of the adrenal glands in patients with malignant disease. *Clin Radiol.* 1994;49: 456–460.

171. Wahl HR. Adrenal cysts. *Am J Pathol* 1951;27:758.
172. Weiner SN, Bernstein RG, Lowy S, et al. Combined adrenal adenoma and myelolipoma. *J Comput Assist Tomogr.* 1981;5:440–442.
173. Welch TJ, Sheedy PJ, van Heerden JA, et al. Pheochromocytoma: value of computed tomography. *Radiology* 1983;148:501–503.
174. Whaley D, Becker S, Presbrey T, et al. CT evaluation. *J Comput Assist Tomogr.* 1985;9:959–960.
175. White EA, Schambelan M, Rost CR, et al. Use of computed tomography in diagnosing the cause of primary aldosteronism. *N Engl J Med.* 1980;303:1503–1508.
176. Wilms G, Baert A, Marchal G, et al. Computed tomography of the normal adrenal glands: correlative study with autopsy specimens. *J Comput Assist Tomogr.* 1979;3:467–469.
177. Wilms G, Marchal G, Baert A, et al. CT and ultrasound features of post-traumatic adrenal hemorrhage. *J Comput Assist Tomogr.* 1987;11:112–115.
178. Wilms GE, Baert AL, Lint EJ, et al. Computed tomographic findings in bilateral adrenal tuberculosis. *Radiology* 1983;146:729–730.
179. Wilson DA, Muchmore HG, Tisdal RG, et al. Histoplasmosis of the adrenal glands studied by CT. *Radiology* 1984;150: 779–783.
180. Wolverson MK, Kannegiesser H. CT of bilateral adrenal hemorrhage with acute adrenal insufficiency in the adult. *AJR Am J Roentgenol.* 1984;142:311–314.
181. Xarli VP, Steele AA, Davis PJ, et al. Adrenal hemorrhage in the adult. *Medicine* 1978;57:211–221.

Pelvis

Julia R. Fielding

Both magnetic resonance imaging (MRI) and computed tomography (CT) have important roles to play in the imaging of disease of the male and female pelvis. Although CT remains preeminent in the evaluation of bowel pathology and advanced cancers of the genitourinary tract, MR has become the test of choice for benign disease of the female pelvis and the staging of early cervical and uterine cancer. Both modalities can be used to image the posttherapy pelvis.

TECHNIQUES

Computed Tomography

The development of helical CT markedly increased its value in the diagnosis of pelvic pathology. Helical, and now multidetector, techniques, allow optimization of both contrast bolus and slice thickness for lesion characterization. An entire pelvic CT examination can be completed in less than 20 seconds and nearly immediately reviewed as both axial and three-dimensional (3D) reformatted images in the coronal and/or sagittal planes. A high-quality pelvic CT still requires meticulous attention to technique. Barium or water-soluble oral contrast agents (800 to 1,000 mL) should be routinely administered. To maximize patient throughput, one half of the oral contrast agent is administered 2 hours prior to scanning, and the second half is given 1 hour before scanning. Rectal contrast may be used when bowel opacification is inadequate in the pelvis. Various intravenous contrast medium injection schemes are acceptable; however, the simplest for a helical CT scanner of any type is probably a single-phase injection of 100 mL of 350 mg I/mL administered at 3 mL per second with a power injector following a 70-second delay. The increased delay may cause suboptimal imaging of the liver when using a single-detector scanner; however, the majority of pelvis disease, including cancers, spreads by local extension. This delay maximizes mass detection and venous opacification in the pelvis. Scanning can be performed beginning at either the diaphragm or pubis. For single detector systems, 5-mm slice increments and a pitch of no greater than 1.5 is usually adequate. For four-row detector systems, 5-mm slice thickness reconstructed at 5- to 7-mm intervals and table speed of 15 mm per rotation resulting in a pitch of 6:1 is optimal. For 16-row detector systems, 1.5-mm collimation and gantry rotation of 0.5 per second is the usual default. Most systems have some sort of dose modulation system that varies mA slice by slice and maintains optimal table speed. Contiguous images 5 mm in thickness are then reconstructed. Delayed images are rarely necessary but may be of some value in outlining bladder tumors. Review of images on a workstation with cine and/or 3D capability makes identification of the bowel and other organs simpler.

Magnetic Resonance Imaging

The unique contrast differentiation among pelvic organs and the ability to generate images in any plane make MRI unique. Both of these attributes should be fully exploited when designing pelvic protocols. Prior to imaging, the patient should fast for 6 hours to diminish bowel peristalsis. Alternatively, 0.5 to 1.0 mg of glucagon can be administered intramuscularly at the beginning of the examination. It is also advisable to have the patient void prior to the examination to limit deformation of adjacent organs by an enlarged bladder.

Although imaging using the body coil is certainly adequate for most diagnoses, the highest resolution images are obtained using a multicoil array. All major vendors have such an array in which several surface coils are contained

1375

within a band that encircles the pelvis. Information from the surface coils is summed to form the final images. Saturation bands can be placed along the anterior and posterior body wall fat to diminish near field artifact. Coronal, sagittal, and axial rapid T1-weighted scout images encompassing the entirety of the abdomen and pelvis should be the first images obtained. These images serve two purposes. The midline structures must be identified so that the subsequent small field of view images can be centered on the organs of interest. Second, identification of the kidneys is necessary to exclude anomalies and hydronephrosis that are common accompaniments to pelvic pathology. Sagittal, axial, and sometimes coronal high-resolution fast T2-weighted images are then obtained. These high-contrast images are almost always diagnostic. A pulse sequence with simultaneous encoding of multiple 180 pulses such as fast spin-echo (FSE) or turbo spin-echo (TSE) yields the highest resolution in a relatively short amount of time (33). A 20-cm field-of-view, 128 phase encoding steps, echo train length of 8, and slices 3 to 5 mm in thickness with minimal gap are good general sequence parameters. After the T2-weighted images are obtained, the need for further imaging is variable. In the case of benign disease of the uterus, no further imaging is necessary. When characterizing a pelvic mass or staging a pelvic malignancy, dynamic, axial, and/or sagittal images of the pelvis should be obtained at 20 seconds, 40 seconds, and 3 to 5 minutes following the administration of intravenous contrast medium. These images should be obtained using a rapid T1-weighted gradient echo series (fast low-angle shot [FLASH] or spoiled gradient recalled acquisition

steady state [GRASS]). Fat saturation should be used during the performance of the contrast-enhanced images to distinguish between the presence of blood and fat.

NORMAL ANATOMY

The pelvis is a complex structure composed of an osseous ring formed by the ischia, ilii, and sacrum, with numerous muscles and fascial condensations attached for support of the pelvis viscera and to enable ambulation. Within the pelvis reside the organs of reproduction, urination, and evacuation, in addition to major blood vessels, lymphatics, and nerves. This section covers the essential CT and MR features of the internal pelvic organs. Information concerning the relationship between the peritoneal and extraperitoneal spaces of the pelvis can be found in Chapter 10.

Computed Tomography

Female Pelvis

Because CT is an x-ray–based technology, all soft tissue structures are of nearly the same, homogeneous soft tissue density. On contrast-enhanced CT scans, there is rapid enhancement of the vagina, uterus, and paravaginal plexus of veins (Fig. 20-1). The cervix, usually located at the level of the roof of the acetabulum, enhances more slowly and often appears hypodense to the uterus. The adjacent venous enhancement makes it nearly impossible to adequately assess cervical volume and small masses cannot be detected. The uterus may be anteverted, upright, lateroflexed, or

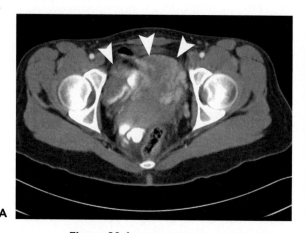
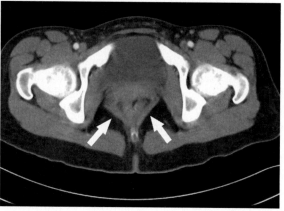

Figure 20-1 Normal female pelvis. **A:** Contrast-enhanced computed tomography shows fundus of uterus anteriorly (*middle and left arrows*), right ovary (*right arrow*) and plexus of densely enhancing veins abutting the left pelvic sidewall. **B:** Image obtained caudal to **A** shows the rectum and vagina held in place by the puborectalis muscle (*arrows*). The bladder is filled with fluid density urine.

retroverted. The endometrial canal is often heart shaped and slightly hypodense to the adjacent myometrium on axial images. In women of menstrual age, the ovaries are usually identified just medial to the iliac vessels and are of soft tissue density with occasional fluid density follicles or cysts. The broad ligaments extend from the ovaries to the pelvic sidewalls and, although not directly visualized, contain the fallopian tubes, ovarian ligaments, uterine and ovarian blood vessels, nerves, lymphatic vessels, and portions of the ureters. The round ligaments extend through the processus vaginalis bilaterally and into the inguinal canals and are usually seen. Posteriorly, the uterosacral ligaments extend from the lower uterine segment to the sacrum. These are usually not identified unless thickened and diseased. The bladder has a smooth wall, with thickness varying with distention. The perivesical fat should be pristine. The urethra appears as a round structure on the most inferior images of the pelvis.

The levator ani is composed of the horizontal, sheetlike iliococcygeus and the puborectalis or levator sling. The sling inserts just adjacent to the symphysis bilaterally and compresses the rectum, vagina, and bladder neck anteriorly. The rectosigmoid is located within the presacral space and is tortuous with a thin wall and pliable appearance. The psoas and iliacus muscles are the lateral most soft tissue structures within the pelvis. Just medial to these are the internal and external iliac vessels, artery anterior to vein. Lymph nodes in the iliac chain should not exceed 1cm in greatest dimension or number greater than three in close proximity. Posteriorly the sciatic nerve travels just anterior to the pyriformis muscle.

Male Pelvis

On axial contrast-enhanced CT images, the organs of the male pelvis are of homogeneous soft tissue density, similar to the female pelvis. There may be a slight difference in density of central and peripheral zones of the prostate, the peripheral zone being slightly hypodense. Central zone calcifications are common. When the prostate exceeds 5 cm in diameter on an axial image or when it abuts the medial portion of the obturator internus muscle, hypertrophy is usually present. The enlarged prostatic median lobe may also impress on the posterior and inferior aspects of the bladder. Patients who have undergone transurethral prostate reduction procedures will often have a central prostatic defect containing urine. The seminal vesicles have a bow-tie appearance and rest posterior and superior to the base of the prostate gland (Fig. 20-2). They are usually hypodense to the prostate because they are fluid-filled and separated from the prostate by a plane of fat. At the apex of the prostate is the root of the penis. If images are taken in the early venous phase, the corpora of the penis will enhance very brightly. The testicles are usually not imaged using CT scan. The bladder and pelvic muscles are of the same appearance as those in the female.

Magnetic Resonance Imaging

Female Pelvis

Because of the unique contrast differences among the viscera, T2-weighted MR images are often superior to CT in assessing the female pelvis (94). A small amount of high T2-signal free fluid is often seen in the cul-de-sac and is a

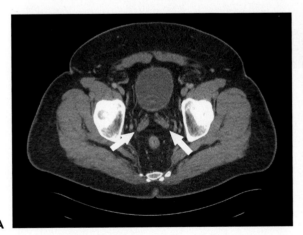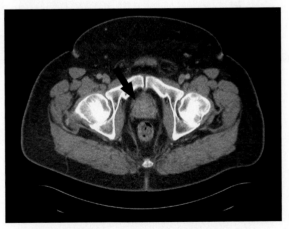

Figure 20-2 Normal male pelvis. **A:** Contrast-enhanced computed tomography shows ovoid seminal vesicles posterior to the bladder (*arrows*) and an abundance of presacral fat. **B:** Image obtained caudal to **A** shows the intermediate density prostate (*arrow*) anterior to the rectum. The bandlike muscles on each side are portions of the iliococcygeus.

normal variant in a woman of menstrual age. The uterus has three distinct zones, the high T2-signal endometrium, the low T2-signal junctional zone and the intermediate T2-signal myometrium (83). The endometrium, composed of high signal glands, may measure up to 1.5 cm in women of menstrual age and 5 mm in postmenopausal women (11). The junctional zone, located just adjacent to the endometrium, has been shown to consist of compacted myometrial cells with a high nuclear to cytoplasmic ratio. The junctional zone should measure no more than 11 mm in thickness (50,77). It may atrophy and become difficult to identify in elderly women and those women taking oral contraceptives. Inferiorly, the junctional zone widens to become the low T2 signal intensity cervical stroma (Fig. 20-3). Within the cervical stroma, two zones can be identified. There is a central very high signal area likely consisting of

mucus and glandular tissue. Just adjacent to this is the frondlike plicae palmitae (cervical glands) (84). On sagittal and axial images, the vaginal fornices delineate the external os. On axial images the vagina is an intermediate signal intensity H or butterfly-shaped organ that is closed at rest and is bordered anteriorly by the urethra and posteriorly by the rectum. It contains a high-signal mucosal layer surrounded by an intermediate muscular layer (86). A high T2 signal plexus of veins surrounds the vagina. Following the administration of intravenous gadolinium-DTPA (Gd-DTPA), on T1-weighted images this plexus and the uterus are the first structures to enhance followed by the vagina and finally, the cervix. In women of menstrual age, the ovaries should be identified in virtually every case. They are ovoid structures of intermediate signal containing high-signal follicles (73). In postmenopausal women the

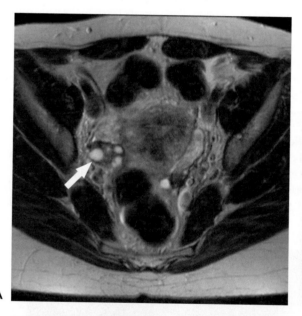

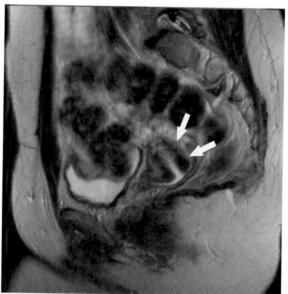

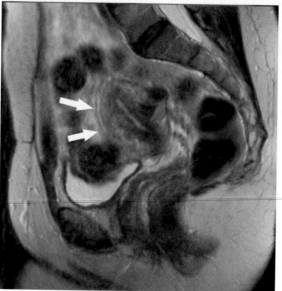

Figure 20-3 Normal female pelvis. **A:** Axial T2-weighted half Fourier turbo spin-echo (HASTE) (90/4.4) magnetic resonance (MR) image of the pelvis shows the anteverted uterus centered at the midline. The right ovary is identified by high-signal follicles (*arrow*). **B:** Sagittal T2-weighted MR image to the left of midline using the same pulse sequence shows the low signal intensity of the cervical stroma (*arrows*). Just posterior to the cervix the high signal glands extend into the vaginal fornices. **C:** Sagittal image at the midline shows the uterus with arrows pointing to the serosa. From external to internal, the myometrium is of intermediate signal, the junctional zone dark signal and the endometrium bright signal.

ovaries are atrophied and identified in only 40% of cases. The ovaries enhance homogenously and quickly, slightly later than the myometrium. The bladder usually contains high-signal urine and has a low T2 signal muscular wall. The urethra is a round structure of intermediate signal with a central low signal lumen. Normal lymph nodes should measure less than 1 cm in longest diameter, have smooth borders, and enhance homogeneously. On T1- and T2-weighted images flowing blood within the iliac vessels is of low signal. Following administration of intravenous Gd-DTPA, flowing blood is bright. The levator ani and muscles of the pelvic sidewall are of intermediate signal intensity. As with CT, fascial condensations supporting the pelvic organs are usually not identified.

Male Pelvis

Similar to the female, the varying contrast and multiple planes of MRI allow better characterization of the male pelvic organs. The prostate gland can be imaged using a wrap-around torso or pelvis surface coil alone or in combination with an endorectal coil. The base of the gland is the most cephalad aspect and the apex extends to the pelvic floor. The prostate is divided into two major zones on T2-weighted MRI—central and peripheral (40). The central zone encircles the urethra and is of low to intermediate signal intensity. It may contain some lobulated areas of heterogeneous signal that are usually benign adenomas. The peripheral zone is of homogeneous high T2 signal intensity and is horseshoe shaped encompassing the central zone (Fig. 20-4). The higher signal intensity has been attributed to its more abundant glandular components and its more loosely interwoven muscle bundles. The peripheral zone is separated from the adjacent fat and vessels by a thin very low T2 signal capsule, the posterior aspect of which encompasses Denonvillier's fascia. Assuming anterior midline to be the 12 o'clock position, the neurovascular bundles arise from the prostate at the 5 and 7 o'clock positions near the base of the gland. These should be round and of intermediate signal on axial T2-weighted images and separated from the gland by triangles of high signal fat. Near the apex of the gland a bright periprostatic plexus of veins is present and surrounds the prostate.

On axial and coronal images, the ejaculatory ducts can be seen extending superiorly from the level of the verumontanum to connect with the seminal vesicles. On axial images the vasa deferentia appear as slightly thick-walled tubular structures in the midst of the high signal seminal vesicle (40). They extend laterally and inferiorly to become a portion of the spermatic cord. On T2-weighted images, the seminal vesicles are paired primarily high signal fluid structures that contain numerous, gracile septa. Following the administration of intravenous Gd-DTPA on T1-weighted images the prostate gland demonstrates moderate enhancement and the septa of the seminal vesicles enhance brightly.

The root of the penis is composed of low to intermediate signal intensity tissue. Similar to CT, the corpora enhance densely and quickly following the administration of Gd-DTPA intravenously. The bladder contains high T2 signal urine. The wall is of varying thickness with trabeculation and diverticula common in the elderly. The testicles are usually not included on routine pelvic imaging but are of homogeneous high T2 signal intensity. The iliac vessels are of low T2 signal and the skeletal muscles of intermediate T2 signal intensity.

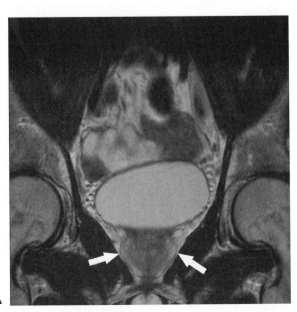
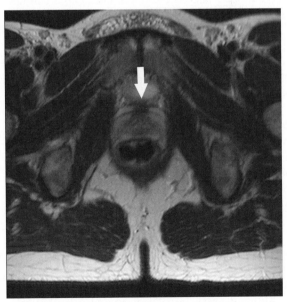

Figure 20-4 Normal male pelvis. **A:** Coronal T2-weighted half Fourier turbo spin-echo (HASTE) (90/4.4) magnetic resonance (MR) image shows high T2-signal bladder superior and anterior to the heart-shaped prostate gland (*arrows*). **B:** Axial image using the same pulse sequence as **A**, show the low signal urethra (*arrow*) is surrounded by high signal peripheral zone of the prostate gland.

BENIGN AND MALIGNANT DISEASE OF THE FEMALE PELVIS

MRI and CT are important tools in the diagnosis of benign and malignant diseases of the female pelvis. Although ultrasound (US) and hysterosalpingography remain the primary forms of imaging, MRI is now routinely used in the diagnostic evaluation of infertility, including Müllerian anomalies, and chronic pelvic pain. Both CT and MR can be used to define the origin of and characterize an adnexal mass. Staging of gynecologic malignancies can also be performed with both modalities. In obstetrics, MRI is used to assess maternal complications of pregnancy and to identify or confirm fetal anomalies.

Magnetic Resonance Imaging of Benign Gynecologic Disease and Infertility

Diagnostic images of the female pelvic organs may be obtained with the body coil; however, a multicoil array is preferred because smaller fields-of-view (20 cm) can be used and higher spatial resolution obtained without loss of signal to noise. In the evaluation of benign disease, the two most important pulse sequences are sagittal and axial T2-weighted images that encompass the uterus and ovaries. A rapid imaging technique such as FSE or TSE yields the highest quality images although ultra-fast pulse sequences such as half Fourier turbo spin-echo (HASTE) or single-shot fast spin echo (SSFSE) with 192 lines of phase encoding are often sufficient for diagnosis. In the case of Müllerian anomalies it is often useful to oblique the plane of the axial images to parallel that of the long axis of the uterus to best visualize the fundal contour. For evaluation of Müllerian anomalies, fibroids and adenomyosis, intravenous contrast medium is not necessary. For characterization of an adnexal mass, a fat saturation sequence and dynamic gradient echo based axial images following administration of contrast medium are recommended. In all cases of pelvic imaging, a large-field-of-view coronal image encompassing the abdomen should be performed to assess for renal anomalies.

Müllerian Anomalies

The müllerian ducts are paired structures that fuse between weeks 8 and 15 of gestation. They form the uterus, cervix, fallopian tubes, and upper one third of the vagina (21). The lower two thirds of the vagina arises from the urogenital sinus. Anomalies occur in less than 1% of the general population but are present in approximately 20% of patients who present with multiple spontaneous first trimester abortions (31,90). Anomalies occur because of failure of development or fusion of the müllerian ducts as well as failure of septal resorption once fusion has occurred. Although often initially diagnosed using hysterosalpingography, MRI should be performed when surgical therapy is considered to more accurately characterize the anomaly. It is particularly important to differentiate a sep-

tate from a bicornuate uterus, each of which requires different therapy. Anomalies should be classified according to the American Fertility Society (13).

The most common müllerian anomalies remain those due to *in utero* exposure to diethylstilbestrol (DES). This medication, intended to thwart premature labor, was last given in 1972. It is estimated that 60% of exposed individuals will have an abnormal hysterosalpingogram (51). Abnormal findings include a squared off uterine contour (resulting from myometrial hypertrophy), uterine hypoplasia, and fallopian tube diverticula (51,98). An appropriate medical history and abnormal hysterosalpingogram are usually all that is needed to make the diagnosis. MRI is rarely required.

Failure of development of the müllerian ducts may be partial or complete and unilateral or bilateral. Complete failure of development results in uterine agenesis. This finding in association with congenital anomalies, usually of the skeleton, comprises Rokitansky-Meyer-Kuster-Hauser syndrome (76,92). The external vagina is of normal appearance. Failure of development of one duct leads to unicornuate uterus. This anomaly is identified as a small, lateroflexed uterine cavity on both HSG and MRI. Once diagnosed, MR images should be thoroughly scrutinized for the presence of a rudimentary horn (12). This horn may be separate from or connected to the contralateral horn and may contain endometrial tissue. The presence of endometrial tissue in an isolated rudimentary horn usually leads to chronic pelvic pain with symptoms similar to endometriosis.

Complete failure of fusion of the müllerian ducts yields uterus didelphys. Two widely separated uterine cavities are identified, each with its own cervix and cephalad portion of the vagina (Fig. 20-5). In the minority of cases, a transverse septum will obstruct one of the uterine canals, leading to hematometrocolpos. Again, the external vagina is of normal appearance. Partial failure of müllerian duct fusion forms the bicornuate uterus. This anomaly is characterized by a concave external fundal contour and two uterine canals divided by a septum (74,102). The septum may be composed of a mixture of fibrous tissue and myometrium. In most cases, a single cervix and vagina will be present. This anomaly, when treated, usually requires an open metroplasty. Minimal failure of fusion leads to the arcuate uterus with a U-shaped internal contour at the fundal portion of the endometrial canal. This is an entirely benign variant and has no effect on fertility.

Once fusion of the müllerian ducts has occurred, the septum will resorb from caudalmost extent within the proximal vagina cephalad. Failure of septal resorption is the cause of the septate uterus (Fig. 20-6). This is the second most common uterine anomaly. In contradistinction to the bicornuate uterus, the external contour is flat or minimally (less than 1 cm) concave. The septum may be of variable length and contain fenestrations. Again, the septum often contains a mixture of low T2 signal fibrous and intermediate T2 signal myometrial tissue; however, in most cases the caudal most aspect will be of homogeneous low T2 signal

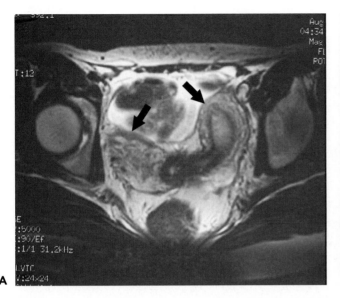

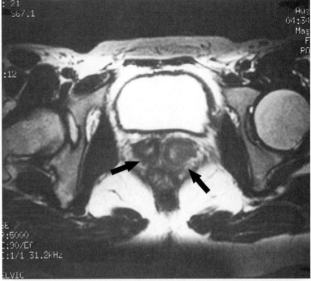

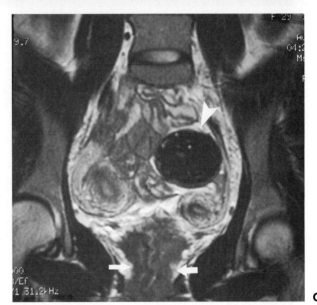

Figure 20-5 Uterus didelphys. **A:** Axial T2-weighted fast spin-echo (FSE) (4902/132) magnetic resonance (MR) image shows both uterine horns extending laterally (*arrows*). No obstruction is identified. **B:** Caudally, image demonstrates the presence of two low signal cervices (*arrows*). **C:** Coronal T2-weighted MR image using the same pulse sequence as **A** shows both uterine horns and two vertical high signal vaginal canals (*arrows*). The low signal mass superior to the left horn is a pedunculated fibroid (*arrowhead*).

indicating a fibrous nature. This anomaly is often treated with hysteroscopic metroplasty, a day surgery procedure.

Failure of development of the urogenital sinus leads to an absence of the caudal two thirds of the vagina and an obstructed cervix and uterus. The differential diagnosis is imperforate hymen. On axial T2-weighted MR images of the pelvic floor, the vagina is absent. A small low T2 signal scar may be present. Hematometrocolpos manifests as a heterogeneous but predominantly high T2 signal filling the uterine canal often markedly thinning the myometrium. Treatment in the young female often involves the formation of a neo-vagina.

Fibroids

Fibroids, or leiomyomata, are present in an estimated 40% of women older than 40 years and are particularly common in the black population (18). Symptoms associated with fibroids include bleeding, pain, and urinary incontinence. Their presence can also contribute to infertility. US, either transabdominal or transvaginal, in combination with physical examination, is most often used to diagnose the presence and monitor the growth of fibroids. On CT images, fibroids are usually of soft tissue density but may exhibit coarse peripheral or central calcification (Fig 20-7). They enlarge and distort the usually smooth uterine contour. Enhancement pattern is variable (see Fig. 20-7B and C). MRI is of value in the symptomatic patient when surgery and uterine salvage therapy is considered (22,100). This includes myomectomy, focal endometrial curettage, hormone administration, and uterine artery embolization. Using axial and sagittal T2-weighted imaging, most fibroids, including pedunculated ones, can be identified with confidence (109). They should be described in terms of size, location, and signal intensity. Any fibroid that

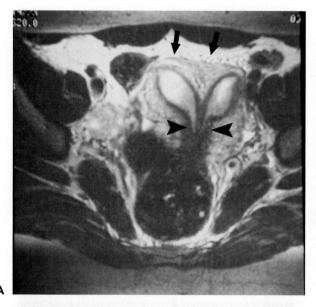

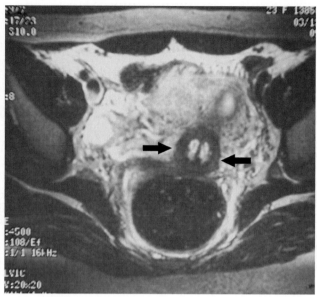

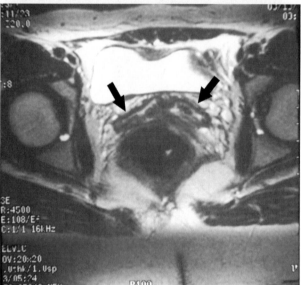

Figure 20-6   Septate uterus. **A:** Axial T2-weighted fast spin-echo (FSE) (4500/108) magnetic resonance image shows a convex uterine fundal contour (*arrows*) and two endometrial canals with a septum (*arrowheads*). **B:** At a lower level, the low signal fibrous septum is seen to extend into the cervix (*arrows*). **C:** Two proximal vaginal canals are present (*arrows*).

impresses on the endometrial canal is considered to have a submucosal component and can be a source of bleeding.

Using T2-weighted MRI, fibroids can be further classified into three groups, depending on their degree of cellularity (105). The most common group is the ordinary fibroids, of relatively homogeneous low T2 signal and composed of collagenous material (Fig. 20-8). Cellular fibroids contain less collagen and are of intermediate T2 signal intensity. These fibroids will often respond to hormonal therapy. Degenerating fibroids are of very bright T2 signal intensity (see Fig. 20-8) but often contain thick septation or wall nodules. When large or pedunculated, they can be difficult to differentiate from an ovarian neoplasm. These fibroids do not respond well to uterine artery embolization because of central necrosis (20,66). There are no discriminating features between large degenerating fibroids and leiomyosarcoma.

Adenomyosis

Adenomyosis is a common cause of pelvic pain in women of menstrual age. It is defined as extension of endometrial glandular tissue more than one third of the depth of the myometrium with adjacent muscular hypertrophy (4). Adenomyosis cannot be diagnosed using CT. With meticulous US technique, it appears as heterogeneous and cystic areas (65,75). Because of its accuracy and ease, MRI remains the test of choice (1). On T2-weighted MR images, adenomyosis appears as poorly defined low T2-signal intensity confluent with and widening the junctional zone (greater than 11 mm) (77). High T2-signal intensity glands are often seen within the diseased area (Fig. 20-9). Occasionally, focal adenomyosis will form a cavity with a very low T2-signal intensity hemosiderin rim (72). Treatment options have traditionally been limited to hysterectomy;

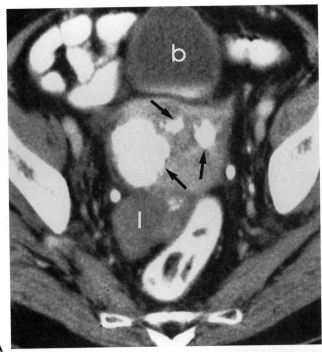

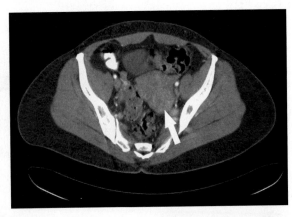

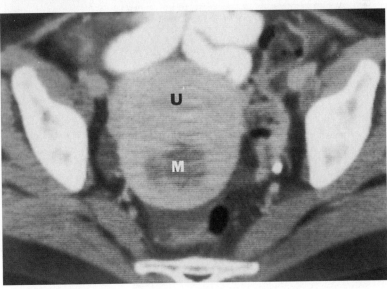

Figure 20-7   Fibroid uterus. **A:** Calcified uterine leiomyomata. Contrast-enhanced computed tomography (CT) scan through the pelvis shows the uterus to be lobulated, containing several calcified leiomyomata (*arrows*) as well as a pedunculated noncalcified leiomyoma (l) in the right cul-de-sac. b, bladder. **B:** Axial contrast-enhanced CT scan shows a round mass arising from the dorsal aspect of the myometrium, slightly increased in density compared with the adjacent uterine tissue (*arrow*). **C:** Uterine leiomyoma. An irregular mass (M) with central low attenuation enlarges the posterior uterine fundus (U) in this contrast-enhanced CT image. By CT criteria, this leiomyoma is indistinguishable from uterine malignancy.

however, recently there has been some reported success with uterine artery embolization (47).

Polycystic Ovarian Disease

The triad of hirsutism, obesity, and amenorrhea comprises Stein-Leventhal syndrome. Although the biochemical underpinnings of this syndrome are variable, most patients have elevated levels of luteinizing hormone. The classic imaging appearance of a polycystic ovary is that of increased central stroma with peripheral location of follicles (Fig. 20-10) (68). The presence of multiple peripheral cysts alone is not specific for polycystic ovarian disease (54). The ovary is enlarged (>4 cm maximal diameter) in one third of cases. There is a strong association with endometrial hyperplasia and these

patients are at increased risk for development of endometrial carcinoma.

Computed Tomography and Magnetic Resonance Imaging of Benign Adnexal Masses

Computed Tomography

The differential diagnosis for benign cystic lesions of the ovary includes simple cysts of various origins, dermoids, endometriomas, cystadenomas, and tuboovarian abscess. On CT scan, the ovary should measure no more than 4 cm in maximum diameter. It is usually of soft tissue density; however, small follicles may be seen, particularly follow-

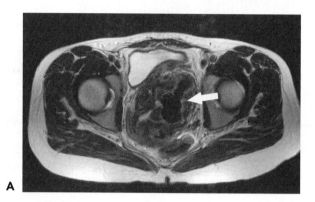

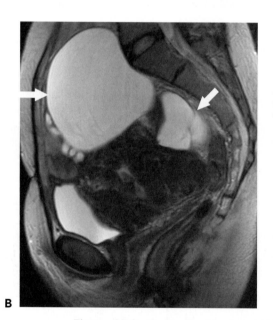

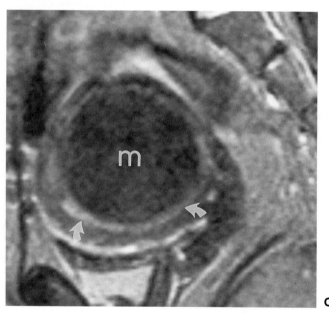

Figure 20-8   Uterine fibroids. **A:** Axial T2-weighted turbo spin-echo (TSE) (4902/132) magnetic resonance (MR) image shows an enlarged, ovoid shaped uterus. The high signal endometrial canal is distorted and deviated to the right by a conglomerate mass of predominantly low signal, collagenous fibroids (*arrow*). **B:** Sagittal T2-weighted TSE (4902/132) MR image of the same patient demonstrates that the normal intermediate signal myometrium has been nearly entirely replaced by low-signal fibroids. There are bilateral hydrosalpinges (*arrows*). **C:** Sagittal T2-weighted SE image (2100/90) shows low-signal-intensity mass (m) compressing endometrial stripe (*arrows*) inferiorly.

ing the administration of intravenous contrast agents. Simple cysts may represent a dominant follicle or corpus luteum cyst (Fig. 20-11). They are of fluid density and have no internal architecture. In women of childbearing age, any cyst less than 4 cm in diameter does not merit follow-

up, with the exceptions of those patients with known malignancies in which metastases are a consideration (88). In postmenopausal women, all cysts greater than 1 cm should probably be followed with US because of the higher likelihood of malignancy.

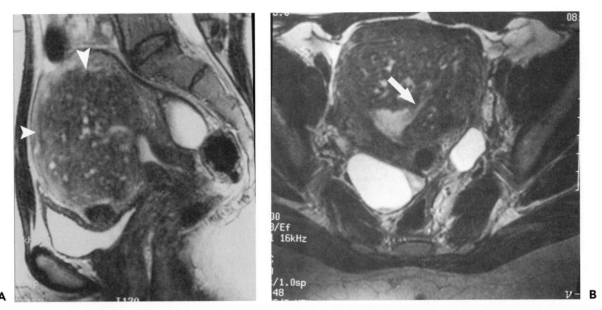

Figure 20-9 Adenomyosis. **A:** Sagittal T2-weighted fast spin-echo (FSE) (4500/108) magnetic resonance image shows enlargement of the uterus and a markedly thickened low signal junctional zone (*arrowheads*). Multiple foci of high T2 signal are present. **B:** Axial image using the same technique shows the high T2 foci to be endometrial glands extending into the adenomyoma (*arrow*). Bilateral high T2 signal ovarian cysts are present.

Dermoid

Mature teratoma or dermoid is an ovarian mass composed of tissue arising from the endo-, meso-, and ectoderm. It is a benign lesion that is bilateral in approximately 25% of cases. Identification is usually straightforward. An echogenic mass with dense posterior shadowing (the tip of the iceberg sign) is seen on US. On CT, a fat density mass with or without a fat–fluid level is present (Fig. 20-12). The high-density Rokitansky nodule, composed of hair and other components, may float within the center of the mass and calcification is often present. Dermoids without macroscopic fat have been reported, are rare, and cannot be confidently diagnosed using any modality. Most asymptomatic dermoids smaller than 4 cm are left in place. Those larger

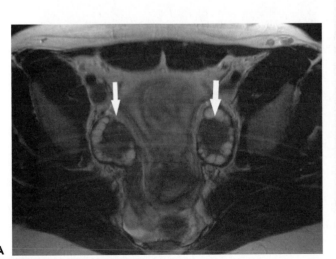

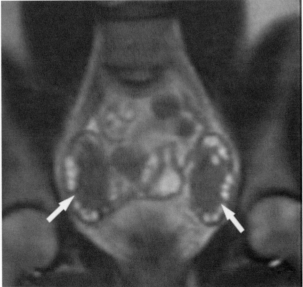

Figure 20-10 Polycystic ovaries. Axial (**A**) and coronal (**B**) T2-weighted fast spin-echo (FSE) (4500/108) magnetic resonance image shows enlarged ovaries bilaterally with an increased volume of central stroma (*arrows*) displacing the follicles peripherally.

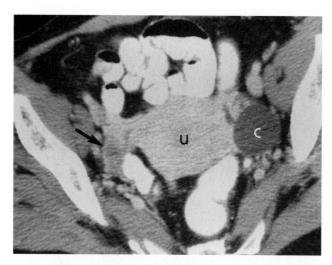

Figure 20-11 Benign ovarian cyst. Contrast-enhanced computed tomography scan of the pelvis shows a well-circumscribed, nonenhancing structure of water density (c) arising from the left ovary consistent with benign cyst. Note right ovary (*arrow*) and uterus (u).

than 4 cm are often removed because of the higher risk of ovarian torsion.

Endometriosis

Laparoscopy remains the test of choice for diagnosing and staging endometriosis because the majority of disease consists of small solid implants in the uterine cul-de-sac, along the fallopian tubes, and adjacent to the ovaries. CT, transvaginal US, and MRI are of use only when the diagnosis of an endometrioma is suspected. On contrast-enhanced CT images, endometriomas may be uni- or multilocular and are often higher in density than clear fluid (Fig. 20-13). Intermediate density debris is often seen within the dependent portion of the endometrioma. No inflammatory stranding of fat surrounds this adnexal mass. The main differential diagnosis is that of a hemorrhagic cyst and endovaginal US is often of use in distinguishing between the two entities.

Cystadenoma

Ovarian cystadenomas often are quite large when they first present. They appear as well-defined, uni- or multilocular, low-density masses. The walls and internal septa are of varying thickness and regularity (Fig. 20-14). Papillary projections of soft tissue density may be seen within the tumor. Whereas serous cystadenoma has a CT density approaching that of water, mucinous cystadenoma has a density slightly less than that of soft tissue. Amorphous, coarse calcifications sometimes can be seen in the wall or within the soft tissue component of a serous cystadenoma. Although the presence of a thick, irregular wall, irregular septa, and enhancing soft tissue projections or nodules suggests malignancy, malignant ovarian cystadenocarcinomas cannot be reliably distinguished from benign cystadenomas unless metastases are present (99,62). In one study, 69% of benign serous cystadenomas and 62% of benign mucinous cystadenomas were correctly characterized based on CT findings (99).

Tuboovarian Abscess

Usually a sequela of pelvic inflammatory disease or gynecologic instrumentation, formation of tuboovarian complex is secondary to infection with gonorrhea or chlamydia. The fallopian tube becomes dilated and obstructed, usually

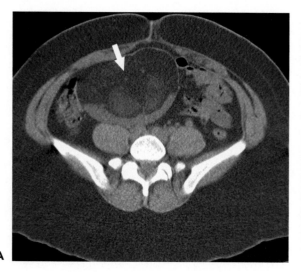
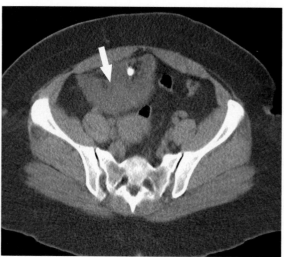

Figure 20-12 Ovarian dermoid. **A:** Axial contrast-enhanced computed tomography images show a large mass within the right side of the pelvis that contains fat (*arrow*), soft tissue and calcific densities. In **B**, the mass is seen to arise from the right ovarian pedicle (*arrow*).

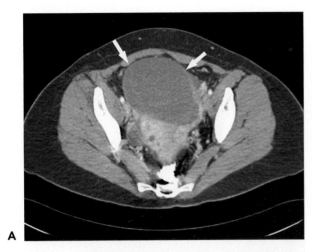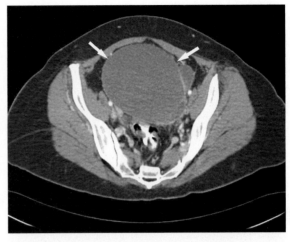

Figure 20-13 Endometrioma. **A** and **B:** Axial contrast-enhanced computed tomography images show a large cystic lesion anterior and superior to the uterus (*arrows*) with density slightly higher than urine and containing at least one septation.

by a combination of blood and pus. The ovary is often involved in the resultant inflammatory mass, sometimes called a tuboovarian complex. The process may be uni- or bilateral. On contrast-enhanced CT imaging, tuboovarian complex has the appearance of an enhancing mass with cystic and solid components (Fig. 20-15). There is extensive stranding of adjacent fat. Differential diagnosis includes torsion, diverticulitis, appendicitis, and ovarian neoplasm; however, the presence of fever, cervical motion tenderness,

and appropriate history will usually point to the correct diagnosis. Primary treatment is antibiotic therapy for 48 to 72 hours. If this regimen fails, percutaneous or surgical drainage is usually performed.

Ovarian Torsion

Rotation of the ovary on its long axis with resultant vascular and lymphatic obstruction constitutes ovarian torsion. It most commonly occurs in children and adolescents.

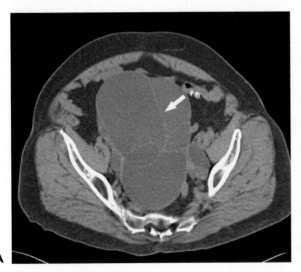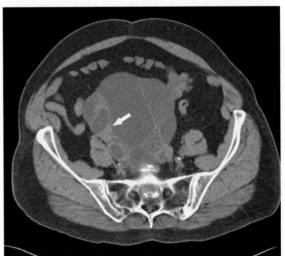

Figure 20-14 Cystadenoma. **A** and **B:** Axial contrast-enhanced computed tomography images show a large fluid density cystic mass with multiple predominantly thin septations (*arrows*) and no associated ascites.

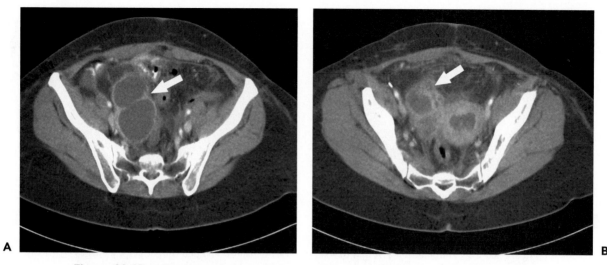

Figure 20-15 Tuboovarian abscess. Axial contrast-enhanced computed tomography images at two levels, **A** and **B**, in the pelvis show a bilobed cystic and solid mass arising from the right adnexa (*arrow*, **A**). There is extensive stranding in the adjacent fat (*arrow*, **B**) and fluid and debris within the endometrial canal.

The cause is usually an ovarian mass such as a cyst or dermoid. Because the ovary has two arterial blood supplies, one arising from the uterus, and the second, the gonadal artery, associated hemorrhage is common. The appearance on CT scans is that of a hemorrhagic solid or, in late cases, cystic mass (78). The engorged ovary is usually large enough to displace adjacent organs (Fig. 20-16). There is often an associated dilated or hemorrhagic fallopian tube.

Treatment is emergent salpingo-oophorectomy. Traditionally, an adnexal mass larger than 4 cm in a young female has been removed prophylactically because of the presumed higher incidence of torsion.

Magnetic Resonance Imaging
Similar to CT, the normal ovarian stroma is of intermediate signal intensity. High T2-signal follicles are dispersed

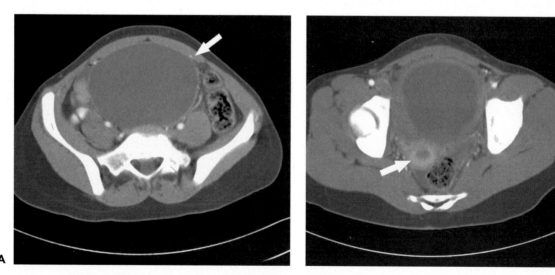

Figure 20-16 Ovarian torsion. Axial contrast-enhanced computed tomography images at two levels, **A** and **B**, in the pelvis show a large cystic structure (*arrow*, **A**) displacing the uterus posteriorly (*arrow*, **B**). The patient had been catheterized to decompress the bladder. Free fluid is seen within the cul-de-sac.

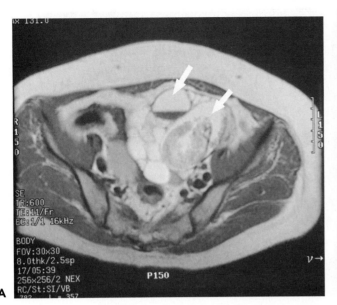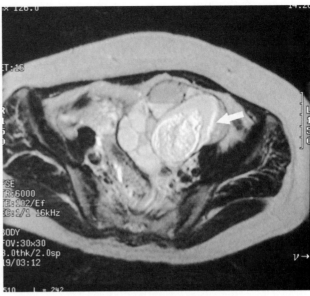

Figure 20-17 Ovarian dermoid. **A:** Axial T1-weighted spin echo (800/11) magnetic resonance (MR) image shows a complex pelvic mass containing signal similar to that of the abdominal wall fat as well as multiple fluid levels (*arrows*). **B:** Axial T2-weighted fast spin-echo (FSE) (600/102) MR image demonstrates both the chemical shift (*arrow*) and internal speckling artifacts diagnostic of dermoid.

throughout. The differential diagnosis for a simple cyst remains the same; however, internal architecture cannot be adequately discerned on T2-weighted images alone and review of the contrast-enhanced images is necessary to ascertain the absence of septa and nodules (69).

Dermoid
On T1- and T2-weighted images, the fat within the dermoid will follow the signal changes of fat within the subcutaneous tissues. Fat can be definitely identified and separated from high T1 signal blood using fat suppression pulse sequences (95). The chemical shift artifact consisting of an adjacent black and white line at the edge of the teratoma in the frequency encoding direction (usually right to left on axial images) is also diagnostic of macroscopic fat (Fig. 20-17). On T2-weighted images, the speckling artifact within the Rokitansky nodule is virtually diagnostic of a dermoid. It is composed of myriad chemical shift artifacts involving hair and adjacent fat. In some cases, a dermoid mimics adjacent bowel and the sigmoid colon must be carefully reviewed to separate it from the adnexa.

Endometriosis
Endometriomas may be uni- or multilocular and are of predominantly high signal on T1- and T2-weighted images. On T2-weighted images, intermediate signal shading, resulting from T2 shortening of blood products, is often seen within the mass. Recurrent bleeding may lead to a very low signal hemosiderin rim (Fig. 20-18). Adjacent bowel loops may be tethered to the mass. Confident diagnosis

can be difficult when some of the above MRI features are absent. Differentiation from a dermoid can be particularly difficult when the latter contains a large amount of high-T2-signal debris (70,91).

Cystadenoma
Ovarian cystadenomas often appear as large pelvic masses (34,62). The signal characteristics of these masses differ depending on the chemical composition of the cyst fluid and the amount of solid components contained within the tumor (Fig. 20-19). Although the accuracy for distinguishing between benign and malignant ovarian lesions improves with the addition of Gd-enhanced MR images (34,62,104), malignant ovarian cystadenocarcinomas cannot be reliably differentiated from benign cystadenomas unless metastases are present.

Tuboovarian Abscess
Although it is extremely unusual for diagnosis of tuboovarian abscess to require MRI, findings include free pelvic fluid, a dilated fallopian tube, and complex cystic mass (96). It is possible that a large abscess may mimic an ovarian neoplasm. Both masses consist of cystic and solid components and have thick capsules and septa (71). Ascites may also be present in both clinical scenarios. In this case, clinical history should be taken into consideration and a careful search made for inflammatory stranding of the pelvic fat. Stranding almost always heralds the presence of an inflammatory rather than a neoplastic process.

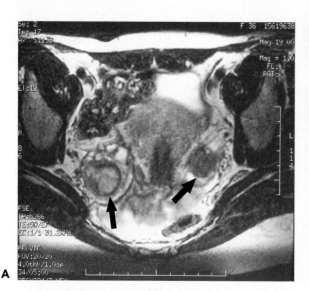

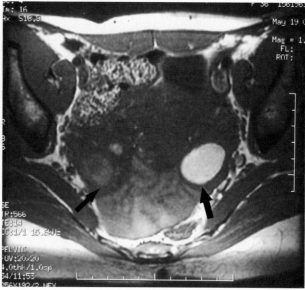

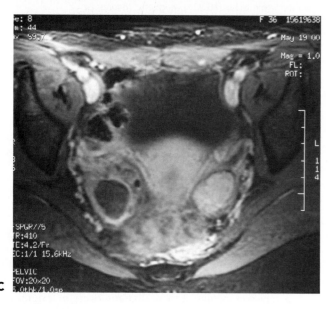

Figure 20-18 Bilateral endometriomas. **A:** Axial T2-weighted fast spin-echo (FSE) (5266/90) magnetic resonance (MR) image shows bilateral adnexal masses of low to intermediate signal (*arrows*). A low-signal hemosiderin ring surrounds the right mass. **B:** Axial T1-weighted (566/14) MR image demonstrates that the left mass is now of high signal (*arrow*) whereas the right is of low signal (*arrow*), indicating the presence of blood products. **C:** Axial contrast-enhanced (410/4.2) MR image with fat saturation shows no wall nodularity to suggest malignancy.

Gynecologic Neoplasms

Most gynecologic oncologists stage pelvic neoplasms according to the International Federation of Gynecology and Obstetrics (FIGO) system. This form of clinical staging relies on a high-quality physical examination performed under general anesthesia. Numerous radiologic tests are then performed, including chest radiograph, barium enema, and intravenous pyelogram. Hardesty et al. (37) demonstrated that, when staging endometrial cancer, performing a single MR examination of the pelvis can replace all of the ancillary examinations (with the exception of the chest radiograph) at a similar cost (37). The preoperative use of MRI was also found to decrease the number of unnecessary lymph node dissections.

Gynecologic oncologists argue that once a significant gynecologic mass is detected imaging is unnecessary because

the presumed tumor must be removed using an extensive oncologic type resection that is both diagnostic and therapeutic. There is agreement that CT or MRI is of particular value in the case of advanced disease in which the primary therapy should be chemotherapy and not surgery and should precede or replace the second-look operation in identification of recurrent metastases. Staging criteria for the gynecologic malignancies using both the TNM and FIGO systems are delineated in Tables 20-1 to 20-3.

Optimal CT technique requires excellent bowel opacification. Introduction of rectal contrast medium, although not essential, can be of help in difficult cases such as those with multiple masses or invasion of the colon. Intravenous contrast should be administered at a rapid rate and scans 5 mm in thickness obtained following a delay of 70 to 80 seconds. This delay allows good characterization of the

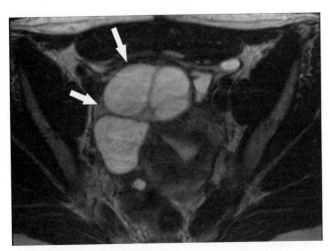

Figure 20-19 Cystadenoma. Axial T2-weighted turbo spin-echo (TSE) (4902/82) magnetic resonance image of the pelvis shows a high-signal multilocular cystic mass without wall nodularity (*arrows*). This appearance suggests benignity.

pelvic mass and opacification of both pelvic arteries and veins, facilitating identification of abnormal lymph nodes. MRI should consist of sagittal and axial T2-weighted images, optimally obtained with a multicoil array and fast-pulse sequences and dynamic images immediately postintravenous administration of Gd-DTPA. These contrast-enhanced images better characterize cervical and ovarian masses and can separate them from adjacent structures such as the bladder and rectum.

Using either CT or MRI, it is best to approach gynecologic malignancies in a systematic way. The source of the pelvic mass should be identified whenever possible. Because gynecologic malignancies spread via direct extension and the lymphatics, all images should be scrutinized for the presence of ascites, peritoneal metastases, and enlarged lymph nodes. Ascites extends along the path of least resistance posteriorly into the cul-de-sac, along the right paracolic gutter, and over the top of the liver. Peritoneal implants also follow this route first and then extend to the left paracolic gutter and medial to the spleen. Direct extension may occur anteriorly to the greater omentum. Lymphatic spread occurs laterally to the pelvic sidewalls, posteriorly to the presacral space and superiorly to the level of the renal arteries. Lymph nodes greater than 1 cm in diameter indicate metastatic disease in approximately 65% of cases (106). Finally, hydronephrosis is a common complication of gynecologic malignancy and surgical therapy. It is important that it be identified early to salvage the kidney before the onset of chemotherapy. Visceral and chest metastases occur only in extremely advanced disease.

TABLE 20-1
STAGING OF CERVICAL CARCINOMA

TNM Categories	FIGO Surgical Stages	Criteria
TX		Primary tumor cannot be assessed.
T0		No evidence of primary tumor.
Tis	0	Carcinoma *in situ.*
T1	I	Cervical carcinoma confined to uterus (extension to corpus should be disregarded).
	IA	Preclinical invasive carcinoma, diagnosed by microscopy only.
T1a1	IA1	Minimal microscopic stromal invasion 3 mm or less in depth, taken from the base of the epithelium and 7 mm or less in horizontal spread.
T1a2	IA2	Tumor with invasive component 5 mm or less in depth, taken from the base of the epithelium, and 7 mm or less in horizontal spread.
T1b	IB	Tumor larger than T1a2.
T2	II	Cervical carcinoma invades beyond uterus but not to pelvic wall or to lower third of the vagina.
T2a	IIA	Without parametrial invasion.
T2b	IIB	With parametrial invasion.
T3	III	Cervical carcinoma extends to pelvic wall and/or involves the lower third of the vagina and/or causes hydronephrosis or nonfunctioning kidney.
T3a	IIIA	Tumor involves lower third of the vagina; no extension to pelvic wall.
T3b	IIIB	Tumor extends to the pelvic wall and/or causes hydronephrosis or nonfunctioning kidney.
T4	IVA	Tumor extends outside true pelvis or has involved mucosa of the bladder or rectum.

Used with the permission of the American Joint Committee on Cancer (AJCC), Chicago. The original source for this material is Greene FL, Fleming ID, Page DL, et al., eds. *AJCC cancer staging manual*, 6th ed. New York: Springer-Verlag, 2002, www.springer-ny.com

Computed Tomography

Cervical Cancer

Cervical cancer is a usually a disease of women of menstrual age that plateaus at age 40 years in American women. Approximately 13,000 new cases are diagnosed each year (48). Causality by human papilloma virus has been generally accepted and the vast majority of tumors are of squamous cell origin (79). Patients are usually asymptomatic and detection is usually via the Papanicolaou smear. The majority of cancers are confined to the cervical canal when discovered. They are treated with a variety of local therapies including

TABLE 20-2
STAGING OF ENDOMETRIAL CARCINOMA

TNM Categories	FIGO Surgical Stages	Criteria
TX		Primary tumor cannot be assessed.
T0		No evidence of primary tumor.
Tis	0	Carcinoma in situ.
T1	I	Tumor confined to corpus.
T1a	Ia	Tumor limited to endometrium.
T1b	Ib	Invasion of inner half of myometrium.
	Ic	Invasion of outer half of myometrium.
T2	II	Tumor invades cervix but does not extend beyond uterus.
T2a	IIa	Cervical stroma not invaded.
T2b	IIb	Cervical stroma invaded.
T3	III	Tumor extends beyond uterus but not outside true pelvis.
T3a	IIIa	Tumor invades serosa and/or adnexa; peritoneal cytology.
T3b	IIIb	Vaginal metastases.
T3c	IIIc	Regional lymph nodes.
T4	IVa	Tumor extends outside true pelvis or has involved mucosa of the bladder or rectum.
M1	IVb	Distant metastases

Used with the permission of the American Joint Committee on Cancer (AJCC), Chicago. The original source for this material is Greene FL, Fleming ID, Page DL, et al., eds. *AJCC cancer staging manual*, 6th ed. New York: Springer-Verlag, 2002, www.springer-ny.com

TABLE 20-3
STAGING OF OVARIAN CARCINOMA

TNM Categories	FIGO Stage	Criteria
TX		Primary tumor cannot be assessed.
T0		No evidence of primary tumor.
T1	I	Tumor limited ovaries (one or both).
T1a	IA	Tumor limited to one ovary; capsule intact, no tumor on ovarian surface. No malignant cells in ascites or peritoneal washings.
T1b	IB	Tumor limited to both ovaries; capsules intact, no tumor on ovarian surface. No malignant cells in ascites or peritoneal washings.
T1c	IC	Tumor limited to one or both ovaries with any of the following: capsule ruptured, tumor on ovarian surface, malignant cells in ascites or peritoneal washings.
T2	II	Tumor involves one or both ovaries with pelvic extension and/or implants.
T2a	IIA	Extension and/or implants on uterus and/or tube(s). No malignant cells in ascites or peritoneal washings.
T2b	IIB	Extension and/or implants on other pelvic tissues. No malignant cells in ascites or peritoneal washings.
T2c	IIC	Pelvic extension and/or implants (T2a or T2b) with malignant cells in ascites or peritoneal washings.
T3	III	Tumor involves one or both ovaries with microscopically confirmed peritoneal metastasis outside the pelvis.
T3a	IIIA	Microscopic peritoneal metastasis beyond pelvis (no macroscopic tumor).
T3b	IIIB	Macroscopic peritoneal metastasis beyond pelvis 2 cm or less in greatest dimension.
T3c	IIIC	Peritoneal metastasis beyond pelvis more than 2 cm in greatest dimension and/or regional lymph node metastasis.

Used with the permission of the American Joint Committee on Cancer (AJCC), Chicago. The original source for this material is Greene FL, Fleming ID, Page DL, et al., eds. *AJCC cancer staging manual*, 6th ed. New York: Springer-Verlag, 2002, www.springer-ny.com

laser ablation. Any cervical mass that is greater than 1.5 cm or presumed to extend beyond the cervix should be examined using MRI. CT scanning lacks the contrast resolution necessary for primary staging of relatively low volume disease, with overall staging accuracy reportedly ranging from 60% to 80% (16,53). In cases of advanced disease, CT is preferred (Fig. 20-20). It is quick to perform and read and has a higher spatial resolution than MRI. The cervix is often enlarged in the anterior-posterior direction and may contain gas (Fig. 20-21). Images should be scrutinized for extension into the pelvic sidewall manifested by encasement of the iliac vessels and/or separation the vessels from the mass by a fat plane measuring less than 3 mm in width. Increased number and enlargement of pelvic and retroperitoneal lymph nodes should be noted. CT and MRI are equivalent in the detection of involved lymph nodes. Using 1 cm as the upper limits of normal, Yang et al. (106) found a 65% accuracy with CT and a 70% accuracy with MR. Thickening of the uterosacral ligaments also manifests extension of disease, although this can also be a result of radiation (23). The development of hydronephrosis is often the result of bladder wall or ureteric invasion and upstages the disease to IIIB. Finally, using CT, a survey of the other abdominal organs for the presence of metastases can be accomplished without requiring extra scanning time.

Endometrial Cancer

The most common of the gynecologic malignancies, endometrial cancer also has the best prognosis. Of the 38,000 new cases diagnosed each year, 75% of patients present with stage I disease confined to the endometrial canal and curable by hysterectomy (48). Presentation is usually painless vaginal bleeding in a postmenopausal woman and

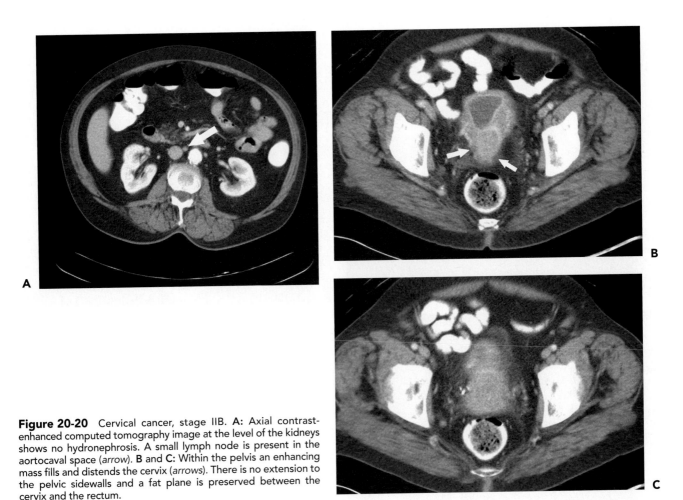

Figure 20-20 Cervical cancer, stage IIB. **A:** Axial contrast-enhanced computed tomography image at the level of the kidneys shows no hydronephrosis. A small lymph node is present in the aortocaval space (*arrow*). **B** and **C:** Within the pelvis an enhancing mass fills and distends the cervix (*arrows*). There is no extension to the pelvic sidewalls and a fat plane is preserved between the cervix and the rectum.

diagnosis is usually made by a combination of US and pipette biopsy. In addition to age, risk factors include obesity and prolonged exposure to unopposed estrogens. The endometrial thickness of a postmenopausal woman should not exceed 5 mm (11). Women with bleeding and thickened endometrial linings on US examination merit biopsy. However, even in the presence of vaginal bleeding, endometrial thickness of less than 5 mm excludes endometrial cancer (11). Women taking hormone replacement therapy or tamoxifen may have slightly thicker endometrial linings and polyps; however, 5 mm should still be taken as the upper limit of normal because these women are at a higher risk for endometrial carcinoma (2,3).

Most women with endometrial carcinoma do not require imaging. Treatment is predicated on physical examination and low-stage disease confined to the endometrium. Women with disease confined to the endometrium or superficial myometrium have a better prognosis than those with deep invasion (10,64). Gynecologic oncologists rely heavily on clinical staging; however, enlarged lymph nodes and depth of primary tumor invasion may not be appreciated. Creasman et al. (19) recently reported that, using clinical staging, only 35 of 148 (24%) of patients with

presumed stage II endometrial cancer actually had disease confined to the uterus. In the minority of patients, endometrial carcinoma will present as an obstructing lower uterine segment mass with associated hemato- or pyometra. On contrast-enhanced CT scans, the nodules of tumor usually abut the walls of the dilated endometrial canal and completely fill the lower uterine segment (Fig. 20-22). Metastases can extend via the fallopian tubes to the ovaries, causing development of an adnexal mass. Findings of advanced disease are similar to those of cervical cancer and consist of extension of lymphatic extension of disease to the pelvic sidewall chains and retroperitoneum. In cases in which these pathways are blocked by tumor, extension via the processus vaginalis to the inguinal nodes may occur. Peritoneal and mesenteric metastases may also occur. There is a paucity of data on the accuracy of helical CT for the staging of endometrial cancer. In the sole published study of 25 patients, single detector row helical CT was found less sensitive than MRI for the detection of deep myometrial invasion (42% and 83%, respectively) (36). However, in a meta-analysis performed by Kinkel et al. (56), CT, US, and MRI were found to perform equally well in the overall staging of endometrial cancer. Sarcomas of the uterus usually

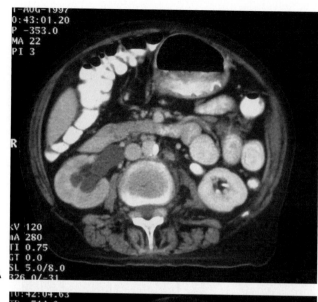

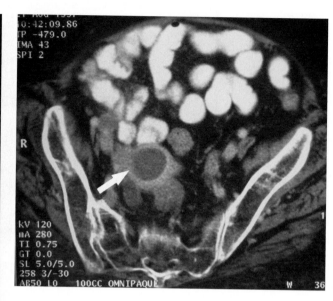

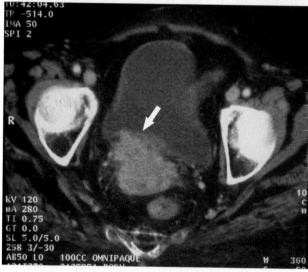

Figure 20-21 Advanced cervical cancer, stage IIIB. **A:** Axial contrast-enhanced computed tomography image at the level of the kidneys shows right hydronephrosis and a diminished nephrogram. **B:** The uterine canal is obstructed and filled with fluid (*arrow*). **C:** The cervix is markedly enlarged, invades the posterior wall of the bladder at the level of the ureterovesical junction (*arrow*).

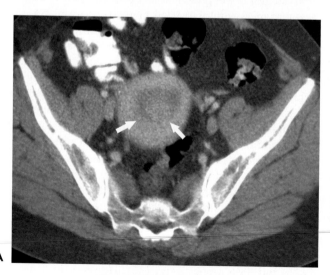

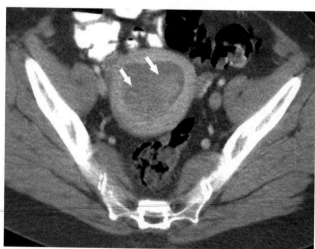

Figure 20-22 Endometrial cancer, stage IB. **A:** Axial contrast-enhanced computed tomography image of the pelvis shows abnormal soft tissue with invasion of the posterior aspect of the myometrium (*arrows*). **B:** Tumor is present within a dilated endometrial canal (*arrows*). No enlarged lymph nodes are seen.

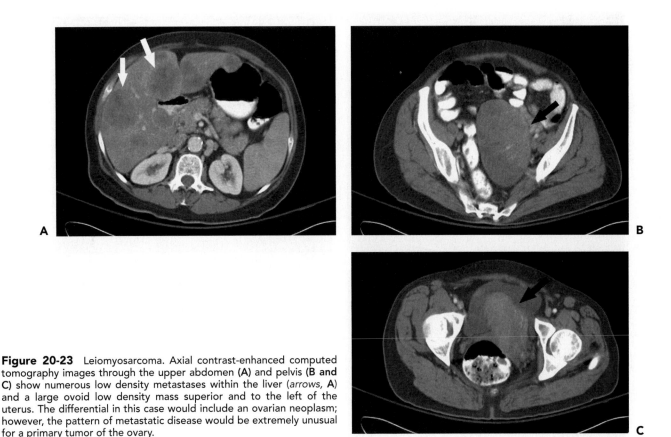

Figure 20-23 Leiomyosarcoma. Axial contrast-enhanced computed tomography images through the upper abdomen (**A**) and pelvis (**B and C**) show numerous low density metastases within the liver (*arrows*, **A**) and a large ovoid low density mass superior and to the left of the uterus. The differential in this case would include an ovarian neoplasm; however, the pattern of metastatic disease would be extremely unusual for a primary tumor of the ovary.

mimic either endometrial carcinoma (two thirds) or degenerating fibroids (one third) (Fig. 20-23).

Ovarian Cancer

Ovarian cancer is a disease of perimenopausal women with its peak between ages 45 and 55 years. Approximately 23,000 new cases are identified each year (48). Risk factors include a family history of ovarian carcinoma and, in some cases, breast cancer. Most tumors are of epithelial origin and are serous or mucinous cystadenocarcinomas. Unfortunately, no effective screening examination exists, and the majority of women (60%) present with advanced disease extending beyond the pelvis. A recent radiologic diagnostic oncologic trial showed that US, CT, and MRI are equal in the overall staging of ovarian cancer, approximately 87% to 95% (59). Both CT and MRI have excellent positive and negative predictive values (greater than 90%) for tumor resectability (27). MRI has a slightly higher detection rate for peritoneal metastases. In routine practice, CT is usually preferred because it is well accepted by the patient and gives an overall view of the abdomen and pelvis well understood by referring physicians. MRI, however, is particularly useful in the detection of recurrent disease because its tremendous contrast sensitivity yields excellent identification of even very small high signal cystic implants on fat-suppressed T2-weighted images.

Cystadenocarcinoma usually appears on contrast-enhanced CT images as a large, predominantly cystic mass with a nodular, enhancing wall and thick, enhancing septa. Ascites, hydronephrosis, and omental and peritoneal implants are common accompaniments (Fig. 20-24). Enlarged lymph nodes are less common but do occur.

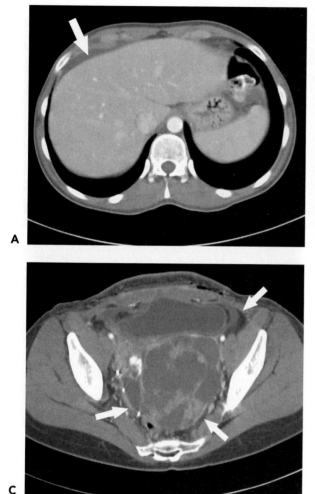

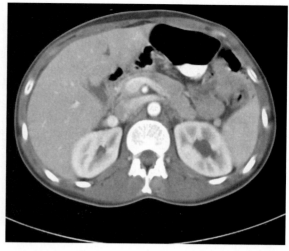

Figure 20-24 Recurrent ovarian carcinoma. Axial contrast-enhanced computed tomography scans at the level of the upper abdomen (**A** and **B**) show ascites rimming the liver (*arrow*) and left hydronephrosis. **C:** An image of the pelvis, reveals a large mixed cystic and solid mass filling the cul-de-sac and extending into the right paracolic gutter (*posterior arrows*). Ascites is also present in the left gutter adjacent to the bladder (*anterior arrow*).

Cystadenocarcinoma with ascites and minimal implant formation is treated with an extensive surgery. The procedure comprises hysterectomy, bilateral salpingo-oophorectomy, lymphadenectomy, ascites and peritoneal sampling, omentectomy, and manual examination of the surface of the liver. On imaging examinations, it is important to identify solid implants prior to therapy, because a large solid tumor burden is best treated with chemotherapy rather than primary debulking surgery (63).

Magnetic Resonance Imaging

Cervical Cancer

Although cervical cancer has been reported as being equally well identified using both the body and surface coils and also using lower field strength magnets, lesion conspicuity is improved using the surface coils (108). On MR images, cervical cancer is usually hyperintense to the dark cervical stroma on T2-weighted images. The preservation of the black ring of the cervical stroma, no matter how thin, virtually excludes parametrial extension. These patients are candidates for surgical cure. Those in whom the black line is broken and a mass extends beyond the expected confines of the cervix have an 85% likelihood of parametrial invasion and are usually treated primarily with brachytherapy (41,80,85). It is generally agreed that the administration of intravenous Gd-DTPA improves staging accuracy to between 85% and 90% (41,81,82). In cases of advanced disease, sagittal T2-weighted and/or Gd-DTPA enhanced T1-weighted images will show invasion of the rectum, bladder, and vaginal fornices (Fig. 20-25). Lymph nodes greater than 1 cm in size are positive for tumor in 70% of cases (106). Several small (less than 1 cm) lymph nodes in a chain are also suspicious for extension of disease.

Endometrial Cancer

MRI is recommended when locally advanced disease is expected based on physical examination findings and in the patient with a difficult physical examination due to obesity or prior radiation or surgery. Sagittal and axial T2-weighted

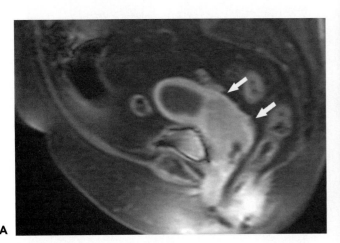

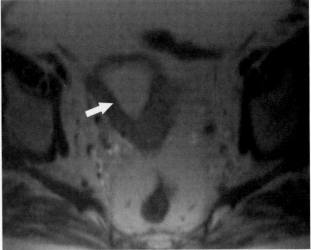

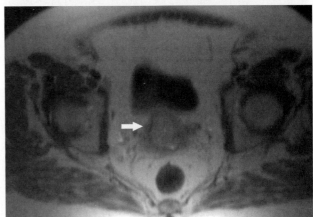

Figure 20-25 Cervical carcinoma, stage IIB. **A:** Sagittal T1-weighted contrast-enhanced (147/4.1) magnetic resonance image of the pelvis shows the characteristic barrel shape of a large cervical carcinoma (*arrows*). There is normal enhancement of the stroma surrounding the tumor; however, there is extension posteriorly into the vaginal fornix. **B** and **C:** Axial T2-weighted (90/4.4) images of the cervix show obstructed high signal uterine canal (*arrow,* **B**), and tumor filling the entirety of the cervical canal (*arrow,* **C**). Note loss of low signal stroma at 5 o'clock position.

images as well as contrast-enhanced images should be performed and scrutinized for extension of hyperintense tumor into or through the myometrium (Fig. 20-26). Preservation of a subendometrial band of enhancement 120 seconds postinjection of intravenous contrast virtually excludes myometrial extension (103). In a recent meta-analysis, intravenous Gd-DTPA was also shown to be of significant value in identifying deep invasion (28). Invasion of greater than 50% of the myometrium is strongly indicative of lymph node metastases and a poorer overall prognosis. Unfortunately, because of excretion of fluorodeoxyglucose into the urine and bladder, positron emission tomography (PET) imaging has not yet been proved to be of value in detecting adjacent involved lymph nodes (101).

Ovarian Cancer

Although equal to CT scanning in accurate staging of disease, MRI of the entire abdomen and pelvis requires at least 45 minutes. This can be difficult for an ill patient. In addi-

tion, the presence of ascites often yields artifacts, particularly on the ultrafast-pulse sequences (Fig. 20-27). For this reason, CT is the preferred examination for staging of ovarian cancer. MRI can be particularly useful when searching for small-volume recurrent disease. It has also been shown that recurrent tumor may be present and visible on MRI despite a normal CA-125 level and physical examination (61). Axial fat-saturated T2-weighted images have exquisite sensitivity in detecting small cystic implants.

Magnetic Resonance Imaging of Pelvic Floor Relaxation

Approximately 50% of parous women in the United States have pelvic floor relaxation, and 20% of that group is symptomatic enough to seek treatment. Symptoms include urinary and fecal incontinence and protrusion of tissue, usually the cervix or uterus, through the pelvic floor. Pelvic floor relaxation is usually the result of a combination of

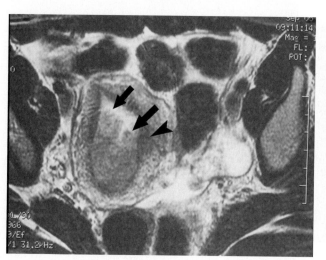

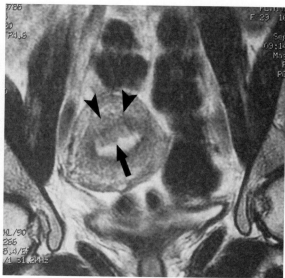

Figure 20-26   Endometrial carcinoma, stage IA. Axial T2-weighted turbo spin-echo (TSE) (4902/132) magnetic resonance image of the uterus in the axial (**A**) and coronal (**B**) planes show intermediate signal tumor rimming the endometrial canal (*arrows*). The low signal junctional zone is intact (*arrowheads*) indicating that no invasion of the myometrium has taken place.

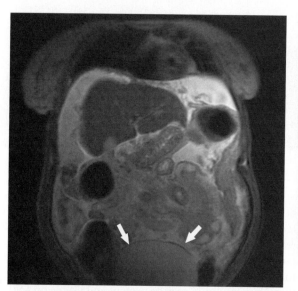

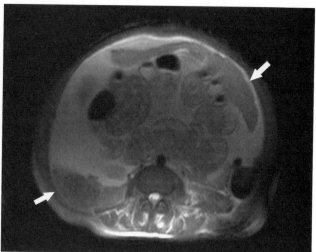

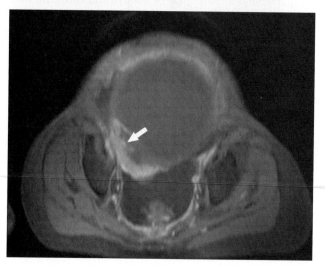

Figure 20-27   Advanced ovarian cancer. **A:** Coronal T2-weighted (90/4.4) magnetic resonance (MR) image shows massive high signal ascites and a large, midline, high-signal pelvic mass (*arrows*). Motion causes the low signal artifact seen within the ascites. **B:** Axial image at the level of the midabdomen using the same pulse sequence demonstrates intermediate soft tissue solid implants in the right paracolic gutter and replacing the omentum (*arrows*). **C:** Contrast-enhanced T1-weighted (147/4.1) MR image of the pelvis shows a large pelvic mass with an intensely enhancing nodular component along the right anterior wall (*arrow*). The peritoneum is also thickened and enhances abnormally brightly, suggesting diffuse disease.

muscle damage and fascial stretching or tearing sustained during childbirth. Most women with urinary incontinence can be diagnosed and treated based on physical examination findings and office urodynamics. Pelvic floor imaging using MRI is indicated when multiple compartments of the pelvic floor are involved and prior to repeat surgeries. It can also often replace fluoroscopic defecography. Sagittal midline images using an ultrafast T2-weighted pulse sequence with the woman at rest and at maximal strain quantify the descent of all three compartments at once and can be used to identify enterocele, sigmoidocele, and anterior urethral rotation and kinking (Fig. 20-28). Thin, axial, high-resolution T2-weighted images detail muscle atrophy and tears. Lateral deviation of the vagina usually indicates a paravaginal fascial tear (24,45).

Pregnancy

Imaging of the pregnant mother or fetus is done only for the diagnosis of specific disease entities and following a clear discussion of possible risks and benefits to the mother and fetus. This discussion should involve the mother, the referring physician, and the radiologist.

Computed Tomography

In the case of significant maternal trauma, contrast-enhanced CT scan is the test of choice. It can be done quickly and is extremely reliable in the detection of hemoperitoneum and visceral injury (Fig. 20-29). The most common cause of fetal death is maternal death, followed by placental abruption. All scan parameters should be recorded and given to the departmental physicist, who will

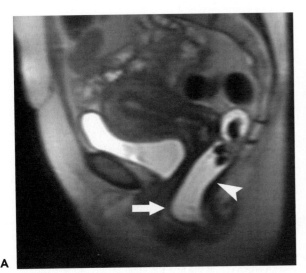

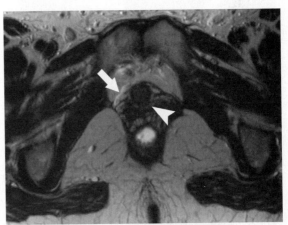

Figure 20-28 Pelvic floor damage in a middle-aged woman **A:** Sagittal T2-weighted half Fourier turbo spin-echo (HASTE) (140/4.5) magnetic resonance (MR) image of the female pelvis obtained during maximum downward strain reveals a small anterior rectocele (*arrow*) as well as abnormal caudal angulation of the levator plate (*arrowhead*). **B:** Axial T2-weighted turbo spin-echo (TSE) (4902/132) MR image shows thinning of the right aspect of the puborectalis, transection of the compressor urethrae muscle (*arrow*) and an abnormal contour of the vagina (*arrowhead*). **C:** Coronal T2-weighted TSE MR image using the same pulse sequence as in **B** shows thin, gracile fibers of the usually thick band like iliococcygeus (*arrows*).

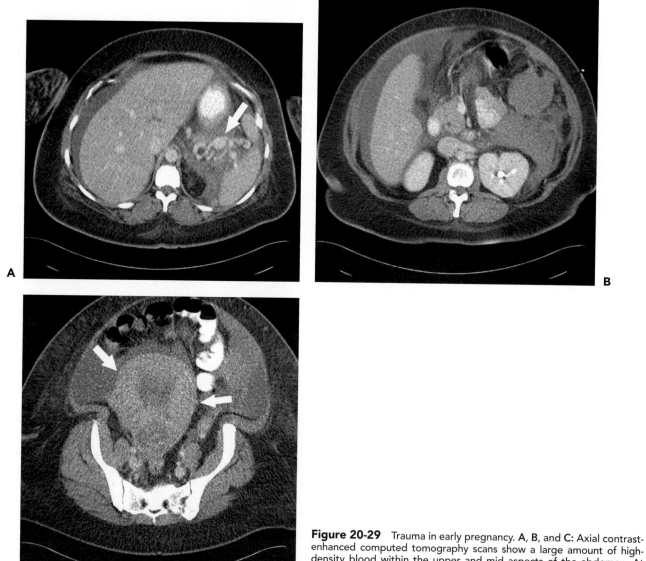

Figure 20-29 Trauma in early pregnancy. **A, B,** and **C:** Axial contrast-enhanced computed tomography scans show a large amount of high-density blood within the upper and mid aspects of the abdomen. At surgery, a ruptured splenic artery aneurysm was identified (*arrow,* **A**). **C:** Mild enlargement of the first trimester uterus (*arrows,* **C**).

then make an estimate of maternal dose. In general, a dose of greater than 10 rads should generate a consideration of abortion in a first trimester pregnancy (35). CT may also be used to diagnose obstructing maternal ureteral stones, particularly in the third trimester when the absorbed dose to the fetus decreases significantly.

Magnetic Resonance Imaging

MRI is often requested for evaluation of maternal pathology ranging from headaches and back pain to cancer staging. Although no teratogenic effects have been reported secondary to pulse sequences routinely used in human imaging, it is still prudent to discuss the possible maternal benefits and the unknown long-term risk of MRI to the fetus. One of the

more common requests is the characterization of a maternal pelvic mass identified on US examination. In most cases, imaging should be done in the second trimester because the corpus luteum cyst has resolved and it is the optimal time for surgery. The radiologist should monitor all scans. Pulse sequences should be kept to a minimum and Gd-DTPA administered only when absolutely necessary (49). It is critically important that the origin of any mass be identified (Fig. 20-30). A pedunculated fibroid will be left in place, whereas a presumed ovarian malignancy will be operatively removed (52,67). MRI should also be the test of choice when staging cancer in the abdomen and pelvis. Detection rates for liver metastases and enlarged lymph nodes are approximately equal to those of CT and no ionizing radiation

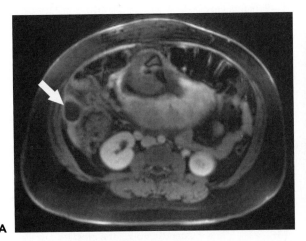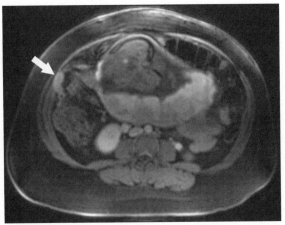

A

B

Figure 20-30 Appendicitis in a pregnant woman. **A** and **B:** Axial T1-weighted (147/4.1) contrast-enhanced magnetic resonance images at two levels in the abdomen show fluid collection with an enhancing rim in the right paracolic gutter (*arrow*) diagnostic of an abscess. Inferior to the fluid collection is an intensely enhancing tubular structure, the inflamed appendix (*arrow*).

is involved, although intravenous administration of Gd-DTPA will likely be required.

CT and MRI are both useful in the peripartum state. Flow sensitive gradient echo MRI pulse sequences through the pelvis are a particularly fast and accurate way to exclude pelvic or ovarian vein thrombosis (97). CT scan is usually the test of choice for identification of abscess secondary to endometritis or wound infection. This usually appears as an enlarged uterus with gas inside the uterine cavity and extensive stranding of adjacent fat. The ovary and fallopian tube may also be involved similar to a tuboovarian abscess. MRI is particularly useful in imaging gestational trophoblastic disease. This appears as a distended uterine cavity containing a relatively high T2 signal mass that often invades the myometrium (7).

Fetal Anomalies

With the advent of ultrafast T2-weighted pulse sequences such as HASTE and SSFSE, it has become possible to image the fetus without the blurring associated with motion. An MR image is first obtained parallel to the fetal spine. Each set of images then serves as the scout for the next, including fetal axial and coronal planes. Although US remains the mainstay in the detection of fetal anomalies, MR has proved of value in confirming visceral and musculoskeletal anomalies and identifying cranial anomalies (Fig. 20-31). Imaging is usually done as part of a complete clinical workup in a woman known to carry a second trimester fetus with an abnormal karyotype or US

(60). The most common indication is myelomeningocele. Findings can be used to plan for *in utero* surgery or to counsel parents on prognosis and the need for further genetic testing.

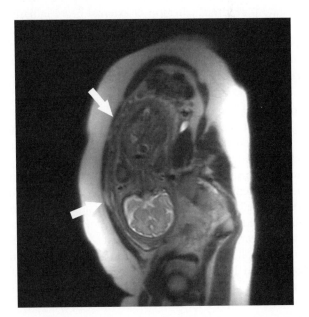

Figure 20-31 Potter's syndrome in a third trimester fetus. Sagittal T2-weighted half Fourier turbo spin-echo (HASTE) (147/4.1) image parallel to the long axis of the fetus in vertex position demonstrates severe oligohydramnios (*arrows*). Kidneys were not identified on any projection.

NEOPLASMS OF THE MALE PELVIS

CT and MR protocols for the male pelvis are the same as those for the female pelvis. Cancers of the testes and prostate are primarily identified using US. CT and MRI are reserved for staging of disease. For CT imaging, both oral and intravenous contrast media should be administered in all cases. In MRI of the prostate, intravenous administration of Gd-DTPA is necessary only when seminal vesicle extension is suspected. Recently, some authors have reported the value of ultrasmall paramagnetic iron particles in the identification of lymph nodes involved with prostate cancer; however, these have not yet been approved for human use by the U.S. Food and Drug Administration (38,39).

Prostate Carcinoma

Prostate adenocarcinoma is primarily a disease of the elderly male. Approximately 200,000 new cases are diagnosed each year (48). It is usually detected by an elevated (greater than 4 ng/dL) prostate-specific antigen (PSA) or abnormal digital rectal examination. Transrectal US is then used to direct biopsy of suspicious, hypoechoic regions, usually in the peripheral zone. Because of the high incidence of multifocality, sextant biopsies are performed. Pathologic specimens are graded using the Gleason scale, which is the sum of the most prevalent and second most prevalent types of dysplasia, each on a scale of 1 to 5, with 5 being the most dysplastic. In general, patients with a Gleason grade of less than 7 and a PSA of less than 10 ng/L are considered to have potentially curable disease. These patients undergo prostatectomy, brachytherapy, or external beam radiation. Patients that do not meet these criteria will usually undergo a combination of hormone therapy and external beam radiation. The TNM staging system for prostate cancer is listed in Table 20-4.

Computed Tomography

In most institutions, no pelvic imaging is performed prior to radical prostatectomy. CT scans of the abdomen and pelvis are ordered prior to the onset of radiation therapy to identify bony landmarks for planning. At the same time, the abdomen and pelvis can be screened for comorbidities, although this has been shown to be an extremely low yield procedure (26). In advanced disease, CT scan is the test of choice to identify enlarged pelvic and retroperitoneal lymph nodes and hydronephrosis (Fig. 20-32). Images should be examined using bone windows for the presence of osteoblastic metastases, particularly in the lower lumbar spine.

TABLE 20-4
STAGING OF PROSTATE CANCER

T—Primary tumor
Clinical

TX	Primary tumor cannot be assessed.
T0	No evidence of primary tumor.
T1	Clinically inapparent tumor neither palpable nor visible by imaging.
T1a	Tumor incidental histologic finding in 5% or less of tissue resected.
T1b	Tumor incidental histologic finding in more than 5% of tissue resected.
T1c	Tumor identified by needle biopsy (e.g., because of elevated PSA).
T2	Tumor confined within prostate.
T2a	Tumor involves one half of one lobe or less.
T2b	Tumor involves more than one half of one lobe but not both lobes.
T2c	Tumor involves both lobes.
T3	Tumor extends through the prostate capsule.
T3a	Extracapsular extension (unilateral or bilateral).
T3b	Tumor invades seminal vesicle(s).
T4	Tumor is fixed or invades adjacent structures other than seminal vesicles: bladder neck, external sphincter, rectum, levator muscles, and/or pelvic wall.

N—Regional lymph nodes
Clinical

NX	Regional lymph nodes were not assessed.
N0	No regional lymph node metastasis.
N1	Metastasis in regional lymph node(s).

PSA, prostate-specific antigen.
Used with the permission of the American Joint Committee on Cancer (AJCC), Chicago. The original source for this material is Greene FL, Fleming ID, Page DL, et al., eds. *AJCC cancer staging manual*, 6th ed. New York: Springer-Verlag, 2002, www.springer-ny.com

Magnetic Resonance Imaging

Small field-of-view, T2-weighted MRI, using a multicoil array or an endorectal coil, or both, can be of value in the patient with conflicting signs and symptoms, such as a high PSA and a small, smooth prostate (17,82). On T2-weighted FSE images prostate cancer usually appears as a region of low to intermediate signal within the peripheral zone. Most significant cancers occur along the posterior portion of the gland at the 5 and 7 o'clock positions. Direct extension of disease through the low T2-signal capsule is indicative of extracapsular extension and likely incurable disease. Images should also be scrutinized for asymmetry of the neurovascular bundles, obliteration of the rectoprostatic angle, involvement of the urethra at the apex of the gland, and extension into the seminal vesicles (Fig. 20-33)

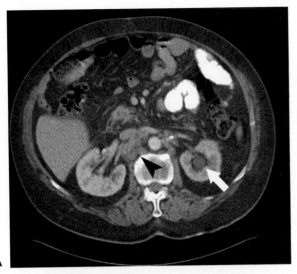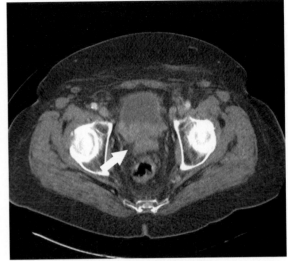

Figure 20-32 Advanced prostate cancer. **A:** Axial contrast-enhanced computed tomography image through the level of the kidneys shows right retroperitoneal lymphadenopathy (*arrowhead*) and left hydronephrosis (*arrow*). **B:** At a lower level, tumor has invaded the bladder wall and seminal vesicle (*arrow*).

(107). An experienced reader will accurately stage prostate carcinoma in 68% of cases (93). Lymph node metastases can be seen if the involved nodes are enlarged. Lymphadenopathy is best appreciated on T1-weighted images. Unfortunately, tissue characterization based on MR signal is not possible. Lymphadenopathy from benign causes cannot be distinguished from malignant disease. The ability to detect small nodal metastasis is significantly improved with MR lymphangiography that uses an intravenous contrast agent consisting of ultrasmall super paramagnetic iron oxide particles (USPIO). In one phase III clinical trial of patients with prostate carcinoma (39), post-USPIO

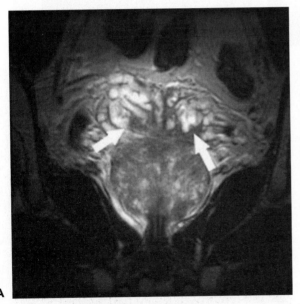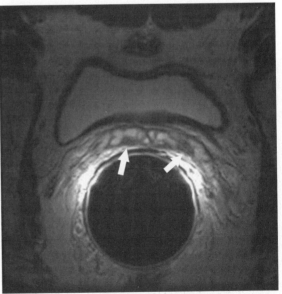

Figure 20-33 Advanced prostate cancer. **A:** Coronal T2-weighted fast spin-echo (FSE) image (4000/108) of the prostate obtained using an endorectal coil shows diffuse abnormal low signal throughout the peripheral zone. These are multiple sites of adenocarcinoma. The ejaculatory ducts are also thickened (*arrows*). **B:** Axial T2-weighted FSE image using the same pulse sequence as in **A** shows thickening of the normally gracile seminal vesicle septa indicating tumor invasion (*arrows*). (Images courtesy of Dr. Clare Tempany, Boston, MA.)

MRI had a sensitivity of 90.5% in detecting metastasis in lymph nodes between 5 to 10 mm in size (versus 35% for noncontrast scans) and a sensitivity of 41% in nodes less than 5 mm in size (versus 0% for noncontrast scans). Following radical prostatectomy, patients with elevated PSA should be examined using MRI. Similar to the patient status postabdominoperineal resection, viewing the pelvic floor with high-contrast T2-weighted or contrast-enhanced images makes it much easier to separate tumor from nor-

mal tissue (87). CT and MR images can also be of value in diagnosing inflammatory processes of the prostate and adjacent organs. Prostate abscess is usually secondary to infection, with either *Chlamydia* or *Neisseria gonorrhoeae* in the sexually active or *Escherichia coli* in the elderly with prostatic outlet obstruction. The normal gland is replaced with low-density fluid on CT scans or high T2-signal fluid that often forms multiple abscesses and extends into the adjacent seminal vesicles. Treatment is generally intra-

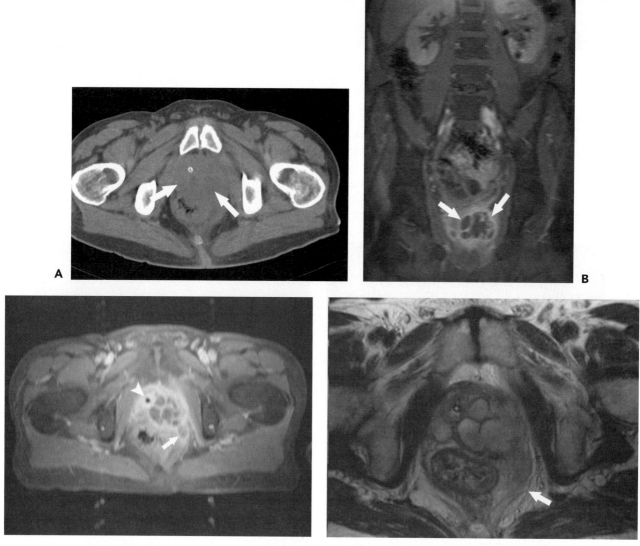

Figure 20-34 Prostate abscess. **A:** Axial non-contrast-enhanced computed tomography scan of the lower pelvis performed to diagnose presumed renal colic shows an enlarged prostate gland containing low-density areas (*arrows*). **B:** Coronal T1-weighted contrast-enhanced (147/4.1) magnetic resonance (MR) image demonstrates normal appearance of the kidneys with exception of a few cysts and a multiseptated mass replacing the majority of the prostate (*arrows*). **C:** Axial image obtained using the same parameters as **B** better defines the inflammatory mass that replaces the prostate, displaces the urethra to the right (*arrowhead*) and extends into the left seminal vesicle (*arrow*). **D:** Axial T2-weighted turbo spin-echo (TSE) (4902/132) MR image at the same level as **C** demonstrates extensive fat stranding radiating posteriorly from the left side of the prostate (*arrow*).

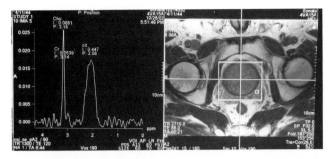

Figure 20-35 Prostate cancer. Axial T2-weighted turbo spin-echo (TSE) (4902/132) magnetic resonance image of the prostate shows an enlarged central zone that virtually obliterates the peripheral zone. Previous biopsies had demonstrated diffuse intermediate grade carcinoma. Spectra obtained within the peripheral zone (*box*) show elevated choline levels correlating with the presence of carcinoma.

venous antibiotics and incision and drainage, usually via a transrectal route (Fig. 20-34).

The addition of spectroscopy to fast T2-weighted imaging is a new area of research that holds significant promise for the detection of primary and recurrent disease. A virtual grid is superimposed on a 3D acquisition and nuclear magnetic resonance spectra obtained within each square of tissue (Fig. 20-35). The normal prostate produces a large of amount of citrate from the peripheral zone. Tumors do not produce citrate. Using the MR spectra, elevated choline-to-citrate ratios can be used to identify sites of tumor (58).

Testicular Cancer

Computed Tomography

Testicular malignancies occur predominantly in young men and are relatively uncommon with approximately 7,000 new cases diagnosed each year (48). These malignancies are almost always diagnosed by a combination of physical examination and US. Tumors are divided into the more common seminomatous tumors and the relatively rare germ cell tumors. The majority of tumors are mixed cell type with seminoma predominant and smaller amounts of other cell types including yolk sac, embryonal cell, and teratoma. Following the standard treatment of orchiectomy, contrast-enhanced CT scans of the abdomen and pelvis are performed to search for metastatic disease. The lymphatic drainage of the testicles is to the renal hila. Secondary drainage to the aortoiliac bifurcation also occurs, particularly on the right. Involved lymph nodes are of soft tissue density with dense enhancement (Fig. 20-36). The enlarged nodes may encase the renal vessels and compress and occasionally invade the inferior vena cava (IVC). Particularly large and low-density nodes indicate the presence of teratoma. Unfortunately, node density does not correlate with the degree of cell kill following chemotherapy. Residual cystic appearing nodes often undergo surgical débridement to maximize potential for cure. On follow-up scans, all nodes greater than 5 mm are considered suspicious for metastasis (44). Imaging findings should be correlated with biochemical tumor markers to further direct therapy.

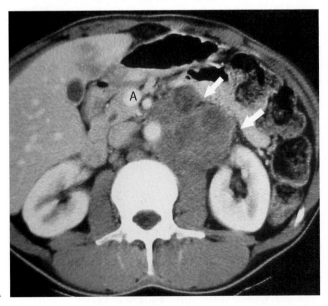

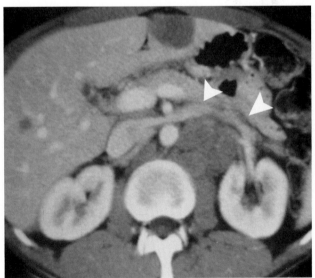

A   B

Figure 20-36 Testicular cancer. **A** and **B:** Axial contrast-enhanced computed tomography images of the abdomen show large lymph nodes at the level of left renal hilum (*arrows*) partially encase aorta (A). **B:** The patent renal vein is draped anteriorly over the enlarged lymph nodes (*arrowheads*). (Images courtesy of Dr. Jeffrey Klein, Williamsburg, VA.)

Magnetic Resonance Imaging

Magnetic resonance imaging is rarely performed for the primary diagnosis of testicular cancer. T2-weighted MRI, using a loop or shoulder coil placed over the scrotum, can be useful in identifying masses when US is indeterminate. Tumors appear as low-signal masses within the normal very high T2-signal intensity tissue. It is difficult to identify calcifications; however, capsular involvement can often be determined.

Undescended Testes

During embryogenesis the testes migrate from the level of the kidneys inferiorly and through the inguinal canal into the scrotum. When a testicle fails to descend properly, it is located within the inguinal canal 90% of the time. In children, US is often used to make this diagnosis and an orchiopexy is performed. In the adult presenting with an empty scrotum, thin-section CT or T2-weighted MR images extending from the level of the kidneys to the scrotum should be performed. On CT scans, the testicle appears as a small almond-shaped soft tissue density structure along the migration path (Fig. 20-37) (29). On MR images, the testicle is of variable signal intensity. In young adults and when fertility remains an issue, an orchiopexy will be performed. When the patient is older than 35 years, the undescended testicle is usually removed. All previously undescended testicles are at risk for

sarcomatous transformation and must be monitored for change in size, usually by physical examination.

PELVIC NEOPLASMS COMMON TO BOTH SEXES

Bladder Cancer

More than 50,000 new cases of bladder cancer are diagnosed each year, the majority in males older than 60 years (48). Risk factors include smoking, chronic infection, and exposure to aromatic amines and cyclophosphamide.

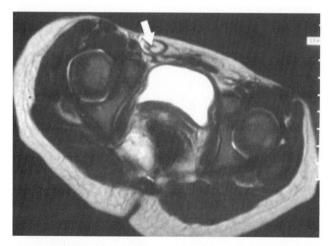

Figure 20-37 Undescended testicle. Axial T2-weighted half Fourier turbo spin-echo (HASTE) (90/4.5) image shows a high signal ovoid testicle within the right inguinal canal (*arrow*).

TABLE 20-5

STAGING OF URINARY BLADDER CANCER

Primary tumor (T)

TX	Primary tumor cannot be assessed.
T0	No evidence of primary tumor.
Ta	Noninvasive papillary carcinoma.
Tis	Carcinoma *in situ*: "flat tumor."
T1	Tumor invades subepithelial connective tissue.
T2	Tumor invades muscle.
pT2a	Tumor invades superficial muscle (inner half).
pT2b	Tumor invades deep muscle (outer half).
T3	Tumor invades perivesical tissue.
pT3a	Microscopically.
pT3b	Macroscopically (extravesical mass).
T4	Tumor invades any of the following: prostate, uterus, vagina, pelvic wall, abdominal wall.
T4a	Tumor invades prostate, uterus, vagina.
T4b	Tumor invades pelvic wall, abdominal wall.

Regional lymph modes (N)
Regional lymph nodes are those within the true pelvis; all others are distant lymph nodes.

NX	Regional lymph nodes cannot be assessed.
N0	No regional lymph node metastasis.
N1	Metastasis in a single lymph node, 2 cm or less in greatest dimension.
N2	Metastasis in a single lymph node, more than 2 cm but not more than 5 cm in greatest dimension; or multiple lymph nodes, none more than 5 cm in greatest dimension.
N3	Metastasis in a lymph node, more than 5 cm in greatest dimension.

Distant metastasis (M)

MX	Distant metastasis cannot be assessed.
M0	No distant metastasis.
M1	Distant metastasis.

Used with the permission of the American Joint Committee on Cancer (AJCC), Chicago. The original source for this material is Greene FL, Fleming ID, Page DL, et al., eds. *AJCC cancer staging manual*, 6th ed. New York: Springer-Verlag, 2002, www.springer-ny.com

Ninety-five percent of bladder tumors are transitional cell carcinomas, with the rest comprising a mix of squamous cell carcinoma, adenosquamous cell carcinoma, and the rare sarcoma. Seventy percent of bladder cancers are superficial in origin. Patients do not usually require imaging because disease is treated cystoscopically with fulguration, snaring, and topical chemotherapy. Some radiologic groups have experimented with virtual cystoscopy using CT images of an air-filled bladder; however, this is not yet accepted as routine practice (25,89). The remaining 30% of bladder cancers are invasive when discovered. To determine whether a potentially curative cystectomy should be attempted, the surgeon needs to know whether the disease is confined to the bladder wall (stage II) or extends into the perivesical fat (stage III). This is done using a combination of cystoscopic biopsy and CT or MRI. The

TNM staging system for bladder cancer is presented in Table 20-5.

Computed Tomography

CT should be performed using oral and intravenous contrast with thin sections through the bladder with both a 70-second and a 5-minute delay. The early images will serve to demonstrate hypervascular areas of tumor and the later images are sometimes valuable in outlining the tumor extent along the wall surface. Tumors may be polypoid or sessile and often extend to involve a large area of the bladder wall, including the ureterovesical junction.

Because transitional cell carcinoma is often multifocal, evaluation of the entirety of the urothelial tract should be attempted. Using multidetector CT scans with rapid refor-

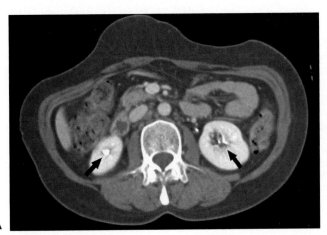
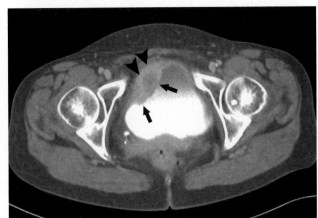
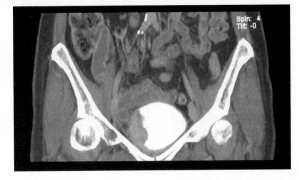

Figure 20-38 Bladder cancer with computed tomography urogram (CTU). **A and B:** Axial contrast-enhanced images with extrinsic compression device in place show (**A**) normal symmetric enhancement of kidneys and normal appearance of intrarenal collecting systems (*arrows*) and (**B**) a large mass arising from the right anterior bladder wall (*arrows*). There is associated stranding of the perivesical fat suggesting invasion and advanced disease (*arrowheads*). **C:** A coronal reformatted image 5 mm in thickness again shows the bladder mass arising from the right aspect of the wall. The intrarenal collecting systems and both ureters were enhanced and identified on other coronal images.

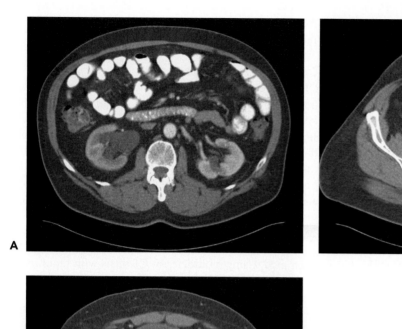

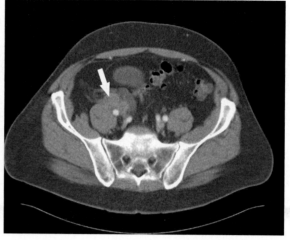

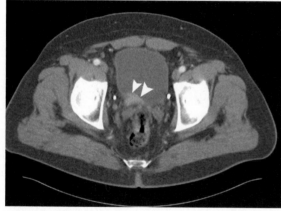

Figure 20-39 Advanced bladder cancer. **A:** Axial contrast-enhanced computed tomography image at the level of the kidneys shows right hydronephrosis with a diminished nephrogram as well as a left renal cyst. **B** and **C:** Images of the pelvis show enlarged right external iliac lymph nodes (*arrow*, **B**) and a small bladder mass involving the right ureterovesical junction (*arrowheads*, **C**).

matting, coronal images can be used to check the renal pelves and ureters for the presence of strictures and masses (Fig. 20-38). It is not known whether the spatial resolution of reformatted CT scans images is adequate for identification of very small ureteral tumors, although recent work suggests this may be the case (15). Fortunately, only 1% of transitional cell carcinoma occurs primarily in the ureter. All images should also be evaluated for the presence of increased number and size of pelvic and retroperitoneal lymph nodes and distant disease (Fig. 20-39). In cases of advanced disease, CT is probably preferred because of its rapid acquisition and ease of interpretation. Because postbiopsy inflammatory changes in the perivesical fat can mimic tumor, a definite diagnosis of perivesical extension of tumor can sometimes be difficult to make. Definitive diagnosis of stage III disease is possible when an enhancing mass is present.

Magnetic Resonance Imaging

On T2-weighted MRI, the muscular wall of the bladder is of homogeneously dark signal. Extension into but not through the muscular wall is Stage II disease (Fig. 20-40). Extension of high signal mass through the wall indicates Stage III disease. Metastasis to a lymph node can be recognized if it leads to nodal enlargement (Fig. 20-41). Using 1.5 T systems and Gd-DTPA intravenous contrast agent, overall staging accuracy is approximately 85% (6,42). For local extension, T1-weighted, dynamic, post-Gd-DTPA enhanced images may be of help in delineating a mass from adjacent inflammatory stranding. Coronal images of the upper urinary tract, similar to those with CT or intravenous urography (IVU), can be obtained using a heavily T2-weighted coronal series, obtained either as a volume or comprising multiple slices. MRI has also been advocated for assessing response to chemotherapy, with de-

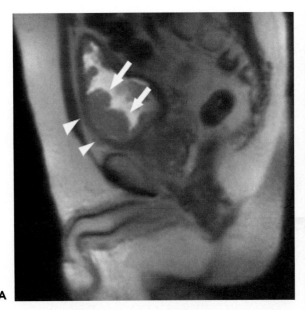
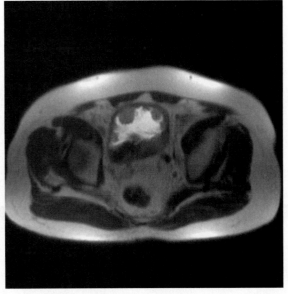

Figure 20-40 Multifocal superficial bladder cancer. **A:** Sagittal T2-weighed half Fourier turbo spin-echo (HASTE) (90/4.5) magnetic resonance image of the bladder shows multiple intermediate signal masses arising from the wall (*arrows*). The low signal muscular wall appears intact in this image (*arrowheads*), suggesting that these are superficial type tumors. **B:** Using the same pulse sequence in an axial plane, the muscular wall again appears intact. The left posterior aspect of the wall was seen to better advantage on other images.

layed enhancement of responding lymph nodes identified after four cycles of methotrexate, vinblastine, adriamycin, and cisplatin (5).

An unusual tumor of the pelvis arises from the urachal remnant. This tumor, located at the bladder dome, is usually an adenocarcinoma. The classic, although uncommon, clinical presentation is that of mucus in the urine. Appearance on CT and MR images is that of a solid, enhancing mass arising from the bladder dome (Fig. 20-42). Tumor may extend superiorly and anteriorly toward the umbilicus. Differential diagnosis includes an urachal abscess and treatment is always surgical.

Recurrent Colorectal Cancer Following Abdominoperineal Resection

Aggressive rectal cancers are treated with surgical resection, closure of the rectum, and the formation of a colostomy. The pelvic floor is often packed with fat, sometimes obtained from the omentum. The remaining pelvic organs rotate posteriorly and descend inferiorly, significantly changing their appearance on cross-sectional imaging. In males, on axial images the prostate is often heart shaped

with the apex directed at the symphysis. The seminal vesicles extend posteriorly and can be mistaken for tumor. In the female, similar changes occur with descent and rotation of the uterus. The ovaries usually remain located laterally within the pelvis.

Computed Tomography

Following abdominoperineal resection, it is common to see soft tissue density within the presacral space. When this material remains plaque-like, fibrosis is likely. The development of an enhancing rounded solid or necrotic mass is often indicative of recurrent disease (Fig. 20-43). PET scanning or biopsy should then be performed.

Magnetic Resonance Imaging

T2-weighted MRI offers high-contrast differentiation between residual fat and bowel from recurrent usually intermediate to high-signal disease. Recurrent disease usually occurs as a mass at the resection site near the pelvic floor and demonstrates enhancement on Gd-DTPA–enhanced images within the first 90 seconds postinjection (55,57).

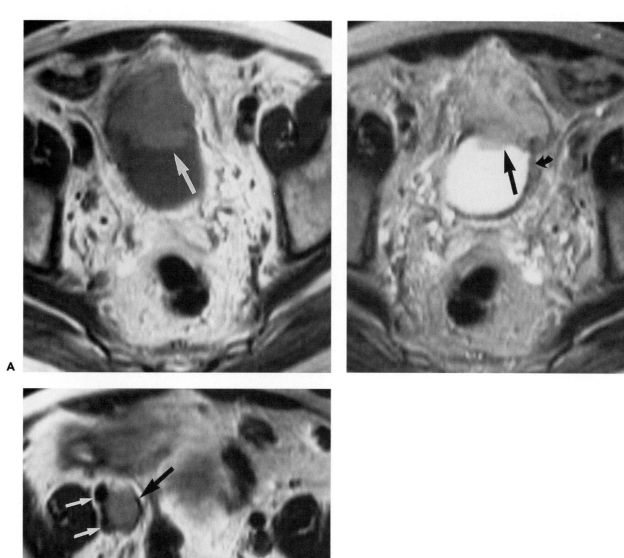

Figure 20-41 Adenocarcinoma of the bladder. **A:** Transaxial T1-weighted SE image (600/15) shows a mass (*arrow*) slightly hyperintense to urine arising from the anterior bladder wall and extending into the perivesical fat. **B:** The mass (*straight arrow*) is hyperintense to normal bladder wall (*curved arrow*) on this T2-weighted SE image (2500/90). **C:** Transaxial T1-weighted SE image (600/15) several centimeters cephalad shows right external iliac adenopathy. The nodal mass (*black arrow*) can be distinguished easily from adjacent high-signal fat and flow voids of the iliac vessels (*white arrows*).

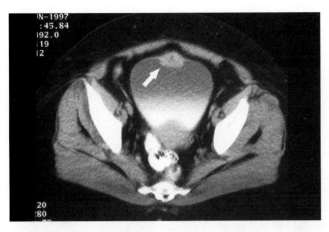

Figure 20-42 Urachal carcinoma. Axial contrast-enhanced computed tomography image at the level of the bladder dome shows an enhancing mass (*arrow*). Although these tumors often appear to be locally confined, the prognosis is extremely poor and the vast majority of patients succumb to metastatic disease.

It is important to assess the adjacent muscles and peritoneal surfaces for abnormal, increased enhancement, which usually indicates extension of disease beyond the presacral space (Fig. 20-44).

OTHER ABNORMALITIES OF THE TREATED PELVIS

Surgical and radiation therapy causes numerous abnormalities in the pelvis. The majority of these can be identified using either CT or MRI. Findings associated with radiation therapy include bright enhancement of the peritoneum, thickening and tethering of large and small bowel loops, and thickening of the bladder wall and uterosacral ligaments (46). Soft tissue edema of the presacral space, pelvic muscles, and subcutaneous fat may persist for up to 18 months posttreatment (9). Ureteral dilation may be found in up to 50% of cases (8). Radiation may also cause fatty replacement and thinning of the pyriformis muscle, yielding increased T2 signal on MR images. Associated damage to the sciatic nerve with resulting leg pain is sometimes called pyriformis syndrome.

Fistula formation between the bowel and bladder or, in the case of the female, cervix or vagina and bladder are uncommon but devastating complications of surgical or radiation therapy. These can be identified using either intravenous or oral contrast, but not simultaneously, and demonstrating extension of contrast from one organ to the other (43) (Fig. 40-45).

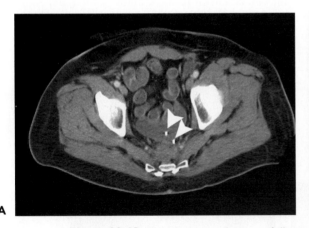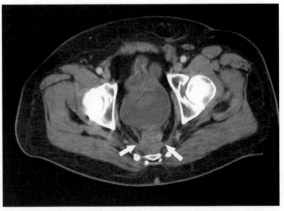

A B

Figure 20-43 Recurrent rectal cancer following abdominoperineal resection. Axial contrast-enhanced computed tomography images of the pelvis (**A** and **B**) show the bladder to be displaced posteriorly and to contain a left ureteral stent (*arrowheads*, **A**). A round mass located in the presacral space (*arrows*, **B**) was later biopsied and found to be recurrent disease. This could also have been confirmed using positron emission tomography imaging.

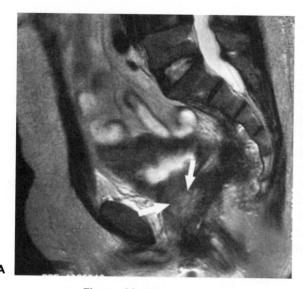

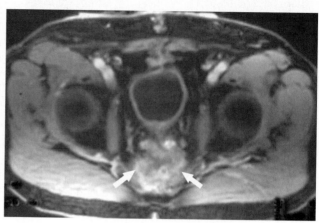

Figure 20-44 Recurrent rectal cancer following surgical resection. **A:** Sagittal T2-weighted half Fourier turbo spin-echo (HASTE) (90/4.5) image of the pelvis shows an intermediate signal intensity mass (*arrow*) just inferior and posterior to the bladder. **B:** Axial T1-weighted contrast-enhanced image of the presacral mass (*arrows*) demonstrates it to be inseparable from the seminal vesicles.

Finally, fluid collections may result from therapy including seromas, urinomas, lymphoceles, and abscesses. Seromas and urinomas have no central and minimal peripheral enhancement. No air bubbles are seen within them. Large lymphoceles most commonly occur following cystectomy or prostatectomy. They usually contain gracile septa and extend into the retroperitoneum. Abscesses contain fluid density material and often have a thick, enhancing wall. Small air pockets, many of them dependent, may also be present (Fig. 20-46).

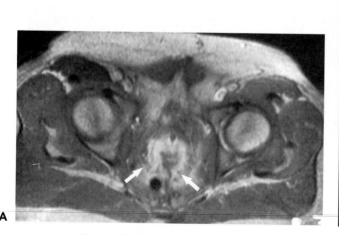

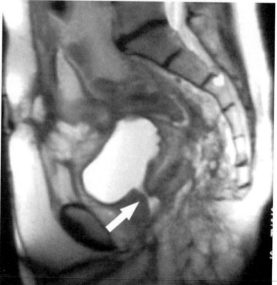

Figure 20-45 Recurrent rectal tumor with fistula formation. **A:** Axial T1-weighted contrast-enhanced image demonstrates an enhancing mass at the resection site near the pelvic floor (*arrows*). **B:** Sagittal T2-weighted half Fourier turbo spin-echo (HASTE) (90/4.5) magnetic resonance image shows a high signal fistula between the bladder and tumor mass (*arrow*).

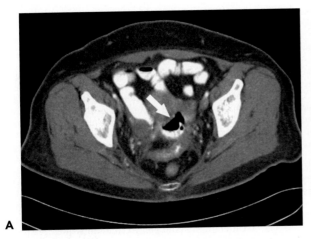

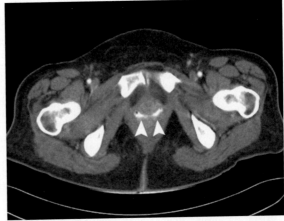

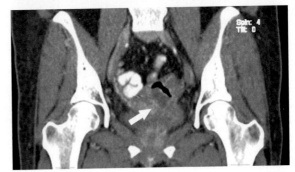

Figure 20-46 Enterovaginal abscess and fistula following a hysterectomy. Axial computed tomography images of the pelvis obtained following the ingestion of oral contrast demonstrate an abnormal collection of gas and contrast material interposed between a small bowel loop and the vagina (*arrow*, **A**). High-density contrast is present within the vaginal canal confirming the presence of a fistula (*arrowheads*, **B**). **C:** coronal reformatted maximum intensity projection 5 mm in thickness again shows the abscess (*arrow*) and its relation to the left vaginal fornix.

REFERENCES

1. Ascher SM, Arnold LL, Patt RH, et al. Adenomyosis: prospective comparison of MR imaging and transvaginal sonography. *Radiology* 1994;190:803–806.
2. Ascher SM, Imaoka I, Lage JM. Tamoxifen-induced uterine abnormalities: the role of imaging. *Radiology* 2000;214:29–38.
3. Ascher SM, Johnson JC, Barnes WA, et al. MR imaging appearance of the uterus in postmenopausal women receiving tamoxifen therapy for breast cancer: histopathologic correlation. *Radiology* 1996;200:105–110.
4. Azziz R. Adenomyosis: current perspectives. *Obstet Gynecol Clin North Am* 1989;16:221–235.
5. Barentsz JO, Berger-Hartog O, Witjes JA, et al. Evaluation of chemotherapy in advanced urinary bladder cancer with fast dynamic contrast-enhanced MR imaging. *Radiology* 1998;207:791–797.
6. Barentsz JO, Jager GJ, van Vierzen Peter BJ, et al. Staging urinary bladder cancer after transurethral biopsy: value of fast dynamic contrast-enhanced MR imaging. *Radiology* 1996;201:185–193.
7. Barton JW, McCarthy SM, Kohorn EI, et al. Pelvic MR imaging findings in gestational trophoblastic disease, incomplete abortion, and ectopic pregnancy: are they specific? *Radiology* 1993;186:163–168.
8. Blomlie V, Rofstad EK, Tropé C, et al. Critical soft tissues of the female pelvis: serial MR imaging before, during, and after radiation therapy. *Radiology* 1997;203:391–397.
9. Blomlie V, Rofstad EK, Tverå K, et al. Noncritical soft tissues of the female pelvis: serial MR imaging before, during, and after radiation therapy. *Radiology* 1996;199:461–468.
10. Boronow RC, Morrow CP, Creasman WT, et al. Surgical staging in endometrial cancer: clinical-pathologic finding of a prospective study. *Obstet Gynecol* 1984;63:852–832.
11. Bree RL, Carlos RC. US for postmenopausal bleeding: consensus development and patient-centered outcomes. *Radiology* 2002;222:595–598.
12. Brody JM, Koelliker SL, Frishman GN. Unicornuate uterus: imaging appearance, associated anomalies, and clinical implications. *AJR Am J Roentgenol* 1998;171:1341–1347.
13. Buttram VC. Müllerian anomalies and their management. *Fertil Steril* 1983;40:159–163.
14. Buy JN, Moss AA, Guinet C, et al. MR staging of bladder carcinoma: correlation with pathologic findings. *Radiology* 1988;169:695–700.
15. Caoili EM, Cohan RH, Korobkin M, et al. Urinary tract abnormalities: initial experience with multi-detector row CT urography. *Radiology* 2002;222:353–360.
16. Cobby M, Browning J, Jones A, et al. Magnetic resonance imaging, computed tomography and endosonography in the local staging of carcinoma of the cervix. *Br J Radiol* 1990;63:673–679.
17. Cornud F, Flam T, Chauveinc L, et al. Extraprostatic spread of clinically localized prostate cancer: factors predictive of pT3 tumor and of positive endorectal MR imaging examination results. *Radiology* 2002;224:203–210.
18. Creasman WT. Disorders of the uterine corpus. In: Soutt JR, DiSaia PH, Hammand CCB, Spellacy WN, eds. *Dansforth's obstetrics and gynecology.* Philadelphia: Lippincott; 1994:925–955.
19. Creasman WT, DeGeest K, DiSaia PJ, et al. Significance of true surgical pathologic staging: a Gynecologic Oncology Group Study. *Am J Obstet Gynecol* 1999;181:31–34.
20. deSouza NM, Williams AD. Uterine arterial embolization for leiomyomas: perfusion and volume changes at MR imaging and relation to clinical outcome. *Radiology* 2002;222:367–374.
21. Doyle M. Magnetic resonance imaging in müllerian fusion defects. *J Reprod Med* 1992;37:33–38.
22. Dudiak CM, Turner DA, Patel SK, et al. Uterine leiomyomas in the infertile patient: preoperative localization with MR imaging versus US and hysterosalpingography. *Radiology* 1988;167:627–630.

23. Feong YY, Kang HK, Chung TW, et al. Uterine cervical carcinoma after therapy: CT and MR imaging findings. *Radiographics* 2003;23:969–981.

24. Fielding JR. Practical MR imaging of female pelvic floor weakness. *Radiographics* 2002;22:295–304.

25. Fielding JR, Hoyte LX, Okon SA, et al. Tumor detection by virtual cystoscopy with color mapping of bladder wall thickness. *J Urol* 2002;167[2 Pt 1]:559–562.

26. Forman HP, Heiken JP, Brink JA, et al. CT screening for comorbid disease in patients with prostatic carcinoma: is it cost-effective. *AJR Am J Roentgenol* 1994;162:1125–1128; discussion 1129–1130.

27. Forstner R, Hricak H, Occhipinti KA, et al. Ovarian cancer: staging with CT and MR imaging. *Radiology* 1995;197:619–626.

28. Frei KA, Kinkel K, Bonél HM, et al. Prediction of deep myometrial invasion in patients with endometrial cancer: clinical utility of contrast-enhanced MR imaging—a meta-analysis and bayesian analysis. *Radiology* 2000;216:444–449.

29. Friedland GW, Chang P. The role of imaging in the management of the impalpable undescended testis. *AJR Am J Roentgenol* 1988;151:1107–1111.

30. Ghossain MA, Buy JN, Ligneres C, et al. Epithelial tumors of the ovary: comparison of MR and CT findings. *Radiology* 1991;181:863–870.

31. Golan A, Langer R, Bukovsky I, et al. Congenital anomalies of the müllerian system. *Fertil Steril* 1989;51:747–755.

32. Greene FL, Fleming ID, Page DL, et al., eds. *AJCC Cancer Staging Handbook*, 6th ed. New York: Springer-Verlag, 2002.

33. Gryspeerdt S, Van Hoe L, Bosmans H, et al. T2-weighted MR imaging of the uterus: comparison of optimized fast spin-echo and HASTE sequences with conventional fast spin-echo sequences. *AJR Am J Roentgenol* 1998;171:211–215.

34. Hamlin DJ, Fitzsimmons JR, Pettersson H, et al. Magnetic resonance imaging of the pelvis: evaluation of ovarian masses at 0.15T. *AJR Am J Roentgenol* 1985;145:585–590.

35. Hammer-Jacobsen E. Therapeutic abortion on account of x-ray examination during pregnancy. *Dan Med Bull* 1959;6:113–121.

36. Hardesty LA, Sumkin JH, Hankim C, et al. The ability of helical CT to preoperatively stage endometrial carcinoma. *AJR Am J Roentgenol* 2001;176:603–606.

37. Hardesty LA, Sumkin JH, Nath ME, et al. Use of preoperative MR imaging in the management of endometrial carcinoma: cost analysis. *Radiology* 2000;215:45–49.

38. Harisinghani MG, Barentsz JO, Hahn PF, et al. MR lymphangiography for detection of minimal nodal disease in patients with prostate cancer. *Acad Radiol* 2002;9[Suppl 2]:S312–313.

39. Harisinghani MG, Barentsz J, Hahn PF, et al. Noninvasive detection of clinically occult lymph-node metastases in prostate cancer. *N Engl J Med* 2003;348:2491–2499.

40. Harris RD, Schned AR, Heaney JA. Staging of prostate cancer with endorectal MR imaging: lessons from a learning curve. *Radiographics* 1995;15:813–829.

41. Hawighorst Hans, Knapstein PG, Weikel W, et al. Cervical carcinoma: comparison of standard and pharmacokinetic MR imaging. *Radiology* 1996;201:531–539.

42. Hayashi N, Tochigi H, Shiraishi T, et al. A new staging criterion for bladder carcinoma using gadolinium-enhanced magnetic resonance imaging with an endorectal surface coil: a comparison with ultrasonography. *BJU Int* 2000;85:32–36.

43. Healy JC, Phillips RR, Reznek RH, et al. The MR appearance of vaginal fistulas. *AJR Am J Roentgenol* 1996;167:1487–1489.

44. Hilton S, Herr HW, Teitcher JB, et al. CT detection of retroperitoneal lymph node metastases I patients with clinical stage I testicular nonseminomatous germ cell cancer: assessment of size and distribution criteria. *AJR Am J Roentgenol* 1997;169:521–525.

45. Hoyte L, Schierlitz L, Zou K, et al. Two- and 3-dimensional MRI comparison of levator ani structure, volume, and integrity in women with stress incontinence and prolapse. *Am J Obstet Gynecol* 2001;185:11–19.

46. Iyer RB, Jhingran A, Sawaf H, et al. Imaging findings after radiotherapy to the pelvis. *AJR Am J Roentgenol* 2001;177:1083–1089.

47. Jha RC, Takahma J, Imaoka I, et al. Adenomyosis: MRI of the uterus treated with uterine artery embolization. *AJR Am J Roentgenol* 2003;181:851–856.

48. Jemal A, Murray T, Samuels A, et al. Cancer statistics, 2003. *CA Cancer J Clin* 2003;53:5–26.

49. Kanal E, Borgstede JP, Barkovich AJ, et al. American College of Radiology White Paper on MR safety. *AJR Am J Roentgenol* 2002;178:1335–1347.

50. Kang S, Turner DA, Foster GS, et al. Adenomyosis: specificity of 5 mm as the maximum normal uterine junctional zone thickness in MR images. *AJR Am J Roentgenol* 1996;166:1145–1150.

51. Kaufman RH, Noller K, Adam E, et al. Upper genital tract abnormalities and pregnancy outcome in diethylstilbestrol-exposed progeny. *Am J Obstet Gynecol* 1984;148:973–984.

52. Kier R, McCarthy SM, Scoutt LM, et al. Pelvic masses in pregnancy: MR imaging. *Radiology* 1990;176:709–713.

53. Kim SH, Choi BI, Lee HP, et al. Uterine cervical carcinoma: comparison of CT and MR findings. *Radiology* 1990;175:45–51.

54. Kimura I, Togashi K, Kawakami S, et al. Polycystic ovaries: implications of diagnosis with MR imaging. *Radiology* 1996;201:549–552.

55. Kinkel K, Ariche M, Tardivon AA, et al. Differentiation between recurrent tumor and benign conditions after treatment of gynecologic pelvic carcinoma: value of dynamic contrast-enhance subtraction MR imaging. *Radiology* 1997;204:55–63.

56. Kinkel K, Kaji Y, Yu KK, et al. Radiologic staging in patients with endometrial cancer: a meta-analysis. *Radiology* 1999;212:711–718.

57. Kinkel K, Tardivon AA, Soyer P, et al. Dynamic contrast-enhanced subtraction versus T2-weighted spin-echo MR imaging in the follow-up of colorectal neoplasm: a prospective study of 41 patients. *Radiology* 1996;200:453–458.

58. Kurhanewicz J, Vigneron DB, Males RG, et al. The prostate: MR imaging and spectroscopy. *Radiol Clin North Am* 2000;38:115–138.

59. Kurtz AB, Tsimikas JV, Tempany CMC, et al. Diagnosis and staging of ovarian cancer: comparative values of Doppler and conventional US, CT, and MR imaging correlated with surgery and histopathologic analysis—report of the Radiology Diagnostic Oncology Group. *Radiology* 1999;212:19–27.

60. Levine D, Barnes PD, Edelman RR. Obstetric MR imaging. *Radiology* 1999;211:609–617.

61. Low RN, Saleh F, Song SYT, et al. Treated ovarian cancer: comparison of MR imaging with serum CA-125 level and physical examination—a longitudinal study. *Radiology* 1999;211:519–528.

62. Mitchell DG, Minta MC, Spritzer CE, et al. Adnexal masses: MR imaging observations at 1.5T, with US and CT correlation. *Radiology* 1987;162:319–324.

63. Meyer JI, Kennedy AW, Friedman R, et al. Ovarian carcinoma: value of CT in predicting success of debulking surgery. *AJR Am J Roentgenol* 1995;165:875–878.

64. Morrow CP, Bundy BN, Kurman RJ, et al. Relationship between surgical-pathological risk factors and outcome in clinical stage I and II carcinoma of the endometrium Gynecologic Oncology Group study. *Gynecol Oncol* 1991;40:55–65.

65. Mostafa A, Reinhold C, Mehio AR, et al. Adenomyosis: US features with histologic correlation in an in vitro study. *Radiology* 2000;215:783–790.

66. Murase E, Siegelman ES, Outwater EK, et al. Uterine leiomyomas: histopathologic features, MR imaging findings, differential diagnosis, and treatment. *Radiographics* 1999;19:1179–1197.

67. Nagayama M, Watanabe Y, Okumura A, et al. Fast MR imaging in obstetrics. *Radiographics* 2002;22:563–582.

68. Occhipinti KA, Frankel SD, Hricak H. The ovary: computed tomography and magnetic resonance imaging. *Radiol Clin North Am* 1993;31:1115–1132.

69. Outwater EK, Mitchell DG. Normal ovaries and functional cysts: MR appearance. *Radiology* 1996;198:397–402.

70. Outwater E, Schiebler ML, Owen RS, et al. Characterization of hemorrhagic adnexal lesions with MR imaging: blinded reader study. *Radiology* 1993;186:489–494.

71. Outwater EK, Siegelman ES, Chiowanich P, et al. Dilated fallopian tubes: MR imaging characteristics. *Radiology* 1998;208:463–469.

72. Outwater EK, Siegelman ES, Van Deerlin V. Adenomyosis: current concepts and imaging considerations. *AJR Am J Roentgenol* 1998;170:437–441.

73. Outwater EK, Talerman A, Dunton C. Normal adnexa uteri specimens: anatomic basis of MR imaging features. *Radiology* 1996;201:751–755.

74. Pellerito JS, McCarth SM, Doyle MB, et al. Diagnosis of uterine anomalies: relative accuracy of MR imaging, endovaginal sonography, and hysterosalpingography. *Radiology* 1992;183:795–800.

75. Reinhold C, Atri M, Mehio A, et al. Diffuse uterine adenomyosis: morphologic criteria and diagnostic accuracy of endovaginal sonography. *Radiology* 1995;197:609–614.

76. Reinhold C, Hricak H, Forstner R, et al. Primary amenorrhea: evaluation with MR imaging. *Radiology* 1997;203:383–390.

77. Reinhold C, McCarthy S, Bret PM, et al. Diffuse adenomyosis: comparison of endovaginal US and MR imaging with histopathologic correlation. *Radiology* 1996;199:151–158.

78. Rha SE, Byun FY, Seung EJ, et al. CT and MR imaging features of adnexal torsion. *Radiographics* 2002;22:283–294.

79. Rubin SC. Cervical cancer: successes and failures. *CA Cancer J Clin* 2001;51:92–114.

80. Saez F, Urresola A, Larena JA, et al. Endometrial carcinoma: assessment of myometrial invasion with plain and gadolinium-enhanced MR imaging. *J Magn Reson Imaging* 2000;12:460–466.

81. Scheidler J, Heuck AF. Imaging of cancer of the cervix. *Radiol Clin North Am* 2002;40:577–590.

82. Schwartz LH, LaTrenta LR, Bonaccio E, et al. Small cell and anaplastic prostate cancer: correlation between CT findings and prostate-specific antigen level. *Radiology* 1998;208:735–738.

83. Scoutt LM, Flynn SD, Luthringer DJ, et al. Junctional zone of the uterus: correlation of MR imaging and histologic examination of hysterectomy specimens. *Radiology* 1991;179:403–407.

84. Scoutt LM, McCauley TR, Flynn SD, et al. Zonal Anatomy of the cervix: correlation of MR imaging and histologic examination of hysterectomy specimens. *Radiology* 1993;186:159–162.

85. Seki H, Takano T, Sakai K. Value of dynamic MR imaging in assessing endometrial carcinoma involvement of the cervix. *AJR Am J Roentgenol* 2000;175:171–176.

86. Siegelman ES, Outwater EK, Banner MP, et al. High-resolution MR imaging of the vagina. *Radiographics* 1997;17:1183–1203.

87. Silverman JM, Krebs TL. MR imaging evaluation with a transrectal surface coil of local recurrence of prostatic cancer in men who have undergone radical prostatectomy. *AJR Am J Roentgenol* 1997;168:379–385.

88. Slanetz PJ, Hahn PF, Hall DA, et al. The frequency and significance of adnexal lesions incidentally revealed by CT. *AJR Am J Roentgenol* 1997;168:647–650.

89. Song JH, Francis IR, Platt JF, et al. Bladder tumor detection at virtual cystoscopy. *Radiology* 2001;218:95–100.

90. Sørensen SS. Estimated prevalence of müllerian anomalies. *Acta Obstet Gynecol Scand* 1988;67:441–445.

91. Stevens SK, Hricak H, Campos Z. Teratomas versus cystic hemorrhagic adnexal lesions: differentiation with proton-selective fat-saturation MR imaging. *Radiology* 1993;186:481–488.

92. Strübbe EH, Willemsen WNP, Lemmens JAM, et al. Mayer-Rokitansky-Küster-Hauser syndrome: distinction between two forms based on excretory urographic, sonographic, and laparoscopic findings. *AJR Am J Roentgenol* 1993;160:331–334.

93. Tempany CM, Zhou X, Zerhouni EA, et al. Staging of prostate cancer: results of Radiology Diagnostic Oncology Group project comparison of three MR imaging techniques. *Radiology* 1994;192:47–54.

94. Togashi K, Nakai A, Sugimura K. Anatomy and physiology of the female pelvis: MR imaging revisited. *J Magn Reson Imaging* 2001;13:842–849.

95. Togashi K, Nishimura K, Itoh K, et al. Ovarian cystic teratomas: MR imaging. *Radiology* 1987;162:669–673.

96. Tukeva TA, Aronen HJ, Karjalainen PT, et al. MR imaging in pelvic inflammatory disease: comparison with laparoscopy and US. *Radiology* 1999;210:209–216.

97. Twickler DM, Setiawan AT, Evans RS, et al. Imaging of puerperal septic thrombophlebitis: prospective comparison of MR imaging, CT, and sonography. *AJR Am J Roentgenol* 1997;169:1039–1043.

98. Van Gils APG, Tham RTOTA, Falke THM, et al. Abnormalities and pregnancy outcome in diethylstilbestrol exposure: correlation of findings on MR and hysterosalpingography. *AJR Am J Roentgenol* 1989;153:1235–1238.

99. Walsh JW, Rosenfield AT, Jaffe CC, et al. Prospective comparison of ultrasound and computed tomography in the evaluation of gynecologic pelvic masses. *AJR Am J Roentgenol* 1978;131:955–960.

100. Weinreb JC, Barkoff ND, Megibow A, et al. The value of MR imaging in distinguishing leiomyomas from other solid pelvic masses when sonography is indeterminate. *AJR Am J Roentgenol* 1990;154:295–299.

101. Williams AD, Cousins C, Soutter WP, et al. Detection of pelvic lymph node metastases in gynecologic malignancy: a comparison of CT, MR imaging, and positron emission tomography. *AJR Am J Roentgenol* 2001;177:343–348.

102. Woodward PJ, Wagner BJ, Farley TE. MR imaging in the evaluation of female infertility. *Radiographics* 1993;13:293–310.

103. Yamashita Y, Harada M, Sawada T, et al. Normal uterus and FIGO stage I endometrial carcinoma: dynamic gadolinium-enhanced MR imaging. *Radiology* 1993;186:495–501.

104. Yamashita Y, Torashima M, Hatanaka Y, et al. Adnexal masses: accuracy of characterization with transvaginal US and precontrast and postcontrast MR imaging. *Radiology* 1995;194:557–565.

105. Yamashita Y, Torashima M, Takahashi M, et al. Hyperintense uterine leiomyoma at T2-weighted MR imaging: differentiation with dynamic enhanced MR imaging and clinical implications. *Radiology* 1993;189:721–725.

106. Yang WT, Lam WWM, Yu MY, et al. Comparison of dynamic helical CT and dynamic MR imaging in the evaluation of pelvic lymph nodes in cervical carcinoma. *AJR Am J Roentgenol* 2000;175:759–766.

107. Yu KK, Hricak H, Alagappan R, et al. Detection of extracapsular extension of prostate carcinoma with endorectal and phased-array coil MR imaging: multivariate feature analysis. *Radiology* 1997;202:697–702.

108. Yu KK, Hricak H, Subak LL, et al. Preoperative staging of cervical carcinoma: phased array coil fast spin-echo versus body coil spin-echo T2-weighted MR imaging. *AJR Am J Roentgenol* 1998;171:707–711.

109. Zawin M, McCarthy S, Scoutt LM, et al. High-field MRI and US evaluation of the pelvis in women with leiomyomas. *J Magn Reson Imaging* 1990;8:371–376.

Computed Tomography of Thoracoabdominal Trauma

Paul L. Molina   *Michele T. Quinn*   *Edward W. Bouchard*   *Joseph K. T. Lee*

Trauma is the fifth leading cause of death in the United States (1), and it is the leading cause of death in persons under the age of 40 years (319). Potential life years lost as a result of trauma exceed those resulting from heart disease and cancer (424). Trauma also results in more than 100,000 permanent disabilities annually (158).

Blunt trauma, also called wide impact trauma, accounts for the majority of injuries and is most commonly the result of motor vehicle accidents. Other frequent causes include home and work-related accidents such as crush injuries, blast injuries, and falls from a height. Multisystem trauma is a characteristic of motor vehicle accidents, with the extremities involved most frequently, followed by injury to the head (70%), chest (50%), abdomen (30%), and pelvis (25%) (424).

Improved triage using telecommunication and expedited transport to designated trauma centers has enhanced survival of major trauma victims (16). Trauma centers effectively reduce morbidity and mortality of the accident patient, and the nationwide development of the Emergency Medical Service System, which identifies trauma centers by a process of categorization, regionalization, and verification, has markedly improved the care of trauma patients (271). Another significant advancement in modern trauma care has been the intensive use of computed tomography (CT) for immediate patient evaluation. Over the last several decades, improvements in CT scanner hardware and software have provided increased scanning speed and faster data acquisition, as well as improved spatial resolution (319). The continuing evolution in CT technology from conventional to helical scanning, and then from single-detector CT (SDCT) to multidetector CT (MDCT) has led to unprecedented speed and quality of CT imaging. As a consequence, CT has solidified its role as the primary diagnostic tool in the evaluation of the hemodynamically stable blunt trauma victim.

The newest generation of MDCT scanners provides several advantages for the trauma patient. The fast scanning time of MDCT makes larger patient coverage possible in a single breath-hold with thinner slices and greater spatial resolution, allowing for the rapid performance of several, sequential examinations in a patient with injuries to multiple body parts (466). Motion artifacts are significantly reduced with MDCT and contrast bolus imaging is improved, leading to better intravenous (IV) contrast material opacification of blood vessels and improved IV contrast material enhancement of solid organs (319). Additionally, high-quality multiplanar reformations and three-dimensional (3D) reconstructions with preservation of spatial resolution are made possible by the near-isotropic imaging provided by the thinner collimation used with MDCT (436).

1417

BLUNT THORACIC TRAUMA

Blunt chest trauma is much more common than penetrating chest trauma and is responsible for almost 90% of the chest injuries that occur in civilian populations (160). Chest injury, alone or in combination with other injuries, accounts for nearly half of all traumatic deaths. The overall death rate is 2% to 12% for isolated chest injuries. For patients with chest injuries associated with polytrauma, the mortality rate rises to 35% (158). Most patients with blunt chest trauma have associated extrathoracic injuries. In a representative large series of 515 cases of blunt chest trauma, 431 patients (84%) had extrathoracic injuries, and nearly half of these patients had involvement of two or more extrathoracic sites (401). The most common associated injuries were head trauma, extremity fractures, and intraabdominal injuries. These extrathoracic injuries in conjunction with thoracic trauma can lead to additional impairment of respiratory function. Head injuries, for example, can result in aspiration or neurogenic pulmonary edema. Skeletal trauma combined with hypovolemic shock can produce the fat embolism syndrome. Abdominal injuries resulting in hemorrhagic shock (i.e., hepatic or splenic lacerations) may also compound the effects of blunt chest trauma (425).

Blunt chest injury results from the transfer of kinetic energy to the chest wall and thoracic contents through a number of synergistic mechanisms including (a) direct impact, (b) sudden inertial deceleration, (c) spallation, and (d) implosion. *Direct impact*, as occurs with forceful, direct blows to the chest, causes a sudden release of local kinetic energy that may fracture bony structures and contuse, crush, and shear underlying soft tissues. If the chest wall is compressed substantially by the force of the impact, the resultant increase in intrathoracic pressure may also lead to rupture of alveoli and supporting structures. *Sudden inertial deceleration* at the time of impact is a major injury factor in high-speed motor vehicle accidents. Inertial deceleration imparts differential moments of rotation to chest tissues and causes mobile or elastic structures to rotate about points of fixation. The resulting torsional deformation and shearing stresses at internal thoracic interfaces (i.e., interface between the relatively mobile alveolar tissues and the more fixed bronchovascular interstitium) can cause microscopic tears or gross lacerations. *Spallation* occurs when a broad kinetic shock wave from sudden compression is partially reflected at gas-fluid interfaces, such as at the alveolocapillary surface. The resulting release of energy causes local disruption of tissue near the point of shock-wave impact. Spallation injury is typically manifest in the anterior lung during sudden compression of the anterior chest wall in steering wheel injuries. *Implosion* is the low-pressure decompressive wave that follows the high-pressure compressive shock wave of spallation, causing disruption of lung tissue through rebound overexpansion of gas bubbles within alveoli. In most cases, blunt thoracic injury is the result of a combination of these major energy transfer mechanisms (144,158).

INDICATIONS

Although CT is the examination of choice in trauma of the head and abdomen, its precise role in the evaluation of blunt chest trauma continues to evolve. This is largely because of the remarkable amount of information provided by chest radiography, which remains the principal diagnostic screening examination in patients with blunt thoracic trauma. Many traumatic abnormalities of the thorax (e.g., tension pneumothorax, hemothorax, pulmonary contusion) can be diagnosed or suggested with reasonable confidence by conventional radiographic methods. In stable posttraumatic patients, thoracic CT can be performed to confirm or, more precisely, define the full extent of thoracic injury, which is often underestimated by chest radiography (218,263,273,296,362,412,443,458). CT can be particularly beneficial in patients with equivocal radiographic findings or technically inadequate radiographic examinations. CT may also be used to diagnose radiographically inapparent or clinically unsuspected injuries, such as parenchymal lacerations or occult pneumothoraces. CT is fast becoming the primary imaging modality following chest radiography for evaluation of patients with suspected traumatic aortic injury. In the later postinjury stage, additional indications for use of CT include demonstration of sites of thoracic infection (292), differentiation of pleural from parenchymal abnormalities (154), and guidance of therapeutic interventions such as empyema drainage (35) or revision of malpositioned and occluded thoracostomy tubes (292).

In general, magnetic resonance imaging (MRI) is not used routinely to assess acute chest or abdominal trauma, because prolonged scan times and decreased access to patients requiring continuous monitoring limit its practicality in the imaging of trauma patients (492). Occasionally, in select hemodynamically stable patients, MRI may be of use in the initial evaluation of suspected injuries to the spine and diaphragm (151,396).

TECHNIQUE

Posttraumatic thoracic SDCT examinations are generally performed at 5-mm collimation, a pitch of 1.0 to 1.5, and 5-mm intervals through the entire thorax following the bolus administration of IV contrast material. Typically, 90 to 120 mL of nonionic contrast material with an iodine concentration of 240 to 300 mg/mL is administered using a power injector at 2 to 4 mL per second through a 20-gauge or larger peripheral venous catheter. Injection of the right antecubital fossa is preferred to the left to avoid contrast artifact from the left brachiocephalic vein, which can limit evaluation of the mediastinum (319). Scanning is initiated after a delay of 20 to 25 seconds during a single breath-hold and images are reviewed at lung, soft-tissue, and bone window settings. When multiplanar or 3D reformations are indicated, images are reconstructed at 1- to 3-mm spacing. Cardiac-gating may further improve image quality by limiting cardiovascular motion artifact and improving reconstructions (366). Parameters such as slice collimation, pitch, and reconstruction interval may vary depending on the number of CT scanner detectors. For the 16-channel scanners, typical collimation choices are 1.5 mm and 0.75 mm. With the 64-channel scanners, 1.2- to 0.6-mm collimation is achievable.

Whenever performing trauma CT, the patient should be closely monitored throughout the examination by trained medical personnel, and emergency resuscitative equipment must be immediately available in the CT scanning room. If possible, the patient's arms should be positioned above the head rather than along the sides so as to reduce streak artifacts. Artifacts can also be minimized by removing as many nonessential tubes and other foreign objects from the scanning field as possible prior to imaging.

SPECIFIC TRAUMA SITES

Chest Wall

Trauma to the chest often results in injury to the bony thorax and soft tissues of the chest wall, increasing patient morbidity and mortality (64). For the majority of chest wall injuries, a combination of physical examination and radiographs is sufficient to define their nature and extent. Chest wall contusion, with or without rib fracture, can produce a reticular pattern of higher density within the usually homogeneous subcutaneous fat. Soft tissue hematomas can obliterate fat-tissue planes between muscles and produce a focal mass-like bulge (242) (Fig. 21-1). Both contusions

and hematomas of the chest wall are readily demonstrated by CT, but are generally of little clinical significance.

Subcutaneous or intramuscular chest wall emphysema is also readily demonstrated by CT because of the significant contrast difference between air and soft tissue. Subcutaneous emphysema appears on CT as bands of air within the subcutaneous fat and along or between the chest wall muscles. Following blunt chest trauma, the finding of subcutaneous emphysema can indicate the presence of underlying pneumothorax or pneumomediastinum, particularly if skin lacerations or open soft tissue wounds are absent. Detection of mottled subcutaneous air and/or soft tissue swelling days to weeks following trauma should suggest the possibility of an abscess, the extent of which can be easily delineated with CT (154).

Rib fractures occur in over 50% of patients with significant chest trauma and most commonly affect the fourth through ninth ribs (424). Although rib fractures are a common sequela of blunt chest trauma, major internal thoracic injury can occur in the absence of rib fractures or other evident injury to the chest wall, particularly in younger individuals with compliant chest walls. There is a much greater incidence of rib fractures in older adults, whose ribs are relatively inelastic, than in children, whose ribs are generally more pliable and resilient (160).

Rib fractures, in and of themselves, are usually of little clinical significance and are not accurate predictors of serious injury. However, they do reflect the magnitude of force imparted and can provide clues as to the type and location of underlying injuries (158). Fractures of the first three ribs indicate significant energy transfer because these ribs are protected by the shoulder girdles and by heavy surrounding musculature. Their association with aortic or tracheobronchial injury is not as constant as previously believed, however, and they are not, as isolated findings, reliable predictors of aortic rupture (126,239,484). Extrapleural

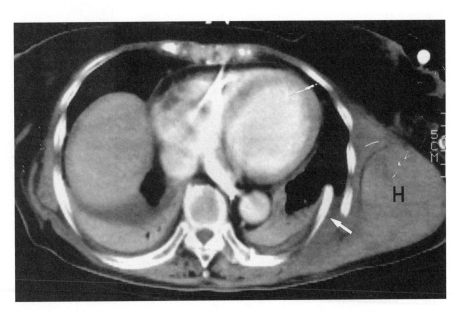

Figure 21-1 Chest wall hematoma secondary to lacerated thoracodorsal artery following blunt trauma. Note large left chest wall hematoma (H) and adjacent displaced rib fracture (*arrow*). Bilateral lower lobe atelectasis is also present.

hematomas may accompany fractures of the upper ribs or trauma to the subclavian vessels over the apex of the lung. Such extrapleural hematomas or "pleural caps" can mimic a large hemothorax on supine chest radiographs. CT readily distinguishes between an extrapleural collection of blood over the apex of the lung and a hemothorax. Fractures of the lower ribs, particularly the tenth through twelfth ribs, should increase suspicion of hepatic, splenic, or renal injury, as well as associated intraperitoneal and retroperitoneal hemorrhage. Confirmation of such injuries should then be sought by appropriate diagnostic investigations, such as CT (242).

Fractures of three or more sequential ribs or costal cartilages in multiple places can lead to an unstable, isolated segment of chest wall that exhibits paradoxical respiratory motion, the so-called flail chest. The flail segment of chest wall is sucked in with inspiration and blown out with expiration, moving in a direction opposite to the usual and leading to impaired pulmonary ventilation. The diagnosis of flail chest is made clinically and it represents a very severe form of chest wall injury. Because significant force is needed to produce a flail segment, multiple associated injuries are frequently encountered, many of which can be documented by CT if necessary (e.g., lung contusion, lung laceration, sternal fracture) (424). Rarely, a segment of lung may herniate through a defect in the chest wall created by the flail segment, and this too can be easily detected by CT (295).

Additional fractures of the bony thorax discovered by CT, including scapular (Fig. 21-2), sternal (Fig. 21-3), or thoracic spine fractures (Fig. 21-4), may be of considerable value in clarifying radiographic findings, elucidating the mechanism of injury, and initiating investigation for important associated injuries. Thoracic spine fractures most often involve the

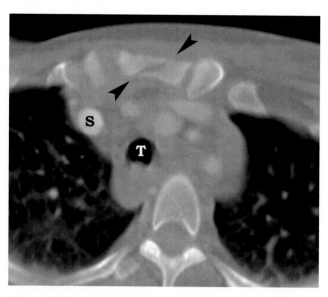

Figure 21-3 Sternal fracture. Computed tomography image through the upper sternum demonstrates an oblique fracture of the sternum (*arrowheads*). Associated retrosternal and mediastinal hematoma resulted in mediastinal widening, S, superior vena cava; T, trachea.

lower thoracic spine (T-9 through T-11 vertebrae) and are of particular clinical significance because the thoracic spinal cord is unusually susceptible to injury. In comparison with the cervical or lumbar spinal cord, the thoracic spinal cord occupies a greater percentage of the total cross-sectional area of its surrounding spinal canal, and it is easily injured by displaced fragments of bone or disk material. The blood supply to the midthoracic spinal cord is also very tenuous and, when disrupted, can result in devastating neurologic deficits. CT can accurately determine the presence, extent,

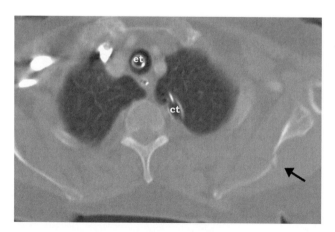

Figure 21-2 Scapular fracture. Computed tomography image through the upper chest reveals a scapular fracture (*arrow*) not appreciated on the chest radiograph. High-attenuation intravenous contrast material is present in the right axillary and brachiocephalic veins from right arm injection. et, endotracheal tube; ct, chest tube.

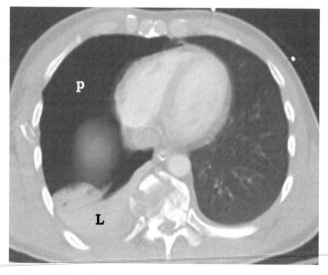

Figure 21-4 Thoracic spine fracture. Computed tomography image through the lower chest demonstrates a burst fracture of the thoracic vertebral body. Note also the large right pneumothorax (p) with right lung collapse (L).

and stability of thoracic spine fractures. Vertebral body fractures are readily demonstrated on CT, as are the relationships of fracture fragments and displaced disk material to the spinal cord (160).

Sternal fractures, occurring in 8% to 10% of patients after severe blunt trauma, are more easily diagnosed on CT than on supine chest radiographs. CT is also superior for detection of retrosternal hematoma, which may result from laceration of the internal mammary vessels by sternal fracture fragments. Sternal fractures should elicit concern about associated myocardial injury, such as myocardial contusion, which can lead to significant arrhythmias and hemodynamic instability (424).

Posterior dislocation of the clavicle at the sternoclavicular joint is another injury best visualized by CT. Although less common than anterior dislocations, posterior dislocations of the sternoclavicular joint are more difficult to diagnose clinically and can result in compression or laceration of the trachea, esophagus, and great vessels (247,426). Prompt reduction of such dislocations can decrease the likelihood of visceral injury (142).

Pleural Space

Pneumothorax

Pneumothorax, with or without an associated rib fracture, is a frequent complication of blunt chest trauma, occurring in up to 40% of blunt trauma victims (96). Pneumothoraces secondary to trauma are often bilateral and associated with hemothorax (158). When a rib fracture is present with a pneumothorax (70% of cases), laceration of the visceral pleura by rib fragments is usually the cause. When no fracture is present (30% of cases), the mechanism is likely that of parenchymal lung injury, including laceration, with subsequent interstitial emphysema. Pneumomediastinum and subcutaneous emphysema may also develop (242,424). Additional causes of posttraumatic pneumothorax include alveolar compression in crushing injuries, tracheobronchial or esophageal tears, and barotrauma.

The supine chest radiograph can detect most pneumothoraces large enough to require immediate thoracostomy. However, it has been reported that as many as 30% of pneumothoraces in critically ill patients are not detected on supine radiographs and that half of these progress to tension pneumothoraces (440). In the supine position, small amounts of pleural air tend to collect in the anteromedial and subpulmonic pleural spaces and may be difficult to detect on supine chest radiographs. The use of lateral decubitus radiography of the uppermost lung with a horizontal beam, as well as chest CT, has been recommended to improve detection of pneumothoraces.

CT is an exquisitely sensitive method for detecting a pneumothorax in the supine position. Occult pneumothorax, defined as pneumothorax evident by CT but not by clinical examination or chest radiography, has been reported in 2% to 12% of patients undergoing abdominal

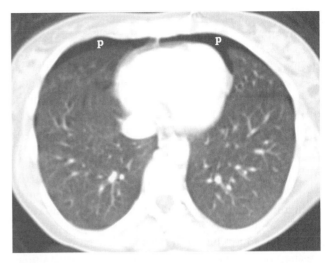

Figure 21-5 Bilateral occult pneumothoraces. Computed tomography image through the lower chest reveals small, bilateral pneumothoraces (p) that were not identified on an anteroposterior supine chest radiograph.

CT scanning for blunt trauma (356,463,479) (Fig. 21-5). A much higher percentage of occult pneumothorax (44%) has been reported in a select group of patients with severe head trauma undergoing limited chest CT examination in addition to cranial CT scanning (441).

Although CT is capable of demonstrating pneumothoraces that are not evident on clinical examination or plain radiographs, the clinical significance of, and definitive indications for, CT detection of occult pneumothorax are not entirely clear (32,180,313,480). As a general rule, a careful search for pneumothoraces in major trauma patients with seemingly normal supine chest radiographs is appropriate. In patients already undergoing abdominal CT scanning for blunt trauma, images of the upper abdomen (lower thorax) should be viewed at lung windows in addition to the usual soft tissue windows to enhance detection of small pneumothoraces (463).

Recognition of even a small, occult pneumothorax is sometimes critical, particularly in patients requiring mechanical ventilation or general anesthesia for emergent surgery. Barotrauma from mechanical ventilation and induction of anesthesia may produce enlargement of a pneumothorax resulting in significant respiratory or cardiovascular compromise (101,195). Animal studies have shown that inspiration of 75% nitrous oxide will double a 300-mL pneumothorax in 10 minutes and triple it in 45 minutes (101). To prevent progression to a tension pneumothorax, prophylactic tube thoracostomy is generally recommended for occult pneumothoraces in trauma patients needing to undergo mechanical ventilation or general anesthesia (34,441). Patients with a small, occult pneumothorax who are hemodynamically stable and not ventilated may be followed with close clinical observation and serial chest radiography to detect an increase in size of the pneumothorax. Tube thoracostomy may then be performed when appropriate (34,65,136,180,313,479,480).

In patients treated with a chest tube for pneumothorax, CT may be helpful in assessing the adequacy of chest tube placement and pneumothorax drainage. A large percentage of thoracostomy tubes placed for acute chest trauma lie within a pleural fissure, but they may still function as effectively as those located elsewhere in the pleural space (77). At times, unsuspected extrapleural location of a chest tube and/or significant residual pneumothorax is detected on CT (141). In such situations, CT can be used to guide chest tube repositioning or additional chest tube insertion.

CT may also be of value in characterizing a number of potentially confusing posttraumatic air collections noted on chest radiography. Medial pneumothorax, for example, can be distinguished from pneumomediastinum, paramediastinal pneumatocele, or air within the pulmonary ligament on CT. A narrow air collection with a fluid level occurring after blunt trauma suggests medial pneumothorax, whereas a broad or spherical gas collection without a fluid level suggests posterior pneumomediastinum, particularly when it occurs in association with respiratory distress and mechanical ventilation (149). Underlying pneumothorax in patients with extensive subcutaneous emphysema can also be reliably identified with CT.

Pleural Effusion/Hemothorax

Posttraumatic pleural effusions may be composed of transudate, exudate, blood, or chyle, or some mixture of these fluids. Transudative effusions can occur with acute pulmonary atelectasis or with vigorous resuscitation and overhydration of the patient (383). Exudative effusions are often a result of infection of the pleural space. Chylous pleural fluid may follow a crush or penetrating injury to the thorax or neck with resultant damage to the thoracic duct. The overwhelming majority of pleural effusions developing after trauma represent hemothorax (Fig. 21-6).

Hemothorax occurs in 50% of patients with blunt thoracic trauma and is often bilateral. It can be caused by many different injuries, such as lung contusion, lung laceration, intercostal vessel laceration, and mediastinal or diaphragmatic tears (158). When hemothorax is caused by bleeding from the lung (e.g., lung contusion), it is usually mild and self-limited. The low perfusion pressures and rich thromboplastin content of the lung favor hemostasis, as does the tamponade effect of associated collapsed lung (30). A large, rapidly expanding hemothorax is more likely a result of injury to higher-pressure arterial sources in the chest wall, diaphragm, or mediastinum. Laceration of systemic vessels, such as the intercostal arteries, internal mammary arteries, aorta, and great vessels, can lead to massive hemothorax and resultant shock.

CT and sonography are more sensitive than radiographs to the presence of pleural fluid collections. In a study evaluating the frequency and significance of tho-

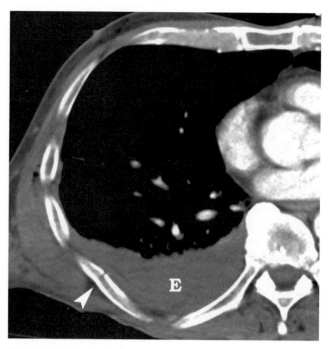

Figure 21-6 Hemothorax. Computed tomography image demonstrates high-attenuation (50 Hounsfield units) effusion (E) representing hemothorax. Note nondisplaced posterolateral rib fracture (*arrowhead*).

racic injuries detected on abdominal CT scans of multiple trauma patients, hemothorax was recognized by CT alone in 23 (88%) of 26 patients (356). Although most pleural fluid collections apparent only at CT are small and may not require emergent drainage, possible increases in their size need to be assessed, and they may require sampling to determine their cause. The CT density of the fluid collection sometimes can suggest its origin. Acute hemothorax, for example, can measure 70 to 80 Hounsfield units (HU), compared with 10 to 20 HU for most transudates (443). Because of the tendency for hemothorax to produce pleural fibrosis, chest tube drainage is often indicated.

Occasionally, even large pleural effusions, particularly if symmetric and bilateral, may not be apparent on supine chest radiographs. The same is true of fluid collections located at the bases or trapped behind stiff, noncompliant lung [such as develops with posttraumatic acute respiratory distress syndrome (ARDS)]. Both CT and sonography can readily identify such collections as well as guide their aspiration and/or drainage (428). In patients treated with catheter or thoracostomy tube drainage, CT may be particularly beneficial in assessing the adequacy of pleural drainage. Persistent loculated collections and/or malpositioned chest tubes can be reliably detected with CT (141) (Fig. 21-7). When appropriate, CT can be used to guide chest tube repositioning or additional chest tube insertion (292,423). CT is also of value

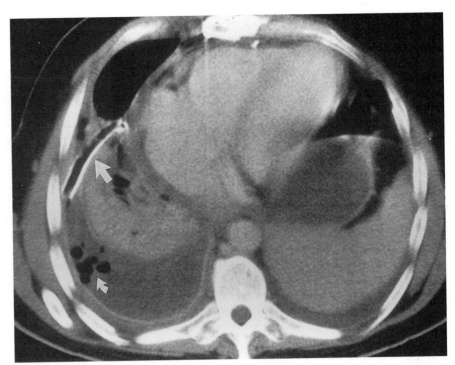

Figure 21-7 Malpositioned chest tube. Computed tomography image through the lower chest demonstrates that the right chest tube (*straight arrow*) is well anterior to the right pleural fluid collection. Locules of air (*curved arrow*) within the pleural fluid collection were introduced at the time of chest tube placement.

in the detection and drainage of associated complications such as empyema (Fig. 21-8) or lung abscess. CT can better delineate complex pleuroparenchymal opacities, distinguishing pleural fluid from other components causing radiographic density such as atelectasis, consolidation, or contusion (295).

Lung Parenchyma

Pulmonary Contusion

Pulmonary contusion is the most common injury resulting from blunt chest trauma (477), occurring in 30% to 75% of patients sustaining blunt trauma to the chest (225).

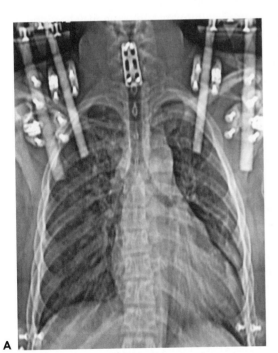

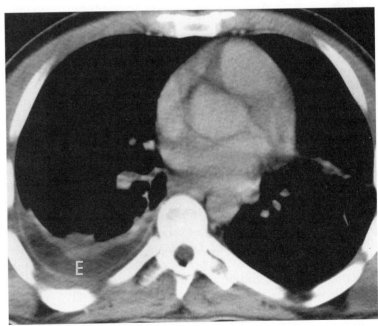

A

B

Figure 21-8 Occult empyema in a febrile patient following blunt trauma. **A:** Scout view from the computed tomography (CT) examination is unremarkable except for hardware related to a halo fixation device that overlies the upper chest. **B:** CT image through the lower chest reveals an occult empyema (E).

Contusion results in exudation of blood and/or edema fluid into the air spaces and interstitium of the lung. Although often mild and localized, pulmonary contusion may be widespread and associated with respiratory failure. Massive contusion can lead to the development of ARDS (63). The mortality rate from pulmonary contusion ranges from 14% to 40%, depending on the severity and extent of lung damage and other injuries (158,225).

Radiologically, pulmonary contusion generally results in nonsegmental, air–space consolidation, which may vary from patchy, faint, ill-defined areas of increased parenchymal density to extensive homogeneous opacification in one or both lungs. Contusions are frequently peripheral in distribution and tend to occur near the site of blunt impact and adjacent to solid structures such as the ribs, spine, heart, or liver (354). Contusions may also be seen in areas remote from the injured site because of the contrecoup effect (353,477). Usually, contusions appear within four to six hours after injury and clear within three to eight days. The abrupt onset and relatively rapid clearing of areas of parenchymal opacification are characteristic of pulmonary contusion. Contusions may increase in size and become more visible for up to 48 hours after injury. Progressive increase in parenchymal opacification after 48 hours or delayed resolution beyond six to ten days suggests either the wrong initial diagnosis or superimposition of another pathologic process, such as pneumonia, atelectasis, aspiration, or ARDS (242,295,425,430). Intra-alveolar blood and edema fluid within contused lung, coupled with impaired clearance of secretions and regional diminished lung compliance, provide a nidus for the development of infection and sepsis. In addition, because of disruption of alveolar/capillary membranes, contused lung is more susceptible to pulmonary edema (175). Administration of large amounts of IV fluids may accentuate the degree of edema and result in worsening radiographic opacification (158,175).

The overall severity and extent of contusion are often underestimated at initial clinical and radiographic examination (28). Rib fractures or other external signs of chest wall injury may be absent, even when extensive life-threatening contusion has occurred. Animal studies suggest that contusion involving up to one third of the lung may go undetected with plain radiography (103).

CT is much more sensitive than chest radiography in determining the presence and extent of pulmonary contusion (380,459,461). On CT, contusion appears as an ill-defined area of hazy ground-glass density or consolidation, usually with a peripheral, nonsegmental distribution (Fig. 21-9). As with chest radiography, the CT appearance of contusion initially may be indistinguishable from that of other causes of consolidation such as aspiration, edema, and pneumonia. CT demonstration of localized, patchy infiltrates neighboring a rib fracture or chest-wall hematoma suggests contusion, whereas infiltrates predominantly located in the superior segments of both lower lobes and other dependent segments suggest aspiration (438).

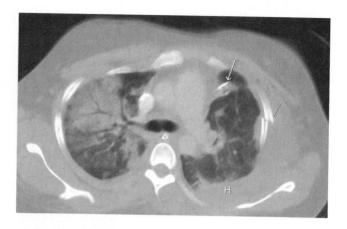

Figure 21-9 Pulmonary contusion. Computed tomography image through the carina of a young woman struck by an automobile demonstrates nonsegmental areas of parenchymal consolidation and ground-glass density in the right lung. *Thick arrow*, left chest tube; *thin arrow*, rib fracture; H, hemothorax.

Although CT is capable of demonstrating earlier, as well as more extensive, pulmonary contusion than chest radiography, several investigators have questioned the clinical significance of this improved detection (346,415). In some studies, only those contusions diagnosed by chest radiography proved clinically significant (415), and it has been stated that the detection of pulmonary contusion on CT should not dictate a change in clinical management in the absence of hypoxemia or other respiratory disturbances (346). Nevertheless, other investigators have shown that CT quantitation of pulmonary contusion may be useful in the management of patients with blunt chest injury. In a review of 69 patients with severe blunt chest trauma examined by CT within 24 hours of admission, it was found that when there was CT evidence of pulmonary contusion involving greater than 28% of the total lung volume, ventilatory support was invariably required (460). Another report found that patients with greater than or equal to 20% pulmonary contusion volume were at significantly higher risk of developing ARDS (281).

Pulmonary Laceration, Pneumatocele, and Hematoma

Pulmonary laceration is a tear in the lung parenchyma that develops through any of the four major mechanisms of blunt injury described earlier (i.e., direct impact, inertial deceleration, spallation, implosion) or from any penetrating injury, such as from sharp, depressed rib fragments. The initial linear or stellate tear of a laceration tends to form an ovoid- or elliptical-shaped postlaceration space because of elastic recoil of the adjacent intact lung (300). Concomitant tears of bronchi and blood vessels may fill the postlaceration space with air (pneumatocele), blood (hematoma), or both (hematopneumatocele) (158). Pathologically, lacerations are lined by compressed alveoli and connective tissue remnants, and may be uni- or multilocular, generally varying from 2 cm to 14 cm in diameter (291,300).

Radiographically, pulmonary lacerations appear as circumscribed areas containing air, fluid, or both. They are often obscured initially by surrounding pulmonary contusion and may become more apparent as the contusion resolves. If the laceration becomes filled with blood and a pulmonary hematoma forms, it can present as a focal mass on chest radiography, mimicking a primary lung cancer.

CT is considerably more sensitive than chest radiography in detecting pulmonary laceration. In a series of 85 consecutive chest trauma victims, CT detected 99 lacerations compared with only 5 detected by radiography (459). Because of the frequent CT identification of pulmonary laceration following blunt trauma, it has been suggested that pulmonary laceration is the basic mechanism of injury in pulmonary contusion, pulmonary hematoma, and traumatic pulmonary cyst, as well as the cause of most cavities in areas of pulmonary contusion (459) (Fig. 21-10). In cases of severe blunt chest trauma, multiple traumatic lacerations and air cysts may be seen within an area of air–space consolidation, giving rise to the so-called "pulverized" lung appearance on CT images (233) (Fig. 21-11).

Pulmonary lacerations can be divided into four types on the basis of CT criteria and mechanism of injury (233,436,454,459). Type 1 lacerations, the most common type seen on CT, result from sudden compression of a pliable chest wall, causing rupture of air-containing lung. They usually appear on CT as intraparenchymal cavities with or without an air–fluid level (Fig. 21-12). On occasion, they may appear as air-filled linear structures extending through the visceral pleura, resulting in a pneumothorax. Type 2 lacerations are relatively uncommon and present as air-containing cavities or intraparenchymal air–fluid levels

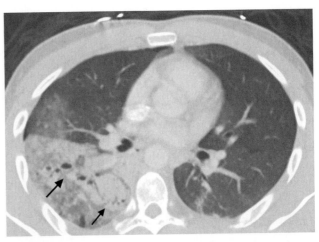

Figure 21-11 Pulverized lung. Computed tomography image in a young man who sustained severe blunt chest trauma demonstrates multiple traumatic lacerations and air cysts (*arrows*) within an area of right lower lobe consolidation, resulting in the so-called "pulverized" lung appearance. A small right pneumothorax is also present.

within the basilar paravertebral lung (Fig. 21-13). They result from sudden compression of the more pliable lower chest wall, which causes the lower lobe to shift suddenly across the spine, producing a shearing-type injury. Type 3 lacerations appear as small peripheral cavities or linear lucencies neighboring a fractured rib that has punctured the underlying lung. These lacerations are usually associated with a pneumothorax. Type 4 lacerations are rare and occur at sites of pleuroparenchymal adhesion, which causes the lung to tear when the overlying chest wall is violently moved inward or is fractured. These lacerations can be diagnosed only surgically or at autopsy (459).

Most pulmonary lacerations resolve completely in a period of several weeks to months after injury, with air-filled lacerations (pneumatoceles) resolving more quickly than blood-filled lacerations (hematomas) (54). In mechanically ventilated patients, postlaceration spaces/pneumatoceles can progressively enlarge and communicate with the pleural space, resulting in pneumothorax. Rarely, they can become infected. CT has been shown to be superior to chest radiography in identifying and following the evolution of these lesions and in establishing the presence of complications such as infection or hemorrhage (26,211, 400) (Fig. 21-14).

Aorta and Great Vessels

Laceration of the thoracic aorta and brachiocephalic arteries is a significant cause of morbidity and mortality secondary to blunt chest trauma. The majority of these injuries result from high-speed motor vehicle accidents. Most of the remainder are a result of falls from heights and crush or blast injuries. Of all autopsied auto-accident victims, about 16% have aortic laceration (157). Laceration is thought to result from shearing stress on the aorta produced by differential

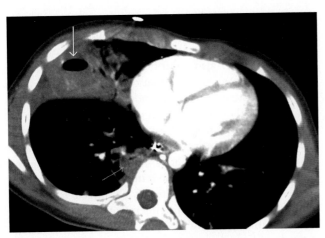

Figure 21-10 Pulmonary laceration and contusion. Computed tomography image through the lower chest in a 7-year-old girl involved in a motor vehicle accident demonstrates an air-filled cavity (*thick arrow*) representing pulmonary laceration within an area of pulmonary contusion. An additional area of contusion is noted in the right paraspinal area (*thin arrow*).

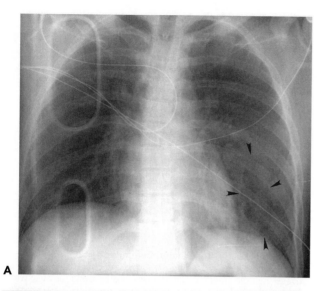

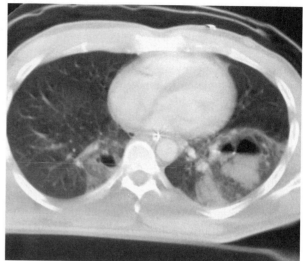

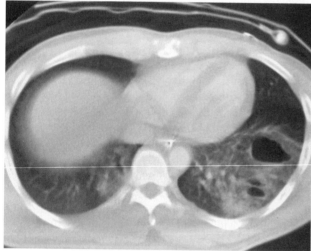

Figure 21-12 Pulmonary lacerations following blunt chest trauma. **A:** Supine chest radiograph demonstrates subtle, focal air lucency (*arrowheads*) at the left lung base. **B, C:** Computed tomography images reveal multiple, bilateral lower lobe intraparenchymal cavities containing air–fluid levels. Surrounding parenchymal contusion is also evident.

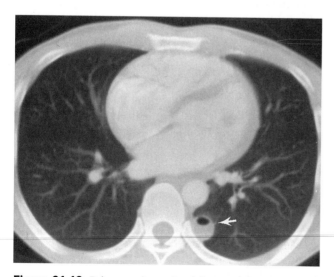

Figure 21-13 Pulmonary laceration following fall from a height. Computed tomography image demonstrates intraparenchymal air-fluid level (*arrow*) within the basilar paravertebral lung.

deceleration (whiplash) of the aortic root, aortic arch, and descending aorta at the time of impact. Sudden increases in intraaortic pressure produced by chest or abdominal wall compression may also contribute to aortic injury (256). Another hypothesis suggests that compression of the aorta between the sternum and the thoracic spine results in an "osseous pinch" of the aorta that causes laceration (61,62,73). Whatever the mechanism of injury, the result is that one or more layers of the aortic wall are torn, usually in a transverse fashion. Though the tear may be short (few millimeters) and superficial (limited to the intima), most are circumferential and transmural, constituting a complete transection. When only part of the aortic circumference is involved, the tear tends to be posterior (335).

In clinical series, over 90% of aortic tears occur at the aortic isthmus (i.e., the distal aortic arch at the insertion of the ligamentum arteriosum just after the origin of the left subclavian artery), which is the site of maximum aortic wall shear stress. Approximately 5% of tears involve the ascending aorta,

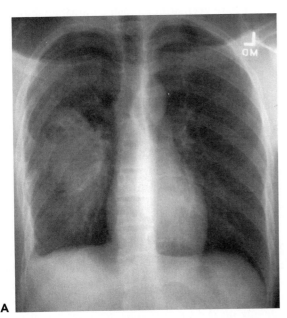
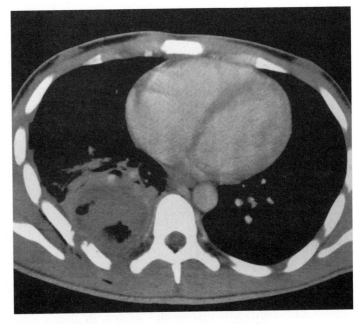

Figure 21-14 Infected hematoma. **A:** Chest radiograph in febrile patient three weeks after rollover motor vehicle accident demonstrates multiple right rib fractures and a large, rounded opacity containing multiple locules of air in the right midlung field. **B:** Computed tomography image shows large intraparenchymal mass containing fluid and air compatible with an infected hematoma or lung abscess. A small amount of subcutaneous air is present in the right posterior chest wall.

usually just above the aortic valve (78,223,255,372). In autopsy series, the incidence of ascending aortic tears is higher (20% to 25%), reflecting the fact that tears of the ascending aorta are almost always immediately fatal (335,431). Death is usually a result of associated cardiac injuries. Severe cardiac injuries, such as myocardial contusion, aortic valve rupture, coronary artery laceration, and hemopericardium with cardiac tamponade, are present in 75% of patients with ascending aortic laceration, compared with only 25% of patients with aortic isthmus laceration (335). Most victims of combined ascending aortic laceration and cardiac injury have been pedestrians, ejected passengers, or sufferers of falls, including airplane crashes and elevator accidents (157,335,431). Injuries to the descending aorta from blunt trauma are rare. When laceration of the descending aorta does occur, it is usually at the level of the aortic hiatus, where the distal descending aorta exits the thorax through the diaphragm (425). Multiple aortic tears occur in 6% to 19% of cases (157,335), and associated injury or avulsion of the brachiocephalic arteries has been reported in 4% of cases (125). Brachiocephalic injuries are often multiple, occurring much more commonly in association with other aortic or brachiocephalic lacerations than as single-artery insults (125).

Eighty percent to ninety percent of all patients with aortic laceration die at the scene of the accident or before they can be transported to a hospital and treated (335). For the remaining 10% to 20% who arrive at a hospital alive, expedient diagnosis and immediate surgical repair generally are essential to prevent exsanguinating hemorrhage at the site of the aortic tear. The importance of rapid diagnosis and treatment in this group of patients is underscored by the fact that survival rates ranging from 68% to 80% have been reported if timely surgical repair can be performed (58,68,223,227,381). Without treatment, it is estimated that less than 5% of patients survive. These are usually patients with only partial aortic transection, in whom the pulsating hematoma is contained by the adventitia or the periaortic tissues (335).

Clinical findings in patients with traumatic aortic laceration are frequently absent, and the possibility of aortic injury is often initially raised solely on the basis of a history of trauma involving significant deceleration (i.e., high-speed motor vehicle accident). More than 50% of patients with aortic laceration may have no visible external signs of chest trauma. Furthermore, it may be impossible to elicit symptoms in a substantial number of these patients because of altered mental status resulting from concomitant head trauma (231). The most common complaint in the immediate postinjury period is retrosternal or interscapular pain, thought to be a result of mediastinal dissection of blood. Less frequently encountered signs and symptoms include dyspnea, dysphagia, upper extremity hypertension, lower extremity hypotension, and a harsh systolic murmur over the precordium or interscapular area (because of turbulent flow across the area of transection). Unfortunately, none of these clinical findings are sufficiently sensitive or specific to be considered diagnostic of aortic injury (223).

The diagnosis of aortic injury is usually suggested by findings on chest radiography and then confirmed by MDCT and/or thoracic aortography. Radiographic findings suggestive of acute aortic trauma primarily reflect the presence of mediastinal hematoma and may include (a) widening of the superior mediastinum; (b) fullness, deformity, or obscuration of the aortic contour, particularly in the region of the aortic arch, isthmus, or aortopulmonary window; (c) deviation of the trachea or nasogastric tube in the esophagus to the right; (d) caudal displacement of the left main stem bronchus; (e) widening of the right paratracheal stripe; (f) widening of the paravertebral stripes; and (g) extrapleural extension of hemorrhage over the lung apex (apical cap) (284,406,437,485). Of these numerous findings, widening of the mediastinum with loss of the aortic contour is the most sensitive predictor of aortic injury, and the most frequent indication for aortography (15,162, 231,389). Isolated fractures of the first and/or second ribs, once thought to indicate severe mediastinal trauma, do not correlate with aortic rupture and are not, by themselves, an indication for aortography in the absence of radiographic or CT evidence of mediastinal hematoma (126,239,484).

Although the chest radiograph has a high sensitivity for mediastinal hematoma, it is frequently falsely positive as a result of a variety of factors, including shallow inspiration, supine anteroposterior positioning, vascular ectasia, pulmonary disease adjacent to the mediastinum, and mediastinal fat. It is important to note that, even when mediastinal hemorrhage is correctly diagnosed, it is most commonly caused by disruption of small arteries and veins in the mediastinum, rather than by aortic injury (10,328). Mediastinal hematoma may also result from nonaortic hemorrhage associated with other mediastinal injuries, such as tracheobronchial tears or fractures of the lower cervical and upper thoracic spine (86). A completely normal chest radiograph is of greater diagnostic significance than an abnormal chest radiograph, since it has a 98% negative predictive value for traumatic aortic or brachiocephalic artery rupture (264,285,483).

Aortography is a well-established method of diagnosing traumatic aortic laceration and of defining its anatomic extent. It is used liberally in trauma patients because the consequences of missing an aortic rupture are grave, the clinical findings are frequently absent, and the radiographic findings are nonspecific. Only 10% to 20% of patients with clinical and radiographic findings suggestive of aortic trauma have angiographic confirmation of an aortic tear (162,285,433,454). Angiographically, lacerations appear as sharply defined linear lucencies, produced by the infolded, torn edges of the intima. Associated irregularity of the aortic wall and/or a false aneurysm may also be seen. Conventional aortography has been reported to have a 100% sensitivity and 99% specificity for the diagnosis of traumatic aortic injury, with a positive predictive value of 97% and a negative predictive value of 100% (433). Similar

success rates have been achieved using intraarterial digital subtraction aortography, which, in comparison to conventional aortography, can reduce both the amount of time and the amount of intravascular contrast material needed to obtain a diagnostically accurate study (290).

The role of CT in the evaluation of patients with suspected injury of the aorta continues to evolve. Initially, CT was used primarily as an adjunct to chest radiography in determining the need for aortography (4,260,289,307,352,357). Some questioned the accuracy of CT findings and the validity of CT usage in this regard, stating that CT only delayed performance of aortography or definitive treatment with surgery (279,471). CT has typically been performed on hemodynamically stable patients with a clinical suspicion of aortic tear in whom chest radiographic findings are equivocal (307). In such patients, CT can accurately exclude the presence of mediastinal hemorrhage or provide alternative explanations for equivocal radiographic findings, thus eliminating the need for aortography. Apparent mediastinal widening on chest radiographs, for example, may be shown on CT to represent excessive mediastinal fat (Fig. 21-15), paravertebral pleural effusion, atelectatic/contused lung adjacent to the mediastinum, vascular ectasia, or congenital vascular anomalies such as right aortic arch, persistent left superior vena cava, or hemiazygous continuation of the inferior vena cava (373,419,439,442). Chest CT has also been used as an ancillary screening modality for aortography in clinically stable patients requiring CT examination for another indication (e.g., evaluation of intracranial or abdominal trauma) (307,352). In a meta-analysis evaluating the cost-effectiveness of using CT to triage patients to aortography, the addition of chest CT in patients requiring head or abdominopelvic CT for evaluation of other injuries was found to be both medically effective and cost reducing (105,194).

Most studies to date suggest that an unequivocally normal chest CT reliably excludes aortic injury, with an overall false–negative CT rate of approximately 1% (4,122,124, 260,279,289,307,352,357,472). False–negative CT studies have been attributed to contained intimal and/or medial tears unassociated with mediastinal hemorrhage, or to technically suboptimal examinations degraded by motion artifact or inadequate contrast material administration (307). By excluding mediastinal hemorrhage or providing alternative explanations for mediastinal widening, CT has been reported in a number of studies to reduce the need for aortography in selected trauma patients by 50% to 73% (198,260,289,307,352,357). Another study, however, reported that the "absolute exclusion" of mediastinal hemorrhage by CT was often difficult and resulted in only a 25% reduction in the use of aortography (124).

CT can demonstrate both direct and indirect (i.e., mediastinal hemorrhage) evidence of aortic injury. Some authors consider the presence of mediastinal hemorrhage on CT to be an indication for aortography, even in the absence of direct signs of aortic injury (289,307,357,492).

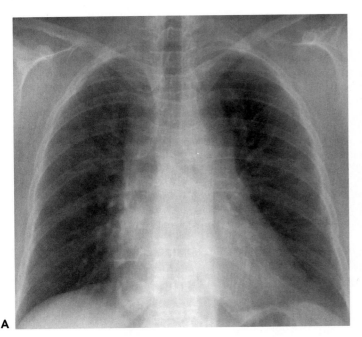

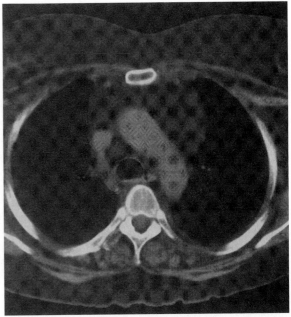

Figure 21-15 Mediastinal lipomatosis. **A:** Chest radiograph demonstrates mediastinal widening in a 40-year-old woman following a motor vehicle accident. **B:** Computed tomography image at the level of the aortic arch demonstrates abundant mediastinal fat accounting for the mediastinal widening.

The mediastinal hemorrhage may be focal or diffuse and appears on CT as homogeneous areas of fluid within the mediastinum or as streaky tissue-density fluid infiltrating the mediastinal fat (124,307,352) (Fig. 21-16). Difficulties in interpretation may arise because of the confusion of mediastinal hemorrhage with thymic tissue in the anterior mediastinum, partial volume averaging of the pulmonary artery in the aortopulmonary window, periaortic atelectasis in the left lower lobe, or motion artifact producing haziness in the mediastinum (351,357,471). The majority of patients with CT evidence of mediastinal hemorrhage do not have angiographic evidence of an aortic tear (124,307,352,357). As mentioned previously, mediastinal hemorrhage is merely a marker of significant mediastinal trauma and is not specific for aortic injury. Most commonly, the bleeding is from disruption of mediastinal veins and/or small arteries rather than from aortic rupture (10).

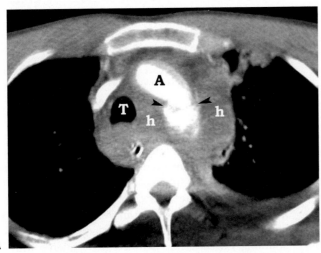

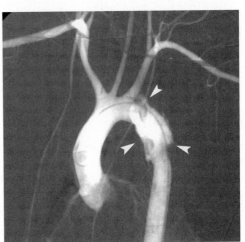

Figure 21-16 Mediastinal hemorrhage secondary to aortic laceration. **A:** Computed tomography image through the level of the aortic arch (A) demonstrates extensive periaortic mediastinal hematoma (h) and irregular tears (*arrowheads*) in the aortic wall. The trachea (T) and the nasogastric tube within the esophagus are shifted to the right. **B:** Digital subtraction angiographic image confirms the presence of extensive aortic laceration (*arrowheads*), beginning just distal to the origin of the left subclavian artery.

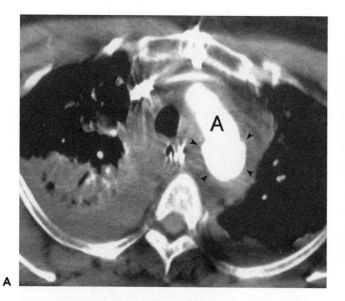

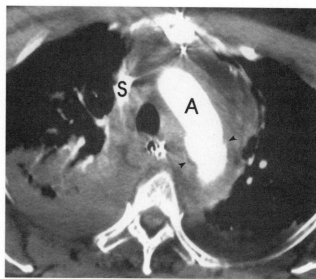

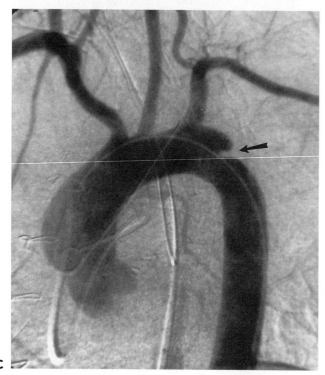

Figure 21-17 Aortic laceration in a 56-year-old woman involved in a motor vehicle accident. **A, B:** Computed tomography sections through the aortic arch (A) and proximal descending thoracic aorta demonstrate periaortic mediastinal hemorrhage and a focal increase in caliber of the aortic lumen with marked irregularity of the aortic margins (*arrowheads*). Right lung contusion and small left pleural effusion are also evident. There is streak artifact from the nasogastric tube in the esophagus and from multiple median sternotomy suture wires. S, superior vena cava. **C:** Angiography confirms the presence of aortic laceration (*arrow*) just distal to the origin of the left subclavian artery.

Direct CT findings of aortic injury include pseudoaneurysm, intimal flap, aortic contour deformity (Fig. 21-17), abrupt tapering of the descending aorta relative to the ascending aorta ("pseudocoarctation"), and active extravasation of contrast material (127,137,138,172,174,265,378, 468,492). The pseudoaneurysm may be focal or circumferential, and can be identified on CT as a saccular outpouching or increase in caliber of the aortic lumen compared with the more proximal normal aorta (Fig. 21-18). An intimal flap produced by the torn edge of the aortic wall appears on CT as a small, linear, low-density intraluminal filling defect within the opacified aortic lumen (Fig. 21-19). In injuries in

which the aortic adventitia is breached, extravasation of contrast material can occur, ranging from small leaks to gross extravasation. In a prospective series examining the efficacy of CT for direct detection of traumatic aortic injury, helical CT was found to have an overall diagnostic accuracy of nearly 100% (293). In a separate large series using helical scanning exclusively to screen 1,518 patients with blunt chest trauma, helical CT with thin overlapping reconstruction was found to be 100% sensitive and 81.7% specific in detecting aortic injury (138). Advances in MDCT technology are likely to further improve our ability to evaluate the aorta for direct signs of injury (6).

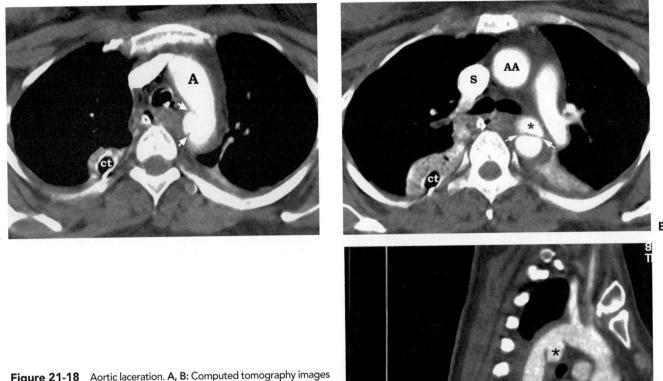

Figure 21-18   Aortic laceration. **A, B:** Computed tomography images through the aortic arch (A) and proximal descending aorta at the level of the carina demonstrate a tear (*arrows*) in the aortic wall and an associated pseudoaneurysm (*asterisk*). There is a right chest tube (ct) with adjacent hematoma and atelectatic lung. AA, ascending aorta; S, superior vena cava. **C:** Sagittal reconstruction better separates the true aortic lumen from the pseudoaneurysm (*asterisk*).

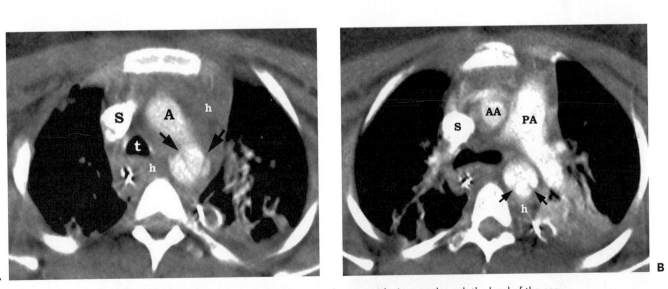

Figure 21-19   Aortic laceration. **A, B:** Computed tomography images through the level of the aortic arch (A) and main pulmonary artery (PA) demonstrate periaortic mediastinal hemorrhage (h), irregularity of the aortic contour, and linear lucencies (*arrows*) within the opacified aortic lumen, representing intimal flaps produced by the torn edges of the aortic wall. The trachea (t) and esophagus (containing a nasogastric tube) are shifted to the right by the mediastinal hematoma. A left chest tube and adjacent parenchymal atelectasis are also present. AA, ascending aorta; S, superior vena cava.

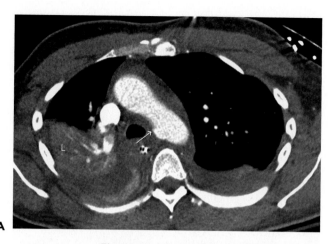

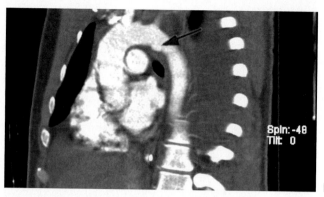

Figure 21-20 Aortic laceration. **A:** Transaxial computed tomography image at the level of the aortic arch demonstrates marginal irregularity of the aortic wall (*arrow*) with adjacent periaortic hemorrhage. Blood is noted in both pleural cavities. L, consolidated lung parenchyma. **B:** Sagittal image confirms the subtle focal abnormality (*arrow*).

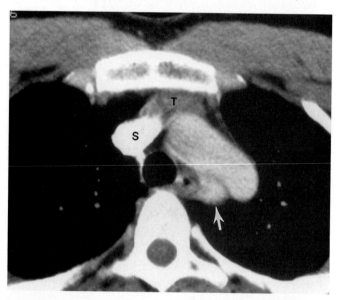

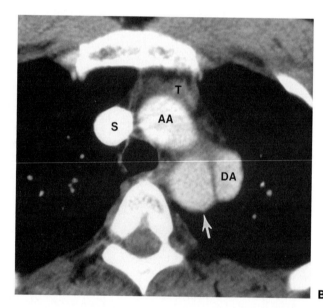

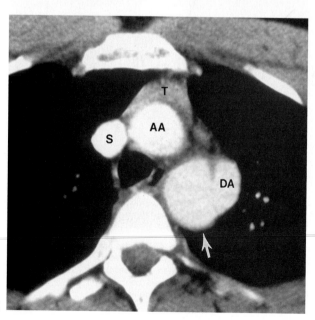

Figure 21-21 Posttraumatic aortic pseudoaneurysm in a 21-year-old man approximately two years following a motor vehicle accident and repair of a ruptured left hemidiaphragm. **A–C:** Computed tomography images demonstrate a pseudoaneurysm (*arrow*) projecting medially from the proximal descending aorta (DA). The distal aortic arch and descending aorta are displaced superiorly and laterally by the pseudoaneurysm. The patient underwent successful surgical repair with placement of an aortic tube graft. AA, ascending aorta; S, superior vena cava; T, thymus.

Patients with obvious direct signs of aortic injury on CT may be taken directly to surgery without confirmatory aortography (100,137,351,382,445). Subtle contour abnormality seen on a transaxial section may be better demonstrated on sagittal or coronal images (Fig. 21-20). Equivocal or less specific CT findings, such as marginal irregularity of the aortic wall or isolated periaortic hematoma, generally still warrant aortography.

If the aorta is only partially transected following blunt trauma and the patient survives without recognition and treatment, a localized false (pseudo) aneurysm may subsequently develop over a period of months to years. These lesions, which continue to communicate with the aortic lumen through the tear and tend to expand with time, are most commonly found immediately distal to the origin of the left subclavian artery, in the region of the aortic isthmus. They have been estimated to occur in 2% to 5% of patients with aortic injury and may be detected incidentally on plain chest radiography or because of symptoms related to their expansion (20,123,335). Contrary to the assessment of acute traumatic injury of the aorta, either CT or MRI usually is adequate for diagnostic confirmation of a chronic traumatic pseudoaneurysm suspected on plain chest radiography, and aortography is rarely required. On CT or MRI, a chronic traumatic pseudoaneurysm appears as saccular or fusiform dilatation of the aortic isthmus (Fig. 21-21). Peripheral calcification of the wall of the pseudoaneurysm may be seen on CT (53) (Fig. 21-22). Sagittal MR images have been reported to be helpful in defining the exact relationship of the pseudoaneurysm to the left subclavian artery and in determining the size of its communication with the aortic lumen (302). Because of the persistent risk of rupture of these posttraumatic aneurysms, endovascular stent graft repair or elective surgical excision is generally performed (6,20,123,176).

Heart and Pericardium

Blunt chest trauma can result in a spectrum of cardiac injuries, ranging in severity from inconsequential, asymptomatic lesions that are detectable only by serial electrocardiograms (ECGs) to rapidly fatal cardiac rupture. Acute heart injuries include contusion, transmural myocardial necrosis, and laceration or rupture of the pericardium, myocardium, septa, papillary muscles, cardiac valves, and coronary arteries (97,225,334). Although the exact incidence of cardiac injury from blunt chest trauma is unknown, autopsy series have demonstrated that greater than 10% of highway fatalities have evidence of cardiac damage, and that in approximately 5%, the cardiac injury is lethal (326,414). In clinical series, estimates of cardiac injury as high as 76% have been reported among selected groups of severely injured patients (405).

Myocardial contusion represents the most common manifestation of cardiac trauma and has been reported to occur in 8% to 76% of patients following severe chest injury (181). It results in myocardial edema, hemorrhage, and necrosis, and an increase in the MB fraction of the enzyme creatine phosphokinase (CPK). ECG changes are similar to those of myocardial ischemia and infarction. Delayed onset of right ventricular contractions, localized wall-motion abnormalities, and depressed ejection fraction on ECG-gated radionuclide blood pool scans have also been observed (240,369). The right ventricle is the most frequently injured because it makes up the majority of the exposed anterior surface of the heart directly behind the sternum. Clinically, myocardial contusion usually is well tolerated. However, the resultant myocardial damage

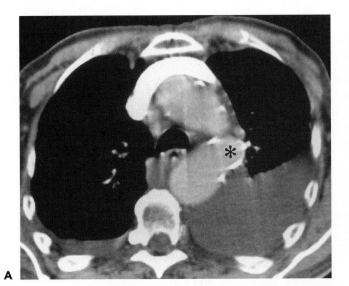

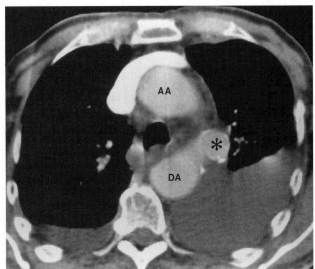

A   B

Figure 21-22 Posttraumatic aortic pseudoaneurysm in a patient with a remote history of a motor vehicle accident requiring hospitalization. **A, B:** Computed tomography images demonstrate focal aortic pseudoaneurysm with peripheral calcification (*asterisk*). There are bilateral pleural effusions, left greater than right. AA, ascending aorta; DA, descending aorta.

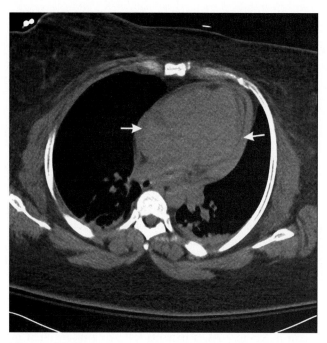

Figure 21-23 Acute traumatic hemopericardium. Noncontrast computed tomography image demonstrates high-attenuation pericardial effusion (*arrows*) consistent with acute pericardial hemorrhage.

multisystem injuries and because routine tests, such as ECGs and CPK isoenzyme determinations, are nonspecific following severe trauma (28,369). Chest radiography and CT play only a minor role in the evaluation of myocardial injury. Radiographic findings may include evidence of congestive failure, such as cardiac enlargement and pulmonary edema. The presence of anterior rib fractures and sternal fractures should increase clinical suspicion of myocardial injury, although there is no clear relationship between the extent of chest wall injury and the degree of underlying cardiac damage (295). Ventricular aneurysms may develop as a sequela of cardiac injury such as contusion or infarction, and can be detected on CT or conventional chest radiographs by a change in cardiac contour and by the presence of calcification within the wall of the aneurysm (154).

Acute hemopericardium can occur following injury to the heart or pericardium. CT is very sensitive for detecting pericardial space fluid and may indicate the presence of pericardial hemorrhage by the high CT attenuation (i.e., near soft tissue density) of the fluid (429) (Fig. 21-23). Small hemorrhagic pericardial effusions of no functional significance are sometimes seen as incidental findings on posttraumatic CT examinations. Rapid accumulation of blood in the pericardial space can lead to cardiac tamponade and severe hemodynamic compromise. The diagnosis of acute tamponade is usually established by the presence of clinical signs such as tachycardia, elevated central venous pressure, distended neck veins, muffled cardiac sounds, and diminished cardiac output. Emergency bedside sonographic evaluation of the heart can document the presence of pericardial effusion prior to prompt pericardiocentesis or pericardiotomy. CT findings of acute tamponade following blunt trauma include hemorrhagic

can lead to functional cardiac abnormalities such as diminished cardiac output or acute cardiac arrhythmias in up to 20% of patients (187).

Cardiac dysfunction resulting from blunt trauma is frequently missed or detected late because the cardiac injury (e.g., contusion) is often masked by other more obvious

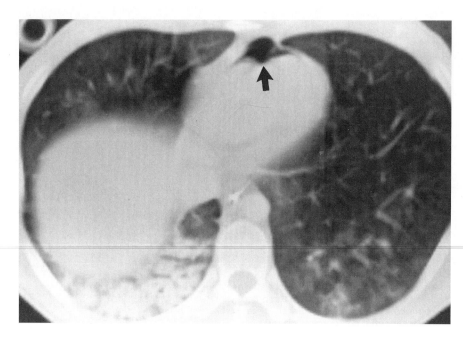

Figure 21-24 Posttraumatic pneumopericardium. Computed tomography image at the level of the right hemidiaphragm demonstrates a small amount of pericardial air (*arrow*). Parenchymal contusion is evident at both lung bases, right greater than left.

pericardial fluid, distended central veins (e.g., vena cavae, hepatic veins, renal veins), and periportal lymphedema within the liver (152).

Pneumopericardium is an uncommon manifestation of blunt chest trauma and is thought to result from dissection of air along perivascular and/or peribronchial sheaths into the pericardium. Air from ruptured alveoli, for example, can track along the adventitia of the pulmonary veins and enter the pericardial space (258,262). Moderately small amounts of pericardial air are generally of little clinical significance, and may be detected incidentally on CT (Fig. 21-24). Rarely, larger amounts of air can compress the heart and lead to the development of tension pneumopericardium. Radiographically this is manifested by a sudden, substantial decrease in size of the cardiac silhouette in the presence of pneumopericardium and clinical signs of cardiac tamponade (287). Prolonged positive airway pressure in combination with pulmonary contusion, pneumothorax, or tracheobronchial tear may increase the development of this complication.

Pericardial rupture is a rare sequela (less than 0.5%) of severe blunt chest trauma (135). Rupture may involve the diaphragmatic pericardium and/or the pleuropericardium, most commonly on the left. The diagnosis is usually made intraoperatively or at autopsy. Antemortem diagnosis may be suggested by chest radiographic or CT findings of herniation of air-containing abdominal viscera into the pericardium accompanying diaphragmatic rupture (295). Additional CT findings that have been reported in patients with traumatic pericardial rupture include pneumopericardium, posterolateral rotation of the cardiac apex, and extrusion of the heart through the pericardial tear (222).

Trachea and Bronchi

Tracheobronchial tear is an uncommon but serious complication of blunt chest trauma, with an estimated overall mortality of 30% (224). Most tears involve the distal trachea (15%) or proximal mainstem bronchi (80%) (477), with more than 80% of all tears occurring within 2.5 cm of the carina (224). The clinical and radiographic findings vary, depending on the site and extent of the tear. Complete tears of the right mainstem and distal left mainstem bronchi generally manifest as pneumothorax. The pneumothorax tends to be large and unrelieved by chest tube drainage. Tears of the trachea and proximal left mainstem bronchus usually result in pneumomediastinum. The pneumomediastinum is often severe, persistent, and progressive, with widespread dissection of air into the neck and subcutaneous tissues. Incomplete tracheobronchial tears with intact peritracheal and peribronchial adventitia may not be associated with pneumothorax, pneumomediastinum, or other radiographic findings. This is because the integrity of the airway is initially maintained, preventing passage of air into the mediastinum or pleura. Such partial tears may remain occult until subsequent high-pressure mechanical ventilation causes mediastinal emphysema or delayed massive pneumothorax (158).

Although the findings of tracheobronchial tear are sometimes subtle and overshadowed by other injuries, the diagnosis is usually suggested by the presence of dyspnea, persistent pneumothorax or air leak following chest tube drainage, and massive or rapidly increasing mediastinal or subcutaneous emphysema (182). Abnormalities in position and configuration of an endotracheal tube, including overdistention of the balloon cuff or extraluminal position of the tip, may be seen in patients with tracheal rupture (365,451). In complete bronchial tear with associated pneumothorax, the collapsed lung may fall away from the hilum toward the most dependent portion of the hemithorax, giving rise to the so-called "falling lung sign" (Fig. 21-25) (234,322,435,476). This is the reverse of the usual finding in uncomplicated pneumothorax, in which the lung is tethered by the hilum and collapses toward it. The disrupted bronchus may be deformed (i.e., sharply angulated) or obstructed. Both the presence of the "falling lung sign" and endotracheal tube abnormalities such as an overdistended balloon cuff are considered reliable though uncommon indicators of airway injury (451).

CT can be used to diagnose tracheal tears in patients with indwelling endotracheal tubes by demonstrating extraluminal tip position or by showing an overdistended balloon protruding through the tracheal tear into the mediastinum (52,438). The actual rent in the tracheal wall may be seen even in the absence of endotracheal tube abnormality (329). Associated mediastinal and subcutaneous emphysema are also well depicted on CT. Bronchial rupture has been recognized on CT by abrupt tapering of the injured bronchus, coupled with shift of the mediastinum toward the compromised lung and retraction of the trachea in the opposite direction (465). Although CT is capable of demonstrating tracheobronchial injury, the standard chest radiograph and appropriate clinical findings are usually enough to suggest urgent bronchoscopy, which generally is required for definitive diagnosis prior to surgery (154). In a few select cases of tracheal rupture, diagnostic findings on CT examination have led to immediate surgical repair without bronchoscopy (438).

Esophagus

Injury to the esophagus from blunt chest trauma is extremely uncommon. When it does occur, it is usually secondary to severe chest and/or abdominal compression and is frequently associated with other thoracic injuries, such as aortic rupture and cardiac contusion (455). Proposed mechanisms of esophageal injury in blunt trauma include sudden elevation in esophageal hydrostatic pressure, crushing of the esophagus between the spine and trachea, tearing resulting from hyperextension (particularly at the level of the diaphragmatic hiatus), and direct penetration by cervical spine fracture fragments (291). Other causes of esophageal injury in the acute trauma setting include inadvertent esophageal intubation and traumatic nasogastric tube placement. The vast majority of traumatic esophageal perforations

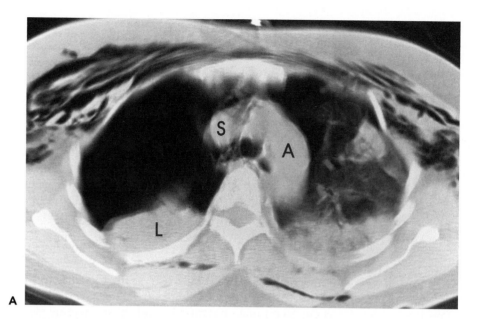

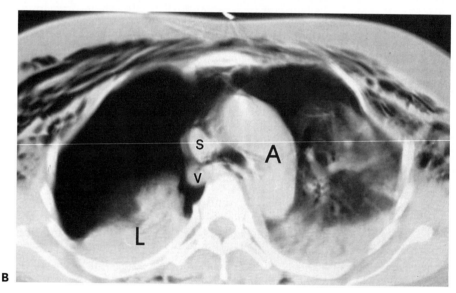

Figure 21-25 Traumatic rupture of the right main stem bronchus. **A, B:** Computed tomography images at the level of the aortic arch (A) demonstrate bilateral pneumothoraces, pneumomediastinum, and extensive subcutaneous emphysema. The collapsed right lung (L) has fallen away from the hilum toward the most dependent portion of the hemithorax. Patchy areas of parenchymal contusion are noted in the left lung. S, superior vena cava; V, azygous vein arch. (Case courtesy of Paul Barry, M.D., Greensboro, North Carolina.)

are caused by iatrogenic interventions such as endoscopy, tube placement, or esophageal dilatation (154).

Radiologic manifestations of esophageal rupture include pneumomediastinum, cervical emphysema, pneumothorax, pleural effusion, and an abnormal mediastinal contour resulting from hemorrhage or leakage of gastroesophageal contents into the mediastinum. Early recognition and prompt medical and surgical intervention is critical, as esophageal rupture may rapidly progress to fulminant mediastinitis and septic shock (486). If there is associated rupture of the mediastinal pleura, acute empyema may also develop (159). Occasionally, a tracheoesophageal fistula develops either from the initial trauma or as a sequela of the acute mediastinitis. In such cases, the fistula may protect against mediastinal abscess formation by providing a route of drainage for

esophageal contents (486). Contrast esophagography is over 90% sensitive in the diagnosis of esophageal rupture, and is the procedure of choice for establishing its presence and extent (27). Esophagoscopy has similar diagnostic sensitivity and may provide complementary diagnostic information in select cases (291).

CT scanning has been reported to be useful in suggesting the diagnosis of esophageal perforation in patients with atypical or confusing clinical signs and symptoms (12,467). CT findings indicative of esophageal perforation include esophageal thickening, periesophageal fluid, extraluminal air, and pleural effusion (Fig. 21-26). Identification of extraesophageal air is the most useful finding and is demonstrated on CT with greater sensitivity than on plain chest radiographs (467). In some cases, leakage of oral contrast material from the disrupted esophagus into the mediastinum or pleural space may be seen (295). CT is also useful for defining extraluminal manifestations of esophageal rupture, such as mediastinitis, mediastinal abscess, and empyema (467). Such information often has important implications for medical and/or surgical management.

Diaphragm

Diaphragmatic rupture occurs in approximately 5% of patients who have experienced major blunt trauma (277), and 65% to 85% of diaphragmatic ruptures are on the left side (215,277,305,363,469). Left-sided injury predominates because of the protective effect of the liver on the right hemidiaphragm and/or underdiagnosis of right-sided injuries (104,177). Proposed mechanisms of injury in blunt diaphragmatic rupture include shearing of a stretched membrane, avulsion of the diaphragm from its points of attachment, and abrupt increase in transdiaphragmatic pressure following severe compression of the upper abdomen and lower thorax (215). Injury can also result from direct laceration of the diaphragm by fractures of the lower thoracic ribs. The diaphragm most frequently ruptures in the area of the central tendon or at its transition to the muscular portion of the diaphragm. The posterior and posterolateral diaphragmatic segments are most commonly involved (383,425). With laceration of the left hemidiaphragm, the omentum, stomach, spleen, and small and large bowel can herniate into the thorax. With tears of the right hemidiaphragm, the liver is usually the offending organ.

Diaphragmatic rupture is often unrecognized at the time of trauma because of lack of early herniation of abdominal organs into the thorax and because the diaphragmatic injury is often obscured or overshadowed by other associated injuries. Diaphragmatic rupture rarely occurs in isolation, and a high percentage of patients sustain serious concomitant intraabdominal (59%) or intrathoracic (45%) injuries (305). In the absence of characteristic clinical signs and radiologic findings at the time of injury, the correct initial diagnosis may be made in less than 50% of cases. The diagnosis is most readily made when the injury is recent and the tear is large and left sided with herniation of hollow abdominal organs. If the trauma is remote or unknown and the tear is right sided with herniation of solid organs such as the liver, the diagnosis is less likely to be made (13). Not uncommonly, recognition of diaphragmatic tears may be delayed for hours to years, allowing time for progressive herniation of abdominal contents into the thorax. Such tears may only be discovered when the patient presents with complications of posttraumatic herniation, such as intestinal obstruction, visceral strangulation, and respiratory impairment (71,76, 155,171). Delayed presentation of diaphragmatic rupture with visceral herniation and strangulation is associated with higher morbidity and mortality (30%) than when the diagnosis is made and managed acutely (71,425).

The diagnosis of diaphragmatic rupture is usually suggested on the basis of abnormalities on chest radiography or is made incidentally at the time of an exploratory laparotomy (160). Diagnostic or strongly suggestive radiographic findings include the presence of air-filled viscera (i.e., stomach, bowel) and the tip of a nasogastric tube above the diaphragm. The nasogastric tube may be seen to extend inferiorly below the normal gastroesophageal junction and then form an upward curve into herniated gastric fundus within the left hemithorax (340). Other abnormalities suggestive but not diagnostic of diaphragmatic injury are more commonly seen and include an indistinct or elevated hemidiaphragm, an irregular or lumpy diaphragm contour, a persistent basilar opacity that resembles atelectasis or a supradiaphragmatic mass, an unexplained pleural effusion, and fractures of the lower ribs (8,143,282). The nonspecificity of these findings results in the chest radiograph being inconclusive for diaphragmatic injury in most cases. Diaphragmatic rupture

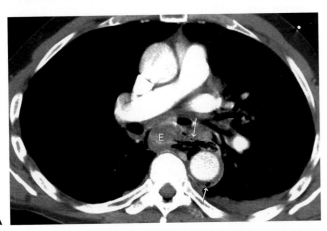
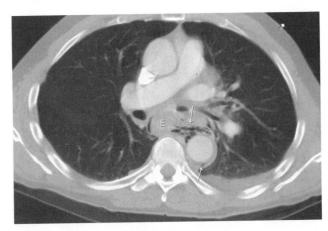

A   **B**

Figure 21-26 Esophageal rupture. **A:** Computed tomography image on soft tissue window demonstrates a fluid-filled esophagus (E) and periesophageal mediastinal air (*arrows*) tracking into the left pleural space. A small left pleural effusion is also present. **B:** Same image as (**A**) on lung window setting.

with herniation of abdominal contents can be mimicked or masked by concurrent pulmonary abnormalities such as multiple traumatic lung cysts, lower lobe contusion and/or atelectasis, pleural effusion, loculated hemopneumothorax, phrenic nerve paresis, and total or partial eventration of the hemidiaphragm (143,295).

CT has been used to diagnose diaphragmatic rupture in patients with nonspecific or equivocal chest radiographs. On transverse CT images, the diaphragm appears as a thin, curvilinear structure of soft tissue density outlined centrally by subdiaphragmatic fat and peripherally by lung. The posterolateral portions of the diaphragm are usually best demonstrated, and tears at those sites are readily detected. Tears involving the dome of the diaphragm or portions of the diaphragm in contact with structures of similar density, such as the liver, spleen, and stomach, are more difficult to detect, unless there is associated herniation of abdominal contents (173). CT has been reported to have 61% to 71% sensitivity and 87% to 100% specificity in the diagnosis of acute traumatic diaphragmatic rupture (219,310)

CT findings of diaphragmatic rupture include abrupt discontinuity of the diaphragm, herniation of abdominal viscera or fat into the thorax, and focal waist-like constriction of the stomach or bowel at the site of herniation (CT "collar sign") (Fig. 21-27) (219,310,391,487). A large gap between the torn ends of the diaphragm may be seen, giving rise to the "absent diaphragm sign" (454). A diagnosis of herniation is indicated by the presence of abdominal viscera and/or fat posterolateral (i.e., peripheral) to the diaphragm and thus within the thoracic cavity. On occasion, CT can demonstrate diaphragmatic disruption before visceral herniation, leading to early surgical intervention and averting the potentially life-threatening complications of an undiagnosed herniation (179). Other CT findings of diaphragmatic rupture include thickening of the diaphragm as a result of edema or hematoma (244) and herniated abdominal viscera layering dependently in the thorax against the posterior ribs ("dependent viscera" sign) (Fig. 21-28) (22). One series reported that a positive "dependent viscera" sign in which the upper one third of the liver abutted the posterior right ribs or the bowel or stomach lay in contact with the posterior left ribs was identified in 100% of patients with left-sided diaphragmatic rupture and 83% of patients with right-sided diaphragmatic rupture (22).

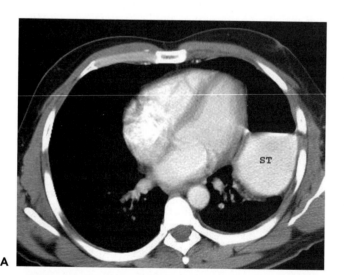

A

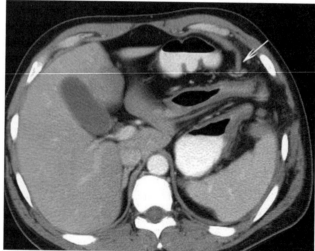

B

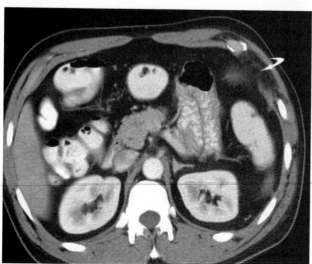

C

Figure 21-27 Diaphragmatic rupture. **A:** Computed tomography (CT) image at the level of the heart demonstrates an air–contrast level within stomach (ST), which is herniated into the thorax. **B, C:** CT images more caudally demonstrate thickened, disrupted left hemidiaphragm (*straight arrow*) with herniated intraabdominal fat (*curved arrow*) located lateral to the diaphragm. (Case courtesy of Kevin Smith, MD, Birmingham, Alabama.)

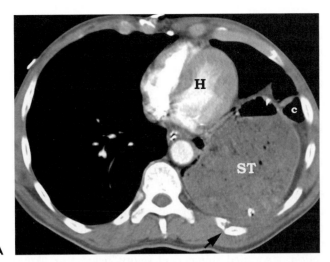

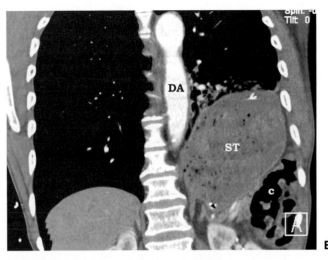

A   B

Figure 21-28   Diaphragmatic rupture. **A:** Computed tomography image at the level of the heart (H) reveals a debris-filled stomach (ST) laying dependently in the left hemithorax against the posterior ribs (dependent viscera sign). Note associated rib fracture (*arrow*). c, colon. **B:** Coronal reconstruction at the level of the descending aorta (DA) demonstrates stomach (ST) and colon (c) within the left hemithorax.

In patients with suboptimal diaphragmatic visualization or equivocal findings of diaphragmatic rupture, use of thin-section helical CT (e.g., 3 to 5 mm) with overlapping reconstructed images obtained at 2- or 3-mm intervals for generation of sagittal and coronal reformations may help improve diagnostic accuracy (Fig. 21-29) (391). In a retrospective study to determine the sensitivity and specificity of helical CT in diagnosing blunt diaphragmatic injury, reformatted sagittal and coronal images helped detect subtle right-sided visceral herniation and to delineate the outline of the diaphragm in 17 patients with suspicious chest radiographic findings but an intact diaphragm (391). Targeted helical CT of the diaphragm with sagittal and coronal reformatted images has also been shown to increase the sensitivity of CT in the detec-

tion of diaphragmatic injury from 73% to 92% in a prospective controlled animal model (199). It is possible that use of MDCT scanners with 1- to 3-mm collimation and rapid multiplanar reformatting will further improve the diagnosis of blunt diaphragmatic rupture, especially for small defects (312).

In a small number of stable trauma patients, direct coronal and sagittal MRI has also been performed to demonstrate traumatic diaphragmatic rupture (29,288,396). On T1-weighted and gradient-echo MR sequences, the normal diaphragm is seen as a continuous hypointense band, outlined by high-signal-intensity fat on the left and the liver on the right. Injuries to the diaphragm appear on MRI as an abrupt defect in the low-signal-intensity diaphragm. Intrathoracic herniation of abdominal fat and/or viscera

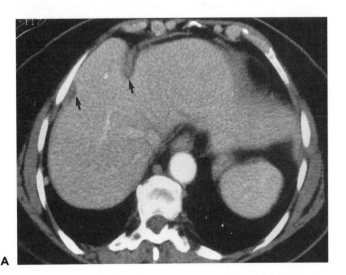

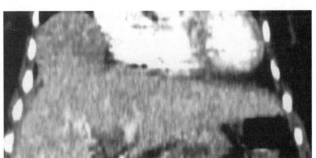

A   B

Figure 21-29   Diaphragmatic rupture. **A:** A 5-mm helical computed tomography section demonstrates herniation of a portion of the right lobe of the liver through the diaphragmatic defect (*arrows*). A small, incidental pulmonary nodule is noted in the right posterolateral lung base. **B:** Coronal reformation demonstrates herniated liver in the right lower chest.

through the diaphragm rupture can also be accurately demonstrated by MRI (197,396).

BLUNT ABDOMINAL TRAUMA

Approximately 10% of all trauma deaths are a result of abdominal injuries (318,478). Trauma most often results from traffic accidents, with falls (mainly on the work site), recreational accidents, and violence accounting for the other causes (475). Two different mechanisms may cause injury with blunt abdominal trauma: compression forces and deceleration forces. Compressive forces result from blows or external compression against a fixed object, such as the spine. These forces can cause lacerations and subcapsular hematomas of solid parenchymal organs such as the spleen and liver, or they can deform and increase the intraluminal pressure in hollow organs such as the bowel, resulting in rupture. Deceleration injuries cause stretching and linear shearing forces between fixed and more freely movable objects, resulting in injuries to structures such as the renal arteries and mesenteric blood vessels (318,466). The patient's chance for survival increases the earlier trauma care is instituted after the injury; thus, the common goal of management of patients with blunt abdominal trauma is the rapid identification of life-threatening lesions and their causes, and the prompt initiation of appropriate treatment (241,466).

CT has become increasingly valuable and is extensively used in the early clinical management of blunt abdominal trauma (249,448). CT has proved to be a highly sensitive and specific method for the detection of abdominal injury, and is the method of choice for the initial evaluation of patients with hemodynamically stable and unstable trauma (92,342,344,478). The accuracy of CT in the diagnosis of blunt abdominal trauma has been reported to be as high as 97% (92,319). Abdominal CT can also help evaluate coexisting extra-abdominal injuries, such as pneumothorax, as well as pelvic and spinal fractures that may be clinically unsuspected (474). The more recent development of MDCT technology has further enhanced the role of CT in the evaluation of blunt abdominal trauma. As in thoracic trauma, the advantages of MDCT in the context of abdominal trauma include not only increased speed of image acquisition and overall improved resolution but also the ability to obtain multiplanar reconstructions and immediate online interpretation of images at the workstation (344). MDCT allows for complete scanning in a single breath-hold, and faster scanning speeds and narrow collimation increase contrast opacification in the mesenteric, retroperitoneal, and portal vessels, as well as in parenchymal organs. This improves identification of organ injury and, additionally, sites of active arterial bleeding. Breath holding may not be possible in trauma CT, and the speed of multislice scanning further reduces breathing artifact (318,466,470).

The use of CT in the initial and follow-up evaluations of trauma victims has played a pivotal role in decreasing the rates of unnecessary exploratory laparotomies and increasing conservative nonoperative management of abdominal injuries (9,59,355,379).

INDICATIONS

In the past, the major indication for CT examination of abdominal trauma was in patients with suspected abdominal injuries who were sufficiently hemodynamically stable for transportation from the trauma suite to the CT scanner (318,342,466). Additional indications included an equivocal physical examination, associated head injury or intoxication, associated spinal cord injury, hematoma with a significant mechanism of injury, decreasing hematocrit, elevated amylase, or associated pelvic fracture (113,338). Recently, CT has been increasingly used in patients with suspected active internal bleeding, and is now a recognized method for evaluation and decision making in patients with hemodynamically unstable trauma, provided that it is available without delay and that life-support measures are not interrupted during examination (342).

Before the widespread use of CT, diagnostic peritoneal lavage (DPL) was the gold standard for the detection of hemoperitoneum (266). More recently, DPL has been reserved for hemodynamically unstable patients who may require immediate surgery (478). While DPL is very sensitive for detecting hemorrhage, is quick and simple to perform, and does not require sophisticated equipment, it has several important limitations. It cannot differentiate inconsequential from significant bleeding, which may result in unnecessary laparotomies. DPL does not provide information on location or extent of injuries and it often fails to detect bleeding in the retroperitoneum. It is an invasive procedure, and traumatic cannula insertion can result in false–positive examinations (113,153,478). Futhermore, retained lavage fluid may simulate intraperitoneal blood on subsequent CT examination.

The advantages of CT over DPL include its high sensitivity and specificity for visceral lacerations, its noninvasive nature, the capability to localize the source of hemoperitoneum, and the ability to assess both intraperitoneal and retroperitoneal injuries (113). DPL has fallen into disfavor with many trauma surgeons because abdominal injuries that can be managed nonoperatively following CT examination would require operative intervention based on currently accepted guidelines for DPL (153).

CT examination of the abdomen for trauma has largely replaced other imaging techniques, such as radionuclide scintigraphy, angiography, and ultrasound (US) (153). The bedside four-quadrant abdominal US examination for trauma has been referred to as focused abdominal sonogram for trauma (FAST) (280,318). FAST is a noninvasive method for the identification of blunt abdominal trauma and is similar to DPL in that its purpose is to identify hemoperitoneum (153,280). Many trauma centers have incorporated the use of FAST for the evaluation of blunt abdominal trauma (3,280,466). It was originally suggested that the routine use of FAST could result in a reduction in the number of abdominal CT scans, and therefore a reduction in the cost of treatment of blunt abdominal trauma (368). However, as with DPL, FAST does not identify the source of the bleeding, evaluate the retroperitoneum, or detect hollow organ injuries or occult fractures. FAST also has the disadvantage of being operator dependent, and the quality of the examination can be affected by obesity, ileus, and subcutaneous emphysema. Furthermore, the absence of hemoperitoneum does not exclude the presence of organ injuries. Because of these limitations, CT is felt to be superior to US as the initial screening examination for blunt abdominal trauma (280,466).

TECHNIQUE

Proper patient preparation and scanning technique is critical for accurate abdominal CT examination in patients with blunt abdominal trauma. Extraneous objects such as ECG leads, IV lines, and other monitoring or support apparatus should be repositioned out of the scanning field whenever possible because the streak artifacts they produce degrade image quality and may simulate or obscure traumatic lesions (113). The patient's arms should be placed over the chest or above the head. If this cannot be done, then the arms should be positioned next to the trunk because allowing an air gap to remain between the arm and the body causes worse artifact than securing the limb against the abdomen (140). If the arms must remain over the abdomen, a larger scanning field of view may be used to decrease artifact (114). Restraints or sedation may be necessary to avoid motion artifacts in patients unable to maintain proper position.

The routine use of oral contrast material in CT examination of abdominal trauma is controversial. In some trauma centers, dilute (1% to 2%), water-soluble contrast material is administered orally or via a nasogastric tube prior to CT scanning, while in others, it is not a part of the trauma protocol. Oral contrast material can aid in the identification of bowel loops, delineation of the mesentery, and differentiation of bowel from hematoma, hemorrhage, and pancreatic injury. Disadvantages of oral contrast material include risk of aspiration, vomiting, and additional time requirements for its dispersal, which may delay diagnosis and treatment of injuries. Several recent studies suggest that oral contrast material is unnecessary, as no diagnoses were missed in its absence (84,402,420). As time is one of the most important factors in the early management of trauma victims, many of whom have injuries involving multiple organ systems, the delay needed for the dispersal of oral contrast material may not be justified, especially if there is no significant added benefit.

Posttraumatic abdominal CT examinations should be performed using IV contrast material, unless contraindicated by known major contrast allergy or severe renal insufficiency. IV infusion of contrast material maximizes the difference between contrast-enhancing parenchyma and nonenhancing hematomas and lacerations (113). It also aids in detection of extravasation of contrast-opacified urine (113) and in visualization of sites of active arterial hemorrhage (202,395). IV contrast material is best administered with an automated power injector via a large-bore peripheral venous line or central venous catheter. A total of approximately 120 to 180 mL of 60% contrast material can be given IV at a rate of 2 to 4 mL per second (318,403,470). Scanning is usually initiated 70 to 90 seconds after the start of contrast infusion (403,466). The timing of the scan after the contrast injection is important, since early scanning can produce artifacts that may simulate injury, especially in the spleen and kidneys, and late scanning can decrease sensitivity to injuries that may be present. With the increasing use of MDCT and faster acquisitions, the timing of contrast material delivery becomes even more critical. In general, shorter acquisition times may reduce the total amount of contrast material needed, but at the same time may require higher injection rates (129).

Scanning should span from the dome of the diaphragm to the inferior aspect of the ischium. With SDCT, scanning is generally performed with 5- to 8-mm-thick sections and a pitch of 1 to 2. Technical factors with MDCT vary with the number of detectors. In MDCT, the thickness of the x-ray beam is determined by the detector row collimation, as opposed to the x-ray beam collimation, so the definition of pitch is extended. For example, a 4-slice CT scan using 5-mm row collimation (and therefore 20-mm x-ray beam collimation) and a 15-mm table translating distance per rotation will result in a helical pitch of 3 (i.e., 15/5) rather than 0.75 (i.e., 15/20) (190). MDCT offers unparalleled speed of acquisition, spatial resolution, and anatomic coverage. However, it also brings with it the challenge of assessing a significant increase in number of rapidly generated, reconstructed cross sections. Additional techniques available on clinical workstations include multiplanar reformation, maximum intensity projection, shaded surface display, and volume rendering (371).

Patients should be closely monitored throughout the examination, and adequate equipment and personnel for emergency resuscitation should be readily available (475,478). Ideally, the CT scanning area should be located as near as possible to the trauma room to allow rapid transport to and from the scanner. Whether viewed on film or on the console video monitor, all images should be reviewed with multiple window settings (lung, bone, and standard soft tissue) to detect not only organ injury but also pneumothorax, pneumoperitoneum, and bone injury (403).

HEMOPERITONEUM

Hemoperitoneum is a common result of blunt abdominal trauma, and its identification on CT should prompt a thorough search for injury to visceral organs (19,325,403, 466,478). At times, small quantities of hemoperitoneum may be the only sign of subtle or occult visceral injury, particularly those involving the bowel or mesentery. CT is highly sensitive and specific for diagnosing hemoperitoneum (121), which initially tends to collect near the source of bleeding and then spills over into more dependent portions of the peritoneal cavity. Morison's pouch (also known as the hepatorenal fossa or posterior subhepatic space), the most dependent peritoneal recess in the upper abdomen, is the most common site of blood collection seen on CT in upper abdominal trauma (Fig. 21-30) (113). Other common sites of blood accumulation include the perihepatic (right subphrenic) and perisplenic (left subphrenic) spaces, the paracolic gutters (peritoneal recesses lateral to the ascending and descending colon) (Fig. 21-31), and the pelvis, particularly adjacent to the urinary bladder. Blood from any intraabdominal source typically flows down along the root of the mesentery and the right paracolic gutter into the pelvis (278). With extensive hemorrhage, large collections of blood may fill the pelvis, even when relatively little blood is seen in the paracolic gutters or other upper abdominal sites (121) (Fig. 21-32); this is because the pelvis is the most dependent portion of the peritoneal cavity and contains up to one third of its volume. It is important, therefore, that the entire pelvis be scanned in patients following blunt abdominal trauma to accurately assess the presence and extent of hemoperitoneum (113).

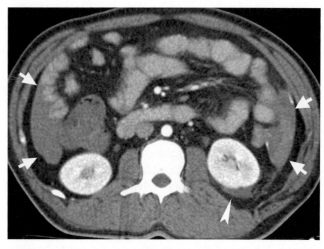

Figure 21-31 Hemoperitoneum. Computed tomography image demonstrates blood tracking along both paracolic gutters (*arrows*) in this patient following blunt abdominal trauma. A small left perinephric hematoma (*arrowhead*) is also present.

The CT appearance of blood in the peritoneal cavity is variable and depends on the location, age, and physical state (clotted versus lysed) of extravasated blood. Immediately after hemorrhage, intraperitoneal blood has the same attenuation as circulating blood, but within hours, its attenuation increases as hemoglobin is concentrated during clot formation (315,317). Clotted blood usually measures between 50 and 75 HU attenuation, whereas lysed blood flowing freely within the peritoneal cavity has attenuation values generally ranging from 30 to 45 HU. Densely clotted blood may have attenuation values of greater than 100 HU (114). Clots within the peritoneal cavity tend to lyse rapidly because of repetitive respiratory motion and adjacent bowel peristalsis, whereas clots within solid viscera, such as the liver, remain intact for longer periods (121). In most cases, the attenuation value of blood begins to decrease within several days as

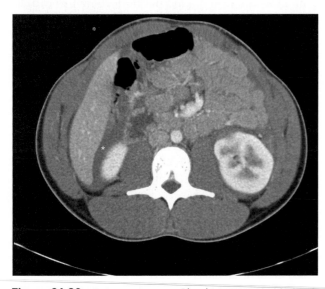

Figure 21-30 Hemoperitoneum. Blood is present in Morison's pouch (*asterisk*), the most dependent peritoneal recess in the upper abdomen. Note that the acute hemoperitoneum appears relatively low in attenuation compared with the attenuation of enhanced liver and renal parenchyma.

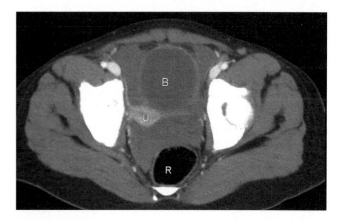

Figure 21-32 Hemoperitoneum secondary to splenic laceration. Computed tomography (CT) image through the lower pelvis demonstrates a large amount of blood pooling in the pelvis. If CT sections through the pelvis had not been obtained, the extent of hemoperitoneum would have been grossly underestimated. U, uterus; R, rectum; B, urinary bladder.

clot lysis takes place. The attenuation value continues to decrease steadily with time and often approaches that of water (0 to 20 HU) after 2 to 3 weeks (229).

Recent intraperitoneal hemorrhage can exhibit a variety of morphologic features. The fluid collection may be homogeneously hyperdense or it may be inhomogeneous, with linear or nodular areas of high attenuation intermixed with lower attenuation fluid. The inhomogeneity may result from irregular clot resorption or intermittent bleeding, leading to repeated episodes of clot formation and retraction (481). Occasionally, fresh blood within a hematoma or confined within a peritoneal space may demonstrate a hematocrit effect, with layering of serous fluid on dependent, sedimented erythrocytes and clot (121) (Fig. 21-33). More frequently, a localized collection of high-attenuation clotted blood, referred to as the sentinel clot, is seen in close proximity to a site of visceral injury (325) (Fig. 21-34). The sentinel clot is a sensitive sign of visceral injury, and it may be the only sign indicating the source of peritoneal hemorrhage in a significant percentage of cases. When present, it should prompt careful examination of the adjacent viscera for subtle or occult injury. In some patients, especially those with small capsular lacerations, the localized perivisceral hematoma may be more evident than the underlying intraparenchymal hematoma or laceration (121). As such, the sentinel clot sign has been noted to be particularly useful in the diagnosis of subtle bowel, mesenteric, and splenic injuries (140,325).

It must be remembered that the presence of hemoperitoneum on CT does not necessarily indicate that active hemorrhage is present. Rather, the quantity of hemoperitoneum on a single CT study merely reflects the amount of blood lost since the time of injury. Serial CT evaluation of hemoperitoneum may be useful in documenting resolution or in detecting new hemorrhage (131). Hemoperitoneum should resolve significantly in most cases by 1 week after injury. Persistence of hemoperitoneum without change for 3 to 7 days after injury suggests continued intraperitoneal bleeding, even though the patient may remain hemodynamically stable (131).

Active arterial hemorrhage can be identified on contrast-enhanced CT as focal or diffuse high-attenuation areas of extravasated contrast-enhanced blood (Fig. 21-35) (202,395). The areas of extravasation range in attenuation from 80 to 370 HU (higher attenuation than free or clotted blood) and typically are isodense or hyperdense to the abdominal aorta and adjacent major arteries. The areas of extravasation are often surrounded by a large hematoma that is lower in attenuation than the extravasated contrast material. With the increasing use of MDCT, detection of active bleeding sites in patients with blunt abdominal trauma is becoming increasingly more common. The faster data acquisition and higher spatial resolution afforded by MDCT enable visualization of active hemorrhage as a focal jet of extravasated contrast material, or as a focal or diffuse collection of high-attenuation extravasated contrast material surrounded by low-attenuation hematoma. In patients with significant blood loss resulting in hypovolemia, several CT signs may be seen. These include a small, constricted aorta (399), a flattened or collapsed inferior vena cava (203), and abnormally intense contrast enhancement of the bowel wall and kidneys (411).

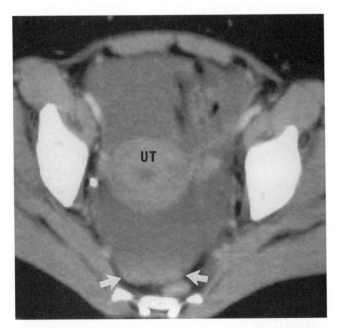

Figure 21-33 Hemoperitoneum with hematocrit effect. Computed tomography scan through the lower pelvis demonstrates a large amount of blood filling the pelvis. Note hematocrit effect with blood elements layering dependently (*arrows*). UT, uterus.

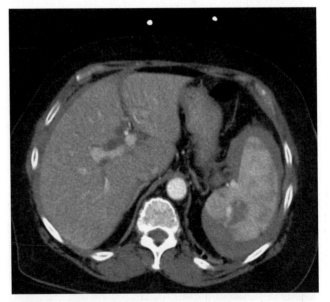

Figure 21-34 Splenic lacerations with hemoperitoneum and sentinel clot. Contrast-enhanced computed tomography image demonstrates multiple splenic lacerations and high-attenuation clotted perisplenic blood, or so-called sentinel clot. Lower-attenuation lysed blood is also present in the perihepatic space.

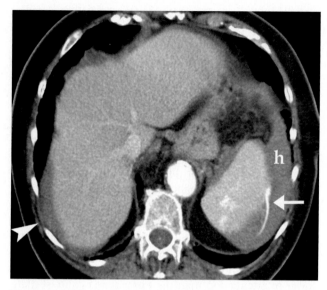

Figure 21-35 Active arterial hemorrhage. Contrast-enhanced multidetector computed tomography image demonstrates a linear focus of extravasated contrast-enhanced blood (*arrow*) originating from the spleen. This focus of active hemorrhage is surrounded by a large perisplenic hematoma (h) that is lower in attenuation than the extravasated contrast-enhanced blood. Perihepatic blood (*arrowhead*) is also evident.

SPECIFIC TRAUMA SITES

Spleen

In blunt abdominal trauma, the spleen is the most frequently affected organ, accounting for approximately 40% of abdominal organ injuries (19,318,344,403,466,478). Traumatic injuries to the spleen must always be considered in patients who have suffered blows to the left lower chest or left upper abdomen, whether from motor vehicle accidents, sports accidents, falls, or nonaccidental trauma. The presence of left lower rib fractures is highly suggestive of the simultaneous presence of splenic injury (19,403,466).

Contrast-enhanced CT is the modality of choice for evaluation of splenic trauma and has been reported to be up to 98% sensitive for detecting blunt splenic injury (318,344,403). Following rapid IV injection of contrast material, the spleen may initially exhibit a heterogeneous pattern of parenchymal opacification, reflecting variable blood flow within different compartments of the spleen (145) (Fig. 21-36). Care must be taken not to misinterpret this early postinjection heterogeneity as representing splenic injury. In questionable cases, repeat scans should be obtained following equilibration of the contrast material. In normal cases, the splenic parenchyma achieves a uniform, homogeneous appearance with no surrounding hemorrhage.

Injury to the spleen can take the form of laceration, intrasplenic hematoma, subcapsular hematoma, or infarction (344,466). Splenic laceration typically appears as an irregular linear area of hypodensity on contrast-enhanced CT (Fig. 21-37). Intrasplenic hematoma appears as a broader area of hypodense, nonperfused splenic parenchyma (Fig. 21-38). The intraparenchymal hematoma may be homogeneous or inhomogeneous, and may contain a higher attenuation clot (19,318,403,478). Subcapsular hematomas appear as crescentic or oval collections of fluid that flatten or indent the underlying splenic parenchyma (113,318, 478) (Fig. 21-39). Splenic infarcts may occur following injury to the splenic vasculature and appear as wedge-shaped areas of nonperfusion that extend to the splenic capsule. Unenhancing portions of the spleen should suggest injury or thrombosis of the artery of the affected segment (478), although perfusion defects may also be a result of contusion or may correspond to reversible local reactive hypoperfusion secondary to hypotension (19). In cases of severe trauma, the spleen may be shattered into multiple small fragments. Multiple lacerations

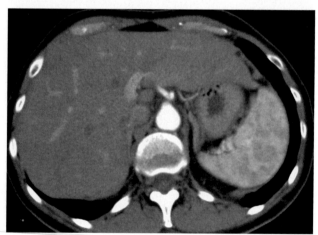

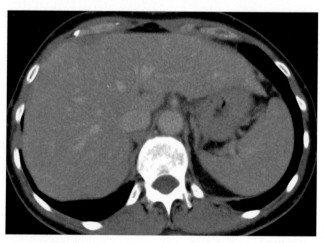

A   B

Figure 21-36 Heterogeneous early splenic enhancement. **A:** Early arterial phase contrast-enhanced computed tomography image demonstrates heterogeneous enhancement of the splenic parenchyma that could be mistaken for splenic injury. Note the absence of perisplenic hematoma. **B:** Delayed scan during equilibrium phase demonstrates homogeneous splenic parenchyma without evidence of splenic injury.

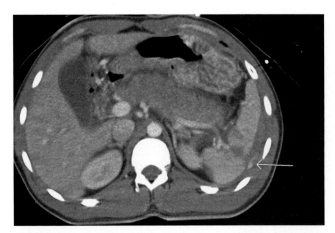

Figure 21-37 Splenic laceration. Contrast-enhanced computed tomography scan demonstrates irregular, low-attenuation splenic laceration extending to the splenic hilum. There is a small amount of perisplenic blood and an active extravasation site (*arrow*).

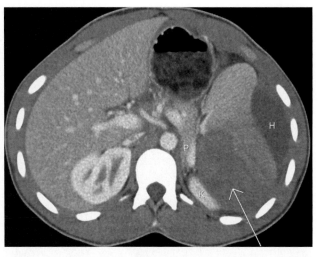

Figure 21-39 Subcapsular splenic hematoma. Contrast-enhanced computed tomography image demonstrates a lenticular-shaped subcapsular hematoma (H) that indents the underlying splenic parenchyma. A higher attenuation perisplenic hematoma (*arrow*) is seen posteriorly. P, pancreatic tail; K, left kidney.

connecting opposed visceral surfaces defines a shattered spleen (318,403,466,478).

Streak artifact from nasogastric tubes or ECG leads may mimic splenic laceration, and ideally these objects should be repositioned or removed prior to scanning. Beam-hardening artifact from ribs and streak artifact from an air–contrast interface in the stomach may also simulate splenic injury. Such artifacts generally are better defined and more regular in appearance than true lacerations, and often extend beyond the margin of the spleen. Splenic clefts, most commonly located in the superomedial aspect of the spleen, can mimic laceration but typically are more smoothly contoured in appearance (Fig. 21-40). The absence of associated perisplenic blood is also helpful in distinguishing clefts from true lacerations (113). Enhancing atelectatic lung, as well as a prominent left lobe of the liver draping around the spleen, may on occasion simulate splenic injury and perisplenic hematoma (55).

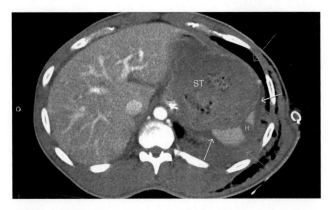

Figure 21-38 Splenic hematoma and hemoperitoneum. Contrast-enhanced computed tomography scan demonstrates a broad area of hypodense, nonperfused splenic parenchyma representing intrasplenic hematoma (H). Lower attenuation perisplenic blood (*thick arrows*) is present. The patient also has a left hemopneumothorax (*thin arrows*) and subcutaneous emphysema. ST, stomach.

Hemoperitoneum is present in nearly all patients with clinically important splenic injury. In cases in which there is significant intraabdominal fluid, the presence of local perisplenic clot, the so-called sentinel clot, suggests splenic injury as the site of bleeding (Figs. 21-34, 21-38, and 21-41) (325). Such a clot usually appears denser and more heterogeneous than the remainder of the intraabdominal blood (120). The sentinel clot is a valuable adjunct in the CT evaluation of splenic trauma, being both sensitive and specific for identification of the injured organ. While CT demonstrates the parenchymal injury itself in a large percentage of cases, there are a significant number of cases in which perisplenic clot is the principal finding indicating the spleen as the source of the hemoperitoneum. In a smaller percentage of cases, the sentinel clot may be the only clue to the source of the hemorrhage (120,325).

Active bleeding can be identified on contrast-enhanced CT as intra- or extrasplenic areas of bright vascular enhancement with an attenuation similar to or greater than that of the aorta or an adjacent major artery (Fig. 21-35 and 21-42). The appearance may vary with the rate of hemorrhage and the CT technique used. With the introduction of faster MDCT protocols, earlier data acquisition may allow smaller amounts of active hemorrhage to be detected before the high-density contrast material is diluted by surrounding hematoma, especially in a perisplenic location (246,325).

Pseudoaneurysm formation can occur following trauma and appears as a focal well-circumscribed area of vascular enhancement within the splenic parenchyma that is larger than the normal vessels (Fig. 21-43). Surrounding hematoma is frequently noted (139,178). The CT attenuation of a pseudoaneurysm may be affected by several mechanisms. Higher rates of IV contrast material injection will raise con-

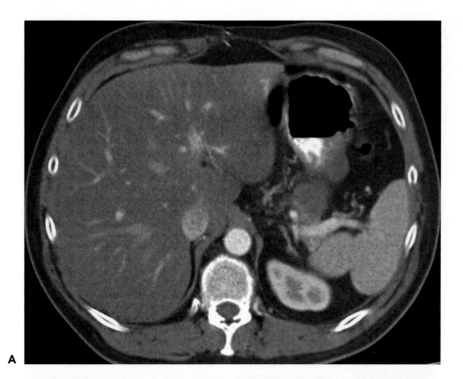

A

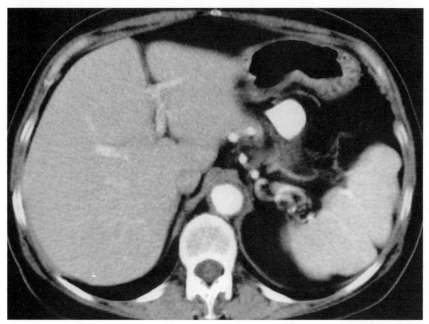

B

Figure 21-40 Congenital splenic clefts. A: Computed tomography image demonstrates a sharply marginated cleft in the posterior tip of the spleen. The smooth, rounded contour of the cleft as it meets the margin of the spleen, as well as the absence of perisplenic hematoma, is helpful in distinguishing a congenital cleft from a parenchymal laceration. B: Another patient with multiple splenic clefts along the lateral margin of the spleen.

trast media levels and therefore the attenuation of the abnormality. Poor cardiac output, vasodilatation, and hypotension may decrease perfusion, resulting in decreased attenuation of the pseudoaneurysm (246).

CT findings that indicate ongoing hemorrhage and the possible need for more immediate angiographic intervention or surgery include active contrast material extravasation, seen as a focal jet or "contrast blush," a pseudoaneurysm, or an arteriovenous fistula (325,470). Although some posttraumatic vascular lesions, particularly those of small size, may thrombose spontaneously, many trauma sur-

geons feel that the presence of a contrast blush or a pseudoaneurysm should automatically prompt either operative or angiographic intervention. Identification of a contrast blush on contrast-enhanced CT may be predictive of failure of nonoperative conservative management. At the least, close medical observation is required should intervention be deferred (92,118,139,324,385,394).

Major changes have occurred in the past two to three decades in the treatment of traumatic injuries to the spleen, with a continuing trend away from immediate splenectomy and toward conservative therapy (374,452). Splenectomy

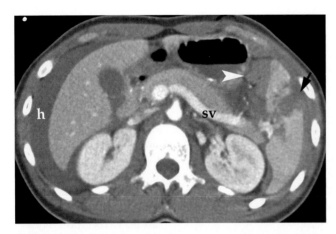

Figure 21-41 Splenic fracture with hemoperitoneum and perisplenic sentinel clot. Computed tomography image at the level of the splenic vein (SV) demonstrates an irregular splenic fracture (*arrow*) and adjacent high-attenuation sentinel clot (*arrowhead*). Note lower attenuation lysed blood (h) around the liver.

can permanently increase susceptibility to infections, the most devastating of which is overwhelming postsplenectomy sepsis, a rare complication characterized by fulminant and often fatal bacterial infection (355,374,427, 434,452).

Attempts have been made by several investigators to grade the CT appearance of splenic injuries to identify those patients who can be treated successfully nonoperatively. The desirability of such a predictive grading system is increased by the fact that early surgical intervention more often results in splenic salvage than does delayed operation (355,379, 450). Most CT grading systems assess the integrity of the splenic capsule, the size of hematoma, the length and number of lacerations, involvement of segmental or hilar vessels, and extent of parenchymal devascularization (41,118,301, 318,394). Two of the more well-known classification systems include those by Buntain et al. (Table 21-1) (41) and

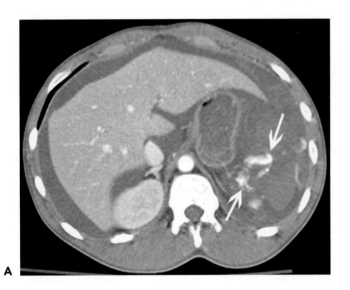

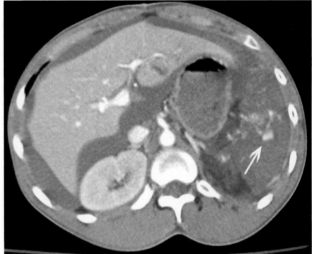

Figure 21-42 Partial transection of the splenic hilum with active bleeding and massive hemoperitoneum. **A, B:** Computed tomography (CT) scans through the upper pole of the right kidney demonstrate a large amount of hemoperitoneum, virtually absent perfusion of the splenic parenchyma, and active bleeding (*arrows*) from disrupted hilar vessels. **C:** CT scan through the lower margin of the spleen (S) shows some preservation of splenic enhancement consistent with partial hilar transection. A small laceration is noted in the left kidney. (Case courtesy of Christine O Menias, M.D., St. Louis, Missouri.)

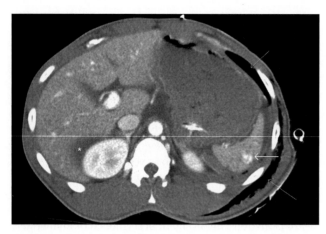

Figure 21-43 Splenic pseudoaneurysm (*thick arrow*) in a 22-year-old man involved in a motor vehicle accident. Blood is present in the perisplenic space and Morison's pouch (*asterisk*). *Thin arrows* point to a left pneumothorax and chest wall emphysema.

the American Association for the Surgery of Trauma (AAST) (Table 21-2) (394).

Early reports suggested that the use of these grading systems would be useful in predicting which patients would benefit from nonoperative management versus urgent surgical intervention, with the need for surgery indicated by the score of the given system. These systems have met with only variable success. Young patients under 20 years of age may do well with even severe degrees of injury, whereas patients over 55 years of age may require surgery for the lowest grades of injury (318,355,379,416). Several more recent studies have shown that while CT is highly accurate in delineating the extent of splenic injury, this determination cannot reli-

TABLE 21-2

AMERICAN ASSOCIATION FOR THE SURGERY OF TRAUMA SPLENIC INJURY SCALE (1994 REVISION)

Grade[a]	Type	Description of injury
I	Hematoma	Subcapsular, less than 10% surface area.
	Laceration	Capsular tear, less than 1 cm parenchymal depth.
II	Hematoma	Subcapsular, 10% to 50% surface area; intraparenchymal, less than 5 cm in diameter.
	Laceration	1 to 3 cm parenchymal depth; does not involve a trabecular vessel.
III	Hematoma	Subcapsular, greater than 50% surface area or expanding; ruptured subcapsular or parenchymal hematoma.
	Laceration	Greater than 3 cm parenchymal depth or involved trabecular vessels.
IV	Laceration	Laceration involving segmental or hilar vessels and producing major devascularization (greater than 25% of spleen).
V	Laceration	Completely shattered spleen.
	Vascular	Hilar vascular injury that devascularizes spleen

[a]Advance one grade for multiple injuries up to grade III.
From Shanmuganathan K, Mirvis SE, Boyd-Kranis R, et al. Nonsurgical management of blunt splenic injury: use of CT criteria to select patients for splenic arteriography and potential endovascular therapy. *Radiology* 2000;217:75–82, with permission.

TABLE 21-1

BUNTAIN CLASSIFICATION OF SPLENIC INJURY

Class I   Localized capsular disruption or subcapsular hematoma, without significant parenchymal injury.

Class II   Single or multiple capsular and parenchymal disruptions, transverse or longitudinal, that do not extend into the hilum or involve major vessels. Intraparenchymal hematoma may or may not coexist.

Class III   Deep fractures, single or multiple, transverse or longitudinal, extending into the hilum and involving major blood vessels.

Class IV   Completely shattered or fragmented spleen, or separated from its normal blood supply at the pedicle.

A. Without other intraabdominal injury.

B. With other associated intraabdominal injury.

B1. solid viscus

B2. hollow viscus

C. With associated extraabdominal injury.

Adapted from Buntain WL, Gould HR, Maull KI. Predictability of splenic salvage by computed tomography. *J Trauma* 1988;28:24–34.

ably predict the success or failure of nonsurgical management of blunt splenic trauma. Regardless of which parameters are used in the grading systems, a small, but significant, number of patients with low scores or even a negative CT experience nonsurgical failure or delayed splenic rupture. Clinical signs in these patients include falling hematocrit, sudden increase in pain, and hypotension. Furthermore, higher grades of splenic injury are not necessarily associated with an increased risk of nonoperative failure (228,297,450). Most recent investigators agree that, while CT is valuable for initial documentation, and sometimes for monitoring the progression, of splenic injuries, the decision for surgery should be based principally on hemodynamic variables, laboratory studies, and serial bedside clinical assessments (9,228,297,374,434,450).

Delayed splenic rupture is a rare but well-recognized and potentially dangerous clinical entity that has been reported in patients in whom the initial CT scan showed no evidence of splenic abnormality (333,450). No exact data exist regarding its true incidence. Delayed rupture may be secondary to splenic fracture in which there is little initial hemorrhage or in which poor contrast opacification of the spleen renders hematoma isodense with splenic parenchyma (333,450). Several mechanisms have been proposed, including delayed rupture of a subcapsular hematoma as a result of increased osmotic pressure developing in the course of clot lysis and free rupture of an initially confined perisplenic hematoma into the peritoneal cavity (19,478).

Splenic injuries may take several months to almost a year to fully resolve on follow-up CT examinations, depending on the grade of injury (21,348). Typically, intraperitoneal blood and perisplenic hematoma resolve in 1 to 3 weeks. Intrasplenic hematomas gradually decrease in density and become more sharply defined as the clots mature. They may go on to complete resolution, leaving only a slightly deformed splenic margin, or they may form a posttraumatic splenic pseudocyst (89,107). Infection may complicate hematoma resolution and produce a splenic abscess. Splenic lacerations usually resolve in a few weeks to a few months depending on their depth and severity. Splenic infarcts generally resolve over several months. Although it has been suggested by some authors that follow-up CT may be valuable in demonstrating healing, and hence allow earlier return to normal physical activity (116), others report that routine follow-up CT evaluation is not necessary or useful in clinically stable patients treated conservatively (21,116,238,449).

Liver

The liver is the second most frequently injured organ in blunt abdominal trauma, and the most common abdominal injury leading to death (113,318,403). Mortality tends to increase with increasing number and severity of associated extrahepatic injuries. As with splenic trauma, associated injury to other abdominal organs is a common occurrence.

Concomitant injuries to the head, chest, and extremities also are frequently present (114).

Traumatic liver injury most frequently involves the right hepatic lobe, particularly the posterior segment (131,422). This is because the right lobe constitutes most of the volume of the liver and because the posterior segment of the right lobe is readily accessible to blunt impact from the ribs and spine (392,403). Right-sided rib fractures have been reported in up to 33% of patients with injuries to the right lobe of the liver (392). Relative fixation of the liver to the undersurface of the diaphragm and to the posterior abdominal wall by the coronary ligaments may also contribute to the predilection for right lobe injury (392). Left hepatic lobe injuries are much less common than injuries to the right lobe and tend to occur with a forceful, direct blow to the epigastrium. Left lobe injuries have a much higher association with injuries to the pancreas, duodenum, and transverse colon (205).

CT is highly sensitive, specific, and accurate in defining and characterizing hepatic injury (19,318,344,392,403). The CT findings of hepatic injury are similar to those seen in the spleen and include laceration or fracture through the hepatic parenchyma, intraparenchymal hematoma, and subcapsular hematoma. Lacerations are the most common injury and appear as irregular linear, branching, or rounded areas of low attenuation within the normally enhancing liver parenchyma (113,392) (Fig. 21-44). High-attenuation foci of freshly clotted blood may be seen in the areas of laceration (Fig. 21-45). Lacerations commonly parallel the hepatic or portal venous vasculature and often extend to the periphery of the liver. Lacerations that extend through the liver capsule are usually associated with hemoperitoneum (113,318). Parallel, linear lacerations on the surface of the liver or radiating out from the hilar region may assume a configuration that has been termed the

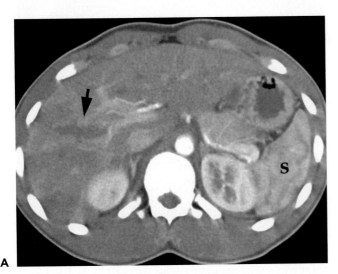

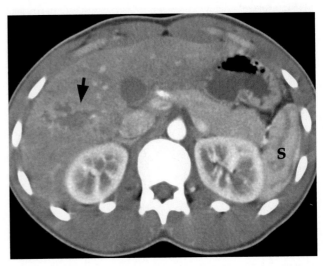

A   B

Figure 21-44 Hepatic laceration. **A, B:** Computed tomography images demonstrate an irregular, low-attenuation laceration (*arrow*) in the right hepatic lobe. Note heterogeneous early arterial phase contrast enhancement of the spleen (S).

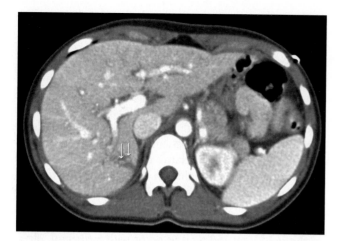

Figure 21-45   Hepatic laceration. Note irregular, low-attenuation laceration in the posterior right lobe of the liver. High-attenuation foci of clotted blood *(arrows)* are seen within the area of laceration.

two visceral surfaces, may result in fragmentation of the liver, producing isolated nonperfused fragments. Partial hepatic devascularization can occur from laceration of blood vessels in the perihilar region or complete avulsion of the dual blood supply of the liver, producing wedge-shaped, nonenhancing regions that extend to the periphery (395,489). Lacerations extending into the perihilar region of the liver have an increased incidence of bile duct injury and associated complications such as biloma and hemobilia (205,392). Disruption of the biliary tree is only rarely detectable on an initial CT examination, but may become manifest on delayed scans in the form of a loculated intrahepatic biloma or an extrahepatic bile collection with attenuation values typically near 0 HU. Although small bilomas usually resolve spontaneously, large or increasing bilomas may indicate the need for percutaneous drainage or surgical repair (19).

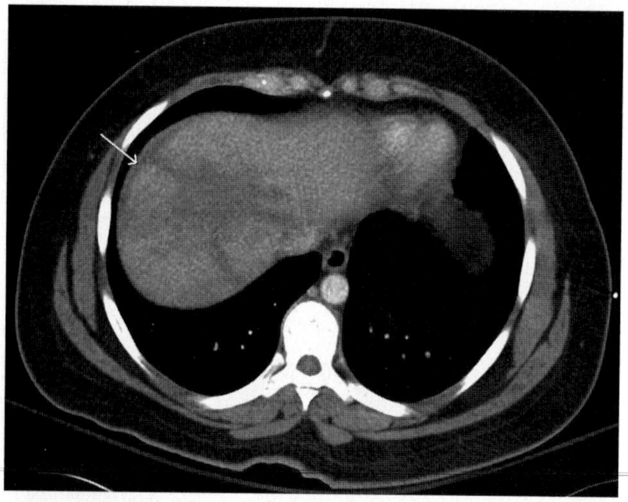

Intrahepatic hematomas appear as poorly marginated, confluent areas of low attenuation within the hepatic parenchyma (Figs. 21-47 and 21-48). They tend to be rounded or oval in configuration and often display a central high-attenuation area of clotted blood surrounded by a larger low-attenuation region of lysed clot and contused liver parenchyma (205,392). On pathologic examination, intrahepatic hematomas have been found to represent areas of microscopic hemorrhage, necrosis, and edema.

Subcapsular hematomas occasionally result from blunt trauma, but more frequently are the result of iatrogenic injuries such as percutaneous liver biopsy. Subcapsular hematomas usually appear on CT as peripheral, well-marginated, lenticular or crescent-shape fluid collections

bear claw pattern because of its radiating, parallel, and jagged appearance (205,392) (Fig. 21-46). On occasion, hepatic lacerations may demonstrate a branching pattern that simulates the appearance of unopacified portal or hepatic veins, or dilated bile ducts (113,392). This resemblance is usually limited to a single CT section, and in most cases, careful analysis of contiguous sections allows correct diagnosis.

Lacerations may be anatomically localized to lobes and segments, and further classified as superficial, perihilar, or deep. Deep lacerations, or lacerations extending between

Figure 21-46   Bear claw type laceration of the right hepatic lobe. Note roughly parallel, radiating, low-attenuation lacerations involving the dome of the liver. A small amount of perihepatic blood is present *(arrow)*.

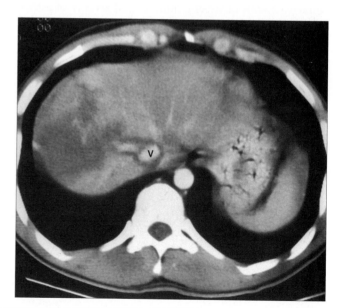

Figure 21-47   Intrahepatic hematoma. Contrast-enhanced computed tomography scan demonstrates a poorly marginated, confluent area of low attenuation within the dome of the liver consistent with an intraparenchymal hematoma. Dissection of blood along the right hepatic vein and around the inferior vena cava (V) is also noted.

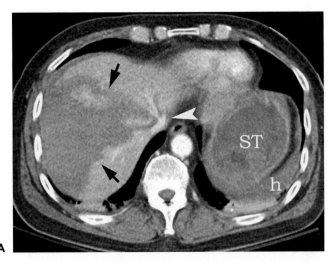
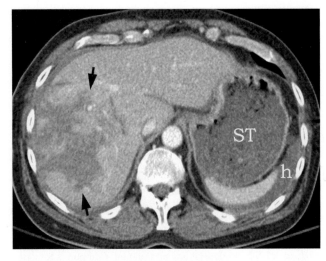

A

B

Figure 21-48 Hepatic laceration and hematoma. A, B: Computed tomography images demonstrate extensive, irregular laceration and intraparenchymal hematoma (*arrows*), occupying much of the right lobe of the liver. The injury extends centrally to the confluence of the hepatic veins and inferior vena cava (*arrowhead*). Note associated perihepatic and perisplenic hemorrhage (h). ST, stomach.

that characteristically flatten or indent the underlying liver parenchyma. Most subcapsular hematomas occur along the parietal surface of the liver, particularly along the anterolateral aspect of the right hepatic lobe (361). The attenuation of the collection depends on the age of the hematoma, generally being of higher attenuation early when clotted blood is present and then decreasing in attenuation over time as clot lysis takes place (113,205,392).

Occasionally, hepatic parenchymal or subcapsular gas may be seen in areas of hepatic laceration or hematoma within 2 to 3 days following blunt abdominal trauma

(2,331) (Fig. 21-49). Although the presence of hepatic gas often indicates the presence of infection, such gas may also be a manifestation of severe blunt trauma without infection. It has been postulated that the gas arises from hepatic ischemia and necrosis (283). In the appropriate clinical setting, such gas-containing injuries can be treated conservatively without the need for surgical or percutaneous intervention (2,331,403).

Periportal low attenuation surrounding portal venous branches (periportal tracking) is seen in up to 22% of patients with blunt abdominal trauma (259,337,392,393,403,

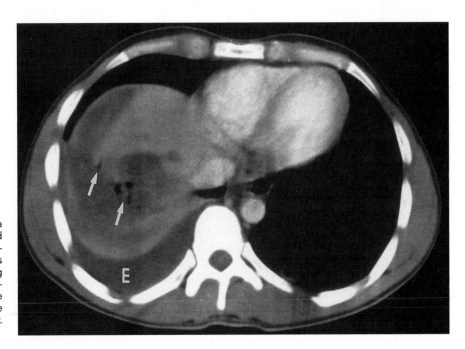

Figure 21-49 Intrahepatic hematoma with sterile necrosis. Contrast-enhanced computed tomography scan 3 days following blunt abdominal trauma demonstrates intraparenchymal hematoma containing several small bubbles of gas (*arrows*), presumably secondary to necrosis within the area of injury. The patient had no evidence of infection and recovered uneventfully. E, pleural effusion.

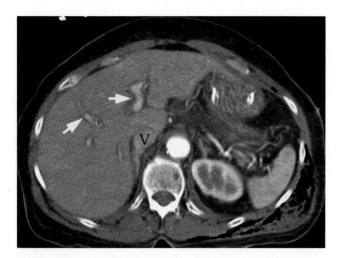

Figure 21-50 Periportal low attenuation. Computed tomography image demonstrates periportal low attenuation (*arrows*) surrounding the portal triads. A small amount of fluid is seen adjacent to the inferior vena cava (V).

478) (Fig. 21-50). In patients with hepatic injury, the periportal low attenuation has been attributed to dissection of blood along the course of the portal veins (259). In the absence of CT evidence of hepatic disruption, however, the finding of diffuse periportal low attenuation after blunt trauma should not be taken as de facto evidence of underlying hepatic parenchymal injury (393). In most trauma patients, periportal tracking most likely represents distension of periportal lymphatics and lymphedema associated with elevated central venous pressure produced by rapid expansion of intravascular volume during vigorous fluid resuscitation (69,393). Other trauma-related pathologic changes leading to elevated central venous pressure, such as tension pneumothorax, pericardial tamponade, or hematoma obstructing hepatic venous outflow, also may result in diffuse periportal low attenuation (230,393).

Lacerations or hematomas of the hepatic parenchyma can be simulated by beam-hardening artifact from adjacent ribs or streak artifacts from air–contrast interfaces. Rib artifacts can usually be identified by their typical location deep to the rib and by their tendency to fade and become more diffuse as they proceed into the liver (140). Artifacts from air–contrast interfaces in stomach and bowel generally are more regular and linear in appearance than true lacerations. Lacerations also can be simulated by congenital hepatic clefts or fissures (Fig. 21-51).

A laceration or hematoma can be missed in cases of fatty liver in which the low-attenuation fatty-infiltrated parenchyma, even when enhanced, remains isodense with the areas of low-attenuation injury. Associated hemoperitoneum should remain evident, however, and may be the only readily identifiable sign suggesting hepatic injury. In such cases, it may be helpful to view images of the liver with narrow window widths (100 to 200 HU) to enhance

detection of subtle parenchymal findings, such as alteration of the course of intrahepatic vessels and ducts within the areas of parenchymal injury (114,361).

Intrahepatic vascular injuries have been reported in association with injuries of higher CT grade and severity (343,344). Specific vascular structures that may be affected include the major hepatic veins, the inferior vena cava (IVC), and the hepatic artery (392). As with vascular injuries to the spleen, there are several CT signs of hepatic vascular injury. Active bleeding may be identified on contrast-enhanced CT as irregular, round, or oval areas of bright vascular enhancement in the hepatic parenchyma with CT attenuation values usually within 10 HU of an adjacent artery. Active subcapsular or extrahepatic bleeding appears as an irregular blush of high-density contrast material extending from the liver periphery into a surrounding hematoma (343,392). More recently, a number of authors have reported contrast pooling on CT as a sign of active hemorrhage (110,111). The increasing visualization of this sign may be a result of faster scanning with MDCT, which allows smaller amounts of active hemorrhage to be detected before the high-density contrast material is diluted by surrounding hematoma. The presence of pooling of contrast material within the peritoneal cavity indicates active and massive bleeding. Patients with this CT scan finding show rapid deterioration of hemodynamic status, and may require emergency surgery. Pooling of contrast material in ruptured hepatic parenchyma also indicates active bleeding, requiring at least close monitoring and possibly emergent angiography and intervention. The status of the liver capsule, either intact or ruptured, may help predict which patients will deteriorate hemodynamically and which patients will be successfully treated conservatively (110).

Hepatic vein damage has been noted to occur in 10% to 15% of liver injuries, often as a result of avulsion of the right hepatic vein from the IVC. Lacerations near the confluence of the hepatic veins or the intrahepatic IVC should suggest the potential for hepatic vein or IVC laceration. Such injuries are of particular concern because they can result in rapid exsanguination, particularly when the liver is mobilized at the time of surgical inspection (24,205). The recognition of active hemorrhage in these cases is of major clinical importance as it indicates the need for possible surgical or interventional treatment because conservative therapy is unlikely to be successful (205).

Pseudoaneurysms of the hepatic artery may result from hepatic lacerations extending across the hepatic arteries. They represent contained arterial perforations and usually appear as discrete, oval or round lesions within the hepatic parenchyma that are isodense with adjacent major arterial structures (205). Not infrequently, hematoma will be noted to surround the pseudoaneurysm.

Although a significant percentage of patients with hepatic injury have obvious signs of shock or peritonitis at the time of admission and require immediate surgery without preliminary imaging studies, there are also a large number of patients with significant hepatic trauma who

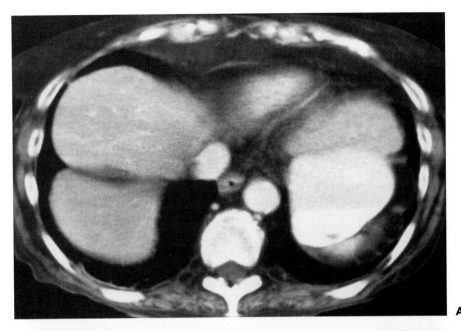

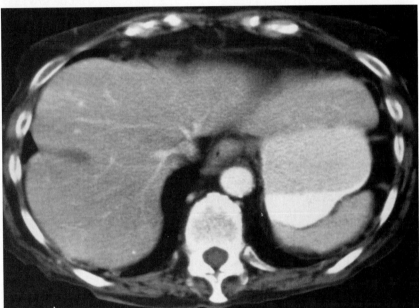

Figure 21-51 Congenital hepatic cleft. **A:** Computed tomography (CT) scan through the dome of the liver demonstrates a deep cleft in the hepatic parenchyma. **B:** On a CT image 1 cm caudal to (**A**), the peripheral cleft mimics a parenchymal laceration. Note the absence of perihepatic blood.

are hemodynamically stable that may be best managed nonoperatively. Nonoperative management of liver injuries in hemodynamically stable patients can be expected to be successful in up to 90% of patients in whom it is used (75,131,269,303,343,478). Keys to successful nonoperative management include constant hemodynamic monitoring, serial clinical and laboratory assessment, blood replacement as necessary, and ready availability of nursing, surgical, and imaging facilities in the event of hemodynamic deterioration (131,298).

Several attempts have been made to grade liver injury by means of CT to help guide clinical management. A CT-based grading system adapted from the AAST (Table 21-3) (343)

assesses the location of hepatic lacerations and hematomas, as well as the presence and extent of tissue destruction and devascularization (298,343,344). Although reflective of the degree of hepatic parenchymal damage, this CT grading system, as well as others, does not reliably predict the need for surgical or interventional treatment, nor does it help predict the outcome of conservative treatment (17,298,343,344). The surgical organ injury scale of the AAST includes some criteria that cannot be assessed with CT, and wide discrepancies have been found between the CT injury grade and operative findings (74,344). Some lower grade injuries (grades 1 or 2) may require surgical intervention, possibly because of severe associated injury

TABLE 21-3

COMPUTED TOMOGRAPHY–BASED INJURY SEVERITY OF HEPATIC TRAUMA

Grade I   Capsular avulsion, superficial laceration(s) less than 1 cm deep, subcapsular hematoma less than 1 cm in maximum thickness, periportal blood tracking only.

Grade II   Laceration(s) 1 to 3 cm deep, central-subcapsular hematoma(s) 1 to 3 cm in diameter.

Grade III Laceration greater than 3 cm deep, central-subcapsular hematoma(s) greater than 3 cm in diameter.

Grade IV   Massive central-subcapsular hematoma greater than 10 cm, lobar tissue destruction (maceration) or devascularization.

Grade V   Bilobar tissue destruction (maceration) or devascularization.

From Poletti PA, Mirvis SE, Shanmuganathan K, et al. CT criteria for management of blunt liver trauma: correlation with angiographic and surgical findings. *Radiology* 2000;216:418–427, with permission.

to the falciform ligament not detected using CT. In addition, the majority of patients with even high-grade injuries (grades 3 or 4) and major hemoperitoneum may respond favorably to conservative treatment (17,74,344).

CT can be useful in monitoring the healing of hepatic injuries, confirming the resorption of hemoperitoneum, and detecting complications such as hepatic infarction, enlarging hematoma, biloma, or abscess formation (17,39, 131). Hemoperitoneum normally is resorbed from the peritoneal cavity, and in most cases is either significantly reduced or absent by 1 week after injury. Persistence of hemoperitoneum or increase in the volume of intraperitoneal fluid on repeat CT scans 3 to 7 days after injury suggests either ongoing intraperitoneal bleeding or bile leakage (131). Delayed hemorrhage, or progression of initially stable parenchymal injuries, is less common with hepatic trauma than with splenic injury (201,298).

Subcapsular liver hematomas usually resolve in 6 to 8 weeks. Intraparenchymal hematomas heal much more slowly, often requiring 6 months to several years to resolve completely, because bile in the hematoma prolongs clot resorption and adversely affects parenchymal healing (377). Lacerations heal more rapidly, with evidence of significant healing generally noted on serial CT examinations over a 2- to 3-week period (131) (Fig. 21-52). Hepatic lacerations and hematomas typically demonstrate a decrease in CT attenuation value, as well as a slight increase in size on initial follow-up CT studies (i.e., 7 days postinjury), probably as a result of osmotic absorption of fluid. Irregular margins of lacerations and hematomas become better defined with healing and tend to assume a rounded or ovoid configuration with resolution (131). Such lesions may progressively decrease in size or they may persist as well-defined hepatic cysts or bilomas (377).

Gallbladder

The gallbladder is infrequently injured in blunt abdominal trauma, with a reported incidence of 2% to 6% (392). The low incidence of gallbladder injury may be because of the protective effect of the liver (42). Gallbladder injury is usually associated with injuries to other organs, most commonly the liver, spleen, and duodenum (52). Traumatic injuries to the gallbladder include contusion, laceration, perforation, and complete avulsion (392,403). CT findings include pericholecystic fluid (most common), blurring of the contour of the gallbladder, focal thickening or discontinuity of the gallbladder wall, an enhancing mucosal flap within the lumen, mass effect on the adjacent duodenum, and high-density intraluminal blood (19,392,403). A collapsed gallbladder, coupled with additional imaging signs of gallbladder injury, should raise the possibility of gallbladder perforation or avulsion (163). Avulsion of the gallbladder may involve variable portions of the gallbladder, cystic duct, and cystic artery and may lead to major blood loss (52).

Pancreas

Pancreatic injuries from trauma are relatively uncommon, accounting for only 3% to 12% of all abdominal injuries (11,95,132,208). Depending on patient demographics, blunt or penetrating trauma accounts for the majority of pancreatic injuries (5,130). Generally, penetrating pancreatic injuries arise from gunshot wounds or stab wounds (5). The mechanism of injury to the pancreas in blunt trauma is thought to be compression of the pancreas between the vertebral column and the anterior abdominal wall, often as a result of direct steering wheel injury (in adults) or bicycle handlebar injury (in children) to the midepigastrium (95,209). In 50% to 98% of cases, pancreatic injuries are associated with injuries to other intraabdominal organs (119,473), and this combination of injuries results in a mortality rate of approximately 20%, as compared with a mortality rate of 3% to 10% for isolated pancreatic injuries (473). Most deaths within the first 48 hours are a result of hemorrhage from extrapancreatic injuries (132,209). Delays in diagnosis can lead to increased late (greater than 48 hours postinjury) morbidity and mortality related to the pancreatic injuries alone (248). In general, increasing severity of pancreatic injury is correlated with increasing severity and extent of extrapancreatic injury (130).

The diagnosis of pancreatic injury can be extremely difficult because the clinical, laboratory, and radiographic findings are highly variable and nonspecific (11). Clinical manifestations of pancreatic injury, such as abdominal pain and leukocytosis, frequently are mild, absent, or masked by associated injuries (72,314). Serum amylase levels may be elevated, but this is not invariably the case, and initial serum amylase determinations have been reported to be normal in up to 40% of patients with pancreatic in-

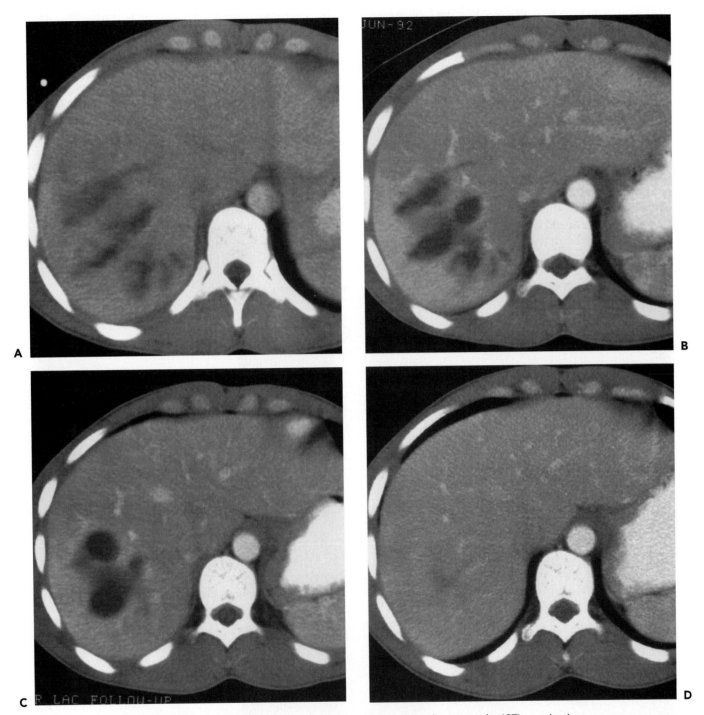

Figure 21-52 Healing hepatic lacerations on serial computed tomography (CT) examinations. **A:** Initial scan demonstrates bear claw–type laceration in the right lobe of the liver. **B:** Scan 4 days later shows decrease in CT attenuation value and slight increase in size of the hepatic lacerations, probably a result of osmotic absorption of fluid. **C:** On a scan 3 weeks later, the lacerations have assumed a more rounded configuration, and the margins of the lacerations are better defined. **D:** Follow-up scan 3 months after the initial injury demonstrates virtually complete resolution of the liver lacerations.

jury (209). Even with total disruption of the pancreatic ductal system, amylase levels may not be elevated until 24 to 48 hours postinjury. In addition, the degree of serum amylase elevation does not correlate with the degree of pancreatic injury (132). Because pancreatic injuries may be clinically occult or unrecognized, they often are discovered at the time of laparotomy for other known intraabdominal injuries (60,207,327).

Pancreatic injuries can range from minor parenchymal contusions and hematomas to major lacerations or fractures with associated pancreatic duct disruption. CT has been reported to diagnose pancreatic injury in 67% to

85% of cases (204,410), with a specificity of 98% (25,130, 196). The sensitivity of CT for diagnosis of traumatic pancreatic injury is likely to improve in the future with the use of MDCT, thinner collimation, and high-quality multiplanar reconstruction.

On contrast-enhanced CT, contusions generally appear as focal low-attenuation areas within the normally enhancing pancreatic parenchyma. Lacerations or fractures appear as linear, irregular regions of low attenuation, often oriented perpendicular to the long axis of the pancreas (323) (Figs. 21-53 and 21-54). Fractures most commonly occur in the pancreatic neck or body where the pancreas overlies the spine, although some fractures have been reported in the pancreatic head or tail (25,91,252). Hematomas, pseudocysts, and abscesses are often seen communicating with the pancreas at the site of fracture or transection (163). The rare appearance of active pancreatic bleeding is pathognomonic of pancreatic injury (25). Additional suggestive but nonspecific signs of pancreatic injury include focal enlargement of the pancreas, infiltration of the peripancreatic fat and mesentery, thickening of the left anterior renal fascia (204), tracking of fluid between the splenic vein and pancreas (236), and fluid in the anterior pararenal space or lesser sac (408).

Pancreatic laceration or fracture may be difficult to identify acutely (less than 12 hours postinjury) with CT because of obscuration of the fracture plane by hemorrhage and/or close apposition of the lacerated parenchymal fragments (204). As the time from injury progresses, edema, inflammation, and autodigestion by exuded pancreatic enzymes

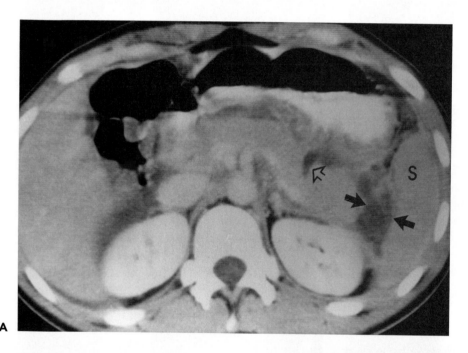

A

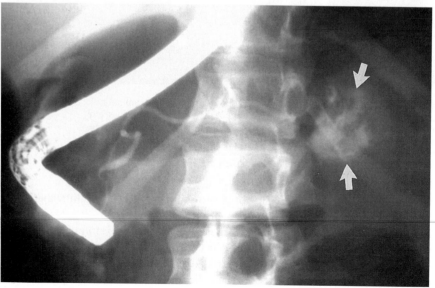

B

Figure 21-53 Pancreatic laceration with disruption of the pancreatic duct. **A:** Computed tomography scan demonstrates laceration through the tail of the pancreas (*open arrow*). Fluid is seen about the tail of the pancreas (*solid arrows*) adjacent to the spleen (S). **B:** Endoscopic retrograde cholangiopancreatography (ERCP) demonstrates disruption of the main pancreatic duct in the tail of the pancreas with extravasation of contrast material (*arrows*).

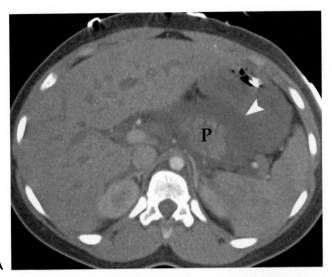
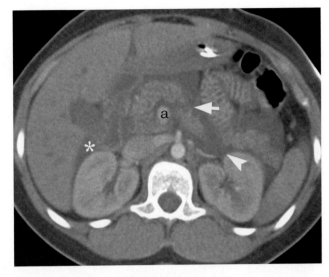

Figure 21-54 Pancreatic laceration. **A, B:** Computed tomography images through the pancreas (P) demonstrate peripancreatic fluid (*arrowheads*) tracking into the left anterior pararenal space. Note irregular, low-attenuation laceration (*arrow*) extending through the body of the pancreas. Adjacent fluid surrounds the superior mesenteric vein (a). Fluid is also present in the hepatorenal fossa (*asterisk*).

often make the CT findings of pancreatic injury more apparent. Thus, if suspicion of pancreatic injury persists despite initially normal CT findings, repeat CT scans in 12 to 24 hours may be warranted (91,275).

One retrospective review of the CT findings in patients with traumatic pancreatic injury suggested that most cases of missed diagnosis could be averted with careful scrutiny of the images, decreased CT slice thickness (5 mm or less), and appropriate CT technique, including proper administration of IV contrast material (25). Also stressed was the need to thoroughly examine the pancreas despite the distracting presence of profound extrapancreatic injuries. When pancreatic injury is evident on CT, it may be difficult to accurately grade the severity of the injury. There are varying reports on the efficacy of CT for grading pancreatic injury, with some reports noting underestimation of injury severity (5,196,336) while others report overestimation (482).

False–positive diagnosis of pancreatic laceration or fracture may result from streak artifacts, physiologic thinning of the pancreatic neck (Fig. 21-55), or misinterpretation of unopacified proximal jejunal loops as the pancreatic body, separated from the pancreatic head and neck region by a fat plane around the mesenteric vessels (114). In questionable cases, repeat delayed scans with additional oral contrast material usually demonstrates changes in shape and opacification of the bowel loops, allowing correct diagnosis.

CT cannot directly assess the integrity of the pancreatic duct, which is the principal determinant in the management of pancreatic injuries (66). One study assessing CT grading of blunt pancreatic injuries suggested that ductal disruption was likely to be present if CT scans demonstrated a deep laceration or transection of the pancreas (482). In general, however, definitive determination of

pancreatic duct integrity requires either endoscopic retrograde cholangiopancreatography (ERCP), intraoperative evaluation (51,119), or, more recently, MR pancreatography (336). MR pancreatography has the advantage of being noninvasive, faster, and more readily available than ERCP (163). In addition to identifying the main pancreatic duct in most cases (134), MR pancreatography is helpful in assessing parenchymal injury, and in demonstrating fluid collections associated with pancreatic duct laceration or transection (418).

Bowel and Mesentery

Injuries to the bowel and mesentery are reported to occur in 3% to 5% of patients sustaining blunt abdominal trauma (37,397). They are most often associated with motor vehicle accidents, and their prevalence has increased with the use of lap-type seat-belt restraints, particularly in children (79,390,413). Mechanisms of injury include direct compression of the bowel between the vertebral column and the anterior abdominal wall, a sudden marked increase in intraluminal pressure, and shearing-type injury near sites of mesenteric fixation, such as the ligament of Treitz and the ileocecal junction (70,85,193). Bowel injuries can range from focal mural contusions or hematomas to complete transections. They most commonly involve the duodenum, usually the second and third portions, although this predilection over other small bowel injuries does vary with geographic location (50,193). Colonic injuries following blunt abdominal trauma are less common than either duodenal or other small bowel injuries (188). Traumatic injuries to the colon are more likely to involve the more vulnerable transverse and

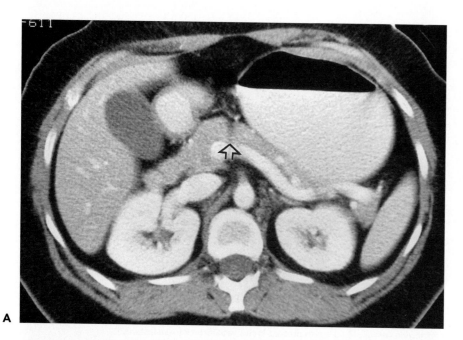

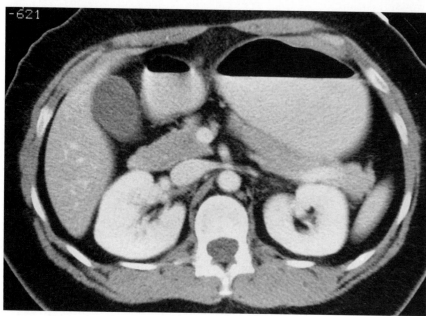

Figure 21-55 Pseudofracture of the pancreas due to physiologic thinning of the pancreatic neck. **A:** Computed tomography (CT) scan at the level of the superior mesenteric vein–splenic vein confluence demonstrates apparent fracture of the pancreatic neck (*open arrow*). **B:** CT scan 1 cm caudal to (**A**) shows fat in the region of the neck consistent with physiologic thinning. Note also the absence of peripancreatic fluid.

sigmoid colon, with damage to the right colon accompanied by multiple other injuries and rectal injury associated with pelvic fracture (193,206).

Prompt diagnosis of intestinal or mesenteric injury is often difficult because signs and symptoms may be delayed and physical examination is neither sensitive nor specific (43,93). Early clinical findings are frequently subtle, and the classic triad of tenderness, rigidity, and absent bowel sounds only occurs in about 30% of patients (43). Abdominal wall bruising, or the "seat-belt sign," should increase suspicion for bowel and mesenteric injury (193). Children presenting with iliac wing fractures from improperly positioned lap belts are at high risk for such injuries (102).

Clear-cut peritoneal signs and symptoms can take hours or days to develop in stable patients with intestinal injury because of minimal blood loss, contained retroperitoneal involvement in some duodenal and colonic injuries, and the nonirritative composition (i.e., neutral pH) and low bacterial counts of small bowel chyme (93,397). Changes in laboratory values also develop over time. One study found correlation between an increased base deficit and small bowel and mesenteric injuries (133). Another study found that significantly more patients with small bowel injury developed leukocytosis within 3 hours of presentation than did patients with other intraabdominal injuries (170).

As previously discussed, diagnostic peritoneal lavage (DPL) is highly sensitive for hemoperitoneum but not at all specific for the source of the bleeding, and may miss retroperitoneal hemorrhage (7,344). One study found that although DPL was sensitive for intraabdominal injuries in general, it was not as useful in identifying isolated small bowel and mesenteric injuries (133). US has been shown, in the hands of an experienced operator, to be highly sensitive in the rapid detection of intraperitoneal fluid (491), and in many centers, has replaced DPL. In addition, sonography has been found to be useful in identifying intramural bowel hematomas (253,490) and solid organ parenchymal injuries. If undiagnosed, bowel perforation can lead to fatal peritonitis. A delay of more than 24 hours in diagnosis and surgical repair of bowel perforation results in a significant increase in morbidity (146,254,360). Whether or not there is an increase in mortality, however, has been recently debated in the literature, with some studies finding delayed diagnosis to have no impact on death rates (7,14,133). One study focusing on small bowel injury found that a delay in diagnosis of longer than 8 hours did result in significantly increased mortality (108). Undiagnosed mesenteric injuries can lead to intestinal stenosis presenting weeks after the initial trauma (80,251,447). In general, undiagnosed bowel and mesenteric injuries evolve with time, affecting the patient's physical condition. In many cases of missed diagnosis with onset of new signs and symptoms, a repeat CT scan will show more definitive evidence of injury (7,156) (Fig. 21-56).

CT has been shown to be useful for detecting bowel and mesenteric injuries caused by blunt trauma, but careful inspection and meticulous scanning technique are required to detect often subtle findings (286,316,344,397). In a retrospective study of blunt duodenal injury, the authors found that CT findings of bowel injury were present in 83% of patients with missed diagnoses, and they surmised that these findings were overlooked in the context of multiple associated injuries (7). Although many earlier studies found poor sensitivity of CT for detection of bowel injuries (48,66,216,266,276,398), more recent studies have reported higher sensitivity of CT for diagnosing bowel and mesenteric injuries and for distinguishing those injuries that are likely to require surgical intervention (40,94,98, 286, 359,397). One study found that CT differentiated surgical from nonsurgical injuries in 86% of bowel cases and 75% of mesenteric cases (220), while another reported a 75% success rate at differentiation (200).

Current studies report sensitivities of CT for the diagnosis of bowel and mesenteric injuries ranging from 64% to 96% (18,44,192,200,220,261,268), but these have all involved retrospective reviews, most have analyzed small cohorts of patients, and often the CT reviewers were not blinded to the patients' surgical diagnosis. Furthermore, in these studies, the CT findings considered diagnostic of bowel and mesenteric injury varied, and some used conventional CT while others used helical CT and still others used a combination of both technologies. Larger, prospective studies with consistently defined diagnostic criteria are needed to accurately assess the sensitivity of modern CT in the diagnosis of bowel and mesenteric injury.

The use of MDCT promises to greatly improve the sensitivity and specificity of CT for traumatic bowel and mesenteric injuries. The increased speed, which eliminates motion artifact, higher z-axis resolution, and thinner collimation allow superior visualization of the bowel and mesenteric vasculature (184,185). Slices as thin as 0.5 mm and speeds of eight slices per second are obtainable on the eight-detector scanners, and this collimation and speed is surpassed by scanners with additional detectors (186). Typically, slices of

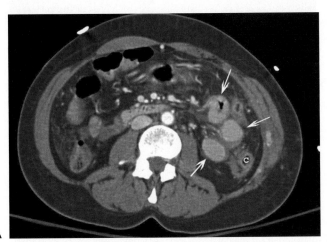
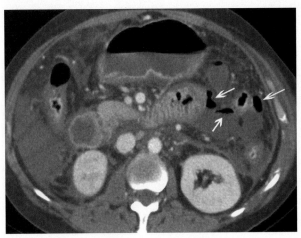

Figure 21-56 Missed jejunal perforation. **A:** Computed tomography (CT) scan of the midabdomen demonstrates thickened jejunal loops (*arrows*) in the left upper quadrant. Small amount of fluid/blood also is noted surrounding these loops and adjacent to the descending colon (c). No extraluminal gas was found. **B:** Repeat CT scan 2 days after (**A**) shows marked increase in the amount of intraperitoneal fluid. Extraluminal gas collections (*arrows*) are now clearly visible. Surgery confirmed jejunal perforation. (Case courtesy of Christine O Menias, M.D., St. Louis, MO.)

1.25 mm are used to evaluate the bowel and mesentery. MDCT angiography can generate detailed views of the mesenteric arteries and veins, and MDCT colonoscopy provides a noninvasive means to examine the colon lumen. Individual loops of small bowel can be visualized using 3D reconstruction (186). When MDCT is immediately available in the trauma department, obtaining CT evaluation is feasible in even unstable patients (466).

CT signs of bowel and mesenteric injury include extraluminal air, extravasation of oral contrast material, free intraabdominal fluid, thickened and/or discontinuous bowel wall, high-attenuation clot (sentinel clot) adjacent to the involved bowel, and streaky soft tissue infiltration of the mesenteric fat (94,252,286,316,325,344,359) (Fig. 21-57). Free air in either the peritoneal cavity or the retroperitoneum is a relatively specific sign of bowel perforation but is seen in only 50% of cases (87,146,359). The volume of air may be quite small and subtle (245). To optimize detection of extraluminal air and to facilitate its differentiation

from intraluminal air and from fat, images should be viewed at wide window settings (i.e., lung windows) (see Fig. 21-57) (70,397). Pneumoperitoneum is most commonly seen in the subdiaphragmatic area, along the anterior peritoneal surfaces of the liver and spleen. Extraluminal air also may be present within the leaves of the mesentery (Fig. 21-58) or in the retroperitoneum, particularly in the anterior pararenal space (316,478). Occasionally, intraperitoneal or retroperitoneal gas results from extraperitoneal dissection of air from traumatic injuries of the thorax (pneumothorax, pneumomediastinum) or bladder (bladder rupture) and is not related to bowel trauma (40,66,344). Additionally, pneumoperitoneum may occur iatrogenically, following diagnostic peritoneal lavage or chest tube placement (18). Extravasation of oral contrast material from the bowel lumen is considered diagnostic of bowel perforation but is seen in only a minority of cases (70,87,359) (Fig. 21-59). There has been some controversy over the use of oral contrast material in trauma patients, with some authors claiming an in-

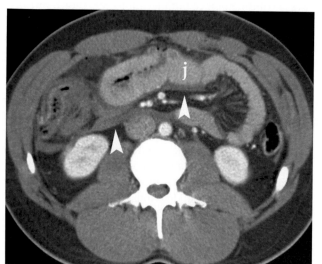

A

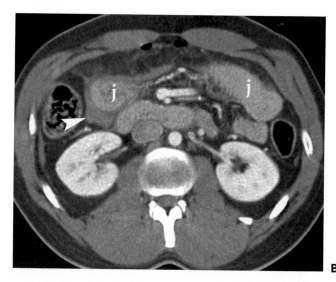

B

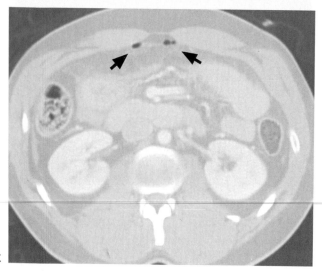

C

Figure 21-57 Jejunal perforation. **A:** Computed tomography image demonstrates a markedly thickened loop of jejunum (j), with free fluid (*arrowheads*) tracking along the posterior aspect of the jejunum and into the mesentery. **B, C:** Images at a slightly higher level demonstrate additional perijejunal fluid (*arrowhead*) on soft tissue window settings, and several foci of extraluminal air (*arrows*) on lung window settings.

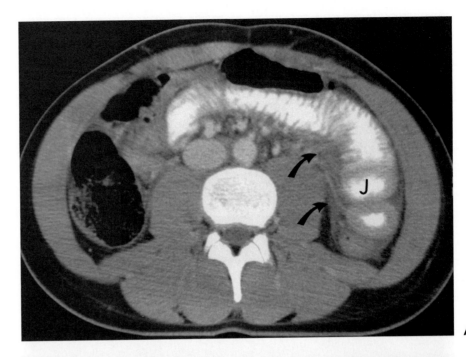

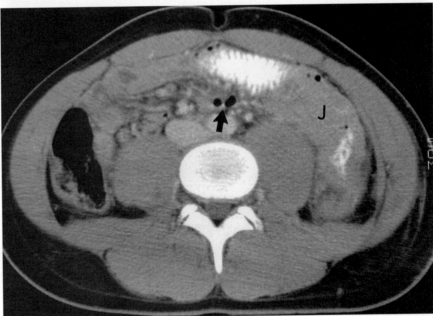

Figure 21-58 Jejunal perforation. Computed tomography images through the lower abdomen **(A, B)** demonstrate thick-walled jejunum (J), soft tissue infiltration of the adjacent mesenteric fat (*curved arrows*), and extraluminal mesenteric air (*straight arrow*).

creased risk of vomiting and aspiration without improved diagnostic capability (57,446), while others assert that oral contrast material is safe and improves visualization of bowel injuries (117,286,311,316). A recent retrospective study found that MDCT without oral contrast material was adequate for depiction of bowel and mesenteric injuries requiring surgical repair, and that their results were comparable to previously reported data for single-detector row helical CT with oral contrast material (432). Both positive oral contrast agents, such as sodium amidotrizoate/meglumine amidotrizoate (Gastrografin) or barium, and neutral agents, such as water, are commonly used (186). Water allows for

better distinction between the opacified vasculature, the enhanced bowel wall, and the bowel lumen, but does not provide as much bowel distension as the positive agents because of a higher bowel transit time (186). Water is often used for MDCT because positive agents may degrade non-axial reconstructed images (367).

Intraabdominal fluid is a very common but nonspecific CT finding of bowel or mesenteric injury (286,359). The fluid may be of low attenuation, representing extravasated small bowel contents, or of intermediate to high attenuation from acute hemorrhage. Free intraperitoneal fluid in the absence of an apparent solid visceral source of hemor-

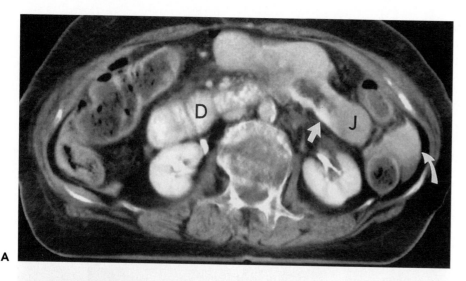

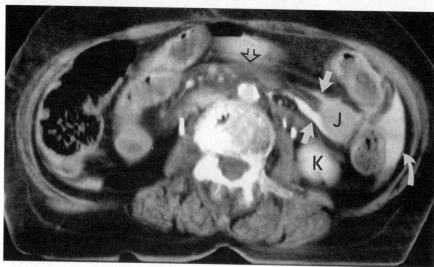

Figure 21-59 Small bowel laceration at the ligament of Treitz with extravasation of oral contrast material. Computed tomography images at the level of the transverse duodenum (A) and lower pole of the left kidney (B) demonstrate extravasated oral contrast material along the small bowel mesentery (*straight arrows*) and in the left paracolic gutter (*curved arrow*). Ill-defined hemorrhage is noted at the root of the mesentery (*open arrow*). D, opacified transverse duodenum; J, unopacified jejunum; K, lower pole of left kidney.

rhage should heighten suspicion of a bowel or mesenteric injury (33,170, 286,359). Occasionally, small quantities of intraperitoneal fluid, particularly when localized in the small bowel mesentery or between loops of bowel, may be the only CT sign of bowel perforation. Moderate or large amounts of fluid are less common as the sole CT abnormality but have a higher likelihood of being associated with bowel or mesenteric injury (246). Other suggestive but nonspecific abnormalities, such as focal bowel wall thickening or strandy soft tissue infiltration of the mesenteric fat, can improve diagnostic accuracy when combined with other CT scan findings (40,94, 245,344). One study, including over 2,000 patients with small bowel injury (SBI), used a logistic regression model to identify CT signs that best predict SBI. The final model included free fluid, pneumoperitoneum, and bowel wall thickening, resulting in a sensitivity for SBI of 75% and a specificity of 79.1% (109). In another study, the CT findings of mesenteric

bleeding and bowel wall thickening associated with mesenteric hematoma or infiltration indicated a high likelihood of a mesentery-bowel injury requiring surgical intervention (99) (Fig. 21-60).

Intramural hemorrhage is detected in most patients with bowel injury as circumferential or eccentric thickening of the bowel wall on CT, often with associated luminal narrowing (191,235). Intense enhancement of the bowel wall has also been reported as a sign of bowel injury (168,409). When combined with bowel wall thickening and free peritoneal fluid, intense bowel wall enhancement suggests bowel perforation and peritonitis (168). It should be noted, however, that increased contrast enhancement of the bowel wall is not a specific sign of bowel rupture because it can also be seen in children with the hypoperfusion complex and in adults with compromised central venous return or prolonged hypoperfusion resulting in so-called shock bowel (294,364).

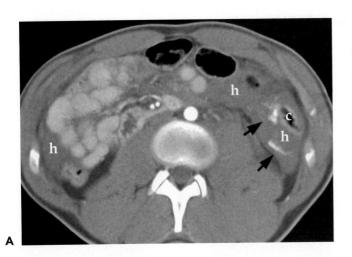

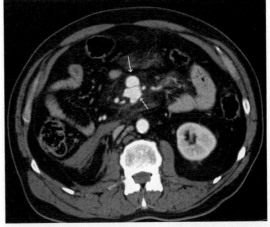

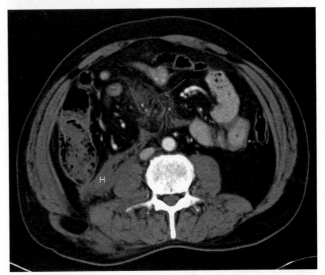

Figure 21-60 Mesenteric arterial hemorrhage. **A:** Computed to-mography (CT) image demonstrates hemoperitoneum (h) secondary to surgically proven mesenteric arterial bleeding at the level of the mid descending colon (c). Note active arterial extravasation of con-trast material (*arrows*). **B, C:** In another patient with recent abdominal trauma, CT images demonstrate irregular collections of iodinated contrast material (*thick arrows*) in the mesentery, repre-senting pseudoaneurysms. Non–contrast-enhanced acute blood is seen in the mesentery (*thin arrow*) and right anterior pararenal space (H).

Kidney

Trauma to the kidney can occur either as an isolated event or, more frequently, as concomitant injury in patients with acute abdominal trauma. Worldwide, blunt trauma is re-sponsible for 80% of renal injuries, but the number attrib-utable to penetrating wounds increases dramatically in urban settings with a high rate of violent crime (167). Most closed renal injuries are a result of motor vehicle ac-cidents, with contact sports, falls, fights, and assaults ac-counting for the remainder. With blunt trauma, the kidney may be injured by a direct blow, lacerated by the lower ribs, or torn by rapid acceleration–deceleration (31,345).

Penetrating injuries are usually secondary to gunshot or stab wounds. Interventional procedures, such as percuta-neous nephrostomy and renal biopsy, constitute another group of penetrating injuries. A diseased or anomalous kidney is more susceptible to injury than a healthy one. Minor or trivial trauma may lead to disruption of a

hydronephrotic renal pelvis, fracture of a fragile, infected kidney, or laceration of a poorly protected ectopic or horseshoe kidney (Fig. 21-61). Preexisting renal disease should be suspected whenever the inciting trauma seems disproportionately trivial to the patient's clinical findings (36,128). Children are more likely than adults to sustain traumatic injuries to the kidney because the pediatric kid-ney is less well protected, larger with respect to the body, and frequently retains fetal lobulations, which increase susceptibility to parenchymal laceration (350).

Renal injuries can be divided into four broad categories, originally described by Federle, based on a combination of clinical and imaging findings (115,212). Category I lesions include contusions, nonexpanding subcapsular hemato-mas, and small corticomedullary lacerations that do not communicate with the collecting system. They account for 75% to 85% of all renal injuries. Category II lesions con-sist of deep lacerations that extend into the medulla, with or without communication with the renal collecting

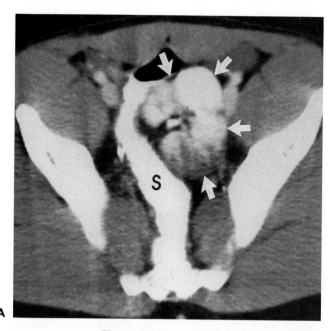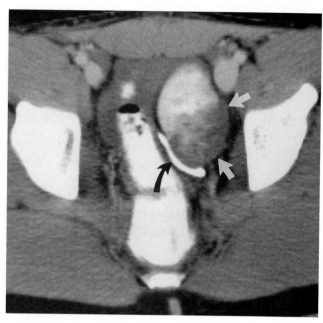

A

B

Figure 21-61 Devascularization injury of a pelvic kidney. **A:** Pelvic kidney (*straight arrows*) is identified just to the left of the sigmoid colon (S). Ill-defined region of low attenuation along the posterior margin of the kidney represents the superior aspect of an area of devascularization involving the lower pole. **B:** Computed tomography image 2 cm caudal to (A) demonstrates a well-demarcated area of hypoperfusion involving the posterior half of the lower pole of the pelvic kidney (*straight arrows*). *Curved arrow,* ureter from pelvic kidney.

system, and account for about 10% of cases. Lesions in category III consist of shattered kidneys and injuries to the renal vascular pedicle. They comprise about 5% of the total. Category IV was established for the relatively uncommon entity of ureteropelvic junction (UPJ) avulsion and laceration of the renal pelvis. The AAST developed an alternate renal injury scale that includes five grades and is based on depth and number of parenchymal lacerations. Both systems of categorization appear in the CT literature.

Most surgeons agree that category I injuries are best managed nonoperatively, whereas category IV injuries require prompt surgery (161,166). Controversy exists as to the proper management of category II and III lesions, with opinions ranging from extreme conservatism to aggressive intervention (46,106,169,488). In a study of conservative management of category II and III injuries with urinary extravasation, the authors reported decreased morbidity and shorter hospital stays for patients who did not exhibit devitalized renal segments (308). Those patients with devascularized parenchyma often required eventual surgical intervention. These findings have been confirmed in additional reports (358,376). In other studies, successful superselective transarterial embolization for renovascular injuries, including shattered kidney, has been reported (88,166). These injuries may increasingly be treated with minimally invasive means. Main renal vein injury and severe bilateral renal trauma remain consistent indications for surgical intervention (166).

Unlike closed renal injuries, which generally are managed more conservatively, penetrating renal trauma usually is an indication for surgery. Gunshot wounds almost invariably require surgical exploration and debridement because of the prevalence of associated injuries, contamination by foreign material (e.g., clothing), and extensive tissue necrosis produced by their blast effects (161). One study of selective management of gunshot wounds reported successful kidney preservation with conservative management in patients who presented without hilar involvement or persistent hemorrhage (457). Stab wounds of the kidney, once an incontrovertible indication for surgery, are now being managed by watchful expectancy in selected cases because of the precise information provided by noninvasive imaging methods (161,417).

In the absence of associated injuries, clinical findings of the patient with a renal injury are dictated by the type and severity of renal trauma. Renal injury must be presumed in every patient with abdominal trauma who has gross or microscopic hematuria. In one report of 38 children after blunt abdominal trauma, the amount of hematuria correlated better than hypotension with the severity of renal injury (421). However, in another report of 254 children, only 51% of those sent for surgical exploration for severe renal injuries presented with gross hematuria (350). In 10% to 28% of patients with renal trauma, hematuria may be absent, especially those with injuries to the renal pedicles (270). Because rapid deceleration is a common cause of renal pedicle injury, it is prudent to subject all patients with deceleration injuries (e.g., head-on motor vehicle collision, fall from a height) to renal imaging, regardless of the presence or absence of hematuria (31).

The role of the radiologist in assessing patients with suspected renal trauma is to accurately define the nature and extent of renal damage so that the maximum amount of functioning renal parenchyma can be preserved with the fewest complications. The choice of imaging studies depends upon the condition of the patient, the availability of imaging resources and personnel, and the surgeon's approach to management of renal trauma.

CT is the most informative radiologic study in renal trauma. A complete CT examination of the abdomen and pelvis can be completed with ease and speed using state-of-the-art CT scanners. The use of CT is no longer limited to the evaluation of patients with severe renal trauma, suspected multiorgan trauma, or penetrating trauma. CT is commonly used as the initial imaging study in all stabilized patients with abdominal and renal trauma (226,474, 488), in every setting from major trauma centers to rural emergency departments (150). IV urography is useful in the gross assessment of kidney status in unstable patients (212) and still is used occasionally in some institutions to evaluate stable, asymptomatic patients with a history of minor, localized renal trauma. A normal urogram obviates further imaging evaluation in this clinical setting. CT is performed only in patients with persistent hematuria or a falling hematocrit. CT also is performed if the prior urogram suggests major injury or is inconclusive.

Ultrasonography and radionuclide scintigraphy generally are not used as initial imaging studies in renal trauma. Color Doppler ultrasonography can demonstrate subcapsular or perinephric hematomas and vascular injuries, but has limited capacity to evaluate the renal parenchyma and cannot demonstrate urinary extravasation (213,272,341, 456). Radionuclide imaging can be used to assess residual renal function after conservative treatment of renal injury (488). Arteriography is reserved for preoperative road mapping and for therapeutic interventions, such as embolization of bleeding vessels and arteriovenous fistulas. As the quality of 3D reconstruction of CT images continues to improve, MDCT with 3D multiplanar reconstruction may provide a noninvasive alternative to perioperative angiography in the future (165,384). In spite of its ability to demonstrate vascular patency and parenchymal abnormalities (contusions and lacerations), MRI offers few advantages over well-performed contrast-enhanced CT and is not used in acute situations (232,243).

A complete CT evaluation of renal trauma includes both early and delayed enhanced scans (213,456). The early contrast-enhanced scans acquired during the corticomedullary phase optimize vascular opacification and visualization of contrast material extravasation. Delayed scans performed at 5 to 15 minutes following IV contrast material administration capture the excretory phase of the

kidney, allowing assessment of the collecting system. Arterial-phase scans can improve visualization of traumatic pseudoaneurysms, which occur more commonly with penetrating trauma but can be associated with blunt injuries (299). The capability of CT to evaluate renal trauma will undoubtedly improve with the increased speed and thinner collimation of MDCT. The use of MDCT urography to evaluate nontraumatic urinary tract abnormalities has yielded excellent results, particularly in imaging of the collecting system and the small, pediatric kidney (45,49, 274,349). In one study, the authors compared MDCT urography and traditional IV urography and reported as good or better opacification of the entire collecting system and ureters with MDCT (274).

CT is capable of demonstrating virtually the entire spectrum of renal injury and effectively reveals preexisting renal abnormalities. The mildest form of renal injury is a contusion (Fig. 21-62). Renal contusion appears on unenhanced scans as diffuse or focal swelling containing scattered foci of high-density fresh blood intermixed with normally homogeneous soft tissue attenuation renal parenchyma. The involved area often exhibits delayed and decreased enhancement after IV administration of iodinated contrast medium (345). A striated nephrogram, presumably resulting from stasis of urine in blood-filled tubules, also has been encountered (370).

Parenchymal lacerations likewise can be recognized on CT. They appear as unenhanced areas disrupting the normally enhancing renal parenchyma on contrast-enhanced scans (Fig. 21-63). Both contusions and small parenchymal lacerations are often accompanied by a small subcapsular or perirenal hemorrhage. Whereas subcapsular hematomas generally appear as lenticular collections that

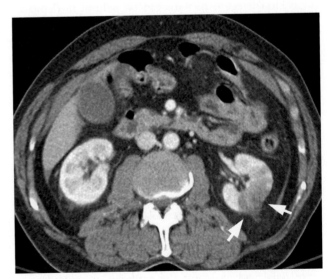

Figure 21-62 Renal contusion. Computed tomography image demonstrates a focal area of low attenuation in the posterior aspect of the left kidney representing renal contusion (*arrows*).

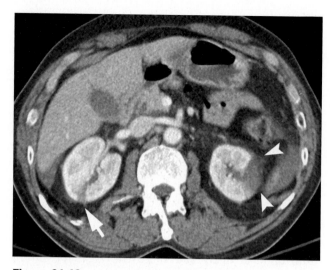

Figure 21-63   Renal laceration. Computed tomography image at the level of the renal veins demonstrates an irregular, linear, low-attenuation renal laceration (*arrow*) extending from the right renal hilum to the renal capsule. A left renal contusion (*arrowheads*) is also present. The hemoperitoneum was related to concomitant splenic injury.

flatten the underlying renal contour, perirenal hematomas infiltrate or displace perirenal fat and may extend to the renal (Gerota's) fascia (Fig. 21-64).

Category II injuries are easily detected on enhanced CT as parenchymal defects extending from the renal surface into the medulla, where they may enter the collecting system and/or transect the kidney (Fig. 21-65). Typically, such renal "fractures" parallel intervascular tissue planes, often without tearing major arteries or veins (386). The parenchymal margins often enhance inhomogeneously, producing a mottled appearance (386). Two- and three-dimensional reconstructions can be helpful in depicting the topography of renal lacerations (384).

Category II injuries are almost always accompanied by perirenal hemorrhage. Extravasation of opacified urine, into either renal parenchyma or the perirenal space, frequently occurs (see Fig. 21-65). An admixture of urine and blood also may be seen in the leaves of renal fascia as well as the anterior pararenal space (404).

Catastrophic renal injuries (category III) include shattered kidney and renal vascular pedicle injury. A shattered or pulverized kidney is recognized on CT as multiple fracture planes separating enhancing or nonenhancing renal fragments (Fig. 21-66). In contradistinction to the "fractures" in category II lesions, fractures associated with a shattered kidney generally shear across segmental renal blood vessels. A large perirenal hematoma is invariably present with a shattered kidney.

In renal pedicle injury, the occluded or avulsed main renal artery can be depicted on contrast-enhanced helical CT (56,267,321). In such an injury, a normal-sized, nonenhancing kidney is identified (Fig. 21-67). A rim of cortical

tissue may be perfused by subcapsular collateral vessels (147,257), although this finding may not be noted acutely. Other associated findings include hematoma surrounding the renal hilus, abrupt cutoff of the contrast-filled renal artery, small perinephric hematoma, and retrograde filling of the renal vein (47). Disruption of a branch vessel results in a segmental infarct that appears as a wedge- or hemispheric-shaped zone of underperfused renal parenchyma subtending the distribution of the occluded vessel. A wedge-shaped infarct is typically oriented with its base directed toward the renal capsule and its apex toward the renal hilus (147).

Thrombosis of the renal artery is preceded by intimal tearing. Disruption of the intima leads to dissection, arterial stenosis, and, finally, clot formation. Often the injury is detected only after the occlusion. Contrast-enhanced helical CT has been reported to detect asymmetric renal enhancement secondary to renal artery dissection, enabling stenting or reconstruction of the lesion prior to thrombosis (90,320).

Renal vein injury occurs in 20% of patients with solitary pedicle injury (112). Acute renal vein occlusion may produce an enlarged rather than a normal-sized kidney, and associated cortical rim enhancement is usually thicker than with arterial obstruction (148). Demonstration of thrombus within a dilated renal vein on CT confirms the diagnosis (23). Venography may be required to detect venous lacerations (213).

CT findings of massive accumulation of extravasated urine in the medial rather than dorsolateral aspect of the perirenal space, absence of renal parenchymal injury, and lack of ureteral opacification should suggest the diagnosis of UPJ disruption (category IV injury) (214,217,388). One

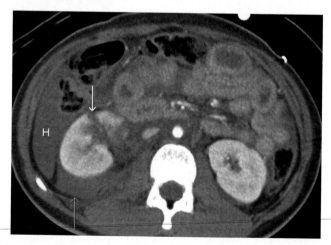

Figure 21-64   Renal laceration with perirenal hematoma. Contrast-enhanced computed tomography scan demonstrates a right renal laceration (*thick arrow*) with associated perirenal hematoma confined by the posterior renal (Gerota's) fascia (*thin arrow*). The patient also has intraperitoneal blood (H) from a ruptured spleen.

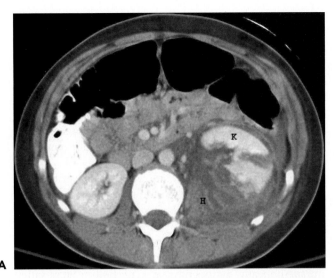

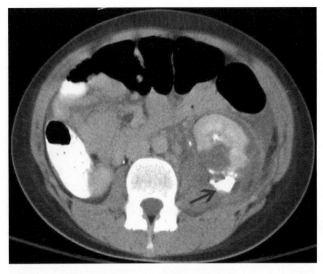

A B

Figure 21-65 Renal fracture. **A:** Contrast-enhanced computed tomography scan demonstrates fractured left lower renal pole (K) with large perirenal hematoma (H). **B:** Delayed scan shows extravasation of opacified urine into the perirenal space (*arrow*).

study found that UPJ injury was missed at the authors' institution because the scan delay following IV contrast material administration was too short (approximately 45 to 60 seconds) to allow for opacification of the renal collecting system (38). Repeat scans upon completion of the initial scans consistently revealed the UPJ disruptions. Thus, delayed scans at 5 to 15 min after the IV administration of contrast material are recommended to adequately evaluate for UPJ injury (213,309,347,462). Retrograde ureteropyelography should be performed to confirm the diagnosis prior to surgical correction.

Ureter

Iatrogenic trauma secondary to surgical procedures is the leading cause of ureteral injury (237). Penetrating and blunt trauma account for a relatively small number of ureteral injuries. When present, they commonly are associated with renal parenchymal, arterial, and venous injuries (444). Most reported cases are hyperextension injuries sustained by children in motor vehicle collisions. CT findings of isolated ureteral disruption in adults include nonvisualization of the ureter distal to the point of disruption, intact

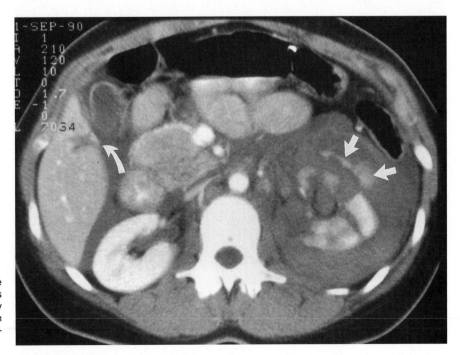

Figure 21-66 Shattered kidney with large perirenal hematoma. Active bleeding is noted in the left perirenal space anteriorly (*straight arrows*). Small liver laceration (*curved arrow*) and blood in the hepatorenal fossa are also evident.

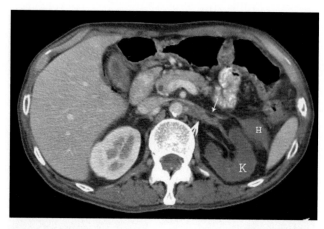

Figure 21-67 Renal pedicle injury with devascularization of the left kidney. Computed tomography scan at the level of the left renal hilum demonstrates absent perfusion of the left kidney **(K)**. Blood tracks along an unenhanced left renal artery (*thick arrow*). A diminutive left renal vein (*thin arrow*) and a small amount of hemorrhage **(H)** in the left anterior pararenal space are also noted. (Case courtesy of Kevin Smith, M.D., Birmingham, Alabama.)

renal parenchyma, and confinement of extravasated urine to the medial perirenal space (217). In children, however, the urine extravasation also expands into leaves of the renal fascia, anterior pararenal space, and the psoas compartment (404).

Bladder

Bladder injuries may occur as a result of blunt, penetrating, or iatrogenic trauma. The susceptibility of the bladder to injury varies with the degree of distension; a distended urinary bladder is much more prone to injury than a nearly empty one. Most patients with bladder rupture complain of suprapubic pain or tenderness; however, the discomfort associated with a fractured bony pelvis often obscures the pain associated with the urinary tract injury. Gross hematuria almost invariably accompanies bladder injury. In one reported series (330), 95% of patients with bladder rupture had gross hematuria and the remainder had microscopic hematuria.

The type of urine extravasation (intraperitoneal or extraperitoneal) is dependent on the location of the bladder tear and its relationship to the peritoneal reflections (375). With an anterosuperior perforation, extravasation may be either intraperitoneal, into the prevesical space (space of Retzius), or both. With a posterosuperior tear, fluid can spread intraperitoneally, retroperitoneally, or both. Extravasation may also extend inferiorly into the perineum, the scrotum, and the thigh, if the urogenital diaphragm is disrupted.

Intraperitoneal rupture usually results from a direct blow (often a kick) to a distended bladder and requires surgical repair. Extraperitoneal rupture often results from a shearing injury at the base of the bladder and is best treated with suprapubic cystostomy (67). If extraperitoneal rupture occurs in the setting of pelvic fracture requiring internal fixation, however, the rupture may be surgically repaired to protect the orthopedic hardware from extravasated urine and potential infection (83).

Radiographic evaluation of the lower urinary tract is warranted in cases of gross hematuria with pelvic fracture, gross hematuria with unexplained pelvic fluid, or signs of

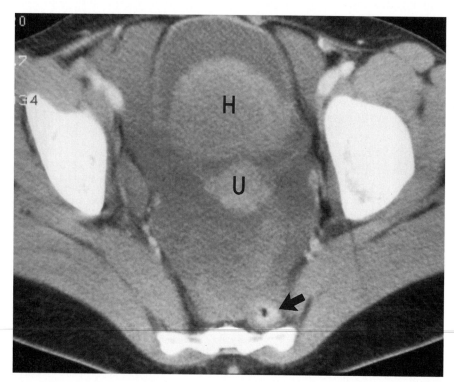

Figure 21-68 Bladder hematoma. There is a large mural hematoma **(H)** involving the bladder base. A large amount of blood is also seen filling the pelvis. Note the hematocrit effect with denser blood elements layering posteriorly adjacent to the rectum (*arrow*). The patient had multiple liver lacerations on computed tomography scans of the abdomen. U, uterus.

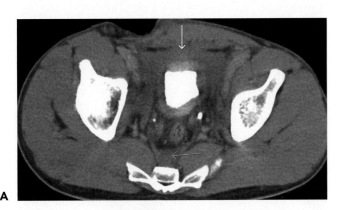

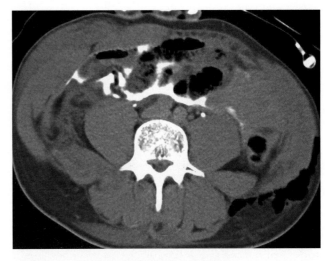

Figure 21-69 Intraperitoneal bladder rupture. **A:** Image through the pelvis from a computed tomography cystogram demonstrates diffusely thickened bladder wall. Blood is seen both in the presacral space (*thin arrow*) and prevesical space (*arrow*). **B:** Image through the lower abdomen shows extravasated iodinated contrast material outlining the bowel loops.

perineal trauma, such as voiding difficulties, bleeding from the urethra, perineal hematoma, or elevation of the prostate on digital exam (304,306,462). One study found that certain pelvic fractures, including pubic symphysis diastasis, sacroiliac diastasis, and sacral, iliac, and pubic rami fractures, were significantly associated with bladder rupture (306). CT cystography has replaced conventional cystography as the study of choice for suspected bladder injury and can be done in concert with CT evaluation of associated injuries. If urethral trauma is suspected, a retrograde urethrogram should precede CT cystography.

Although conventional CT has performed poorly in the diagnosis of bladder rupture (164,189,332), several studies have demonstrated that properly executed CT cystography is as sensitive for detecting bladder injuries as conventional cystography (183,210,250,339,453). In one cohort of 316 patients, the authors reported overall sensitivity and specificity of CT cystography as 95% and 100% respectively for detection of surgically-confirmed bladder rupture (82,83). Intraperitoneal rupture was diagnosed with a sensitivity of 78% and a specificity of 99%. Reasons for a false–negative CT cystogram include inadequate bladder distension, the presence of hematoma or tissue edema preventing extravasation, misinterpretation, overly dilute contrast material, and poor quality scans (82,164). To minimize false–negative CT diagnosis of bladder rupture, scans of the pelvis should be obtained with the urinary bladder fully distended either by retrograde or antegrade means (183,210,250). Antegrade distension is facilitated by clamping the urinary catheter once satisfactory urine output has been established (462). Retrograde bladder filling can be accomplished by instillation of 300 to 400 mL of 2% to 4% contrast material. Filling with less than 250 mL can result in false–negative

scans. Both delayed scans and repeat scanning of the pelvis after bladder drainage have been used to help detect subtle bladder injury (183,210,407), although their usefulness and practicality have been debated (306).

MDCT has been used in nontrauma patients to perform virtual cystoscopy. One recent study compared the findings of virtual cystoscopy with those of conventional cystoscopy in patients with gross hematuria (221). The sensitivity and specificity of virtual cystoscopy were 95% and 93% for detecting abnormal bladders. This technology may prove useful for detecting subtle bladder injury.

Angiography plays no role in the primary assessment of bladder injury but may be of considerable value in the diagnosis and management of arterial bleeding associated with pelvic fractures. Radionuclide scintigraphy can detect small amounts of extravasation with great sensitivity, but because of its inferior spatial resolution compared with conventional radiography and CT it is rarely used in assessing cases of bladder trauma. Although ultrasonography also may demonstrate lacerations of the urinary bladder (464), it is not widely used in the United States for this purpose. Testing diagnostic peritoneal lavage fluid for elevated creatinine has been useful in the diagnosis of intraperitoneal rupture that may be overlooked on CT (81).

Different types of bladder injuries can be identified and differentiated from one another on CT (453). Bladder contusion or hematoma appears as focal or diffuse wall thickening without extravasation of contrast medium (Fig. 21-68). With intraperitoneal rupture of the bladder, extravasated urine and contrast medium can be found surrounding the bladder or bowel and pooling in the paracolic gutters (375) (Fig. 21-69). Extraperitoneal rupture results in extravasation of

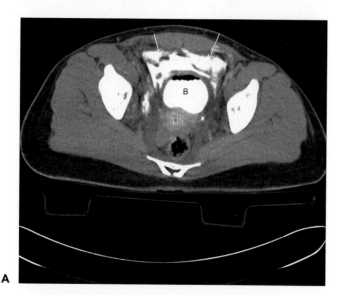

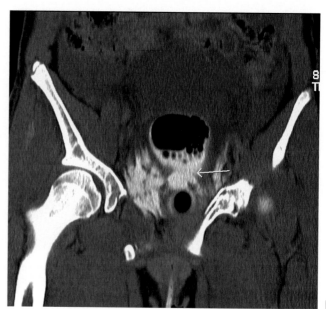

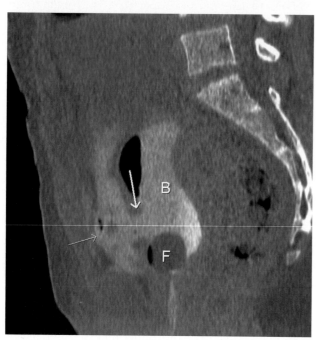

Figure 21-70   Extraperitoneal bladder rupture. **A:** Transaxial image from a computed tomography cystogram demonstrates extravasation of iodinated contrast material (*arrows*) from the urinary bladder (B) into the extraperitoneal prevesical space. U, uterus. **B:** Coronal image demonstrates the site of bladder rupture (*arrow*). Multiple pelvic fractures are present. **C:** Sagittal image clearly shows the size and site (*thick arrow*) of the contrast extravasation from the urinary bladder (B) into the prevesical space (*thin arrow*). F, Foley balloon.

contrast medium and urine into the prevesical fat, anterior thigh, scrotum, penis, and abdominal wall (Fig. 21-70). Contrast medium also can extend cephalad to the perirenal and pararenal spaces (375). Distinguishing intraperitoneal from extraperitoneal rupture can be difficult in some cases. Care must be taken when posteriorly extravasated contrast media from extraperitoneal rupture appears contiguous with intraperitoneal pelvic fluid because the separating peritoneum is so thin (387).

REFERENCES

1. National Center for Injury Prevention and Control. Available at: http://webapp.cdc.gov/cgi-bin/broker.exe.
2. Abramson SJ, Berdon WE, Kaufman RA, et al. Hepatic parenchymal and subcapsular gas after hepatic laceration caused by blunt abdominal trauma. *AJR Am J Roentgenol* 1989;153:1031–1032.
3. Abu-Zidan FM, Sheikh M, Jadallah F, et al. Blunt abdominal trauma: comparison of ultrasonography and computed tomography in a district general hospital. *Australas Radiol* 1999;43: 440–443.

4. Agee CK, Metzler MH, Churchill RJ, et al. Computed tomographic evaluation to exclude traumatic aortic disruption. *J Trauma* 1992;33:876–881.

5. Akhrass R, Yaffe MB, Brandt CP, et al. Pancreatic trauma: a ten-year multi-institutional experience. *Am Surg* 1997;63:598–604.

6. Alkadhi H, Wildermuth S, Desbiolles L, et al. Vascular emergencies of the thorax after iatrogenic trauma: multi-detector row CT and three-dimensional imaging. *Radiographics* 2004;24:1239–1255.

7. Allen GS, Moore FA, Cox CS Jr, et al. Delayed diagnosis of blunt duodenal injury: an avoidable complication. *J Am Coll Surg* 1998;187:393–399.

8. Aronchick JM, Epstein DM, Gefter WE, et al. Chronic traumatic diaphragmatic hernia: the significance of pleural effusion. *Radiology* 1988;168:675–678.

9. Aseervatham R, Muller M. Blunt trauma to the spleen. *Aust N Z J Surg* 2000;70:333–337.

10. Ayella RJ, Hankins JR, Turney SZ, et al. Ruptured thoracic aorta due to blunt trauma. *J Trauma* 1977;17:199–205.

11. Bach RD, Frey CF. Diagnosis and treatment of pancreatic trauma. *Am J Surg* 1971;121:20–29.

12. Backer CL, LoCicero J, Hartz RS, et al. Computed tomography in patients with esophageal perforation. *Chest* 1990;98:1078–1080.

13. Ball T, McCrory R, Smith JO, et al. Traumatic diaphragmatic hernia: errors in diagnosis. *AJR Am J Roentgenol* 1982;138:633–637.

14. Ballard RB, Badellino MM, Eynon CA, et al. Blunt duodenal rupture: a 6-year statewide experience. *J Trauma* 1997;43:229–232; discussion 233.

15. Barcia TC, Livoni JP. Indications for angiography in blunt thoracic trauma. *Radiology* 1983;147:15–19.

16. Baxt WG, Moody P. The impact of a rotorcraft aeromedical emergency care service on trauma mortality. *JAMA* 1983;249:3047–3051.

17. Becker CD, Gal I, Baer HU, et al. Blunt hepatic trauma in adults: correlation of CT injury grading with outcome. *Radiology* 1996;201:215–220.

18. Becker CD, Mentha G, Schmidlin F, et al. Blunt abdominal trauma in adults: role of CT in the diagnosis and management of visceral injuries. Part 2: gastrointestinal tract and retroperitoneal organs. *Eur Radiol* 1998;8:772–780.

19. Becker CD, Mentha G, Terrier F. Blunt abdominal trauma in adults: role of CT in the diagnosis and management of visceral injuries. Part 1: liver and spleen. *Eur Radiol* 1998;8:553–562.

20. Bennett, DE, Cherry, JK. The natural history of traumatic aneurysms of the aorta. *Surgery* 1967;61:516–523.

21. Benya EC, Bulas DI, Eichelberger MR, et al. Splenic injury from blunt abdominal trauma in children: follow-up evaluation with CT. *Radiology* 1995;195:685–688.

22. Bergin D, Ennis R, Keogh C, et al. The "dependent viscera" sign in CT diagnosis of blunt traumatic diaphragmatic rupture. *AJR Am J Roentgenol* 2001;177:1137–1140.

23. Berkovich GY, Ramchandani P, Preate DL Jr, et al. Renal vein thrombosis after martial arts trauma. *J Trauma* 2001;50:144–145.

24. Berland LL. CT of blunt abdominal trauma. In: Fishman EK, Federle MP, eds. *Body CT categorical course syllabus.* New Orleans, LA: American Roentgen Ray Society, 1994:207–214.

25. Bigattini D, Boverie JH, Dondelinger RF. CT of blunt trauma of the pancreas in adults. *Eur Radiol* 1999;9:244–249.

26. Black WC, Gouse JC, Williamson BR, et al. Computed tomography of traumatic lung cyst: case report. *J Comput Tomogr* 1986;10:33–35.

27. Bladergroen MR, Lowe JE, Postlethwait RW. Diagnosis and recommended management of esophageal perforation and rupture. *Ann Thorac Surg* 1986;42:235–239.

28. Blair E, Topuzlu C, Davis JH. Delayed or missed diagnosis in blunt chest trauma. *J Trauma* 1971;11:129–145.

29. Boulanger BR, Mirvis SE, Rodriguez A. Magnetic resonance imaging in traumatic diaphragmatic rupture: case reports. *J Trauma* 1992;32:89–93.

30. Boyd AD. Pneumothorax and hemothorax. In: Hood RM, Boyd AD, Culliford AT, eds. *Thoracic trauma,* ed.[SD4] Philadelphia, PA: WB Saunders, 1989:133–148.

31. Brandes SB, McAninch JW. Urban free falls and patterns of renal injury: a 20-year experience with 396 cases. *J Trauma* 1999;47:643–649; discussion 649–650.

32. Brasel KJ, Stafford RE, Weigelt JA, et al. Treatment of occult pneumothoraces from blunt trauma. *J Trauma* 1999;46:987–990; discussion 990–991.

33. Breen DJ, Janzen DL, Zwirewich CV, et al. Blunt bowel and mesenteric injury: diagnostic performance of CT signs. *J Comput Assist Tomogr* 1997;21:706–712.

34. Bridges KG, Welch G, Silver M, et al. CT detection of occult pneumothorax in multiple trauma patients. *J Emerg Med* 1993;11:179–186.

35. Brooks AP, Olson LK. Computed tomography of the chest in the trauma patient. *Clin Radiol* 1989;40:127–132.

36. Brower P, Paul J, Brosman SA. Urinary tract abnormalities presenting as a result of blunt abdominal trauma. *J Trauma* 1978;18:719–722.

37. Brown RA, Bass DH, Rode H, et al. Gastrointestinal tract perforation in children due to blunt abdominal trauma. *Br J Surg* 1992;79:522–524.

38. Brown SL, Hoffman DM, Spirnak JP. Limitations of routine spiral computerized tomography in the evaluation of blunt renal trauma. *J Urol* 1998;160:1979–1981.

39. Bulas DI, Eichelberger MR, Sivit CJ, et al. Hepatic injury from blunt trauma in children: follow-up evaluation with CT. *AJR Am J Roentgenol* 1993;160:347–351.

40. Bulas DI, Taylor GA, Eichelberger MR. The value of CT in detecting bowel perforation in children after blunt abdominal trauma. *AJR Am J Roentgenol* 1989;153:561–564.

41. Buntain WL, Gould HR, Maull KI. Predictability of splenic salvage by computed tomography. *J Trauma* 1988;28:24–34.

42. Burgess P, Fulton L. Gallbladder and extrahepatic biliary duct injury following abdominal trauma. *Injury* 1992;23:413–414.

43. Burney RE, Mueller GL, Coon GL, et al. Diagnosis of isolated small bowel injury. *Ann Emerg Med* 1983;12:71–74.

44. Butela ST, Federle MP, Chang PJ, et al. Performance of CT in detection of bowel injury. *AJR Am J Roentgenol* 2001;176:129–135.

45. Caoili EM, Cohan RH, Korobkin M, et al. Urinary tract abnormalities: initial experience with multi-detector row CT urography. *Radiology* 2002;222:353–360.

46. Cass AS. Discussion. In: Guerriero, WG, ed. *Problems in urology,* Philadelphia, PA: Lippincott Williams & Wilkins, 1988:184.

47. Cates JD, Foley WD, Lawson TL. Retrograde opacification of renal vein: a CT sign of renal artery avulsion. *Urol Radiol* 1986;8:92–94.

48. Ceraldi CM, Waxman K. Computerized tomography as an indicator of isolated mesenteric injury: a comparison with peritoneal lavage. *Am Surg* 1990;56:806–810.

49. Chai RY, Jhaveri K, Saini S, et al. Comprehensive evaluation of patients with haematuria on multi-slice computed tomography scanner: protocol design and preliminary observations. *Australas Radiol* 2001;45:536–538.

50. Champion MP, Richards CA, Boddy SA, et al. Duodenal perforation: a diagnostic pitfall in non-accidental injury. *Arch Dis Child* 2002;87:432–433.

51. Chapman WC, Morris JA. Diagnosis and management of blunt pancreatic injury. *J Tenn Med Assoc* 1989;82:84–85.

52. Chen X, Talner LB, Jurkovich GJ. Gallbladder avulsion due to blunt trauma. *AJR Am J Roentgenol* 2001;177:822.

53. Chew FS, Panicek DM, Heitzman ER. Late discovery of a posttraumatic right aortic arch aneurysm. *AJR Am J Roentgenol* 1985;145:1001–1002.

54. Chiles C, Putman CE. Acute thoracic trauma. In: Goodman LR, Putman CE, eds. *Critical care imaging,* 3rd ed. Philadelphia, PA: WB Saunders, 1992:199–212.

55. Cholankeril JV, Zamora BO, Ketyer S. Left lobe of the liver draping around the spleen: a pitfall in computed tomography diagnosis of perisplenic hematoma. *J Comput Tomogr* 1984;8:261–267.

56. Chowdhary SK, Pimpalwar A, Narasimhan KL, et al. Blunt injury of the abdomen: a plea for CT. *Pediatr Radiol* 2000;30:798–800.

57. Clancy TV, Ragozzino MW, Ramshaw D, et al. Oral contrast is not necessary in the evaluation of blunt abdominal trauma by computed tomography. *Am J Surg* 1993;166:680–684; discussion 684–685.

58. Clark DE, Zeiger MA, Wallace KL, et al. Blunt aortic trauma: signs of high risk. *J Trauma* 1990;30:701–705.

59. Cogbill TH, Moore EE, Jurkovich GJ, et al. Nonoperative management of blunt splenic trauma: a multicenter experience. *J Trauma* 1989;29:1312–1317.

60. Cogbill TH, Moore EE, Morris JAJ, et al. Distal pancreatectomy for trauma: a multicenter experience. *J Trauma* 1991;31:1600–1606.

61. Cohen AM, Crass JR. Traumatic aortic injuries: current concepts. *Semin Ultrasound CT MR* 1993;14:71–84.

62. Cohen AM, Crass JR, Thomas HA, et al. CT evidence for the "osseous pinch" mechanism of traumatic aortic injury. *AJR Am J Roentgenol* 1992;159:271–274.

63. Cohn SM. Pulmonary contusion: review of the clinical entity. *J Trauma* 1997;42:973–979.

64. Collins J. Chest wall trauma. *J Thorac Imaging* 2000;15:112–119.

65. Collins JC, Levine G, Waxman K. Occult traumatic pneumothorax: immediate tube thoracostomy versus expectant management. *Am Surg* 1992;58:743–746.

66. Cook DE, Walsh JW, Vick CW, et al. Upper abdominal trauma: pitfalls in CT diagnosis. *Radiology* 1986;159:65–69.

67. Corriere JN, Sandler CM. Mechanisms of injury: patterns of extravasation and management of extraperitoneal bladder rupture due to blunt trauma. *J Urol* 1987;139:43–44.

68. Cowley RA, Turney SZ, Hankins JR, et al. Rupture of thoracic aorta caused by blunt trauma. A fifteen-year experience. *J Thorac Cardiovasc Surg* 1990;100:652–661.

69. Cox JF, Friedman AC, Radecki PD, et al. Periportal lymphedema in trauma patients. *AJR Am J Roentgenol* 1990;154:1124–1125.

70. Cox TD, Kuhn JP. CT scan of bowel trauma in the pediatric patient. *Radiol Clin North Am* 1996;34:807–818.

71. Cozacov C, Krausz L, Freund U. Emergencies in delayed diaphragmatic herniation due to blunt trauma. *Injury* 1984;15:370–371.

72. Craig MH, Talton DS, Hauser CJ, et al. Pancreatic injuries from blunt trauma. *Am Surg* 1995;61:125–128.

73. Crass JR, Cohen AM, Motta AO, et al. A proposed new mechanism of traumatic aortic rupture: the osseous pinch. *Radiology* 1990;176:645–649.

74. Croce MA, Fabian TC, Kudsk KA, et al. AAST organ injury scale: correlation of CT-graded liver injuries and operative findings. *J Trauma* 1991;31:806–812.

75. Croce MA, Fabian TC, Menke PG, et al. Nonoperative management of blunt hepatic trauma is the treatment of choice for hemodynamically stable patients: results of a prospective trial. *Ann Surg* 1995;221:744–755.

76. Cruz CJ, Minagi H. Large-bowel obstruction resulting from traumatic diaphragmatic hernia: imaging findings in four cases. *AJR Am J Roentgenol* 1994;162:843–845.

77. Curtin JJ, Goodman LR, Quebbeman EJ, et al. Thoracostomy tubes after acute chest injury: relationship between location in a pleural fissure and function. *AJR Am J Roentgenol* 1994;163:1339–1342.

78. Daniels DL, Maddison FE. Ascending aortic injury: an angiographic diagnosis. *AJR Am J Roentgenol* 1981;136:812–813.

79. Dauterive AH, Flancbaum L, Cox EF. Blunt intestinal trauma: a modern day review. *Ann Surg* 1985;201:198–203.

80. De Backer AI, De Schepper AM, Vaneerdeweg W, et al. Intestinal stenosis from mesenteric injury after blunt abdominal trauma. *Eur Radiol* 1999;9:1429–1431.

81. Deck AJ, Porter JR. Diagnostic peritoneal lavage as sole indicator of intraperitoneal bladder rupture: case report. *J Trauma* 2000;49: 946–947.

82. Deck AJ, Shaves S, Talner L, et al. Computerized tomography cystography for the diagnosis of traumatic bladder rupture. *J Urol* 2000;164:43–46.

83. Deck AJ, Shaves S, Talner L, et al. Current experience with computed tomographic cystography and blunt trauma. *World J Surg* 2001;25:1592–1596.

84. Delgado Millan MA, Deballon PO. Computed tomography, angiography, and endoscopic retrograde cholangiopancreatography in the nonoperative management of hepatic and splenic trauma. *World J Surg* 2001;25:1397–1402.

85. Denis R, Allard M, Atlas H, et al. Changing trends with abdominal injury in seatbelt wearers. *J Trauma* 1983;23:1007–1008.

86. Dennis LN, Rogers LF. Superior mediastinal widening from spine fractures mimicking aortic rupture on chest radiographs. *AJR Am J Roentgenol* 1989;152:27–30.

87. Desai KM, Dorward IG, Minkes RK, et al. Blunt duodenal injuries in children. *J Trauma* 2003;54:640–645; discussion 645–646.

88. Dinkel HP, Danuser H, Triller J. Blunt renal trauma: minimally invasive management with microcatheter embolization experience in nine patients. *Radiology* 2002;223:723–730.

89. Do HM, Cronan JJ. CT appearance of splenic injuries managed nonoperatively. *AJR Am J Roentgenol* 1991;157:757–760.

90. Dobrilovic N, Bennett S, Smith C, et al. Traumatic renal artery dissection identified with dynamic helical computed tomography. *J Vasc Surg* 2001;34:562–564.

91. Dodds WJ, Taylor AJ, Erickson SJ, et al. Traumatic fracture of the pancreas: CT characteristics. *J Comput Assist Tomogr* 1990;14:375–378.

92. Dondelinger RF, Trotteur G, Ghaye B, et al. Traumatic injuries: radiological hemostatic intervention at admission. *Eur Radiol* 2002;12:979–993.

93. Donohue JH, Crass RA, Trunkey DD. The management of duodenal and other small intestinal trauma. *World J Surg* 1985;9:904–913.

94. Donohue JH, Federle MP, Griffiths BG, et al. Computed tomography in the diagnosis of blunt intestinal and mesenteric injuries. *J Trauma* 1987;27:11–17.

95. Donovan AJ, Turrill F, Berne CJ. Injuries of the pancreas from blunt trauma. *Surg Clin North Am* 1972;52:649–665.

96. Dougall AM, Paul ME, Finley RJ, et al. Chest trauma: current morbidity and mortality. *J Trauma* 1977;17:547–553.

97. Dow RW. Myocardial rupture caused by trauma. *Surgery* 1982;91: 246–247.

98. Dowe MF, Shanmuganathan K, Mirvis SE, et al. CT findings of mesenteric injury after blunt abdominal trauma: implications for surgical intervention. *AJR Am J Roentgenol* 1997;168:425–428.

99. Dowe MF, Shanmuganathan K, Mirvis SE, et al. CT findings of mesenteric injury after blunt trauma: implications for surgical intervention. *AJR Am J Roentgenol* 1997;168:425–428.

100. Downing SW, Sperling JS, Mirvis SE, et al. Experience with spiral computed tomography as the sole diagnostic method for traumatic aortic rupture. *Ann Thorac Surg* 2001;72:495–501; discussion 501–502.

101. Eger EI, Saidman LJ. Hazards of nitrous oxide anesthesia in bowel obstruction and pneumothorax. *Anesthesiology* 1965;26:61–66.

102. Emery KH. Lap belt iliac wing fracture: a predictor of bowel injury in children. *Pediatr Radiol* 2002;32:892–895.

103. Erickson DR, Shinozaki T, Beekman E, et al. Relationship of arterial blood gases and pulmonary radiographs to the degree of pulmonary damage in experimental pulmonary contusion. *J Trauma* 1971;11:689–696.

104. Estrera AS, Landay MJ, McClelland RN. Blunt traumatic rupture of the right hemidiaphragm: experience in 12 patients. *Ann Thorac Surg* 1985;39:525–530.

105. Evens RG. *Radiology* decision making: the importance of cost-effectiveness analysis. *AJR Am J Roentgenol* 1995;165:37.

106. Evins SC, Thomason WB, Rosenblaum R. Non-operative management of severe renal lacerations. *J Urol* 1980;123:247–249.

107. Faer MJ, Lynch RD, Lichtenstein JE, et al. Traumatic splenic cyst. *Radiology* 1980;134:371–376.

108. Fakhry SM, Brownstein M, Watts DD, et al. Relatively short diagnostic delays (<8 hours) produce morbidity and mortality in blunt small bowel injury: an analysis of time to operative intervention in 198 patients from a multicenter experience. *J Trauma* 2000;48:408–414; discussion 414–405.

109. Fakhry SM, Watts DD, Luchette FA, et al. Current diagnostic approaches lack sensitivity in the diagnosis of perforated blunt small bowel injury: analysis from 275,557 trauma admissions from the east multi-institutional HVI trial. *J Trauma* 2003;54:295–306.

110. Fang JE, Chen RJ, Wong YC, et al. Classification and treatment of pooling of contrast material on computed tomographic scan of blunt hepatic trauma. *J Trauma* 2000;49:1083–1088.

111. Fang JE, Chen RJ, Wong YC, et al. Pooling of contrast material on computed tomography mandates aggressive management of blunt hepatic injury. *Am J Surg* 1998;176:315–319.

112. Fanney DR, Casillas J, Murphy BJ. CT in the diagnosis of renal trauma. *Radiographics* 1990;10:29–40.

113. Federle MP. Computed tomography of blunt abdominal trauma. *Radiol Clin North Am* 1983;21:461–475.

114. Federle MP. CT of abdominal trauma. In: Federle MP, Brant-Zawadzki M, eds. *Computed tomography in the evaluation of trauma*, 2nd ed. Baltimore: Williams and Wilkins, 1986:191–273.

115. Federle MP. Evaluation of renal trauma. In: Pollack HM, ed. *Clinical urography*, Philadelphia, PA: WB Saunders, 1990:1472–1494.

116. Federle MP. Splenic trauma: is follow-up CT of value? *Radiology* 1995;194:23–24.

117. Federle MP. Diagnosis of intestinal injuries by computed tomography and the use of oral contrast medium. *Ann Emerg Med* 1998;31:769–771.

118. Federle MP, Courcoulas AP, Powell M, et al. Blunt splenic injury in adults: clinical and CT criteria for management, with emphasis on active extravasation. *Radiology* 1998;206:137–142.

119. Federle MP, Crass RA, Jeffrey RB, et al. Computed tomography in blunt abdominal trauma. *Arch Surg* 1982;117:645–650.

120. Federle MP, Griffiths B, Minagi H, et al. Splenic trauma: evaluation with CT. *Radiology* 1987;162:69–71.

121. Federle MP, Jeffrey RB. Hemoperitoneum studied by computed tomography. *Radiology* 1983;148:187–192.

122. Fenner MN, Fisher KS, Sergel NL, et al. Evaluation of possible traumatic thoracic aortic injury using aortography and CT. *Am Surg* 1990;56:497–499.

123. Finkelmeier BA, Mentzer RMJ, Kaiser DL, et al. Chronic traumatic thoracic aneurysm, influence of operative treatment on natural history: an analysis of reported cases, 1950-1980. *J Thorac Cardiovasc Surg* 1982;84:257–266.

124. Fisher RG, Chasen MH, Lamki N. Diagnosis of injuries of the aorta and brachiocephalic arteries caused by blunt chest trauma: CT vs aortography. *AJR Am J Roentgenol* 1994;162:1047–1052.

125. Fisher RG, Hadlock F, Ben-Menachem Y. Laceration of the thoracic aorta and brachiocephalic arteries by blunt trauma: report of 54 cases and review of the literature. *Radiol Clin North Am* 1981;19:91–110.

126. Fisher RG, Ward RE, Ben-Menachem Y, et al. Arteriography and the fractured first rib: too much for too little? *AJR Am J Roentgenol* 1982;138:1059–1062.

127. Fishman JE, Nunez D Jr, Kane A, et al. Direct versus indirect signs of traumatic aortic injury revealed by helical CT: performance characteristics and interobserver agreement. *AJR Am J Roentgenol* 1999;172:1027–1031.

128. Fitzgerald JB, Crawford ES, deBakey ME. Surgical considerations of nonpenetrating abdominal injuries. *Am J Surg* 1960;100:22–29.

129. Fleischmann D. Present and future trends in multiple detector-row CT applications: CT angiography. *Eur Radiol* 2002;12:S 11–S15.

130. Fleming WR, Collier NA, Banting SW. Pancreatic trauma: universities of Melbourne HPB Group. *Aust N Z J Surg* 1999;69:357–362.

131. Foley WD, Cates JD, Kellman GM, et al. Treatment of blunt hepatic injuries: role of CT. *Radiology* 1987;164:635–638.

132. Frey CF. Trauma to the pancreas and duodenum. In: Blaisdell FW, Trunkey DD, eds. *Abdominal trauma*, 1st ed. New York: Thieme-Stratton, 1982:87–122.

133. Frick EJ Jr, Pasquale MD, Cipolle MD. Small-bowel and mesentery injuries in blunt trauma. *J Trauma* 1999;46:920–926.

134. Fulcher AS, Turner MA, Capps GW, et al. Half-Fourier rare MR cholangiopancreatography in 300 subjects. *Radiology* 1998;207:21–32.

135. Fulda G, Rodriguez A, Turney SZ, et al. Blunt traumatic pericardial rupture: a ten-year experience 1979 to 1989. *J Cardiovasc Surg* 1990;31:525–530.

136. Garramone RR, Jacobs LM. An objective method to measure and manage occult pneumothorax. *Surg Gynecol Obstet* 1991;173:257–261.

137. Gavant ML, Flick P, Menke P, et al. CT aortography of thoracic aortic rupture. *AJR Am J Roentgenol* 1996;166:955–961.

138. Gavant ML, Menke PG, Fabian T, et al. Blunt traumatic aortic rupture: detection with helical CT of the chest. *Radiology* 1995;197:125–133.

139. Gavant ML, Schurr M, Flick PA, et al. Predicting clinical outcome of nonsurgical management of blunt splenic injury: using CT to reveal abnormalities of splenic vasculature. *AJR Am J Roentgenol* 1997;168:207–212.

140. Gay SB, Sistrom CL. Computed tomographic evaluation of blunt abdominal trauma. *Radiol Clin North Am* 1992;30:367–388.

141. Gayer G, Rozenman J, Hoffmann C, et al. CT diagnosis of malpositioned chest tubes. *Br J Radiol* 2000;73:786–790.

142. Gazak S, Davidson SJ. Posterior sternoclavicular dislocations: two case reports. *J Trauma* 1984;24:80–82.

143. Gelman R, Mirvis SE, Gens D. Diaphragmatic rupture due to blunt trauma: sensitivity of plain chest radiographs. *AJR Am J Roentgenol* 1991;156:51–57.

144. Gerblich AA, Kleinerman J. Blunt chest trauma and the lung. *Am Rev Respir Dis* 1977;115:369–370.

145. Glazer GM, Axel L, Goldberg HI, et al. Dynamic CT of the normal spleen. *AJR Am J Roentgenol* 1981;137:343–346.

146. Glazer GM, Buy JN, Moss AA, et al. CT detection of duodenal perforation. *AJR Am J Roentgenol* 1981;137:333–336.

147. Glazer GM, Francis IR, Brady TM, et al. Computed tomography of renal infarction: clinical and experimental observations. *AJR Am J Roentgenol* 1983;140:721–727.

148. Glazer GM, Francis IR, Gross BH, et al. Computed tomography of renal vein thrombosis. *J Comput Assist Tomogr* 1984;8:288–293.

149. Godwin JD, Merten DF, Baker ME. Paramediastinal pneumatocele: alternative explanations to gas in the pulmonary ligament. *AJR Am J Roentgenol* 1985;145:525–530.

150. Goff CD, Collin GR. Management of renal trauma at a rural, level I trauma center. *Am Surg* 1998;64:226–230.

151. Goldberg AL, Rothfus WE, Deeb ZL, et al. The impact of magnetic resonance on the diagnostic evaluation of acute cervicothoracic spinal trauma. *Skeletal Radiol* 1988;17:89–95.

152. Goldstein L, Mirvis SE, Kostrubiak IS, et al. CT diagnosis of acute pericardial tamponade after blunt chest trauma. *AJR Am J Roentgenol* 1989;152:739–741.

153. Gonzalez RP, Ickler J, Gachassin P. Complementary roles of diagnostic peritoneal lavage and computed tomography in the evaluation of blunt abdominal trauma. *J Trauma* 2001;51:1128–1134; discussion 1134–1126.

154. Goodman PC. CT of chest trauma. In: Federle MP, Brant-Zawadzki M, eds. *Computed tomography in the evaluation of trauma*, 2nd ed. Baltimore, MD: Lippincott Williams & Wilkins, 1986:168–190.

155. Graivier L, Freeark RJ. Traumatic diaphragmatic hernia. *Arch Surg* 1963;86:363–373.

156. Grassi R, Pinto A, Rossi G, et al. Conventional plain-film radiology, ultrasonography and CT in jejuno-ileal perforation. *Acta Radiol* 1998;39:52–56.

157. Greendyke RM. Traumatic rupture of aorta: special reference to automobile accidents. *JAMA* 1966;195:119–122.

158. Greene R. Blunt thoracic trauma. In: Radiological Society of North America, ed. *Syllabus: a categorical course in diagnostic radiology—chest radiology*. Oak Brook, IL: RSNA Publications, 1992:297–309.

159. Grimes OF. Nonpenetrating injuries to the chest wall and esophagus. *Surg Clin North Am* 1972;52:597–609.

160. Groskin SA. Selected topics in chest trauma. *Radiology* 1992;183:605–617.

161. Guerriero WG. Genitourinary trauma. In: Guerriero WG, ed. *Problems in urology*. Philadelphia, PA: Lippincott Williams & Wilkins,[SD10] 1988:186–187.

162. Gundry SR, Williams S, Burney RE, et al. Indications for aortography. Radiography after blunt chest trauma: a reassessment of the radiographic findings associated with traumatic rupture of the aorta. *Invest Radiol* 1983;18:230–237.

163. Gupta A, Stuhlfaut JW, Fleming KW, et al. Blunt trauma of the pancreas and biliary tract: a multimodality imaging approach to diagnosis. *Radiographics* 2004;24:1381–1395.

164. Haas CA, Brown SL, Spirnak JP. Limitations of routine spiral computerized tomography in the evaluation of bladder trauma. *J Urol* 1999;162:51–52.

165. Haas CA, Newman J, Spirnak JP. Computed tomography three-dimensional reconstruction in the diagnosis of traumatic renal artery thrombosis. *Urology* 1999;54:559–560.

166. Hagiwara A, Sakaki S, Goto H, et al. The role of interventional *radiology* in the management of blunt renal injury: a practical protocol. *J Trauma* 2001;51:526–531.

167. Hai MA, Pontes JE, Pierce JM. Surgical management of major renal trauma: a review of 102 cases treated by conservative surgery. *J Urol* 1977;118:7–9.

168. Hara H, Babyn PS, Bourgeois D. Significance of bowel wall enhancement on CT following blunt abdominal trauma in childhood. *J Comput Assist Tomogr* 1992;16:94–98.

169. Harris AC, Zwirewich CV, Lyburn ID, et al. CT findings in blunt renal trauma. *Radiographics* 2001;21:S201–S214.

170. Harris HW, Morabito DJ, Mackersie RC, et al. Leukocytosis and free fluid are important indicators of isolated intestinal injury after blunt trauma. *J Trauma* 1999;46:656–659.

171. Hegarty MM, Bryer JV, Angorn IB, et al. Delayed presentation of traumatic diaphragmatic hernia. *Ann Surg* 1978;188:229–233.

172. Heiberg E, Wolverson MK. CT of traumatic injuries of the aorta. *Semin Ultrasound CT MR* 1985;6:172–180.

173. Heiberg E, Wolverson MK, Hurd RN, et al. CT recognition of traumatic rupture of the diaphragm. *AJR Am J Roentgenol* 1980;135:369–372.

174. Heiberg E, Wolverson MK, Sundaram M, et al. CT in aortic trauma. *AJR Am J Roentgenol* 1983;140:1119–1124.

175. Henry DA. Thoracic trauma: radiologic triage of the chest radiograph. In: American Roentgen Ray Society. *Syllabus, categorical course on chest radiology.* American Roentgen Ray Society 1986:13–22.

176. Heystraten FM, Rosenbusch G, Kingma LM, et al. Chronic post-traumatic aneurysm of the thoracic aorta: surgically correctable occult threat. *AJR Am J Roentgenol* 1986;146:303–308.

177. Hill LD. Injuries of the diaphragm following blunt trauma. *Surg Clin North Am* 1972;52:611–624.

178. Hiraide A, Yamamoto H, Yahata K, et al. Delayed rupture of the spleen caused by an intrasplenic pseudoaneurysm following blunt trauma: case report. *J Trauma* 1994;36:743–744.

179. Holland DG, Quint LE. Traumatic rupture of the diaphragm without visceral herniation: CT diagnosis. *AJR Am J Roentgenol* 1991;157:17–18.

180. Holmes JF, Brant WE, Bogren HG, et al. Prevalence and importance of pneumothoraces visualized on abdominal computed tomographic scan in children with blunt trauma. *J Trauma* 2001;50:516–520.

181. Holness R, Waxman K. Diagnosis of traumatic cardiac contusion utilizing single photon-emission computed tomography. *Crit Care Med* 1990;18:1–3.

182. Hood RM, Sloan HE. Injuries of the trachea and major bronchi. *J Thorac Cardiovasc Surg* 1959;38:458–480.

183. Horstman WG, McClennan BL, Heiken JP. Comparison of computed tomography and conventional cystography for detection of traumatic bladder rupture. *Urol Radiol* 1991;12:188–193.

184. Horton KM, Fishman EK. Multi-detector row CT of mesenteric ischemia: can it be done? *Radiographics* 2001;21:1463–1473.

185. Horton KM, Fishman EK. Volume-rendered 3D CT of the mesenteric vasculature: normal anatomy, anatomic variants, and pathologic conditions. *Radiographics* 2002;22:161–172.

186. Horton KM, Fishman EK. The current status of multidetector row CT and three-dimensional imaging of the small bowel. *Radiol Clin North Am* 2003;41:199–212.

187. Hossack KF, Moreno CA, Vanway CW, et al. Frequency of cardiac contusion in nonpenetrating chest injury. *Am J Cardiol* 1988;61:391–394.

188. Howell HS, Bartizal JF, Freeark RJ. Blunt trauma involving the colon and rectum. *J Trauma* 1976;16:624–632.

189. Hsieh CH, Chen RJ, Fang JF, et al. Diagnosis and management of bladder injury by trauma surgeons. *Am J Surg* 2002;184:143–147.

190. Hu H. Multi-slice helical CT: scan and reconstruction. *Med Phys* 1999;26:5–18.

191. Hughes JJ, Brogdon BG. Computed tomography of duodenal hematoma. *J Comput Tomogr* 1986;10:231–236.

192. Hughes TM. The diagnosis of gastrointestinal tract injuries resulting from blunt trauma. *Aust N Z J Surg* 1999;69:770–777.

193. Hughes TM, Elton C, Hitos K, et al. Intra-abdominal gastrointestinal tract injuries following blunt trauma: the experience of an Australian trauma centre. *Injury* 2002;33:617–626.

194. Hunink MGM, Bos JJ. Triage of patients to angiography for detection of aortic rupture after blunt chest trauma: cost-effectiveness analysis of using CT. *AJR Am J Roentgenol* 1995;165:27–36.

195. Hunter AR. Problems of anesthesia in artificial pneumothorax. *Proc R Soc Med* 1955;48:765–768.

196. Ilahi O, Bochicchio GV, Scalea TM. Efficacy of computed tomography in the diagnosis of pancreatic injury in adult blunt trauma patients: a single-institutional study. *Am Surg* 2002;68:704–707; discussion 707–708.

197. Iochum S, Ludig T, Walter F, et al. Imaging of diaphragmatic injury: a diagnostic challenge? *Radiographics* 2002;22:S103–S116; discussion S116–S118.

198. Ishikawa T, Nakajima Y, Kaji T. The role of CT in traumatic rupture of the thoracic aorta and its proximal branches. *Semin Roentgenol* 1989;24:38–46.

199. Israel RS, McDaniel PA, Primack SL, et al. Diagnosis of diaphragmatic trauma with helical CT in a swine model. *AJR Am J Roentgenol* 1996;167:637–641.

200. Janzen DL, Zwirewich CV, Breen DJ, et al. Diagnostic accuracy of helical CT for detection of blunt bowel and mesenteric injuries. *Clin Radiol* 1998;53:193–197.

201. Jeffrey RB. CT diagnosis of blunt hepatic and splenic injuries: a look to the future. *Radiology* 1989;171:17–18.

202. Jeffrey RB, Cardoza JD, Olcott EW. Detection of active intraabdominal arterial hemorrhage: value of dynamic contrast-enhanced CT. *AJR Am J Roentgenol* 1991;156:725–729.

203. Jeffrey RB, Federle MP. The collapsed inferior vena cava: CT evidence of hypovolemia. *AJR Am J Roentgenol* 1988;150:431–432.

204. Jeffrey RB, Federle MP, Crass RA. Computed tomography of pancreatic trauma. *Radiology* 1983;147:491–494.

205. Jeffrey RB, Olcott EW. Imaging of blunt hepatic trauma. *Radiol Clin North Am* 1991;29:1299–1310.

206. Johnson D, Hamer DB. Perforation of the transverse colon as a result of minor blunt abdominal trauma. *Injury* 1997;28:421–423.

207. Jones RC. Management of pancreatic trauma. *Am J Surg* 1985;150:698–704.

208. Jones RC, Shires GT. Pancreatic trauma. *Arch Surg* 1971;102:424–430.

209. Jurkovich GJ. Injuries to the duodenum and pancreas. In: Feliciano DV, Moore EE, Mattox KL, eds. *Trauma*, 3rd ed. Stamford, CT: Appleton and Lange, 1996:573–594.

210. Kane NM, Francis IR, Ellis JH. The value of CT in the detection of bladder and posterior urethral injuries. *AJR Am J Roentgenol* 1989;153:1243–1246.

211. Kato R, Horinouchi H, Maenaka Y. Traumatic pulmonary pseudocyst. Report of twelve cases. *J Thorac Cardiovasc Surg* 1989;97:309–312.

212. Kawashima A, Sandler CM, Corl FM, et al. Imaging of renal trauma: a comprehensive review. *Radiographics* 2001;21:557–574.

213. Kawashima A, Sandler CM, Corl FM, et al. Imaging evaluation of posttraumatic renal injuries. *Abdom Imaging* 2002;27:199–213.

214. Kawashima A, Sandler CM, Corriere JN Jr, et al. Ureteropelvic junction injuries secondary to blunt abdominal trauma. *Radiology* 1997;205:487–492.

215. Kearney PA, Rouhana SW, Burney RE. Blunt rupture of the diaphragm: mechanism//diagnosis//and treatment. *Ann Emerg Med* 1989;18:1326–1330.

216. Kearney PA, Vahey T, Burney RE, et al. Computed tomography and diagnostic peritoneal lavage in blunt abdominal trauma. *Arch Surg* 1989;124:344–347.

217. Kenney PJ, Panicek DM, Witanowski LS. Computed tomography of ureteral disruption. *J Comput Assist Tomogr* 1987;11:480–484.

218. Kerns SR, Gay SB. CT of blunt chest trauma. *AJR Am J Roentgenol* 1990;154:55–60.

219. Killeen KL, Mirvis SE, Shanmuganathan K. Helical CT of diaphragmatic rupture caused by blunt trauma. *AJR Am J Roentgenol* 1999;173:1611–1616.

220. Killeen KL, Shanmuganathan K, Poletti PA, et al. Helical computed tomography of bowel and mesenteric injuries. *J Trauma* 2001;51:26–36.

221. Kim JK, Ahn JH, Park T, et al. Virtual cystoscopy of the contrast material-filled bladder in patients with gross hematuria. *AJR Am J Roentgenol* 2002;179:763–768.

222. Kirsch JD, Escarous A. CT diagnosis of traumatic pericardium rupture. *J Comput Assist Tomogr* 1989;13:523–524.

223. Kirsh MM, Behrendt DM, Orringer MB, et al. The treatment of acute traumatic rupture of the aorta: a 10-year experience. *Ann Surg* 1976;184:308–316.

224. Kirsh MM, Orringer MB, Behrendt DM, et al. Management of tracheobronchial disruption secondary to nonpenetrating trauma. *Ann Thorac Surg* 1976;22:93–101.

225. Kirsh MM, Sloan H. *Blunt chest trauma: general principles of management.* Boston, MA: Little, Brown, and Company, 1977:247.

226. Kisa E, Schenk WG. Indications for emergency intravenous pyelography (IVP) in blunt abdominal trauma: a reappraisal. *J Trauma* 1986;26:1086–1089.

227. Kodali S, Jamieson WRE, Leia-Stephens M, et al. Traumatic rupture of the thoracic aorta. A 20-year review: 1969-1989. *Circulation* 1991;84:40–46.

228. Kohn JS, Clark DE, Isler RJ, et al. Is computed tomographic grading of splenic injury useful in the nonsurgical management of blunt trauma? *J Trauma* 1994;36:385–390.

229. Korobkin M, Moss AA, Callen PW, et al. Computed tomography of subcapsular splenic hematoma: clinical and experimental studies. *Radiology* 1978;129:441–445.

230. Koslin DB, Stanley RJ, Berland LL, et al. Hepatic perivascular lymphedema: CT appearance. *AJR Am J Roentgenol* 1988;150: 111–113.

231. Kram HB, Appel PL, Wohlmuth DA, et al. Diagnosis of traumatic thoracic aortic rupture: a 10-year retrospective analysis. *Ann Thorac Surg* 1989;47:282–286.

232. Ku JH, Jeon YS, Kim ME, et al. Is there a role for magnetic resonance imaging in renal trauma? *Int J Urol* 2001;8:261–267.

233. Kuhlman JE, Pozniak MA, Collins J, et al. Radiographic and CT findings of blunt chest trauma: aortic injuries and looking beyond them. *Radiographics* 1998;18:1085–1106; discussion 1107–1108.

234. Kumpe DA, Oh KS, Wyman SM. A characteristic pulmonary finding in unilateral complete bronchial transection. *AJR Am J Roentgenol* 1970;110:704–706.

235. Kunin JR, Korobkin M, Ellis JH, et al. Duodenal injuries caused by blunt abdominal trauma: value of CT in differentiating perforation from hematoma. *AJR Am J Roentgenol* 1993;160: 1221–1223.

236. Lane MJ, Mindelzun RE, Sandhu JS, et al. CT diagnosis of blunt pancreatic trauma: importance of detecting fluid between the pancreas and the splenic vein. *AJR Am J Roentgenol* 1994;163: 833–835.

237. Lang EK. Ureteral injuries. In: Pollack HM, ed. *Clinical urography.* Philadelphia, PA: WB Saunders, 1990:1495–1504.

238. Lawson DE, Jacobson JA, Spizarny DL, et al. Splenic trauma: value of follow-up CT. *Radiology* 1995;194:97–100.

239. Lazrove S, Harley DP, Grinnell VS, et al. Should all patients with first rib fracture undergo arteriography? *J Thorac Cardiovasc Surg* 1982;83:532–537.

240. Lee VW, Allard JC, Berger P, et al. Right ventricular tardokinesis in cardiac contusion: a new observation on phase images. *Radiology* 1988;167:737–741.

241. Leidner B, Adiels M, Aspelin P, et al. Standardized CT examination of the multitraumatized patient. *Eur Radiol* 1998;8:1630–1638.

242. Leitman BS, Birnbaum BA, Naidich DP. Radiologic evaluation of thoracic trauma. In: Hood RM, Boyd AD, Culliford AT, eds. *Thoracic trauma.* Philadelphia, PA: WB Saunders, 1989: 67–100.

243. Leppaniemi A, Lamminen A, Tervahartiala P, et al. MRI and CT in blunt renal trauma: an update. *Semin Ultrasound CT MR* 1997;18:129–135.

244. Leung JC, Nance ML, Schwab CW, et al. Thickening of the diaphragm: a new computed tomography sign of diaphragm injury. *J Thorac Imaging* 1999;14:126–129.

245. Levine CD, Gonzales RN, Wachsberg RH, et al. CT findings of bowel and mesenteric injury. *J Comput Assist Tomogr* 1997;21: 974–979.

246. Levine CD, Patel UJ, Wachsberg RH, et al. CT in patients with blunt abdominal trauma: clinical significance of intraperitoneal fluid detected on a scan with otherwise normal findings. *AJR Am J Roentgenol* 1995;164:1381–1385.

247. Levinsohn EM, Bunnell WP, Yuan HA. Computed tomography in the diagnosis of dislocations of the sternoclavicular joint. *Clin Orthop Relat Res* 1979;140:12–16.

248. Linos DA, King RM, Mucha P, et al. Blunt pancreatic trauma. *Minn Med* 1983;66:153–160.

249. Linsenmaier U, Krotz M, Hauser H, et al. Whole-body computed tomography in polytrauma: techniques and management. *Eur Radiol* 2002;12:1728–1740.

250. Lis LE, Cohen AJ. CT cystography in the evaluation of bladder trauma. *J Comput Assist Tomogr* 1990;14:386–389.

251. Loberant N, Szvalb S, Herskovits M, et al. Posttraumatic intestinal stenosis: radiographic and sonographic appearance. *Eur Radiol* 1997;7:524–526.

252. Lopez PP, LeBlang S, Popkin CA, et al. Blunt duodenal and pancreatic trauma. *J Trauma* 2002;53:1195.

253. Lorente-Ramos RM, Santiago-Hernando A, Del Valle-Sanz Y, et al. Sonographic diagnosis of intramural duodenal hematomas. *J Clin Ultrasound* 1999;27:213–216.

254. Lucas CE, Ledgerwood AM. Factors influencing outcome after blunt duodenal injury. *J Trauma* 1975;15:839–846.

255. Lundell CJ, Quinn MF, Finck EJ. Traumatic laceration of the ascending aorta: angiographic assessment. *AJR Am J Roentgenol* 1985;145:715–719.

256. Lundevall J. The mechanism of traumatic rupture of the aorta. *Acta Pathol Microbiol Scand* 1964;62:34–46.

257. Lupetin AR, Mainwaring BL, Daffner RH. CT diagnosis of renal artery injury caused by blunt abdominal trauma. *AJR Am J Roentgenol* 1989;153:1065–1068.

258. Macklin CC. Transport of air along sheaths of pulmonic blood vessels from alveoli to mediastinum. *Arch Intern Med* 1939;64: 913–926.

259. Macrander SJ, Lawson TL, Foley WD, et al. Periportal tracking in hepatic trauma: CT features. *J Comput Assist Tomogr* 1989;13: 952–957.

260. Madayag MA, Kirshenbaum KJ, Nadimpalli SR, et al. Thoracic aortic trauma: role of dynamic CT. *Radiology* 1991;179: 853–855.

261. Maniatis V, Chryssikopoulos H, Roussakis A, et al. Perforation of the alimentary tract: evaluation with computed tomography. *Abdom Imaging* 2000;25:373–379.

262. Mansfield PB, Graham CB, Beckwith JB, et al. Pneumopericardium and pneumomediastinum in infants and children. *J Pediatr Surg* 1973;8:691–699.

263. Manson D, Babyn PS, Palder S, et al. CT of blunt chest trauma in children. *Pediatr Radiol* 1993;23:1–5.

264. Marnocha KE, Maglinte DDT. Plain-film criteria for excluding aortic rupture in blunt chest trauma. *AJR Am J Roentgenol* 1985;144:19–21.

265. Marotta R, Franchetto AA. The CT appearance of aortic transection. *AJR Am J Roentgenol* 1996;166:647–651.

266. Marx JA, Moore EE, Jorden RC, et al. Limitations of computed tomography in the evaluation of acute abdominal trauma: a prospective comparison with diagnostic peritoneal lavage. *J Trauma* 1985;25:933–937.

267. Master VA, Franks J, McAninch JW. Grade v renal injury: avulsion of the renal pedicle. *J Am Coll Surg* 2002;195:425.

268. Mathonnet M, Peyrou P, Gainant A, et al. Role of laparoscopy in blunt perforations of the small bowel. *Surg Endosc* 2003;17: 641–645.

269. Maull KI. Current status of nonoperative management of liver injuries. *World J Surg* 2001;25:1403–1404.

270. McAninch JW. *Urogenital trauma.* New York: Thieme-Stratton, 1985.

271. McCort JJ. Caring for the major trauma victim: the role for *radiology. Radiology* 1987;163:1–9.

272. McGahan JP, Richards JR, Jones CD, et al. Use of ultrasonography in the patient with acute renal trauma. *J Ultrasound Med* 1999;18:207–213.

273. McGonigal MD, Schwab CW, Kauder DR, et al. Supplemental emergent chest computed tomography in the management of blunt torso trauma. *J Trauma* 1990;30:1431–1435.

274. McTavish JD, Jinzaki M, Zou KH, et al. Multi-detector row CT urography: comparison of strategies for depicting the normal urinary collecting system. *Radiology* 2002;225:783–790.

275. Meredith JW, Trunkey DD. CT scanning in acute abdominal injuries. *Surg Clin North Am* 1988;68:255–268.

276. Meyer DM, Thal ER, Weigelt JA, et al. Evaluation of computed tomography and diagnostic peritoneal lavage in blunt abdominal trauma. *J Trauma* 1989;29:1168–1172.

277. Meyers BF, McCabe CJ. Traumatic diaphragmatic hernia: occult marker of serious injury. *Ann Surg* 1993;218:783–790.

278. Meyers MA. Intraperitoneal spread of infections. In: Meyers MA, ed. *Dynamic radiology of the abdomen: normal and pathologic anatomy*, 4th ed. New York: Springer-Verlag, 1994:55–113.

279. Miller FB, Richardson JD, Thomas HA, et al. Role of CT in diagnosis of major arterial injury after blunt thoracic trauma. *Surgery* 1989;106:596–603.

280. Miller MT, Pasquale MD, Bromberg WJ, et al. Not so FAST. *J Trauma* 2003;54:52–59; discussion 59–60.

281. Miller PR, Croce MA, Bee TK, et al. ARDS after pulmonary contusion: accurate measurement of contusion volume identifies high-risk patients. *J Trauma* 2001;51:223–228; discussion 229–230.

282. Minagi H, Brody WR, Laing FC. The variable roentgen appearance of traumatic diaphragmatic hernia. *J Can Assoc Radiol* 1977;28:124–128.

283. Mindelzun RE. Abnormal gas collections. In: McCort JJ, ed. *Abdominal radiology*. Baltimore, MD: Williams and Wilkins, 1981:204–206.

284. Mirvis SE, Bidwell JK, Buddemeyer EU, et al. Imaging diagnosis of traumatic aortic rupture. A review and experience at a major trauma center. *Invest Radiol* 1987;22:187–196.

285. Mirvis SE, Bidwell JK, Buddemeyer EU, et al. Value of chest radiography in excluding traumatic aortic rupture. *Radiology* 1987;163:487–493.

286. Mirvis SE, Gens DR, Shanmuganathan K. Rupture of the bowel after blunt abdominal trauma: diagnosis with CT. *AJR Am J Roentgenol* 1992;159:1217–1221.

287. Mirvis SE, Indeck M, Schorr RM, et al. Posttraumatic tension pneumopericardium: the "small heart" sign. *Radiology* 1986;158:663–669.

288. Mirvis SE, Keramati B, Buckman R, et al. MR imaging of traumatic diaphragmatic rupture. *J Comput Assist Tomogr* 1988;12:147–149.

289. Mirvis SE, Kostrubiak I, Whitley NO, et al. Role of CT in excluding major arterial injury after blunt thoracic trauma. *AJR Am J Roentgenol* 1987;149:601–605.

290. Mirvis SE, Pais SO, Gens DR. Thoracic aortic rupture: advantages of intraarterial digital subtraction angiography. *AJR Am J Roentgenol* 1986;146:987–991.

291. Mirvis SE, Rodriguez A. Diagnostic imaging of thoracic trauma. In: Mirvis SE, Young JWR, eds. *Imaging in trauma and critical care*. Baltimore, MD: Lippincott Williams & Wilkins, 1992:93–147.

292. Mirvis SE, Rodriguez A, Whitley NO. CT evaluation of thoracic infections after major trauma. *AJR Am J Roentgenol* 1985;144:1183–1187.

293. Mirvis SE, Shanmuganathan K, Buell J, et al. Use of spiral computed tomography for the assessment of blunt trauma patients with potential aortic injury. *J Trauma* 1998;45:922–930.

294. Mirvis SE, Shanmuganathan K, Erb R. Diffuse small-bowel ischemia in hypotensive adults after blunt trauma (shock bowel): CT findings and clinical significance. *AJR Am J Roentgenol* 1994;163:1375–1379.

295. Mirvis SE, Templeton P. Imaging in acute thoracic trauma. *Semin Roentgenol* 1992;27:184–210.

296. Mirvis SE, Tobin KD, Kostrubiak I, et al. Thoracic CT in detecting occult disease in critically ill patients. *AJR Am J Roentgenol* 1987;148:685–689.

297. Mirvis SE, Whitley NO, Gens DR. Blunt splenic trauma in adults: CT-based classification and correlation with prognosis and treatment. *Radiology* 1989;171:33–39.

298. Mirvis SE, Whitley NO, Vainwright JR, et al. Blunt hepatic trauma in adults: CT-based classification and correlation with prognosis and treatment. *Radiology* 1989;171:27–32.

299. Mizobata Y, Yokota J, Fujimura I, et al. Successful evaluation of pseudoaneurysm formation after blunt renal injury with dual-phase contrast-enhanced helical CT. *AJR Am J Roentgenol* 2001;177: 136–138.

300. Moolten SE. Mechanical production of cavities in isolated lungs. *Arch Pathol Lab Med* 1935;19:825–832.

301. Moore EE, Shackford SR, Pachter HL, et al. Organ injury scaling: spleen, liver, and kidney. *J Trauma* 1989;29:1664–1666.

302. Moore EH, Webb WR, Verrier ED, et al. MRI of chronic posttraumatic false aneurysms of the thoracic aorta. *AJR Am J Roentgenol* 1984;143:1195–1196.

303. Moore FA, Moore EE, Seagraves AS. Nonresectional management of major hepatic trauma. *Am J Surg* 1985;150:725–729.

304. Morey AF, Iverson AJ, Swan A, et al. Bladder rupture after blunt trauma: guidelines for diagnostic imaging. *J Trauma* 2001;51: 683–686.

305. Morgan AS, Flancbaum L, Esposito T, et al. Blunt injury to the diaphragm: an analysis of 44 patients. *J Trauma* 1986;26:565–568.

306. Morgan DE, Nallamala LK, Kenney PJ, et al. CT cystography: Radiographic and clinical predictors of bladder rupture. *AJR Am J Roentgenol* 2000;174:89–95.

307. Morgan PW, Goodman LR, Aprahamian C, et al. Evaluation of traumatic aortic injury: does dynamic contrast-enhanced CT play a role? *Radiology* 1992;182:661–666.

308. Moudouni SM, Patard JJ, Manunta A, et al. A conservative approach to major blunt renal lacerations with urinary extravasation and devitalized renal segments. *BJU Int* 2001;87:290–294.

309. Mulligan JM, Cagiannos I, Collins JP, et al. Ureteropelvic junction disruption secondary to blunt trauma: excretory phase imaging (delayed films) should help prevent a missed diagnosis. *J Urol* 1998;159:67–70.

310. Murray JG, Caoili E, Gruden JF, et al. Acute rupture of the diaphragm due to blunt trauma: diagnostic sensitivity and specificity of CT. *AJR Am J Roentgenol* 1996;166:1035–1039.

311. Nastanski F, Cohen A, Lush SP, et al. The role of oral contrast administration immediately prior to the computed tomographic evaluation of the blunt trauma victim. *Injury* 2001;32: 545–549.

312. Nchimi A, Szapiro D, Ghaye B, et al. Helical CT of blunt diaphragmatic rupture. *AJR Am J Roentgenol* 2005;184:24–30.

313. Neff MA, Monk JS Jr, Peters K, et al. Detection of occult pneumothoraces on abdominal computed tomographic scans in trauma patients. *J Trauma* 2000;49:281–285.

314. Nelson MG, Jones DR, Vasilakis A, et al. Computed tomographic diagnosis of acute blunt pancreatic transection. *W V Med J* 1994;90:274–278.

315. New PF, Aronow S. Attenuation measurements of whole blood and blood fractions in computed tomography. *Radiology* 1976;121: 635–640.

316. Nghiem HV, Jeffrey RB, Mindelzun RE. CT of blunt trauma to the bowel and mesentery. *AJR Am J Roentgenol* 1993;160:53–58.

317. Norman D, Price D, Boyd D, et al. Aspects of computed tomography of the blood and cerebrospinal fluid. *Radiology* 1977;123: 335–338.

318. Novelline RA, Rhea JT, Bell T. Helical CT of abdominal trauma. *Radiol Clin North Am* 1999;37:591–612, vi–vii.

319. Novelline RA, Rhea JT, Rao PM, et al. Helical CT in emergency radiology. *Radiology* 1999;213:321–339.

320. Novotny AR, Brauer RB, Brandl R, et al. Successful renal transplantation after intimal dissection of the renal artery secondary to trauma. *Transplantation* 2003;75:1077–1079.

321. Nunez D, Becerra JL, Fuentes D, et al. Traumatic occlusion of the renal artery: helical CT diagnosis. *AJR Am J Roentgenol* 1996;167: 777–780.

322. Oh KS, Fleischner FG, Wyman SM. Characteristic pulmonary finding in traumatic complete transection of a main-stem bronchus. *Radiology* 1969;92:371–372.

323. O'Hanlon DM, Shaw C, Fenlon HM, et al. Traumatic transection of the pancreas. *Am J Surg* 2002;183:191.

324. Omert LA, Salyer D, Dunham CM, et al. Implications of the "contrast blush" finding on computed tomographic scan of the spleen in trauma. *J Trauma* 2001;51:272–277; discussion 277–278.

325. Orwig D, Federle MP. Localized clotted blood as evidence of visceral trauma on CT: the sentinel clot sign. *AJR Am J Roentgenol* 1989;153:747–749.

326. Osborn GR, Meld MB. Findings in 262 fatal accidents. *Lancet* 1943;245:277–284.

327. Pachter HL, Hofstetter SR, Liang HG, et al. Traumatic injuries to the pancreas: the role of distal pancreatectomy with splenic preservation. *J Trauma* 1989;29:1352–1355.

328. Pais SO. Assessment of vascular trauma. In: Mirvis SE, Young JWR, eds. *Imaging in trauma and critical care.* Baltimore, MD: Williams and Wilkins, 1992:485–515.

329. Palder SB, Shandling B, Manson D. Rupture of the thoracic trachea following blunt trauma: diagnosis by CAT scan. *J Pediatr Surg* 1991;26:1320–1322.

330. Palmer JK, Benson GS, Corriere JN. Diagnosis and initial management of urological injuries associated with 200 consecutive pelvic fractures. *J Urol* 1983;130:712–714.

331. Panicek DM, Paquet DJ, Clark KG, et al. Hepatic parenchymal gas after blunt trauma. *Radiology* 1986;159:343–344.

332. Pao DM, Ellis JH, Cohan RH, et al. Utility of routine trauma CT in the detection of bladder rupture. *Acad Radiol* 2000;7:317–324.

333. Pappas D, Mirvis SE, Crepps JT. Splenic trauma: false-negative CT diagnosis in cases of delayed rupture. *AJR Am J Roentgenol* 1987;149:727–728.

334. Parmley LF, Manion WC, Mattingly TW. Nonpenetrating traumatic injury of the heart. *Circulation* 1958;18:371–396.

335. Parmley LF, Mattingly TW, Manion WC, et al. Nonpenetrating traumatic injury of the aorta. *Circulation* 1958;17:1086–1101.

336. Patel SV, Spencer JA, el-Hasani S, et al. Imaging of pancreatic trauma. *Br J Radiol* 1998;71:985–990.

337. Patrick LE, Ball TI, Atkinson GO, et al. Pediatric blunt abdominal trauma: periportal tracking at CT. *Radiology* 1992;183:689–691.

338. Peitzman AB, Makaroun MS, Slasky BS, et al. Prospective study of computed tomography in initial management of blunt abdominal trauma. *J Trauma* 1986;26:585–592.

339. Peng MY, Parisky YR, Cornwell EE 3rd, et al. CT cystography versus conventional cystography in evaluation of bladder injury. *AJR Am J Roentgenol* 1999;173:1269–1272.

340. Perlman SJ, Rogers LF, Mintzer RA, et al. Abnormal course of nasogastric tube in traumatic rupture of left hemidiaphragm. *AJR Am J Roentgenol* 1984;142:85–88.

341. Perry MJ, Porte ME, Urwin GH. Limitations of ultrasound evaluation in acute closed renal trauma. *J R Coll Surg Edinb* 1997;42:420–422.

342. Petridis A, Pilavaki M, Vafiadis E, et al. CT of hemodynamically unstable abdominal trauma. *Eur Radiol* 1999;9:250–255.

343. Poletti PA, Mirvis SE, Shanmuganathan K, et al. CT criteria for management of blunt liver trauma: correlation with angiographic and surgical findings. *Radiology* 2000;216:418–427.

344. Poletti PA, Wintermark M, Schnyder P, et al. Traumatic injuries: role of imaging in the management of the polytrauma victim (conservative expectation). *Eur Radiol* 2002;12:969–978.

345. Pollack HM, Wein AJ. Imaging of renal trauma. *Radiology* 1970;172:297–308.

346. Poole GV, Morgan DB, Cranston PE, et al. Computed tomography in the management of blunt thoracic trauma. *J Trauma* 1993;35:296–302.

347. Powell MA, Nicholas JM, Davis JW. Blunt ureteropelvic junction disruption. *J Trauma* 1999;47:186–188.

348. Pranikoff T, Hirschl RB, Schlesinger AE, et al. Resolution of splenic injury after nonoperative management. *J Pediatr Surg* 1994;29:1366–1369.

349. Puig S, Schaefer-Prokop C, Mang T, et al. Single- and multi-slice spiral computed tomography of the paediatric kidney. *Eur J Radiol* 2002;43:139–145.

350. Radmayr C, Oswald J, Muller E, et al. Blunt renal trauma in children: 26 years clinical experience in an alpine region. *Eur Urol* 2002;42:297–300.

351. Raptopoulos V. Chest CT for aortic injury: Maybe not for everyone. *AJR Am J Roentgenol* 1994;162:1053–1055.

352. Raptopoulos V, Sheiman RG, Phillips DA, et al. Traumatic aortic tear: screening with chest CT. *Radiology* 1992;182:667–673.

353. Rashid MA. Contre-coup lung injury: evidence of existence. *J Trauma* 2000;48:530–532.

354. Ratliff JL, Fletcher JR, Kopriva CJ, et al. Pulmonary contusion: a continuing management problem. *J Thorac Cardiovasc Surg* 1971;62:638–644.

355. Resciniti A, Fink MP, Raptopoulos V, et al. Nonoperative treatment of adult splenic trauma: development of a computed tomographic scoring system that detects appropriate candidates for expectant management. *J Trauma* 1988;28:828–831.

356. Rhea JT, Novelline RA, Lawrason J, et al. The frequency and significance of thoracic injuries detected on abdominal CT scans of multiple trauma patients. *J Trauma* 1989;29:502–505.

357. Richardson P, Mirvis SE, Scorpio R, et al. Value of CT in determining the need for angiography when findings of mediastinal hemorrhage on chest radiographs are equivocal. *AJR Am J Roentgenol* 1991;156:273–279.

358. Richter ER, Shriver CD. Delayed nephrectomy in grade V renal injury with two interesting anatomic variations. *Urology* 2001;58:607.

359. Rizzo MJ, Federle MP, Griffiths BG. Bowel and mesenteric injury following blunt abdominal trauma: evaluation with CT. *Radiology* 1989;173:143–148.

360. Robbs, JV Moore, SW Pillary, SP. Blunt abdominal trauma with jejunal injury: a review. *J Trauma* 1980;20:308–311.

361. Roberts JL, Dalen K, Bosanko CM, et al. CT in abdominal and pelvic trauma. *Radiographics* 1993;13:735–752.

362. Roddy LH, Unger KM, Miller WC. Thoracic computed tomography in the critically ill patient. *Crit Care Med* 1981;9:515–518.

363. Rodriguez-Morales G, Rodriguez A, Shatney CH. Acute rupture of the diaphragm in blunt trauma: analysis of 60 patients. *J Trauma* 1986;26:438–444.

364. Rogers FB, Osler TM, Healey MA. "Shock" bowel. *J Trauma* 2002;53:1029.

365. Rollins RJ, Tocino I. Early radiographic signs of tracheal rupture. *AJR Am J Roentgenol* 1987;148:695–698.

366. Roos JE, Willmann JK, Weishaupt D, et al. Thoracic aorta: motion artifact reduction with retrospective and prospective electrocardiography-assisted multi-detector row CT. *Radiology* 2002;222:271–277.

367. Ros PR, Ji H. Special focus session: multisection (multidetector) CT: applications in the abdomen. *Radiographics* 2002;22:697–700.

368. Rose JS, Levitt MA, Porter J, et al. Does the presence of ultrasound really affect computed tomographic scan use? A prospective randomized trial of ultrasound in trauma. *J Trauma* 2001;51:545–550.

369. Rosenbaum RC, Johnston GS. Posttraumatic cardiac dysfunction: assessment with radionuclide ventriculography. *Radiology* 1986;160:91–94.

370. Rubin BE, Schliftman R. The striated nephrogram in renal contusion. *Urol Radiol* 1979;1:119–121.

371. Rubin GD. Data explosion: The challenge of multidetector-row CT. *Eur J Radiol* 2000;36:74–80.

372. Sanborn JC, Hietzman ER, Markarian B. Traumatic rupture of the thoracic aorta. Roentgen-pathological correlations. *Radiology* 1970;95:293–298.

373. Sanchez FW, Greer CF, Thomason DM, et al. Hemiazygous continuation of a left inferior vena cava: misleading radiographic findings in chest trauma. *Cardiovasc Intervent Radiol* 1985;8:140–142.

374. Sanders MN, Civil I. Adult splenic injuries: treatment patterns and predictive indicators. *Aust N Z J Surg* 1999;69:430–432.

375. Sandler CM, Hall JT, Rodriguez MB, et al. Bladder injury in blunt pelvic trauma. *Radiology* 1986;158:633–638.

376. Santucci RA, McAninch JM. Grade IV renal injuries: evaluation, treatment, and outcome. *World J Surg* 2001;25:1565–1572.

377. Savolaine ER, Grecos GP, Howard J, et al. Evolution of CT findings in hepatic hematoma. *J Comput Assist Tomogr* 1985;9:1090–1096.

378. Scaglione M, Pinto A, Pinto F, et al. Role of contrast-enhanced helical CT in the evaluation of acute thoracic aortic injuries after blunt chest trauma. *Eur Radiol* 2001;11:2444–2448.

379. Scatamacchia SA, Raptopoulos V, Fink MP, et al. Splenic trauma in adults: impact of CT grading on management. *Radiology* 1989;171:725–729.

380. Schild HH, Strunk H, Weber W, et al. Pulmonary contusion: CT vs plain radiograms. *J Comput Assist Tomogr* 1989;13:417–420.

381. Schmidt CA, Wood MN, Razzouk AJ, et al. Primary repair of traumatic aortic rupture: a preferred approach. *J Trauma* 1992;32:588–592.

382. Schnyder P, Chapuis L, Mayor B, et al. Helical CT angiography for traumatic aortic rupture: correlation with aortography and surgery in five cases. *J Thorac Imaging* 1996;11:39–45.

383. Schnyder P, Gamsu G, Essinger A, et al. Trauma. In: Moss AA, Gamsu G, Genant HK, eds. *Computed tomography of the body with magnetic resonance imaging*, 4th ed. Philadelphia, PA: WB Saunders, 1992:311–323.

384. Schreyer HH, Uggowitzer MM, Ruppert-Kohlmayr A. Helical CT of the urinary organs. *Eur Radiol* 2002;12:575–591.

385. Schurr MJ, Fabian TC, Gavant M, et al. Management of blunt splenic trauma: computed tomographic contrast blush predicts failure of nonoperative management. *J Trauma* 1995;39:507–513.

386. Sclafani SJA, Becker JA. Radiological diagnosis of renal trauma. *Urol Radiol* 1985;7:192–200.

387. Scott MH, Porter JR. Extraperitoneal bladder rupture: pitfall in CT cystography. *AJR Am J Roentgenol* 1997;168:1232.

388. Sebastia MC, Rodriguez-Dobao M, Quiroga S, et al. Renal trauma in occult ureteropelvic junction obstruction: CT findings. *Eur Radiol* 1999;9:611–615.

389. Sefczek DM, Sefczek RJ, Deeb ZL. Radiographic signs of acute traumatic rupture of the thoracic aorta. *AJR Am J Roentgenol* 1983;141:1259–1262.

390. Shalaby-Rana E, Eichelberger M, Kerzner B, et al. Intestinal stricture due to lap-belt injury. *AJR Am J Roentgenol* 1992;158:63–64.

391. Shanmuganathan K, Killeen K, Mirvis SE, et al. Imaging of diaphragmatic injuries. *J Thorac Imaging* 2000;15:104–111.

392. Shanmuganathan K, Mirvis SE. CT scan evaluation of blunt hepatic trauma. *Radiol Clin North Am* 1998;36:399–411.

393. Shanmuganathan K, Mirvis SE, Amoroso M. Periportal low density on CT in patients with blunt trauma: association with elevated venous pressure. *AJR Am J Roentgenol* 1993;160:279–283.

394. Shanmuganathan K, Mirvis SE, Boyd-Kranis R, et al. Nonsurgical management of blunt splenic injury: use of CT criteria to select patients for splenic arteriography and potential endovascular therapy. *Radiology* 2000;217:75–82.

395. Shanmuganathan K, Mirvis SE, Sover ER. Value of contrast-enhanced CT in detecting active hemorrhage in patients with blunt abdominal or pelvic trauma. *AJR Am J Roentgenol* 1993;161:65–69.

396. Shanmuganathan K, Mirvis SE, White CS, et al. MR imaging evaluation of hemidiaphragms in acute blunt trauma: experience with 16 patients. *AJR Am J Roentgenol* 1996;167:397–402.

397. Sherck J, Shatney C, Sensaki K, et al. The accuracy of computed tomography in the diagnosis of blunt small-bowel perforation. *Am J Surg* 1994;168:670–675.

398. Sherck JP, Oakes DD. Intestinal injuries missed by computed tomography. *J Trauma* 1990;30:1–7.

399. Shin MS, Berland LL, Ho K-J. Small aorta: CT detection and clinical significance. *J Comput Assist Tomogr* 1990;14:102–103.

400. Shin MS, Ho K-J. Computed tomography evaluation of posttraumatic pulmonary pseudocysts. *Clin Imaging* 1993;17:189–192.

401. Shorr RM, Crittenden M, Indeck M, et al. Blunt thoracic trauma. Analysis of 515 patients. *Ann Surg* 1987;206:200–205.

402. Shreve WS, Knotts FB, Siders RW, et al. Retrospective analysis of the adequacy of oral contrast material for computed tomography scans in trauma patients. *Am J Surg* 1999;178:14–17.

403. Shuman WP. CT of blunt abdominal trauma in adults. *Radiology* 1997;205:297–306.

404. Siegel MJ, Balfe DM. Blunt renal and ureteral trauma in childhood: CT patterns of fluid collections. *AJR Am J Roentgenol* 1989;152:1043–1047.

405. Sigler LH. Traumatic injuries of the heart incidence of its occurrence in 42 cases of severe accidental bodily injury. *Am Heart J* 1945;30:459–478.

406. Simeone JF, Minagi HM, Putman CE. Traumatic disruption of the thoracic aorta: significance of the left apical extrapleural cap. *Radiology* 1975;117:265–268.

407. Sivit CJ, Cutting JP, Eichelberger MR. CT diagnosis and localization of rupture of the bladder in children with blunt abdominal trauma: significance of contrast material extravasation in the pelvis. *AJR Am J Roentgenol* 1995;164:1243–1246.

408. Sivit CJ, Eichelberger MR. CT diagnosis of pancreatic injury in children: significance of fluid separating the splenic vein and the pancreas. *AJR Am J Roentgenol* 1995;165:921–924.

409. Sivit CJ, Eichelberger MR, Taylor GA. CT in children with rupture of the bowel caused by blunt trauma: diagnostic efficacy and comparison with hypoperfusion complex. *AJR Am J Roentgenol* 1994;163:1195–1198.

410. Sivit CJ, Eichelberger MR, Taylor GA, et al. Blunt pancreatic trauma in children: CT diagnosis. *AJR Am J Roentgenol* 1992;158:1097–1100.

411. Sivit CJ, Taylor GA, Bulas DI, et al. Posttraumatic shock in children: CT findings associated with hemodynamic instability. *Radiology* 1992;182:723–726.

412. Sivit CJ, Taylor GA, Eichelberger MR. Chest injury in children with blunt abdominal trauma: evaluation with CT. *Radiology* 1989;171:815–818.

413. Sivit CJ, Taylor GA, Eichelberger MR, et al. Significance of periportal low-attenuation zones following blunt trauma in children. *Pediatr Radiol* 1993;23:388–390.

414. Slatis P. Injuries in fatal traffic accidents. *Acta Chir Scand* 1962;297(suppl):9–39.

415. Smejkal R, O'Malley KF, David E, et al. Routine initial computed tomography of the chest in blunt torso trauma. *Chest* 1991;100:667–669.

416. Smith JS, Wengrovitz MA, Delong BS. Prospective validation of criteria, including age, for safe, nonsurgical management of the ruptured spleen. *J Trauma* 1992;33:363–369.

417. Sofer M, Kaver I, Kluger Y, et al. Conservative management of an uncommon renal foreign body secondary to explosion injury. *J Trauma* 2001;51:594–596.

418. Soto JA, Alvarez O, Munera F, et al. Traumatic disruption of the pancreatic duct: diagnosis with MR pancreatography. *AJR Am J Roentgenol* 2001;176:175–178.

419. Spouge AR, Burrows PE, Armstrong D, et al. Traumatic aortic rupture in the pediatric population. Role of plain film CT and angiography in the diagnosis. *Pediatr Radiol* 1991;21:324–328.

420. Stafford RE, McGonigal MD, Weigelt JA, et al. Oral contrast solution and computed tomography for blunt abdominal trauma: a randomized study. *Arch Surg* 1999;134:622–626; discussion 626–627.

421. Stalker HP, Kaufman RA, Stedje K. The significance of hematuria in children after blunt abdominal trauma. *AJR Am J Roentgenol* 1990;154:569–571.

422. Stalker HP, Kaufman RA, Towbin R. Patterns of liver injury in childhood: CT analysis. *AJR Am J Roentgenol* 1986;147:1199–1205.

423. Stark DD, Federle MP, Goodman PC. CT and radiographic assessment of tube thoracostomy. *AJR Am J Roentgenol* 1983;141:253–258.

424. Stark P. *Radiology* of thoracic trauma. *Invest Radiol* 1990;25:1265–1275.

425. Stark P. *Radiology* of thoracic trauma. Boston, MA: Andover Medical Publishers, 1993.

426. Stark P, Jaramillo D. CT of the sternum. *AJR Am J Roentgenol* 1986;147:72–77.

427. Starnes S, Klein P, Magagna L, et al. Computed tomographic grading is useful in the selection of patients for nonoperative management of blunt injury to the spleen. *Am Surg* 1998;64:743–748; discussion 748–749.

428. Stavas J, van Sonnenberg E, Casola G, et al. Percutaneous drainage of infected and noninfected thoracic fluid collections. *J Thorac Imaging* 1987;2:80–87.

429. Stern EJ, Frank MS. Acute traumatic hemopericardium. *AJR Am J Roentgenol* 1994;162:1305–1306.

430. Stevens E, Templeton AW. Traumatic nonpenetrating lung contusion. *Radiology* 1965;85:247–252.

431. Strassmann G. Traumatic rupture of the aorta. *Am Heart J* 1947;33:508–515.

432. Stuhlfaut JW, Soto JA, Lucey BC, et al. Blunt abdominal trauma: performance of CT without oral contrast material. *Radiology* 2004;233:689–694.

433. Sturm JT, Hankins DG, Young G. Thoracic aortography following blunt chest trauma. *Am J Emerg Med* 1990;8:92–96.

434. Sutyak JP, Chiu WC, D'Amelio LF, et al. Computed tomography is inaccurate in estimating the severity of adult splenic injury. *J Trauma* 1995;39:514–518.

435. Tack D, Defrance P, Delcour C, et al. The CT fallen-lung sign. *Eur Radiol* 2000;10:719–721.

436. Thoongsuwan N, Kanne JP, Stern EJ. Spectrum of blunt chest injuries. *J Thorac Imaging* 2005;20:89–97.

437. Tisando J, Tsai FY, Als A, et al. A new radiographic sign of acute traumatic rupture of the thoracic aorta: displacement of the nasogastric tube to the right. *Radiology* 1977;125: 603–608.

438. Tocino I, Miller MH. Computed tomography in blunt chest trauma. *J Thorac Imaging* 1987;2:45–59.

439. Tocino IM, Miller MH. Mediastinal trauma and other acute mediastinal conditions. *J Thorac Imaging* 1987;2:79–100.

440. Tocino IM, Miller MH, Fairfax WR. Distribution of pneumothorax in the supine and semirecumbent critically ill adult. *AJR Am J Roentgenol* 1985;144:901–905.

441. Tocino IM, Miller MH, Frederick PR, et al. CT detection of occult pneumothorax in head trauma. *AJR Am J Roentgenol* 1984;143: 987–990.

442. Tomiak MM, Rosenblum JD, Messersmith RN, et al. Use of CT for diagnosis of traumatic rupture of the thoracic aorta. *Ann Vasc Surg* 1993;7:130–139.

443. Toombs BD, Sandler CM, Lester RG. Computed tomography of chest trauma. *Radiology* 1981;140:733–738.

444. Townsend M, DeFalco AJ. Absence of ureteral opacification below ureteral disruption: a sentinel CT finding. *AJR Am J Roentgenol* 1995;164:253–254.

445. Trerotola SO. Can helical CT replace aortography in thoracic trauma? *Radiology* 1995;197:13–15.

446. Tsang BD, Panacek EA, Brant WE, et al. Effect of oral contrast administration for abdominal computed tomography in the evaluation of acute blunt trauma. *Ann Emerg Med* 1997; 30:7–13.

447. Tsushima Y, Yamada S, Aoki J, et al. Ischaemic ileal stenosis following blunt abdominal trauma and demonstrated by CT. *Br J Radiol* 2001;74:277–279.

448. Udekwu PO, Gurkin B, Oller DW. The use of computed tomography in blunt abdominal injuries. *Am Surg* 1996;62:56–59.

449. Uecker J, Pickett C, Dunn E. The role of follow-up radiographic studies in nonoperative management of spleen trauma. *Am Surg* 2001;67:22–25.

450. Umlas S-L, Cronan JJ. Splenic trauma: can CT grading systems enable prediction of successful nonsurgical treatment? *Radiology* 1991;178:481–487.

451. Unger JM, Schuchmann GG, Grossman JE, et al. Tears of the trachea and main bronchi caused by blunt trauma: radiologic findings. *AJR Am J Roentgenol* 1989;153:1175–1180.

452. Uranus S, Pfeifer J. Nonoperative treatment of blunt splenic injury. *World J Surg* 2001;25:1405–1407.

453. Vaccaro JP, Brody JM. CT cystography in the evaluation of major bladder trauma. *Radiographics* 2000;20:1373–1381.

454. Van Hise ML, Primack SL, Israel RS, et al. CT in blunt chest trauma: indications and limitations. *Radiographics* 1998;18: 1071–1084.

455. Van Moore A, Ravin CE, Putman CE. Radiologic evaluation of acute chest trauma. *Crit Rev Diagn Imaging* 1983;19:89–110.

456. Vasile M, Bellin MF, Helenon O, et al. Imaging evaluation of renal trauma. *Abdom Imaging* 2000;25:424–430.

457. Velmahos GC, Demetriades D, Cornwell EE 3rd, et al. Selective management of renal gunshot wounds. *Br J Surg* 1998;85: 1121–1124.

458. Voggenreiter G, Aufmkolk M, Majetschak M, et al. Efficiency of chest computed tomography in critically ill patients with multiple traumas. *Crit Care Med* 2000;28:1033–1039.

459. Wagner RB, Crawford WO, Schimpf PP. Classification of parenchymal injuries of the lung. *Radiology* 1988;167:77–82.

460. Wagner RB, Crawford WO, Schimpf PP, et al. Quantitation and pattern of parenchymal lung injury in blunt chest trauma. Diagnostic and therapeutic implications. *J Comput Tomogr* 1988;12:270–281.

461. Wagner RB, Jamieson PM. Pulmonary contusion. Evaluation and classification by computed tomography. *Surg Clin North Am* 1989;69:31–40.

462. Wah TM, Spence, JA. The role of CT in the management of adult urinary tract trauma. *Clin Radiol* 2001;56:268–277.

463. Wall SD, Federle MP, Jeffrey RB, et al. CT diagnosis of unsuspected pneumothorax after blunt abdominal trauma. *AJR Am J Roentgenol* 1983;141:919–921.

464. Wan YL, Asich H, Lee TY, et al. Wall defect as a sign of urinary bladder rupture in sonography. *J Ultrasound Med* 1988;7: 511–513.

465. Weir IH, Muller NL, Connell DG. CT diagnosis of bronchial rupture. *J Comput Assist Tomogr* 1988;12:1035–1036.

466. Weishaupt D, Grozaj AM, Willmann JK, et al. Traumatic injuries: imaging of abdominal and pelvic injuries. *Eur Radiol* 2002;12: 1295–1311.

467. White CS, Templeton PA, Attar S. Esophageal perforation: CT findings. *AJR Am J Roentgenol* 1993;160:767–770.

468. Wicky S, Capasso P, Meuli R, et al. Spiral CT aortography: an efficient technique for the diagnosis of traumatic aortic injury. *Eur Radiol* 1998;8:828–833.

469. Wiencek RG, Wilson RF, Steiger Z. Acute injuries of the diaphragm. An analysis of 165 cases. *J Thorac Cardiovasc Surg* 1986;92:989–993.

470. Willmann JK, Roos JE, Platz A, et al. Multidetector CT: detection of active hemorrhage in patients with blunt abdominal trauma. *AJR Am J Roentgenol* 2002;179:437–444.

471. Wills JS, Lally JF. Use of CT for evaluation of possible traumatic aortic injury. *AJR Am J Roentgenol* 1991;157:1123–1124.

472. Wilson D, Voystock JF, Sariego J, et al. Role of computed tomography scan in evaluating the widened mediastinum. *Am Surg* 1994;60:421–423.

473. Wilson RH, Moorehead RJ. Current management of trauma to the pancreas. *Br J Surg* 1991;78:1196–1202.

474. Wing VW, Federle MP, Morris JA, et al. The clinical impact of CT for blunt abdominal trauma. *AJR Am J Roentgenol* 1985;145: 1191–1194.

475. Wintermark M, Poletti PA, Becker CD, et al. Traumatic injuries: organization and ergonomics of imaging in the emergency environment. *Eur Radiol* 2002;12:959–968.

476. Wintermark M, Schnyder P, Wicky S. Blunt traumatic rupture of a mainstem bronchus: spiral CT demonstration of the "fallen lung" sign. *Eur Radiol* 2001;11:409–411.

477. Wiot JF. The radiologic manifestations of blunt chest trauma. *JAMA* 1975;231:500–503.

478. Wolfman NT, Bechtold RE, Scharling ES, et al. Blunt upper abdominal trauma: evaluation by CT. *AJR Am J Roentgenol* 1992;158: 493–501.

479. Wolfman NT, Gilpin JW, Bechtold RE, et al. Occult pneumothorax in patients with abdominal trauma: CT studies. *J Comput Assist Tomogr* 1993;17:56–59.

480. Wolfman NT, Myers WS, Glauser SJ, et al. Validity of CT classification on management of occult pneumothorax: a prospective study. *AJR Am J Roentgenol* 1998;171:1317–1320.

481. Wolverson MK, Crepps LF, Sundaram M, et al. Hyperdensity of recent hemorrhage at body computed tomography: incidence and morphologic variation. *Radiology* 1983;148:779–784.

482. Wong YC, Wang LJ, Lin BC, et al. CT grading of blunt pancreatic injuries: prediction of ductal disruption and surgical correlation. *J Comput Assist Tomogr* 1997;21:246–250.

483. Woodring JH. The normal mediastinum in blunt traumatic rupture of the thoracic aorta and brachiocephalic arteries. *J Emerg Med* 1990;8:467–476.

484. Woodring JH, Fried AM, Hatfield DR, et al. Fractures of first and second ribs: predictive value for arterial and bronchial injury. *AJR Am J Roentgenol* 1982;138:211–215.

485. Woodring JH, Pulmano CM, Stevens RK. The right paratracheal stripe in blunt chest trauma. *Radiology* 1982;143: 605–608.

486. Worman LW, Hurley JD, Pemberton AH, et al. Rupture of the esophagus from external blunt trauma. *Arch Surg* 1962;85: 173–178.

487. Worthy SA, Kang EY, Hartman TE, et al. Diaphragmatic rupture: CT findings in 11 patients. *Radiology* 1995;194:885–888.

488. Yale-Loehr AJ, Kramer SS, Quinlan DM, et al. CT of severe renal trauma in children: evaluation and course of healing with conservative therapy. *AJR Am J Roentgenol* 1989;152: 109–113.

489. Yao DC, Jeffrey RB Jr, Mirvis SE, et al. Using contrast-enhanced helical CT to visualize arterial extravasation after blunt abdominal trauma: incidence and organ distribution. *AJR Am J Roentgenol* 2002;178:17–20.

490. Yin WY, Gueng MK, Huang SM, et al. Acute colonic intramural hematoma due to blunt abdominal trauma. Int Surg 2000;85: 51–54.

491. Yutan E, Waitches GM, Karmy-Jones R. Blunt duodenal rupture: complementary roles of sonography and CT. *AJR Am J Roentgenol* 2000;175:1600.

492. Zinck SE, Primack SL. Radiographic and CT findings in blunt chest trauma. *J Thorac Imaging* 2000;15:87–96.

Musculoskeletal System

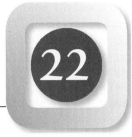

22

Robert Lopez-Ben *Daniel S. Moore* *D. Dean Thornton*

Conventional radiographs are usually the initial imaging choice in the evaluation of musculoskeletal (MSK) complaints. In the setting of trauma, arthritis, metabolic bone disease and bone tumors, radiographs remain the most valuable diagnostic modality. However, if a suspected osseous lesion cannot be identified on radiography, or if a soft tissue abnormality is suspected, additional imaging may be warranted.

Bone scintigraphy is a proven sensitive test in establishing the presence and extent of osseous disease in the setting of normal radiographs. It remains the test of choice in identifying additional osseous lesions throughout the skeleton, like metastases. However, its not as useful in the assessment of the soft tissues, and we seem to turn with increasing frequency to the cross-sectional imaging modalities of CT and MRI to further characterize osseous lesions and define their local extent as well as identify any adjacent soft tissue abnormalities.

Due to its lack of ionizing radiation and low cost, sonography is an attractive first choice for imaging the superficial tendons and soft tissues. Many studies have shown its accuracy in the assessment of these structures. However, the assessment of osseous structures is limited to the cortex. Although there has been increasing interest as the body of information on MSK sonography continues to grow in the radiological literature, it remains underutilized in the United States for various reasons (lack of formal training in most residency programs and operator dependence of the technique, among them).

Because of the capability to directly image in multiple planes as well as its superior soft tissue contrast, MRI has become the mainstay of MSK imaging. By exploiting the differences in the magnetic spin-relaxation times of different tissues, MRI demonstrates exquisite depiction and delineation of the subcutaneous tissues, fasciae, vessels, nerves, muscles, tendons, ligaments, and cartilage. It is particularly sensitive in the depiction of bone marrow abnormalities.

One of the most common questions encountered daily in our practice is choosing between CT and MRI as a cross-sectional modality in the evaluation of (MSK) disease.

The lack of ionizing radiation or iodinated contrast administration contributes to making MRI an attractive choice in light of patient safety. However, the MSK imager is also aware of the limitations of this modality. Patient contraindications like cardiac pacemaker and MR incompatible implanted devices (like certain vascular surgical clips) may prohibit the use of this modality. CT, especially with multi-slice spiral acquisition and high spatial resolution multiplanar reformatted images, may be an imaging option in these cases, as well as the preferred modality in the evaluation of the patient with trauma who may not be able to fully cooperate with the time requirements of MRI, or the patient with orthopedic hardware that may limit MRI evaluation to a greater extent than CT. This chapter will focus on the role of CT in the clinical practice of MSK imaging.

TECHNIQUE

Assessment of the scout view in computed radiography (topogram) is perhaps of more importance in MSK imaging than other aspects of body CT. After proper positioning of the extremity is verified, scanning coverage should be tailored to address the clinical question. Limiting the area covered will decrease radiation dose and increase patient throughput, as well as patient comfort if the extremity is held in a potentially discomforting position (i.e., the outstretched arm over the head position may be chosen to minimize beam hardening artifacts in the assessment of the hand and wrist).

The selection of slice thickness is also tailored to the clinical question and the anatomical area to be studied. Minimizing field of view to the body part of interest, utilizing thin collimation and edge-enhancing filters used in image reconstruction algorithms helps maximize spatial resolution and bone detail. Small joints are best imaged with as thin collimation as possible. With single slice helical CT, different collimation thickness combinations can be performed to assess the pelvis: volume coverage can be maximized in some areas (5 mm through the iliac wings) and detail of the hip articulation emphasized in other anatomic areas (2- to 3-mm thickness through the acetabulum).

The introduction of helical CT has provided a definite advantage over standard axial CT in MSK exams. Minimizing scan times, especially in the patient with MSK trauma, leads to decreased interslice motion artifacts. The improved spatial Z-axis resolution of helical CT allows the reconstruction of complementary anatomic planes without having to reposition the patient. This is especially useful in the assessment of fracture patterns of the pelvis or knee (167). However, positioning with the CT acquisition plane perpendicular to the area of greatest interest is still performed with single-slice CT when the patient is able, as the in-plane resolution of the scanning plane with single slice helical CT is usually better than that available with the reformatted images. In small, complex anatomic areas like the wrist, direct coronal and sagittal images are often acquired in the assessment of intercarpal alignment (15,216). Dedicated scanning planes, like of the longitudinal axis of the scaphoid, may be needed for assessment of fracture healing (269). Positioning of the ankle in axial and direct coronal acquisition planes is also routinely performed, with reformatted sagittal images performed. In some areas, like the shoulder and hip, only axial acquisitions can be acquired and the coronal and sagittal planes can only be evaluated with reformatted images. Overlapping thickness of the helical im-

ages acquired (by decreasing section increment or pitch) improves the subsequent multiplanar reformatted images.

Acquiring volumetric data with helical CT also allows the postprocessing option of changing the displayed FOV. Thus, two sets of images can be reconstructed from the same data without rescanning the patient. For example, a smaller FOV and maximal image overlap may be helpful in the visualization of acetabular fractures, but the assessment of the entire pelvis can be reconstructed with a larger FOV. This technique could also be used for obtaining "comparison" images of the contralateral extremity after the patient has left the CT scanner (provided the body part in question was included on the original scanned FOV).

As in other areas of imaging, the recent introduction of multi-slice helical CT (MSHCT), with increased gantry revolution speed and multiple detector rows, has revolutionized the MSK CT examination (10,125). The faster acquisition of isotropic volumetric CT data has simplified most of our scanning protocols. Because of the marked improvement in the speed of data acquisition, motion artifacts are less common, which is of particular value in the patient with MSK trauma (57). Higher tube current can be maintained with thinner collimation of the scanned area, increasing the resolution and diagnostic accuracy in MSK CT exams of smaller anatomic areas like the wrist and ankle or in the depiction of intra-articular pathology in conjunction with arthrography. Thinner sections as low as 0.5 mm in thickness are now routine, with further improved spatial resolution in the longitudinal or Z-axis. This also allows for decreased partial volume artifacts, which is very beneficial in patients with metallic internal fixation devices (Fig. 22-1).

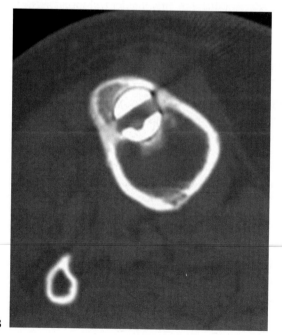
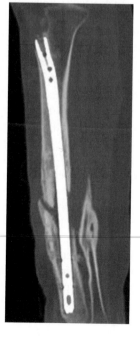

Figure 22-1 MSHCT: decreased metallic artifact. **A:** Axial image acquired with a 16-detector CT with thin collimation (1.5-mm slices) of the proximal tibia with an intramedullary rod in place. There is minimal streak artifact from the hardware; even with using the high detail bone algorithm reconstruction kernel. **B:** Sagittal reformation shows the ununited fracture of the mid tibia best. The metallic artifact is usually decreased on reformations.

A, B

Relatively thinner slices as compared with single slice helical CT exams can now be acquired in the same time. For example, 3-mm images are now used in the pelvis exams when greater coverage is desired, and reconstructed at 1- to 2-mm intervals for greater detail if the 3-mm images are limited (i.e., assessing for suspected intra-articular fragments if an acetabular fracture is detected on the standard 3-mm examination). For most of the 16 or greater slice scanners the maximum detector collimation is 1.25 to 1.5 mm and minimum detector collimation is about 0.5 mm to 0.65 mm. Thicker images are generally reconstructed, but the raw data allows thin direct images or multiplanar reformat reconstruction.

Thinly collimated MSHCT near isotropic volumetric CT data can be reconstructed in different planes without loss of resolution, rivaling the multi-planar capabilities that are usually quoted as one of the intrinsic advantages of MSK MRI over CT. This is possible without a significant loss of scan speed with the new 4, 8 and 16-detector scanners most recently introduced (155). We routinely formulate 2D multiplanar reformatted images in coronal and sagittal planes on most of our MSK studies. By using a small focal spot, small field of view (i.e., 10 cm) and very thin sections (0.5 mm), the Z-axis or longitudinal resolution is near equal to the in-plane (usually axial) resolution (37,241). Thus, when scanning a small part like the wrist or ankle, the multiplanar reformatted (MPR) images in the coronal or sagittal plane will have similar spatial resolution as those obtained in the axial scanned plane. Of course, the thinner sections will be noisier, so radiation dose may need to be increased.

However, by decreasing the need to reposition the small body part for direct coronal CT imaging (for instance, an imaging strategy previously commonly performed in the ankle and foot was the standard CT evaluation of the tibiotalar and subtalar joints in separate coronal and axial plane acquisitions), patient comfort is increased and the overall radiation dose to the patient may be decreased without loss of diagnostic information (241). This is especially useful in patients with limitations in extremity positioning within the gantry due to overlying casts or external fixators.

Because of this ability to create high-resolution MPR images from the volume scanned, precise positioning of the extremity part within the gantry becomes less critical if one is obtaining an isotropic volume of CT data (Fig. 22-2). If near isotropic imaging is not used, due to increased slice width or scanner limitations, the area of interest should be placed in the center of the gantry. A 45-degree obliquity of the scanning plane to the joint surface will allow a larger number of slices to traverse the joint surface and improve the subsequent multiplanar reformations (33).

One limitation to MPR images is in the setting of very displaced fractures where all the structures of interest may not lie on the same plane. Curved planar reformations

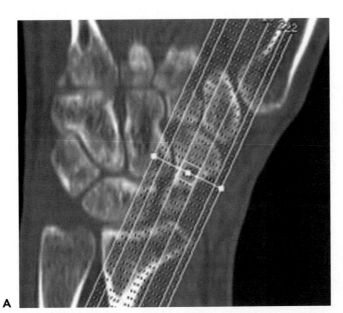
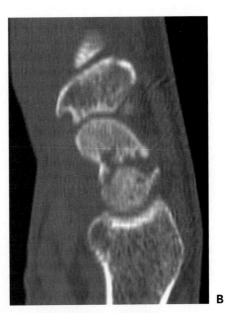

Figure 22-2 Multiplanar reformations: near-isotropic imaging for oblique plane reformations. **A:** Coronal reformation of the wrist from a volumetric MSHCT acquisition (kVp 120, MAs 200) at 0.6 mm is used to prescribe oblique sagittal reformations through the longitudinal plane of the scaphoid. **B:** Oblique sagittal image shows the ununited scaphoid waist fracture. With the near isotropic imaging possible by the initial thin slice acquisitions, the patient did not have to be repositioned and rescanned to view this plane.

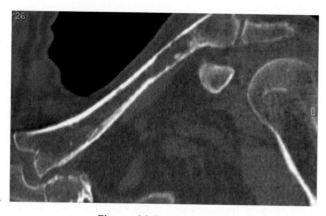

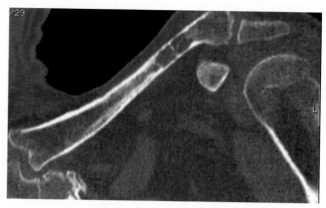

A   **B**

Figure 22-3 Multiplanar reformations: curved reformations. **A** and **B:** Sequential coronal curved reformations of the left clavicle allow visualization of the clavicle in its entirety on each image.

can be performed by manually selecting points of interest to form a 3D "curve image" (47) (Fig. 22-3). However, this approach can be tedious or inaccurate if the selected points are few. Especially when acquiring isotropic MSHCT data, dramatic 3D imaging reconstruction of the datasets is now possible. The postprocessing of data is usually performed at an independent workstation. Although these images usually do not help the radiologist in establishing the presence of fractures or their extent, they do help the surgeon in the visualization of complex fracture patterns, especially in establishing the rotational displacement of major fragments, and may alter surgical planning in complex trauma (2,14,152,153,165,302) (Fig. 22-4).

Two common methods of 3D reconstructions are shaded surface and volume rendering. Surface rendering

shows the contour of the bone surface and may be helpful in fracture characterization (290) (Fig. 22-5). However, the images may be degraded by stair-step artifact and one cannot display subcortical pathology when present. We routinely use volume rendering for our MSK 3D reconstructions as bone and soft tissues can be highlighted separately by altering the opacity of the objects rendered (215) (Fig. 22-6). We believe volume rendering is the most flexible of these techniques; it allows visualizing subcortical skeletal pathology or gross 3D relationships by differing the degree of opacity or transparency of the bones with less artifact formation (135). Visualization of minimally displaced fractures is also possible with this technique, although we do not find it as useful as the 2D multiplanar reformatted images in this regard (72). Because high-frequency image reconstruction kernels

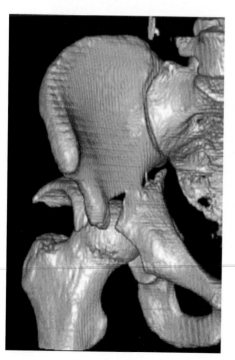

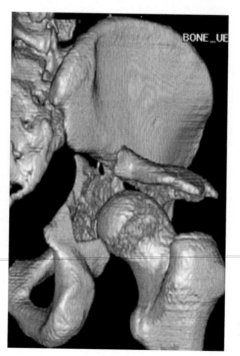

A, B

Figure 22-4 Transverse and posterior wall acetabular fracture: volume 3D Rendering. **A:** Anterior and posterior (**B**) views of this 3D model showing the degree of displacement and rotation of the right acetabular fracture components. (Image courtesy of J. Kevin Smith, MD, PhD, Birmingham, AL.)

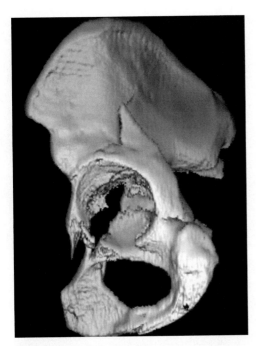

Figure 22-5 Bicolumn acetabular fracture: shaded surface 3D rendering. Left hemipelvis as viewed from a lateral position shows the bicolumn fracture planes. The femur has been removed from the model ("postprocessing disarticulation"), allowing a better look at the fracture distraction of the quadrilateral medial plate. (Image courtesy of J. Kevin Smith, MD, PhD, Birmingham, AL.)

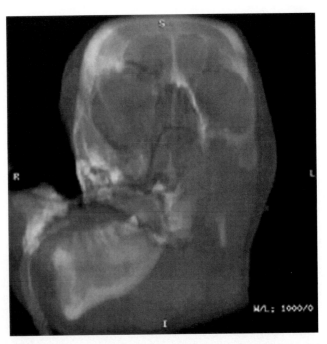

Figure 22-6 Complex facial trauma: volume rendered 3D model displaying different degrees of opacity. Anterior view of the skull shows the marked displacement of the mandible and maxillary fractures. By altering opacity and transparency, the bones and overlying soft tissues are displayed. Note the semitransparent endotracheal tube visualization. (Image courtesy of J. Kevin Smith, MD, PhD, Birmingham, AL.)

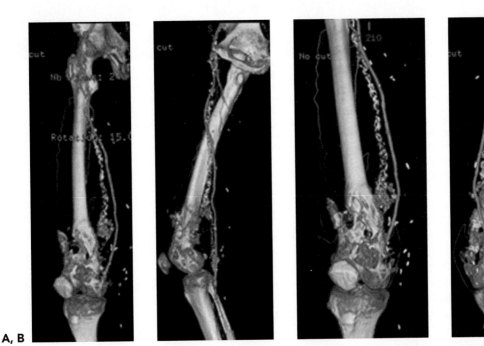

A, B

C, D

Figure 22-7 CT angiography: 3D reconstructions: A 69-year-old man with severe atherosclerotic vascular disease and femoral-popliteal graft revascularization who now presents with an angiosarcoma of the distal right femur. Anterior (**A**) and lateral (**B**) views show the patent femoral-popliteal graft in its entirety, as well as the densely calcified occluded native vessels. Surgical clips from saphenous vein harvesting are noted medially as well. Anterior (**C**) and posterior (**D**) magnified views of the distal femur show the permeative destruction of the distal femur by the angiosarcoma, as well as several feeder vessels recruited from proximal branches.

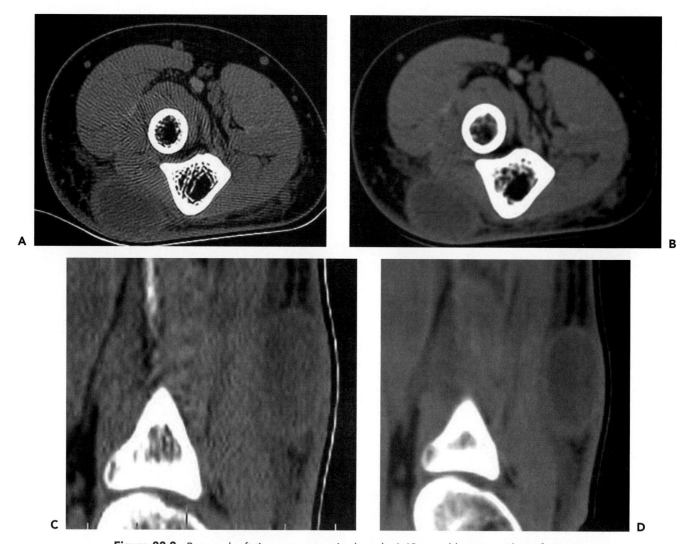

Figure 22-8   Bone and soft tissue reconstruction kernels. A 19-year-old woman with a soft tissue abscess in the dorsum of the proximal forearm. All images were obtained with a 4-channel multidetector CT scanner at contiguous 1.3-mm intervals using the same technique (120 kV, 200 MAs, 512 × 512 matrix). The dataset was reconstructed into true axial and sagittal MPR images with a bone algorithm (**A** and **C**) and with standard soft tissue algorithm (**B** and **D**). Note the beam-hardening artifacts arising from the interface of the radius and ulna that are most noticeable on the bone kernels but not seen with the soft tissue kernels.

typically used in MSK CT for bone detail and sharpness have increased image noise, 3D reconstructions may be less smooth and with inferior low-contrast structure depiction (204). Therefore, in cases where 3D reconstruction is considered, we will also reconstruct the volumetric dataset with standard kernels.

As in other areas of body CT, the decision to use intravenous contrast during imaging must be carefully considered in light of the clinical question that is being asked. If CT is being performed to document the presence or the extent of a fracture, or the presence or imaging pattern of a sclerotic or lytic process of bone, contrast is not usually administered. However, contrast enhancement can be helpful in the evaluation of soft tissue processes like infection and masses. This is particularly true in helping differentiate intramuscular processes. When traumatic vascular injury is suspected, or if a vascular mass is suspected, we obtain a CT angiogram as well (Fig. 22-7). Imaging delay after contrast bolus can be optimized to allow the separation of the arterial and venous phases. We will use 100 to 150 mL of contrast injected at a rate of 3 to 4 mL/sec; for a CT angiogram in the lower extremities, a 30-second delay is usually adequate (less in the upper extremities), and if venous phase is needed, 100- to 120-second

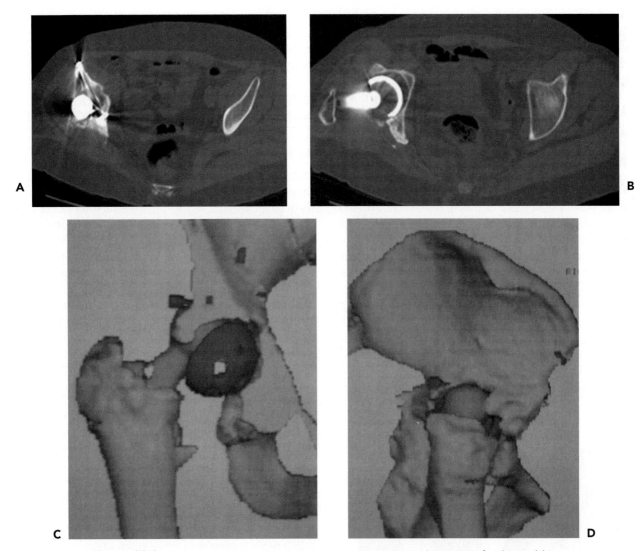

Figure 22-9 Shaded surface rendered 3D reconstruction: aseptic loosening of right total hip arthroplasty. **A** and **B:** Axial CT images shows uncovered superior and laterally subluxed femoral head component and lucency surrounding displaced acetabular cup. **C** and **D:** Shaded surface rendered 3D images in coronal and lateral views with color-coding of the THA components show relationships of displaced acetabular cup best. Note slight stair-stepping artifact seen in proximal femur with this technique.

delay may be used. Because of variability of contrast timing depending on different physiological parameters, we routinely use computer-automated bolus tracking for the timing and triggering of CT acquisition. If this is not available, a small test dose of 10 mL can be injected, with scanning of a vessel in the area of interest performed repeatedly to determine time to peak enhancement.

Finally, the patient with implanted metallic internal fixation devices or joint prostheses can be problematic to image. Star or streak artifacts may compromise the areas surrounding the metallic devices. These artifacts are usually due to beam hardening leading to incomplete filtered

backprojection for image reconstruction (301). The CT scan technique can be altered to improve the ability of the x-ray beam to penetrate the metal. With MSCT, lowering the pitch and using overlapping slices will increase the effective mAs. We prefer to use 140 kVp, and will adjust the mAs depending on the body part scanned. In a small part like the wrist, 200 mAs can be used and 0.5 mm slices can be acquired and reconstructed at 0.2 mm in a 16 row MSCT. For hip prostheses, 2.5-mm slices are scanned and reconstructed at 1-mm intervals utilizing high mAs, especially in obese patients (301). One can also utilize the larger focal spot size of the CT scanner to achieve a greater exposure factor. Image reconstruction is performed not with the edge-enhancing algorithms for traditional bone work resolution as these filters accentuate artifact (301). Using soft tissue or smoothing reconstruction filters helps reduce artifact, at the expense of decreased spatial resolution (Fig. 22-8). Special artifact-reduction reconstruction techniques have been postulated to improve artifact reduction, especially when using an iterative deblurring method (233,294). However, these reconstruction techniques may not be currently available commercially. Utilizing wide windows (4,000 HU window with 1,000 level) or an extended wide window CT scale to view the images can help minimize artifacts (144). Utilizing MPRs reduces the metal-related artifacts as well especially when overlapping source images are utilized and the slice width selected for viewing is the same as the original axial width (83). Three-dimensional reconstructions may also be helpful in the assessment of orthopedic hardware (Fig. 22-9). Volumetric 3D rendering is excellent for assessing the relationship of the metal hardware to the bone (Fig. 22-10). Computer-aided design solid models can be created and machined from the CT data to improve the design and fit of cementless joint prostheses. This may be especially useful in the selection of revision hip arthroplasties, where extensive bone loss can make prosthesis-bone contact and mechanical stability difficult to predict preoperatively (Figs. 22-11 and 22-12).

UPPER EXTREMITY: SHOULDER AND ARM, INCLUDING CLAVICLE/SC JOINT

Anatomy

The upper extremity is connected to the axial skeleton and thoracic cage by the shoulder girdle. The unique arrangement of the skeletal and soft tissue structures of the shoulder allows for the greatest range of motion of any joint in the human body. For these same reasons, the shoulder joint is the least stable of all joints making it prone to dislocation and instability. The osseous structures of the shoulder girdle are the clavicle, scapula, and humerus. Medially, the clavicle articulates with the manubrium of the sternum at the sternoclavicular (SC) joint. This joint serves as the only true articulation between the shoulder girdle and the axial skeleton. The scapulothoracic articulation is not a true joint but is important in stability of the upper extremity. Laterally, the clavicle articulates with the acromion process of the scapula at the acromioclavicular (AC) joint (Fig. 22-13A). The clavicle is further connected to the scapula via the coracoclavicular ligaments, which extend from the undersurface of the distal clavicle to the coracoid process of the scapula. The scapula is a flat, triangular bone with several distinct features. The thin, flat body acts as the primary surface area for scapulothoracic articulation (see Fig. 22-13D, E). This articulation is maintained by overlying soft tissue structures. The posterosuperior acromion process of the scapula provides one half of the AC joint. It also forms most of the osseous portion of the coracoacromial arch, the roof over the rotator cuff. The acromion process is connected to the body of the scapula by the spine (see Fig. 22-13A, B). The anterosuperior coracoid process serves as attachment site for the coracoclavicular and coracoacromial ligaments as well as the short head of the biceps tendon. The glenoid is a shallow, ovoid depression in the lateral scapula. The glenoid cavity is deepened by the cartilaginous glenoid labrum. The glenohumeral (GH) joint is primarily responsible for the tremendous mobility of the upper extremity allowing for extreme abduction/adduction, flexion/extension, and internal/external rotation. The articular surface of the head of the humerus is round and smooth (see Fig. 22-13C). The greater tuberosity is a lateral process that provides the attachment site for most of the rotator cuff tendons. The more anterior lesser tuberosity acts as the attachment site for the subscapularis tendon. Between the tuberosities is the bicipital groove, which accommodates the tendon of the long head of the biceps (see Fig. 22-13D). The anatomic neck of the humerus is the junction between the smooth articular surface of the humeral head and the tuberosities. The

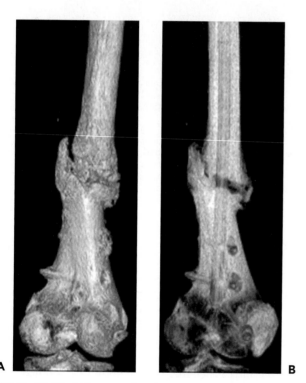

Figure 22-10 Volume rendered 3D reconstructions: nonunion femur fracture. **A** and **B:** Posterior oblique image of the distal femur with intramedullary rod and interlocking screws viewed with different degrees of opacity and transparency of the bone to highlight the nonunion and loosened hardware. Altering the transparency, and using different colors for the hardware and bone can stress different aspects of the nonunion.

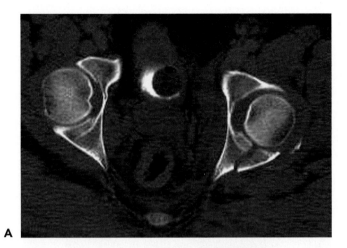

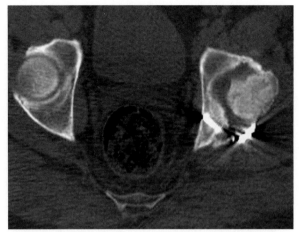

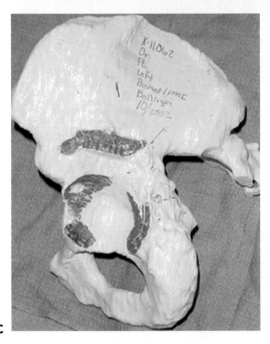

Figure 22-11 Posttraumatic osteonecrosis: machined model of the hemipelvis for preoperative planning. **A:** Axial CT image at time of trauma shows oblique posterior wall left acetabular fracture. **B:** Axial CT image 4 months later shows internal fixation hardware in place but subsequent osteonecrosis of the femoral head that is now sclerotic and fragmented. **C:** 3D model of hemipelvis machined from CT images allows preoperative planning for THA.

surgical neck is slightly more distal between the tuberosities and the proximal shaft of the humerus.

Various muscles also serve to connect the arm to the axial skeleton. Anteriorly, the pectoralis major and minor muscles extend from the sternum and clavicle to the proximal humeral shaft. Posteriorly, the latissimus dorsi muscle arises from the thoracic cage to attach onto the proximal humeral shaft. The great range of motion provided for by the glenohumeral joint is executed in large part by the muscles of the rotator cuff. The supraspinatus muscle arises superior to the scapular spine and attaches to the superior facet of the greater tuberosity (see Fig. 22-13B). The more posterior infraspinatus muscle arises below the spine and inserts onto the posterior facet of the greater tuberosity (see Fig. 22-13D). The teres minor muscle originates and inserts just caudal to the infraspinatus (see Fig.

22-13E). The subscapularis muscle arises from the anterior scapular body to insert onto the lesser tuberosity (see Fig. 22-13D). The long head of the biceps originates at the superior glenoid rim, passes through the rotator cuff interval at the anterosuperior glenohumeral joint, and then follows the bicipital groove between the tuberosities into the upper arm (see Fig. 22-13D, E). The deltoid muscle has a broad origination along the lateral aspect of the acromion from anterior to posterior. It covers the lateral portion of the upper arm before inserting on to the lateral proximal humeral shaft at the deltoid tuberosity (see Fig. 22-13D, E).

Important vascular structures in the shoulder include the subclavian, axillary, and brachial vessels. The brachial plexus provides innervation to the shoulder and the rest of

(*text continues on page 1493*)

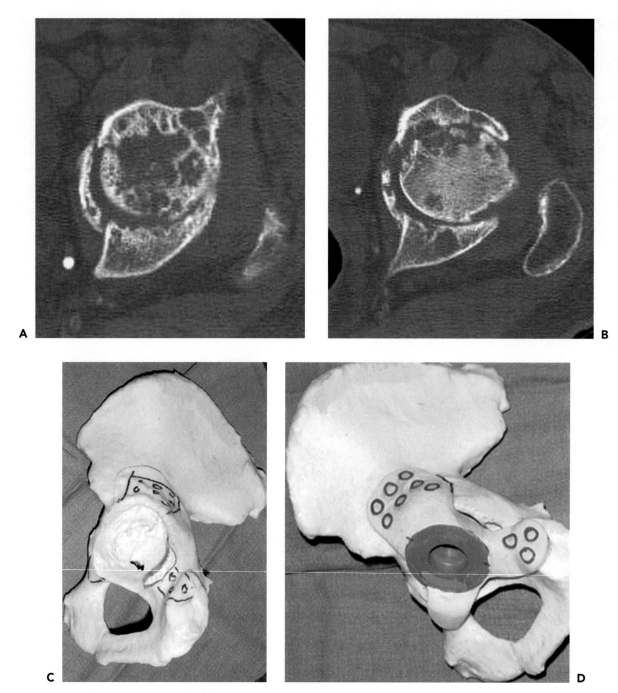

Figure 22-12 Machine modeled hemipelvis for assessment of acetabular press-fit component of THA. **A** and **B**: Axial CT images show marked sclerosis and fragmentation of the femoral head consistent with the history of long-standing osteonecrosis, as well as secondary DJD changes and acetabular protrusio. **C** and **D**: 3D model obtained from CT data without and with a model of the triflanged acetabular component of the subsequently placed THA.

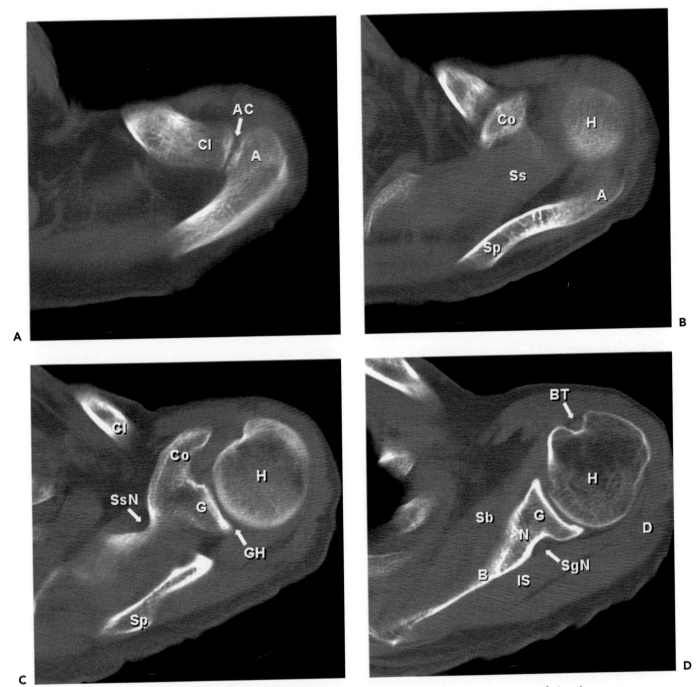

Figure 22-13 Normal shoulder anatomy. Transverse CT images from superior to inferior. **A:** Acromion (A), clavicle (Cl), AC joint (AC). **B:** Coracoid (Co), humerus (H), supraspinatus muscle (Ss), scapular spine (Sp). **C:** Glenoid (G), glenohumeral joint (GH), suprascapular notch (SsN). **D:** Biceps tendon (BT), deltoid muscle (D), subscapularis muscle (Sb), infraspinatus muscle (IS), spinoglenoid notch (SgN), scapular neck (N), scapular body (B). (*continued*)

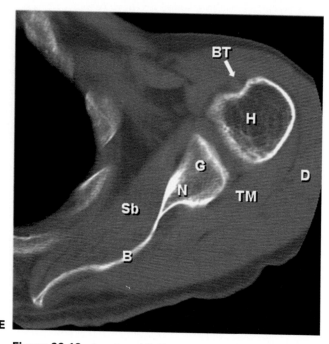

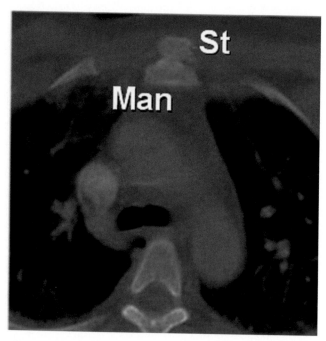

E

Figure 22-13 (*continued*) E: Teres minor muscle (TM).

Figure 22-14 Sternomanubrial dislocation. Transverse CT through the sternomanubrial junction demonstrates posterior displacement of the manubrium (Man) with respect to the body of the sternum (St).

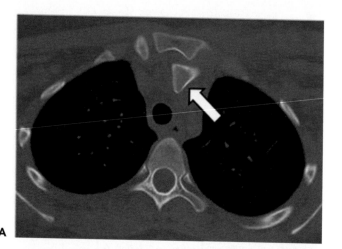

A

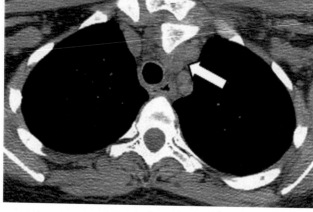

B

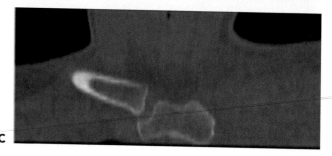

C

Figure 22-15 Posterior clavicular head dislocation. **A:** Transverse CT through the SC joints demonstrates posterior dislocation of the left clavicular head with respect to the sternum. **B:** Soft tissue window at the same level shows impingement, but no direct injury, of the left brachiocephalic vessels (*arrow*). **C, D:** Coronal and sagittal reformatted images demonstrate a normal right SC joint.

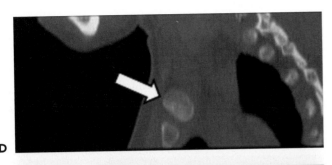

D

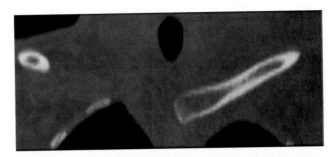

E

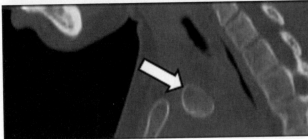

F

Figure 22-15 (*continued*) **E, F:** Coronal and sagittal reformatted images show the posteriorly displaced left clavicular head (*arrows*). Note the excellent resolution of the reformatted images, a consequence of using thin, high-quality sections when obtaining the original data in the transverse plane.

the upper extremity. The axillary nerve travels with the artery in the axilla. The suprascapular nerve crosses over the scapula through the suprascapular notch continuing posteriorly through the spinoglenoid notch (see Fig. 22-13C, D).

Trauma

Any portion of the chain of articulation of the attachment of the upper extremity to the axial skeleton can suffer traumatic injury. Sternal fractures may result from direct impact with the steering wheel in a motor vehicle collision (MVC). Sternomanubrial dislocation (Fig. 22-14) may occur by the same mechanism: if the force is slightly off-center, clavicular or upper anterior rib fractures may result. This same force can result in subluxation or dislocation of the sternoclavicular joint. Most of the injuries at the SC joint occur as a result of direct anterior force applied to the medial clavicle; as a result, most of these injuries involve posterior displacement of the clavicular head (Fig. 22-15). The displaced clavicle can impinge upon and injure the underlying vascular structures, especially on the left side (77). An anterior force applied to the lateral clavicle can result in anterior displacement of the clavicular head at the SC joint, but this is a less common situation. Most clavicular shaft fractures do not require CT for diagnosis or evaluation: the clinical exam and radiographs usually suffice. CT can be useful in cases of markedly displaced fractures which may injure adjacent soft tissue structures or which require more detailed

preoperative planning. CT can also be useful in evaluation of clavicular fracture healing (Fig. 22-16). Complicated injuries of the AC joint may require the greater detail provided by CT to evaluate displaced fracture

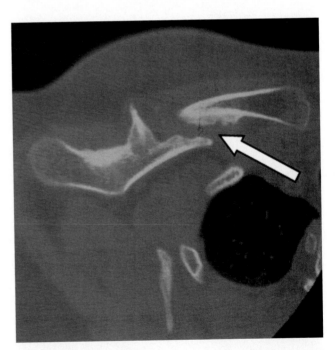

Figure 22-16 Nonunion of right clavicle fracture. Transverse CT demonstrates hypertrophic nonunion of a right clavicle fracture. Note the sclerosis and bony overgrowth along the fracture margins (*arrow*).

fragments and/or the relationship between the distal clavicle and acromion. MR is helpful in these cases for evaluation of the coracoclavicular ligament and underlying rotator cuff (Fig. 22-17). The acromion may fracture anywhere from its base at the spine of the scapula (Fig. 22-18A) to its tip near the AC joint (Fig. 22-18B). The

coracoid process of the scapula may also fracture at its tip or base (102) (Fig. 22-19).

Scapular body fractures are usually managed conservatively because they do not affect a true articulation or a tendoligamentous attachment site. CT can be useful, however, in characterization of such fractures because frag-

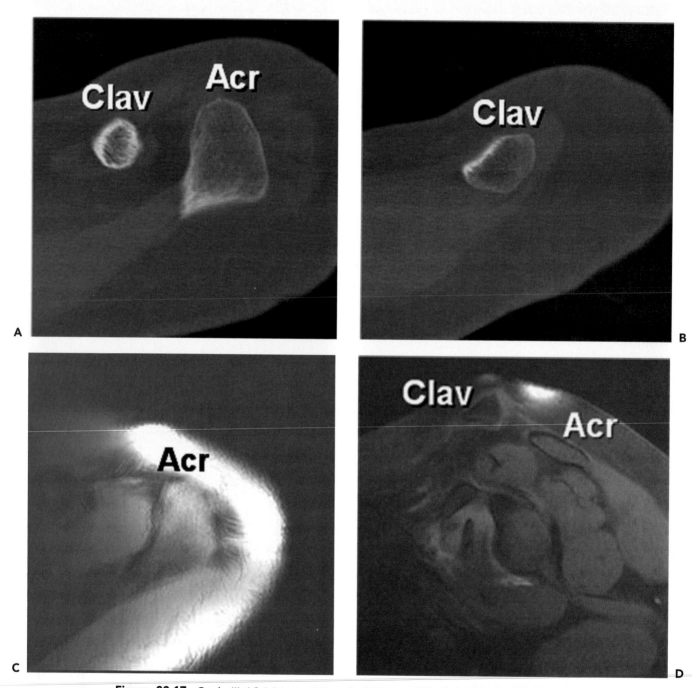

Figure 22-17 Grade III AC joint separation. **A:** Transverse CT of the left shoulder shows a widened AC joint. **B:** On a more superior slice, the end of the distal clavicle (Clav) no longer articulates with the acromion. **C:** Axial T1-weighted MR image again confirms the widened AC joint. **D:** Sagittal PD-weighted fat-suppressed MR image demonstrates the superior displacement of the distal clavicle (Clav) with respect to the acromion (Acr). The distal coracoclavicular ligaments were disrupted as would be expected with this degree of AC separation.

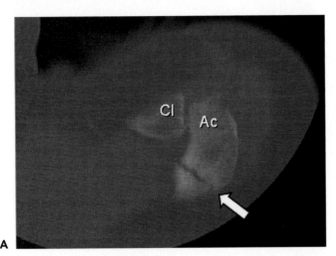

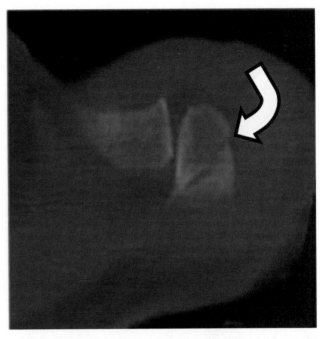

A

B

Figure 22-18   Acromion fracture. **A:** Transverse CT through the left AC joint depicts a fracture through the base of the acromion (Ac) above the level of the scapular spine. The articulation with the clavicle (Cl) is maintained. **B:** Transverse CT through the left AC joint of a different patient shows an oblique fracture near the tip of the acromion. Note the slight widening of the anterior AC joint.

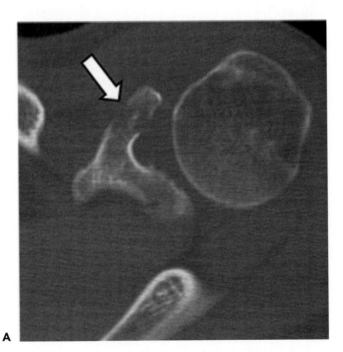

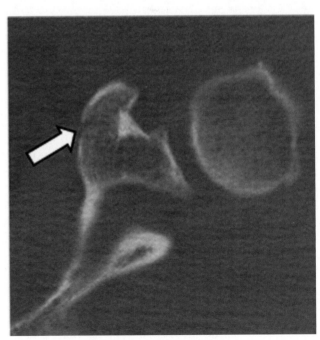

A

B

Figure 22-19   Coracoid process fracture. **A:** Transverse CT through the coracoid shows a transverse fracture through the tip. A superior glenoid fracture is also present. **B:** In a different patient, there is a fracture through the base of the coracoid. (*continued*)

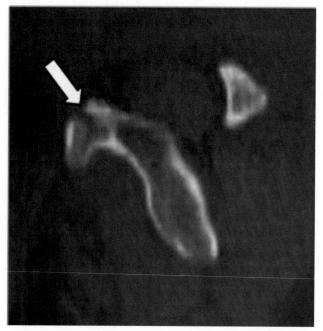

C

Figure 22-19 (*continued*) Coracoid process fracture. C: Sagittal reformatted image shows the coracoid base fracture to better advantage.

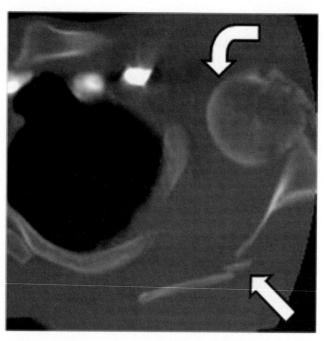

Figure 22-20 Scapular body fracture. Transverse chest computed tomography image depicts a mildly comminuted scapular body fracture (*straight arrow*). The fracture did not extend to the glenoid, scapular spine, or coracoid process. There was an associated anterior shoulder dislocation (*curved arrow*).

ments that are significantly displaced may require reduction. In addition, scapular body fractures noted on radiographs may be associated with acromion, coracoid, or glenoid fractures that do have surgical implications (Fig. 22-20). Fractures that extend to the scapular spine may produce suprascapular nerve injury.

The scapulothoracic articulation is not a true joint, but it is important in maintaining normal motion of the upper extremity with respect to the axial skeleton. Scapulothoracic dissociation is an uncommon manifestation of severe trauma in which the scapula loses its normal broad-based articulation with the thoracic cage. Clinical examination and radiographs may suggest this injury, but CT can be diagnostic (Fig. 22-21).

Fractures involving the glenoid articular surface are of particular concern because these fractures are hard to reduce, making a congruous articular surface difficult to achieve. CT is extremely useful in the evaluation of glenoid fractures. First, the definitive diagnosis of a glenoid fracture can be made with confidence. Radiographic diagnosis can be limited due to difficulty in positioning and the overlying humeral head. CT permits the detection of subtle fractures. Second, the degree of fracture gap and step-off can be accurately assessed, factors which weigh heavily in determining proper management of the fracture (Fig. 22-22). Associated fractures of the scapular neck (Fig. 22-23) and spine should be sought. Most complex glenoid fractures occur due to impaction from the humeral

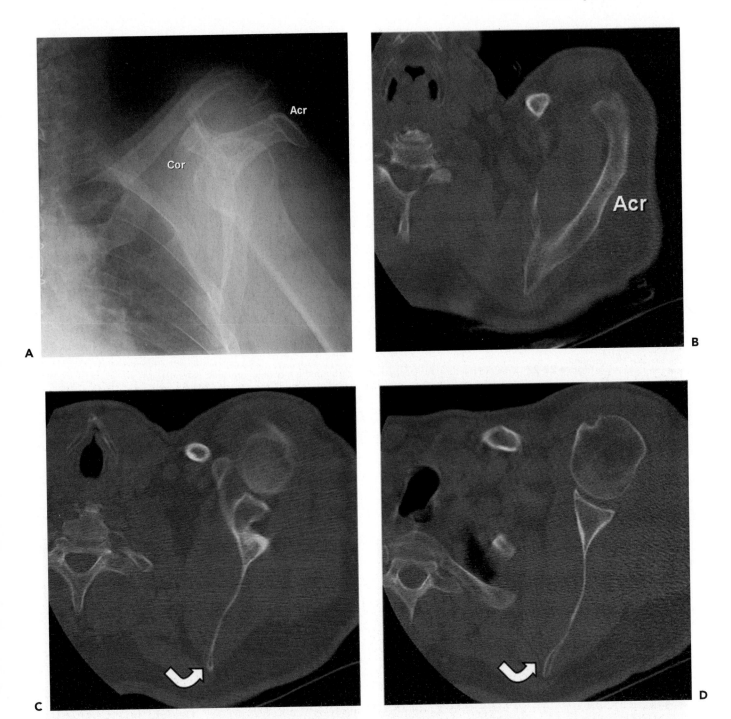

Figure 22-21   Scapulothoracic dissociation. **A:** AP radiograph of the left shoulder has the appearance of a supraspinatus outlet view. **B:** Transverse CT image shows internal rotation of the anterior scapula. The normally oblique acromion (Acr) is now directed in an anteroposterior direction. **C, D.** The posterior scapular body is displaced away from its normal articulation with the thoracic cage (*arrows*). Note also the elevation of the scapula relative to the thoracic cage.

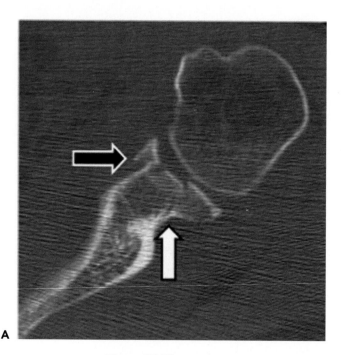
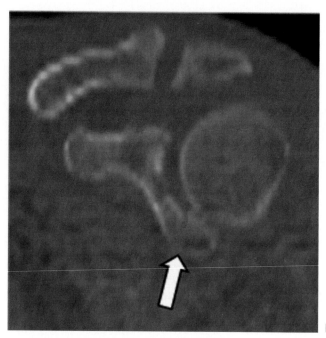

Figure 22-22 Glenoid fracture. **A:** Transverse CT through the glenohumeral joint demonstrates a comminuted glenoid fracture with fracture planes extending through the anterior (*black arrow*) and posterior (*white arrow*) glenoid. Note the slight displacement and rotation of the anterior fragment and the depression of the central glenoid articular surface. **B:** Coronal reformatted image again shows the anterior fracture line (*arrow*) and central glenoid depression. Note the lower quality of the reformatted image, a result of not obtaining thin-section slices in the transverse plane.

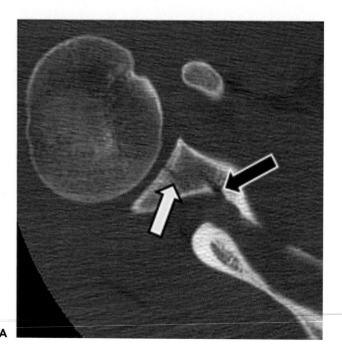
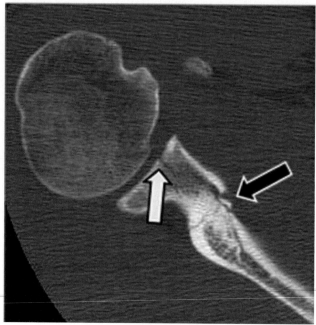

Figure 22-23 Glenoid and scapular neck fracture. **A, B:** Transverse CT images through the glenohumeral joint show a central glenoid fracture (*white arrows*) that extends into the scapular neck (*black arrows*). Note the transverse fracture at the scapular neck that extends from anterior to posterior. (*continued*)

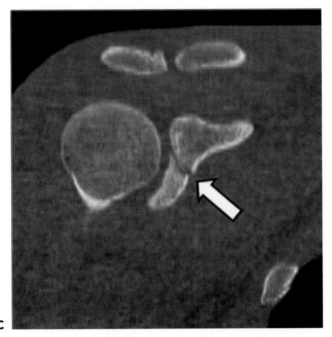

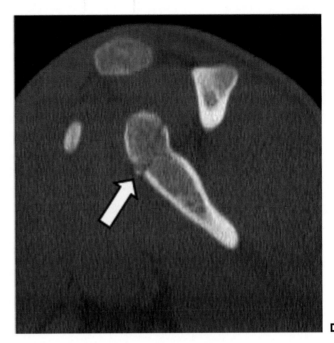

C

D

Figure 22-23 (*continued*) **C:** Coronal reformatted image shows minimal gap and step-off at the glenoid fracture. **D:** Sagittal reformatted image demonstrates the fracture through the scapular neck.

forces directed on the upper arm. The glenoid rim may be fractured after humeral head dislocation. As shoulder dislocations are most often anterior, the anterior glenoid rim is most often affected. As the posterolateral humeral head impacts the anterior glenoid rim, soft tissue or osseous in-

jury may occur (Fig. 22-24). Injury may also take place during relocation efforts as the humeral head makes its way back into position (Fig. 22-25). Such injuries are called Bankart lesions. Osseous Bankart lesions may be detected radiographically, but are better evaluated by CT where

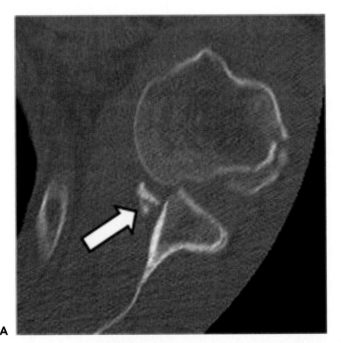

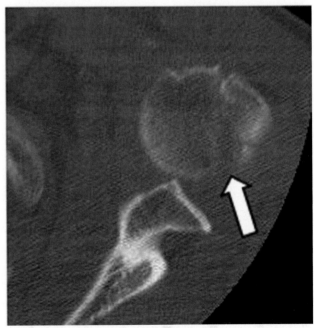

A

B

Figure 22-24 Anterior shoulder dislocation. **A:** Transverse CT image demonstrates anterior dislocation of the humeral head with respect to the glenoid. The anterior rim of the glenoid is fractured with a displaced fragment (*arrow*), the Bankart fracture. A fracture through the base of the greater tuberosity can also be seen. **B:** A more superior image again shows the anterior dislocation. The fracture through the greater tuberosity is better seen (*arrow*).

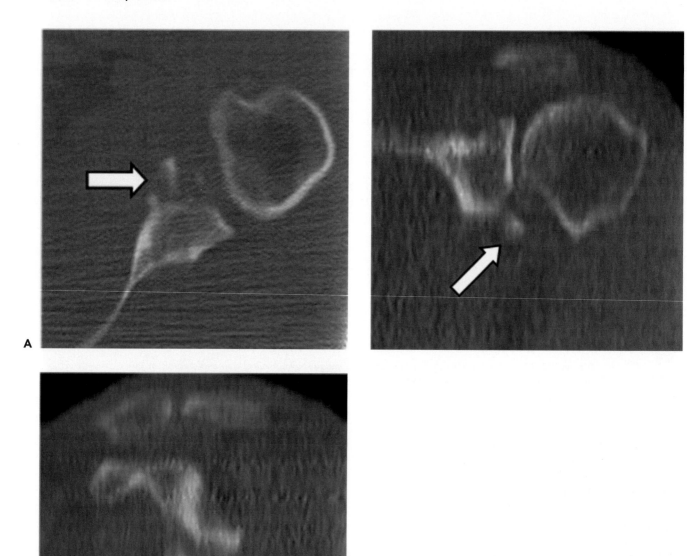

Figure 22-25 Osseous Bankart lesion after anterior shoulder dislocation. **A:** Transverse CT image demonstrates a comminuted fracture of the anterior glenoid rim (*arrow*). **B:** Coronal reformatted CT image shows the inferior and medial displacement of the dominant fracture fragment (*arrow*). **C:** Sagittal reformatted CT image provides a comprehensive depiction of the amount of glenoid articular surface involved by the fracture (*arrow*).

displacement and orientation of fracture fragments is better appreciated. CT can help quantify the amount of glenoid bone loss (105). If a soft tissue Bankart lesion (anterior labral tear) is suspected, MR should be performed, preferably with intra-articular contrast (84) (Figs. 22-26 and 22-27).

Other fractures may occur as a consequence of anterior shoulder dislocation. Most commonly, there may be an impaction fracture on the posterolateral humeral head as it comes into contact with the anterior glenoid rim. This fracture, known as the Hill-Sachs fracture, is often evident on radiographs but is always seen on CT or MR. The top several slices through the humeral head on CT or MR should always be perfectly round; any deformity of the posterolateral humeral head in this area indicates a Hill-Sachs fracture (Fig. 22-28). The more inferior posterolateral humeral head assumes a flat contour that should not be mistaken for a Hill-Sachs fracture. Fracture of the greater tuberosity is also common in the setting of anterior shoulder dislocation due either to avulsion or direct impact (Figs. 22-24 and 22-29).

Posterior shoulder dislocations occur much less frequently than their anterior counterparts. The typical

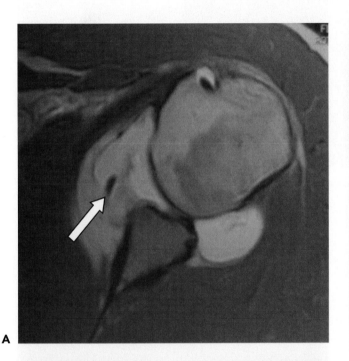

A

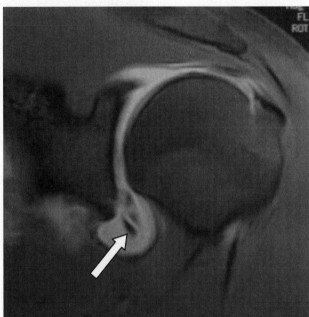

B

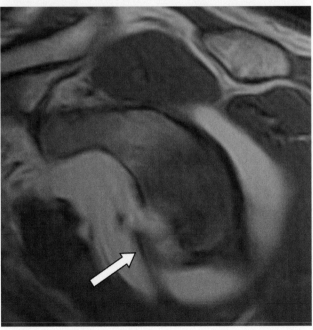

C

Figure 22-26 Osseous Bankart lesion after anterior shoulder dislocation. **A:** Axial T1-weighted MR arthrogram. The cortex of the anterior rim of the glenoid is displaced medially (*arrow*) along with a torn anterior labrum and capsule. **B:** Coronal oblique T1-weighted MR arthrogram with fat suppression. The displaced anterior glenoid fragment (*arrow*) and labrum are again seen. A nondisplaced greater tuberosity fracture is also present. **C:** Sagittal oblique T1-weighted MR arthrogram. The amount of anterior glenoid articular surface involved is best appreciated in this plane. The degree of displacement of the bone and labral fragments (*arrow*) can be determined as well.

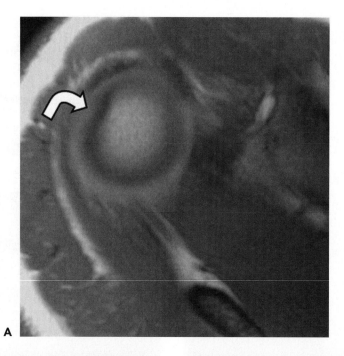

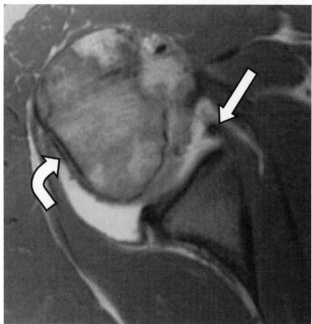

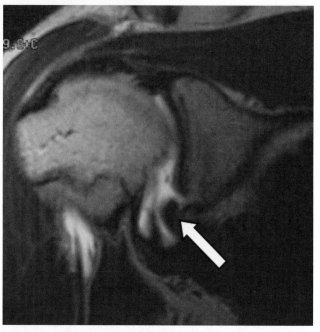

Figure 22-27   Soft tissue Bankart lesion after anterior shoulder dislocation. **A:** Axial T1-weighted MR arthrogram. The posterolateral humeral demonstrates flattening (*curved arrow*) consistent with a Hill-Sachs impaction fracture. **B:** Axial T1-weighted MR arthrogram. A more inferior image through the glenohumeral joint shows an anterior labral tear but no osseous injury. The labrum remains attached to the glenoid periosteum. Note the normal flattening of the posterior humeral head at this level (*curved arrow*), which should not be confused with a Hill-Sachs lesion. **C:** Coronal oblique T2-weighted MR arthrogram. This anterior labral tear (*arrow*) is a Bankart variant called a Perthes lesion.

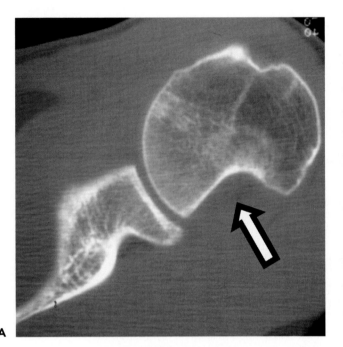

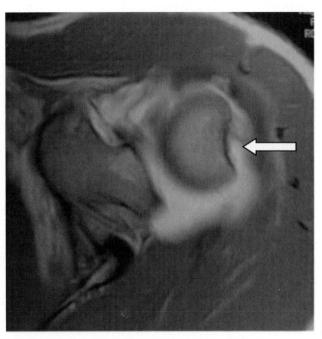

A **B**

Figure 22-28 Hill-Sachs fracture. **A:** Transverse CT demonstrates a large impaction fracture on the posterolateral humeral head (*arrow*). (Image courtesy of Martin L. Schwartz, MD, Birmingham, AL.) **B:** Axial T1-weighted MR arthrogram image from a different patient shows a smaller defect on the lateral humeral head. The exact location of the defect depends on the degree of humeral rotation at the time of injury.

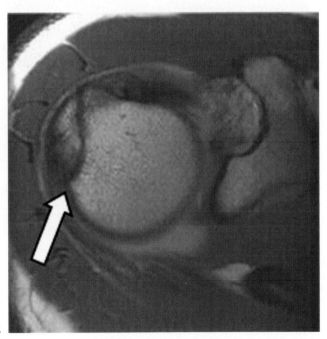

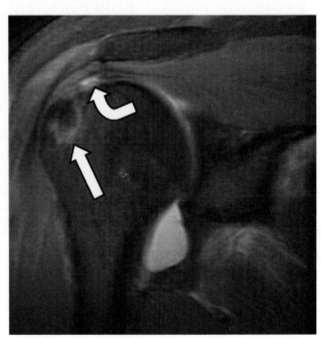

A **B**

Figure 22-29 Greater tuberosity fracture. **A:** Axial T1-weighted MR image shows a nondisplaced fracture through the greater tuberosity (*arrow*) in this patient who had a history of shoulder dislocation. This fracture was not detected on radiographs at the time of dislocation. **B:** Coronal oblique T2-weighted MR arthrogram image with fat suppression. The greater tuberosity fracture is again seen (*arrow*). Note also the partial-thickness undersurface tear of the supraspinatus tendon (*curved arrow*).

mechanism is violent muscle contraction (e.g., seizure) or motor vehicle collision. Many of the same findings described in the anterior dislocation will be present; the findings are simply reversed. The humeral head impaction fracture is located on the anteromedial aspect (Reverse Hill-Sachs fracture). The posterior osseous glenoid rim and cartilaginous labrum may be injured (reverse Bankart lesions) (Figs. 22-30 and 22-31). There may be an associated fracture of the lesser tuberosity (rather than the greater tuberosity seen in anterior dislocations) (see Fig. 22-30).

Fractures through the proximal humerus most often occur at the surgical neck. CT evaluation of these fractures is not usually necessary. The less common anatomic neck fracture may require CT evaluation due to its proximity to the articular surface (Fig. 22-32).

Penetrating injuries of the shoulder girdle (particularly gunshot wounds) often require CT evaluation. The precise location and relationship of bullet and fracture fragments can aid in surgical decision-making and planning (Figs. 22-33 and 22-34).

Joint Abnormality

CT can best contribute to the evaluation of the shoulder girdle joint when abnormalities manifest as osseous changes although some soft tissue abnormalities can certainly be detected. Joint space narrowing can be quantified, chondrocalcinosis and periarticular soft tissue calcifications identified, and subtle articular erosions detected. The addition of intravenous contrast can help identify soft tissue inflammation or infection.

(*text continues on page 1508*)

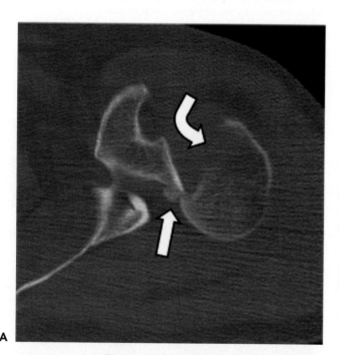 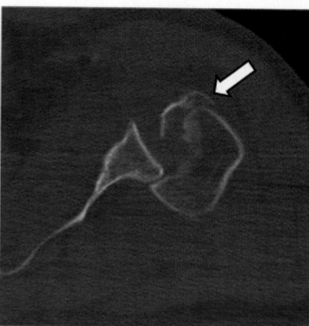

A   B

Figure 22-30 Posterior shoulder dislocation. **A:** Transverse CT image demonstrates posterior dislocation of the humeral head. There is a small bone fragment off of the posterior glenoid rim (*arrow*), which is termed a reverse Bankart fracture. Note also the impaction fracture of the antero-medial humeral head (*curved arrow*), the reverse Hill-Sachs fracture. **B:** A more distal image depicts an associated fracture through the lesser tuberosity (*arrow*).

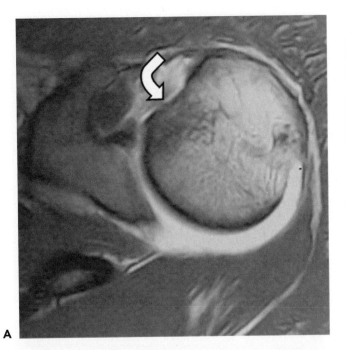

A

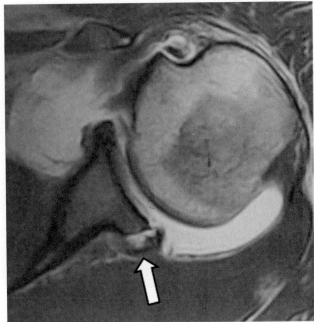

B

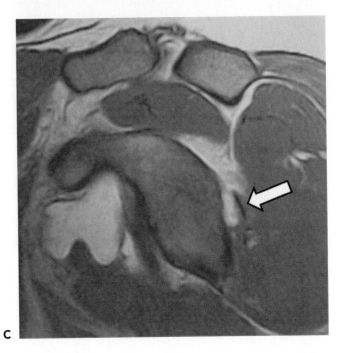

C

Figure 22-31 Reverse osseous Bankart lesion after posterior shoulder dislocation. **A:** Axial T1-weighted MR arthrogram. The humeral head has been reduced. Note the reverse Hill-Sachs fracture (*arrow*). **B:** A lower image shows a fracture fragment from the posterior glenoid rim and the associated posterior labrum (*arrow*) are displaced with intra-articular contrast extending into the defect. **C:** Sagittal oblique T1-weighted MR arthrogram. The glenoid rim fragment is displaced posteriorly (*arrow*).

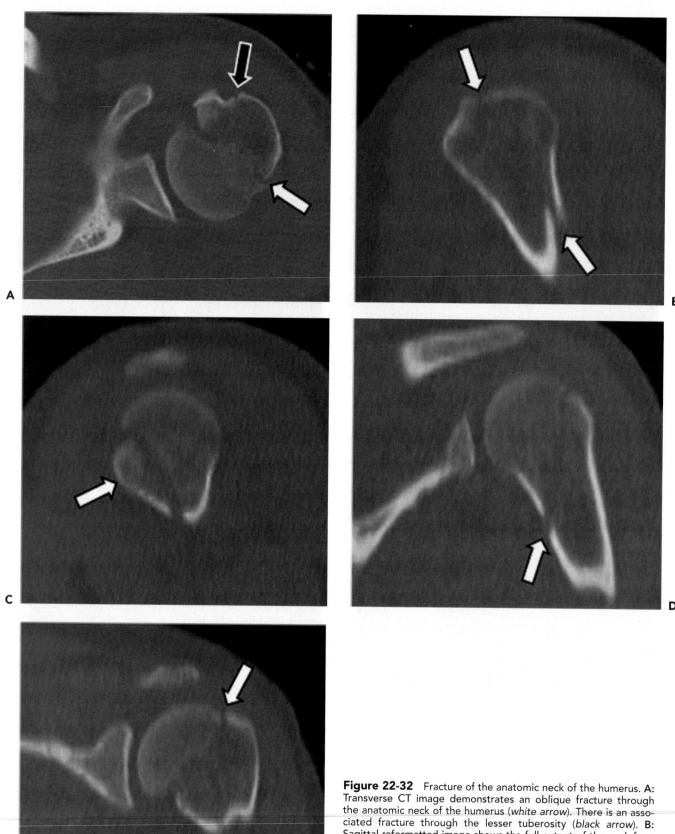

Figure 22-32 Fracture of the anatomic neck of the humerus. **A:** Transverse CT image demonstrates an oblique fracture through the anatomic neck of the humerus (*white arrow*). There is an associated fracture through the lesser tuberosity (*black arrow*). **B:** Sagittal reformatted image shows the full extent of the neck fracture (*arrows*). **C:** A more central sagittal image shows the lesser tuberosity fracture to excellent advantage (*arrow*). **D, E:** Coronal reformatted images confirm the anatomic neck location and demonstrate the preservation of the articular surface of the humeral head (*arrows*).

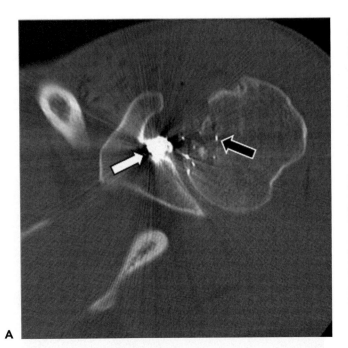
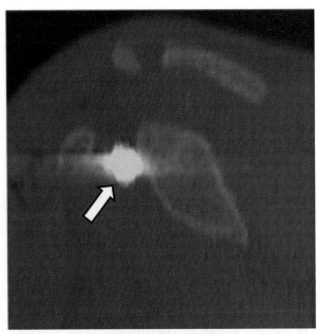

Figure 22-33 Gunshot wound. **A:** Transverse CT demonstrates a fracture of the articular surface of the head of the humerus with small bullet fragments (*black arrow*). The bullet has lodged in the glenoid neck at the base of the coracoid process (*white arrow*). The articular surface of the glenoid is spared. **B:** Sagittal reformatted image confirms the bullet (*white arrow*) is located anterior to the glenoid.

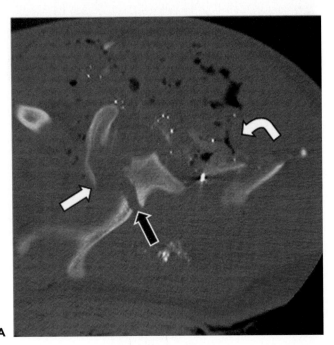
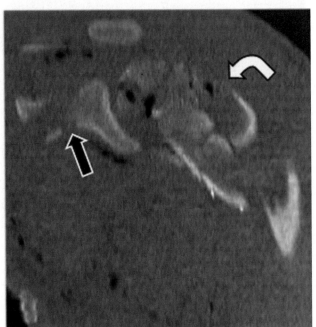

Figure 22-34 Gunshot wound. **A:** Transverse CT accurately demonstrates the extreme severity of the gunshot wound injury. The humeral head fracture is severely comminuted (*curved arrow*). Scapular fractures are also present through the base of the coracoid (*white arrow*) and the glenoid neck (*black arrow*). Note the large amount of soft tissue gas. **B:** Coronal reformatted image shows the extent of the comminuted fracture of the humeral head and neck (*curved arrow*). The glenoid neck fracture is again seen (*black arrow*).

With the difficulty in assessing the sternomanubrial and sternoclavicular joints radiographically, CT can provide valuable information in cases of sternocostoclavicular hyperostosis (45), the SAPHO syndrome (synovitis, acne, pustulosis, hyperostosis, osteitis) (273), or septic arthritis (Fig. 22-35). Radiographic evaluation of the acromioclav-

icular joint is usually sufficient in most cases, but CT can be performed to further evaluate.

The osseous components of the coracoacromial arch (coracoid, distal clavicle, AC joint and acromion) can be evaluated radiographically or with CT; however, the rotator cuff and labroligamentous structures of the shoulder are

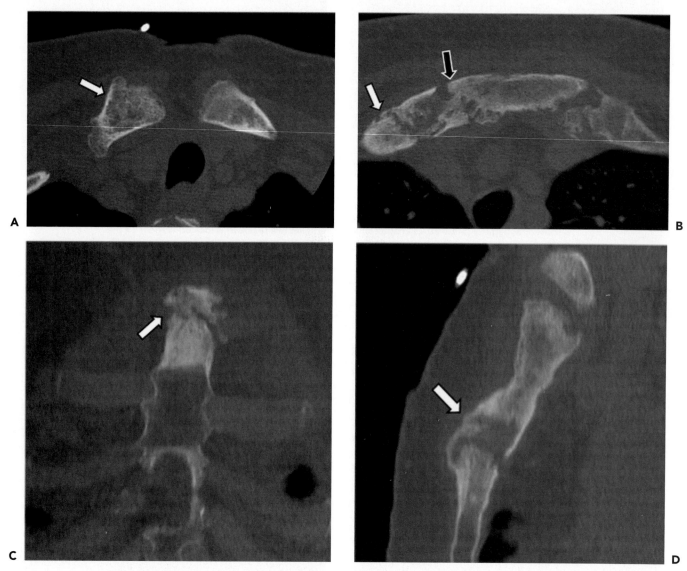

Figure 22-35 Sternocostoclavicular hyperostosis. **A:** Transverse CT image shows sclerosis and overgrowth of the head of the right clavicle (*arrow*). **B:** A more inferior image shows hyperostosis of the anterior right second rib (*white arrow*), its costal cartilage, and the sternocostal articulation (*black arrow*). **C:** Coronal reformatted image demonstrates the marked sclerosis and hypertrophy at the sternomanubrial joint (*arrow*). Note the normal appearance of the lower costal cartilage and sternocostal articulations. **D:** Sagittal reformatted image shows the full extent of the manubrial sclerosis and the sternomanubrial hyperostosis (*arrow*).

best imaged with MRI, often in conjunction with MR arthrography. MR provides a detailed examination of not only the osseous structures but also their relation to the adjacent soft tissue structures (tendons, ligaments, muscles, and cartilage). This ability, coupled with the ease of obtaining multiplanar images, favors MR in cases of suspected impingement or instability. Patients who cannot undergo MRI (pacemaker, severe claustrophobia, etc.) can undergo CT evaluation with some success. Arthrography can be performed using single- or double-contrast technique (Fig. 22-36).

Labral tears can be adequately demonstrated using this CT arthrographic technique (Figs. 22-37 and 22-38), but MR provides a more sensitive, detailed examination (42,60,283) (see Figs. 22-26, 22-27, and 22-31). Shoulder instability related to osseous glenoid rim (rather than labroligamentous) deficiency is best assessed with CT (300). As in most instances, CT provides a more accurate assessment of calcification/ossification. Calcific tendinosis or tendonitis is better seen with CT than MR. Of particular interest in the shoulder is the Bennett le-

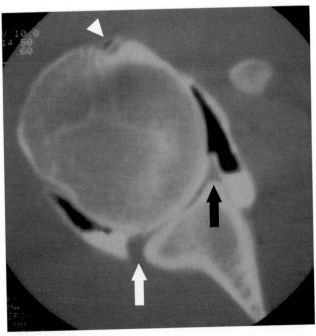

Figure 22-36 Normal double contrast CT arthrogram. Transverse CT image. The small volume of injected contrast outlines the intra-articular structures; the larger volume of injected air provides joint distension. The anterior labrum (*black arrow*) and posterior labrum (*white arrow*) demonstrate normal attachments to the glenoid. Note the small amount of air and contrast tracking down the biceps tendon (*arrowhead*), a normal finding. (Image courtesy of Martin L. Schwartz, MD, Birmingham, AL.)

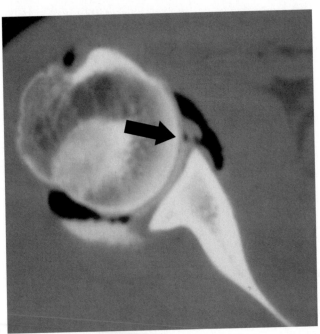

A

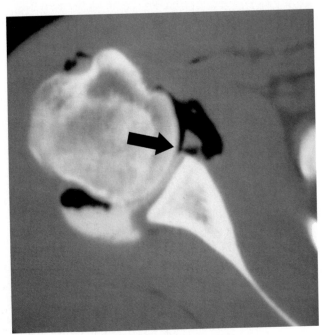

B

Figure 22-37 Anterior labral tear. **A, B:** Transverse images, double contrast CT arthrogram. The anterior labrum is torn at its base with minimal displacement (*arrows*). (Images courtesy of Martin L. Schwartz, MD, Birmingham, AL.)

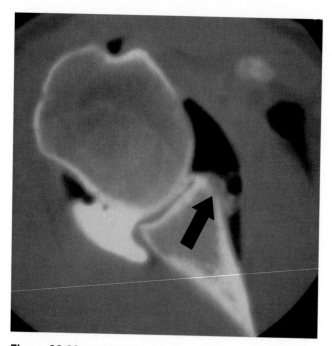

sion in which there is calcification of the posterior capsule near its insertion onto the glenoid. This condition, usually found in throwing athletes, can be detected with MR, but CT allows for a more definitive diagnosis (59) (Fig. 22-39).

Rotator cuff tears, even partial-thickness tears, can be well demonstrated at CT arthrography especially with thin-section images and multi-planar reformatted images (Figs. 22-40 and 22-41). Oblique coronal and sagittal reformatted images can be constructed reproducing the orientation obtained at MRI (223).

Degenerative or inflammatory conditions of the glenohumeral joint do not usually require CT evaluation. Subtle changes such as erosions or intra-articular osteochondral bodies will be better seen at CT than at radiography (Fig. 22-42).

(*text continues on page 1515*)

Figure 22-38 ALPSA lesion. Transverse image, double-contrast CT arthrogram. The anterior labrum is torn but remains attached to the glenoid by a sleeve of periosteum. The torn labrum and periosteum is displaced medially, located anterior to the glenoid (*arrow*). This injury is termed the anterior labroligamentous periosteal sleeve avulsion (ALPSA). (Image courtesy of Martin L. Schwartz, MD, Birmingham, AL.)

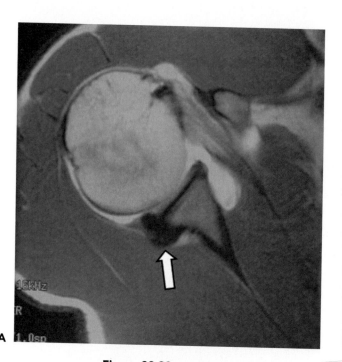

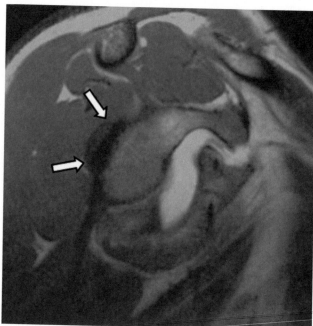

Figure 22-39 Bennett lesion. **A:** Axial T1-weighted MR arthrogram. There is globular low signal intensity suggestive of calcification along the posterior capsular insertion onto the glenoid (*arrow*). The subscapularis tendon is partially torn. **B:** Sagittal T1-weighted MR arthrogram image shows the extent of the posterior capsular low-signal abnormality (*arrows*).

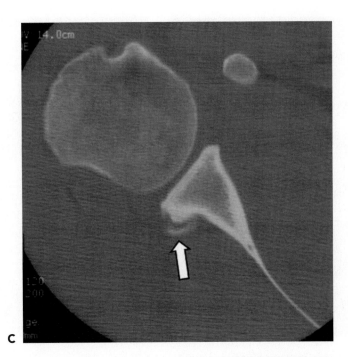

Figure 22-39 *(continued)* **C:** Transverse CT image confirms the presence of calcification of the posterior capsular insertion.

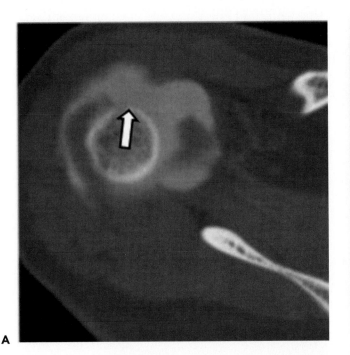

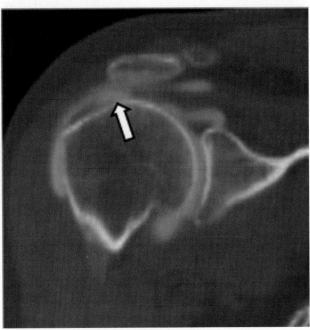

Figure 22-40 Rotator cuff tear. Single contrast CT arthrogram. **A:** Transverse CT image demonstrates a defect on the anterior greater tuberosity at the insertion of the supraspinatus tendon *(arrow)*. **B:** Coronal oblique reformatted image shows a full-thickness tear of the supraspinatus tendon in the critical zone *(arrow)*. *(continued)*

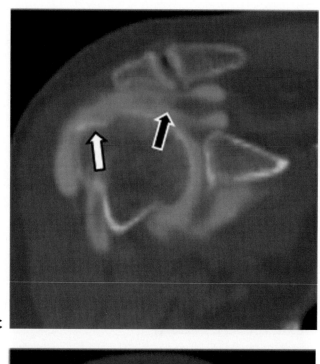

C

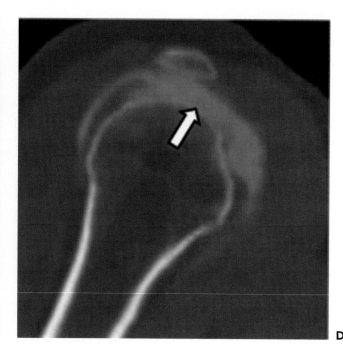

D

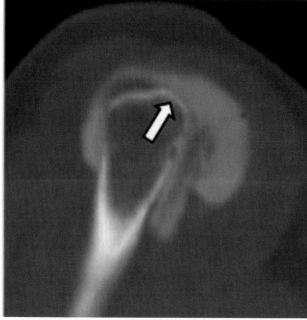

E

Figure 22-40 (*continued*) C: A more anterior coronal oblique image shows the tear to be more extensive. No normal tendon is present at the expected attachment onto the greater tuberosity (*white arrow*). The torn edge of the tendon is slightly retracted (*black arrow*). D: Sagittal oblique reformatted image at the level of the acromion shows absence of the supraspinatus tendon (*arrow*). E: A more lateral image demonstrates absence of the tendon at the greater tuberosity (*arrow*).

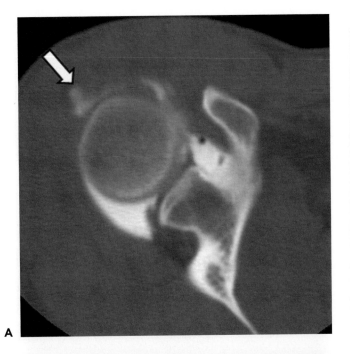

A

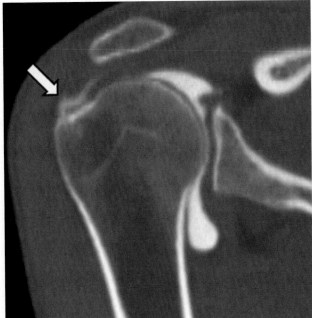

B

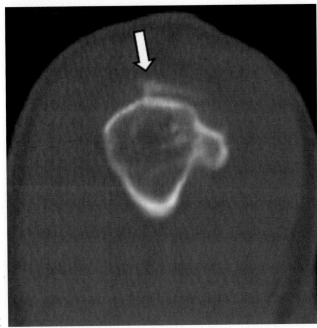

C

Figure 22-41   Rotator cuff tear, partial. Single-contrast CT arthrogram. **A:** Transverse CT image demonstrates a defect in the distal supraspinatus tendon (*arrow*) near the attachment onto the greater tuberosity. **B:** Coronal oblique reformatted image shows the partial undersurface tear of the supraspinatus tendon (*arrow*) to better advantage. **C:** Sagittal oblique reformatted image also shows the partial-thickness tear of the supraspinatus (*arrow*).

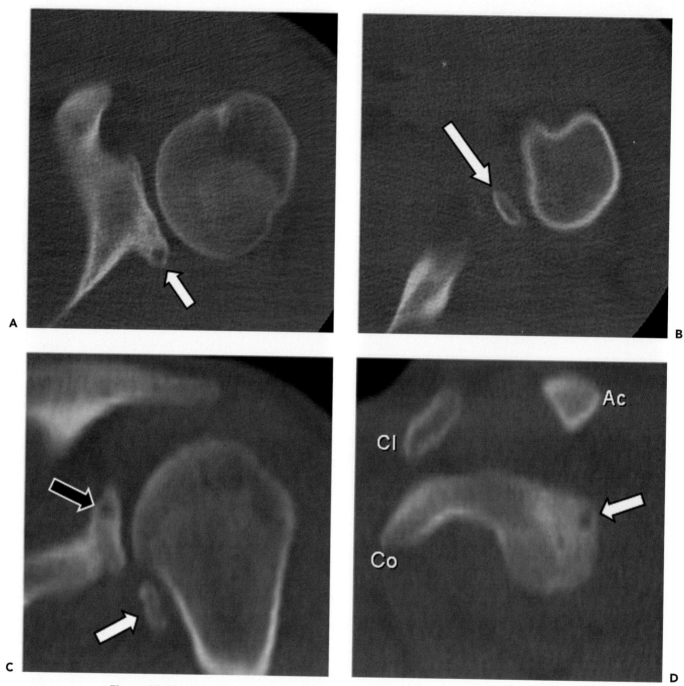

Figure 22-42 Glenohumeral joint osteoarthritis. **A:** Transverse CT image demonstrates sclerosis and remodeling of the posterior glenoid containing a subchondral cyst (*arrow*). **B:** A more inferior image shows an osteochondral body in the axillary recess. **C:** Coronal oblique reformatted image again shows the subchondral cyst (*black arrow*) and osteochondral body in the axillary recess. **D:** Sagittal oblique reformatted image shows the extent of the sclerosis and remodeling of the posterior glenoid (*arrow*). Co, Coracoid; Cl, clavicle; Ac, acromion.

UPPER EXTREMITY: ELBOW

Anatomy

The elbow is primarily a hinge joint allowing flexion and extension, but supination and pronation are also possible due to the construct of the radiocapitellar and proximal radioulnar joints. The medial and lateral epicondyles of the distal humerus serve as attachment sites for the common flexor and extensor tendons respectively (Fig. 22-43B). The distal humerus has two articular surfaces: the trochlea and capitellum. The trochlea is a curved groove that accepts the articular surface of the proximal ulna. This ulnotrochlear joint is the primary hinge of the elbow. Anteriorly, the coronoid process of the ulna is a small osseous extension that resists posterior displacement (Fig. 22-43C). Posteriorly, the much larger olecranon process of the ulna resists anterior displacement. In full elbow extension, the olecranon process fits into posterior olecranon fossa of the distal humerus; in flexion, the coronoid fossa accepts the coronoid process (Fig. 22-43A). The capitellum has a mildly convex articular surface. The head of the radius is a round, slightly concave surface that complements the shape of the capitellum. The radial head also articulates with the radial notch in the proximal ulna forming the proximal radioulnar joint (Fig. 22-43D). The radial head is maintained in this articulation by the circumferential annular ligament. This construct allows for rotation (supination and pronation) at the radiocapitellar joint as well as flexion and extension. Medial elbow joint stability is aided by the ulnar (or medial) collateral ligament (UCL). The radial collateral and lateral ulnar collateral ligaments give lateral support.

The primary flexor of the elbow joint is the brachialis muscle, which originates from the anterior surface of the humerus and inserts on the radial aspect of the proximal ulna. Superficial to the brachialis is the biceps brachii muscle, which aids in flexion. The primary function of the biceps is supination of the forearm. The biceps tendon inserts onto the radial (or bicipital) tuberosity (Fig. 22-43E). The triceps muscle is the principal extensor of the elbow. The triceps tendon inserts on the olecranon process posteriorly. The flexor muscles of the forearm and the pronator have a common tendinous origin from the medial epicondyle of the humerus; likewise, the common extensor and supinator tendon originates from the lateral epicondyle.

Trauma

Evaluation of a subtle or complicated fracture (with or without concomitant subluxation-dislocation) is far and away the most common indication for elbow CT. Given the complex anatomy of the elbow, the precise pattern of injury can be difficult to determine by radiographs alone. Articular surface congruity is better appreciated on CT than on radiographs. The presence, size, and location of intra-articular fragments can also be more readily determined. Identification of fracture fragment displacement and orientation aids in surgical planning.

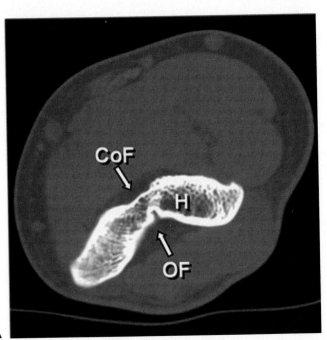

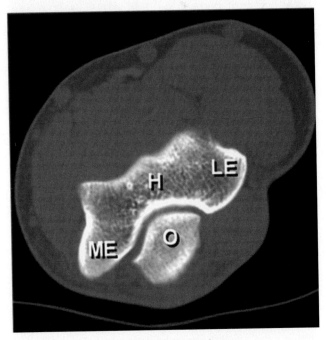

A   B

Figure 22-43 Normal elbow anatomy. Transverse CT images. **A:** Humerus (H), olecranon fossa (OF), coronoid fossa (CoF). **B:** Olecranon process (O), lateral epicondyle (LE), medial epicondyle (ME). (*continued*)

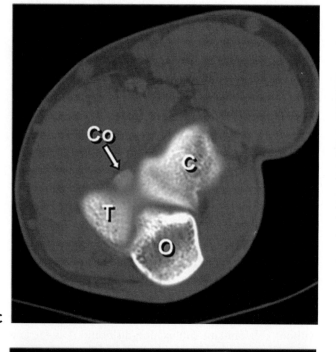

C

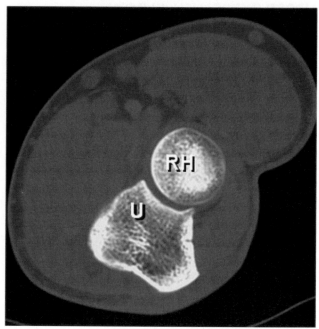

D

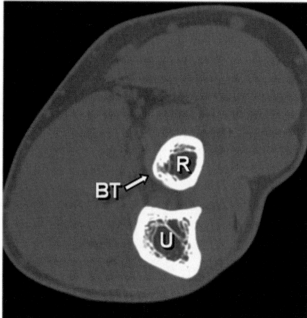

E

Figure 22-43 *(continued)* **C:** Coronoid process (Co), capitellum (C), trochlea (T). **D:** Radial head (RH), ulna (U). **E:** Radius (R), bicipital tuberosity (BT).

Supracondylar humeral fractures occur almost exclusively in children. Fractures of the distal humerus, proximal radius, and proximal ulna can each involve the elbow articular surface. Intercondylar fractures of the distal humerus can affect the epicondyles as well as the articular portions of the capitellum or trochlea (Fig. 22-44). A fall on the outstretched arm can transmit forces to the radiocapitellar articulation resulting in fractures of the capitellum (Fig. 22-45), the radial head, or both (Fig. 22-46). A more substantial force on the forearm may result in elbow

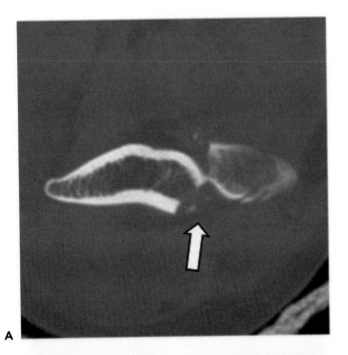

A

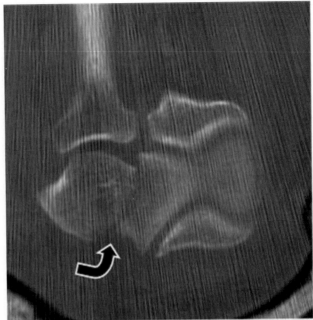

B

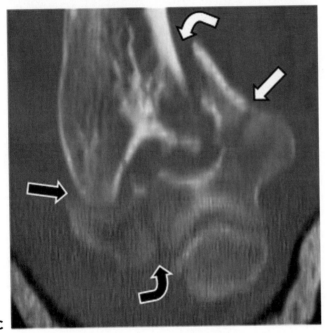

C

Figure 22-44 Intercondylar humeral fracture. **A:** Transverse CT image of the right elbow in 90 degrees of flexion shows a sagittal fracture through the distal humerus (*arrow*) with displacement of the medial epicondyle. **B:** A more distal image demonstrates the fracture extending through the capitellum (*curved arrow*). **C:** Coronal reformatted image shows the intercondylar fracture extending from the medial humerus (*straight white arrow*) between the condyles to the capitellum (*curved black arrow*). The fracture line also extends through the medial (*straight white arrow*) and lateral (*straight black arrow*) epicondyles.

subluxation or dislocation. The proximal radius and ulna most often dislocate posteriorly (Fig. 22-47) but may also displace anteriorly or laterally (Fig. 22-48). Commonly associated fractures include those of the radial head and coronoid process of the ulna (Fig. 22-49). It is important

to perform the elbow CT after reduction of a subluxation-dislocation in order to assess for intra-articular fragments that may have become trapped in the joint and which could prevent complete reduction (Fig. 22-50). Postreduction CT is also useful looking for unreduced fragments or

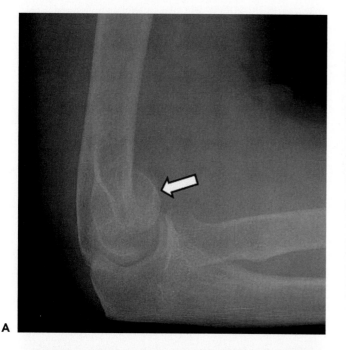

A

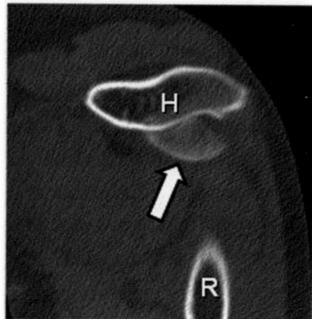

B

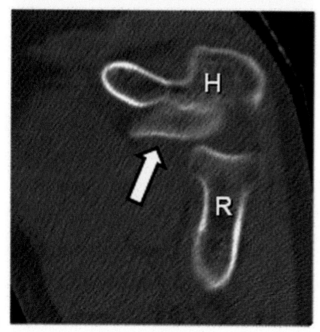

C

Figure 22-45 Capitellum fracture. **A:** Lateral radiograph of the elbow demonstrates a fracture of the capitellum with proximal displacement (*arrow*). **B:** Transverse CT with the elbow in 90 degrees of flexion shows the capitellar fracture fragment (*arrow*) has migrated proximally with respect to the humerus (H). **C:** A more inferior image depicts the donor site of the capitellar fragment (*arrow*) from the humerus (H). Note the incongruity of the capitellar articular surface with the radial head (R).

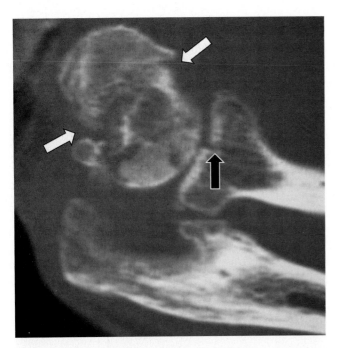

Figure 22-46 Capitellum and radial head fracture. Sagittal reformatted CT image obtained with the elbow in 90 degrees of flexion demonstrates a fracture through the base of the capitellum (*white arrows*). A radial head fracture (*black arrow*) is also present. (Image courtesy of Martin L. Schwartz, MD, Birmingham, AL.)

residual subluxation. Radial head dislocation is associated with a disruption of the forearm ring. This may be due to a proximal ulnar fracture (Monteggia injury) or distal radioulnar joint disruption (Essex-Lopresti injury). Radial head fractures can also be associated with dislocation (Fig. 22-51).

Most radial head fractures do not require CT evaluation. CT scanning is indicated in cases similar to those mentioned above: significant articular surface disruption or intra-articular fragment definition (Fig. 22-52). Radiographically occult elbow fractures will often involve the radial head. CT, especially with multiplanar images, can detect these fractures easily although MR is being advocated for its superior detection of associated soft tissue injury and bone marrow edema. There is debate within the literature whether a traumatic elbow joint effusion is indicative of an occult fracture and whether advanced imaging such as MR should be used in such cases (69,106,157).

Soft tissue injuries of the elbow are best evaluated with MR imaging. The higher soft tissue contrast of MR allows for better visualization of the ligaments, tendons, muscles, and articular cartilage. In those patients who cannot undergo MR scanning, CT evaluation with or without intra-articular contrast is a viable alternative (259,266) (Fig.

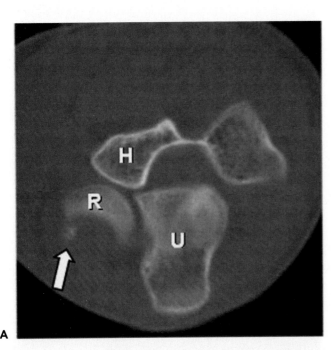

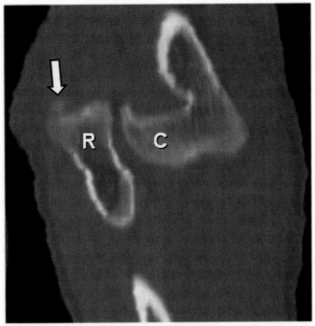

A

B

Figure 22-47 Elbow dislocation, posterior. **A:** Transverse CT image shows displacement of the radial head (R) and proximal ulna (U) posterior to the distal humerus (H). Note the small fracture fragment (*arrow*) adjacent to the radial head. **B:** Coronal reformatted image shows the degree of proximal displacement of the radius (R) with respect to the capitellum (C). The small fracture fragment (*arrow*) came from the radial head (seen on other images). (*continued*)

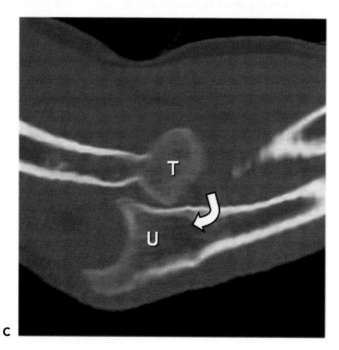

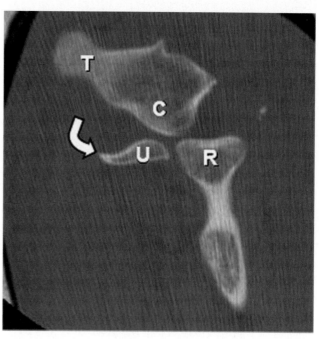

Figure 22-47 (*continued*) Elbow dislocation, posterior. **C:** Sagittal reformatted image shows the posterior dislocation (*arrow*) of the ulna (U) with respect to the trochlea (T).

Figure 22-48 Elbow dislocation, lateral. Coronal CT image with the elbow in flexion demonstrates dislocation of the radius (R) and ulna (U) in a radial direction (*curved arrow*). Note the degree of displacement of the ulna and radius from the trochlea (T) and capitellum (C), respectively.

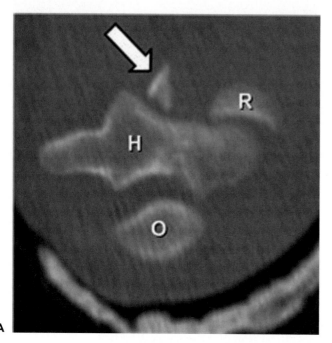

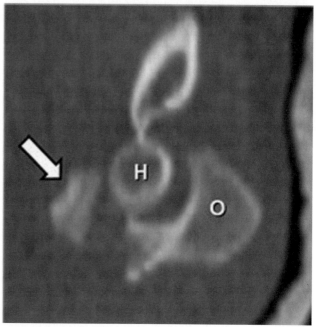

Figure 22-49 Elbow subluxation with coronoid process fracture. **A:** Transverse CT image demonstrates radial and posterior subluxation of the radial head (R) and olecranon process (O). A fracture fragment (*arrow*) is located anterior to the humerus (H). **B:** Sagittal reformatted image shows that the coronoid process is the donor site for the fracture fragment (*arrow*). The posterior olecranon (O) subluxation is again appreciated.

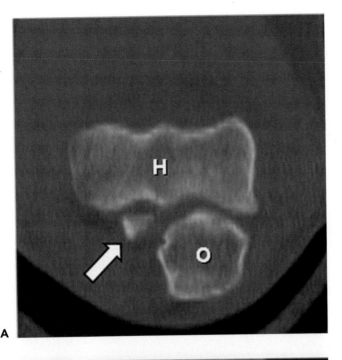

A

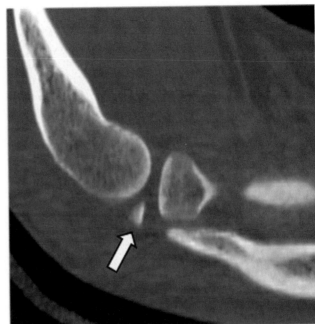

B

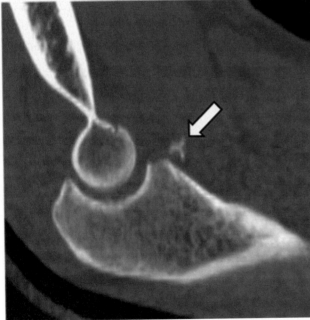

C

Figure 22-50 Coronoid process fracture. **A:** Transverse CT image was obtained with partial elbow flexion (the patient could not straighten the elbow at the time of casting). A fracture fragment (*arrow*) is located within the posterior joint space between the humerus (H) and olecranon (O). **B:** Sagittal reformatted image demonstrates the fragment (*arrow*) located just proximal to the radial head. **C:** A more central sagittal image depicts another fragment (*arrow*) and its donor site, the coronoid process of the ulna.

22-53). In the throwing athlete with medial elbow pain, the primary concern is the integrity of the ulnar collateral ligament (UCL). This can be readily determined with a CT arthrogram using either single or double contrast technique (Figs. 22-54 to 22-56). In the past, direct coronal CT was often obtained with the elbow in 90 degrees of flexion. With today's helical and multi-slice CT scanners, direct axial images are usually obtained which can then produce high quality coronal reformatted images. CT (and radiography) is superior to MR in the detection of calcification or ossification in or around the joint (184) (Fig. 22-57).

(*text continues on page 1524*)

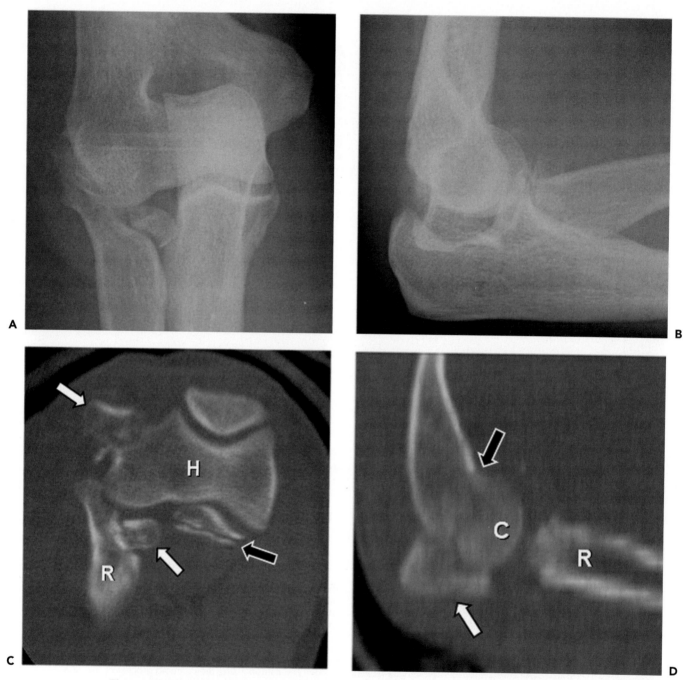

Figure 22-51 Radial head fracture-dislocation. **A, B:** AP and lateral radiographs of the right elbow demonstrate a radial head fracture with posterior dislocation. **C:** Transverse CT image with the elbow in 90 degrees of flexion demonstrates the comminuted fracture of the radial head (R). Two separate fracture fragments (*white arrows*) are present. One fragment remains aligned with the capitellum, whereas the other is dislocated posterior to the humerus (H). An unsuspected fracture of the coronoid process (*black arrow*) is also present. **D:** Sagittal reformatted image again shows the displaced fracture fragment (*white arrow*) from the radius (R) no longer articulating with the capitellum (C). A subtle nondisplaced fracture through the base of the capitellum (*black arrow*) is best seen on the sagittal images because the fracture is in the plane of the transverse images. This radial-head fracture dislocation is associated with disruption of the distal radioulnar joint in the wrist (see Fig. 22-66). This combination of injuries represents the Essex-Lopresti fracture-dislocation.

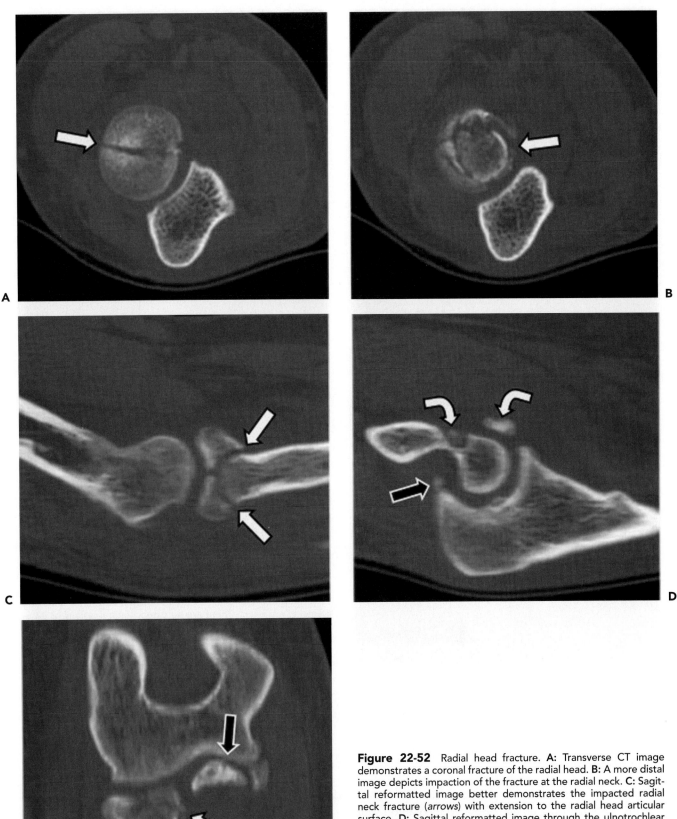

Figure 22-52 Radial head fracture. **A:** Transverse CT image demonstrates a coronal fracture of the radial head. **B:** A more distal image depicts impaction of the fracture at the radial neck. **C:** Sagittal reformatted image better demonstrates the impacted radial neck fracture (*arrows*) with extension to the radial head articular surface. **D:** Sagittal reformatted image through the ulnotrochlear joint shows osteochondral bodies in the anterior joint space (*curved arrows*). These osteochondral bodies are sclerotic and well defined. Note the osteophyte on the tip of the olecranon process (*black arrow*). **E:** Coronal reformatted image again shows the impacted radial fracture (*white arrows*). The large, sclerotic osteochondral body (*black arrow*) was due to osteoarthritis and did not represent a fracture fragment.

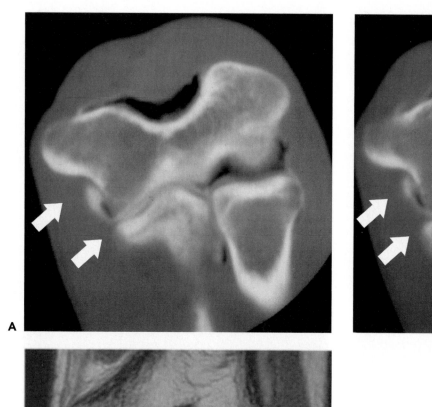

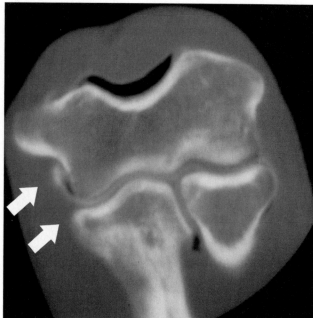

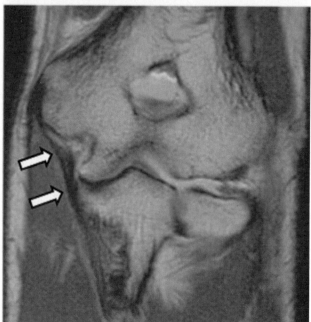

Figure 22-53 Normal elbow arthrogram. **A, B:** Double contrast CT arthrogram. The ulnar collateral (*arrows*) and radial collateral ligaments are intact. There are no osteochondral lesions or intra-articular bodies. **C:** Coronal T1-weighted MR arthrogram in a different patient. The UCL is directly visualized (*arrows*) and appears normal. Note the increased soft tissue contrast. (Images **A** and **B** courtesy of Martin L. Schwartz, MD, Birmingham, AL.)

Joint Abnormality

CT is usually unnecessary in the assessment of elbow arthritis. Osteoarthritis of the elbow is uncommon and readily diagnosed on radiographs when present. If there are complicating or subtle features in question, CT can be of use. CT is excellent at determining the presence of intra-articular osteochondral bodies, especially in the presence of intra-articular contrast (Figs. 22-52 and 22-58). MR is now usually performed for such indications because of its superior soft tissue detail. In the throwing athlete or manual laborer, osteophytes on the olecranon or coronoid process may produce impingement and require resection. CT is well suited to depict such bony abnormalities even when small (Fig. 22-59). Osteochondral defects of the capitellum are better evaluated with MR often in combination with intra-articular contrast (242).

(*text continues on page 1528*)

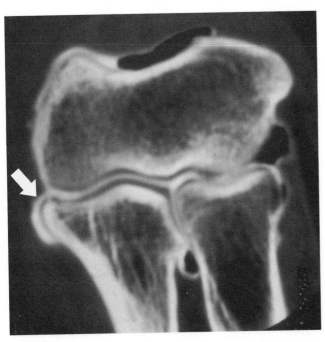

Figure 22-54 Ulnar collateral ligament tear. Coronal double contrast CT arthrogram image shows a full-thickness defect through the distal UCL (*arrow*). (Image courtesy of Martin L. Schwartz, MD, Birmingham, AL.)

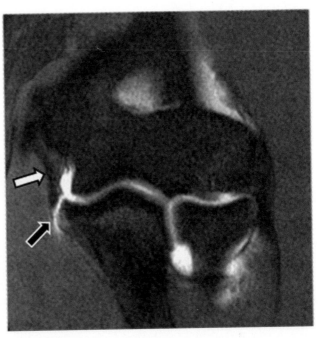

Figure 22-56 UCL tear. Coronal T1-weighted MR arthrogram with fat suppression. With MR imaging, the ligamentous structures such as the UCL (*white arrow*) can be directly visualized. There is a tear of the distal attachment of the UCL onto the ulna (*black arrow*). Note the increased soft tissue contrast as compared to the CT images in Figures 22-54 and 22-55.

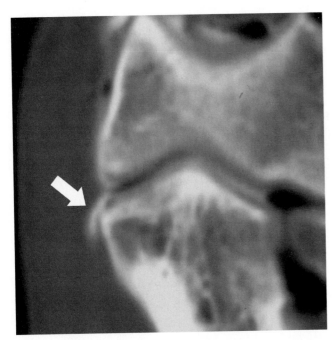

Figure 22-55 Ulnar collateral ligament partial tear. Coronal double contrast CT arthrogram image demonstrates a partial tear of the distal attachment of the UCL (*arrow*). There was no extravasation of contrast beyond the ligament. This appearance of partial tear has been termed the "T" or tau sign. (Image courtesy of Martin L. Schwartz, MD, Birmingham, AL.)

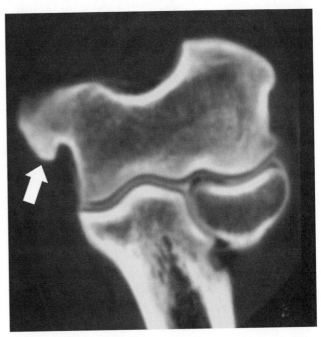

Figure 22-57 Ossification of the proximal ulnar collateral ligament. Coronal double contrast CT arthrogram image demonstrates an intact ulnar collateral ligament. Ossification of the ligament at its proximal attachment onto the medial epicondyle (*arrow*) was likely due to chronic, repetitive stress on the medial elbow in this professional baseball pitcher.

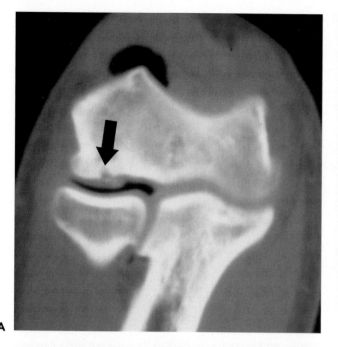

A

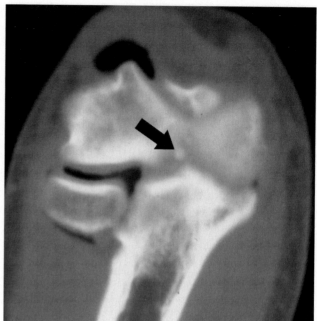

B

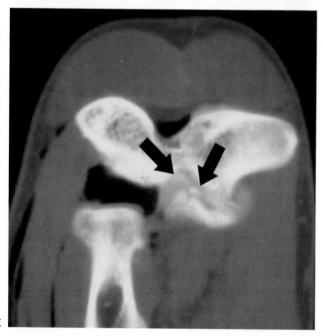

C

Figure 22-58 Intra-articular osteochondral bodies. Direct coronal double contrast CT arthrogram. **A:** A small osteochondral defect is present in the capitellum (*arrow*). There is irregularity of the overlying cartilage. **B, C:** Tiny osteochondral fragments (*arrows*) are located centrally within the joint. (Images courtesy of Martin L. Schwartz, MD, Birmingham, AL.)

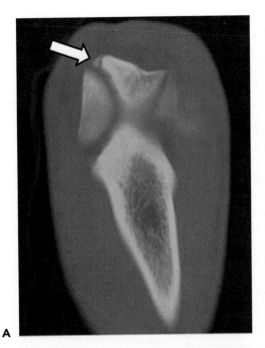

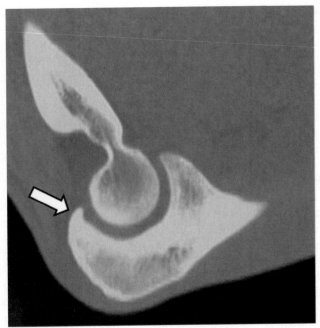

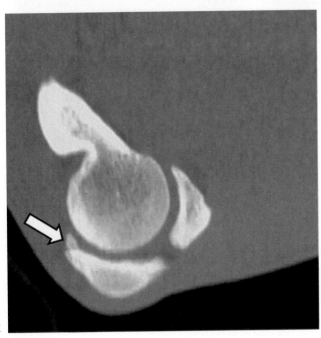

Figure 22-59 Olecranon osteophyte. **A:** Transverse CT with the elbow in 90 degrees of flexion demonstrates an osteophyte on the medial aspect of the tip of the olecranon process. **B, C:** Sagittal reformatted images show the symptomatic olecranon osteophyte (*arrows*). The tip of the olecranon was subsequently resected with relief of the patient's symptoms.

UPPER EXTREMITY: WRIST AND HAND

Anatomy

The wrist is an intricate arrangement of numerous bones and articulations that permits complex and precise motion. The distal radius flares out distally to provide a relatively large surface area for carpal articulation. The distal ulna does not provide a direct articular surface but, instead, offers support for the triangular fibrocartilage. The distal ulna fits into the sigmoid notch of the distal radius at the distal radioulnar joint (DRUJ) (Fig. 22-60A). The carpus is divided into proximal and distal rows. The proximal row consists of the scaphoid, lunate, triquetrum and pisiform (from radial to ulnar) (Fig. 22-60B). The scaphoid and lunate articulate with the radius to form the radiocarpal joint. The triquetrum is positioned over the ulna. The pisiform is situated on the volar aspect of the wrist at the same level as the triquetrum forming the pisotriquetral joint. The distal carpal row

consists of the trapezium, trapezoid, capitate, and hamate (radial to ulnar) (Fig. 22-60C). The articulation between the proximal and distal carpal rows is called the midcarpal joint. The scaphoid articulates with both the trapezium and trapezoid. The lunate supports the capitate; the triquetrum, the hamate. At the carpometacarpal level, the trapezium and trapezoid articulate with the thumb and index finger metacarpals respectively. The capitate supports the middle finger metacarpal. The central stabilizing column of the wrist consists of the distal radius, lunate, capitate, and middle finger metacarpal.

The carpal tunnel is located on the volar aspect of the wrist. It contains most of the flexor tendons of the wrist and the median nerve. The flexor retinaculum forms the roof of the carpal tunnel. Proximally, the retinaculum extends from the distal pole of the scaphoid to the pisiform. Distally, the retinaculum extends from the tubercle of the trapezium to the hook of the hamate. Guyon's canal is a small structure located volar to the carpal tunnel. The ulnar nerve and artery are contained within Guyon's

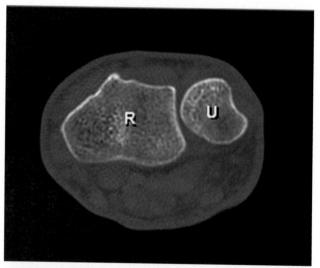

A

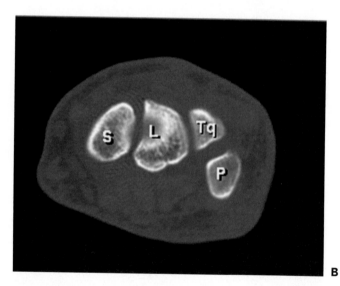

B

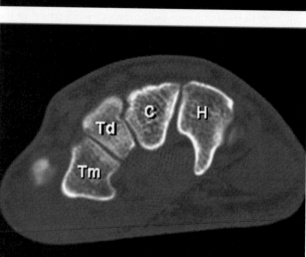

C

Figure 22-60 Normal wrist anatomy. Transverse CT images. **A:** Distal radius (R) and ulna (U). **B:** Proximal carpal row: scaphoid (S), lunate (L), triquetrum (Tq), pisiform (P). **C:** Distal carpal row: trapezium, trapezoid (Tz), capitate (C), hamate (H).

canal. The dorsal wrist tendons are segregated into six compartments.

The triangular fibrocartilage (TFC) extends from the ulnar aspect of the distal radius (where it has a broad attachment) to the base of the styloid process of the ulna. The most important intercarpal ligaments are the scapholunate (SL) and lunotriquetral (LT). The extrinsic ligaments of the wrist are not well visualized by CT.

Trauma

Because of the extremely complex nature of the joints of the wrist and the small size of carpal bones, CT can be very helpful in the evaluation of fractures and dislocations of this region (123,269). Nonarticular fractures of the distal radius, such as those of Colles or Smith, do not usually require CT evaluation. CT is often performed to exclude intra-articular extension of these fractures and to evaluate the congruity of the articular surfaces when present (Fig. 22-61). Distal radius fractures that do involve the articular surface, such as the Barton or reverse Barton, may require CT for evaluation (Fig. 22-62). It is important to determine the number of distal radius fracture fragments just as it is in the better-known concepts regarding the hip and shoulder (172). The die-punch fracture of the distal radius is a depressed fracture of the articular surface (Fig. 22-63).

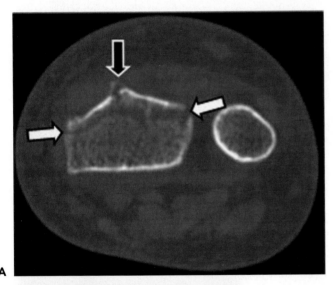

A

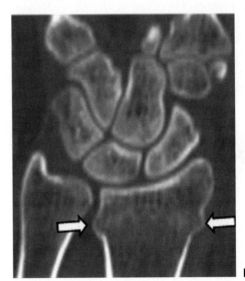

B

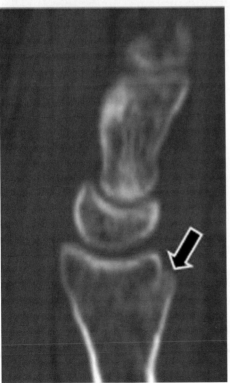

C

Figure 22-61 Buckle fracture of the distal radius. **A:** Transverse CT image reveals a coronal fracture through dorsal distal radius (*white arrows*). The fracture line also extends through the dorsal cortex (*black arrow*). **B:** Coronal reformatted image demonstrates the buckle fracture of the distal radius (*arrows*) and excludes intra-articular extension. **C:** Sagittal reformatted image best displays the dorsal buckle fracture (*arrow*).

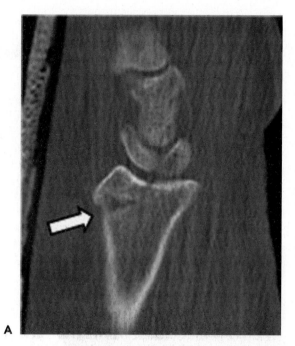

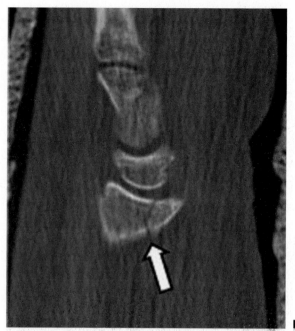

Figure 22-62   Barton fractures, dorsal and volar. **A:** Sagittal CT image at the scapholunate interval demonstrates a fracture of the dorsal lip of the distal radius (*arrow*). **B:** A more ulnar image through the lunate shows a volar lip fracture (*arrow*).

CT can provide an accurate assessment of the degree of step-off and gap at the articular surface. CT is also useful in distal radius fractures to evaluate for the presence of concomitant carpal bone fractures (Fig. 22-64). CT may be performed in postoperative setting if there is concern for residual joint incongruity, malalignment, or intra-articular fracture fragment (Fig. 22-65). The styloid process of the ulna is commonly fractured in the setting of a distal radius fracture. Fractures of the distal ulna are relatively uncommon but can be seen in cases of severe trauma to the wrist.

The distal radioulnar joint (DRUJ) is susceptible to acute or chronic injury. Acute injuries of the DRUJ are often associated with fractures of the distal radius (Galeazzi fracture-dislocation) but ulnar dislocation may occur in isolation. A less common cause of DRUJ injury is the Essex-Lopresti fracture-dislocation in which there is a radial head fracture, interosseous membrane disruption,

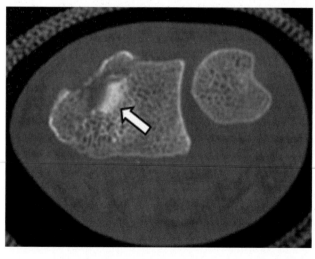

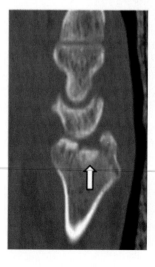

A, B

Figure 22-63 Die-punch distal radius fracture. **A:** Transverse CT image reveals a portion of impacted cortex (*arrow*) from the articular surface. **B:** Sagittal reformatted image displays the focal die-punch defect in the articular surface of the distal radius (*arrow*). There is a step-off of several millimeters at the defect.

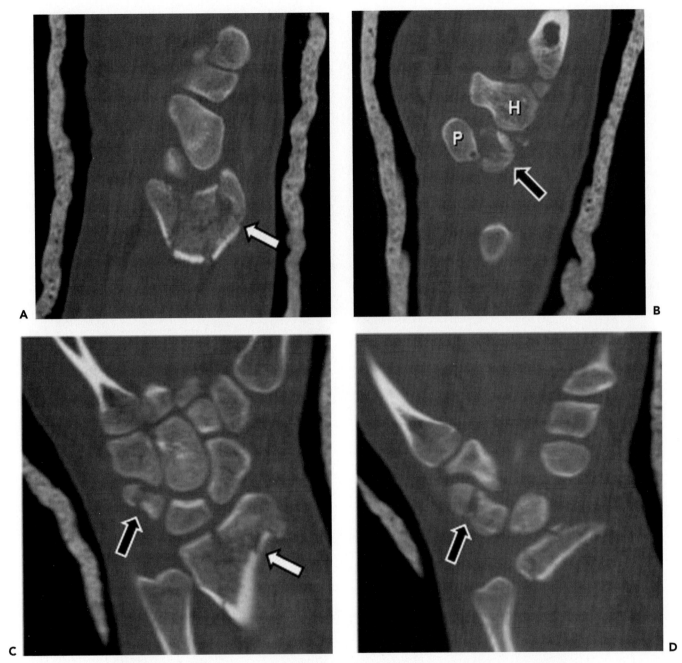

Figure 22-64 Distal radius and triquetrum fractures. **A:** Sagittal CT image through the radio-scaphoid joint shows a transverse fracture of the distal radius (*arrow*) with extension to the articular surface. Note the slight depression of the central fracture fragment. There is no significant dorsal angulation after external reduction. **B:** Sagittal CT image through the ulnar side of the wrist demonstrates a comminuted fracture of the triquetrum (*arrow*). The hamate (H) and pisiform (P) bones are marked for anatomic reference. Note the excellent anatomical detail obtained even with the wrist in a plaster cast. **C:** Coronal reformatted image again shows the distal radius (*white arrow*) and triquetrum (*black arrow*) fractures. **D:** A more volar coronal image better displays the triquetrum fracture (*arrow*). Note the high quality of the reformatted images when the direct CT acquisition is of sufficient technical quality.

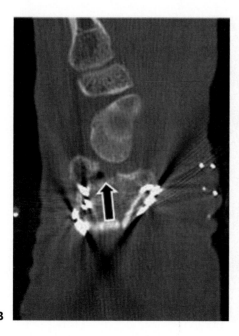 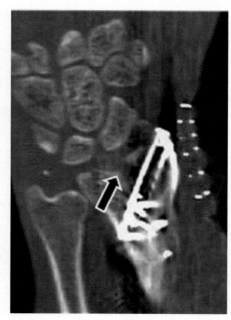

A, B

Figure 22-65 Radial styloid fracture. **A:** Sagittal CT image through the radioscaphoid joint shows a residual gap in the articular surface (*arrow*) of the distal radius after ORIF. **B:** Coronal reformatted image displays the residual articular surface gap (*arrow*). This scan provided clinically significant diagnostic information despite artifact associated with the pins through the radial styloid.

and DRUJ dislocation (Fig. 22-66). In chronic ulnar-sided wrist pain, there may be ligamentous insufficiency resulting in subluxation of the distal ulna with respect to the radius. In cases such as this, it is helpful to scan both wrists together in supination and pronation. The distal ulna will usually displace out of the sigmoid notch of the radius in a dorsal direction (192).

Scaphoid fracture and evaluation of its complications constitute one of the most common indications for wrist CT. A frequently encountered clinical situation is the clinically suspected scaphoid fracture in the face of negative radiographs. CT can identify even extremely subtle

fractures of the scaphoid if proper technique is utilized. Ideally, the scan should be obtained with a direct sagittal acquisition parallel to the long axis of the scaphoid (7) (Fig. 22-67). A scan in the transverse plane should also be acquired directly. Coronal reformatted images can also be helpful. If acquired with a multidetector CT, direct sagittal scanning may not be needed (see Fig. 22-2). Some authors now advocate the use of MR for detection of all radiographically occult fractures (26,71,91,114). MR is more sensitive for bone marrow edema and nondisplaced fractures than is CT. MR also has the advantage of being able to detect soft tissue injuries that

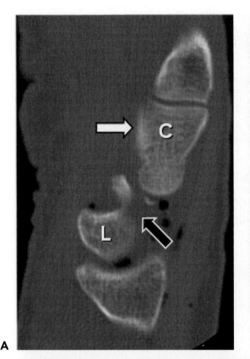

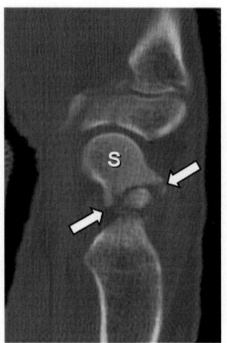

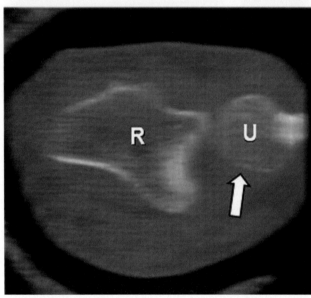

Figure 22-66 Transscaphoid perilunate dislocation with DRUJ injury. **A:** Sagittal CT image reveals dorsal dislocation (*white arrow*) of the capitate (C) with respect to the lunate (L). The lunate remains aligned with the radius. Note the dorsal lunate fracture (*black arrow*). **B:** On a more radial image, there is an associated comminuted scaphoid (S) waist fracture (*arrows*). **C:** Transverse reformatted image demonstrates dorsal dislocation (*arrow*) of the ulna (U) with respect to the radius (R). This is the same case as the radial head fracture-dislocation seen in Figure 22-51. This combination of injuries represents the Essex-Lopresti fracture-dislocation. Note the lower-quality reformatted images when the appropriate parameters are not used on the direct acquisition.

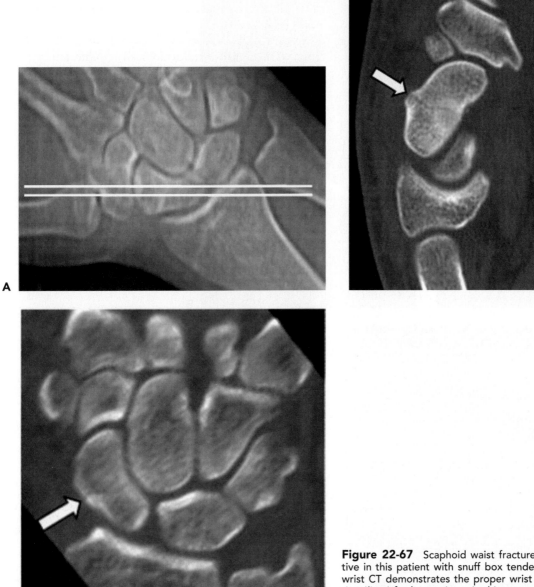

Figure 22-67 Scaphoid waist fracture. Radiographs were negative in this patient with snuff box tenderness. **A:** Scout view for a wrist CT demonstrates the proper wrist alignment and slice selection (*lines*) for long-axis sagittal images of the scaphoid. **B:** Sagittal CT image reveals a nondisplaced scaphoid waist fracture (*arrow*). **C:** Coronal reformatted image also shows the subtle fracture (*arrow*).

may be responsible for the patient's pain. The choice between CT and MR may depend upon factors such as cost and availability of the CT or MR scanner. As is the case elsewhere in the body, uncomplicated scaphoid fractures do not require CT. It is when complicating factors such as angulation, displacement, and comminution are a concern that CT can offer assistance (see Fig. 22-66B). CT is also useful in surveying scaphoid fracture healing, especially if there is a question of bone graft incorporation after internal fixation. CT can detect scaphoid malunion or nonunion that may be difficult to visualize on conventional radiographs or tomography (36). If the distal pole of the scaphoid rotates in a volar (or palmar) direction, there will be a prominent dorsal apex known as a humpback deformity (243). A normal intrascaphoid angle between the proximal and distal poles (less than 35 degrees) is needed for proper scaphoid biomechanical function. An intrascaphoid angle greater than 45 degrees leads to the diagnosis of humpback deformity (Fig. 22-68). Osteonecrosis (avascular necrosis) of the proximal scaphoid fracture fragment is a commonly seen complication of scaphoid fracture. The sclerosis and collapse of the proximal fragment is usually evident radiographically, but CT may detect early changes. MR may be more sensitive for early signs of osteonecro-

sis (bone marrow edema and early subchondral changes). Osteonecrosis can be a complicating factor in other carpal bone fractures such as the lunate or capitate (249) (Fig. 22-69).

Fractures of the carpal bones other than the scaphoid can be difficult to see radiographically. A notoriously difficult carpal bone fracture to see on radiographs is the hook of hamate fracture (Fig. 22-70). These fractures may be well seen on CT, but again, MR is being used more often in cases of radiographically occult fractures. Even when detected, carpal bone fractures may be hard to characterize adequately without CT (see Figs. 22-64, 22-66, and 22-69). Carpal alignment, in the face of subluxation or frank dislocation, may also require CT. The lunate and perilunate dislocations are complex injuries involving numerous carpal structures. In the case of lunate dislocation, the lunate is displaced (usually in a volar direction) but the capitate and distal carpal row remain aligned with the distal radius (Fig. 22-71). In a perilunate dislocation, the lunate and proximal carpal row maintains alignment with the distal radius while the capitate and the distal carpal row are displaced (usually in a dorsal direction). Perilunate dislocations may be accompanied by fractures of the carpal bones, most commonly the scaphoid and/or the capitate (see Fig. 22-66). CT with

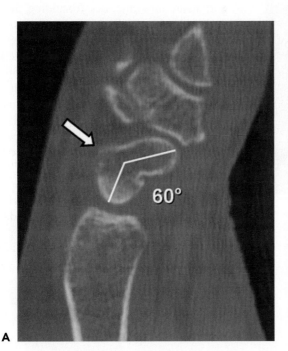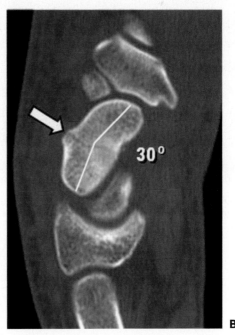

Figure 22-68 Humpback deformity of the scaphoid. **A:** Sagittal reformatted CT image reveals a healing scaphoid waist fracture. There is volar angulation of the distal fracture fragment producing a prominent dorsal apex: the humpback deformity (*arrow*). The intrascaphoid angle is 60 degrees. **B:** Sagittal image in another patient (same image as Fig. 22-67B). The normal intrascaphoid angle between the proximal and distal poles is less than 35 degrees.

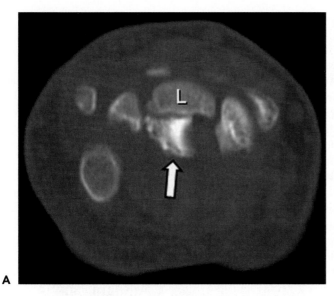

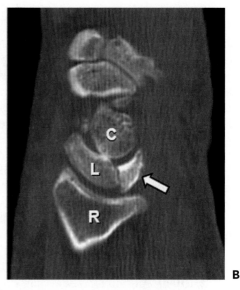

Fig. 22-69 Lunate fracture with osteonecrosis. **A:** Transverse CT image demonstrates a fracture of the lunate (L) in the coronal plane. The volar fracture fragment (*arrow*) is sclerotic. **B:** Sagittal CT image displays the relationship of the coronal fracture of the lunate (L) to the capitate (C) and radius (R). The volar fracture fragment (*arrow*) is slightly displaced and sclerotic. The sclerosis represents developing osteonecrosis.

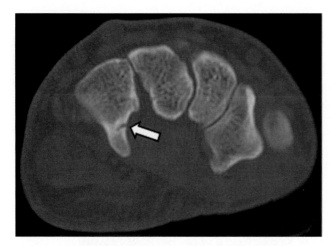

Figure 22-70 Hamate hook fracture. Transverse CT image reveals an incomplete fracture of the hook of the hamate (*arrow*).

multiplanar images can provide necessary information for surgical planning.

Soft tissue abnormalities (including the tendons and ligaments) are best evaluated with MR, again due to its superior soft tissue delineation. Tears of the triangular fibrocartilage and intrinsic wrist ligaments, the scapholunate or lunotriquetral ligaments, are best seen on MR imaging (248) (Fig. 22-72). The carpal tunnel is better evaluated with MR, although CT can visualize the tendon and nerve contents. Kienbock disease is osteonecrosis of the lunate. As mentioned above, CT can be used to evaluate this osteonecrosis, although MR is more sensitive for early findings (66) (Fig. 22-73).

Radiographic assessment of wrist arthropathy is usually sufficient. CT can detect degenerative and inflammatory changes but is not often performed for this indication. CT may detect more erosions of inflammatory arthropathy than radi-

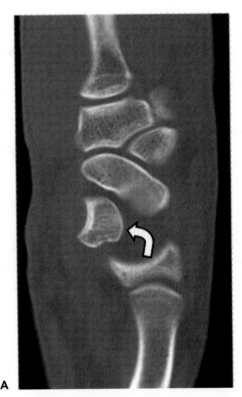

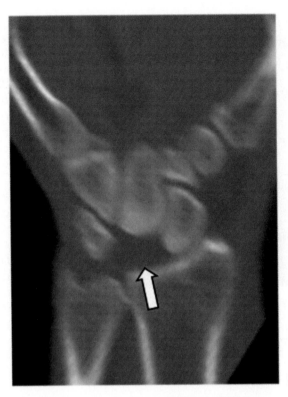

Figure 22-71 Lunate dislocation. **A:** Sagittal CT image demonstrates volar dislocation of the lunate (*arrow*) with 90 degrees of rotation. The distal carpal row remains aligned with the radius. **B:** Coronal reformatted image shows normal alignment of the carpus with the exception of the absent, dislocated lunate (*arrow*).

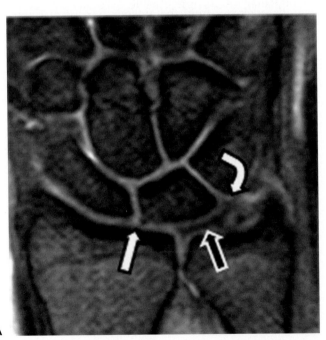

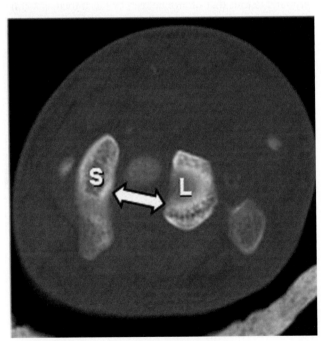

Figure 22-72 Scapholunate ligament tears. **A:** Coronal T2* gradient recalled echo MR image. There is a high-signal defect in the scapholunate ligament (*straight white arrow*) representing a tear. There is no scapholunate widening. The normal lunotriquetral ligament (*curved white arrow*) and triangular fibrocartilage (*black arrow*) are well seen on this MR image. **B:** Transverse CT image in a different patient demonstrates marked traumatic widening (*double arrow*) of the scapholunate (SL) interval. There is rotary subluxation of the scaphoid as evidenced by the fact that the scaphoid (S) lies almost entirely within this transverse plane. These findings imply scapholunate ligamentous insufficiency, although the ligament is not directly visualized on CT.

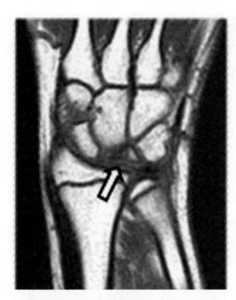

Figure 22-73 Kienbock disease. Coronal T1-weighted MR image in a skeletally immature patient shows low-signal-intensity sclerosis within a partially collapsed lunate (*arrow*). Note the negative ulnar variance, which is thought to be a contributing factor in this disease process.

ographs, but MR and US hold promise for the detection of very early lesions that cannot be seen by CT. If there is a concern for calcification in or around the joint, CT can be helpful.

PELVIS, ACETABULUM, AND HIPS

Anatomy

The osseous pelvis is comprised of three bones: the sacrum and two innominate bones. The innominate bones are composed of three separate ossification centers that converge at the triradiate cartilage of the acetabulum: the ilium, ischium, and pubis. The sacrum articulates with the two innominate bones posteriorly at the sacroiliac joints (Fig. 22-74A to C) with the innominate bones joining anteriorly at the pubic symphysis (see Fig. 22-74F). The sacrum also articulates with the vestigial coccyx distally. The acetabulum (literally "vinegar cup" in Latin) is the bony socket that accepts the femoral head to form the hip joint. The important anatomical components of the acetabulum are the columns, walls, dome, and quadrilateral plate (see Fig. 22-74D, E). The acetabulum is divided into anterior and posterior columns. The anterior column is the larger of the two columns. It begins at the iliac wing extending down the anterior portion of the acetabulum to incorporate the superior pubic ramus. The posterior column begins at the sciatic notch and extends down the posterior acetabulum into the ischium. Both columns are attached to the axial skeleton by the sciatic

buttress that connects the acetabulum to the sacroiliac joint. The posterior wall of the acetabulum is larger than the anterior wall. The lateral portion of either wall is called the acetabular rim. The walls serve to help stabilize the hip joint. The quadrilateral plate is the medial wall of the acetabulum. The dome of the acetabulum is the superior aspect that bears the majority of the weight-bearing forces (see Fig. 22-74D). The obturator ring is an important landmark as some acetabular fractures spare this ring while others disrupt it.

The femoral head articulates with the acetabulum to form the hip joint (see Fig. 22-74E). The articular portion of the femoral head is spherical. The femoral neck is divided into three anatomical regions from proximal to distal: subcapital, mid-cervical, and basicervical. The larger, lateral greater trochanter serves as the attachment site for the abductors and external rotators of the hip: gluteus minimus, gluteus medius and piriformis. The smaller, medial lesser trochanter is the attachment site for the iliopsoas tendon, a hip flexor. Two strong ligaments help provide anterior support for the hip joint, the iliofemoral and pubofemoral ligaments. Posteriorly, the ischiofemoral ligament provides support. The ligamentum teres connects the inferior acetabulum to the fovea capitus of the femoral head.

The sartorius muscle and tensor fascia lata arise from the anterior superior iliac spine (ASIS). The tensor fascia lata gives rise to the lateral iliotibial band. The rectus femoris originates from the anterior inferior iliac spine (AIIS). The gracilis and adductor muscle group arise from the inferior pubic ramus. The hamstring tendons (semimembranosus, semitendinosus, and biceps femoris) arise from the ischial tuberosity. The gluteus maximus has a broad attachment to the posterior iliac wing and sacrum with an insertion on the posterior intertrochanteric line. The anterior vastus medialis, intermedius, and lateralis muscles originate from the proximal femoral shaft.

Within the pelvis, the common iliac vessels and their branches are most important. Around the hip joint, the common femoral and superficial femoral arteries and veins are the key vascular structures. The femoral nerve and its branches join these vessels. The sacral plexus contributes the vast majority of fibers to the sciatic nerve which passes out of the pelvis through the greater sciatic notch, traveling behind to the posterior wall of the acetabulum as it makes it way into the posterior thigh.

Trauma

Pelvic ring fractures occur as the result of high-energy blunt trauma, such as in motor vehicle collisions and falls. Disruption of this ring can lead to pelvic instability with pain and significant loss of function. There are three primary force vectors that lead to pelvic ring fracture: anteroposterior (AP) compression, lateral compression, and vertical shear. Each of these forces leaves its

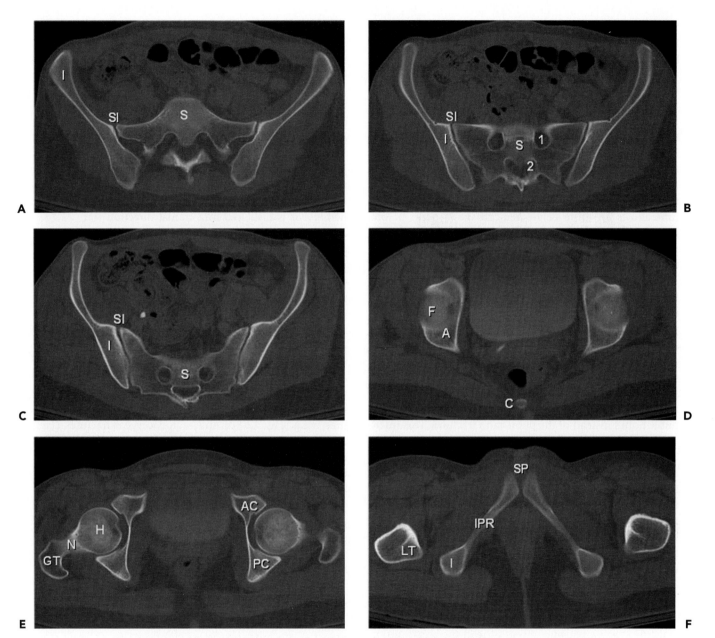

Figure 22-74 Normal pelvic anatomy. Transverse CT images from superior to inferior. **A:** Sacral promontory (S), sacroiliac joint (SI), iliac wing (I). **B:** Sacral body (S), S1 (1) and S2 (2) neural foramina, SI joint (SI), innominate bone (I). **C:** Sacral body (S), SI joint (SI), innominate bone (I). **D:** Acetabular dome (A), femoral head (F), coccyx (C). **E:** Anterior (AC) and posterior (PC) columns of the acetabulum, femoral head (H), femoral neck (N), greater trochanter (GT). **F:** Symphysis pubis (SP), inferior pubic ramus (IPR), ischium (I), lesser trochanter (LT).

mark on the pelvis in a characteristic pattern. Identification of one element of the pattern prompts a search for the remaining elements allowing for identification of all associated injuries (34,53,113,313). Before the advent of helical CT, the pelvis was scanned with 5 mm slices except for the acetabulum that was usually scanned at 3 mm. With today's helical and multislice CT scanners, 3-mm (or less) slices through the entire pelvis are standard. These thin sections acquired with helical technique allow for the production of high quality thin-section 2D and 3D reformatted images.

AP compression injuries most often result from head-on motor vehicle collisions. Such injuries can also be seen in cases of motorcycle wrecks or a pedestrian struck by a vehicle. The force can be directed either anterior to posterior or posterior to anterior. The hallmark of the AP compression injury is pubic symphysis diastasis with or without disruption of the sacroiliac joints (Fig. 22-75). The location and degree of diastasis correlates with the magnitude of force imparted to the pelvis and with the amount of resultant instability. The anteroposterior forces serve to "open" the pelvis; in other words, one or both of the hemipelves undergoes external rotation. In addition, there is diastasis of one or both of the sacroiliac joints. External rotation of the hemipelvis results in an increase in the volume of the pelvic cavity. This increased pelvic volume allows for more pelvic hemorrhage to occur before being tamponaded by osseous and soft tissue structures. Exsanguination due to pelvic hemorrhage is a major potential complication.

Lateral compression injuries usually result from side-impact motor vehicle collisions. Pedestrians struck by motor vehicles from the side will also demonstrate this pattern. The characteristic features of the lateral compression injury are sacral buckle fractures and ipsilateral, horizontal, overlapping pubic rami fractures (Fig. 22-76). The ipsilateral hemipelvis undergoes internal rotation due to the lateral force exerted upon it. Less commonly, there may be disruption of the pubic symphysis with overlap of the pubic bones instead of the pubic rami fractures. This internal rotation results in a decrease in pelvic volume rather than an increase. Consequently, pelvic vascular injuries and resultant hemorrhage are less common. In the most severe lateral compression injuries, the force continues from the ipsilateral hemipelvis across the midline to affect the contralateral side. The ipsilateral hemipelvis sustains a lateral compression injury with associated internal rotation. The contralateral hemipelvis undergoes external rotation and exhibits features of an AP compression injury.

This combined pattern has been described as the "windswept" pelvis (Fig. 22-77). There may be contralateral vertical pubic rami fractures or disruption of the sacrotuberous or sacrospinous ligaments.

Vertical shear injuries typically occur in the setting of a fall from a height, but can also be seen in motor vehicle collisions. A vertically oriented force applied to one hemipelvis, usually by the femur, results in a vertical shear injury. Anteriorly, there are vertically oriented, nonoverlapping fractures of the pubic rami. Posteriorly, there is disruption of the ipsilateral (or occasionally, contralateral) sacroiliac joint and its associated ligaments. The affected hemipelvis is displaced in a cranial direction (Fig. 22-78). There is increased pelvic volume in vertical shear injury, just as in AP compression injury. Occasionally, the forces applied to the pelvis may not conform to the primary vectors described above. Complex fractures involve more than one pattern of injury and are generally the most severe injuries. The specific findings of each pattern will still be present.

There are many fractures of the pelvis that do not significantly disrupt the pelvic ring. Such injuries include avulsion fractures of the anterior iliac spines (Fig. 22-79), iliac crests, and ischial tuberosities (268). Minimally or nondisplaced pubic rami fractures due to a direct blow or straddle injury do not affect pelvic ring stability. Also included are iliac wing (Fig. 22-80) and sacrococcygeal fractures (Fig. 22-81) that do not involve the sacroiliac joints. Sacral fractures are usually vertically oriented and are divided into three zones. Zone 1 fractures involve only the sacral ala. Zone II fractures extend into the neural foramina with potential injury to nerve roots (Fig. 22-82). Zone III fractures pass through the body of the sacrum to involve the sacral spinal canal with potential injury to the cauda equina. Transverse sacral fractures occur less commonly but can have devastating neurologic complications.

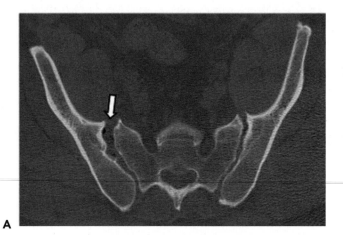

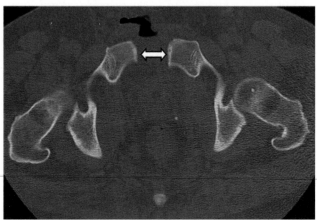

A **B**

Figure 22-75 AP compression pelvic ring injury. **A:** There is diastasis of the right SI joint (*arrow*) with external rotation of the right hemipelvis. **B:** Diastasis of the pubic symphysis (*double arrow*) is also present.

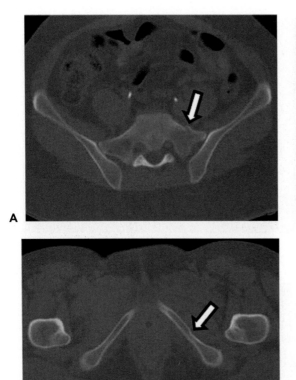

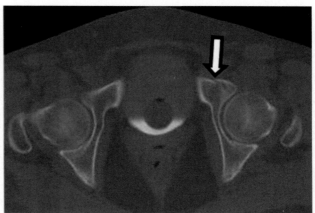

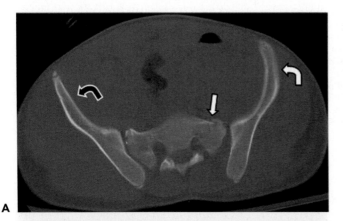

Figure 22-76 Lateral compression pelvic ring injury. **A:** There is a buckle fracture of the left sacral ala (*arrow*). **B:** There is a minimally displaced fracture of the left superior pubic ramus (*arrow*) at the puboacetabular junction. This should not be confused with an anterior column acetabular fracture. **C:** There is also a minimally displaced fracture of the left inferior pubic ramus (*arrow*).

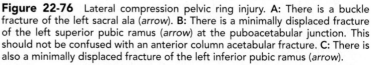

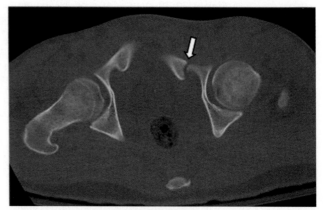

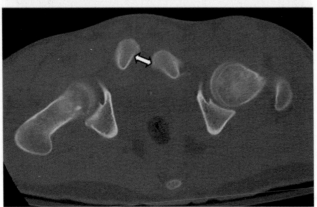

Figure 22-77 Lateral compression pelvic ring injury ("windswept" pelvis). **A:** A buckle fracture of the left sacral ala (*straight arrow*) is seen in conjunction with internal rotation of the left hemipelvis (*curved white arrow*). In addition, there is external rotation of the right hemipelvis (*black curved arrow*) with mild widening of the right SI joint. **B:** An overlapping fracture of the left superior pubic ramus is present (*arrow*). **C:** Pubic symphysis diastasis is also present (*double arrow*). In the "windswept" pelvis, an ipsilateral lateral compression force continues across the pelvis to become an AP compression force on the contralateral side. The pelvis will, therefore, exhibit features of an ipsilateral lateral compression injury and a contralateral AP compression injury.

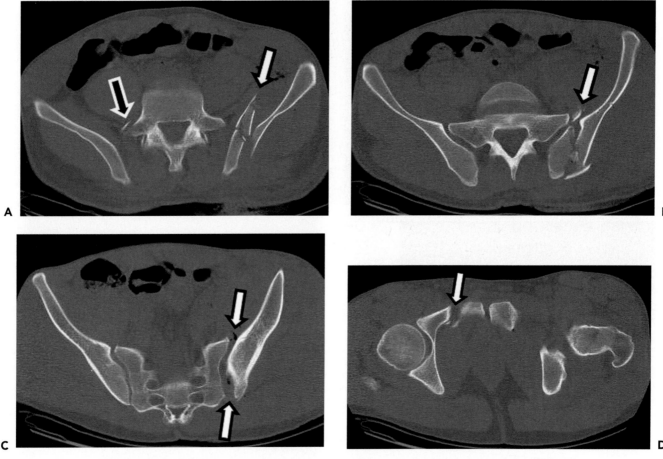

Figure 22-78 Vertical shear pelvic ring injury. **A:** There is a comminuted fracture of the left iliac crest with marked offset (*white arrow*). Note also the avulsion fracture of the right L5 transverse process (*black arrow*) at the attachment of the iliolumbar ligament. Such avulsion fractures are often a sign of pelvic instability. **B:** The left iliac fracture extends to the SI joint (*arrow*) and posteriorly through the posterior iliac crest. **C:** Marked diastasis of the anterior and posterior left SI joint is present (*arrows*). **D:** There is a displaced fracture of the right superior pubic ramus (*arrow*). Anterior ring fractures in vertical shear injuries usually remain ipsilateral but may involve the contralateral side (as in this case). Note also the disparity in the level of the visualized hips. The right femoral head and acetabulum are seen at the same level as the more inferior left femoral neck is seen. This disparity is due to the vertical displacement of the left hemipelvis.

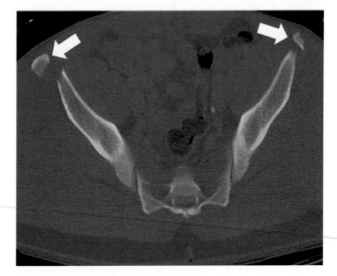

Figure 22-79 Bilateral avulsion fractures of the anterior inferior iliac spines. There have been avulsion fractures (*arrows*) at the attachment sites of both rectus femoris muscles. The pelvic ring was spared.

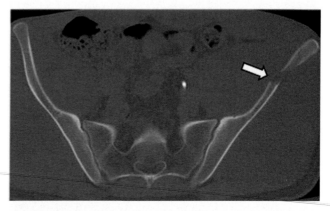

Figure 22-80 Iliac wing fracture. There is an isolated fracture of the left iliac wing (*arrow*). No fracture of the pelvic ring or acetabulum was present.

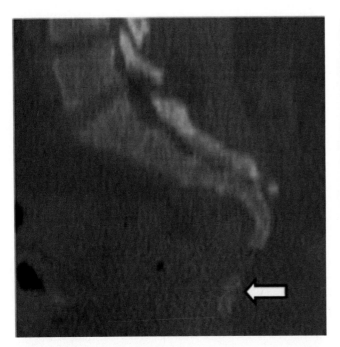

Figure 22-81 Coccyx dislocation. Sagittal reformatted image from a pelvic CT demonstrates displacement of the tip of the coccyx (*arrow*). This injury can be difficult to appreciate on transverse images.

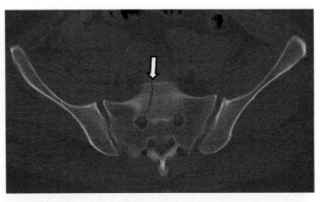

Figure 22-82 Sacral fracture, zone II. A right paramedian sacral body fracture (*arrow*) extends to the right S1 neural foramen.

Acetabular fractures also occur in the setting of significant trauma secondary to either motor vehicle accident or high velocity fall. Blunt force is exerted upon the femur, passes through the femoral head, and is then transferred to the acetabulum. The direction and magnitude of the force and the position of the femoral head determines the pattern of acetabular injury. Determination of the pattern of injury is the key to the classification of acetabular fractures (23,24). Because of their similar underlying mechanisms of injury, pelvic ring fractures and acetabular fractures are often seen in combination.

The function of the acetabulum is to provide a means for the transfer of weight-bearing forces from the appendicular to axial skeleton via its articulation with the femoral head. It is this same femoral head that transfers high-energy forces to the acetabulum in the setting of trauma. The pattern of acetabular injury is determined by the position of the femoral head at the time of the traumatic event. When the femoral head is internally rotated, the force is transferred to the posterior column; when externally rotated, the force is directed toward the anterior column. If the femoral head is adducted, the force is transmitted to the acetabular roof; if abducted, the force is directed inferiorly. The direction of the force also determines which part of the acetabulum will be injured. An anterior force applied to the femoral head will be transmitted to

the posterior wall and column. Conversely, a posterior force will affect the anterior wall and column. A force to the lateral aspect of the femoral head is directed toward the medial wall of the acetabulum often resulting in transverse acetabular fractures.

Fractures of the acetabulum are classified according to the system described by Letournel and Judet (120). The system is based on the orientation of the fractures and the structures involved. The orientation of fractures under this system is based on a lateral view of the acetabulum. There are ten defined patterns of acetabular fracture under this system. These ten patterns are divided into five elementary and five associated patterns. The elementary patterns include those fractures with a single fracture orientation, whereas the associated patterns generally involve combinations of the elementary fractures. The elementary patterns are anterior wall, posterior wall, anterior column, posterior column, and transverse. The associated patterns are both-column, posterior column with posterior wall, transverse with posterior wall, T-shaped, and anterior column with posterior hemitransverse. For simplicity, it is useful to group these 10 patterns into 3 categories: wall, column, and transverse types (24). Some fracture types fall into two of the categories. The three categories of acetabular fractures have a characteristic orientation on CT. Wall fractures occur in an oblique plane. Column fractures

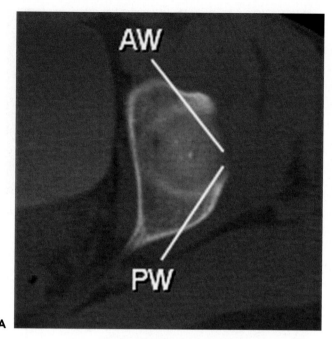
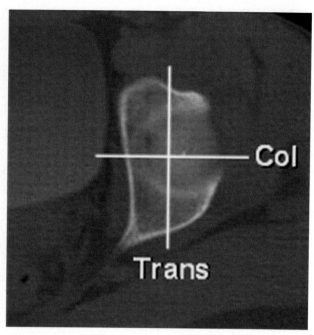

Figure 22-83 Acetabular fracture orientation on transverse CT. **A:** Anterior wall (AW) and posterior wall (PW) fractures occur in an oblique plane. **B:** Column (Col) fractures of the acetabulum occur in the coronal plane. Transverse (Trans) acetabular fractures appear in the sagittal plane. Note that transverse fractures pass through the anterior and posterior walls of the acetabulum.

appear in the coronal plane while transverse fractures occur in the sagittal plane (Fig. 22-83).

Isolated acetabular wall fractures do not typically involve the weight-bearing articular portion of the acetabulum. Fractures of the posterior wall are more common than those of the anterior wall due to the preponderance of poste-

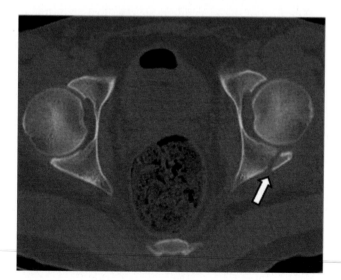

Figure 22-84 Posterior wall acetabular fracture. An oblique fracture passes through the posterior wall of the left acetabulum (*arrow*).

riorly directed forces responsible for acetabular fractures. Posterior wall fractures may be seen in isolation (Fig. 22-84), related to posterior femoral head dislocation (Fig. 22-85), or in combination with posterior column or transverse acetabular fractures. Posterior wall fracture fragments are particularly prone to migrate into the hip joint interposing between the acetabulum and femoral head (Fig. 22-86). Anterior wall fractures are rare in isolation but may be seen in conjunction with other injuries (Fig. 22-87).

Column fractures divide the acetabulum into front and back halves producing their coronal CT orientation. Isolated anterior or posterior column fractures are uncommon. Anterior column fractures involve the iliac wing and anterior acetabulum (Fig. 22-88). Posterior column fractures involve only the posterior portion of the acetabulum and do not affect the iliac wing (Fig. 22-89). Anterior and posterior column fractures pass through the obturator ring to involve the pubic rami. The posterior column with posterior wall fracture displays the features of each of its components (Fig. 22-90). Both-column fractures represent the most common acetabular injury. As the name implies, there is involvement of both the anterior and posterior columns. The sine qua non of the both-column fracture is the "spur" sign. The combination of anterior and posterior column involvement results in an acetabulum that is no longer in continuity with the remainder of the pelvis. A strut of bone extends from the SI joint toward the acetabulum but ends in a posterolateral spur that is virtually

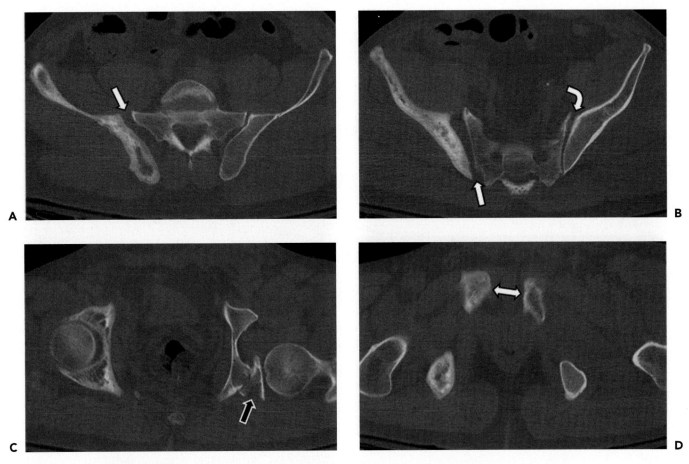

A

B

C

D

Figure 22-85   AP compression pelvic ring injury with posterior left hip dislocation. **A:** The right SI joint is widened (*arrow*). Note also the cortical thickening of the right innominate bone. **B:** On a more inferior image, there is offset at the posterior right SI joint (*straight arrow*). The anterior left SI joint is slightly widened (*curved arrow*). These findings are components of the AP compression injury. **C:** There has been posterior dislocation of the left femoral head, also a result of an anterior force. The posterior wall of the left acetabulum is fractured (*arrow*) with the fracture fragment rotated 90 degrees and interposed between the femoral head and acetabulum preventing complete relocation. Note also the trabecular coarsening of the right acetabulum. The cortical thickening and trabecular coarsening of the right hemipelvis are characteristic of Paget's disease. **D:** Pubic symphysis diastasis (*double arrow*) is another component of the AP compression injury.

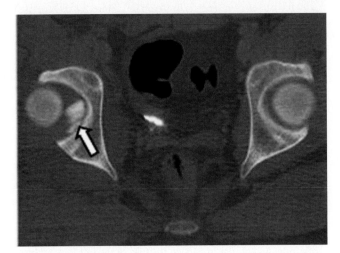

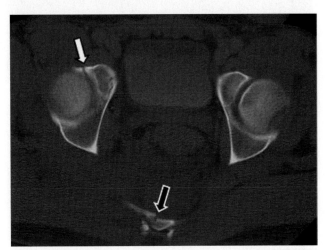

Figure 22-86   Posterior wall acetabular fracture with intra-articular fragment. The right acetabular posterior wall is fractured and the fragment trapped in the joint space preventing relocation of the femoral head.

Figure 22-87   Anterior wall acetabular fracture. A minimally displaced fracture of the anterior wall of the right acetabulum is demonstrated (*white arrow*). These fractures are rarely found in isolation. Note the sagittal fracture of the sacrum (*black arrow*).

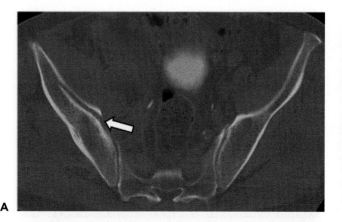

A

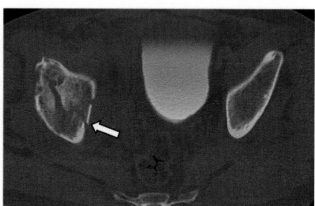

B

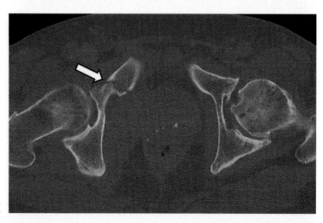

C

Figure 22-88 Anterior column acetabular fracture. **A:** A coronal fracture of the right iliac wing is present (*arrow*). **B:** At the level of the acetabular roof, the coronal orientation of the fracture (*arrow*) indicates a column fracture. **C:** The anterior column fracture extends across the superior pubic ramus (*arrow*) and continues through the obturator ring.

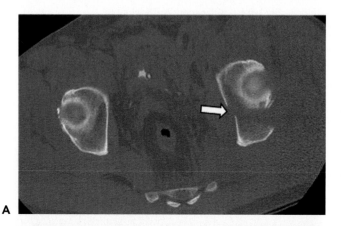

A

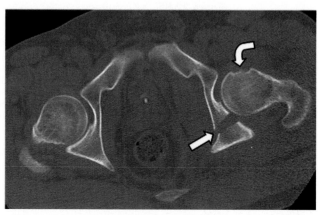

B

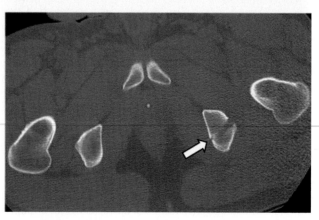

C

Figure 22-89 Posterior column acetabular fracture. **A:** A coronal column-type fracture involves the posterior left acetabulum (*arrow*). **B:** The posterior column fracture (*straight arrow*) extends inferiorly. An anterior impaction fracture of the left femoral head (*curved arrow*) indicates left hip dislocation at the time of initial injury with subsequent relocation. **C:** Posterior column fractures usually extend through the obturator foramen but will sometimes exit through the ischial tuberosity (*arrow*).

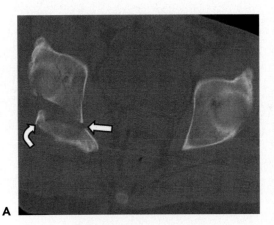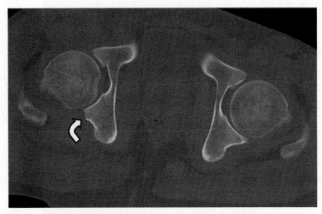

A   B

Figure 22-90 Posterior column with posterior wall acetabular fracture. **A:** A coronally oriented fracture extends through the posterior right acetabulum (*straight arrow*). A bone fragment is seen along the lateral margin of the fracture (*curved arrow*). **B:** A fracture of the posterior wall of the right acetabulum (*curved arrow*) is the donor site for the fragment.

pathognomonic for this injury (Fig. 22-91). The anterior column with posterior hemitransverse fracture is the most complex acetabular fracture to classify. The combination of column and transverse fractures can be difficult to appreciate radiographically. On CT, both the anterior column (including iliac wing) and posterior transverse fracture planes can be appreciated. There is usually no obturator ring fracture and no spur sign present; therefore, this fracture should not be confused with the more common both-column fracture (Fig. 22-92).

Transverse fractures are so called because of their appearance when looking at the acetabulum from the lateral view. On CT, the fracture is vertically oriented in the sagittal plane (Fig. 22-93). The obturator ring is intact in most transverse fractures (except for the T-shaped fracture). The transverse with posterior wall fracture is a common injury that incorporates the features of both elementary fractures (Fig. 22-94). The T-shaped fracture is a fairly common ac-

etabular injury that displays the characteristics of an elementary transverse fracture with the addition of a medial acetabular wall fracture extending through the obturator ring (Fig. 22-95). The anterior column with posterior hemitransverse fracture is discussed above.

In one study (23), the three most common types of acetabular fracture accounted for roughly two thirds of all cases: both-column, transverse with posterior wall, and posterior wall. This figure rose to 90% when the next two most common types were considered: T-shaped and transverse.

An accessory ossification center, the os acetabulum, can mimic an acetabular wall fracture. Differentiating features include its characteristic superolateral location and its well-corticated margins. Fractures of the anterior puboacetabular junction can be seen in pelvic ring fractures. These fractures may extend into the anterior column of the acetabu-

(*text continues on page 1550*)

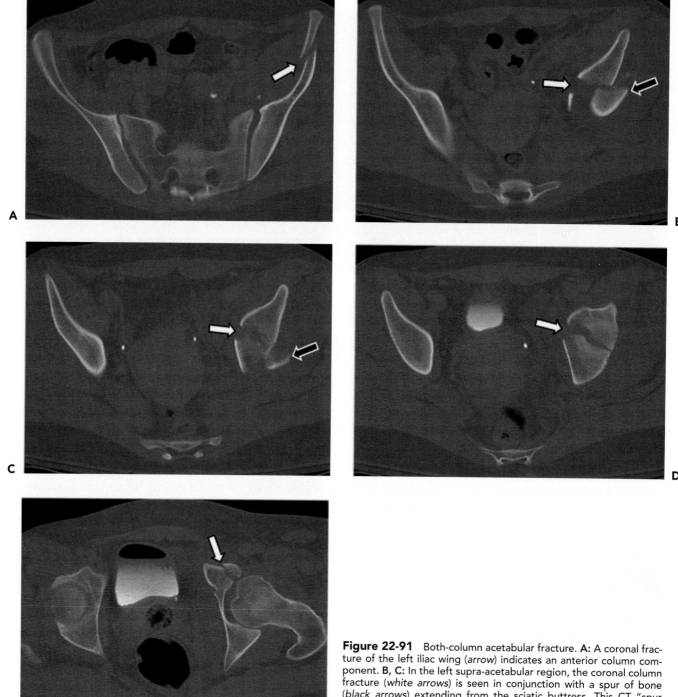

Figure 22-91   Both-column acetabular fracture. **A:** A coronal fracture of the left iliac wing (*arrow*) indicates an anterior column component. **B, C:** In the left supra-acetabular region, the coronal column fracture (*white arrows*) is seen in conjunction with a spur of bone (*black arrows*) extending from the sciatic buttress. This CT "spur sign" is virtually pathognomonic for a both-column fracture. **D, E:** The column fracture continues through the acetabular roof and obturator ring (*white arrows*).

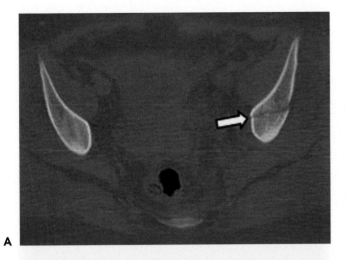

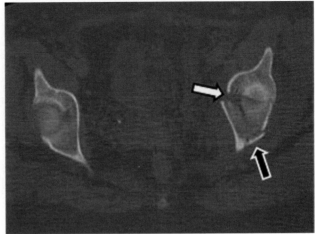

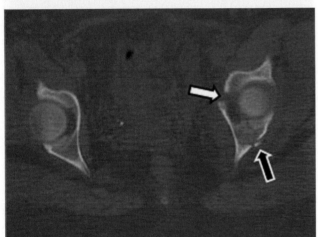

Figure 22-92 Anterior column, posterior hemitransverse acetabular fracture. **A:** An anterior column type fracture (*arrow*) is present in the left iliac wing. **B:** At the level of the acetabular roof, the coronal anterior column fracture is again seen (*white arrow*). A sagittal transverse fracture extends posteriorly (*black arrow*) but not anteriorly. **C:** On a more inferior image, the anterior column (*white arrow*) and posterior hemitransverse (*black arrow*) components are well seen. As is usually the case in this injury, no obturator ring fracture is present (not shown).

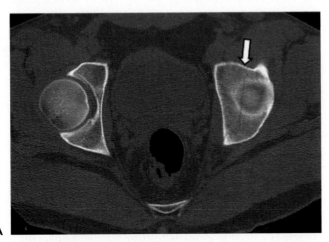

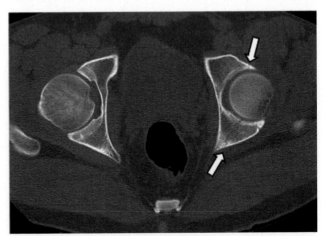

Figure 22-93 Transverse acetabular fracture. There is a nondisplaced fracture of the left acetabulum in the sagittal plane.

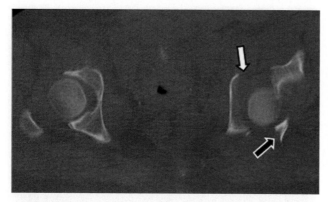

Figure 22-94 Transverse with posterior wall acetabular fracture. A sagittally oriented transverse type fracture involves the left acetabulum (*white arrow*). There is an associated fracture of the posterior wall (*black arrow*).

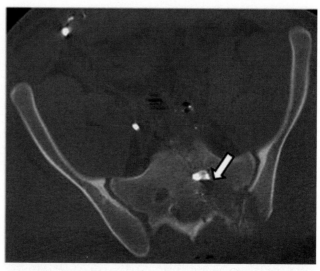

Figure 22-96 Sacral fracture due to gunshot wound. A bullet passed through the posterior left iliac crest, across the left sacroiliac joint, into the sacrum where a fragment lodged. The bullet path crossed the left S1 neural foramen (*arrow*).

lum, but are not anterior column fractures per se. Such fractures are more correctly considered superior pubic rami fractures.

Penetrating trauma, usually due to gunshot injury, may affect the pelvis. As with all gunshot wounds, CT can aid in determining the path of the projectile and in the precise identification of injured structures. Articular surface involvement and neurovascular integrity are of particular interest in the pelvis (Fig. 22-96). Other soft tissue structures (e.g., urinary bladder, rectum) may also be affected.

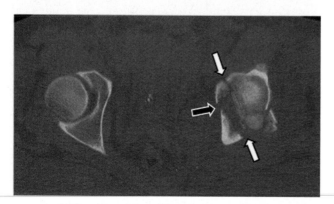

Figure 22-95 T-shaped acetabular fracture. The predominant fracture line has a sagittal orientation (*white arrows*) associated with a transverse-type fracture of the left acetabulum. The second component extends centrally (*black arrow*) from the transverse fracture forming the "T" shape. This component extended through the obturator ring on other slices (not shown).

The same forces that produce pelvic ring and acetabular fractures may also produce femoral head dislocation. The femoral head tends to dislocate posteriorly because the overwhelming majority of forces directed at the pelvis travel in an anterior to posterior direction. This posterior dislocation is in spite of the posterior inclination of the acetabulum that resists posterior displacement of the femoral head. Radiography should be performed prior to hip reduction for diagnosis, but CT should be performed after reduction. The power of CT is its ability to detect subtle associated fractures and intra-articular fracture fragments that may preclude a completely successful reduction. Associated fractures may involve the acetabulum, usually the posterior column and/or wall (see Figs. 22-86 and 22-90), or the femoral head, usually an anterior impaction fracture similar to the Hill-Sachs fracture seen in the shoulder (Fig. 22-97). MR can be used to assess for sciatic nerve injury (213).

Femoral head fractures are uncommon but can be evaluated with CT especially if there is a concern for intra-articular fragments (see Fig. 22-97). Femoral neck, intertrochanteric, subtrochanteric, and shaft fractures are usually sufficiently evaluated with radiography. CT can be utilized if there is a need to evaluate fracture fragment orientation or displacement (Fig. 22-98). If there is a clinical suspicion for a radiographically occult hip fracture, MR is the test of choice (67,107). CT may be unable to detect an acute, nondisplaced femoral neck fracture, especially if the fracture is in the transverse plane of the scan (Fig. 22-99).

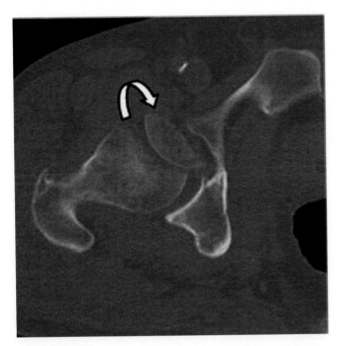

Figure 22-97 Femoral head fracture. The fracture fragment from a right femoral head fracture has flipped 180 degrees (*arrow*).

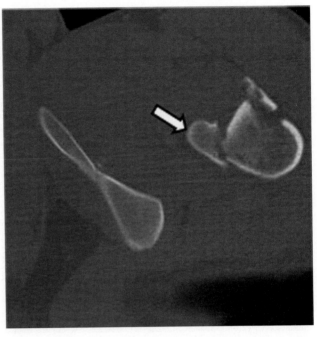

Figure 22-98 Intertrochanteric femur fracture. There is a comminuted fracture of the left femur in the Intertrochanteric region. The lesser trochanter is a separate fragment (*arrow*).

Multiplanar reformatted CT images can be of some use in the patient who is unable to undergo MR imaging. MR can provide immediate visualization of the fracture line and associated bone marrow edema. MR can also detect soft tissue injuries (such as adductor muscle strain) that would be inapparent on CT. These soft tissue injuries may be associated with a fracture or occur in isolation (but could explain the patient's pain) (19).

Once a fracture has been reduced, either with closed technique or open reduction and internal fixation, CT can be used to survey the healing process. Transverse CT scanning with multiplanar reformatted images can provide important information on malunion or nonunion of fractures. CT can accomplish this task even in the presence of metallic instrumentation if performed correctly (Fig. 22-100).

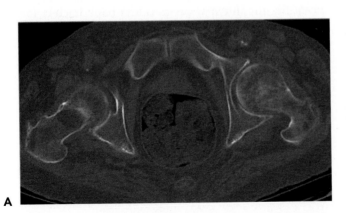

A

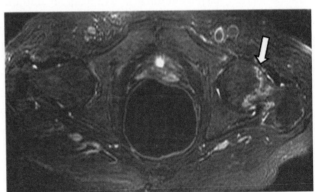

B

Figure 22-99 Subcapital femoral neck fracture. The patient presented to the emergency department with left hip pain after a fall. Conventional radiographs were negative. **A:** Transverse image from a pelvic CT. **B:** Axial T2-weighted MR image with fat suppression. Linear bright T2 signal is seen in the subcapital region of the left femoral neck (*arrow*). (*continued*)

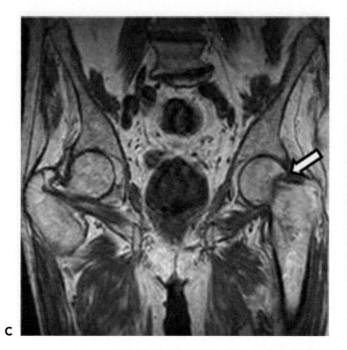

C

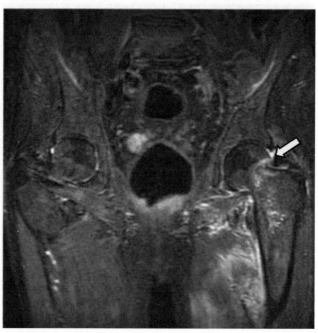

D

Figure 22-99 *(continued)* **C:** Coronal T1-weighted MR image clearly demonstrates a minimally impacted subcapital femoral neck fracture *(arrow)*. **D:** Coronal STIR MR image. The left femoral neck fracture appears bright. Note also the injury to the left adductor muscles consistent with hemorrhage and edema.

Stress fractures are frequently encountered in the pelvis and hips. Common locations include the sacral ala and body, the pubic rami, the supra-acetabular region, and the femoral neck (203). Abnormal forces (e.g., marathon training) placed on normal bones can result in fatigue type stress fractures (Fig. 22-101). Conversely, normal forces (e.g., walking) placed on abnormal bones (osteoporosis) can result in insufficiency-type stress fractures (Figs. 22-102 and 22-103). Radiation necrosis of the pelvic bones can be found in patients who have undergone radiation therapy for a pelvic malignancy. This abnormal bone may lead to the development of insufficiency-type stress fractures (Fig. 22-104). The initial CT finding in stress fracture is sclerosis along the developing fracture line. Cortical thickening and periosteal reaction may then develop (see Fig. 22-101), except in the flat bones of the pelvis where these findings are not often seen. A discrete lucent fracture line may progress to a frank fracture that may then undergo displacement. MR has the advantage of being able to detect bone marrow edema that reflects early stress-related changes before the development of sclerosis on CT or radiographs (18,22,103).

Joint Abnormality

As with arthropathies in any joint, the first imaging test of the sacroiliac joints should be conventional radiography. Most diagnoses can be made without additional

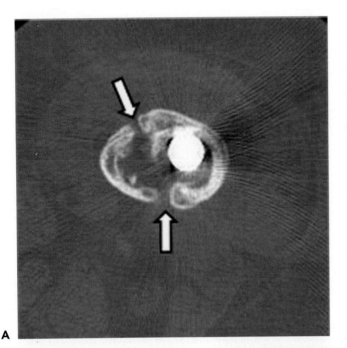

A

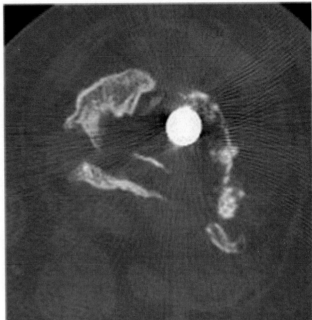

B

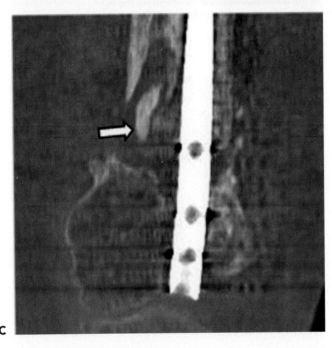

C

Figure 22-100 Femoral shaft fracture nonunion. **A:** Transverse CT image of the distal left femoral shaft shows a defect extending through the anterior and posterior cortex (*arrows*). Note the rounded, dense fracture margins. **B:** A more inferior image demonstrates several nonunited osseous fragments around the intramedullary rod. **C:** Coronal reformatted image demonstrates the extent of the nonunion. Note the sclerotic fragment along the medial fracture line (*arrow*).

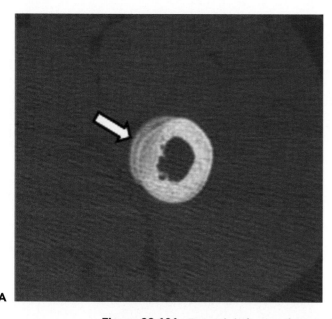

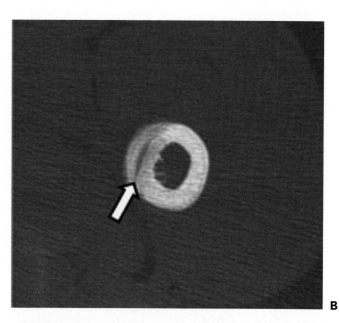

Figure 22-101 Femoral shaft stress fracture, fatigue type ("thigh splints"). **A:** There is a lamellated periosteal reaction (*arrow*) along the medial aspect of the left femoral shaft at the adductor muscle attachment **B:** There is a focal lucency beneath the periosteal reaction representing the actual stress fracture line. This patient began experiencing left thigh pain after beginning a jogging exercise regimen.

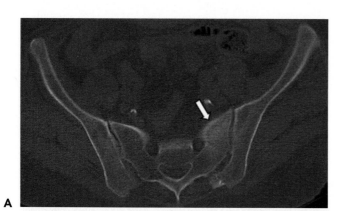

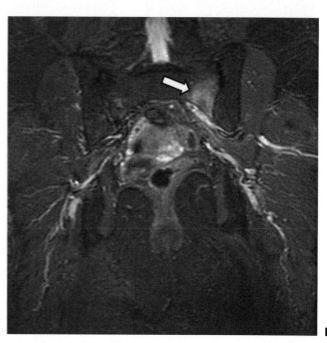

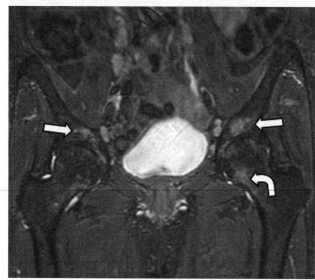

Figure 22-102 Sacral and pelvic stress fractures, insufficiency type. **A:** Transverse CT image shows sclerosis of the left sacral ala. **B:** Coronal STIR MR image demonstrates linear low signal in the left sacral ala with surrounding bright bone marrow edema (*arrow*). **C:** A more anterior image shows additional stress fractures in both supra-acetabular regions (*straight arrows*) and the left femoral neck (*curved arrow*). This patient was on large doses of steroids.

cross-sectional imaging. On occasion, subtle or inconclusive findings at radiography may need to be further evaluated with CT. CT provides an unobstructed look at the SI joints and allows for detailed examination of the anterior and posterior aspects of the joint. Subtle degenerative or inflammatory changes can be visualized more frequently and with greater confidence on MR and CT than on radiographs (217,305). MR with intravenous contrast is useful in suspected cases of infection (272).

The appearance of SI joint osteoarthritis is similar to that in any other joint: irregular joint space narrowing,

subchondral sclerosis and cystic change, and osteophyte formation. In some cases, very large anterior bridging osteophytes may develop. Degenerative disease of the SI joints is often accompanied by disease in the symphysis pubis or hips (Fig. 22-105).

Inflammatory arthropathies such as rheumatoid arthritis produce more uniform joint space narrowing and cortical erosions may be present. With regard to the seronegative spondyloarthropathies, the findings are usually bilateral. Psoriatic arthritis, Reiter disease, and inflammatory bowel disease may all lead to an inflammatory arthropathy of the SI joints, but ankylosing spondylitis is

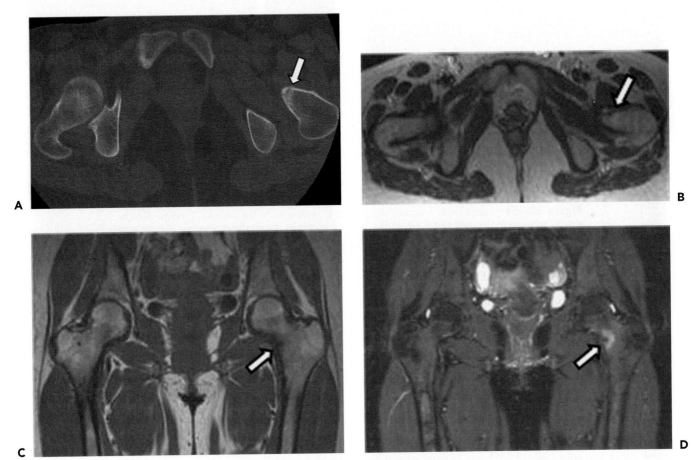

Figure 22-103 Femoral neck stress fracture. **A:** Pelvic CT demonstrates cortical disruption of the medial left femoral neck with surrounding sclerosis (*arrow*). **B:** Axial T1-weighted MR image shows the same cortical break (*arrow*). **C:** Coronal T1-weighted MR image shows the incomplete stress fracture of the medial left femoral neck (*arrow*). **D:** Coronal STIR MR image depicts the surrounding bone marrow edema (*arrow*). This patient had sickle cell anemia.

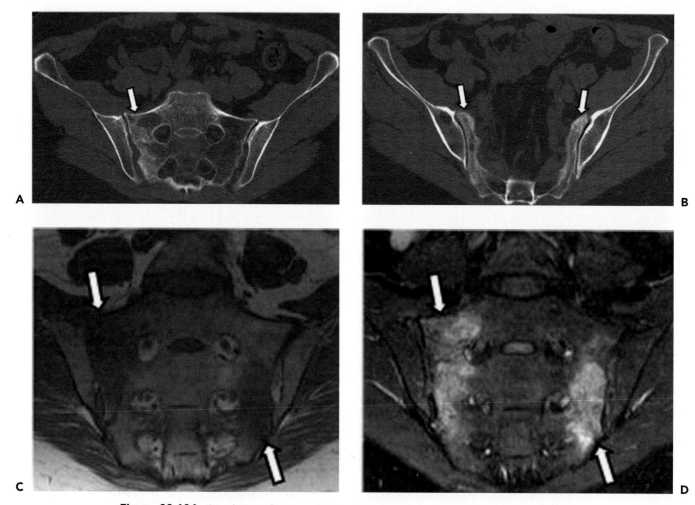

A

B

C

D

Figure 22-104 Sacral stress fractures due to pelvic radiation. **A:** Transverse CT image demonstrates sclerosis of the right sacral ala (*arrow*). **B:** A more inferior image shows sclerosis of both inferior sacral alae (*arrows*). **C:** Coronal T1-weighted MR image demonstrates linear low signal stress fractures of the sacral alae (*arrows*). **D:** Coronal STIR MR image depicts the extent of the bone marrow edema (*arrows*) associated with the stress fractures. This patient had received pelvic radiation therapy for a gynecologic malignancy.

the entity that most commonly leads to SI joint fusion (Fig. 22-106). Crystal deposition diseases are not common in the SI joints, but gout (Fig. 22-107) and calcium pyrophosphate deposition disease should always be considered in cases of SI joint erosive disease. Septic arthritis of the SI joints can mimic an inflammatory arthropathy leading to delayed diagnosis.

The SI joints are a common site for stress-related periarticular changes. Osteitis condensans ilii is a triangular area of sclerosis on the iliac side only of the SI joint; the sacral side is spared. The SI joints themselves are usually normal (Fig. 22-108). Childbirth is most often cited as the etiology for this condition. It is rarely, if ever, seen in men.

Radiographic evaluation of the hip joints is usually sufficient in cases of degenerative or inflammatory arthritis. CT can be useful in cases in which there is complex anatomy or to evaluate the quality and amount of bone prior to an operative procedure. Osteoarthritis of the hips is commonly seen in pelvic CT examinations performed for other reasons (see Fig. 22-105).

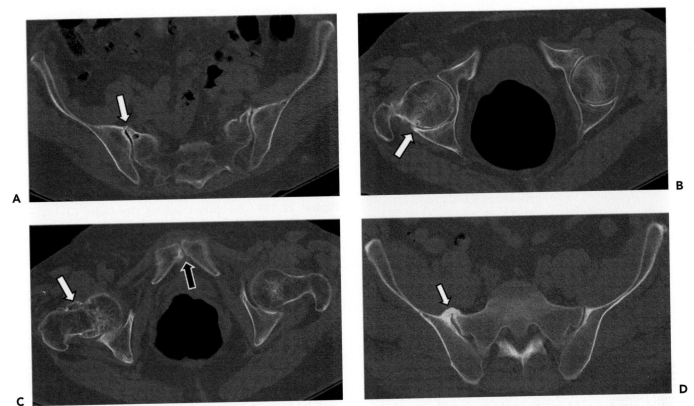

Figure 22-105 Osteoarthritis. **A:** There is sclerosis and narrowing of the right SI joint with small osteophytes (*arrow*). Note the subchondral cyst in the sacral ala. **B:** The right hip degenerative changes are nonuniform: the narrowing and sclerosis are more pronounced posteriorly (*arrow*). **C:** Ring osteophytes of the right femoral neck are prominent (*white arrow*). Degenerative changes are also noted at the symphysis pubis (*black arrow*). **D:** In a different patient, there is a large osteophyte bridging the anterior right SI joint.

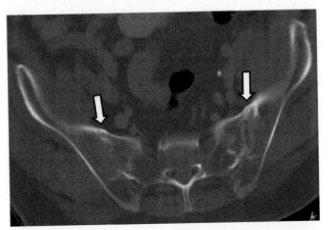

Figure 22-106 Ankylosing spondylitis. Both SI joints demonstrate solid osseous fusion (*arrows*). Ankylosis of the spine was also found in this patient.

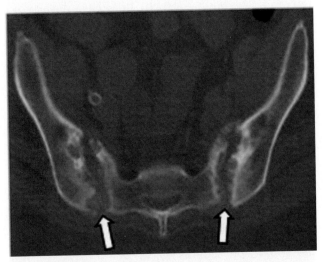

Figure 22-107 Gout. Well-defined erosions with surrounding sclerosis are seen in both SI joints (*arrows*). Aspiration of the joints yielded the urate crystals of gout.

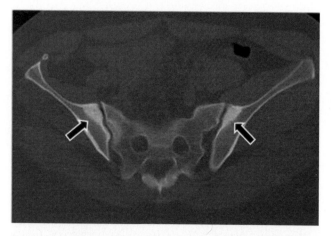

Figure 22-108 Osteitis condensans ilii. There is triangular sclerosis along the iliac sides of both SI joints. The sacral sides and SI joints are normal. This is a stress-related phenomenon usually of no clinical significance.

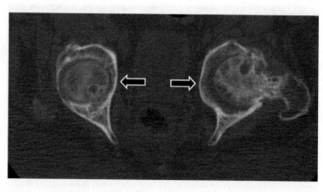

Figure 22-109 Rheumatoid arthritis. Transverse CT image through the hip joints demonstrates marked bilateral joint space narrowing with erosions on the femoral heads. Acetabular protrusion into the pelvis is especially prominent (*arrows*).

Inflammatory arthropathies of the hip include the seropositive and seronegative varieties. The hallmark findings of uniform joint space narrowing and cortical erosions may be better appreciated on CT with more subtle erosions detected (Figs. 22-109 and 22-110). CT may be helpful for preoperative assessment of the osseous acetab-

ulum prior to total joint arthroplasty. Of particular interest is the degree of acetabular protrusion present. A herniation pit is a well-defined lucency near the anterior junction of the femoral head and neck thought to be due to herniation of synovial and fibrous tissue (Fig. 22-111) (212). This lesion is usually asymptomatic and should not be mistaken

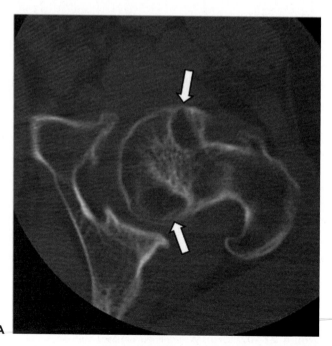

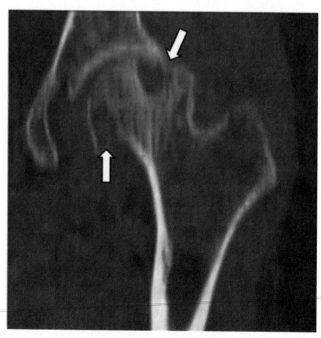

A

B

Figure 22-110 Juvenile chronic arthritis. **A:** Transverse CT image of the left hip of a young adult patient shows large erosions of the femoral head (*arrows*) with joint space narrowing and secondary degenerative changes. **B:** Coronal reformatted image again shows the large erosions (*arrows*) and joint space narrowing.

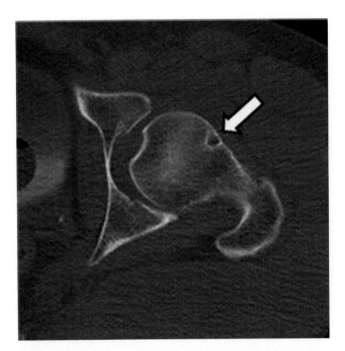

Figure 22-111 Femoral herniation pit. There is a well-defined erosion at the junction of the anterior femoral head and neck (*arrow*).

for an inflammatory erosion. Synovial disorders such as pigmented villonodular synovitis and synovial chondromatosis are best evaluated on MR, but CT may be used to detect calcification.

CT can also be helpful in evaluation of bursitis surrounding the hips although MR is usually performed for such an indication. Such bursae are numerous in the hip region with the iliopsoas and trochanteric bursae being the most constantly present. Most other bursae represent potential spaces. Iliopsoas bursitis can be seen in association with an inflammatory arthropathy such as rheumatoid arthritis. The iliopsoas bursa can communicate with the anterior hip joint in about 15% of patients; therefore, inflammatory joint effusions can be transmitted to the iliopsoas bursa (Fig. 22-112).

Developmental dysplasia of the hips (DDH) should be detected and corrected in childhood, but numerous patients make it into adulthood with this condition. These patients present with degenerative changes of the hips at a relatively young age. Radiographs are adequate in making this diagnosis, but CT with reformatted multiplanar 2D or 3D images can be helpful in preoperative planning (Fig. 22-113). Findings in DDH include a superolaterally displaced, dysplastic femoral head with a

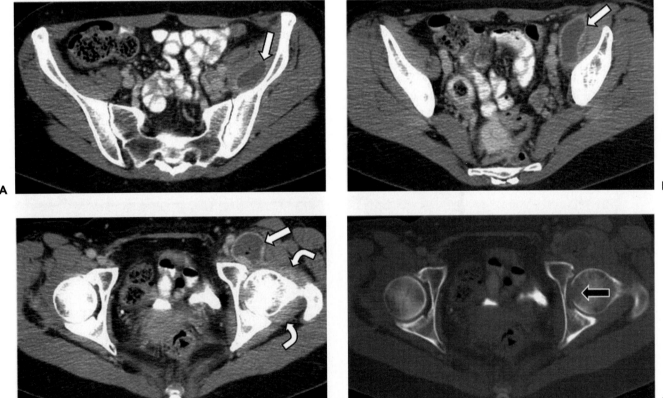

Figure 22-112 Iliopsoas bursitis due to rheumatoid arthritis. **A:** A fluid collection with an enhancing rim is present in the left iliacus muscle (*arrow*). **B:** The fluid collection tracks down the left iliopsoas tendon (*arrow*). **C:** The left iliopsoas bursa is distended (*straight arrow*). As in this case, the iliopsoas bursa can communicate with the hip joint. Note the distention of the left hip joint (*curved arrows*). **D:** At the same level, bone windows demonstrate an erosion of the femoral head (*arrow*) away from the fovea capitis. All of these findings are related to rheumatoid arthritis.

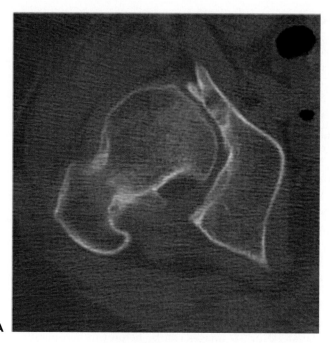
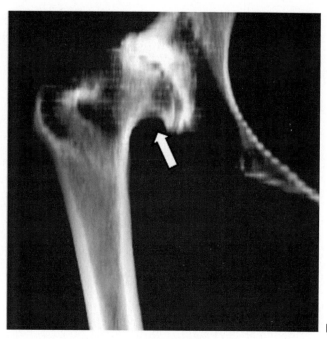

A **B**

Figure 22-113 Developmental dysplasia of the hip with secondary osteoarthrosis. **A:** There are marked degenerative changes of the left hip with joint space narrowing and osteophytes. The acetabulum is shallow with a thick medial wall. **B:** An anterior view from a 3D rendering demonstrates superolateral displacement of the femoral head consistent with developmental dysplasia of the hip.

shallow, malformed acetabulum (190). Other congenital or developmental abnormalities that can be assessed by CT include femoral torsion and femoral anteversion.

CT can be as useful in the postoperative assessment of the patient as it is in the pre-operative evaluation. Assessment of fracture healing and mal-union (or nonunion) is discussed above. CT can also provide useful details regarding the state of joint arthrodesis and instrumentation posi-

tioning (Fig. 22-114). Complications of total hip arthroplasty such as component migration or loosening can be evaluated radiographically, but CT is useful in some circumstances. CT is particularly helpful in suspected cases of polyethylene wear, periprosthetic osteolysis or particle disease (219) (Fig. 22-115). Heterotopic ossification, discussed elsewhere in this chapter, is also commonly found around the postoperative hip.

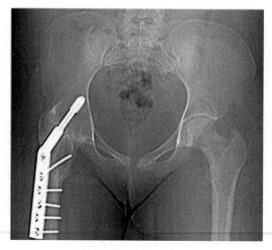
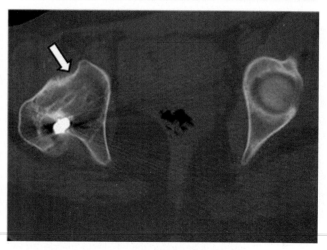

Figure 22-114 Hip fusion. **A:** Scout image of the pelvis demonstrates right hip fusion with a dynamic compression screw and sideplate. **B:** Transverse CT image through the right hip confirms solid osseous fusion from acetabulum to femoral head. Note that the screw is located more posterior than usual due to the presence of prior instrumentation in the femoral neck.

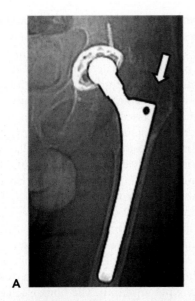

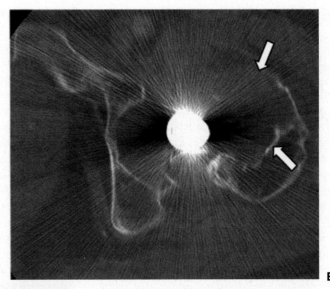

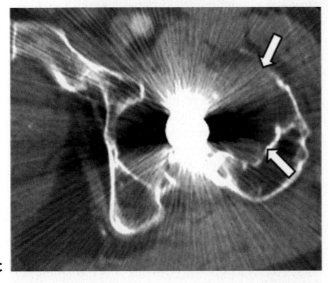

Figure 22-115 Particle disease. A: Scout image of the left hip demonstrates lucency in the greater trochanter (*arrow*) around the hip prosthesis. B, C: Bone and soft tissue windows demonstrate soft tissue density producing well-defined erosion of the greater trochanter (*arrows*).

KNEE

Anatomy

(Figs. 22-116 to 22-118).

The distal femur shaft flares distally to form the medial and lateral femoral condyles, which are separated by the intercondylar notch posteriorly. The anterior-superior portion of the intercondylar area is referred to as the trochlear groove and is the articulating surface with the patella. The patella's articular surface has a vertical bony ridge dividing it into medial and lateral regions. Two horizontal ridges into three facets further subdivide these medially and laterally, with an "extra" odd facet medially. The contact surfaces of the patello-femoral joint will vary between these facets depending on the degree of knee flexion or extension. The tibial plateau is also divided into medial and lateral condyles, separated by an intercondylar area demarcated by the medial and lateral tibial intercondylar eminences. The proximal tibiofibular joint between the lateral tibial condyle and the head of the fibula is very strong, held together by a thick fibrous capsule and ligaments. This joint communicates with the knee joint in approximately 10% of arthrograms (227).

The cruciate ligaments, capsular structures and menisci are not as well appreciated on unenhanced CT axial images as compared with MR but may be better delineated if CT arthrography and multiplanar imaging is performed. The anterior cruciate ligament (ACL) is best seen on the sagittal reformatted images as it attaches proximally into the medial aspect of the lateral femoral condyle and distally fans out attaching to the tibial intercondylar area anteriorly. The posterior cruciate ligament (PCL) is a dense fibrous structure attaching proximally into the posterolateral aspect of the medial femoral condyle and distally into a small inferiorly recessed area in the posterior tibia. The meniscofemoral ligaments extend from the posterior horn of the lateral meniscus to the posterolateral aspect of the medial femoral condyle. The ligament of Humphrey courses anterior to, and the ligament of Wrisberg courses posterior to the PCL. The medial and lateral collateral ligamentous structures are best appreciated on the coronal reformatted images. The medial or tibial collateral ligament has a superficial and a deep component. The former is well seen on CT as it originates from the medial epicondyle of the femur and inserts into the proximal tibia, posterior to the pes anserinus. The fibular collateral ligament arises from the lateral femoral epicondyle and joins the distal tendon of the biceps femoris to form a conjoined tendon inserting into the proximal fibular head. The popliteus tendon contributes to posterolateral knee stability as it inserts into the popliteal hiatus of the lateral femoral condyle. The medial and lateral menisci are also best evaluated on the reformatted images, although tears of these structures are difficult to appreciate on CT without arthrographic contrast. Posteromedially, the semimembranosus tendon inserts mostly into the posteromedial tibia. The oblique ligament represents a thickening of

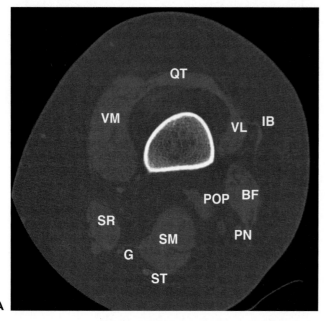
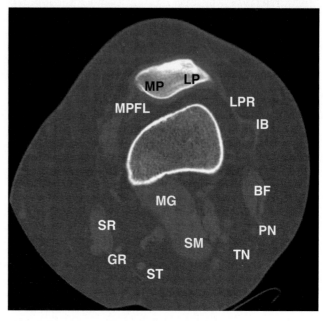

A   **B**

Figure 22-116 **A:** Axial normal anatomy, distal femur shaft. Vastus medialis (VM), vastus lateralis (VL), quadriceps tendon (QT), iliotibial band (IB), biceps femoris (BF), semimembranosus (SM), semitendinosis (ST), sartorius (SR), gracilis (G) popliteal vessels (POP) common peroneal nerve (PN). **B:** Axial anatomy, mid-patella. Medial patellofemoral ligament (MPFL), lateral patellar retinaculum (LPR), medial gastrocnemius (MG), sartorius (SR), gracilis (G), biceps femoris (BF), medial and lateral patellar articular facets (MP and LP), common peroneal nerve (PN) and tibial nerve (TN). (*continued*)

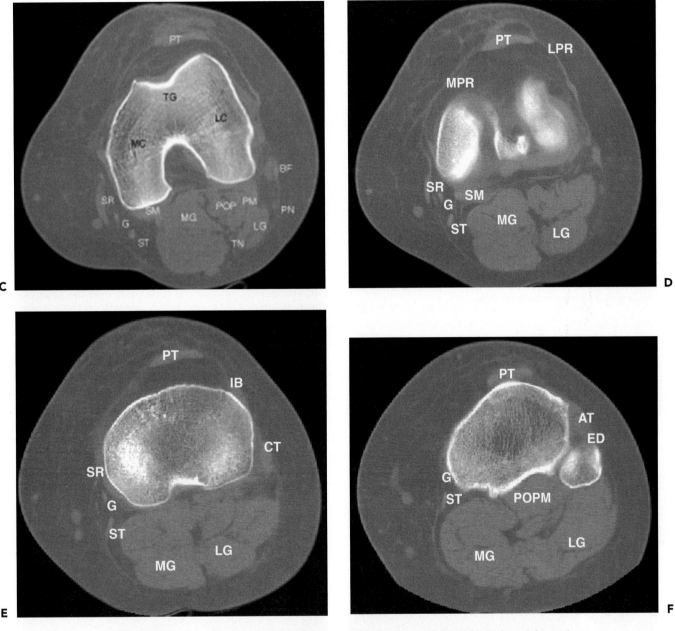

Figure 22-116 (*continued*) **C:** Axial anatomy, intercondylar fossa. Medial and lateral femoral condyles (MC and LC), trochlear groove (TG), patellar tendon (PT), medial and lateral gastrocnemius (MG and LG), popliteal vessels (POP), plantaris muscle (PM), biceps femoris (BF), semitendinosis (ST), sartorius (SR), gracilis (G), tibial (TN) and common peroneal nerve (PN). **D:** Patellar tendon (PT), medial and lateral patellar retinaculum (MPR and LPR), sartorius (SR), gracilis (G), semitendinosis (ST), semimembranosus (SM), medial and lateral gastrocnemius (MG and LG). **E:** Axial anatomy, tibial plateau. Patellar tendon (PT), iliotibial band (IB), sartorius (SR), gracilis (G), semitendinosis (ST), plantaris muscle (PM), conjoined tendon of biceps femoris and fibular collateral ligament (CT). **F:** Axial anatomy, proximal tibiofibular joint. Patellar tendon (PT), anterior tibialis muscle (AT), extensor digitorum muscle (ED), gracilis (G) and semitendinosis (ST), medial and lateral gastrocnemius (MG and LG), popliteus muscle (PopM). (*continued*)

the posterior capsule and also contributes to posteromedial knee stability. The medial and lateral gastrocnemius muscles as they originate from the distal posterior femur also contribute to the posteromedial and posterolateral stability respectively.

Anteriorly, the tendons of vastus lateralis, intermedius and medialis converge on the superior border of the patella as the quadriceps tendon. The patellar tendon originates from a continuation of these fibers from the inferior border of the patella and inserts into

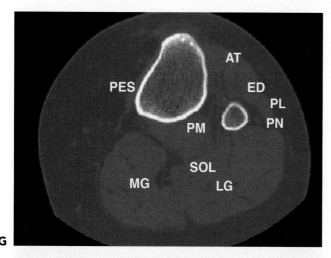

G

Figure 22-116 (*continued*) **G:** Axial anatomy, proximal tibia and fibula. Anterior tibialis and extensor digitorum muscles (AT and ED), peroneal nerve (PN), peroneus longus muscle (PL), popliteus muscle (PM), medial and lateral gastrocnemius (MG and LG) soleus (Sol), Pes anserine tendons (Pes).

the tibial tuberosity anteriorly. Also anteriorly, the iliotibial band inserts into the anterolateral tibia at Gerdy's tubercle. The medial and lateral patellar retinaculum extends from the patella transversely and attach to the femoral and tibial condyles at the sides. These help restrict the transverse motion of the patella as it glides on the trochlear groove of the femur. The medial patellofemoral ligament represents a thickening of the medial patellar retinaculum at the level of the insertion of the vastus medialis fibers and is the strongest static restraint to lateral patellar subluxation. Medially, the posterior tendons of the sartorius, gracilis and semitendinosis merge anteriorly to form the pes anserinus insertion into the proximal anteromedial tibia.

The popliteal artery and vein reside between the two heads of the gastrocnemius, and posterior to the popliteus muscle. The tibial nerve runs posterior to the popliteal artery. The common peroneal nerve is located posterolaterally, and swings anteriorly over the proximal fibula head.

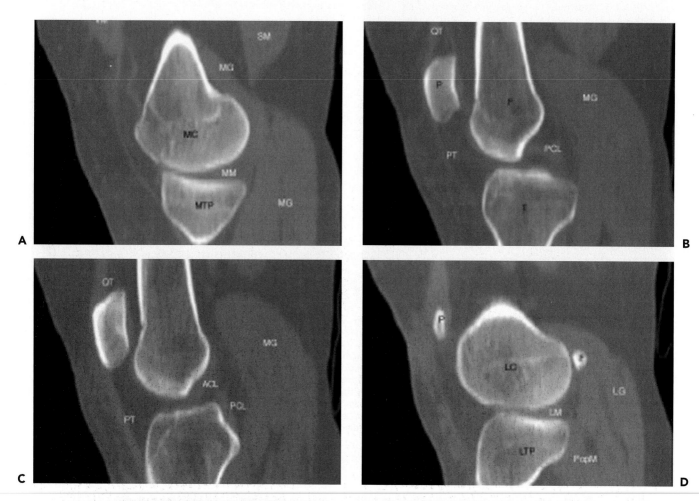

A   **B**   **C**   **D**

Figure 22-117 A: Sagittal reformatted image, medial knee. Medial femoral condyle (MC) and medial tibial plateau (MTP), medial meniscus (MM), medial gastrocnemius (MG), semimembranosus (SM), vastus medialis (VM). **B:** Sagittal reformatted image, medial intercondylar fossa. Femur (F), tibia (T), patella (P), patellar tendon (PT), quadriceps tendon (QT), medial gastrocnemius (MG) and PCL. **C:** Sagittal reformatted image, lateral intercondylar fossa. Patellar tendon (PT), quadriceps tendon (QT), medial gastrocnemius (MG), ACL and PCL. **D:** Sagittal reformatted image, lateral joint. Lateral condyle (LC), Lateral tibial plateau (LTP) patella (P), fabella (Fa) quadriceps tendon (QT), lateral gastrocnemius (LG), popliteus muscle (PopM) and lateral meniscus (LM).

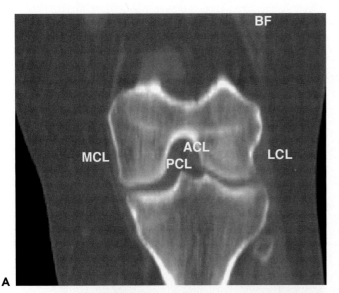
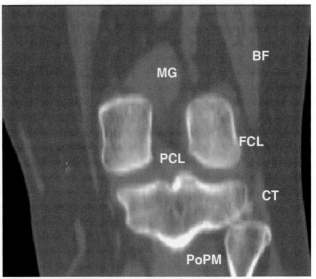

Figure 22-118 **A:** Coronal reformatted image, intercondylar fossa. ACL, PCL, medial collateral ligament (MCL), lateral collateral ligament (LCL), biceps femoris (BF). **B:** Coronal reformatted image, tibiofibular joint. PCL, ACL, Conjoined tendon (CT) of biceps femoris (BF) and fibular collateral ligament (FCL), medial gastrocnemius (MG), popliteus muscle (PopM).

Trauma

As in many other anatomic regions, due to its availability and speed of examination, CT is commonly used as the primary cross-sectional imaging modality to evaluate complex fractures in the setting of acute trauma. The most commonly encountered knee fractures for which CT is utilized include fractures of the distal femoral condyles and of the tibial plateaus.

Fractures of the distal femur are usually supracondylar in location and transverse in orientation (253). These do not require cross-sectional imaging for their routine management. However, fractures may extend into the intercondylar knee in a T- or Y-shaped manner, and the subsequent articular incongruity may be hard to characterize without cross-sectional imaging (Fig. 22-119). Coronal fractures involving primarily the condyles are not common and usually require CT for accurate diagnosis and assessment of displacement (142) (Figs. 22-120 and 22-121).

CT has a well-established role in the diagnosis and management of tibial plateau fractures (41,68,221,303). With the

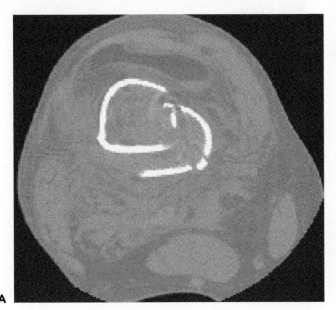
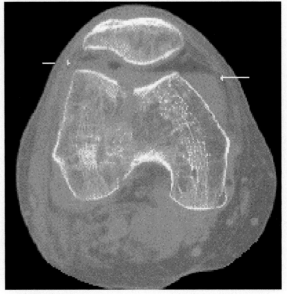

Figure 22-119 Intercondylar femoral fracture. Axial images show fracture of the distal femur shaft (**A**) with extension into the intercondylar region. **B:** Note lipohemarthrosis with fat-fluid level in joint space (*arrow*). (*continued*)

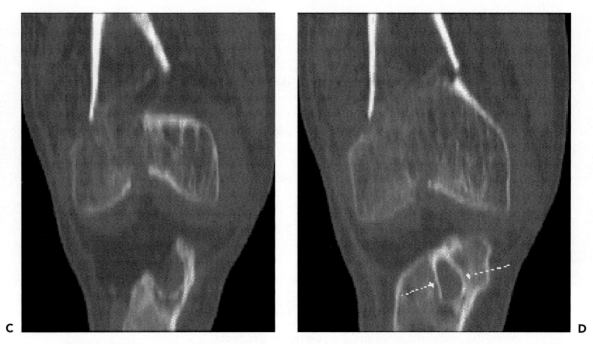

Figure 22-119 (*continued*) **C** and **D:** Coronal reformatted images better depict the Y-shaped configuration of the fracture. Note tibial tunnel from prior intramedullary nail placement (*arrow*).

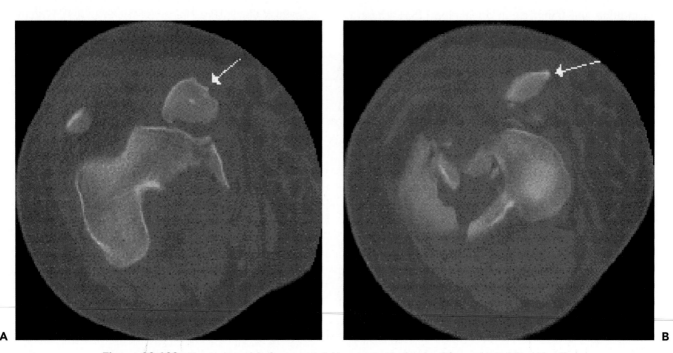

Figure 22-120 Femoral condyle fracture. Axial images at the levels of femoral condyles (**A**) and tibial plateau (**B**). Note the extent of anterior displacement of the posterior medial femoral condyle fragment (*arrow*). There is also an Schatzker 6 type tibial plateau fracture present.

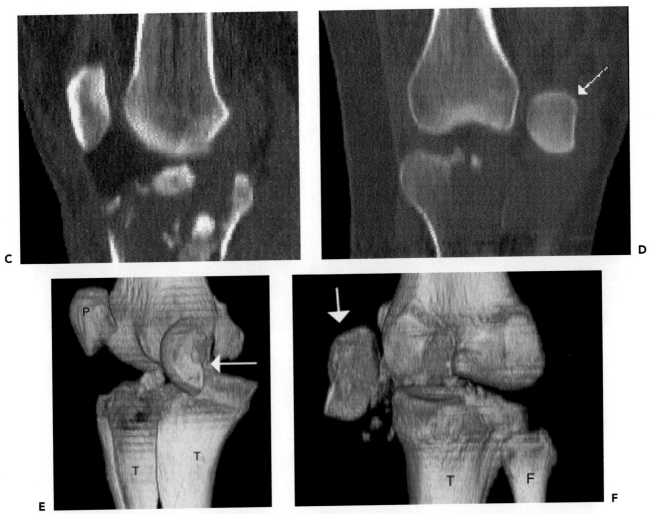

Figure 22-120 (*continued*) **C:** Sagittal reformatted image shows normal position of patella and marked comminution of tibial plateau. **D:** Coronal formatted image shows extent of medial displacement of the posterior medial femoral condyle fragment (*arrow*). Volumetric 3D reconstructions viewed from (**E**) side and (**F**) posteriorly show relationship of fragment (*arrow*) to patella (P), tibia (T) and fibula (F). Note the split component of the tibial fracture.

use of helical and multislice CT, utilizing thin collimation and overlapping reconstructed images (2-mm images at 1-mm intervals are commonly used), the resultant reformatted coronal and sagittal images of the volumetric data allow for accurate fracture evaluation and 3D reformatted images may help in surgical planning (137,148,167,303). However, MRI is being increasingly used in our institutions for the assessment of these fractures, as it also accurately depicts the extent of articular incongruity but may better delineate associated ligamentous and meniscal injuries (29,126,308).

CT images of the axial plane allow determination of extent of plateau comminution. Reconstruction of the coronal and sagittal planes allows characterization of fracture planes. At our institutions, the orthopedic surgeons utilize the Schatzker classification system for these fractures to summarize the extent of articular depression and splitting (diastasis). Type 1 are split fractures of the lateral tibial plateau (Fig. 22-122), type 2 involve a split and depressed lateral plateau fracture (Fig. 22-123), type 3 are depressed lateral plateau fractures (Figs. 22-124 and

(*text continues on page 1571*)

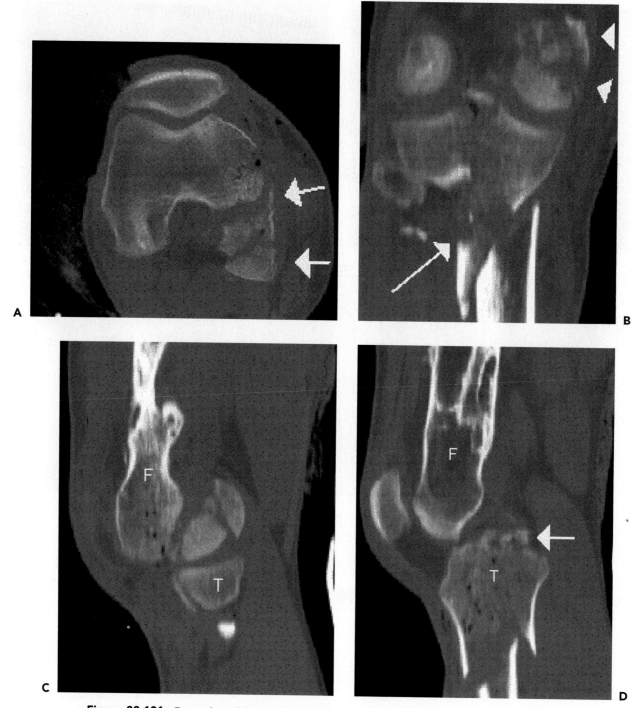

Figure 22-121 Femoral condyle open fracture. **A:** Axial image shows marked comminution of the posterior medial femoral condyle (*arrows*). Note presence of gas within fracture consistent with open communication. **B:** Coronal reformatted image again shows posterior medial condyle fracture (*arrowheads*). There is also a Schatzker 6 type tibial plateau fracture present (*arrow*). **C:** Sagittal reformatted images medially and (**D**) through the intercondylar region show anterior displacement of femur on tibia. Note the PCL avulsion fracture from the posterior intercondylar tibia (*arrow*). Deformity of the distal femoral shaft was from prior trauma.

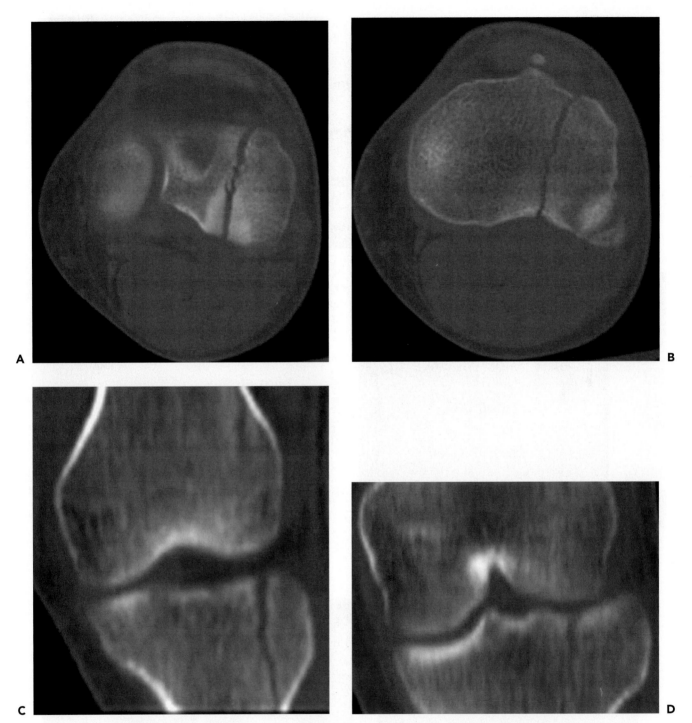

Figure 22-122 Tibial plateau fracture, Schatzker type 1. **A** and **B**: Axial images through the tibial plateau show a fracture line through the lateral tibial plateau directed antero-posteriorly. **C** and **D**: Coronal reformatted images show the lateral plateau split fracture without significant associated depression of the articular surface.

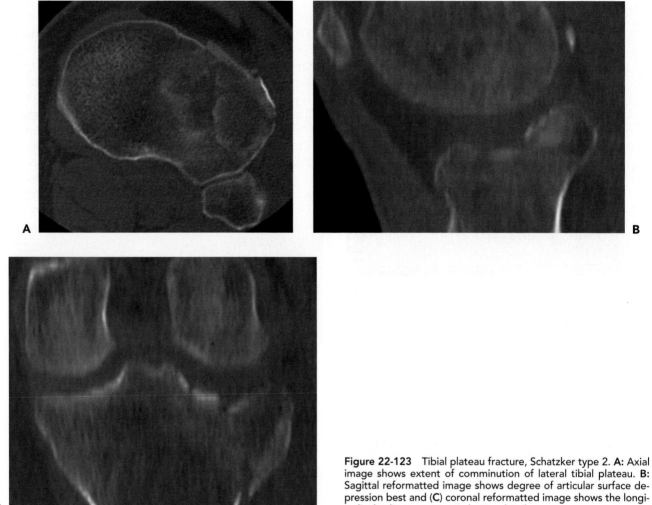

Figure 22-123 Tibial plateau fracture, Schatzker type 2. **A:** Axial image shows extent of comminution of lateral tibial plateau. **B:** Sagittal reformatted image shows degree of articular surface depression best and **(C)** coronal reformatted image shows the longitudinal split component in better detail.

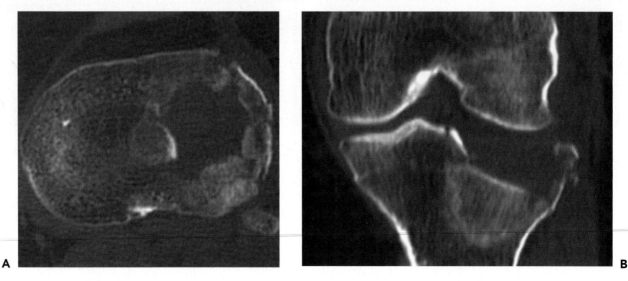

Figure 22-124 Tibial plateau fracture, Schatzker type 3. **A:** Axial image shows comminution and **(B)** coronal and (*continued*)

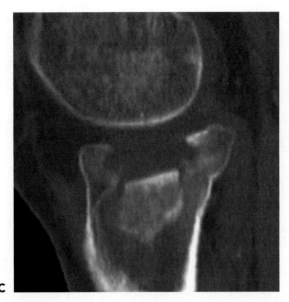

Figure 22-124 (*continued*) (**C**) sagittal images show greater than 1 cm of depression.

22-125), type 4 involves the medial tibial plateau, type 5 are split fractures of both the medial and lateral tibial plateau (Fig. 22-126) and type 6 (Fig. 22-127) implies comminution with no bony continuity of the tibial diaphysis with the plateaus. Thus, the imager needs to report on the accurate measurement of tibial plateau depression from the coronal or sagittal image. The restoration of articular congruity is an important principle of orthopedic management, although the extent of articular depression that warrants surgical intervention is still controversial (122). There is agreement that greater than 1 cm of depression benefits from surgical intervention, although some argue that a depression as small as 3 mm, especially if it involves the medial tibial plateau which is the major weight-bearing surface, should be surgically repaired (122,180,282).

CT can also be used in the assessment of healing, or complications including nonunion, of fractures in the

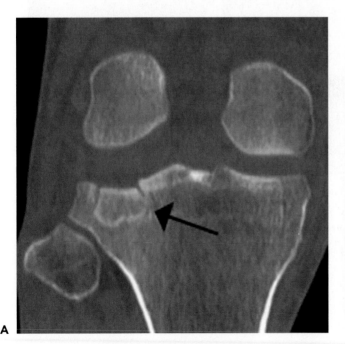
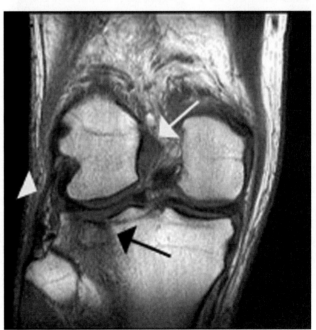

Figure 22-125 Tibial plateau fracture, Schatzker type 3: comparison of MRI and CT. **A:** Coronal reformatted CT shows minimally depressed lateral tibial plateau fragment (*arrow*). **B:** Coronal T1 and (*continued*)

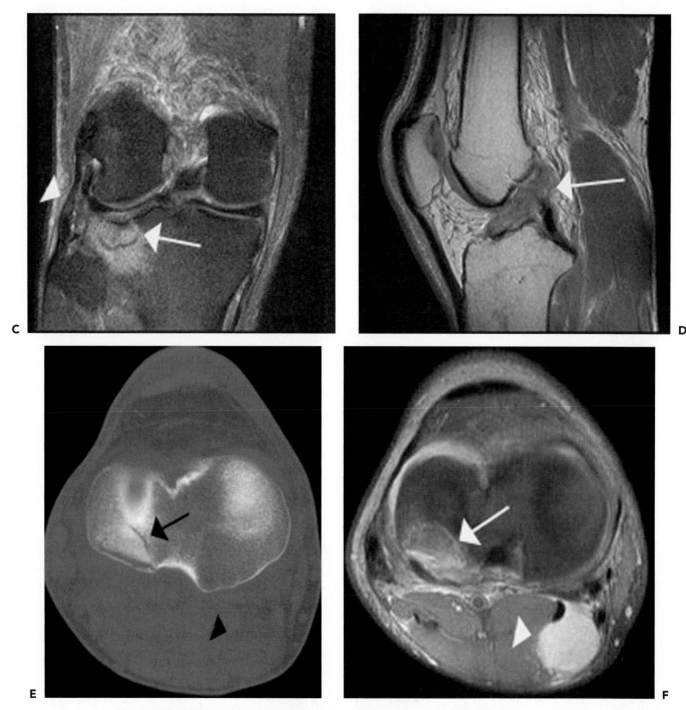

Figure 22-125 (continued) (**C**) T2-weighted images (the latter with fat-suppression technique) show same findings, but CT better depicts the articular depression. However, MRI also identifies ACL rupture (*white arrow* on **B**) and FCL strain (*arrowhead*). **D:** Sagittal proton-density weighted spin echo image clearly depicts ACL rupture (*arrow*). This finding was not appreciated on initial interpretation of CT. **E:** Axial CT image and (**F**) axial fast spin echo T2-weighted image show the fracture equally well (*arrow*), although the distal FCL strain and popliteal cyst (*arrowhead*) are better depicted on the MR.

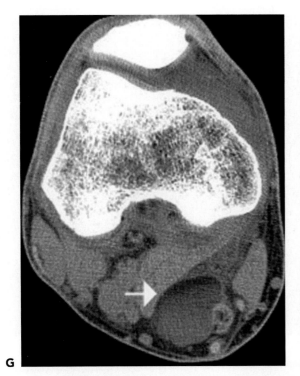
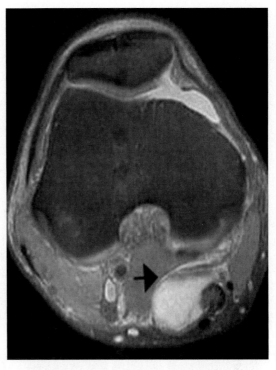

G   H

Figure 22-125 (*continued*) **G:** Axial CT image viewed with soft tissue window and level settings shows a lipohemarthrosis within the popliteal cyst. **H:** Axial MR T2-weighted image at the same level also shows a similar finding.

knee, as well as other locations. Three-dimensional refor-matted images may be helpful in this regard (65).

As in other anatomical areas, CT and MR are used in the diagnosis of osteochondral lesions and defects. In the knee, osteochondritis dissecans most commonly involves the medial femoral condyle (85% of cases) and is usually well depicted on radiography. However, in some patients, it may occur in the lateral anterior femoral sulcus, a loca-tion hard to evaluate on radiography but better appreci-ated with cross-sectional imaging (20). CT will show os-teochondritis dissecans very well, and can help in surgical planning by assessing the size of the defect and if there are any loose bodies within the joint or if the lesion is unstable (presence of subchondral cysts underlying the lesion) (Fig. 22-128). However, MRI may be better in evaluating for instability, and in assessing the overlying cartilage, although CT arthrography may be a good alter-native in patients with contraindications to MRI (61,175).

Internal Joint Derangements

MRI is the exam of choice in the evaluation of internal joint structures like menisci, cruciate ligaments and even articular cartilage due to its superior soft tissue contrast resolution. However, it is important to remember to ac-count for these structures when reviewing CT examina-tions that may have been preformed to evaluate soft tissue processes or osseous lesions that may be due to underlying

(*text continues on page 1577*)

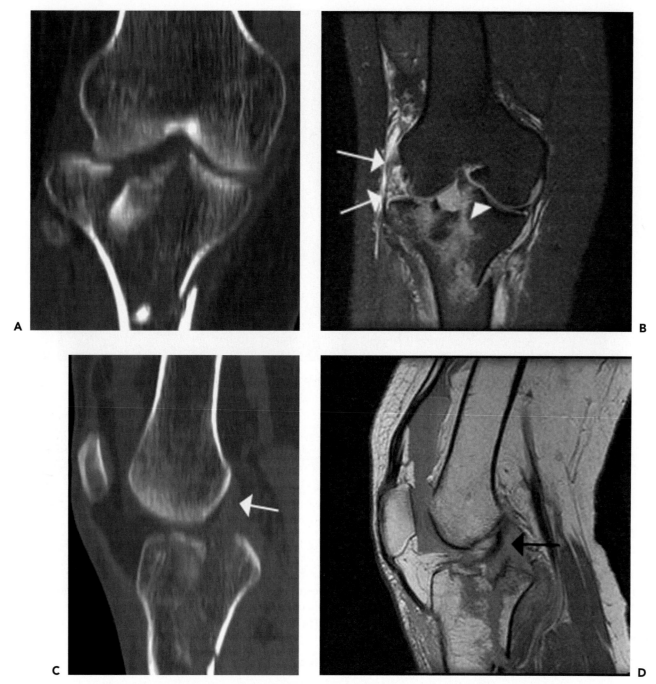

Figure 22-126 Tibial plateau fracture, Schatzker type 5: comparison of MRI and CT. **A:** Coronal reformatted CT image shows the split fractures involving both medial and lateral tibial plateaus. **B:** Coronal T2-weighted fat-suppressed MR image at a comparable location shows similar findings but note the depiction of the tears of the fibular collateral ligament and lateral meniscus (*arrows*), as well as a distally avulsed ACL (*arrowhead*). **C:** Sagittal reformatted CT image and (**D**) PD-weighted spin echo MR image show lipohemarthrosis and fracture delineation equally well, but the abnormal ACL orientation (*arrow*) is better depicted on MR.

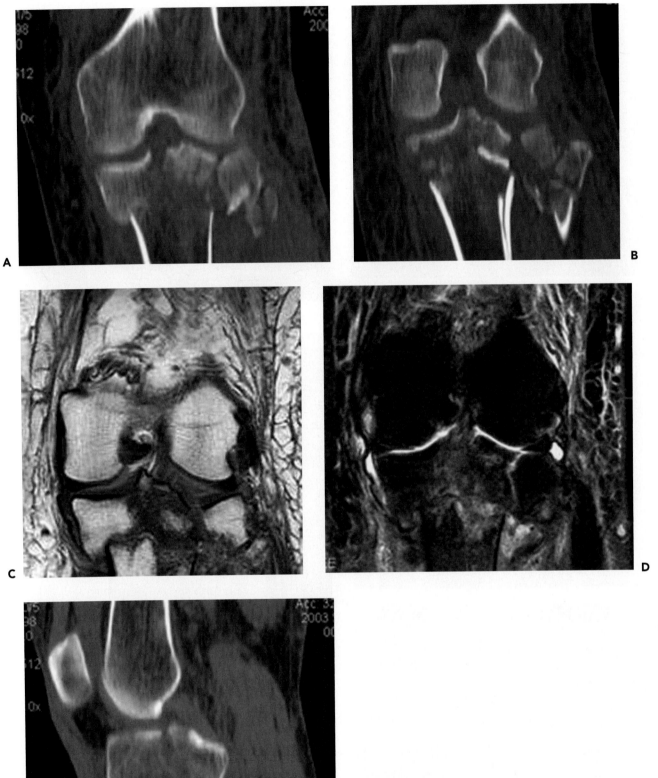

Figure 22-127 Tibial plateau fracture, Schatzker type 6: comparison of MRI and CT. **A** and **B:** Coronal reformatted CT images show bicondylar fractures with discontinuity of tibial plateaus from the proximal tibial shaft. **C:** Coronal T1-weighted spin echo and (**D**) T2-weighted fat-suppressed fast spin echo images show findings similar to CT. **E:** Sagittal reformatted CT image at the level of the PCL and (*continued*)

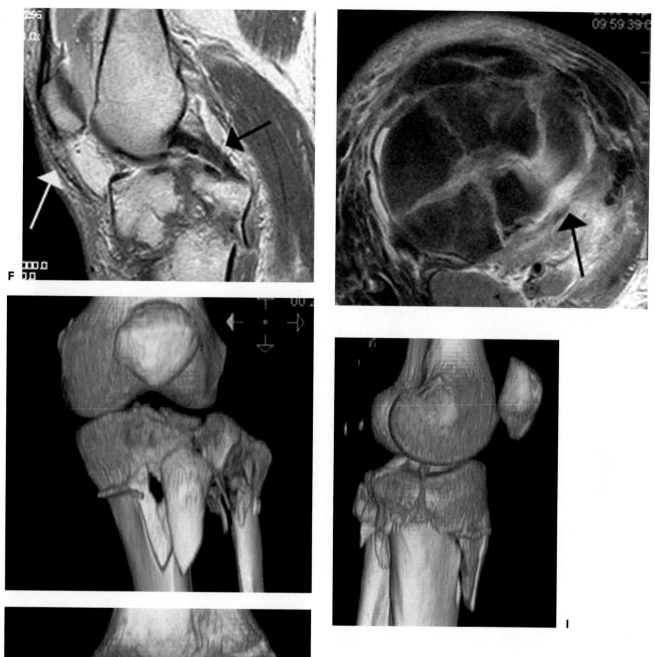

Figure 22-127 (*continued*) (F) sagittal MR PD-weighted spin echo image at the same level. Note the patellar tendon tear (*white arrow*) not appreciated on CT. The PCL has some mild increased signal in the mid body (*black arrow*) but was grossly intact on surgery. **G:** Axial MR PD-weighted fast spin echo image at the level of the tibial plateau also shows disruption of popliteus tendon at musculotendinous junction (*arrow*), a finding not seen on CT at the same level. 3-D volume rendered reconstructions in the anterior (**H**), lateral (**I**) and posterior (**J**) views show best the direction of displacement of the major fragments.

internal joint derangements (Figs. 22-129 and 22-130). An overview of the MRI findings of internal derangement is beyond the scope of this chapter and the reader is referred to the multiple excellent textbooks dedicated to musculoskeletal MRI.

In the patient with contraindications to MRI, or in the patient with internal fixation hardware that may limit MRI's ability to image the joint, CT arthrography may be accurate, especially when thin overlapping images are acquired with a multislice scanner (Fig. 22-131). Multislice CT has been shown to be accurate in the assessment of the native meniscus and ACL injury (285,286). In patients with prior surgery, CT arthrography interpretation may be less impeded by the microscopic metallic debris

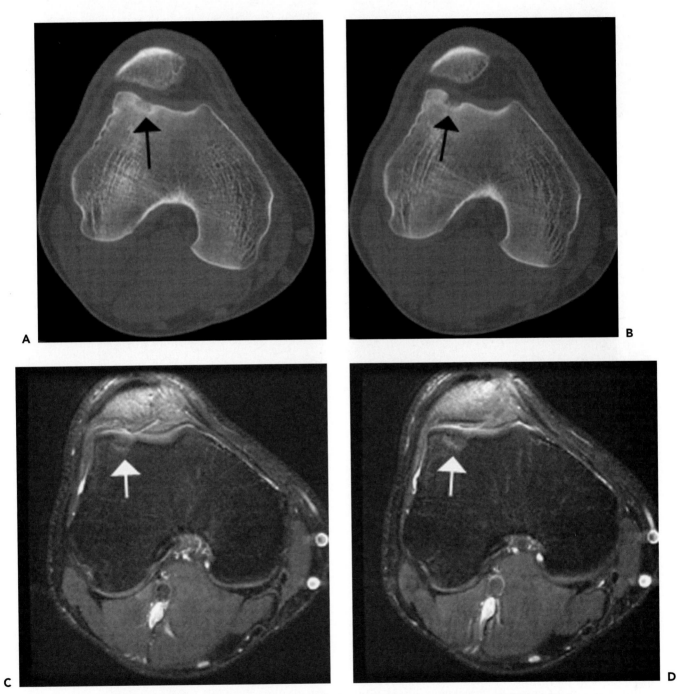

Figure 22-128   A 16-year-old boy with osteochondritis dissecans; comparison of MRI and CT. **A** and **B**: Axial CT images show 6-mm osteochondral defect (*arrows*) in the anterior-medial lateral femoral condyle. **C** and **D**: Axial MR T2-weighted fast spin echo fat-suppressed image shows the defect is not filled with fluid and is harder to appreciate than on the CT images. (*continued*)

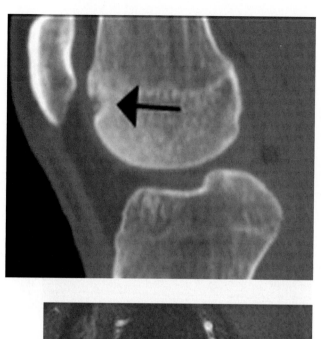

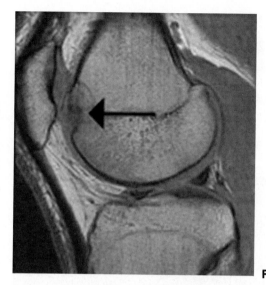

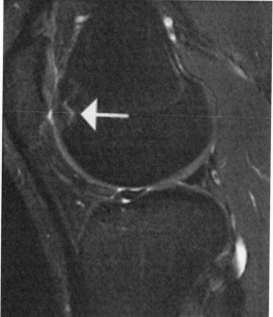

Figure 22-128 (*continued*) **E:** Sagittal reformatted CT image shows some ossific fragments within the osteochondral lesion. **F:** Sagittal MR T1-weighted and (**G**) sagittal MR proton-density-weighted fat-suppressed image show the defect at the same location. Although the overlying cartilage loss is better seen, the fragments within the lesion are not appreciated.

artifacts that may hinder MR interpretation (288). However, CT is limited by the lack of evaluation of marrow abnormalities, and had limited value in the assessment of the cruciate ligaments (particularly the PCL) or the lateral collateral ligamentous structures.

The technique for knee CT arthrography (like in other joints) varies among institutions, with single versus double-contrast technique (air-iodinated contrast) performed depending on operator or institutional preference (Fig. 22-

132). The degree of joint distension is also variable with some injecting large volumes to distend the joint and others advocating that only a small amount (10 mL) of iodinated contrast is needed to coat the articular surfaces (288). Imaging at 20 degrees of knee flexion may improve visualization of the ACL (205).

CT arthrography, like MR arthrography, may be very useful in the setting of prior partial meniscetomy. In this clinical scenario, MR findings like abnormal signal or

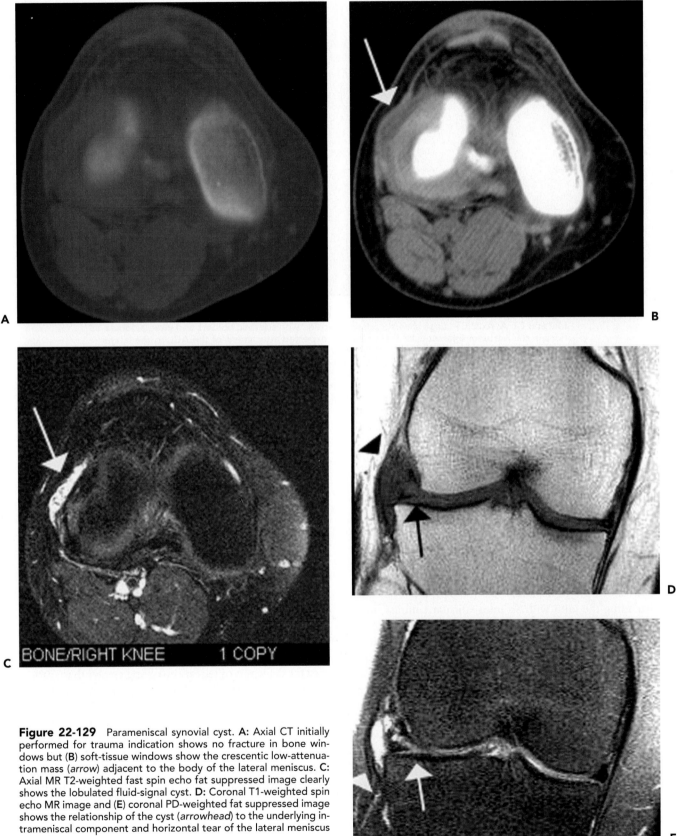

Figure 22-129 Parameniscal synovial cyst. **A:** Axial CT initially performed for trauma indication shows no fracture in bone windows but (**B**) soft-tissue windows show the crescentic low-attenuation mass (*arrow*) adjacent to the body of the lateral meniscus. **C:** Axial MR T2-weighted fast spin echo fat suppressed image clearly shows the lobulated fluid-signal cyst. **D:** Coronal T1-weighted spin echo MR image and (**E**) coronal PD-weighted fat suppressed image shows the relationship of the cyst (*arrowhead*) to the underlying intrameniscal component and horizontal tear of the lateral meniscus (*arrow*).

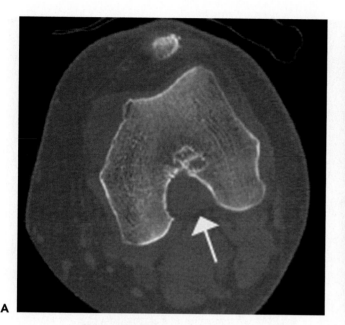
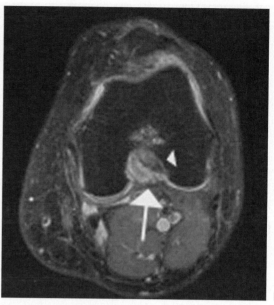

Figure 22-130 Intraosseous and intraarticular extension of ACL ganglion cyst: comparison of MRI and CT. **A:** Axial CT image shows a possible erosion with sclerotic borders and internal lobulations in the posterior intercondylar fossa near the expected attachment of the ACL to the lateral femoral condyle. Note the distension of the posterior capsule at this level (*arrow*). **B:** Axial PD-weighted fast spin echo MR image with fat suppression shows similar findings, however, the proximal ACL is now visualized and appears expanded and with increased signal within it (*arrowhead*) from an intrasubstance ganglion. Note that the distension of the posterior capsule was due to extension of this ganglion posteriorly (*arrow*). A small amount of fluid in the semimembranosus-medial gastrocnemius bursa is incidentally noted. (*continued*)

morphology of the menisci are much less specific in diagnosing a tear than in the nonoperated meniscus, with accuracies of 66% to 80% reported (5,252). However, after distending the joint with an intra-articular contrast injection, identifying linear or globular collections of contrast within the menisci in MR or CT may correlate more accurately with a recurrent or residual tear (5,98,200,252). Recently, retrospective evaluation of a series of patients with spiral CT arthrography of the postoperative meniscus showed a positive predictive value as high as 93% with a negative predictive value of 89% if certain interpretation criteria are used (displaced meniscal fragments, peripheral meniscal separation, with full thickness tear having intrameniscal contrast extending through the entire height or depth of the meniscus and large partial thickness tear involving greater than one third of the height and depth of

the meniscus) (191). Using similar principles of evaluating the abnormal distribution of intra-articular contrast, CT or MR arthrography may be helpful in the evaluation of the stability of osteochondral lesions, in the assessment of cartilage defects or in establishing the presence of loose osteochondral bodies (92,246,287) (Figs. 22-133 to 22-136). Although MR and CT arthrography have equivalent accuracy for detection of lesions involving greater than 50% of cartilage thickness, CT arthrography may have improved specificity for lesions involving less than 50% thickness (287). Distension of the joint with CT arthrography may also help in the visualization of synovial plicae (112). Evaluation of ganglion or synovial cysts around the knee is best accomplished with MRI, but when CT arthrography is used, delayed imaging may prove the cysts' communication to the joint (158).

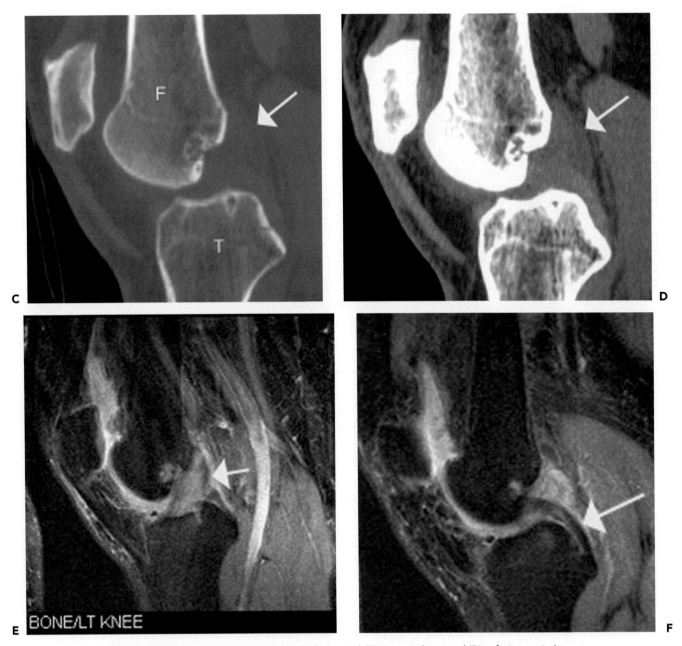

Figure 22-130 *(continued)* C: Sagittal reformatted CT image in bone and (D) soft tissue windows shows the femoral intraosseous ganglion. The soft tissue windows show the low-attenuation ganglion posteriorly better (*arrow*) and the degree of anterior displacement of the femur in relationship to the tibia is better appreciated on the bone windows. E: Sagittal fast spin echo PD-weighted MR image with fat suppression shows the ACL expanded by the increased signal ganglion (*arrow*). Note that the ACL continues to follow the slope of the intercondylar roof, as opposed to the usual ACL tear. F: Sagittal fast spin echo PD-weighted MR image with fat suppression shows the posterior extension of the ganglion causing mass effect on the PCL (*arrow*).

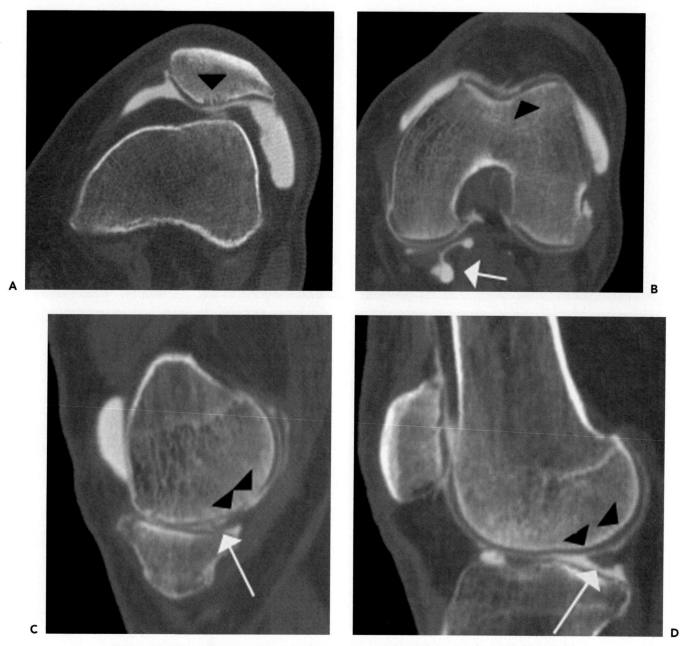

Figure 22-131 A 50-year-old man with knee pain: single contrast arthrography with multidetector CT and overlapping 2-mm images. **A:** Axial CT at level of patella shows marked loss of cartilage mid-patella and underlying subchondral cysts (*arrowhead*). **B:** Axial CT at level of trochlear sulcus shows loss of cartilage (*arrowhead*). Note extension of intra-articular contrast into synovial cyst between medial gastrocnemius and semimembranosus tendons (*arrow*). **C:** Sagittal reformatted image shows medial meniscus degenerative tear of the body and posterior horn medial meniscus (*arrow*) and overlying medial femoral condyle cartilage loss (*arrowheads*). **D:** A more normal appearing cartilage overlying the lateral femoral condyle and posterior horn lateral meniscus is shown for comparison.

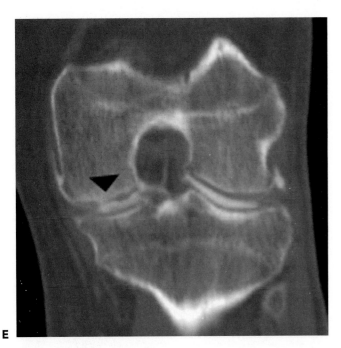

E

Figure 22-131 *(continued)* **E:** Coronal reformatted images shows the loss of medial femoral cartilage *(arrowhead)* best.

Other Conditions Assessed With CT

Patellar Subluxation

Patients with patellofemoral pain and abnormalities of patellar tracking can be evaluated with kinematic CT or MRI. This can be a difficult diagnosis to clinically differentiate from patellar chondromalacia. Malposition of the patella may only be appreciated at the later stages of knee extension (under 20 degrees of flexion), when the patella is not seated fully on the trochlear groove and its central position depends on the balance of lateral and medial quadri-

ceps muscle tension. Axial images through the patellofemoral joint space are performed from the extended knee position through 45 degrees of knee flexion, with the degree of knee flexion usually stabilized by a special thigh holder. The scans are usually performed with incremental positioning, although some advocate continuous scanning with very fast multislice CT acquisitions (183). Patellar subluxation and tilting can be assessed as a measurement of patellofemoral malalignment (Fig. 22-137). Patellar tilt angle is measured between a line parallel to the posterior condyle line and one parallel to the lateral patellar facet. The patellar lateral displacement can be measured either by the bisect offset distance (a line perpendicular to the anterior condyle line at the deepest portion of the trochlear groove will bisect the patellar width, with the amount of patella lateral to this line expressed as a percentage of total patellar width) or the lateral patellar displacement line (measured from the medial border of the patella to a line perpendicular to the posterior condyle line through the most anterior point of the medial femoral condyle). Kinematic MR imaging with ultrafast sequences may give a more accurate depiction of patellar tracking abnormalities, and may be the test of choice when available (183).

Total Knee Arthroplasty

In the patient undergoing total knee arthroplasty with large bony defects of the tibial plateau or femur, CT can be used to determine the level of bone resection for the optimum placement of the components of a total knee replacement. Utilizing 3D imaging and modeling, one could ascertain whether there is adequate bony support after cutting for the prosthesis, as well as providing a solid model on which to carry out the proposed surgery before

(text continues on page 1587)

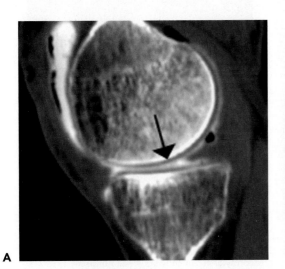

A

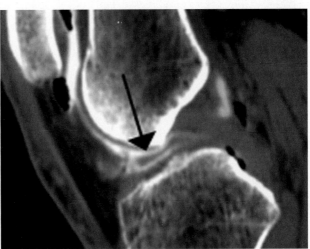

B

Figure 22-132 CT arthrography: bucket handle medial meniscal tear. Images obtained with multidetector CT and thin collimation after intra-articular administration of diluted iodinated contrast and air. **A:** Sagittal reformatted image medially shows absent body of medial meniscus *(arrow)*. The cartilage of the medial femoral condyle appears grossly intact **B:** Sagittal reformatted image through the intercondylar fossa shows displaced meniscal body fragment from a bucket handle tear. *(continued)*

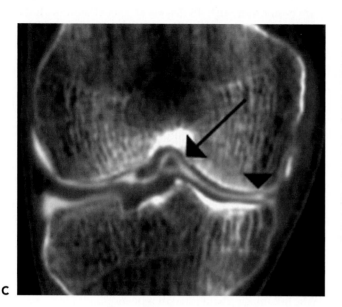

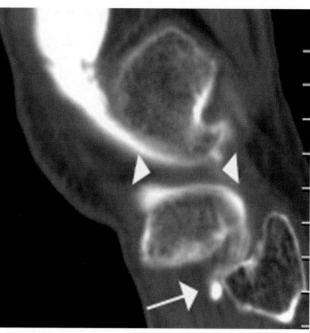

Figure 22-132 *(continued)* **C:** Coronal reformatted image shows displaced fragment *(arrow)* and absent meniscal body *(arrowhead)*. **D:** Sagittal reformatted image laterally shows normal lateral meniscus *(arrowheads)*. Note extension of contrast into the proximal tib-fib joint *(arrow)*, a normal finding. (Case courtesy of Dr. Marc Chitty, Medical Center East Hospital, Birmingham, AL.)

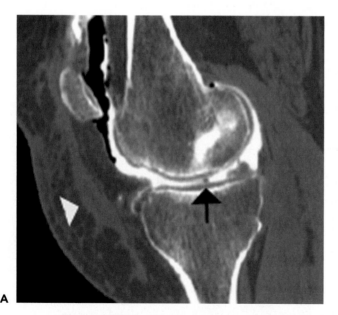

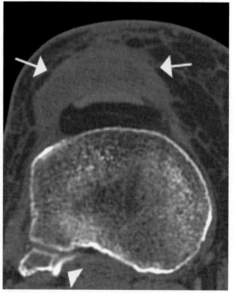

Figure 22-133   CT arthrography: osteochondral body. Images obtained with multidetector CT and thin collimation after intra-articular administration of diluted iodinated contrast and air. **A:** Sagittal reformatted image medial femoral condyle near the intercondylar fossa shows a small nonossified chondral body. A macerated posterior horn of the medial meniscus is present. Note the prepatellar bursa distension *(arrowhead)*. **B:** Axial image at the level of the proximal tibia shows the marked prepatellar bursitis. Normal extension of contract posterior to fibula into popliteal bursa is noted incidentally *(arrowhead)*. (Case courtesy of Dr. Marc Chitty, Medical Center East Hospital, Birmingham, AL.)

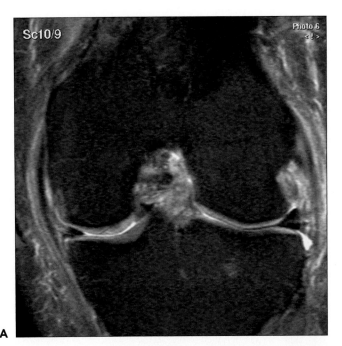
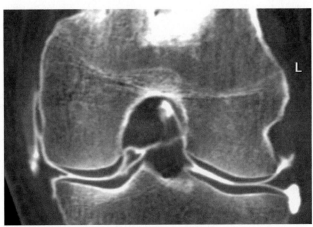

Figure 22-134 CT arthrography: bucket handle medial meniscal tear—correlation with MR and CT. **A:** Coronal fat-suppressed intermediate-weighted spin-echo image and (**B**) coronal reformation obtained after spiral CT arthrography of the left knee of a 27-year-old man shows a tear of the body of the medial meniscus with a meniscal fragment flipped in the intercondylar notch. The lesion was confirmed at arthroscopy. (Case courtesy of Dr. Bruno Vande Berg, Brussels, Belgium.)

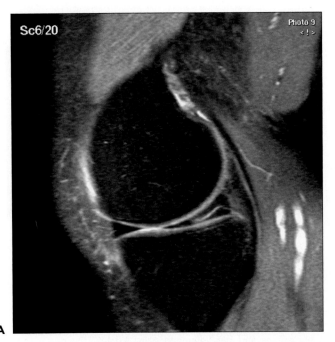
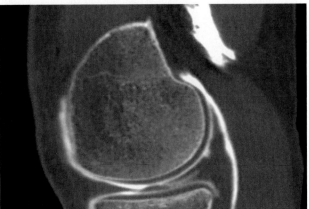

Figure 22-135 CT arthrography: medial meniscal tear—correlation with MR and CT. **A:** Sagittal fat-suppressed intermediate-weighted MR image and (**B**) sagittal reformation obtained after spiral CT arthrography of the right knee of a 47-year-old woman show a tear of the posterior horn of the medial meniscus with a large horizontal component and a short vertical component. A complex unstable tear was found at arthroscopy. (Case courtesy of Dr. Bruno Vande Berg, Brussels, Belgium.)

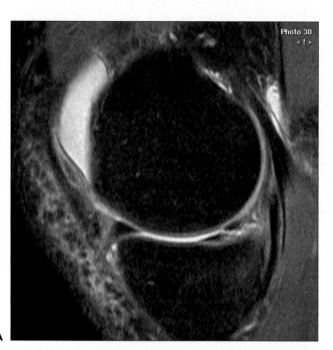

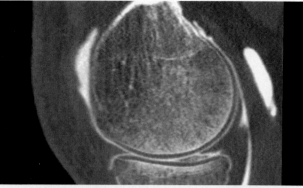

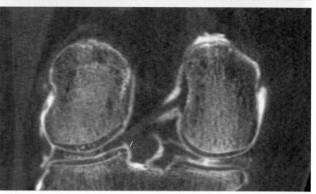

A

B

Figure 22-136 CT arthrography: unstable medial meniscal tear—correlation with MR and CT. **A:** Sagittal fat-saturated intermediate-weighted image shows the cleavage of the posterior horn. **B:** Sagittal and coronal reformations obtained after spiral CT arthrography of the right knee of a 67-year-old woman show a horizontal tear of the posterior horn with a radial component involving the lateral aspect of the posterior horn. Chondrocalcinosis is responsible for the punctuated areas of higher density in the cartilage and in the meniscus. (Case courtesy of Dr. Bruno Vande Berg, Brussels, Belgium.)

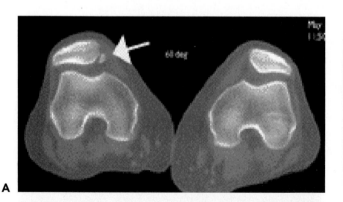

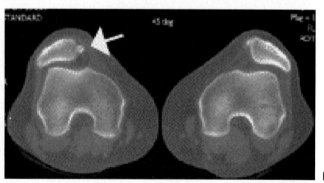

A

B

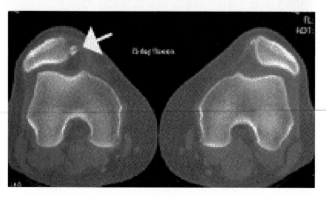

C

Figure 22-137 A 22-year-old woman with patellar tracking abnormalities and patellofemoral pain. Axial CT images of both knees performed at **(A)** 60, **(B)** 45, and **(C)** 15 degrees of flexion show progressive lateral patellar tilt and subluxation during knee extension. Bipartite patella on the right (*arrow*) is incidentally noted as well. The trochelar sulcus is somewhat shallow, which may contribute to the tracking abnormalities. (Case courtesy of Dr. Phillip Lander, Montreal General Hospital.)

undertaking the procedure on the patient (176). Some authors have proposed using CT routinely to preoperatively plan component alignment and soft tissue balance or even to plan robotic surgery (256,270).

With thin sections and wide windows decreasing the extent of metal artifact, CT can be used for assessing particle disease, or to check the alignment of the components in the patient with instability after TKA placement (Fig. 22-138). Although axial malalignment is usually evident on the radiographs, rotational malposition of the femoral or tibial component can be assessed accurately with CT (9,118).

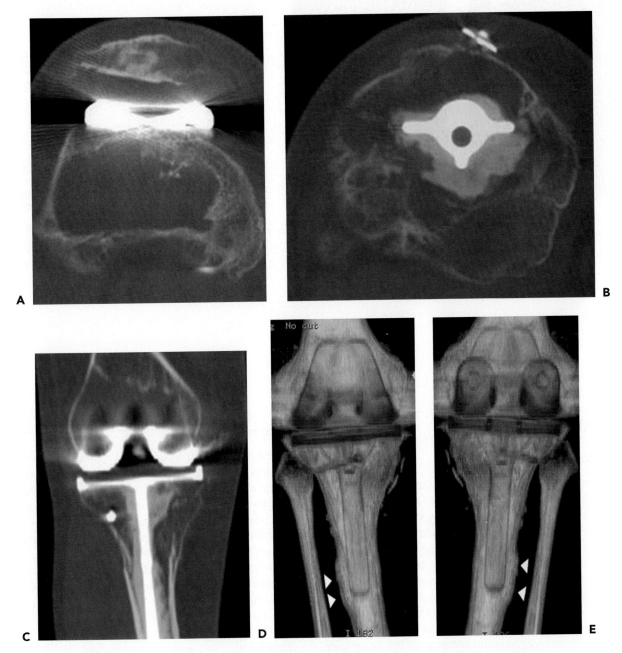

Figure 22-138 A 50-year-old man with knee pain, s/p TKA 12 years ago. **A:** Axial CT image at femoral component level shows large area of osteolysis involving most of the femoral shaft. Note hardware streak artifact from stainless steel TKA component does not significantly impair visualization of femur at this level. An area of osteolysis is also seen involving the medial patella. **B:** Axial CT image at level of the proximal tibial stem component shows osteolysis surrounding the cement-bone interface. The tibial stem component has no significant streak artifact. **C:** Coronal reformatted CT image shows the large degree of osteolysis surrounding the femoral and tibial component, as well as axial malalignment of the components. **D:** Volume-rendered 3-D CT images seen from an anterior and (**E**) posterior viewpoint shows the tibia varus deformity and malalignment of the TKA components. (*continued*)

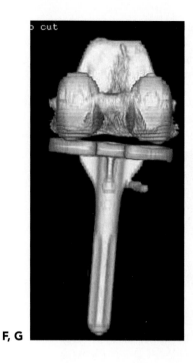 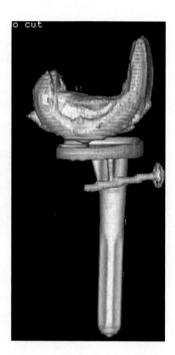

F, G

Figure 22-138 (*continued*) **F:** Volume-rendered 3D CT images seen from a posterior and (**G**) lateral point of view after the TKA components are isolated by postprocessing provides an elegant view of the alignment of the components.

ANKLE AND FOOT

Anatomy

The forefoot includes the metatarsals and phalanges. The midfoot consists of the navicular, cuboid and cuneiforms. The hindfoot is the talus and calcaneus. The Lisfranc joint separates the forefoot and midfoot, with the Chopart joint separating midfoot from hindfoot. The ankle or talocrural joint consists of the talus, distal tibia and fibula. The subtalar joint consists of two separate synovial compartments. The anterior and medial portion, or the sustentacular joint, communicates with the talonavicular joint. The posterior and lateral compartment is the posterior subtalar joint. It occasionally communicates with the ankle joint, about 10% of the time. Either can be a site of coalition (202) (Figs. 22-139 and 22-140).

Congenital Variants

Secondary ossification centers are sometimes confused for fractures. The os trigonum (Fig. 22-141) may be mistaken for the much less common Shepherd fracture of the posterior process of talus. Os trigonum syndrome is a mechanical tenosynovitis caused by tethering of the flexor hallucis longus tendon by the os trigonum (235). An os supranaviculare (Fig. 22-142) can simulate a navicular fracture. Accessory ossicles may be painful. CT features that have been associated with pain include degenerative sclerosis and irregularity, subchondral cyst-like changes and vacuum phenomenon at the synchondrosis (171). A bipartite medial cuneiform is an uncommon variant that is occasionally symptomatic (46) and can be involved in trauma (195) (Fig. 22-143). The corticated nature of sesamoids in the

(*text continues on page 1590*)

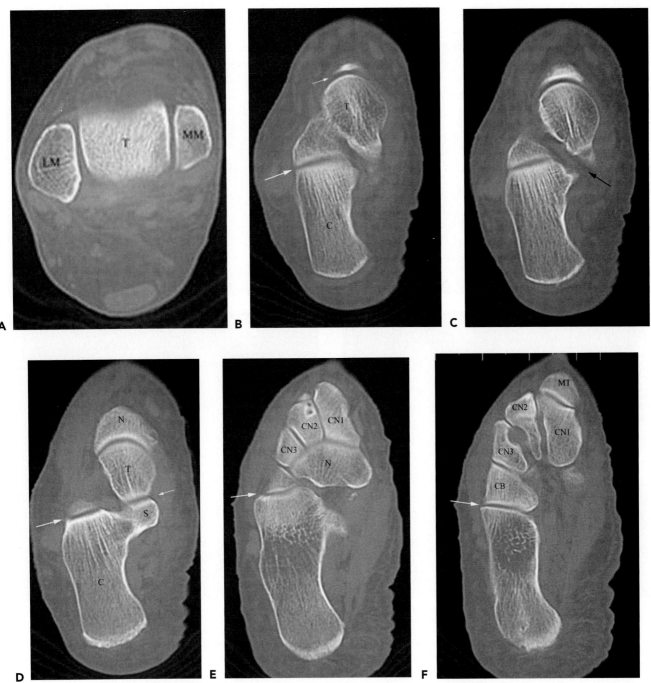

Figure 22-139 Axial anatomy. **A:** The talar dome (T), medial (MM) and lateral malleoli (LM) are the only osseous structures visible. Flexor and extensor tendons are well delineated by surrounding fat in this individual. **B:** More inferiorly, the talar body (T) and calcaneus (C), posterior subtalar joint (large arrow) and upper margin of the talonavicular joint (*small arrow*) are visible. **C:** Slightly more inferiorly, the sinus tarsi (*arrow*) is better seen. **D:** Talus (T), navicular (N), calcaneus (C), sustentaculum tali (S), sustentaculum joint (*small arrow*), posterior subtalar joint (*large arrow*) **E:** Cuneiforms (CN), navicular (N), calcaneocuboid joint (*arrow*). **F:** Base of first metatarsal (MT), cuneiforms (CN), cuboid (CB), calcaneocuboid joint (*arrow*). The rarefaction of trabecular bone in the anterior calcaneus is a common manifestation of osteoporosis.

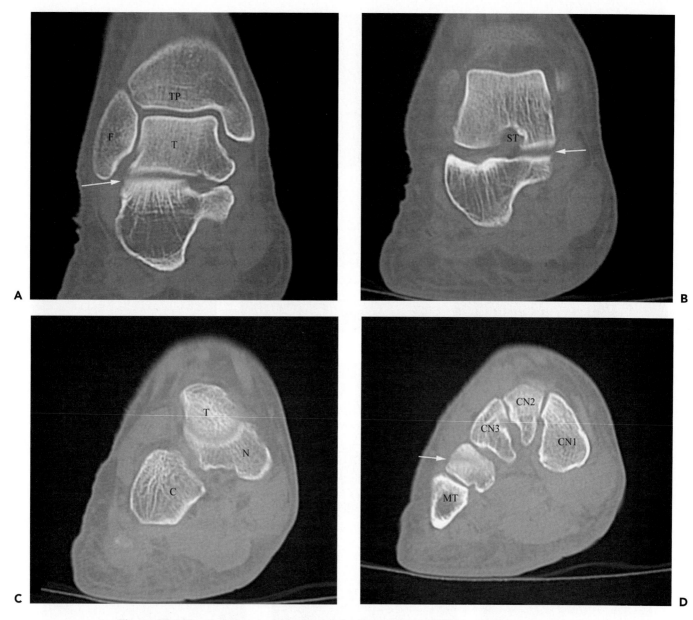

Figure 22-140   Coronal anatomy **A:** Tibial plafond (TP), talus (T), fibula (F), posterior subtalar joint (*arrow*) **B:** Sinus tarsi (ST), sustentaculum joint (*arrow*) **C:** Talus (T), calcaneus (C), navicular (N) **D:** Cuneiforms (CN), fourth tarsometatarsal joint (*arrow*), base of fifth metatarsal (MT).

forefoot distinguishes them from acute fracture fragments and is usually readily apparent on CT. Less noticed are the pathologic and potentially symptomatic entities of these normal structures, including fracture, osteonecrosis and degenerative change.

Tarsal coalition is rare, occurring in less than 2% of the population (210). Symptoms include hindfoot or tarsal pain and stiffness, often precipitated by trauma (193). Adolescents with pain, decreased mobility and deformity

should be evaluated with radiographs and CT. CT is considered to be the best diagnostic method by many authors (210). Coalitions may be fibrous, cartilaginous or osseous. Osseous bridging is readily apparent by CT in the latter form. More subtle osseous hypertrophy and irregularity of the opposing surfaces is seen in fibrous or cartilaginous coalitions (31) (Fig. 22-144). Familiarity with the appearance of tarsal coalitions is useful as they are often incidentally discovered on cross-sectional examinations requested

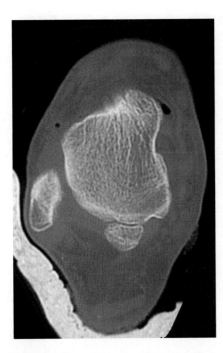

Figure 22-141 Os trigonum. The well-corticated margins of the ununited posterior secondary ossification center distinguish this entity from an acute talar fracture. The intracapsular soft tissue gas in this patient is due to an open ankle injury.

for other reasons (193). The talocalcaneal and calcaneonavicular joints are most commonly involved (210). Talocalcaneal coalition is particularly difficult to diagnose radiographically (193). Talocalcaneal types may involve the middle or posterior portions of the subtalar joint (202), and are usually best seen on coronal images. Calcaneocuboid coalitions (Fig. 22-145) are by comparison very rare (226) with the cubonavicular and naviculocuneiform types rarer still, accounting for only 1% of all coalitions (210).

A lucent lesion in the anterior calcaneus is most commonly a simple bone cyst, (Fig. 22-146) or, less frequently, a calcaneal lipoma (Fig. 22-147). Both of these lesions differ from the rarefaction of trabeculae seen in osteoporosis (see Fig. 22-139F) by the presence of a well-defined, sclerotic border and the absence or scarcity of central trabeculae.

Trauma

For fracture assessment, CT has become an invaluable additional tool, particularly for visualizing complex anatomic regions such as the midfoot and for judging articular surface integrity. The foot and ankle are usually imaged

(*text continues on page 1594*)

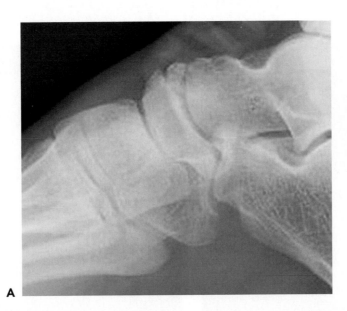

A

Figure 22-142 Os supranaviculare. **A:** Lateral radiograph demonstrates the corticated nature of the ununited ossification center. (*continued*)

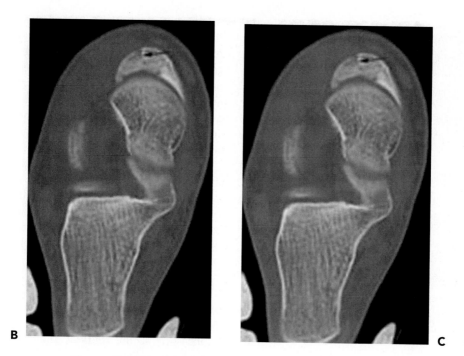

Figure 22-142 (*continued*) **B, C:** CT was requested to better exclude an acute fracture. Volume averaging in the axial plane somewhat hampers visualization, but corticated margins (*arrows*) can still be discerned. Unfortunately, the patient could not tolerate further imaging in the coronal plane, and reformatted images were unsatisfactory.

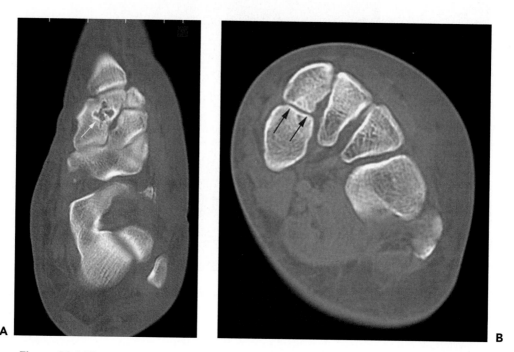

Figure 22-143   Bipartite medial cuneiform. **A:** Axial image reveals a complex cyst-like lesion in the central portion of the medial cuneiform (*arrow*). **B:** Coronal plane imaging better reveals the synchondrosis (*arrows*) dividing the separate ossification centers of the medial cuneiform. **C:** More distally, degenerative-type sclerosis and cyst-like changes are seen to better advantage than on the axial image. These changes can be associated with clinical symptoms.

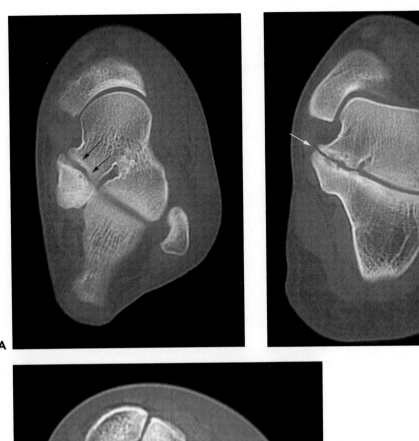

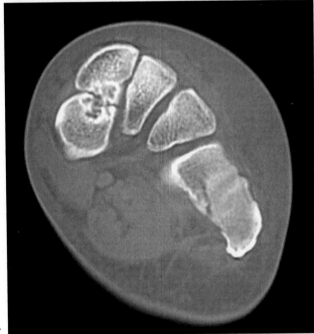

Figure 22-144 Talonavicular coalition of the middle facets. **A:** Axial and (**B**) coronal images. The sustentaculum joint space is narrowed (*arrows*), with irregularity and sclerosis of the articular surfaces in this fibrous or cartilaginous coalition. Compare the appearance to that of the normal adjacent posterior subtalar joint.

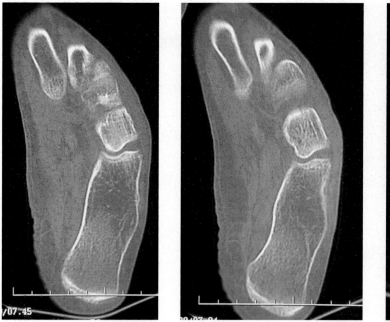
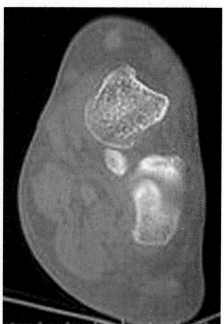

A, B /07:45   C

Figure 22-145 Calcaneocuboid coalition. Fibrous or cartilaginous tarsal coalition of the calcaneocuboid joint results in an elongated, irregular shape of the calcaneal articular surface on axial (**A, B**) and coronal (**C**) images.

with 2- to 3-mm thick sections obtained in the axial plane (axial with respect to the long axis of the body) with the patient supine and the foot in neutral position. Imaging of only the affected extremity is recommended, with the contralateral extremity removed from the scan plane when possible, to minimize streak artifact and optimize field of view and positioning for the area of interest. Including the contralateral side for comparison is occasionally helpful but need not be routinely done. When possible, direct coronal oblique sections are also obtained. With the knee flexed and the foot flat on the scan table, the gantry is tilted towards the knee as far as possible to place the tibia nearly parallel with the plane of section.

Helical CT is useful in the trauma setting due to difficulty positioning caused by pain, splints and concomitant injuries. Helical 1-mm images are obtained in the axial plane with 1:1 pitch, yielding essentially isotropic images and high-quality multiplanar reconstructions (297). Because the tibial plafond and talar dome are nearly parallel to the axial plane of section, direct coronal or multiplanar reformatted images are very helpful for assessment of these articular surfaces. Multiplanar reformatted images are more accurate and offer more information regarding the

degree of articular surface involvement and displacement of fragments than the source axial images (154). Reformatted coronal images have the advantage of no added radiation exposure, an important consideration at a time when CT is estimated to account for more than 60% of the radiation dose to patients in some departments (100). Despite the relative resistance of the extremities to effects of ionizing radiation when compared to the trunk, CT of the extremities should always be performed with the lowest radiation dose possible to arrive at a diagnosis. Alternative imaging methods such as MR or ultrasound can in many circumstances spare the patient any exposure to ionizing radiation. Timing of the exam is also relevant, though often outside the control of the radiologist. While external fixation and traction devices may cause streak artifact and hamper standard positioning, delaying the CT until after initial closed reduction with a traction device may actually improve the exam's quality by aiding in the identification of fracture components when they are reduced to nearer their anatomic positions (296).

In trauma of the skeletally immature distal tibial epiphysis, the Salter-Harris type II lesion is most common (46%), followed by type III (25%), type IV (10%) and type I (6%)

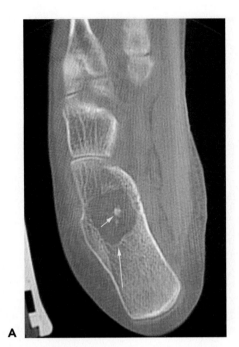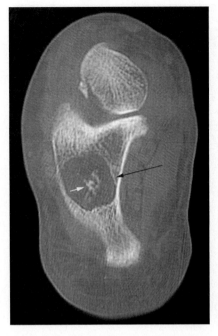

A

B

Figure 22-146 Intraosseous lipoma of anterior calcaneus. **A:** Axial and (**B**) coronal images of a CT performed for trauma reveal an unrelated anterior calcaneal lipoma. The lesional contents are hypodense relative to normal adjacent muscle. A thin, sclerotic margin is visible (*long arrow*). Dystrophic calcification is present centrally (*short arrow*).

injuries. Juvenile Tillaux injury (a form of Salter-Harris type III) constitutes 14% of injuries. The triplane fracture constitutes 10% of distal tibial epiphyseal fractures and defies Salter-Harris classification (151). CT is particularly useful for triplane fractures of the distal tibial epiphysis because of the complex anatomy of this injury pattern, with all three anatomic planes involved. The coronally oriented component involves the posterior tibial metaphysis and a variably sized portion of the epiphysis. The sagittal component is through the epiphysis, usually centrally. The axial component is through the physis itself. Radiographically, the appearance is of a Salter-Harris type II or IV fracture on the lateral radiograph and type III on the frontal projection. More than 2-mm displacement determines the surgical approach, and is best seen by CT. The physeal injury and any joint surface incongruity are best seen with direct coronal imaging. Both the coronal and sagittal components are best seen with axial plane imaging (Fig. 22-148) (48).

Most adult ankle injuries are adequately assessed with conventional radiographs. CT is useful in complex injuries (154,156) especially intra-articular fractures of the tibial plafond or pilon fractures (260). Preoperative CT of pilon fractures changes the operative plan and subjectively de-

creases the length of the procedure in the majority of pilon fractures. Specific details seen best on CT are the number of fragments, presence of impaction and the angle of the major fracture line, which determines the type of surgical incision. The routine CT evaluation of all displaced, intra-articular pilon fractures is recommended by some authors (280).

Distal tibiofibular diastasis implies interosseous ligament disruption and alters surgical repair, especially when it is unexpected, as in the case of a low fibular fracture. Diastasis can be difficult to appreciate radiographically but is readily apparent on axial CT images, sometimes with an associated avulsion fracture at the site of the interosseous ligament (262). Syndesmotic disruption is most easily diagnosed on axial CT scan when the contralateral side is included for comparison. The width of the syndesmosis is measured approximately 1 cm proximal to the level of the plafond. Subluxation of the fibula is a clue to syndesmotic disruption that is apparent on axial CT but virtually impossible to detect radiographically (76).

Calcaneal fractures comprise 60% of all major tarsal injuries (297). CT is extremely helpful to assess the complex anatomy and assist in planning for conservative versus (*text continues on page 1599*)

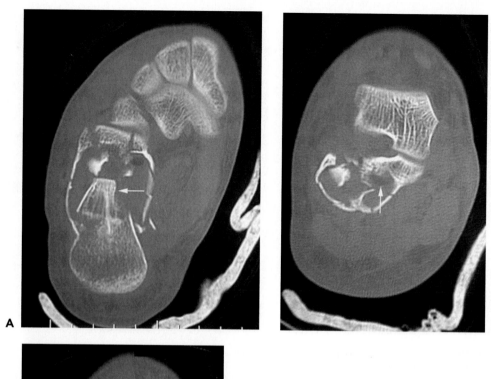

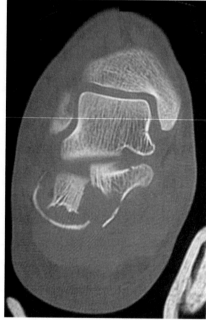

Figure 22-147 Pathologic fracture of calcaneus through a solitary bone cyst. **A:** Axial image demonstrates a depressed subtalar articular surface fragment *(arrow)* and a small amount of free marrow fat within the large anterior calcaneal cyst. **B:** Coronal image through the sustentaculum joint reveals the free fat in the nondependent portion of the cyst *(arrow)*. **C:** Coronal image more posteriorly demonstrates inferior displacement of the large posterior facet fragment.

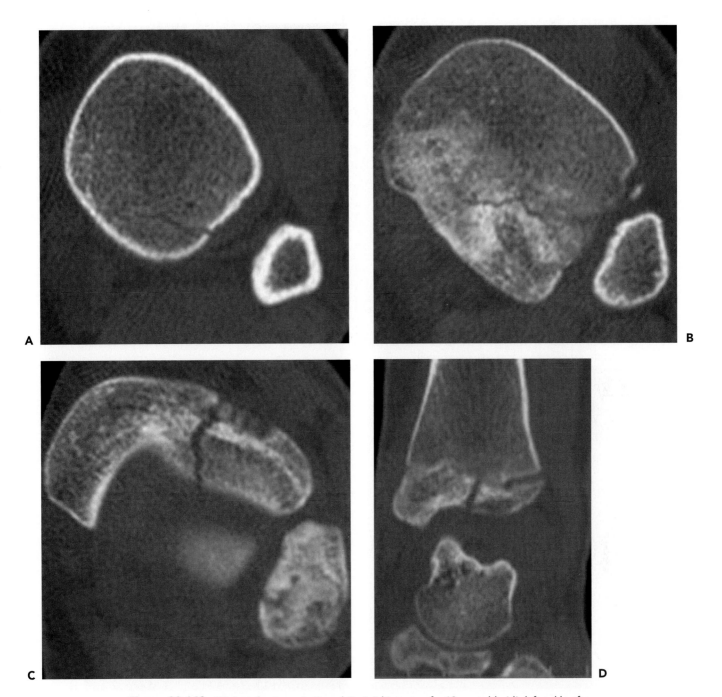

Figure 22-148   Triplane fracture. A, B, and C: Axial images of a 12-year-old-girl's left ankle after trauma were obtained and show the fracture extending into the posterior tibial shaft cortex superiorly, as well as a sagittal component through the anterior epiphysis in the most distal image. D: Coronal reformation shows the vertical epiphyseal fracture best, as well as the widening of the lateral physis, consistent with the axial extent of the fracture. (*continued*)

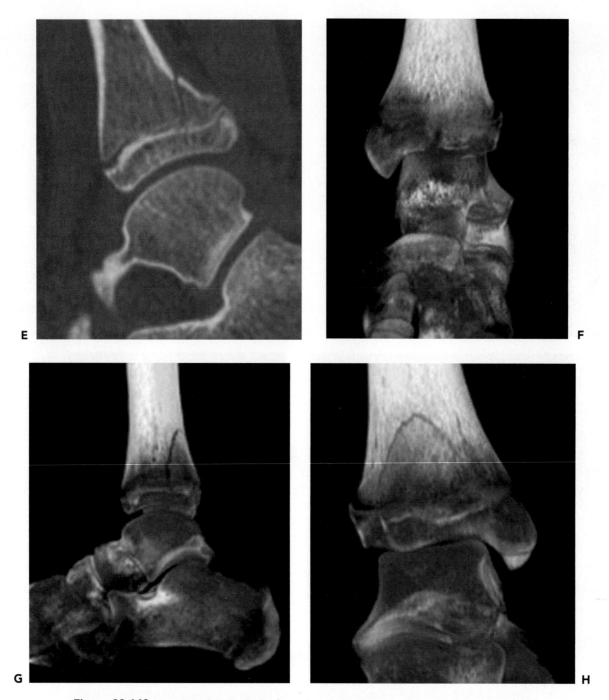

Figure 22-148 (*continued*) **E:** Sagittal reformation shows the posterior coronal component and superior extent of the fracture, and again the physeal fracture component is seen with widening of the anterior physis. Multiple images from a 3D volume rendered reconstruction (the fibula has been removed by postprocessing) as viewed from an anterior (**F**), lateral (**G**), and posterior (**H**) viewpoint show all components of this fracture in great detail. (*continued*)

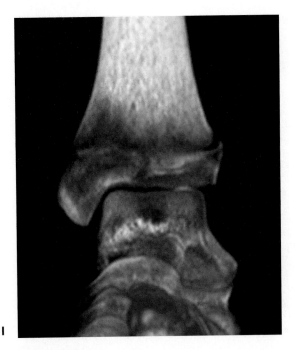

Figure 22-148 (*continued*) A mortise view (I) can be simulated to assess the degree of joint space narrowing laterally.

surgical management. 75% of adults have intra-articular involvement, traditionally mandating open repair (75). Focal points of CT analysis are integrity of the calcaneocuboid and subtalar articular surfaces (Figs. 22-149 to 22-153). When repair is contemplated, the surgical priorities are restoration of calcaneal height, alignment and length and articular surfaces, especially the posterior facet and calcaneocuboid joint (279). Assessment of the anterior facet is relatively unimportant as it is often absent or united with the middle facet and does not sustain surgically significant isolated injuries. The posterior facet is the most important subtalar joint structure (see Fig. 22-149). 3D disarticulated images are useful for illustrating the relationships and displacement of fragments, but may fail to visualize nearly 10% of fractures and must be compared to the more sensitive source axial images (88). Lateral subluxation of the posterior facet is associated with multiple other injuries such as calcaneocuboid joint involvement, lateral collateral ligament injury, peroneal tendon subluxation and fibular fracture and indicates surgical intervention is warranted (76) (see Fig. 22-153). Fractures tend to be less comminuted in adolescents than in adults, and therefore more amenable to operative reduction (32).

(*text continues on page 1602*)

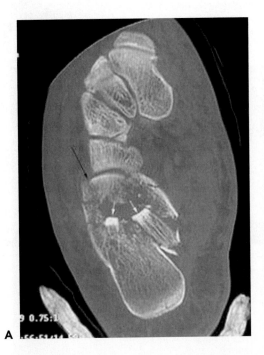

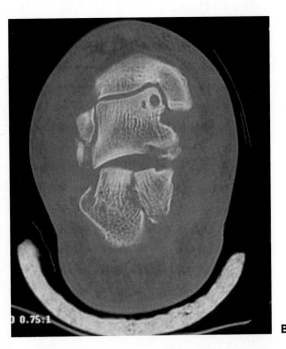

Figure 22-149 Calcaneal fracture. **A:** Axial image. Note impacted articular surface fragments of the posterior facet (*short arrows*) and involvement of the calcaneocuboid joint (*long arrow*). **B:** Coronal image reveals fracture and impaction of the posterior facet, associated fibular fracture and a pre-existing medial talar dome osteochondral lesion. (*continued*)

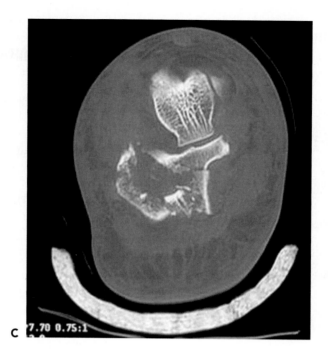

Figure 22-149 (*continued*) **C:** More anterior coronal image demonstrates wide displacement of the lateral calcaneal wall fragments, isolation of the sustentaculum tali and medial subluxation of the middle facet.

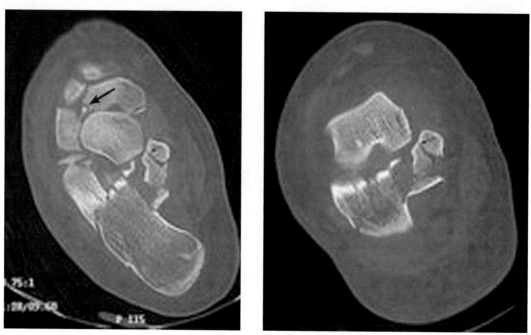

Figure 22-150 Calcaneal and navicular fractures. **A:** Axial and coronal (**B**) images reveal comminution of the calcaneal body, isolation and medial dislocation of the sustentaculum tali with fracture through the middle facet (*small arrow*). Fracture through the mid-portion of the navicular with wide displacement of the fragments (*large arrow*) is also visible on the axial image.

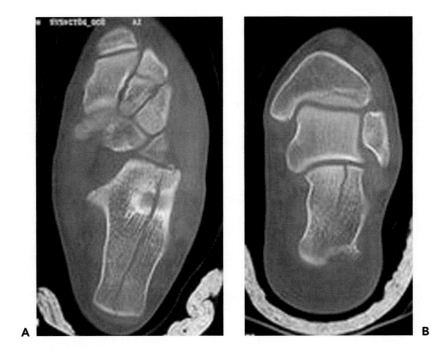

Figure 22-151 Calcaneal fracture. **A:** Axial image reveals a longitudinal fracture extending through the length of the calcaneal body. **B:** Coronal image. The fracture extends into the posterior subtalar joint in a sagittal orientation.

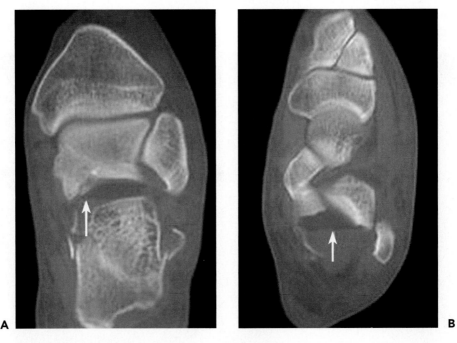

Figure 22-152 Traumatic lipohemarthrosis of the posterior subtalar joint. **A:** Coronal image results in a lipohemarthrosis with the fat-fluid interface (*arrow*) in the axial plane. **B:** Axial image with the leg in extension shifts the fat–fluid interface (*arrow*) into the coronal plane.

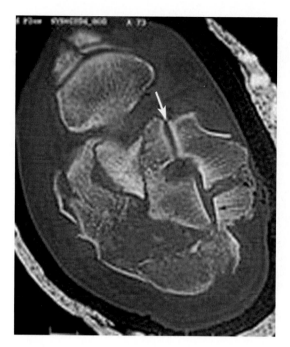

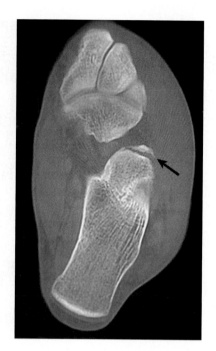

Figure 22-153 Talus and calcaneal fracture. Severe comminu-tion of the talus and calcaneus has resulted in rotation of the sus-tentaculum joint (*white arrow*) and posterior subtalar joint (*black arrow*) articular surfaces into a nearly sagittal orientation on this axial image.

Figure 22-154 Fracture of the anterosuperior process of the calcaneus. Fracture (*arrow*) extends in a semicoronal plane through the uppermost aspect of the calcaneocuboid articular surface. These fractures are often difficult to appreciate radiographically.

Avulsion fractures from the dorsolateral aspect of the cal-caneus result from traction on the extensor digitorum bre-vis muscle during forced inversion. The fragment can be radiographically confused with a normal os peroneum but CT will demonstrate the latter to be plantar in location (194). Fracture of the anterosuperior process of the calca-neus is another radiographically challenging entity that is well demonstrated on CT or MRI (Fig. 22-154).

Most fractures of the talus are avulsion type fractures that may extend into the articular surfaces (Figs. 22-155 and 22-156). Talar neck fractures are infrequent and re-sult from forced dorsiflexion when the foot is in extreme

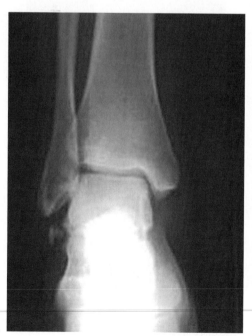

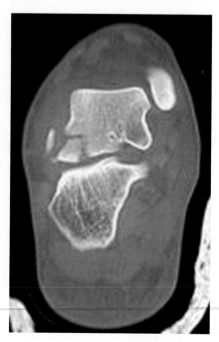

A

B

Figure 22-155 Talus fracture. **A:** AP radiograph demonstrates a fracture fragment lateral to the talar body. **B:** Coronal CT image better demonstrates the size of the fracture fragments and the in-volvement of the posterior subtalar joint articular surface.

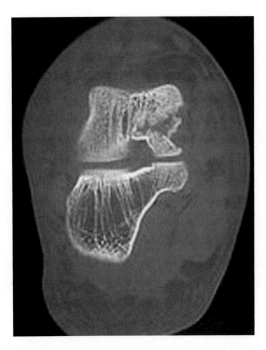

Figure 22-156 Talus fracture. Coronal image demonstrates isolation of the middle facet articular surface.

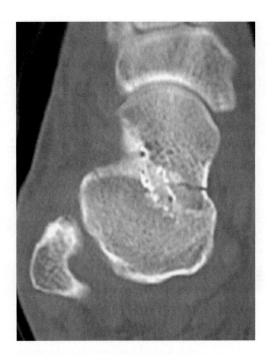

Figure 22-157 Talar neck fracture. Axial image shows a nondisplaced fracture of the proximal talar neck.

plantar flexion, typically in the impact of a motor vehicle collision while the foot is pressed hard against the brake pedal (Fig. 22-157). There is increasing risk of talar dome osteonecrosis with displacement of fracture fragments and subluxation or dislocation of the subtalar, ankle or talonavicular joints respectively (Fig. 22-158). Talar dislocation can occur in the absence of significant talar fracture (Fig.

22-159). Shepherd fracture (Fig. 22-160) of the posterior process of the talus can be distinguished from an os trigonum by the lack of corticated margins.

A Chopart injury often results in fractures of the talus, cuboid and navicular (202). Sagittal reformatted images are helpful to appreciate the anatomy of the Chopart joint (Fig. 22-161). Chopart fracture-dislocations are frequently

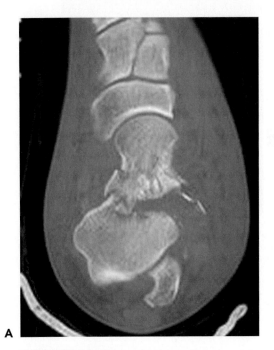

A

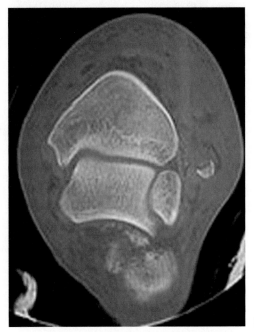

B

Figure 22-158 Talar neck fracture. **A:** Axial image. The talar neck is comminuted. **B:** Coronal image demonstrates dislocation of the posterior subtalar joint with a few comminuted calcaneal fragments visible.

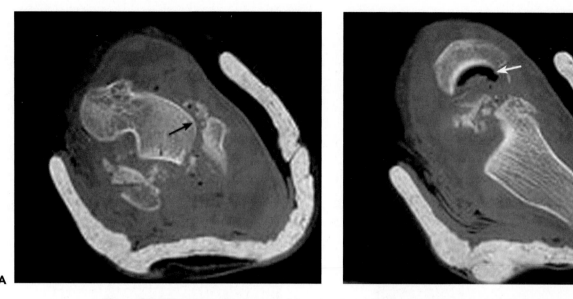

Figure 22-159 Open ankle fracture-dislocation. **A:** Axial image. The talar dome (*large arrow*) and posterior facet of the subtalar joint (*small arrow*) are dislocated, with the body of the talus rotated onto its side. Extensive soft tissue injury and deep soft tissue gas are evident. **B:** The talonavicular joint is dislocated and filled with air (*arrow*).

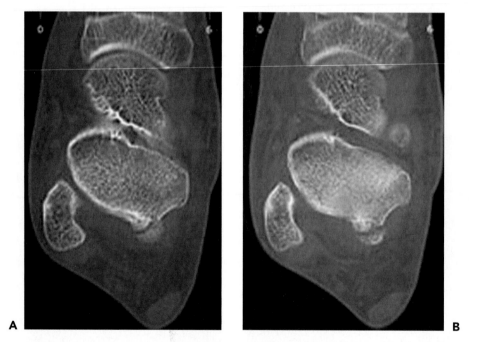

Figure 22-160 Shepherd fracture. **A and B:** Sequential axial images through an acute fracture of the posterior process of the talus. The lack of cortication distinguishes this uncommon fracture from the commonly encountered os trigonum, an ununited accessory ossification center.

reduced prior to obtaining CT or even radiographs. Careful attention to the Chopart joint for fractures or vacuum phenomenon can detect this injury pattern postreduction.

Midfoot fractures result in poorly localized pain. These injuries are often difficult to appreciate radiographically due to overlapping structures, making CT of this region extremely useful (Fig. 22-162). Overlapping the source axial slices is helpful to assure high quality reformatted images through this region (202). Nutcracker fracture of the cuboid (Fig. 22-163) typically occurs when a patient falls with the foot held in exaggerated plantar flexion so that the metatarsals are fixed against the ground during the fall. The weight of the patient is transmitted through the calcaneus, trapping the cuboid between the 4th and 5th metatarsals and the calcaneus and crushing the cuboid (111). Forced abduction of the forefoot by other mechanism could result in this injury (115).

Lisfranc injury involves dorsolateral dislocation of the metatarsals (Fig. 22-164). These may be homolateral, with the first metatarsal remaining aligned or dislocating laterally, or divergent with the first metatarsal dislocating medially (202). CT is exquisitely sensitive for tarsal or metatarsal fractures. Conventional radiographs may miss nearly 40% of tarsal or metatarsal fractures and up to 50% of subluxations at the Lisfranc joint in the setting of high-energy hyperflexion injuries of the foot. CT is the preferred method of evaluation in this population, particularly when obtained in an oblique axial plane, oriented along the metatarsal shafts (214).

Fractures of the proximal aspect of the fifth metatarsal are often misclassified, all being combined under the eponym Jones' fracture. In fact, only a fracture at the proximal diametaphyseal junction should rightly be termed a Jones' fracture, with fractures of the proximal diaphysis

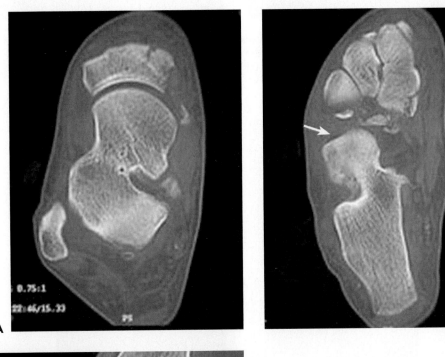

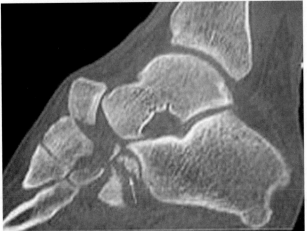

Figure 22-161 Chopart injury. **A:** Axial image reveals a fracture of the navicular. Talonavicular dislocation is not appreciated on this single image. **B:** A more caudal axial image. Note the absence of the cuboid at its expected location (*arrow*) and numerous widely displaced fracture fragments. **C:** Sagittal reformatted image displays the dislocation at the Chopart joint as well as a comminuted cuboid fracture (*arrow*).

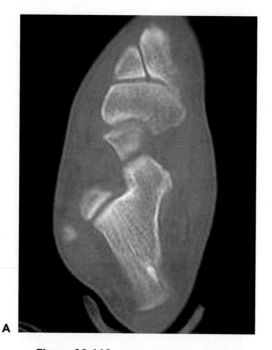
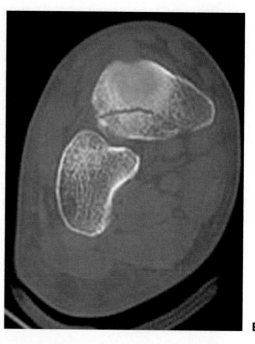

A   B

Figure 22-162 Navicular fracture. **A:** Axial image shows only questionable cortical indistinctness on the medial aspect of the proximal and distal articular surfaces. **B:** Coronal image reveals a minimally displaced navicular fracture in the axial plane, extending into the proximal articular surface.

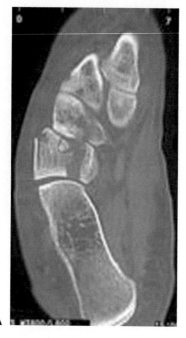
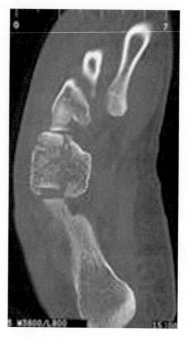

A   B

Figure 22-163 Nutcracker cuboid fracture. **A:** Axial image of the comminuted cuboid body. **B:** with impaction of the proximal articular surface.

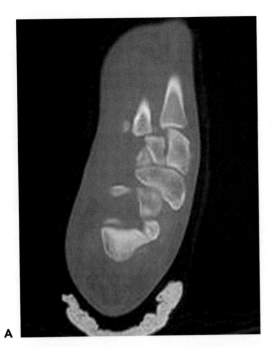 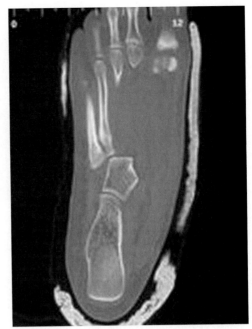

Figure 22-164 Lisfranc injury. **A:** Axial image through the upper midfoot demonstrates lateral subluxation of the first and second metatarsals relative to the medial and middle cuneiforms. **B:** Farther inferiorly, the fourth and fifth metatarsals are also laterally subluxed relative to the cuboid.

and tuberosity considered as separate injuries. Recent evidence suggests that the lateral aspect of the plantar aponeurosis causes avulsion of the tuberosity during forced inversion while weight-bearing (278).

As on radiographs, a fractured sesamoid of the great toe metatarsal head can be distinguished from a multipartite sesamoid by axial tomography. Fracture margins are sharp and can be mentally reassembled into a sesamoid of similar size to its pair. Margins of a multipartite sesamoid are smooth, well corticated, beveled and do not fit together (202).

Feet are especially prone to foreign bodies. Even tiny metallic foreign bodies are readily apparent on conventional radiographs, but the nonmetallic foreign object can pose a diagnostic challenge, particularly if composed of wood. Sonography is the method of choice for detection of a suspected radiolucent foreign body, but the lack of adequate clinical history often results in CT or MR performance instead, because of nonspecific pain, swelling or redness. Of these two methods, CT is superior to MRI in detection of wooden foreign bodies, while MR is better at detecting the inflammation surrounding a foreign body. Longstanding wooden foreign bodies are consistently denser than normal adjacent muscle and fat, and are optimally seen using bone window and level settings (134,207). On occasion, however, wood may be lower attenuation than the soft tissues depending on its water content, which in turn depends on preservative treatments, whether it is fresh or dry wood and how long it is present *in vivo* prior to imaging (169).

Stress Fractures

While MRI is more sensitive for early stress fractures, CT has a useful role in some stress fractures of the foot, particularly the navicular. CT may add additional information when MRI or bone scan is abnormal but nonspecific, by detecting a lucent or sclerotic fracture line or periosteal reaction not visible on radiographs (Fig. 22-165). CT may also visualize the nidus of an osteoid osteoma that can mimic a stress fracture in terms of bone scan uptake, radiographic sclerosis or marrow edema on MRI (264). Axial CT can be helpful in the diagnosis of sesamoid stress fractures in high-performance athletes when radiographs are unremarkable (13).

Most stress fractures of the tibia are the proximal horizontal or oblique type and present little diagnostic difficulty on conventional radiographs. Cross-sectional imaging has resulted in a growing awareness of longitudinal stress fractures of the distal tibia, often invisible on conventional radiographs. CT is more sensitive than MRI for the fracture lucency of a longitudinal stress fracture, al-

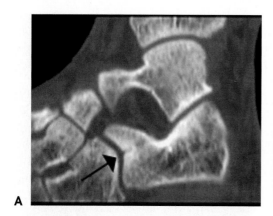
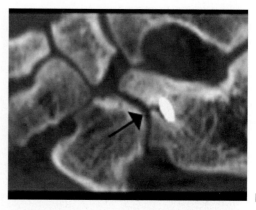

Figure 22-165 Stress fracture of the anterosuperior process of the calcaneus. **A:** Sagittal reformatted image shows a subtle lucent line (*arrow*) extending into the cortex and reactive sclerosis in the anterosuperior process of the lateral calcaneus in this college basketball player. **B:** Sagittal reformatted image of the same area at a later date after internal fixation shows the fracture (*arrow*) failed to unite.

though MR is more sensitive for the accompanying marrow and soft tissue edema. Both modalities may be complementary in this difficult clinical entity (82).

Internal Joint Derangements and Arthritis

MRI is the imaging modality of choice for soft tissue pathology in the ankle and foot region due to high soft tissue contrast, lack of ionizing radiation and ease of multi-

planar capability (235). Not surprisingly, MRI is superior to CT in detection of virtually all tendon and ligament disorders, such as tenosynovitis, peritendinitis, tendinopathy, tendon rupture, dislocation or subluxation (44) and the status of the retinaculum. Unfortunately, both tendon and cortical bone are very low in signal intensity on all MR pulse sequences, so it can be difficult to resolve osseous abnormalities adjacent to a tendon from the tendon itself. In comparison, CT provides exquisite osseous anatomic

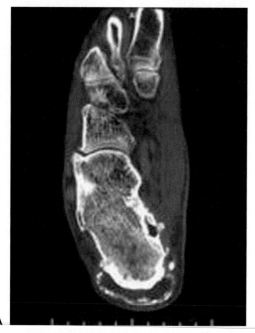
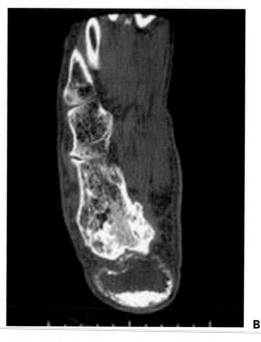

Figure 22-166 Adventitial bursa with hydroxyapatite crystals. **A:** Axial image. Calcaneal body is deformed due to a healed comminuted fracture from trauma many years before. An adventitial bursa has formed posterior to the calcaneus, with irregular calcification in its walls. **B:** More inferiorly, the calcium hydroxyapatite crystals in the bursa form a fluid–fluid level. (Case is courtesy of Dr. Michael Pitt, University of Alabama at Birmingham Department of Radiology, Birmingham, AL.)

detail (225), making it better suited to detect the presence of calcifications (Fig. 22-166), osteophytes, bone fragments impinging on a tendon or a shallow or convex retromalleolar groove (44,235). For this last entity, comparison to the normal contralateral side is very helpful.

In situations where MR is not readily available, CT arthrography is still a valuable tool for assessing cartilage and pericapsular soft tissue abnormalities (Fig. 22-167). CT arthrography can be helpful in diagnosis of soft tissue impingement in the setting of chronic ankle pain following trauma, important because arthroscopic ablation of the inflammatory soft tissue mass often leads to significant clinical improvement (108). MR arthrography aids the diagnosis of a variety of ankle impingement syndromes as well, particularly posterior impingement, although these are usually clinical rather than imaging diagnoses (234). The relative value of CT versus MR arthrography has not been extensively studied, although the usefulness of each is probably similar for synovial and cartilage abnormali-

ties. With its ability to also directly visualize marrow abnormalities and extrasynovial soft tissue structures, particularly ligaments, MR arthrography will likely prove to ultimately be the superior test in the setting of chronic posttraumatic ankle pain.

Normal tendon is higher attenuation than adjacent muscle, in the 75 to 115 HU range. Tendinopathy can be seen as tendon enlargement, decreased attenuation and heterogeneity. Calcification is occasionally seen in chronic tendinopathy. Tenosynovitis may be seen as a halo of lower attenuation fluid surrounding the high attenuation tendon. CT often does not allow distinction between synovial fluid and an abnormal tendon, a task for which MR is more sensitive (235). Of note, volumetric 3D reconstructions of MSHCT data may show tendon abnormalities with improved accuracy (196).

The different degrees of tendon tear are often visible on CT. A type 1 tendon tear demonstrates tendon enlargement and heterogeneity, with a decrease in attenuation to

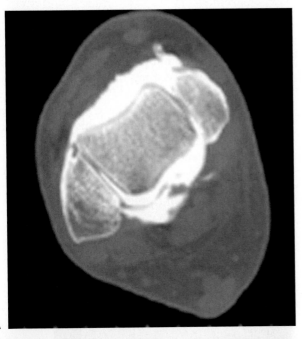

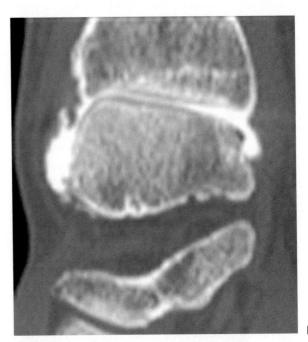

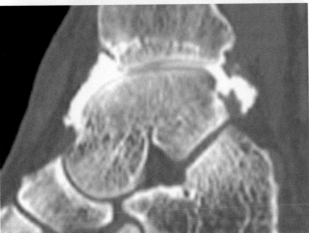

Figure 22-167 CT arthrography: ankle. **A:** Axial CT image and **(B)** coronal and **(C)** sagittal reformation images show normal distribution of intraarticular contrast. There is slight irregularity of the capsule that was felt to represent adhesive capsulitis. (Case courtesy of Dr. Phillip Lander and McGill University Hospital, Montreal, Canada.)

the 30 to 50 HU range. A type 2 tear consists of thinning of the tendon. In a type 3 tear a discontinuity is visible. Vertical splits and tendon heterogeneity are more apparent on MR than on CT. MR is slightly more sensitive and much more accurate for the characterization of posterior tibial tendon tears (235). CT can easily demonstrate tendon dislocation and associated congenital or traumatic osseous abnormalities. It does not visualize adjacent scar, soft tissue disruption or associated partial tendon tear as well as MRI, however (44).

Arthritis

CT is more sensitive than conventional radiographs for the detection of erosions, joint space narrowing, subchondral cyst-like changes, sclerosis and osteophyte formation in inflammatory and degenerative arthropathies of the foot and ankle, particularly in the complex anatomic regions of the midfoot and subtalar joint. Posterior subtalar joint pathology usually results in ankle rather than foot pain. Degenerative change in this location is usually posttraumatic secondary to calcaneal fracture. Inflammatory arthritis in this joint is usually due to rheumatoid arthritis (202). Osteochondral defects of the talar dome can be detected without the use of intra-articular contrast (Figs. 22-168 and 22-169), but with less sensitivity. CT arthrography or MRI only demonstrates the integrity of the overlying cartilage and purely chondral defects.

The Lisfranc joint is the most common site of neuropathic osteoarthropathy in diabetes, although many other sites in the foot and ankle can be affected. CT findings are consistent with severe degenerative joint disease, including osteophyte formation, subchondral sclerosis, cyst-like changes and osteochondral bodies. A combination of atrophic and hypertrophic manifestations is usually present (181).

After primary degenerative joint disease, the next most commonly encountered arthropathy in the forefoot is rheumatoid arthritis. Ninety percent of patients with rheumatoid arthritis (RA) will have some degree of forefoot involvement. Up to 20% of RA patients will have their first manifestation of the disease in this region. The fifth metatarsophalangeal joint is usually the first of the foot or ankle joints to be involved (202). One of the neglected joints of the forefoot is the metatarsal sesamoid joint of the great toe. Subluxation, dislocation and degenerative changes of this joint can be symptomatic and are seen to excellent advantage with coronal CT (202).

When CT demonstrates high attenuation in the joint, the differential considerations include calcification and iron deposition due to pigmented villonodular synovitis (PVNS), hemophilia or other recurrent hemarthroses. While PVNS is usually high attenuation, in the 100 to 120 HU range (236), it may be lower in attenuation than normal muscle. In PVNS, CT is best utilized to assess the degree of bone erosion and cyst formation prior to surgical treatment with synovectomy or total joint replacement (25). A monoarticular process, PVNS is much less common in the ankle than in the knee, where 80% of cases occur. In the foot and ankle region this pathologic entity may take the localized, extra-articular form of giant cell tumor of tendon sheath, also known as nodular tenosynovitis (8).

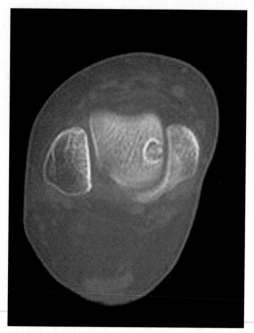
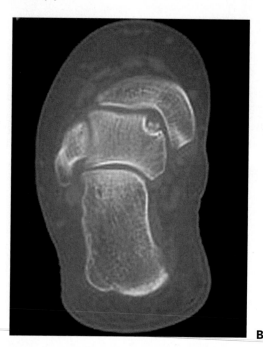

A   B

Figure 22-168 Osteochondral defect (OCD) of the talar dome. **A:** Axial and (**B**) coronal images demonstrate the osteochondral fragment still within a defect of the medial talar dome. Integrity of the overlying cartilage is not assessed, however. (Case is courtesy of Dr. Gina Cho, UT Southwestern Department of Radiology, Dallas, TX.)

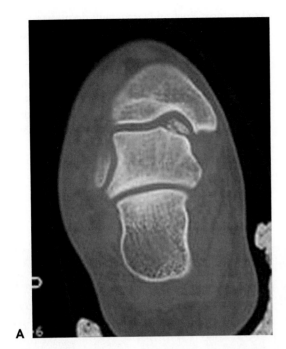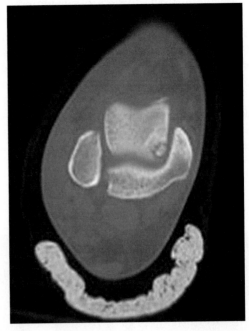

A   B

Figure 22-169   OCD of talar dome. **A:** Coronal and **(B)** axial images demonstrate a large, nondisplaced osseous fragment within the osteochondral defect of the medial talar dome.

NEOPLASMS

The accurate delineation of the extent and staging of musculoskeletal neoplasms of bones and soft tissues is critical for preoperative planning if limb-salvage surgery and neoadjuvant therapy is to be successfully performed. Cross-sectional imaging can establish the location of the origin of the tumor (e.g., bone versus soft tissue) as well as the involvement of adjacent neurovascular structures and joints. MRI has been felt by many to be superior to CT in these assessments because of its improved multiplanar imaging capacities, and increased soft-tissue contrast (1,16,43,63, 208). However, it is worthwhile to note that in a large multi-institutional study comparing contrast-enhanced CT and MR for local staging of primary malignant bone and soft tissue tumors, both modalities were equally accurate in determining degree of tumor involvement of muscle, bone, joints and neurovascular structures (198).

Bone

Even in 2003 at the time of this writing, conventional radiography remains the most useful technique for the diagnosis of osseous lesions. Observations that can be made with

the radiographs include an estimation of aggresivity of the lesion by examining the lesion's margins or zone of transition with the surrounding bone, determining the presence and the type of any associated periosteal reaction. The radiograph will also localize the area of bone affected (intramedullary, cortical) (diaphyseal, metaphyseal, epiphyseal) that, along with knowledge of the patient's age, will help narrow the differential diagnosis. MRI is utilized predominantly to assess tumor extent, and to better evaluate for the presence of any associated soft tissue mass. In our practice, we routinely utilize CT without contrast to better evaluate for the presence and characterization of intralesional mineralized matrix in bone lesions. We prefer it for the evaluation of cortical integrity, although the MR may be able to detect cortical bone destruction as well as CT (54). Thin collimation with reconstruction with bone algorithm will yield improved spatial resolution critical in the assessment for matrix mineralization and endosteal encroachment.

CT can be very helpful in the characterization of intramedullary cartilaginous lesions, especially when they occur in the pelvis or other areas with complex anatomy difficult to evaluate with radiographs. Enchondral ossification as seen with cartilaginous tumors may be identified when central calcifications in a pattern of superimposed rings and arcs are seen.

Enchondromas are composed primarily of dysplastic, hyaline cartilage and usually reside centrally within the intramedullary metaphysis of bones (28). Enchondromas are very common in all age groups, but it may be difficult to differentiate them from bone marrow infarcts radiographically. CT can help in evaluating the pattern of the mineralized matrix. Enchondromas will demonstrate ring and arc-like calcifications of punctuate nodules and a lobulated margin as opposed to the peripheral marginal serpinginous calcification of marrow infarcts (Fig. 22-170). On MRI, they will show increased T2 signal and their lobulated margins may be better depicted, although gradient echo sequences may be needed to improve the visualization of the calcifications (Fig. 22-171). Differentiation between enchondromas

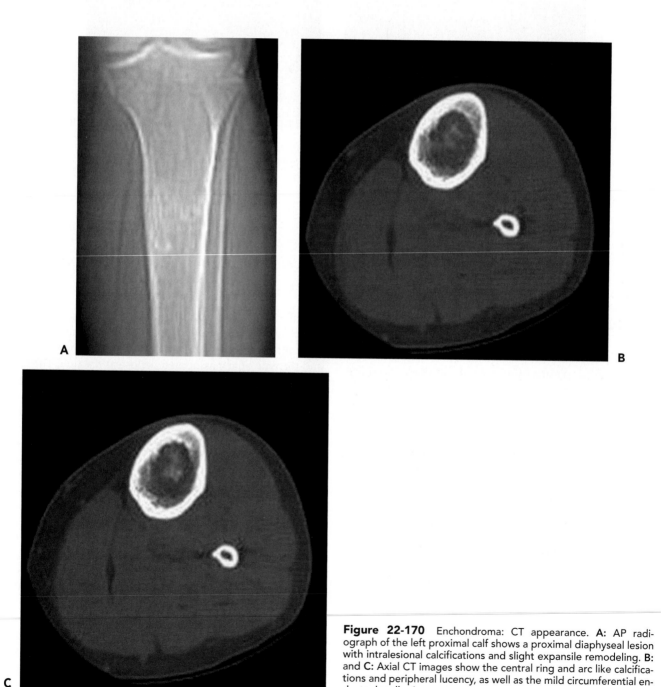

Figure 22-170 Enchondroma: CT appearance. **A:** AP radiograph of the left proximal calf shows a proximal diaphyseal lesion with intralesional calcifications and slight expansile remodeling. **B:** and **C:** Axial CT images show the central ring and arc like calcifications and peripheral lucency, as well as the mild circumferential endosteal scalloping.

and low-grade chondrosarcomas is very difficult histologically, and not infrequently the pathologist will need the MSK imager's input. On CT, enchondromas tend to have evenly distributed central calcifications and usually do not show focal areas of more lysis or endosteal scalloping greater than two thirds of the cortical width. On MR, enchondromas may have normal marrow fat between the dysplastic cartilage nodules and the fibrous septa tend not to enhance (58) (Figs. 22-172 and 22-173). However, the most important differentiating characteristic between these entities continues to be the clinical presentation of pain associated with the malignant lesions. Higher-grade chondrosarcomas are usually easily recognized on radiography, although CT or MR can better demonstrate the areas of lytic destruction, cortical scalloping or thickening and adjacent soft tissue mass (Fig. 22-174).

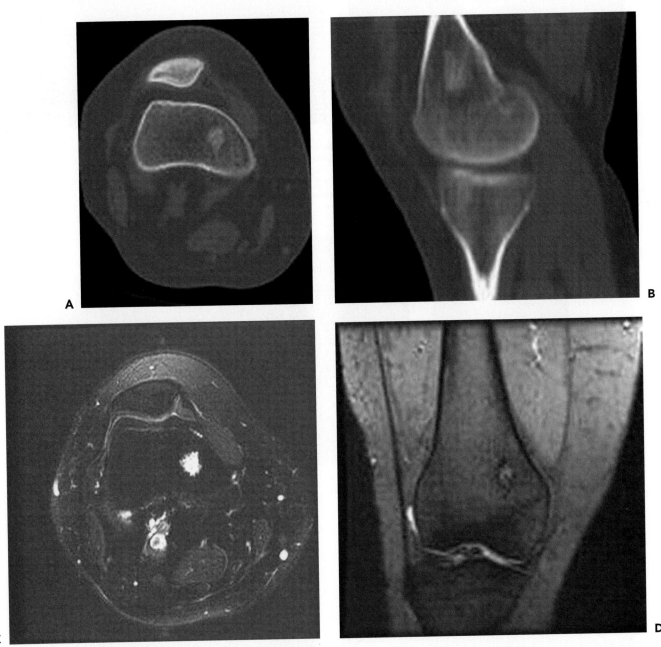

Figure 22-171 Enchondromas: CT and MR appearance. **A:** Axial and (**B**) sagittal reformatted CT image through the distal femoral metaphysis shows medial intramedullary lesion with central calcifications in arc and rings pattern. **C:** Axial T2-weighted fat suppressed fast spin echo image shows the high-signal intensity lesion with lobulated margins and internal septations. **D:** Coronal gradient recalled echo T2*-weighted image shows the intralesional calcifications better than the T2-weighted image, but not as well as CT.

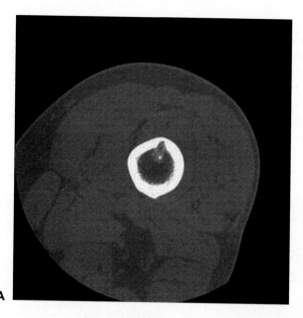

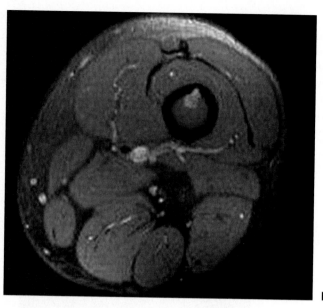

Figure 22-172 Low-grade chondrosarcoma femoral diaphysis. **A:** Axial CT shows an eccentric intramedullary lesion in the femoral shaft with intralesional calcification suggesting cartilaginous matrix and focal endosteal scalloping greater than two thirds of the cortical width. This patient had pain referable to this region. **B:** Axial T1-weighted fat-suppressed spin echo image after fat suppression and gadolinium administration shows similar findings as well as enhancement.

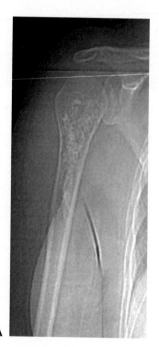

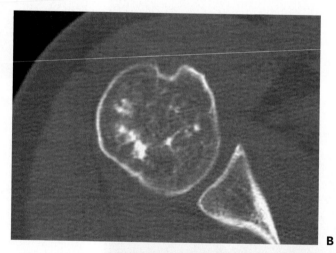

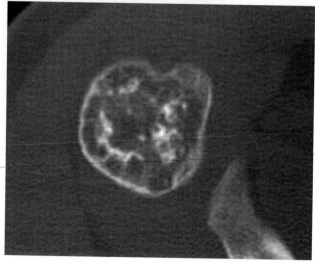

Figure 22-173 Low-grade chondrosarcoma proximal humerus. **A:** AP radiograph shows a long intramedullary lesion with cartilaginous-type intralesional matrix. The patient was having increasing pain. **B** and **C:** Axial CT images through the humeral head show that the calcification pattern is unevenly distributed and there is significant endosteal scalloping but no fracture to explain the increased pain. (*continued*)

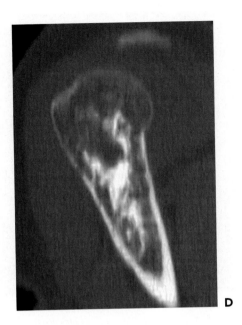
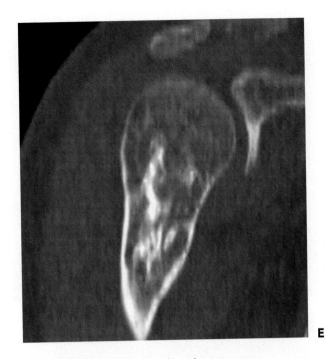

Figure 22-173 *(continued)* **D:** Sagittal and **(E)** coronal reformatted images show the most proximal area of the lesion is relatively radiolucent with respect to the central calcification pattern of the rest of the lesion.

Osteochondromas can be hard to identify when they are sessile or when occurring in areas of overlapping complex anatomical structures like the pelvis or spine. CT will show the continuity of the exostoses' marrow and cortex from the underlying bone and its thin cartilage cap (124) (Fig. 22-175). Pain may be secondary to compression or entrapment of adjacent structures, formation of an adventitial bursa or malignant degeneration, the latter especially of concern in the patient with multiple hereditary exostoses. When there is concern for potential malignant dedifferentiation, the thickness of the overlying cartilage cap in skeletally mature patients is used as an indicator of possible chondrosarcomatous transformation and can be better quantified and separated from overlying bursas by utilizing MRI with cartilage-sensitive gradient echo pulse sequences (Fig. 22-176), although CT can also be used to measure this area (187). A cartilaginous cap greater than 1.5 cm in thickness in an adult is worrisome for malignant transformation (231).

Chondroblastomas are usually well characterized by radiography as well-demarcated lytic lesions in the epiphyses of the skeletally immature. CT may help in identifying an intralesional chondroid calcification pattern that may increase the confidence in this diagnosis, although this may only be seen in about one third of cases (17, 220) (Fig. 22-177). CT can also be helpful in assessing the relationship to the articular surface of these typically epiphyseal lesions, although MRI may be better for depiction of articular invasion. A similar reasoning can be applied to giant cell tumors of bone to evaluate for direct extension into the articular surface (Fig. 22-178). CT can be helpful in identifying other less common cartilaginous lesions like chondromyxoid fibromas. These eccentric intramedullary lesions with lobulated margins and endosteal sclerosis most commonly seen in the proximal tibial metaphysis usually do not show calcification on radiographs but may show it on CT in a minority of cases. The outer cortical margin may be appreciated only on MR or CT (231,309).

CT of unicameral bone cysts will show remodeled bone expansion with thin cortices and fluid-like attenuation, with thin bony septae (Fig. 22-179). CT may be helpful in identifying a "fallen fragment" sign, which is highly suggestive of this diagnosis (164). Fluid–fluid levels on CT, as

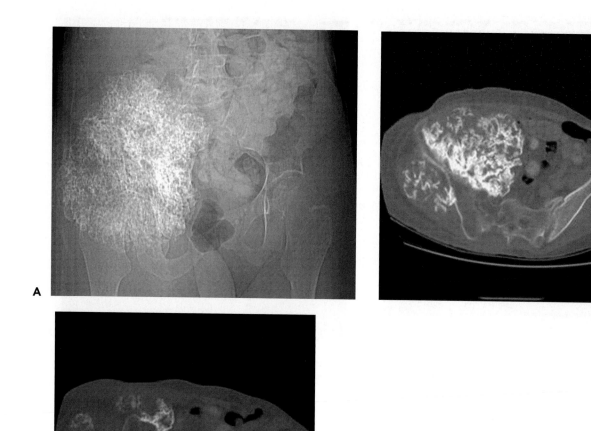

Figure 22-174   Conventional chondrosarcoma pelvis. **A:** AP radiograph shows the large soft tissue mass with cartilaginous-type calcification/ossification. **B** and **C:** Axial CT images again demonstrate the circumferential mass, as well as the radiolucent replaced marrow of the underlying hemipelvis.

on MRI, are typical although not pathognomonic of aneurysmal bone cysts. They have been reported in other tumors including unicameral bone cysts, giant cell tumors and telangiectatic osteosarcomas (35). This CT feature is seen in 80% to 90% of late stage aneurysmal bone cysts (186) (Fig. 22-178 and 22-180).

Although CT is usually not necessary for the assessment of benign fibrous lesions of bone like fibrous dyplasia and fibroxanthomas (nonossifying fibromas), these lesions are not uncommonly seen incidentally in scans obtained for other reasons (e.g., trauma) and should be accurately recognized. Fibrous dyplasia usually have sclerotic margins and may have a matrix of uniform density (Fig. 22-181). Although usually associated with cortical thinning and

bone expansion, CT can reveal areas of cortical breakthrough occasionally that are not appreciated on radiographic views (311).

CT is particularly helpful in the diagnosis of osteoid osteoma. Because of the surrounding reactive sclerosis, the typical small nidus (which may have a central calcification within it) may not be identified on the radiographs but will be evident with thin collimation CT (6) (Fig. 22-182). The use of dynamic contrast-enhanced CT or MRI may help differentiate osteoid osteoma from a focus of osteomyelitis, with the former having a pattern of prominent peak enhancement in the arterial phase, and early washout (149,168).

(*text continues on page 1622*)

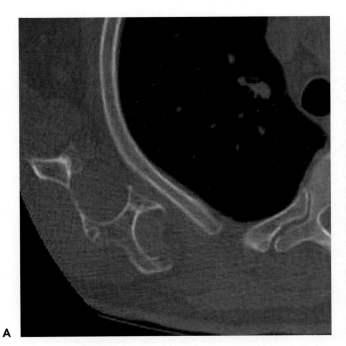
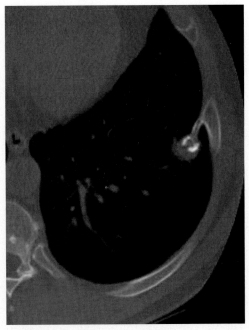

A
B

Figure 22-175 Osteochondromas: chest. **A:** Axial CT of the right chest shows a large osteochondroma projecting anteriorly from the scapular body. Note marrow continuity into the bony excrescence. A cartilage cap is not well seen. The patient noticed a popping sensation with scapulothoracic motion. **B:** Axial CT of the left chest in the same patient shows a pedunculated osteochondroma projecting into the left lower lung. A cartilaginous cap is noted.

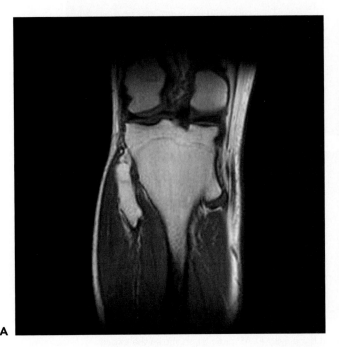
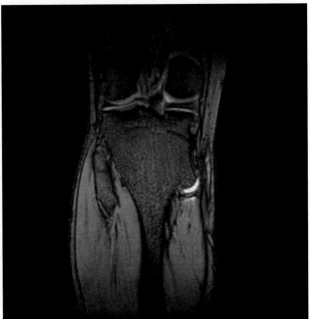

A
B

Figure 22-176 Osteochondroma: MR. **A:** Coronal T1-weighted MR image shows a medial tibial diaphysis osteochondroma. **B:** Coronal gradient recalled echo T2*-weighted image shows the cartilage cap best. The patient was complaining of pain over this area and neoplastic dedifferentiation was a clinical concern but the cartilage cap measured less than 1 cm in thickness.

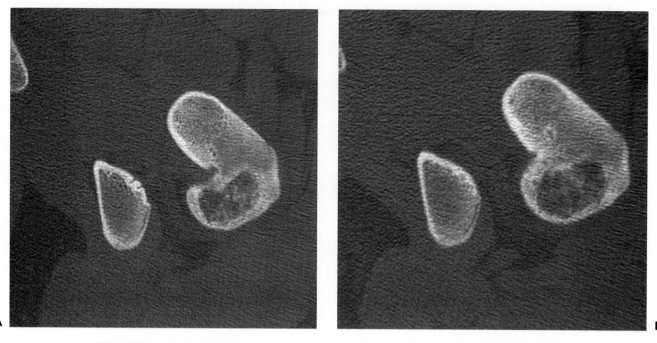

Figure 22-177 Chondroblastoma. **A** and **B:** Axial CT images of the left hip greater trochanter in a skeletally immature person. A lesion with well-demarcated sclerotic margins and chondroid-type calcification has caused expansile remodeling of the trochanter. The location of this tumor in this age group is very suggestive of chondroblastoma. The trochanteric apophyses are epiphyseal equivalents.

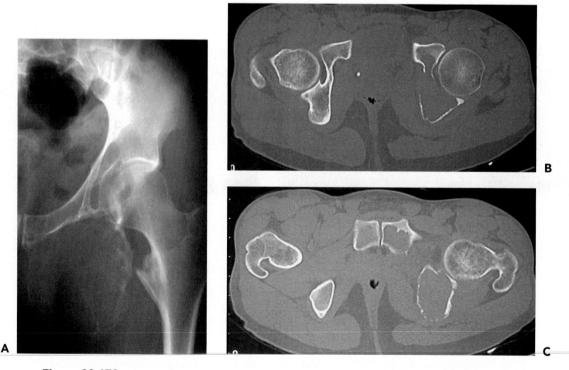

Figure 22-178 Giant cell tumor with aneurysmal bone cyst. **A:** AP radiograph shows the expansile lytic lesion of the left ischium but the most cephalad component of the lesion is not as well appreciated. **B** and **C:** Axial sequential CT images demonstrate a lesion abutting the articular surface with geographic borders, pathologic fracture of the medial acetabular wall (quadrilateral plate) and no mineralized intralesional content.

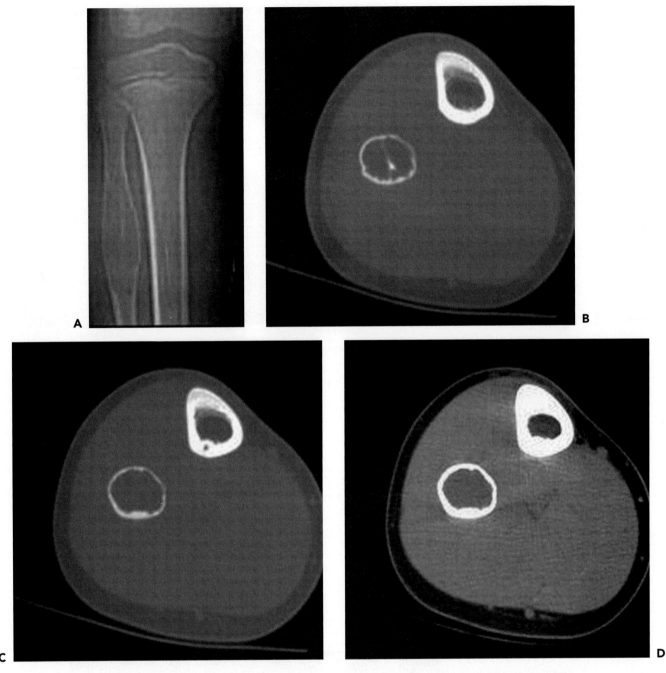

Figure 22-179 Unicameral bone cyst. A: AP radiograph shows the expansile lytic lesion of the proximal fibula. B and C: Axial CT images viewed in bone window settings show a thin bony septa traversing the lesion (B) and no intralesional matrix, periosteal reaction or fracture seen. D: Same image as (C) but viewed in soft tissue windows shows replacement of normal marrow by fluid attenuation.

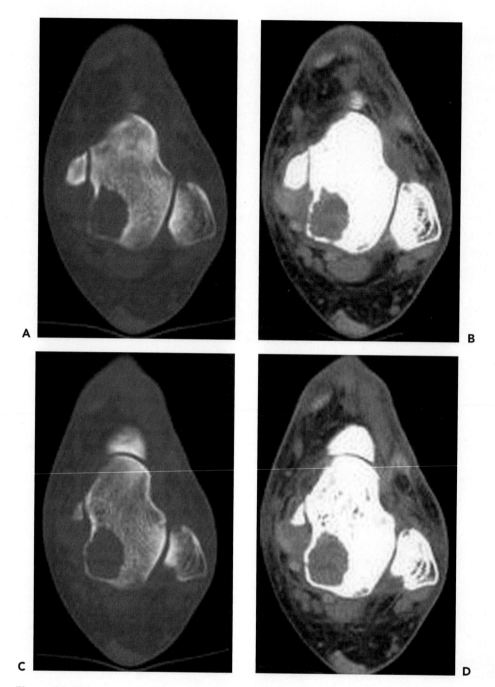

A   B   C   D

Figure 22-180   Aneurysmal bone cyst: fluid-fluid levels. Axial sequential CT images of the proximal talar body seen in bone (**A** and **C**) and soft tissue (**B** and **D**) window settings show a well-demarcated lytic lesion of the posterior talus with marked thinning of the overlying cortex. The soft tissue windows and levels demonstrated several fluid-fluid levels (*arrows*).

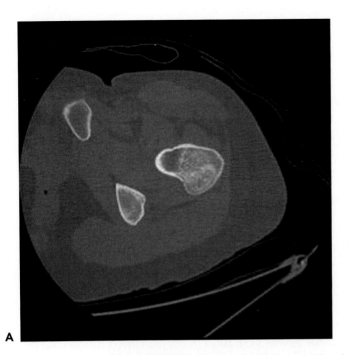

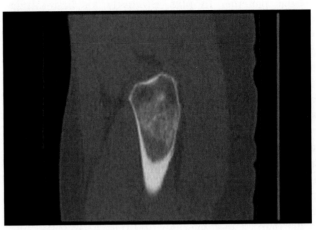

A   B

Figure 22-181   Fibrous dysplasia. **A:** Axial and **(B)** sagittal reformatted CT images of an incidentally discovered asymptomatic lesion of the left proximal hip shaft. Note the subtle expansile remodeling and the uniform density of the faintly sclerotic matrix.

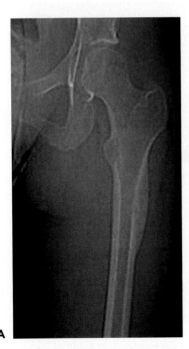

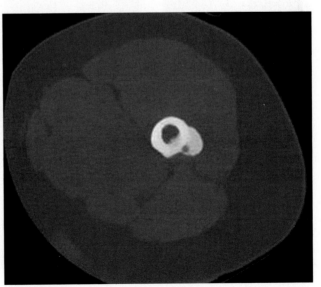

A   B

Figure 22-182   Osteoid osteoma. **A:** AP radiograph of the left femur shows lateral cortical thickening but no nidus is identified. Differential diagnosis would include stress fracture and infection. **B:** Axial CT image demonstrates the small lucent nidus (*arrow*) of the osteoid osteoma adjacent to the cortex and surrounded by reactive sclerosis.

CT may be useful in the evaluation of malignant osseous lesions like osteosarcoma. CT is invaluable in the occasions when radiographs fail to definitely characterize if new bone formation is predominantly reactive or neoplastic. Neoplastic bone is markedly dense and disorganized, whereas reactive bone formation tends to follow trabecular patterns. To plan effectively for limb-salvage surgery and adjuvant radiation, it is important to delineate the tumor as effectively as possible, and maximize the amount of tissue spared. In osteosarcoma, it is important to evaluate the entire length of the affected bone for the presence of skip metastases. CT can evaluate these concerns if performed with thin collimation. As in most osseous neoplasms with a soft tissue component, the administration of intravenous contrast improves tumor margin determination of any associated soft tissue mass and its relationships to any adjacent neurovascular structures (250). However, in our practice, MRI is routinely performed in the staging of these tumors as it may delineate the longitudinal marrow extent and soft tissue mass better than CT in some cases (21) (Fig. 22-183). Because of the sensitivity of MRI to marrow infiltration by tumor, it is also our preferred modality in the evaluation of osseous small cell neoplasms like lymphoma, leukemia and Ewing's sarcoma, as well as in the evaluation of suspected multiple myeloma or osseous metastases when radiographs and radionucleide bone scans are negative (52) (Fig. 22-184). However, PET imaging may be more helpful in assessing the activity of disease and early body marrow infiltration in diffuse processes like myeloma (117) (Fig. 22-185).

Soft Tissues

MRI is the modality of choice for evaluating soft tissue tumors because of its increased soft tissue contrast (1,63,206,277,298). The location and size of the tumor and the age of the patient may be used to great advantage in the differential diagnosis of soft tissue masses (128,129). Most benign soft tissue masses are under 5 cm in length and superficial to the muscular fascia (132). However, most reported series have shown that imaging cannot reliably differentiate benign from malignant soft tissue masses (131,206,274,281). A correct histological diagnosis can be achieved by MR imaging in only 25% to 35% of cases (11,50).

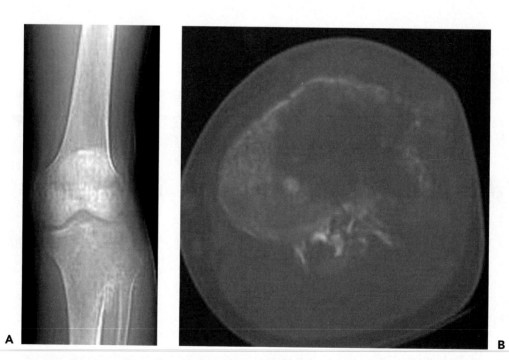

A   B

Figure 22-183   Osteosarcoma. **A:** AP radiograph demonstrates a permeative destruction of the lateral proximal tibia as well as mineralized content suggesting tumor new bone formation. **B:** Axial CT image in bone window settings of the proximal tibial plateau shows marked lytic destruction of the intramedullary lesion and irregular ossification within the intramedullary lesion as well as in its soft tissue extensions. (*continued*)

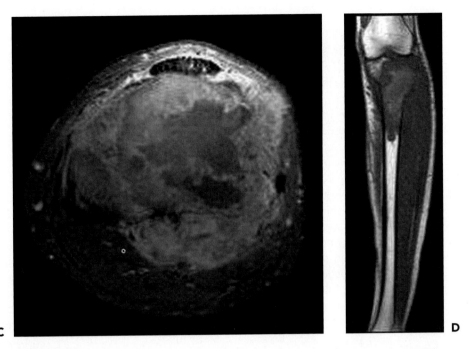

C

D

Figure 22-183. (*continued*) **C:** Axial T1-weighted fat-suppressed MR image after gadolinium administration at the same level as the prior CT image shows the enhancing circumferential soft tissue component best. **D:** Coronal T1-weighted spin echo image was obtained with a larger field of view to determine longitudinal extent of marrow involvement and exclude skip metastases. The marked involvement of the articular surface is well seen on this image as well.

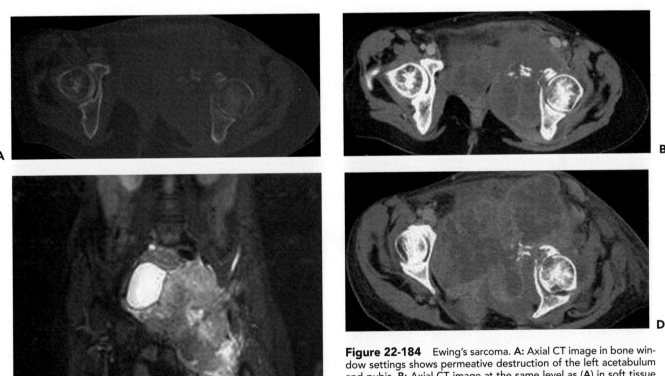

A

B

C

D

Figure 22-184 Ewing's sarcoma. **A:** Axial CT image in bone window settings shows permeative destruction of the left acetabulum and pubis. **B:** Axial CT image at the same level as (**A**) in soft tissue windows after the administration of intravenous contrast shows the large soft tissue component characteristic of Ewing's sarcoma displacing the femoral neurovascular bundle anteriorly. **C:** Coronal T2-weighted STIR MR image shows the cephalolcaudal extent of the mass displacing the bladder cephalad. **D:** Axial CT image with contrast after chemotherapy shows some tumor response with more central low-attenuation suggesting necrosis; however, the size of the mass had increased.

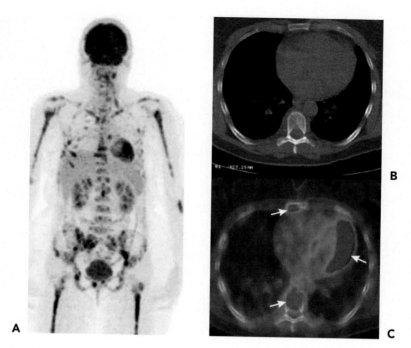

Figure 22-185 Multiple myeloma. **A:** Coronal PET composite image shows whole body marrow burden with numerous foci of tracer uptake in the axial and appendicular skeleton. **B:** Axial CT through the chest and (**C**) CT-PET fusion image through the chest demonstrate areas of active disease in the vertebra and sternum that are not appreciated on the CT. Uptake in the left myocardium is physiologic.

CT is a useful adjunct when radiographs do not adequately characterize the mineralized lesional content or osseous involvement, especially in areas of complex osseous anatomy like the pelvis or shoulder (132). The use of 3D reconstructions of helical CT in soft tissue tumors of the extremities may help preoperative planning (310) (Fig. 22-186). The use of contrast enhancement may be very helpful in increasing lesion conspicuity and margin delineation with CT (Figs. 22-187 and 22-188). As with MRI, CT is most helpful in localizing and staging the lesion, although imaging may suggest histology in some diagnoses. Certain lesions like fibromatosis may have increased attenuation on noncontrast exams due to densely packed fibrous collagen, although this appearance is nonspecific and may be seen with tumors have densely packed cells

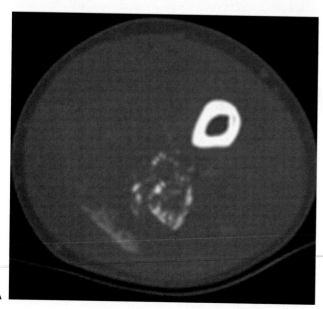

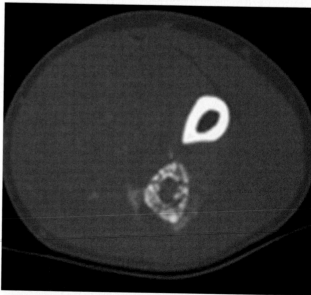

Figure 22-186 Pathologic fracture right ulna shaft from colorectal cancer metastases. **A and B:** Axial CT images in bone window settings demonstrate the permeative destruction of the cortex.

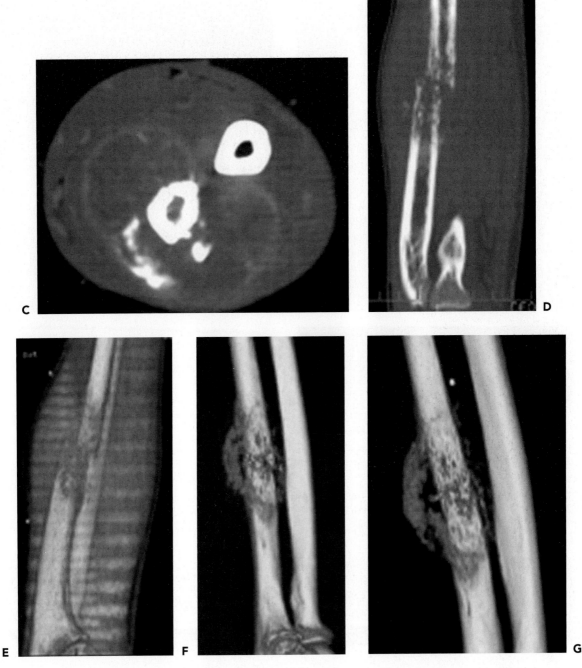

Figure 22-186 (*continued*) C: Axial CT with soft tissue windows shows the associated soft tissue mass and hematoma. D: Sagittal reformatted image shows the transverse fracture best. E: Volume-rendered 3D image shows the soft tissue swelling at the site of the fracture. F: Volume-rendered 3D image with opacities set to delineate bone detail show the permeative destruction and soft tissue calcifications. G: Magnified view of (F) shows similar findings.

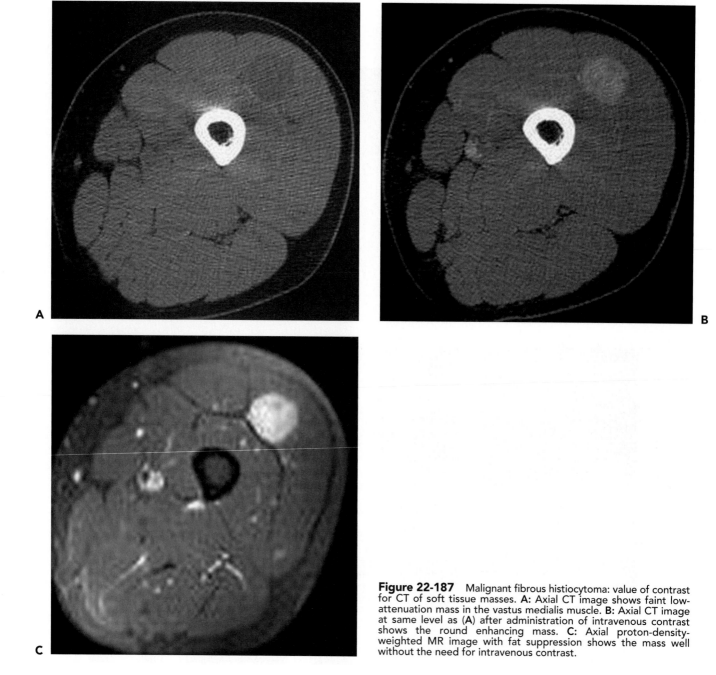

Figure 22-187 Malignant fibrous histiocytoma: value of contrast for CT of soft tissue masses. **A:** Axial CT image shows faint low-attenuation mass in the vastus medialis muscle. **B:** Axial CT image at same level as (**A**) after administration of intravenous contrast shows the round enhancing mass. **C:** Axial proton-density-weighted MR image with fat suppression shows the mass well without the need for intravenous contrast.

with a high nucleus-to-cytoplasm ratio like primitive neuroectodermal tumors (85,232) (Fig. 22-189). Vascular lesions like hemangiomas may be diagnosed when an infiltrating or lobulated soft tissue mass containing phleboliths is identified (188) (Fig. 22-190). Aneurysms and pseudoaneursyms may also be diagnosed with improved confidence after contrast enhancement.

CT is the preferred modality when assessing a soft tissue mass when there is a history of antecedent trauma as it may represent heterotopic ossification. The aggressive appearance of immature heterotopic ossification on MR imaging during the acute and subacute inflammatory phases may mislead the imager (138). CT may be able to visualize the peripheral or zonal pattern of maturity of ossification

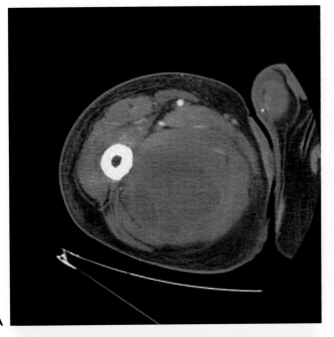

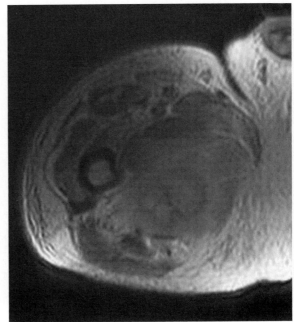

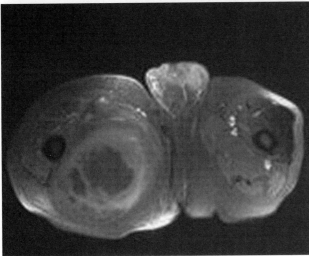

Figure 22-188 Malignant fibrous histiocytoma: margins with CT and MR. **A:** Axial CT image through the proximal right thigh after the administration of intravenous contrast shows the mass with areas of low attenuation consistent with necrosis. The mass is displacing posteriorly the inferior gluteus maximus and is arising from the adductor muscle groups. **B:** Axial proton-density-weighted MR image at a slightly cephalad level shows similar findings. **C:** Axial T1-weighted fat suppressed MR image shows the central area of necrosis, as well as a clear depiction of the enhancing margins of the mass.

within the mass. This may obviate a needle biopsy; a closed biopsy in this situation is to be avoided as areas of the mass may be sampled that could be potentially interpreted as a malignant osteoid-producing tumor. As in bone lesions, when a soft tissue mass has mineralized intratumoral matrix that cannot be adequately characterized as chondroid, ossific or dystrophic type calcification, CT may be able to

help in this differentiation. For example, nonspecific dystrophic calcifications in a soft tissue mass in the extremity of a young adult would be suggestive of a synovial sarcoma, although not diagnostic as other masses like superficial fibromas could have similar calcifications (132).

The location of a soft tissue mass, along with analysis of its morphology, can sometimes suggest the correct diagnosis.

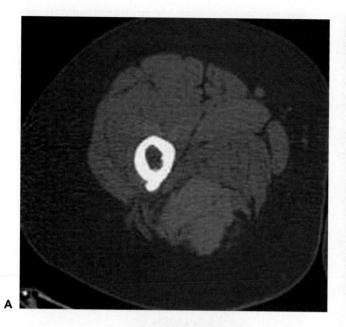

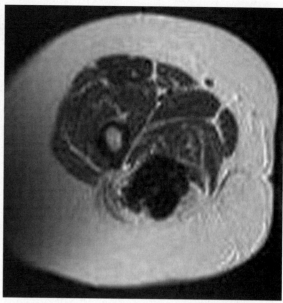

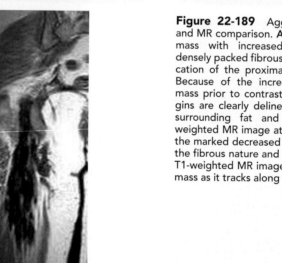

Figure 22-189 Aggressive fibromatosis: CT and MR comparison. **A:** Axial CT image shows a mass with increased attenuation from the densely packed fibrous tissue in the expected location of the proximal biceps femoris muscle. Because of the increased attenuation of the mass prior to contrast administration, the margins are clearly delineated with respect to the surrounding fat and muscles. **B:** Axial T1-weighted MR image at the same location shows the marked decreased signal in the mass due to the fibrous nature and low cellularity. **C:** Coronal T1-weighted MR image shows the length of the mass as it tracks along the biceps femoris plane.

Nerve sheath tumors will occur in continuity with a peripheral nerve and may show a target sign, with central concentric rings of increased attenuation on noncontrast exams (189) (Fig. 22-191). Elastofibromas will appear as homogeneous low-attenuation masses in a periscapular location and may be seen in the chest CT of asymptomatic patients (24). The location of a soft tissue mass with chondroid-type calcified matrix within a joint or a synovial bursa will suggest synovial chondromatosis (Fig. 22-192). If a soft tissue mass is located within a tendon sheath, giant cell tumor of tendon sheath is the primary consideration. A mass that appears to be a simple cyst, with homogeneous low attenuation and thin nonenhancing walls, in close proximity and apparent connection to a joint will

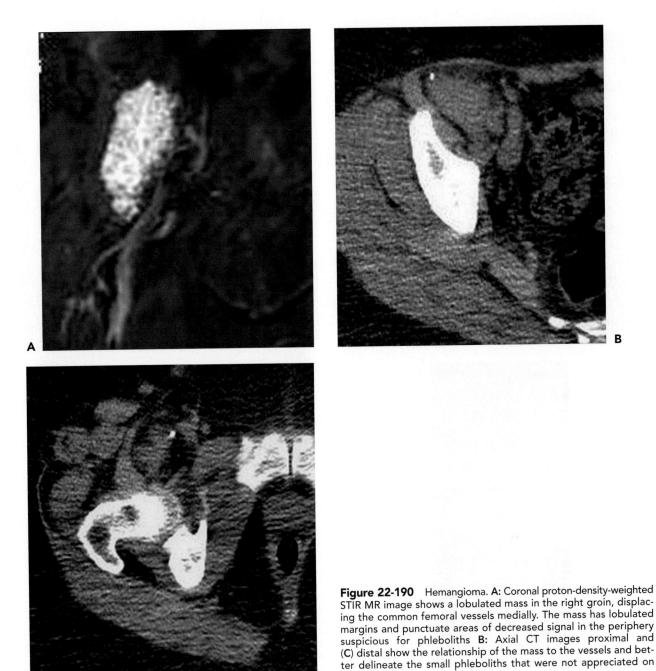

Figure 22-190   Hemangioma. **A:** Coronal proton-density-weighted STIR MR image shows a lobulated mass in the right groin, displacing the common femoral vessels medially. The mass has lobulated margins and punctuate areas of decreased signal in the periphery suspicious for phleboliths **B:** Axial CT images proximal and **(C)** distal show the relationship of the mass to the vessels and better delineate the small phleboliths that were not appreciated on the radiograph.

represent a synovial or ganglion cyst. A fat-containing tumor of homogenous attenuation occurring in the subcutaneous fat layer of the body, superficial to the muscular fascia, will most certainly be a simple lipoma, given the much higher incidence of benign soft tissue masses in this location than malignant tumors (185).

When a predominantly fat-containing tumor is detected, the differential is lipoma, atypical lipoma (the preferred term over well-differentiated liposarcoma when occurring outside the retroperitoneum, reflecting better prognosis) and liposarcoma. It is desirable to utilize

(*text continues on page 1633*)

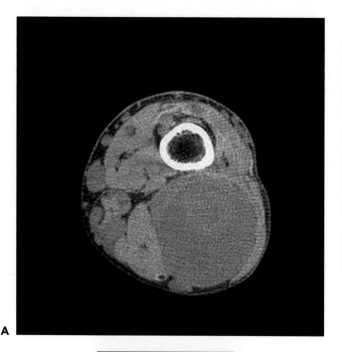

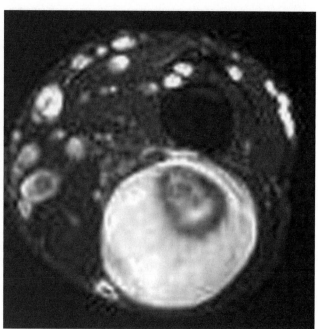

Figure 22-191   Neurofibromatosis. **A:** Axial CT image through the distal left thigh show numerous low attenuation soft tissue masses, with the largest one showing concentric central rings of increased attenuation felt to represent a target sign. **B:** Axial T2-weighted MR image at the same location shows similar findings, with target signs evident in several of the small masses as well. **C:** Coronal T1-weighted MR image shows the fusiform shape of the largest mass, delineated from the surrounding muscles by a thin layer of fat known by the term "fat stripe sign."

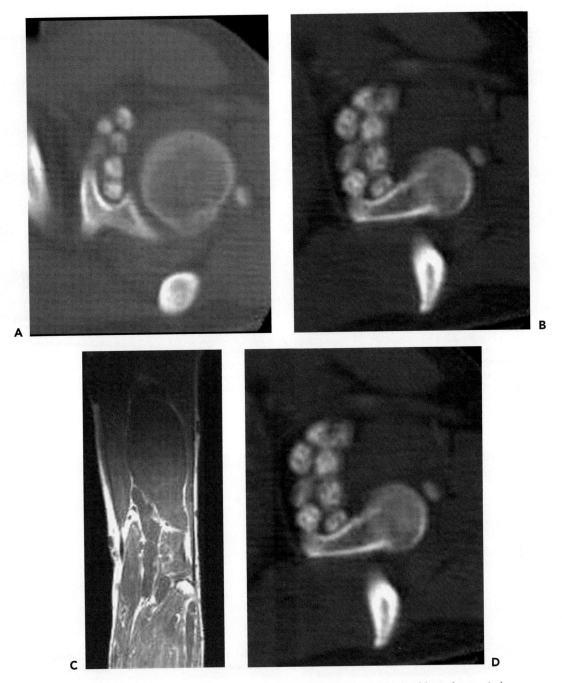

Figure 22-192 Synovial ostochondromatosis. **A:** Axial CT of the left shoulder in bone window settings shows several well-delineated osteochondral bodies adjacent to the coracoid process. **B:** Axial CT image slightly more with more contrasted windows shows the faceted appearance of these osteochondral bodies within the subcoracoid recess. **C:** Sagittal reformatted images and (**D**) coronal reformatted image shows the relationships of these clustered osteochondral bodies in the subcoracoid recess of the joint, as well as in the biceps tendon sheath.

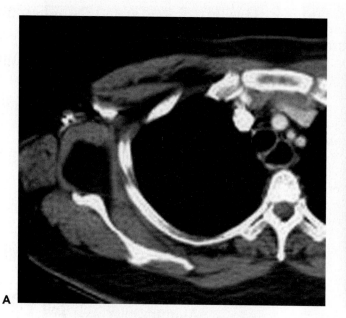
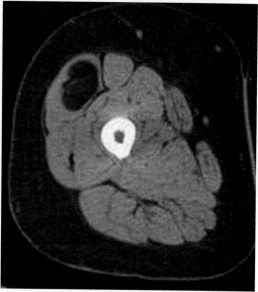

Figure 22-193   Lipomas: CT appearance. **A:** Axial CT image of the chest after intravenous contrast shows a nonenhancing mass of homogenous fat attenuation and well-demarcated margins arising within the right subscapularis muscle. Although contiguous to the scapula, no bone involvement can be identified. **B:** Axial CT image through the proximal thigh shows a similar mass in the right vastus lateralis muscle. A small thin septation is noted within it.

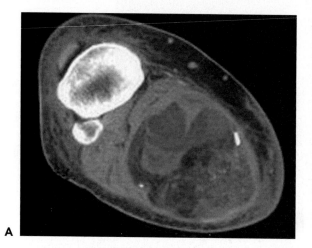
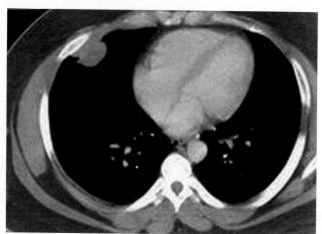

Figure 22-194   Liposarcoma. **A:** Axial CT through the right proximal calf shows a large mass within the posterior compartment with central areas of fat attenuation, as well as areas of more soft tissue attenuation and calcifications intermixed. **B:** Axial CT of the chest shows a pleural-based mass with central decreased attenuation that was liposarcoma metastases in this patient.

imaging features to distinguish between lipoma and atypical lipoma because of the high risk of local recurrence (52%) and somewhat lower risk of malignant degeneration (13%) of the latter tumor type (240). CT features of lipomatous lesions that suggest well-differentiated liposarcoma/atypical lipoma rather than benign lipoma include the presence of thickened septa, nodular or globular areas of soft tissue attenuation or soft tissue masses and higher percentages of soft tissue density components (more than 25% of the lesion) (130) (Figs. 22-193 and 22-194). While CT and MRI can characterize these features, MR is preferred for evaluation of recurrence or malignant dedifferentiation. Dedifferentiation occurs late, so that follow-up for greater than 5 years is recommended (240).

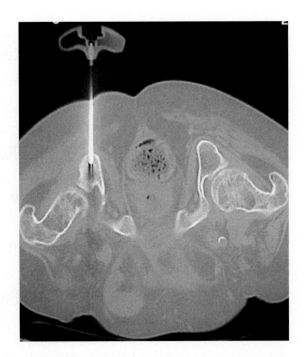

Figure 22-195 CT-guided biopsy of osteomyelitis. Axial image of the lower pelvis with the patient in the prone position. An 11-gauge bone biopsy needle has been advanced into the sclerotic vertical portion of the right ischium to confirm osteomyelitis and provide a sample for culture.

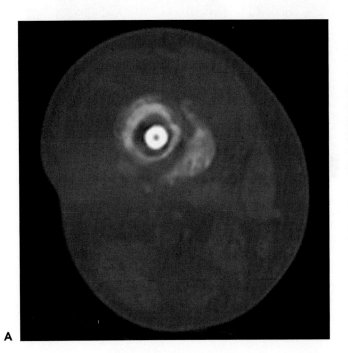

A

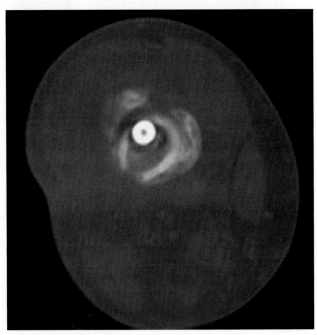

B

Figure 22-196 Nonunion due to infection. A and B: Axial CT images show the fracture as well as the ineffective nonbridging callus and the intramedullary lucency surrounding the retrograde nail.

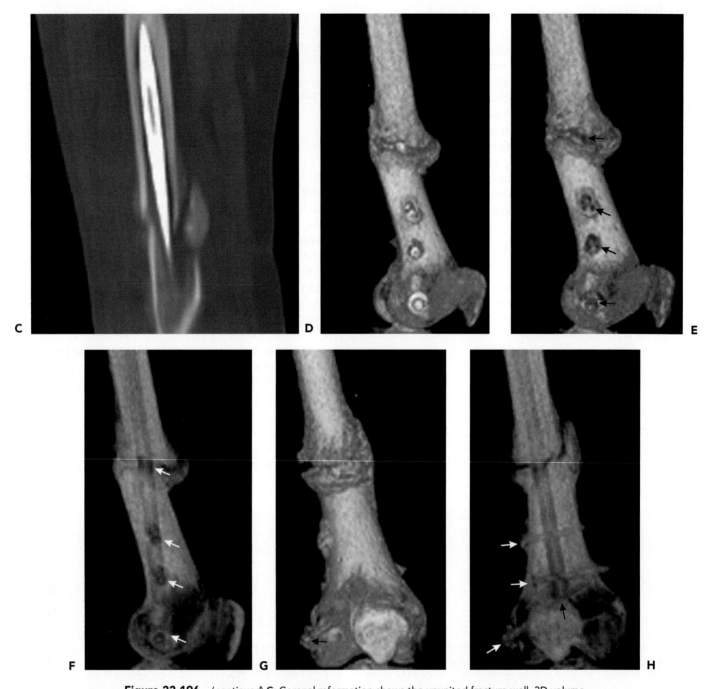

Figure 22-196 (*continued*) **C:** Coronal reformation shows the ununited fracture well. 3D volume-rendered reformations show incredible detail of the ununited fracture and loose hardware. Lateral viewpoint obtained with hardware colored white (**D**) or blue (**E**). Note degree of countersinking of loosened second most distal screw. By varying the transparency of the bone, the hardware position becomes more apparent (**F**). Anterior viewpoint shows similar findings with different degrees of bone opacities (**G** and **H**).

INFECTION AND INFLAMMATION

The infectious conditions of septic arthritis and necrotizing fasciitis represent some of the few true musculoskeletal emergencies because of the need for prompt, aggressive surgical and antimicrobial intervention. CT is less expensive and often more readily available than MRI on an emergent basis. CT can also guide diagnostic or therapeutic aspiration and drainage of suspicious fluid collections. However, MRI with contrast is the preferable method of evaluating most soft tissue infections or inflammatory conditions, if expeditiously available. If CT must be performed instead of MRI, intravenous contrast is strongly recommended (51).

Osteomyelitis

Detection of osteomyelitis while it is still in the early acute stage is critical to improve the probability of cure and decrease morbidity. Because it is less sensitive than MRI for acute osteomyelitis, CT is best reserved for guiding an aspiration or biopsy (Fig. 22-195), if clinically necessary, to confirm osteomyelitis or for culture and antibiotic sensitivity of the organism (245). CT may also be useful in the setting of postoperative infections when extensive orthopedic instrumentation may hamper MRI (Fig. 22-196).

The appearance of osteomyelitis by CT depends on its stage, be it acute, subacute or chronic. In acute osteo-

myelitis, marrow edema is the first imaging finding. Subsequently, periosteal elevation may occur, more commonly in children than in adults, with eventual subperiosteal new bone formation. Subperiosteal abscess may also occur (245). Unenhanced CT is less sensitive than MRI in detecting early periosteal inflammation from osteomyelitis in an animal model (263).

Subacute osteomyelitis is more localized. An example is Brodie's abscess, a pyogenic abscess surrounded by sclerosis and enhancing granulation tissue. Chronic osteomyelitis is characterized by necrotic bone. A focal necrotic bone fragment or sequestrum may be surrounded by granulation tissue or by an involucrum of thick periosteal new bone formation (245). CT shows the sequestrum as an isolated fragment separated from cortical or cancellous bone, free within the medullary cavity or a sinus tract (304). A cloaca or draining defect may be apparent (245). CT of chronic osteomyelitis will typically reveal significant sclerosis, bone deformity and resorption with associated soft tissue scar or granulation tissue (Fig. 22-197). A sinus tract may be demonstrated as a cortical defect leading to a linear soft tissue density in the subcutaneous fat, often with skin defect. Bone or soft tissue abscesses or foreign bodies may also be apparent (Fig. 22-198) (304).

Marrow edema associated with osteomyelitis is best demonstrated with T1 and either T2 fat-suppressed or STIR MR sequences (177), but the extent of osteomyelitis can also be judged, somewhat less accurately, by changes

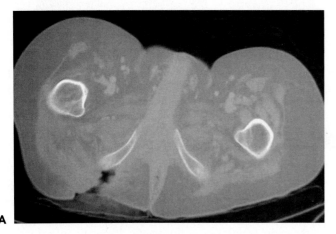
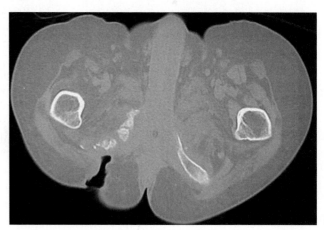

A **B**

Figure 22-197 Chronic osteomyelitis. **A:** Initial CT of a patient with paraplegia demonstrates a deep soft tissue ulcer contacting the intact-appearing right inferior pubic ramus. **B:** Subsequent CT 10 months later. Again demonstrated is the soft tissue ulcer, with interval development of fragmentation, sclerosis and partial resorption of the right inferior pubic ramus.

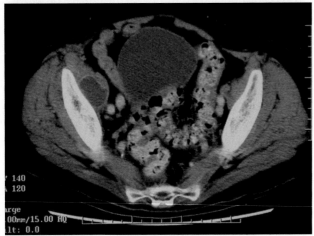

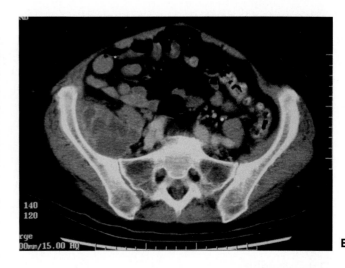

Figure 22-198 Iliacus abscess. **A:** Low attenuation abscess is surrounded by an enhancing rim and contains several enhancing internal septations. **B:** More inferiorly, the abscess is increasingly complex, with thick enhancing walls and septations. Note mass effect on the psoas. **C:** Enhancing rim is apparent next to normal adjacent muscle.

in the CT attenuation of the medullary canal from normal fat to abnormal fluid density. This method is difficult in slender bones such as the fibula, where the marrow space is small. The marrow changes in osteomyelitis are not specific, as they can also be seen in neoplasm, trauma, some anemias, storage diseases and other primary bone marrow disorders such as myelofibrosis. Comparison to the contralateral side may be helpful to see if a marrow-replacing process is systemic or unilateral (133,229).

Gas in the medullary canal is consistent with osteomyelitis but uncommon. It can be seen before the radiographic findings of destruction or new bone formation are apparent. Nontraumatic soft tissue gas is characteristic of infection (224). Fat fluid levels may be seen in the medullary canal or joint in osteomyelitis or septic arthritis, presumably due to fat necrosis (222).

Diabetic neuropathic changes are often indistinguishable from osteomyelitis and septic arthritis by CT. In assessing the diabetic foot for osteomyelitis, an MRI with normal marrow signal has a higher negative predictive value than a normal CT. MR is also more sensitive for

small abscesses and for nonviable soft tissue, especially if gadolinium is given (271). MR can sometimes distinguish between chronic, stable neuropathic osteoarthropathy (when it is low signal on all pulse sequences) and osteomyelitis (162) whereas CT cannot.

Septic Arthritis

Infected joints, bursae and tendon sheaths result in thickened, enhancing synovium, with cellular debris or hemorrhage often seen in the structure. The appearance may mimic an abscess (271). Infectious arthritis can be either pyogenic (septic) or nonpyogenic. Pyogenic infections are most commonly due to *Staphylococcus aureus, Neisseria gonorrhoeae, Klebsiella pneumoniae, Candida albicans,* and *Serratia marcescens.* Nonpyogenic infections include tuberculous arthritis, fungi such as actinomycosis, cryptococcosis, coccidioidomycosis, histoplasmosis, and sporotrichosis, viruses (smallpox) and spirochetes (syphilis, yaws).

The first imaging modality for suspected septic arthritis should be conventional radiography. Arthrography is use-

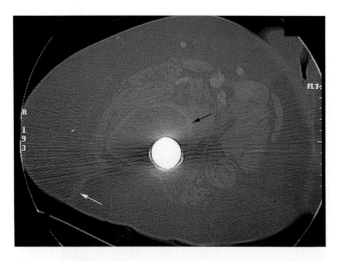

Figure 22-199 Infected hip prosthesis. Low-attenuation fluid with enhancing rim (*black arrow*) surrounds the revision type femoral stem of a total hip arthroplasty. The surrounding femoral shaft has been almost entirely resorbed by osteolysis. Fistulous tract (*white arrow*) extends posterolaterally through the subcutaneous fat.

ful only in conjunction with imaging-guided diagnostic aspiration of the joint. Ultrasound is sensitive for fluid but not specific for infection. It can also be useful for guiding joint aspiration. Likewise, CT is more useful for guidance of joint aspiration than for evaluation of infectious arthritis. CT is particularly helpful in the diagnostic aspiration of fluid around infected components of prosthetic joints (Fig. 22-199).

CT findings of early infectious arthritis are nonspecific, including synovial thickening, fluid in the joint and erosions. Gas in the joint is also nonspecific. Small bubbles may be seen with gas-forming organisms but gas from vacuum phenomenon can also be seen following a traumatic dislocation in adults or nontraumatic traction on the joints of children, effectively excluding a septic arthritis when present. MRI is much more specific for septic arthritis than CT (104). CT is more sensitive for joint effusion and bursal fluid than plain films (228). MR is more sensitive than either CT or ultrasound for detection of fluid in complex anatomic sites such as the iliopsoas bursa (307).

Osteoarticular TB occurs in less than 5% of patients with TB, and diagnosis is often delayed in the United States due to a decline in frequency and physician awareness. Worldwide, however, TB continues to infect 1.9 billion people and risks resurgence in the United States due to immigration and HIV co-infection. Infectious arthritis from TB is usually monostotic and is classically seen in large weight-bearing joints but may be peripheral in children and the elderly. Findings include soft tissue swelling and regional osteopenia, often severe. Marginal erosions follow. Cartilage loss is a late finding because of the lack of proteolytic enzymes. Osseous fusion is rare. Tuberculous osteomyelitis is presumed to result from hematogenous spread (178).

Cellulitis, Myositis, Fascitis, Abscess

Cellulitis is characterized on CT by thickening of the skin and underlying fascia, edema outlining fat lobules and variable degrees of enhancement (Fig. 22-200) (271).

Pyomyositis is a tropical disease uncommon in temperate climates, although it is becoming more frequent due to HIV infection. Multiple abscesses are often present in this condition, an otherwise uncommon finding. MR is more sensitive and should be the imaging modality of choice if pyomyositis is suspected (271). CT findings of pyomyositis include muscle enlargement with low attenuation, heterogeneity, focal fluid collections and rim enhancement (Fig. 22-201). Most have associated cellulitis (101).

Necrotizing fasciitis may demonstrate gas formation in the presence of irregular fascial thickening. MRI is especially superior to CT for this disorder as iodinated IV contrast may be contraindicated due to hypotension (271). CT findings of early necrotizing fasciitis include asymmetric thickening of fascia and strandy fluid density changes in fat, similar to cellulitis. Necrotizing fasciitis tends to spare the epidermis, a finding atypical for cellulitis. Later complications of myonecrosis and abscess

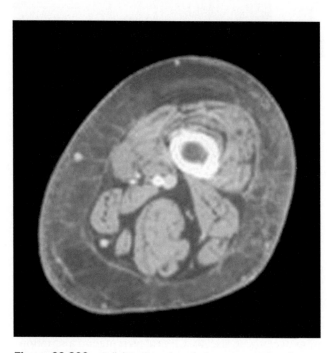

Figure 22-200 Cellulitis. Strandy, soft tissue attenuation changes are present in the subcutaneous fat. The soft tissues deep to the fascia are not affected.

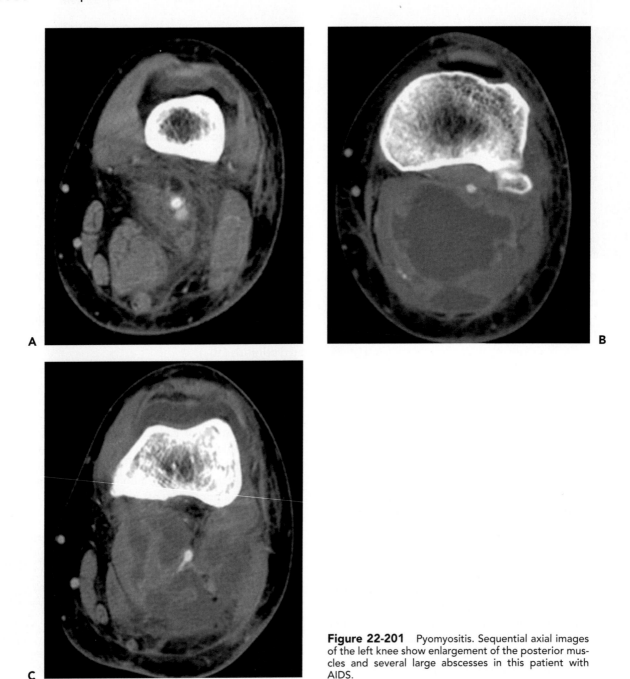

A

B

C

Figure 22-201 Pyomyositis. Sequential axial images of the left knee show enlargement of the posterior muscles and several large abscesses in this patient with AIDS.

formation may be subtly visible as low attenuation regions within muscle or loss of normal muscle architecture. The presence of gas is helpful but inconstant. CT is more sensitive for soft tissue gas than plain films or MRI. In the latter, gas will appear as a signal void that may be misinterpreted as calcification or paramagnetic artifact. Postoperative changes are very difficult to differentiate from necrotizing fasciitis. Clinical presentation and follow-up imaging to assess for resolution versus progression should help resolve uncertainty (51).

An abscess typically manifests as low attenuation fluid with an enhancing rim although blood products or proteinaceous fluid may be high attenuation. Thick, irregular walls are typical, often with enhancing septations (see Fig. 22-198). Multiplanar capability, either by MRI or reformatted CT, is helpful to delineate the extent of involvement. CT is much more sensitive for abscess than conventional radiographs. The presence of adjacent joint fluid may indicate a sterile sympathetic effusion rather than a septic joint (271).

Atypical Infections

CT of cat scratch disease demonstrates markedly enlarged lymph nodes that manifest as an enhancing soft tissue mass with marked surrounding edema and sometimes a nonenhancing area of central necrosis (271). Acute cystercercosis, caused by ingestion of eggs of the tapeworm *Taenia solium*, sometimes results in muscular pseudohypertrophy. CT of widely disseminated living cysticerci may demonstrate a honeycomb appearance of the involved skeletal muscle, with innumerable nonenhancing cysts and little surrounding edema (292). More often, CT reveals the calcified cystercerci of prior infection as 5- to 7-mm rice-shaped bodies lying parallel to the muscle fascicles. Echinococcosis, caused by the dog tapeworm *Echinococcus granulosus*, rarely involves the musculoskeletal system. When it does, unilocular or multilocular low attenuation cysts may be seen (271). When echinococcosis affects skeletal muscle, it forms an abscess-like appearance with enhancing rim and may not exhibit the classic curvilinear calcification or daughter cysts (174). Trichinosis, from ingesting the nematode *Trichinella spiralis*, causes painful muscle swelling acutely, followed by tiny calcifications that are better seen on CT than on conventional radiographs (271).

Idiopathic Inflammatory Myopathy

In the idiopathic inflammatory myopathies such as dermatomyositis, CT is more useful for the assessment of pulmonary changes than for muscle involvement. MR is more sensitive for the muscle edema of active myopathy, although CT may demonstrate areas of muscle atrophy and diffuse or patchy, moth-eaten low attenuation within an affected muscle. CT is more sensitive than MR for calcinosis, which occurs in about 30% of patients, usually with longstanding or untreated disease (Fig. 22-202). For whole body screening, scintigraphy with technetium-99m methylene diphosphonate (MDP) may very well be as sensitive as CT and more expedient (230).

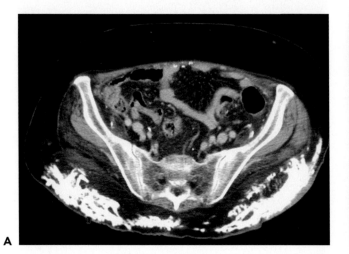
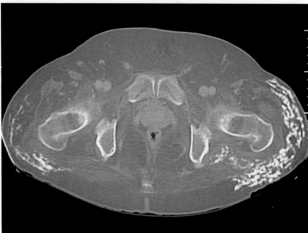

A   B

Figure 22-202 Dermatomyositis. **A:** Soft tissue and (**B**) bone algorithm and windowing reveal extensive soft tissue calcifications.

METABOLIC

The radiologist interpreting a CT may encounter any of the usual manifestations of osteoporosis or other metabolic causes of osteopenia, including cortical tunneling, loss of trabecula or subchondral lucencies. Cortical tunnels are distinguished from nutrient foramina by their smaller size and parallel course relative to the cortex, as opposed to the obliquely oriented nutrient foramen. Disuse osteopenia is often most severe distal to the fracture site. It can simulate the appearance of an aggressive neoplasm (166). CT has little advantage over radiographs in the detection of hyperparathyroidism except in complex articulations such as the sacroiliac joints (109) (Fig. 22-203). CT can be helpful in excluding cystic transformation in brown tumors of hyperparathyroidism, which could lead to pathologic fracture. If the lesional contents enhance, cystic transformation is excluded and risk of pathologic fracture is lessened (70,86).

MRI is the imaging technique of choice for early osteonecrosis (Fig. 22-204). CT is very useful for subsequent staging and follow-up, however, as it is much more sensitive for subchondral fracture (Fig. 22-205). If MR alone is performed, patients with stage III disease will tend to be misclassified as stage II, significantly affecting patient management (267).

Computed Tomography and Magnetic Resonance Bone Densitometry

At the time of this writing, bone mineral density (BMD) measurement is still considered to be the only reliable method to assess fracture risk clinically (140). The most common modalities for BMD assessment in current clinical practice are dual energy x-ray absorptiometry (DXA) and quantitative ultrasound (QUS). Quantitative CT (QCT) is a technique that can be performed on most clinical CT scanners with the addition of a special calibration phantom (80), necessary to compensate for beam hardening and scanner drift (81). Performing densitometry with QCT has an advantage over DXA and QUS in its ability to specifically measure the trabecular bone mineral content with excellent precision. Trabecular bone is often considered to be more labile than cortical bone due to greater surface area, such that it is thought to be about eight times

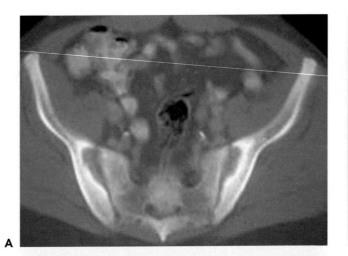

A

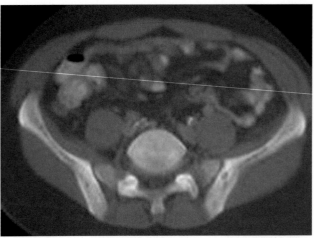

B

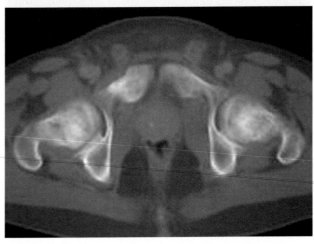

C

Figure 22-203 Hyperparathyroidism. **A:** SI joint resorption predominately affects the iliac sides of the joints. **B:** Indistinct trabecular pattern, patchy sclerosis and lucencies are noted in the pelvis (**C**) and in the hip regions.

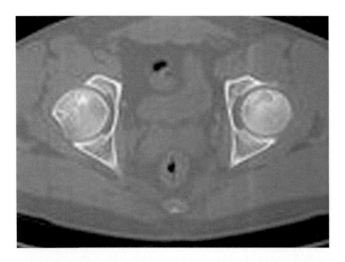

Figure 22-204. Osteonecrosis of the femoral heads bilaterally. Axial image reveals abnormal sclerosis and lucency in the weight-bearing portions of both femoral heads. On the left, the lesion has a better-defined sclerotic, serpentine border.

more sensitive to bone loss than cortical bone, although in truth this is likely a gross oversimplification (199). A more important advantage of QCT over DXA is that QCT is unaffected by degenerative osteophytes, endplate sclerosis or aortic calcification (145). Lumbar spine BMD as de-

termined by QCT is an excellent predictor of osteoporotic fractures (146). A disadvantage of QCT is a much higher ionizing radiation dose than DXA, 200 to 250 mrem to the upper abdomen for a lumbar examination in one study (96) compared to 1 to 5 mrem for most DXA methods (254). Low energy CT technique (80 kVp, 146 mAs) can significantly reduce the QCT effective dose into a range comparable to that of DXA, however (145).

There is growing awareness that the strength of bone is dependent on bone quality as well as bone density. Bone quality is in turn dependent on its architecture, turnover rate and damage accumulation. It stands to reason that assessment of the microarchitecture of trabecular bone can also be a useful tool in the prediction of fracture risk for patients with osteoporosis. Osteoporosis results not only in loss of thickness of cortical and trabecular bone, but also in loss of trabecular cross-linking and subsequent mechanical weakening. For example, the loss of 1 trabecular crosstie would increase the total length of a vertical trabecula by 2 but decrease its strength by a factor of 4 (64).

The two major methods for "virtual bone biopsy" to assess trabecular architecture *in vivo* are 3D-peripheral quantitative computed tomography (pQCT) that can acquire 165 micron resolution at acceptable radiation doses and high resolution MRI which has a 2D resolution that is sim-

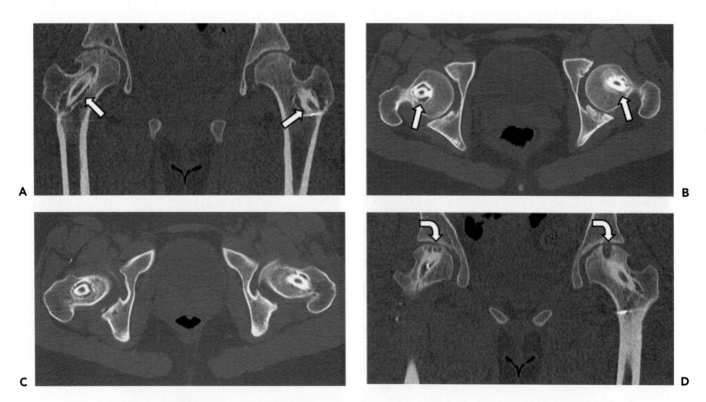

Figure 22-205 Femoral head osteonecrosis with vascularized fibular strut grafts. **A:** Transverse CT image through the femoral heads shows the fibular strut grafts in place (I). **B:** A more inferior image shows the strut grafts extending through the femoral necks. **C:** Coronal reformatted image demonstrates the bilateral femoral head sclerosis, subchondral cysts, and flattening associated with osteonecrosis (I). **D:** The fibular strut grafts are placed through the femoral necks (I) into the heads. Microvascular surgery is performed at the femoral insertion site with the expectation that this blood supply with then be conveyed through the graft to the femoral head.

ilar to pQCT with no exposure to ionizing radiation (211). Both rely on special software to compensate for the fact that individual trabeculae are barely visualized at the achieved spatial resolutions. The former uses a dedicated, low dose peripheral CT device with a skin dose of 0.8 mGy and exam time of 10 minutes (136).

High resolution MR provides better correlation than CT with in vitro studies of trabecular architecture, but with long scan times at typical high field clinical magnet strengths (1.5 T), requiring nearly an hour to acquire 3-mm-thick slices in one study (147). The growing availability of 3 Tesla magnets may improve the clinical practicality of these exams in the near future by improving spatial resolution and scan time. High resolution MR of trabecular architecture in the distal radius performs similar to QCT of the lumbar spine in predicting osteoporotic fractures. Combining the two modalities does not seem to offer significant benefit (146). MRI holds tremendous future potential for predicting fracture risk, not only in analysis of trabecular architecture but also in measuring other bone parameters such as vertebral marrow fat content, which increases in osteoporosis and is an independent measure of fracture risk (299).

Heterotopic Ossification

CT is both sensitive and specific for mature heterotopic ossification (Fig. 22-206). An early lesion, on the other hand, has the nonspecific appearance of a low attenua-tion soft tissue mass, an asymmetrically enlarged muscle belly or the loss of soft tissue plane definition. Prominent contrast enhancement will be present at this stage. Over time, faint and disorganized mineralization appears in the immature osteoid. Eventually, a characteristic zonal architecture develops, with robust peripheral cortical bone and even central fatty marrow elements (27), with little or no discernable contrast enhancement.

Fragility Fractures

Fragility fractures (also referred to as insufficiency fractures) are stress fractures resulting from bone that is of insufficient strength to withstand normal activity, most commonly in the setting of osteoporosis. MR is more sensitive than CT for sacral and acetabular insufficiency fractures in the early subacute phase, particularly with the use of fat-suppressed T2 weighted images or gadolinium (103) (see Figs. 22-102 and 22-104). Sacral fractures are often associated with parasymphyseal fractures of the pubic symphysis. Fragility fractures can have an aggressive appearance on CT while in the reparative phase. If an expansile, mixed lytic and sclerotic lesion is discovered in a typical location and in the appropriate clinical setting for insufficiency fracture, biopsy should be avoided (56,170). Subchondral insufficiency fractures of the femoral head can have a similar appearance to osteonecrosis on CT and MR, with a serpentine border of sclerosis (284).

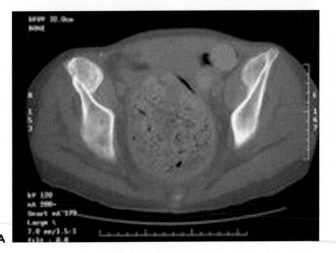 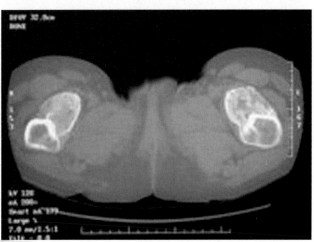

A   B

Figure 22-206 Mature heterotopic ossification following spinal cord injury. **A:** Well-corticated ossification is seen bilaterally in the iliacus region. **B:** Mature ossification also extends from the lesser trochanters.

INTERVENTIONS

Biopsies

Percutaneous biopsies of osseous and soft tissue musculoskeletal lesions are routinely performed at our institutions with a variety of guiding imaging modalities. Fluoroscopy, ultrasound, CT and even MR (with special grids and nonferromagnetic needles) can all be used to safely guide the needle path into the area of concern and avoiding any adjacent neurovascular structures or unaffected muscle compartments in the extremities (12,141,179,315). At our institutions, CT is the preferred imaging modality for percutaneous bone biopsy guidance or for biopsies of deep soft tissue masses, although some of us prefer sonography with its real time needle visualization, especially when the lesion is superficial. With CT, the muscle compartment boundaries and neurovascular structures are always clearly depicted, and small bone lesions are more confidently sampled. Like MR, CT may visualize areas of abnormal attenuation or enhancement of a soft tissue mass that appear more cellular or worrisome for viable tumor, and CT guidance of the needle biopsy may be directed at these areas (Fig. 22-207).

CT fluoroscopy can be very helpful in maneuvering past close neurovascular structures, although potential for increased radiation dose necessitates careful attention to technique (40,201). Intermittent CT fluoroscopy to check needle tip placement is preferred, and decreasing milliamperage allows for adequate needle localization (55,89,257,276). CT fluoroscopy can also dramatically decrease procedure time (40,99,201,255,257).

Like in other organ systems, biopsies should only be considered after a careful review of the clinical history and radiographs and imaging studies fails to elicit a diagnosis (97). Some common osseous lesions like subchondral cysts in the setting of degenerative joint disease or bone islands, herniation pits of the femoral neck (Fig. 22-111), [N1] or common soft tissue masses like lipomas (see Fig. 22-193) may be confidently diagnosed on imaging alone.

The most common malignant osseous lesions in adults are metastases. In a patient who has a known neoplasia, with the onset of multiple osseous lesions, it is usually not necessary to biopsy these lesions to conclude that they are likely metastases. However, biopsy may be needed when histological confirmation is required prior to radiation or chemotherapy protocol initiation, or when the original neoplastic diagnosis either occurred a long time

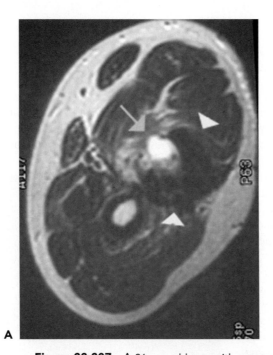
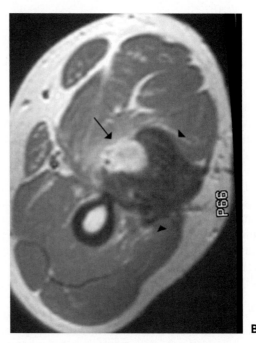

A

B

Figure 22-207 A 36-year-old man with aggressive fibromatosis in left thigh and increased pain. **A:** Axial T2-weighted MR image of the left thigh shows the predominantly low signal mass (*arrowheads*) consistent with fibromatosis in the biceps femoris muscle with a medial area of increased T2 signal (*white arrow*) concerning for dedifferentiation. **B:** Axial T1-weighted MR image after gadolinium administration shows enhancement in this medial area (*black arrow*).

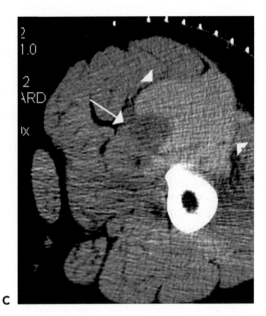

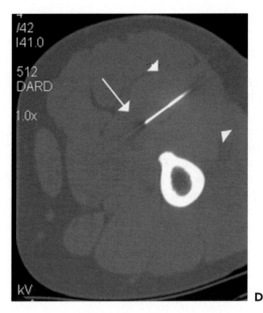

C   D

Figure 22-207 (*continued*) **C:** CT image of the same region shows the bulk of the fibrous tumor to have increased attenuation (*arrowheads*) but an area of decreased attenuation medially (*arrow*) corresponds to the same region on MR with more fluid-type signal. Notice the overlying radiopaque grid markers for biopsy localization. **D:** Using direct CT guidance, the coaxial needle was advanced through the more fibrous region (*arrowheads*) and into the area of decreased attenuation (*arrow*) and core biopsies were obtained throughout this area. The final histological diagnosis in this area remained aggressive fibromatosis.

ago (i.e., 5 to 10 years previously) or the appearance of the lesions is atypical for the usual primary tumor osseous metastases (i.e., lytic lesions in a patient with a history of prostate cancer) (Fig. 22-208) (97). In the setting of a single lesion in a patient with no other known metastases, biopsy is usually performed, although the increasing use of PET imaging, especially when the functional imaging data is cross-registered with the anatomical localizing information of concurrent CT scans, may obviate the need for some biopsies as the experience with this technique in musculoskeletal neoplasia continues to grow (Fig. 22-209) (62,116).

In the adult patient with no history of neoplasia, even after careful review of the history and imaging, it may be very difficult to differentiate between benign but aggressive lesions like infection and aneurismal bone cysts and malignant lesions like metastases without a biopsy. Soft tissue masses that cannot be confidently diagnosed as benign also usually require biopsy. When surgery is needed due to the degree of bone destruction and danger of impending pathological fracture, or if a soft tissue mass is compressing a vital structure, some surgeons may chose to perform an open biopsy at the time of resection.

Percutaneous CT guided biopsy is very accurate in the diagnosis of soft tissue and osseous lesions, with low complication rates of about 1% noted in several series

(73,119). Although the accuracy is best for metastatic lesions or local recurrence, it is also highly accurate in the diagnosis of primary bone tumors (Fig. 22-210) (119,312). Percutaneous needle biopsy, as compared to open biopsy,

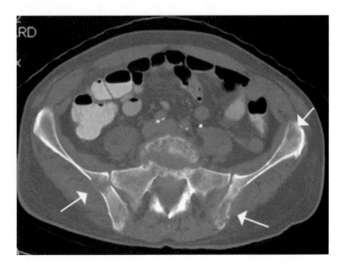

Figure 22-208 A 62-year-old man with history of prostate cancer and new multiple osseous lesions. Axial CT image shows several predominantly lytic lesions in the pelvis (*arrows*), unusual for prostate cancer metastases that usually have prominent sclerotic components. Subsequent CT guided biopsy of left posterior iliac crest lesion confirmed metastatic prostate adenocarcinoma.

A, B

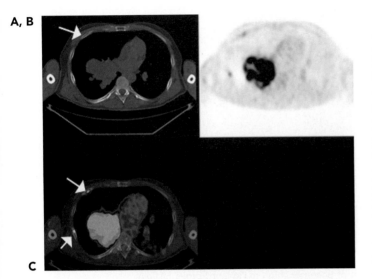

C

Figure 22-209 A 55-year-old man with small cell lung cancer and right chest wall pain and CT-PET imaging. **A:** Axial CT image shows large right hilar nodal mass and subtle intramedullary radiolucency involving the right most anterior rib (*arrow*). **B:** Axial F-18 PET image at the same level shows marked increased activity in the hilar mass, as well as focal increased tracer uptake in several of the right ribs. **C:** Fusion image of the CT and PET combines the anatomic specificity of CT with the functional information of PET, and clearly shows rib uptake (*arrows*) in prior area of subtle anterior rib radiolucency as well as in more posterior rib.

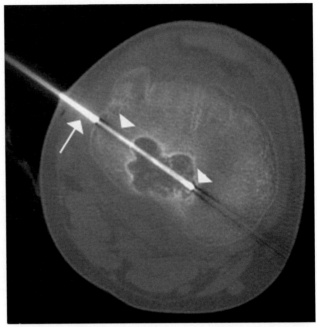

Figure 22-210 A 14-year-old girl with a right knee chondroblastoma. Single axial CT image shows the lesion in the tibial epiphysis with chondroid-type intralesional matrix and sclerotic borders. Using a lateral approach, a coaxial bone biopsy system (RADI Medical Systems, Uppsala, Sweden) has been placed with 14-gauge outer needle (*arrow*) penetrating cortex allowing multiple passes with a 17-gauge bone biopsy needle (*arrowhead*) to ensure adequate sampling.

has also been shown to be a more cost-effective technique by several studies (87,261), We routinely perform fine needle aspiration as well as core biopsies in the same setting with a coaxial needle system, as these techniques can be complementary (73,251,295).

For lesions that are markedly sclerotic or cystic, or soft tissue masses that are markedly heterogeneous, we tend to sample different areas and increase the number of samples obtained in order to increase the diagnostic yield (119,139) (Fig. 22-211). We may also opt to acquire a larger diameter core (Fig. 22-212). In patients with sclerotic bone lesions or intact overlying thick cortices, bigger gauge bone biopsy needles may be needed (8 to 11 gauge) or a hand drill may be used. In these more difficult situations, we may use the expertise of our pathologists to provide frozen section analysis or rapid cytological interpretation to ensure adequacy of material prior to procedure termination (295). For soft tissue tumors that are deep, or all bone biopsies, but especially those with intact cortices, we use conscious sedation techniques with doses of intravenous midazolam and fentanyl citrate titrated to maximize patient comfort (182).

Consultation with the referring surgical orthopedic oncologist for biopsy planning is essential. Bone biopsies may not need to be performed in benign-appearing lesions at risk of fracture that need definitive treatment like curettage and bone grafting (119). If a musculoskeletal sarcoma is a possible diagnostic consideration, discussion with the surgeon who would perform the definitive tumor resection is extremely important, as one would not want to alter the staging of the tumor by intercompartmental seeding or involving muscle compartments that would not be part of the standard surgical approach and thus preclude limb salvage surgery (159,160,258). Seeding of the needle path with tumor is a potential pitfall of percutaneous biopsy (potentially worse in the setting of sarcomas) and the surgeon may need to resect the needle tract at the time of tumor removal (110,197).

The radiologist should be aware of compartmental anatomy in the extremities when planning the biopsy (3). The muscle origins and insertions, as well as the major fascias separate tissues into different compartments. A tumor that has spread beyond its original compartment and has become extracompartmental may limit limb-salvage surgery options. In the arm, the anterior compartment contains the biceps, brachioradialis, brachialis and coracobrachialis muscles. The posterior compartment contains the triceps muscle. When performing biopsies of the proximal humerus, it is recommended to utilize if possible an approach through the anterior third of the deltoid muscle. Since the deltoid is innervated by the axillary nerve from a posterior to anterior direction, resecting a posterior needle tract may make the anterior deltoid denervated after the definitive resection (Fig. 22-213) (3). The forearm contains a dorsal compartment (extensor muscles) and a volar com-

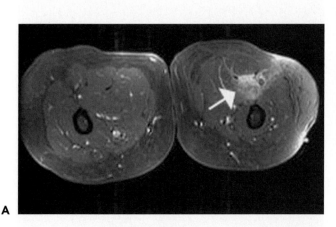 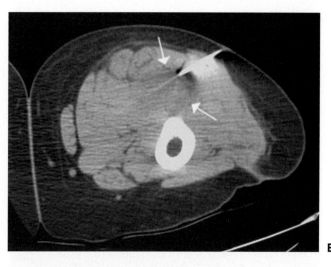

Figure 22-211 A 40-year-old man with resection of posterior thigh malignant fibrous histiocytoma 2 years ago, now with recurrent mass. **A:** Axial MR T1-weighted image with fat suppression after gadolinium enhancement shows a heterogeneously enhancing mass (*arrow*) in the posterior compartment of the thigh. **B:** CT axial image at comparable level shows needle placement into mass (*arrows*). Fine-needle aspiration and core biopsy confirmed tumor recurrence.

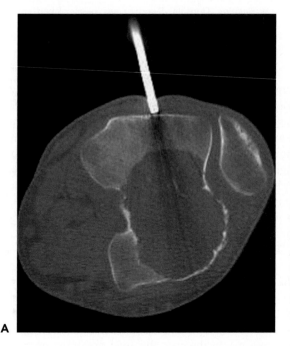 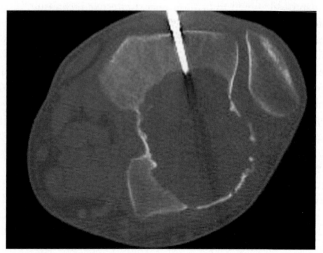

Figure 22-212 A 22-year-old man with giant cell tumor of knee. Prior needle biopsy with 18-gauge core had yielded nondiagnostic tissue. **A:** Axial CT image shows outer guide needle placed at medial femoral condyle. **B:** Axial CT image shows inner trephine needle acquiring 2-mm diameter bone core coaxially of wall of cystic lesion. This specimen yielded the final diagnosis.

partment (flexor muscles). In the pelvis, a transgluteal biopsy path may jeopardize the use of the gluteus maximus as a muscle flap after resection and should not be attempted unless no other path is viable and consultation with the referring oncologic surgeon has been performed (Fig. 22-214). In the thigh, there is an anterior compartment (containing the quadriceps muscle group, tensor fascia muscle, and sartorius muscle), a posterior compartment (containing the hamstring muscles and including the sciatic nerve) and a medial compartment (containing the gracilis and adductor muscles). Biopsy path to the distal femur through the rectus femoris muscle or quadriceps tendon should be avoided if possible. The lower leg contains an anterior (tibialis anterior, extensor digitorum and extensor hallucis longus muscles), lateral (peroneal muscles and nerves), deep posterior (tibialis posterior, flexor digitorum and flexor hallucis longus muscles along with the posterior tibial nerve) and superficial posterior compartment (gastrocnemius and soleus muscles). In the foot, the plantar compartments are medial (abductor hallucis and flexor hallucis brevis muscles), central (flexor digitorum brevis, quadratus plantae, lumbricals and adductor hallucis muscles) and lateral compartments (abductor digiti minimi and flexor digiti minimi brevis) (3).

Image-Guided Ablation of Osseous Lesions

Osteoid Osteoma

There is much interest currently in the application of image-guided tumor ablations to musculoskeletal lesions. At our institutions, radiofrequency thermal coagulation of the vascular nidus of osteoid osteomas is the most common MSK indication for this procedure (Fig. 22-215). There are large series of over 200 patients that have established the efficacy of this technique (237). We prefer to use CT guidance in enabling to localize the lucent nidus (which, due to its small size, may be difficult to distinguish from surrounding sclerosis by fluoroscopy) (239,291). CT guidance also is very helpful in the careful placement of the active tip of the electrode at least 1 cm away from any adjoining major neurovascular structures (the zone of thermal necrosis is 1 cm in diameter when using an electrode with a 5-mm exposed tip) (238). We perform these procedures under general anesthesia, although spinal anesthesia is a pain control option in adults. To ensure adequate coagulation of the nidus, an electrode tip temperature of 90 degrees centigrade for 6 minutes has been advocated (237). The success rate for this procedure has ranged from 75% to 95% (143,237,289). Recurrences

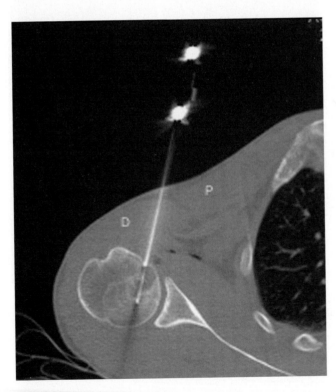

Figure 22-213 A 30-year-old man with lymphoma of bone: utilizing the anterior deltoid pathway. Coaxial needle biopsy was performed through anterior humeral head lesion. The needle was placed within the anterior third of the deltoid muscle as close to the deltopectoral interval as possible as that was the possible surgical approach. Deltoid, D; pectoralis major, P.

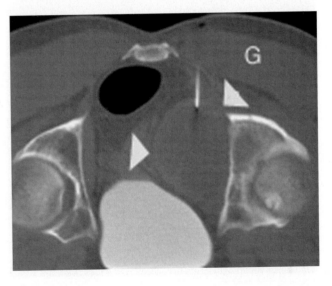

Figure 22-214 A 72-year-old man with myxoid chondrosarcoma of the right acetabulum: hazards of posterior pelvic approach. Axial CT obtained with the patient prone shows a needle biopsy being obtained of the large soft tissue component (*arrowheads*) arising from the acetabular lesion. The posterior approach hindered the future use of the gluteus maximus (G) for flap reconstruction after hemipelvectomy.

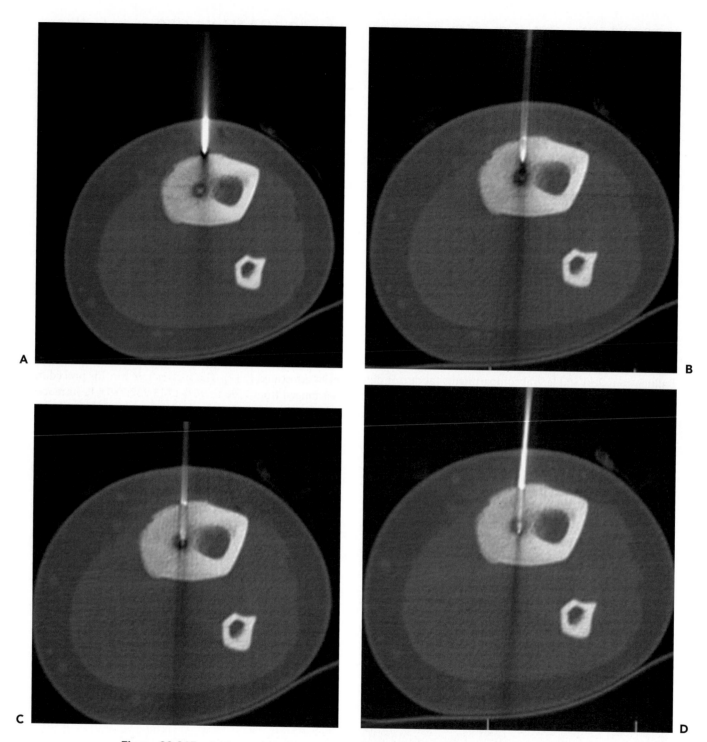

Figure 22-215 A 14-year-old boy with osteoid osteoma of the left tibia: radiofrequency ablation technique. **A:** The small lucent nidus (with central calcification) is localized and a 14-gauge outer guide needle (Bonopty, RADIA, Upsaala, Sweden) inserted into the overlying periosteum. **B:** Hand drill inserted coaxially helps to traverse sclerotic reaction and access nidus. **C:** An 18-gauge core biopsy needle placed coaxially for nidus biopsy. **D:** Thermally insulated electrode with 5-mm active tip (TM-101, Radionics, Boston, MA) was placed directly in nidus. Nidus coagulation at 90 degrees centigrade for 6 minutes was performed. The patient has had complete relief of symptoms for 3 years postprocedure.

are more common in larger lesions, perhaps due to incomplete ablation if the circumference of thermal energy surrounding the electrode tip does not extend completely to the borders of the nidus (306). These recurrences can be amenable to repeat ablation although the success rate of repeat RF ablation can be as low as 60% (237). Other techniques reported for osteoid osteoma ablation include overdrilling and extracting the nidus with large hollow needles, CT-guided laser photocoagulation of the nidus, and instillation of sclerosing agents like ethanol into the nidus (244).

Other Lesions

CT-guided radiofrequency ablation has also been described as a successful joint-sparing treatment alternative for chondroblastomas in a small series (78). Given the epiphyseal location of these tumors, and their potential for local recurrence after surgical resection, radiofrequency ablation may be an effective minimally invasive treatment for local control and potentially curative.

CT-guided radiofrequency ablation has also been recently proposed as an effective pain management technique in the terminally ill patient with painful osteolytic bone metastases (74). In a recently reported small series of patients who had failed prior chemotherapy or radiation therapy, there was a statistically significant decrease in pain scores and use of analgesics at short-term follow-up (38). There is currently an American College of Radiology Imaging Network (ACRIN) sponsored multi-institutional prospective trial being performed at the time of this writing on this subject (Fig. 22-216). Hopefully more data will soon be available to evaluate the efficacy of this treatment in the common clinical scenario of painful osteolytic metastases. There have also been reports combining the use of radiofrequency ablation and percutaneous instillation of acrylic cement using CT and fluoroscopic combined guidance as a minimally invasive treatment for pathologic fractures (247).

CT-Guided Aspirations and Therapeutic Injections

We perform most of our joint aspirations under fluoroscopy but CT guidance can be very helpful in areas of complex overlapping anatomy like the sacroiliac joints or the sternoclavicular joints (Fig. 22-217) (161,218). Although fluoroscopy can be used for the therapeutic injection of local anesthetic and corticosteroid into the sacroiliac joints, we find in patients with noninflammatory and degenerative sacroiliitis that the narrowed joints often have posterior near bridging osteophytes that may impede joint access and are best visualized with CT. Thus, we prefer CT guidance for these injections (Fig. 22-218). When joint fluid is noted to be loculated from prior imaging, CT can be helpful in directing the needle to the fluid pocket and thus increasing the yield of the aspiration. CT guidance is also helpful when attempting aspiration and therapeutic injections of synovial cysts that are deep, as in the pericruciate region of the knee or in a paralabral location like the shoulder's spinoglenoid notch (Fig. 22-219) (4,39,209).

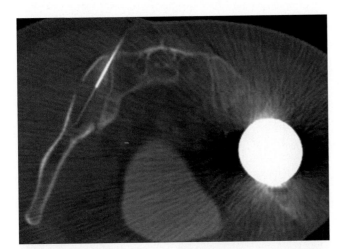

Figure 22-216 A 43-year-old man with metastatic renal cell carcinoma: radiofrequency (RF) ablation for palliation of osseous metastases. This patient had prior custom right hip prosthesis for a pathologic fracture due to metastatic disease and now has severe left pelvis pain from left iliac wing lesion despite prior radiation therapy. CT axial image shows the electrode with active 3-cm tip placed via a posterior approach through an outer guide needle. The length of the tumor was covered with sequential overlapping RF treatments. The patient had excellent pain relief postprocedure.

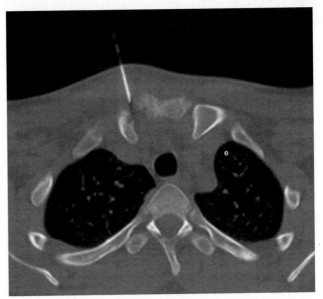

Figure 22-217 A 23-year-old man with history of intravenous drug abuse and septic right sternoclavicular joint: CT guidance for sternoclavicular joint aspiration. CT axial image shows placement of an 18-gauge needle. Pus was subsequently aspirated.

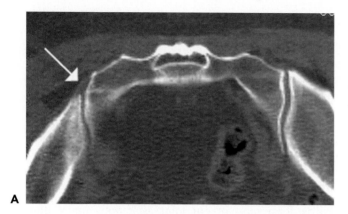
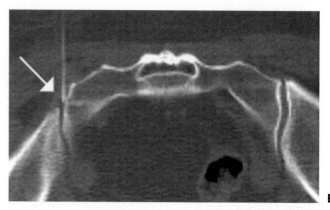

A   B

Figure 22-218 A 50-year-old woman with left sacroiliac pain: CT guidance for sacroiliac joint therapeutic injection. **A:** Prone axial CT image through the inferior portions of the sacroiliac joints shows mild narrowing of the left as compared with the right joint. Note posterior joint capsule (*arrow*). **B:** Prone axial CT image after insertion of 22-gauge spinal needle into posterior left sacroiliac joint (*arrow*). Intraarticular administration of 1 mL of 1% preservative-free lidocaine and 0.5 mL of betamethesone acetate (Celestone Soluspan) was performed.

Facet injections in the spine are usually performed with fluoroscopy, although CT can be used as well (265). Decompression of symptomatic facet synovial cysts can also be performed (127,150). Selective nerve root blocks with anesthetic and corticosteroid injections into the epidural space are traditionally performed under fluoroscopy, although CT and especially fluoroscopy may also be used (293) (Fig. 22-

220). Percutaneous periradicular steroid and anesthetic injection into the epidural space of a symptomatic nerve root within the thoracic spine is best performed with CT guidance (93) (Fig. 22-221). In patients with visceral abdominal pain, regional analgesia with neurolytic block (neurolysis) can be performed for pain management with careful CT guidance into the celiac or splanchnic plexus (90,94,173)

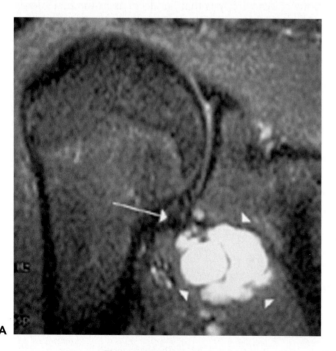
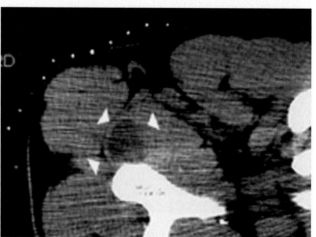

A   B

Figure 22-219 A 30-year-old man with paralabral cyst and atypical shoulder pain: CT guidance for paralabral cyst aspiration. The orthopedic surgeon wanted to determine if the pain pattern arose from the cyst. **A:** Coronal T2-weighted MR image shows large lobulated paralabral cyst (*arrowheads*) with increased T2 signal arising from tear of the inferior labrum (*arrow*). **B:** Axial CT image shows cyst as a low-attenuation rounded structure (*arrowheads*) anterior to the inferior glenoid.

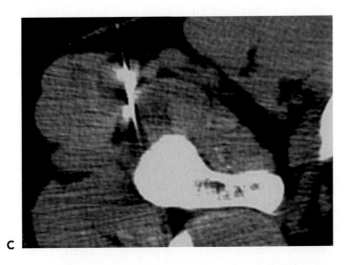

C

Figure 22-219 *(continued)* **C:** Axial CT image shows 18-gauge needle placed into the lateral aspect of the cyst. A small amount of viscous material was inserted and a mixture of lidocaine and corticosteroid was instilled into it. The patient had temporary improvement of pain. Subsequent surgical decompression and labral repair was performed with excellent results.

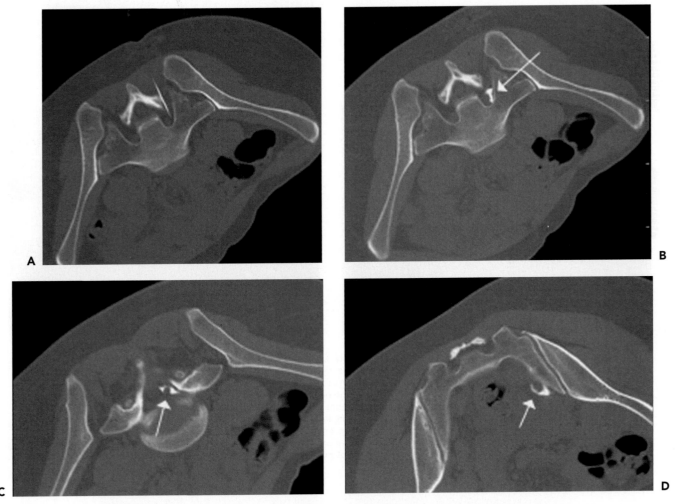

Figure 22-220 A 55-year-old woman with radicular pain in a left S1 distribution: CT guidance for left S1 selective nerve root block. **A:** Axial CT image shows placement of a 22-gauge spinal needle via a posterior approach through the sacral foramina into the epidural space adjacent to the left S1 nerve root. **B:** Axial CT image at same level after contrast material *(arrow)* had been placed, along with a mixture of lidocaine and corticosteroid, into the epidural space. **C:** Axial CT image cephalad to **(B)**. **D:** Axial CT image caudal to **(B)**. Note the contrast material travels in the epidural space in both directions, outlining the nerve *(arrow)*. The patient had complete relief of pain after the injection.

(Fig. 22-222). CT-guided lumbar sympathectomy for the palliation of pain has also been reported to be effective in patients with inoperable peripheral vascular disease (275). Finally, CT guided injection is preferred for the diagnosis and treatment of the piriformis muscle syndrome (Fig. 22-223). Piriformis muscle syndrome can present as buttock pain or sciatica and may be difficult to diagnose. Injection of local anesthetic into the muscle belly may be diagnostic if it relieves the pain (30). More recently, injection of botulinic toxin into the muscle has been performed under CT guidance with some success in a series of patients (79).

Image-Guided Placement of Orthopedic Hardware and Cement

Unstable pelvic ring fractures are usually internally fixed in the operating room suite under general anesthesia using fluoroscopy as a guide for the placement of orthopedic hardware. Intraoperative visualization of iliosacral screw position may be difficult during this procedure and lead to misplaced screws. Recently, an alternative has been reported utilizing CT guidance for the placement of iliosacral screws under local anesthesia with excellent results (314).

Percutaneous vertebroplasty for the palliation of painful osteoporotic or pathological vertebral body fractures was initially reported best performed under combined CT and fluoroscopy guidance (95). However, like others, we now prefer to use solely fluoroscopic guidance. CT post-procedure may be very helpful in assessing for complications including the presence of new fractures or leakage of cement into the spinal canal and neural foramina (121) (Fig. 22-224). Percutaneous cementoplasty of pelvic and acetabular lytic lesions with combined CT and fluoroscopy guidance may be helpful in the palliative therapy of these patients, especially if they fail to respond to radiation therapy (49,163).

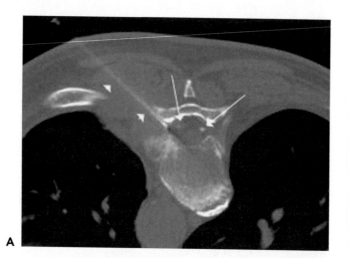

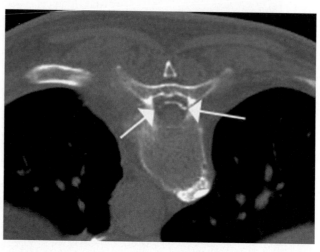

A   B

Figure 22-221 A 67-year-old man with metastatic lung cancer and T7 radicular pain: CT guidance for selective nerve root block at T7. A selective nerve root block was performed to determine whether the patient would benefit from more permanent neurolysis (radiofrequency ablation) for pain control. **A:** Axial CT image shows 22-gauge needle (*arrowheads*) with tip placed at the left T7 foramina. Small amount of contrast material has been injected to confirm positioning with the epidural space, surrounding the dorsal root ganglia bilaterally (*arrows*), before injection of the mixture of anesthetic and corticosteroid. **B:** Axial prone CT image at T7 shows distribution of contrast in the posterior epidural space (*arrows*). The patient did not have significant relief of pain after the injection, so more permanent neurolysis was not performed.

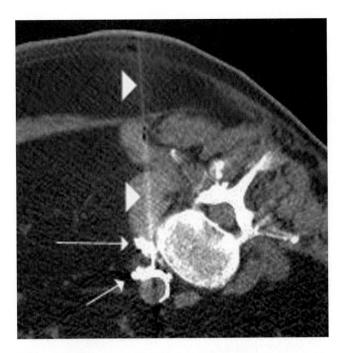

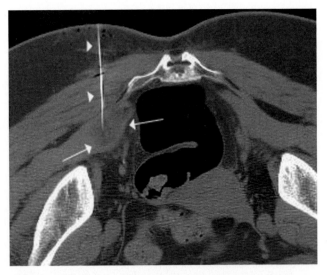

Figure 22-222 A 60-year-old man with complex regional pain syndrome referred for pharmacologic blockade of the lumbar sympathetic plexus: CT guidance for lumbar sympathetic plexus neurologic blockade. Using a left lateral approach, as the patient could not lie on his stomach, a 22-gauge needle was inserted (*arrowheads*) and the tip placed in a periaortic location that was confirmed by a small amount of contrast material (*arrows*). 5 mL of 0.5% bupivicaine was then instilled, with subsequent temporary relief of this pain.

Figure 22-223 A 40-year-old woman with buttock pain and suspected piriformis muscle syndrome: CT guidance for left piriformis muscle injection. Axial CT image with the patient prone demonstrates a 25-gauge needle (*arrowheads*) placed into the left piriformis muscle belly and 5 mL of 1% lidocaine was instilled, which accounts for the low-attenuation region (*arrows*). The patient did not have relief of pain.

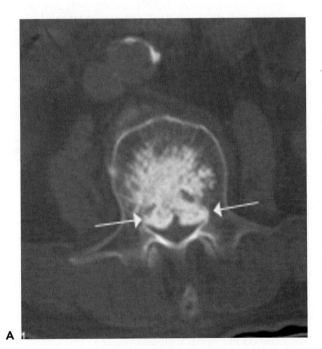

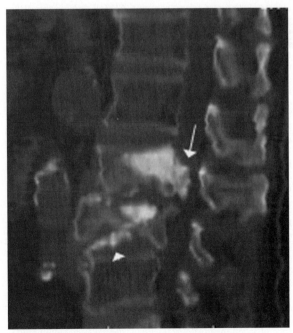

A

B

Figure 22-224 A 91-year-old man with cauda equina syndrome after recent vertebroplasty. **A:** Axial CT at L3 level shows marked posterior extravasation (*arrows*) of polymethylmethacrylate with resultant spinal canal stenosis. **B:** Sagittal reformatted image shows same findings (*arrow*) as well as extravasation of cement into the L4 to L5 disc (*arrowhead*) from prior L4 vertebroplasty.

ACKNOWLEDGMENTS

The authors wish to acknowledge Ms. Trish Thurman for her invaluable help with the reference list and manuscript formatting.

REFERENCES

1. Aisen AM, Martel W, Braunstein EM, et al. MRI and CT evaluation of primary bone and soft-tissue tumors. *Am J Roentgenol* 1986;146(4):749–756.
2. Allon SM, Mears DC. Three-dimensional analysis of calcaneal fractures. *Foot Ankle* 1991;11(5):254–263.
3. Anderson MW, Temple HT, Dussault RG, et al. Compartmental anatomy: relevance to staging and biopsy of musculoskeletal tumors. *Am J Rentgenol* 1999;173(6):1663–1671.
4. Antonacci VP, Foster T, Fenlon H, et al. Technical report: CT-guided aspiration of anterior cruciate ligament ganglion cysts. *Clin Radiol* 1998;53(10):771–773.
5. Applegate GR, Flannigan BD, Tolin BS, et al. MR diagnosis of recurrent tears in the knee: value of intra-articular contrast material. *Am J Roentgenol* 1993;161:821–825.
6. Assoun J, Richardi G, Railhac JJ, et al. Osteoid osteoma: MR imaging versus CT. *Radiology* 1994;191(1):217–223.
7. Bain GI, Bennett JD, Richards RS, et al. Longitudinal computed tomography of the scaphoid: a new technique. *Skeletal Radiol* 1995;24(4):271–273.
8. Bancroft LW, Peterson JJ, Kransdorf MJ, et al. Soft tissue tumors of the lower extremities. *Radiol Clin North Am* 2002;40(5):991–1011.
9. Berger RA, Rubash HE. Rotational instability and malrotation after total knee arthroplasty. *Orthop Clin North Am* 2001;32:639–647.
10. Berland LL, Smith JK. Multidetector-array CT: once again, technology creates new opportunities. *Radiology* 1998;209(2):327–329.
11. Berquist TH, Ehman RL, King BF, et al. Value of MR imaging in differentiating benign from malignant soft-tissue masses: study of 95 lesions. *Am J Roentgenol* 1990;155(6):1251–1255.
12. Bickels J, Jelinek JS, Shmookler BM, et al. Biopsy of musculoskeletal tumors. Current concepts. *Clinical Orthopaedics & Related Research* 1999;368:212–219.
13. Biedert R, Hintermann B. Stress fractures of the medial great toe sesamoids in athletes. *Foot Ankle Int* 2003;24(2):137–141.
14. Billet FP, Schmitt WG, Gay B. Computed tomography in traumatology with special regard to the advances of three-dimensional display. *Arch Orthop Trauma Surg* 1992;111:131–137.
15. Biondetti PR, Vannier MW, Gilula LA, et al. Wrist: coronal and transaxial CT screening. *Radiology* 1987;63(1):149–151.
16. Bland KI, McCoy DM, Kinard RE, et al. Application of magnetic resonance imaging and computerized tomography as an adjunct to the surgical management of soft tissue sarcomas. *Ann Surg* 1987;205(5):473–481.
17. Bloem JL, Mulder JD. Chondroblastoma: a clinical and radiological study of 104 cases. *Skeletal Radiol* 1985;14(1):1–9.
18. Blomlie V, Lien HH, Iversen T, et al. Radiation-induced insufficiency fractures of the sacrum: evaluation with MR imaging. *Radiology* 1993;188(1):241–244.
19. Bogost GA, Lizerbram EK, Crues JB 3rd. MR imaging in evaluation of suspected hip fracture: frequency of unsuspected bone and soft-tissue injury. *Radiology* 1995;197(1):263–267.
20. Boutin RD, Januario JA, Newberg AH, et al. MR imaging features of osteochondritis dissecans of the femoral sulcus. *Am J Roentgenol* 2003;180:641–645.
21. Boyko OB, Cory DA, Cohen MD, et al. MR imaging of osteogenic and Ewing's sarcoma. *Am J Roentgenol* 1987;148(2):317–322.
22. Brahme SK, Cervilla V, Vint V, et al. Magnetic resonance appearance of sacral insufficiency fractures. *Skeletal Radiol* 1990;19(7):489–493.
23. Brandser E, El-Khoury GY, Marsh JL. Acetabular fractures: a systematic approach to classification. *Emergency Radiology* 1995;2:18–28.
24. Brandser E, Marsh JL. Acetabular fractures: easier classification with a systematic approach. *Am J Roentgenol* 1998;171(5):1217–1228.
25. Bravo SM, Winalski CS, Weissman BN. Pigmented villonodular synovitis. *Radiol Clin North Am* 1996;34(2):311–326.
26. Breitenseher MJ, Metz VM, Gilula LA, et al. Radiographically occult scaphoid fractures: value of MR imaging in detection. *Radiology* 1997;203(1):245–250.
27. Bressler EL, Marn CS, Gore RM, et al. Evaluation of ectopic bone by CT. *Am J Roentgenol* 1987;148(5):931–935.
28. Brien EW, Mirra JM, Kerr R. Benign and malignant cartilage tumors of bone and joint: their anatomic and theoretical basis with an emphasis on radiology, pathology and clinical biology. I. The intramedullary cartilage tumors. *Skeletal Radiol* 1997;26(6):325–353.
29. Brophy DP, O'Malley M, Lui D, et al. MR imaging of tibial plateau fractures. *Clin Radiol* 1996;51(12):873–878.
30. Brown JA, Braun MA, Namey TC. Pyriformis syndrome in a 10-year-old boy as a complication of operation with the patient in the sitting position. *Neurosurgery* 1988;23(1):117–119.
31. Brown RR, Rosenberg ZS, Thornhill BA. The C sign: more specific for flatfoot deformity than subtalar coalition. *Skeletal Radiol* 2001;30(2):84–87.
32. Buckingham R, Jackson M, Atkins R. Calcaneal fractures in adolescents. CT classification and results of operative treatment. *Injury* 2003;34(6):454–459.
33. Buckwalter KA, Rydberg J, Kopecky KK, et al. Musculoskeletal imaging with multislice CT. *Am J Roentgenol* 2001;176:979–986.
34. Burgess AR, Eastridge BJ, Young JW, et al. Pelvic ring disruptions: effective classification system and treatment protocols. *J Trauma* 1990;30(7):848–856.
35. Burr BA, Resnick D, Syklawer R, et al. Fluid–fluid levels in a unicameral bone cyst: CT and MR findings. *J Comput Assist Tomogr* 1993;17(1):134–136.
36. Bush CH, Gillespy T 3rd, Dell PC. High-resolution CT of the wrist: initial experience with scaphoid disorders and surgical fusions. *Am J Roentgenol* 1987;149(4):757–760.
37. Caldemeyer KS, Sandrasegaran K, Shinaver CN, et al. Temporal bone: comparison of isotropic helical CT and conventional direct axial and coronal CT. *Am J Roentgenol* 1999;172:1675–1682.
38. Callstrom MR, Charboneau JW, Goetz MP, et al. Painful metastases involving bone: feasibility of percutaneous CT- and US-guided radio-frequency ablation. *Radiology* 2002;224(1):87–97.
39. Campagnolo DI, Davis BA, Blacksin MF. Computed tomography–guided aspiration of a ganglion cyst of the anterior cruciate ligament: a case report. *Archives of Physical Medicine and Rehabilitation* 1996;77(7):732–733.
40. Carlson SK, Bender CE, Classic KL, et al. Benefits and safety of CT fluoroscopy in interventional radiologic procedures. *Radiology* 2001;219(2):515–520.
41. Chan PS, Klimkiewicz JJ, Luchetti WT, et al. Impact of CT scan on treatment plan and fracture classification of tibial plateau fractures. *J Orthop Trauma* 1997;11(7):484–489.
42. Chandnani VP, Yeager TD, DeBerardino T, et al. Glenoid labral tears: prospective evaluation with MRI imaging, MR arthrography, and CT arthrography. *Am J Roentgenol* 1993;161(6):1229–1235.
43. Chang AE, Matory YL, Dwyer AJ, et al. Magnetic resonance imaging versus computed tomography in the evaluation of soft tissue tumors of the extremities. *Ann Surg* 1987;205(4):340–348.
44. Cheung Y, Rosenberg ZS, Magee T, et al. Normal anatomy and pathologic conditions of ankle tendons: current imaging techniques. *Radiographics* 1992;12(3):429–444.
45. Chigira M, Shimizu T. Computed tomographic appearances of sternocostoclavicular hyperostosis. *Skeletal Radiol* 1989;18(5):347–352.
46. Chiodo CP, Parentis MA, Myerson MS. Symptomatic bipartite medial cuneiform in an adult athlete: a case report. *Foot Ankle Int* 2002;23(4):348–351.
47. Cody DD. AAPM/RSNA physics tutorial for residents: topics in CT. Image processing in CT. *Radiographics* 2002;22(5):1255–1268.
48. Cone RO III, Nguyen V, Flournoy JG, et al. Triplane fracture of the distal tibial epiphysis: radiographic and CT studies. *Radiology* 1984;153(3):763–767.
49. Cotten A, Demondion X, Boutry N, et al. Therapeutic percutaneous injections in the treatment of malignant acetabular osteolyses. *Radiographics* 1999;19(3):647–653.

50. Crim JR, Seeger LL, Yao L, et al. Diagnosis of soft-tissue masses with MR imaging: can benign masses be differentiated from malignant ones. *Radiology* 1992;185(2):581–586.

51. Curry CA, Corl FM, Fishman EK. CT diagnosis of necrotizing fasciitis: spectrum of CT findings. *Emergency Radiology* 2000;7:369–375.

52. Daffner RH, Lupetin AR, Dash N, et al. MRI in the detection of malignant infiltration of bone marrow. *Am J Roentgenol* 1986;146(2):353–358.

53. Dalal SA, Burgess AR, Siegel JH, et al. Pelvic fracture in multiple trauma: classification by mechanism is key to pattern of organ injury, resuscitative requirements, and outcome. *J Trauma* 1989;29(7):981–1000.

54. Dalinka MK, Zlatkin MB, Chao P, et al. The use of magnetic resonance imaging in the evaluation of bone and soft-tissue tumors. *Radiol Clin North Am* 1990;28(2) 461–470.

55. Daly B, Krebs TL, Wong-You-Cheong JJ, et al. Percutaneous abdominal and pelvic interventional procedures using CT fluoroscopy guidance. *Am J Roentgenol* 1999;173(3):637–644.

56. Davies AM, Evans NS, Struthers GR. Parasymphyseal and associated insufficiency fractures of the pelvis and sacrum. *Br J Radiol* 1988;61(722):103–108.

57. Dawson P, Lees WR. Multi-slice technology in computed tomography. *Clin Radiol* 2001;56(4):302–309.

58. De Beuckeleer LH, De Schepper AM, Ramon F. Magnetic resonance imaging of cartilaginous tumors: is it useful or necessary? *Skeletal Radiol* 1996;25(2):137–141.

59. De Maeseneer M, Jaovisidha S, Jacobson JA, et al. The Bennett lesion of the shoulder. *J Comput Assist Tomogr* 1998;22(1):31–34.

60. De Maeseneer M, Van Roy F, Lenchik L, et al. CT and MR arthrography of the normal and pathologic anterosuperior labrum and labral-bicipital complex. *Radiographics* 2000; 20:S67–S81.

61. De Smet AA, Fisher DR, Graf BK, et al. Osteochondritis dissecans of the knee: value of MR imaging in determining lesion stability and the presence of articular cartilage defects. *Am J Roentgenol* 1990;155:549–553.

62. Dehdashti F, Siegel BA, Griffeth LK, et al. Benign versus malignant intraosseous lesions: discrimination by means of PET with 2-(F-18)fluoro-2-deoxy-D-glucose. *Radiology* 1996;200(1):243–247.

63. Demas BE, Heelan RT, Lane J, et al. Soft-tissue sarcomas of the extremities: comparison of MR and CT in determining the extent of disease. *Am J Roentgenol* 1988;150(3):615–620.

64. Dempster DW. The impact of bone turnover and bone-active agents on bone quality: focus on the hip. *Osteoporosis International* 2002;13(5):349–352.

65. den Boer FC, Bramer JA, Patka P, et al. Quantification of fracture healing with three-dimensional computed tomography. *Archives of Orthopaedic and Trauma Surgery* 1998;117(6–7):345–350.

66. Desser TS, McCarthy S, Trumble T. Scaphoid fractures and Kienbock's disease of the lunate: MR imaging with histopathologic correlation. *Magnetic Resonance Imaging* 1990;8(4):357–361.

67. Deutsch AL, Mink JH, Waxman AD. Occult fractures of the proximal femur: MR imaging. *Radiology* 1989;170(1):113–116.

68. Dias JJ, Stirling AJ, Finlay DB, et al. Computerized axial tomography for tibial plateau fractures. *J Bone Joint Surg Br* 1987;69(1):84–88.

69. Donnelly LF, Klostermeier TT, Klosterman LA. Traumatic elbow effusions in pediatric patients: are occult fractures the rule? *Am J Roentgenol* 1998;171(1):243–245.

70. Doppman JL, Marx S, Spiegel A, et al. Differential diagnosis of brown tumor vs. cystic osteitis by arteriography and computed tomography. *Radiology* 1979;131(2):339–340.

71. Dorsay TA, Major NM, Helms CA. Cost-effectiveness of immediate MR imaging versus traditional follow-up for revealing radiographically occult scaphoid fractures. *Am J Roentgenol* 2001;177(6):1257–1263.

72. Drebin RA, Magid D, Robertson DD, et al. Fidelity of three-dimensional CT imaging for detecting fracture gaps. *J Comput Assist Tomogr* 1989;13:487–489.

73. Dupuy DE, Rosenberg AE, Punyaratabandhu T, et al. Accuracy of CT-guided needle biopsy of musculoskeletal neoplasms. *Am J Roentgenol* 1998;171(3):759–762.

74. Dupuy DE, Safran H, Mayo-Smith WW, et al. Radiofrequency ablation of painful osseous metastatic disease (abstr). *Radiology* 1998;209(P):389.

75. Eastwood DM, Phipp L. Intra-articular fractures of the calcaneum: why such controversy? *Injury* 1997;28(4):247–259.

76. Ebraheim NA, Elgafy H, Padanilam T. Syndesmotic disruption in low fibular fractures associated with deltoid ligament injury. *Clinical Orthopaedics and Related Research* 2003;409:260–267.

77. Emberg LA, Potter HG. Radiographic evaluation of the acromioclavicular and sternoclavicular joints. *Clinics in Sports Medicine* 2003;22(2):255–275.

78. Erickson JK, Rosenthal DI, Zaleske DJ, et al. Primary treatment of chondroblastoma with percutaneous radio-frequency heat ablation: report of three cases. *Radiology* 2001;221(2):463–468.

79. Fannucci E, Masala S, Sodani G, et al. CT-guided injection of botulinic toxin for percutaneous therapy of piriformis muscle syndrome with preliminary MRI results and denervative process. *Eur Radiol* 2001;11(12):2543–2548.

80. Faulkner KG. Update on bone density measurement. *Rheumatic Diseases Clinics of North America* 2001;27(1):81–99.

81. Faulkner KG, Gluer CC, Grampp S, et al. Cross-calibration of liquid and solid QCT calibration standards: corrections to the UCSF normative data. *Osteoporosis International* 1993;3(1):36–42.

82. Feydy A, Drape J, Beret E, et al. Longitudinal stress fractures of the tibia: comparative study of CT and MR imaging. *Eur Radiol* 1998;8(4):598–602.

83. Fishman EK, Magid D, Robertson DD, et al. Metallic hip implants: CT with multiplanar reconstruction. *Radiology* 1986;160:675–681.

84. Flannigan B, Kursunoglu-Brahme S, Snyder S, et al. MR arthrography of the shoulder: comparison with conventional MR imaging. *Am J Roentgenol* 1990;155(4):829–832.

85. Francis IR, Dorovini-Zis K, Glazer GM, et al. The fibromatoses: CT-pathologic correlation. *Am J Roentgenol* 1986;147(5):1063–1066.

86. Franco M, Bendini JC, Albano L, et al. Radiographic follow-up of a phalangeal brown tumor. *Joint, Bone, Spine: Revue du Rhumatisme* 2002;69(5):506–510.

87. Fraser-Hill MA, Renfrew DL, Hilsenrath PE. Percutaneous needle biopsy of musculoskeletal lesions. 2. Cost-effectiveness. *Am J Roentgenol* 1992;185(4):813–818.

88. Freund M, Thomsen M, Hohendorf B, et al. Optimized preoperative planning of calcaneal fractures using spiral computed tomography. *Eur Radiol* 1999;9(5):901–906.

89. Froelich JJ, Wagner HJ. CT-fluoroscopy: tool or gimmick. *Cardiovascular and Interventional Radiology* 2001;24(5):297–305.

90. Fujita Y. CT-guided neurolytic splanchnic nerve block with alcohol. *Pain* 1993;55(3):363–366.

91. Gaebler C, Kukla C, Breitenseher M, et al. Magnetic resonance imaging of occult scaphoid fractures. *J Trauma* 1996;41(1):73–76.

92. Gagliardi JA, Chung EM, Chandnani VP, et al. Detection and staging of chondromalacia patellae: relative efficacies of conventional MR imaging, MR arthrography, and CT arthrography. *Am J Roentgenol* 1994;163(3):629–636.

93. Gangi A, Dietemann JL, Mortazavi R, et al. CT-guided interventional procedures for pain management in the lumbosacral spine. *Radiographics* 1998;18(3):621–633.

94. Gangi A, Dietemann JL, Schultz A, et al. Interventional radiologic procedures with CT guidance in cancer pain management. *Radiographics* 1996;16(6):1289–1304.

95. Gangi A, Guth S, Imbert JP, et al. Percutaneous vertebroplasty: indications, technique, and results. *Radiographics* 2003;23(2):e10.

96. Genant HK, Cann CE, Ettinger B, et al. Quantitative computed tomography of vertebral spongiosa: a sensitive method for detecting early bone loss after oophorectomy. *Ann Intern Med* 1982;97(5):699–705.

97. Ghelman B. Biopsies of the musculoskeletal system. *Radiol Clin North Am* 1998;36(3):567–580.

98. Ghelman B. Meniscal tears of the knee: evaluation by high resolution CT combined with arthrography. *Radiology* 1985;157:23–27.

99. Gianfelice D, Lepanto L, Perreault P, et al. Effect of the learning process on procedure times and radiation exposure for CT fluoroscopy-guided percutaneous biopsy procedures. *Journal of Vascular and Interventional Radiology* 2000;11(9):1217–1221.

100. Golding SJ, Shrimpton PC. Commentary. Radiation dose in CT: are we meeting the challenge. *Br J Radiol* 2002;75(889):1–4.

101. Gordon BA, Martinez S, Collins AJ. Pyomyositis: characteristics at CT and MR imaging. *Radiology* 1995;197(1):279–286.

102. Goss TP. The scapula: coracoid, acromial, and avulsion fractures. *Am J Orthop* 1996;25(2):106–115.

103. Grangier C, Garcia J, Howarth NR, et al. Role of MRI in the diagnosis of insufficiency fractures of the sacrum and acetabular roof. *Skeletal Radiol* 1997;26(9):517–524.

104. Greenspan A, Tehranzadeh J. Imaging of infectious arthritis. *Radiol Clin North Am* 2001;39(2):267–276.

105. Griffith JF, Antonio GE, Tong CW, et al. Anterior shoulder dislocation: quantification of glenoid bone loss with CT. *Am J Roentgenol* 2003;180(5):1423–1430.

106. Griffith JF, Roebuck DJ, Cheng JC, et al. Acute elbow trauma in children: spectrum of injury revealed by MR imaging not apparent on radiographs. *Am J Roentgenol* 2001;176(1):53–60.

107. Haramati N, Staron RB, Barax C, et al. Magnetic resonance imaging of occult fractures of the proximal femur. *Skeletal Radiol* 1994;23(1):19–22.

108. Hauger O, Moinard M, Lasalarie JC, et al. Anterolateral compartment of the ankle in the lateral impingement syndrome: appearance on CT arthrography. *Am J Roentgenol* 1999;173(3):685–690.

109. Hayes CW, Conway WF. Hyperparathyroidism. *Radiol Clin North Am* 1991;29(1):85–96.

110. Heare TC, Enneking WF, Heare MM. Staging techniques and biopsy of bone tumors. *Orthopedic Clinics of North America* 1989;20(3):273–285.

111. Hermel MB, Gershon-Cohen J. The nutcracker fracture of the cuboid by indirect violence. *Radiology* 1953;60(6):850–854.

112. Hodge JC, Ghelman B, O'Brien SJ, et al. Synovial plicae and chondromalacia patellae: correlation of results of CT arthrography with results of arthroscopy. *Radiology* 1993;186(3):827–831.

113. Hunter JC, Brandser EA, Tran KA. Pelvic and acetabular trauma. *Radiol Clin North Am* 1997;35(3):559–590.

114. Hunter JC, Escobedo EM, Wilson AJ, et al. MR imaging of clinically suspected scaphoid fractures. *Am J Roentgenol* 1997;168(5):1287–1293.

115. Hunter JC, Sangeorzan BJ. A nutcracker fracture: cuboid fracture with an associated avulsion fracture of the tarsal navicular. *Am J Roentgenol* 1996;166(4):888.

116. Ioannidis JP, Lau J. 18F-FDG PET for the diagnosis and grading of soft-tissue sarcoma: a meta-analysis. *J Nucl Med* 2003;44(5):717–724.

117. Jadvar H, Conti PS. Diagnostic utility of FDG PET in multiple myeloma. *Skeletal Radiol* 2002;31(12):690–694.

118. Jazrawi LM, Birdzell L, Kummer FJ, et al. The accuracy of computed tomography for determining femoral and tibial total knee arthroplasty component rotation. *J Arthroplasty* 2000;15(6):761–766.

119. Jelinek JS, Murphey MD, Welker JA, et al. Diagnosis of primary bone tumors with image-guided percutaneous biopsy: experience with 110 tumors. *Radiology* 2002;223(3):731–737.

120. Judet R, Judet J, Letournel E. Fractures of the acetabulum: classification and surgical approaches for open reduction. *J Bone Joint Surg Am* 1964;46:615–1646.

121. Kallmes DF, Jensen ME. Percutaneous vertebroplasty. *Radiology* 2003;229(1):27–36.

122. Kamineni S. Tibial plateau fracture. *Orthopedics* 2002;25(8):858–859.

123. Katz MA, Beredjiklian PK, Bozentka DJ, et al.:Computed tomography scanning of intra-articular distal radius fractures: does it influence treatment. *J Hand Surg [Am]* 2001;26(3):415–421.

124. Kenney PJ, Gilula LA, Murphy WA. The use of computed tomography to distinguish osteochondroma and chondrosarcoma. *Radiology* 1981;139(1):129–137.

125. Kligenbeck-Regn K, Schaller S, Flohr T, et al. Subsecond multislice computed tomography: basics and applications. *Eur J Radiol* 1999;31(2):110–124.

126. Kode L, Lieberman JM, Motta AO, et al. Evaluation of tibial plateau fractures: efficacy of MR imaging compared with CT. *Am J Roentgenol* 1994;163:141.

127. Koenigsberg RA. Percutaneous aspiration of lumbar synovial cyst: CT and MRI considerations. *Neuroradiology* 1998;40(4):272–273.

128. Kransdorf MJ. Benign soft-tissue tumors in a large referral population: distribution of specific diagnoses by age, sex, and location. *Am J Roentgenol* 1995;164(2):395–402.

129. Kransdorf MJ. Malignant soft-tissue tumors in a large referral population: distribution of diagnoses by age, sex, and location. *Am J Roentgenol* 1995;164(1):129–134.

130. Kransdorf MJ, Bancroft LW, Peterson JJ, et al. Imaging of fatty tumors: distinction of lipoma and well-differentiated liposarcoma. *Radiology* 2002;224(1):99–104.

131. Kransdorf MJ, Jelinek JS, Moser RP Jr, et al. Soft-tissue masses: diagnosis using MR imaging. *Am J Roentgenol* 1989;153(3):541–547.

132. Kransdorf MJ, Murphey MD. Radiologic evaluation of soft-tissue masses: a current perspective. *Am J Roentgenol* 2000;175(3):575–587.

133. Kuhn JP, Berger PE. Computed tomographic diagnosis of osteomyelitis. *Radiology* 1979;130(2):503–506.

134. Kuhns LR, Borlaza GS, Seigel RS, et al. An in vitro comparison of computed tomography, xeroradiography, and radiography in the detection of soft-tissue foreign bodies. *Radiology* 1979;132(1):218–219.

135. Kuszyk BS, Heath DG, Bliss DF, et al. Skeletal 3-D CT: advantages of volume rendering over surface rendering. *Skeletal Radiol* 1996;25:207–214.

136. Laib A, Hildebrand T, Hauselmann HJ, et al. Ridge number density: a new parameter for in vivo bone structure analysis. *Bone* 1997;21(6)(Dec):541–546.

137. Lawler LB, Corl FM, Fishman EK. Multi- and single detector CT with 3D volume rendering in tibial plateau fracture imaging and management. *Crit Rev Comput Tomogr* 2002;43(4):251–282.

138. Ledermann HP, Schweitzer ME, Morrison WB. Pelvic heterotopic ossification: MR imaging characteristics. *Radiology* 2002;222(1):189–195.

139. Leffler SG, Chew FS. CT-guided percutaneous biopsy of sclerotic bone lesions: diagnostic yield and accuracy. *Am J Roentgenol* 1999;172(5)(May):1389–1392.

140. Leib ES, Lenchik L, Bilezikian JP, et al. Position statements of the International Society for Clinical Densitometry: methodology. *J Clin Densitom* 2002;5(suppl) S5–S10.

141. Lewin JS, Petersilge CA, Hatem SF, et al. Interactive MR imaging-guided biopsy and aspiration with a modified clinical C-arm system. *Am J Roentgenol* 1998;170(6):1593–1601.

142. Lewis SL, Pozo JL, Muirhead-Allwood WFG. Coronal fractures of the lateral femoral condyle. *J Bone Joint Surg Br* 1989;71(1):118–120.

143. Lindner NJ Ozaki T, Roedl R, et al. Percutaneous radiofrequency ablation in osteoid osteoma. *J Bone Joint Surg Br* 2001;83(3):391–396.

144. Link TM, Berning W, Scherf S, et al. CT of metal implants: reduction of artifacts using an extended CT scale technique. *J Comput Assist Tomogr* 2000;24(1):165–172.

145. Link TM, Majumdar S. Osteoporosis imaging. *Radiol Clin North Am* 2003;41(4):813–839.

146. Link TM, Vieth V, Matheis J, et al. Bone structure of the distal radius and the calcaneus vs BMD of the spine and proximal femur in the prediction of osteoporotic spine fractures. *Eur Radiol* 2002;12(2):401–408.

147. Link TM, Vieth V, Stehling C, et al. High-resolution MRI vs multislice spiral CT: which technique depicts the trabecular bone structure best. *Eur Radiol* 2003;13(4):663–671.

148. Liow RY, Birdsall PD, Mucci B, et al. Spiral computed tomography with two- and three-dimensional reconstruction in the management of tibial plateau fractures. *Orthopedics* 1999;22(10):929–932.

149. Liu PT, Chivers FS, Roberts CC, et al. Imaging of osteoid osteoma with dynamic gadolinium-enhanced MR imaging. *Radiology* 2003;227(3):691–700.

150. Lutz GE, Shen TC. Fluoroscopically guided aspiration of a symptomatic lumbar zygapophyseal joint cyst: a case report. *Arch Phys Med Rehabil* 2002;83(12):1789–1791.

151. MacNealy GA, Rogers LF, Hernandez R, et al. Injuries of the distal tibial epiphysis: systematic radiographic evaluation. *Am J Roentgenol* 1982;138(4):683–689.

152. Magid D, Fishman EK. Imaging of musculoskeletal trauma in three dimensions. An integrated two-dimensional/three-dimensional approach with computed tomography. *Radiol Clin North Am* 1989; 27:945–956.

153. Magid D, Fishman EK, Ney DR, et al. Acetabular and pelvic fractures in the pediatric patient: value of two- and three-dimensional imaging. *J Pediatr Orthop* 1992;12(5):621–625.

154. Magid D, Michelson JD, Ney DR, et al. Adult ankle fractures: comparison of plain films and interactive two- and three-dimensional CT scans. *Am J Roentgenol* 1990;154(5):1017–1023.

155. Mahesh M. Search for isotropic resolution in CT from conventional through multiple-row detector. *Radiographics* 2002;22(4): 949–962.

156. Mainwaring BL, Daffner RH, Riemer BL. Pylon fractures of the ankle: a distinct clinical and radiologic entity. *Radiology* 1988; 168(1):215–218.

157. Major NM, Crawford ST. Elbow effusions in trauma in adults and children: is there an occult fracture. *Am J Roentgenol* 2002; 78(2):413–418.

158. Malghem J, Vande Berg BC, Lebon C, et al. Ganglion cysts of the knee: articular communication revealed by delayed radiography and CT after arthrography. *Am J Roentgenol* 1998;170: 1579–1583.

159. Mankin HJ, Lange TA, Spanier SS. The hazards of biopsy in patients with malignant primary bone and soft-tissue tumors. *J Bone Joint Surg* 1982;64(8):1121–1127.

160. Mankin HJ, Mankin CJ, Simon MA. The hazards of the biopsy, revisited. Members of the Musculoskeletal Tumor Society. *J Bone Joint Surg* 1996 78(5):656–663.

161. Mantle B, Gross P, Lopez-Ben R, et al. Hip pain as the presenting manifestation of acute sacroiliitis. *J Clin Rheumatol* 2001;7: 112–114.

162. Marcus CD, Ladam-Marcus VJ, Leone J, et al. MR imaging of osteomyelitis and neuropathic osteoarthropathy in the feet of diabetics. *Radiographics* 1996;16(6):1337–1348.

163. Marcy PY, Palussiere J, Descamps B, et al. Percutaneous cementoplasty for pelvic bone metastasis. *Support Care Cancer* 2000;8(6): 500–503.

164. Marsh JL, Munk PL, Muller NL. CT of a unicameral bone cyst in a rib. *Br J Radiol* 1992;65(769):74–75.

165. Martinez CR, Di Pasquale TG, Helfet DL, et al. Evaluation of acetabular fractures with two- and three-dimensional CT. *Radiographics* 1992;12:227–242.

166. Mayo-Smith W, Rosenthal DI. Radiographic appearance of osteopenia. *Radiol Clin North Am* 1991;29(1):37–47.

167. McEnery KW, Wilson AJ, Pilgram TK, et al. Fractures of the tibial plateau: value of spiral CT coronal plane reconstructions for detecting displacement in vitro. *Am J Roentgenol* 1994;163(5): 1177–1181.

168. McGrath BE, Bush CH, Nelson TE, et al. Evaluation of suspected osteoid osteoma. *Clin Orthop* 1996;327:247–252.

169. McGuckin JF Jr, Akhtar N, Ho VT, et al. CT and MR evaluation of a wooden foreign body in an in vitro model of the orbit. *Am J Neuroradiol* 1996;17(1):129–133.

170. McNiesh LM. Unique musculoskeletal trauma. *Radiol Clin North Am* 1987;25(6):1107–1132.

171. Mellado JM, Salvado E, Camins A, et al. Painful os sustentaculi: imaging findings of another symptomatic skeletal variant. *Skeletal Radiol* 2002;31(1):53–56.

172. Melone CP Jr. Distal radius fractures: patterns of articular fragmentation. *Orthop Clin North Am* 1993;24(2):239–253.

173. Mercadante S, La Rosa S, Villari P. CT-guided neurolytic splanchnic nerve block by an anterior approach. J Pain Symptom Manage 2002;23(4):268–270.

174. Merkle EM, Schulte M, Vogel J, et al. Musculoskeletal involvement in cystic echinococcosis: report of eight cases and review of the literature. *Am J Roentgenol* 1997;168(6):1531–1534.

175. Mesgarzadeh M, Sapega AA, Bonakdarpour A, et al. Osteochondritis dissecans: analysis of mechanical stability with radiography, scintigraphy, and MR imaging. *Radiology* 1987;165(3): 775–780.

176. Minns RJ, Bibb R, Banks R, et al. The use of a reconstructed three-dimensional solid model from CT to aid the surgical management of a total knee arthroplasty: a case study. *Med Eng Phys* 2003;25:523–526.

177. Mirowitz SA, Apicella P, Reinus WR, et al. MR imaging of bone marrow lesions: relative conspicuousness on T1-weighted, fat-suppressed T2-weighted, and STIR images. *Am J Roentgenol* 1994; 62(1):215–221.

178. Moore SL, Rafii M. Imaging of musculoskeletal and spinal tuberculosis. *Radiol Clin North Am* 2001;39(2):329–342.

179. Moore TM, Meyers MH, Patzakis MJ, et al. Closed biopsy of musculoskeletal lesions. *J Bone Joint Surg* 1979;61(3):375–380.

180. Moore TM, Patzakis MJ, Harvey JP. Tibial plateau fractures: definition, demographics, treatment rationale, and long-term results of closed traction management or operative reduction. *J Orthop Trauma* 1987;1:97–119.

181. Morrison WB, Ledermann HP. Work-up of the diabetic foot. *Radiol Clin North Am* 2002;40(5):1171–1192.

182. Mueller PR, Biswal S, Halpern EF, et al. Interventional radiologic procedures: patient anxiety, perception of pain, understanding of procedure, and satisfaction with medication—a prospective study. *Radiology* 2000;215(3):684–688.

183. Muhle C, Brossmann J, Heller M. Kinematic CT and MR imaging of the patellofemoral joint. *Eur Radiol* 1999;9:508–518.

184. Mulligan SA, Schwartz ML, Broussard MF, et al. Heterotopic calcification and tears of the ulnar collateral ligament: radiographic and MR imaging findings. *Am J Roentgenol* 2000; 175(4):1099–1102.

185. Munk PL, Lee MJ, Janzen DL, et al. Lipoma and liposarcoma: evaluation using CT and MR imaging. *Am J Roentgenol* 1997;169(2):589–594.

186. Muraskin S, Mollabashy A, Bush CH, et al. Tibial lesion in a 12-year-old boy. *Clin Orthop* 2002;400:254–258, 264–267.

187. Murphey MD, Choi JJ, Kransdorf MJ, et al. Imaging of osteochondroma: variants and complications with radiologic-pathologic correlation. *Radiographics* 2000;20(5):1407–1434.

188. Murphey MD, Fairbairn KJ, Parman LM, et al. From the archives of the AFIP. Musculoskeletal angiomatous lesions: radiologic-pathologic correlation. *Radiographics* 1995;15(4):893–917.

189. Murphey MD, Smith WS, Smith SE, et al. From the archives of the AFIP. Imaging of musculoskeletal neurogenic tumors: radiologic-pathologic correlation. *Radiographics* 1999;19(5):1253–1280.

190. Murray KA, Crim JR. Radiographic imaging for treatment and follow-up of developmental dysplasia of the hip. *Semi Ultrasound CT MR* 2001;22(4):306–340.

191. Mutschler C, Vande Berg BC, Lecouvet FE, et al. Postoperative meniscus: assessment at dual-detector row spiral CT arthography of the knee. *Radiology* 2003;228(3) 635–641.

192. Nakamura R, Horii E, Imaeda T, et al. Criteria for diagnosing distal radioulnar joint subluxation by computed tomography. *Skeletal Radiol* 1996;25(7):649–653.

193. Newman JS, Newberg AH. Congenital tarsal coalition: multimodality evaluation with emphasis on CT and MR imaging. *Radiographics* 2000;20(2):321–332.

194. Norfray JF, Rogers LF, Adamo GP, et al. Common calcaneal avulsion fracture. *Am J Roentgenol* 1980;134(1):119–123.

195. O'Neal ML, Ganey TM, Ogden JA. Fracture of a bipartite medial cuneiform synchondrosis. *Foot Ankle Int* 1995;16(1):37–40.

196. Ohashi K, El-Khoury GY, Bennett DL: MDCT of tendon abnormalities using volume-rendered images. *Am J Roentgenol* 2004; 182(1):161–165.

197. Olson PN, Everson LI, Griffiths HJ. Staging of musculoskeletal tumors. *Radiol Clin North Am* 1994;32(1):151–162.

198. Panicek DM, Gatsonis C, Rosenthal DI, et al. CT and MR imaging in the local staging of primary malignant musculoskeletal neoplasms: Report of the Radiology Diagnostic Oncology Group. *Radiology* 1997;202(1):237–246.

199. Parfitt AM. Misconceptions (2): turnover is always higher in cancellous than in cortical bone. *Bone* 2002;30(6):807–809.

200. Passariello R, Trecco F, de Paulis F, et al. Meniscal lesions of the knee joint: CT diagnosis. *Radiology* 1985;157(1):29–34.

201. Paulson EK, Sheafor DH, Enterline DS, et al. CT fluoroscopy-guided interventional procedures: techniques and radiation dose to radiologists. *Radiology* 2001;220(1):161–167.

202. Pavlov H. Imaging of the foot and ankle. *Radiol Clin North Am* 1990;28(5):991–1018.

203. Peh WC, Khong PL, Yin Y, et al. Imaging of pelvic insufficiency fractures. *Radiographics* 1996;16(2):335–348.

204. Pelc JS, Beaulieu CF. Volume rendering of tendon-bone relationships using unenhanced CT. *Am J Roentgenol* 2001;176: 973–977.

205. Periera ER, Ryu kN, Ahn JM, et al. Evaluation of the anterior cruciate positions during MR imaging. *Clin Radiol* 1998;53(8): 574–578.

206. Petasnick JP, Turner DA, Charters JR, et al. Soft-tissue masses of the locomotor system: comparison of MR imaging with CT. *Radiology* 1986;160(1):125–133.

207. Peterson JJ, Bancroft LW, Kransdorf MJ. Wooden foreign bodies: imaging appearance. *Am J Roentgenol* 2002;178(3):557–562.

208. Pettersson H, Gillespy T 3rd, Hamlin DJ, et al. Primary musculoskeletal tumors: examination with MR imaging compared with conventional modalities. *Radiology* 1987;164:237–241.

209. Piatt BE, Hawkins RJ, Fritz RC, et al. Clinical evaluation and treatment of spinoglenoid notch ganglion cysts. *J Shoulder Elbow Surg* 2002;11(6):600–604.

210. Piqueres X, de Zabala S, Torrens C, et al. Cubonavicular coalition: a case report and literature review. *Clin Orthop* 2002;396: 112–114.

211. Pistoia W, van Rietbergen B, Lochmuller EM, et al. Estimation of distal radius failure load with micro-finite element analysis models based on three-dimensional peripheral quantitative computed tomography images. *Bone* 2002;30(6):842–848.

212. Pitt MJ, Graham AR, Shipman JH, et al. Herniation pit of the femoral neck. *Am J Roentgenol* 1982;138(6):1115–1121.

213. Potter HG, Montgomery KD, Heise CW, et al. MR imaging of acetabular fractures: value in detecting femoral head injury, intraarticular fragments, and sciatic nerve injury. *Am J Roentgenol* 1994;163(4):881–886.

214. Preidler KW, Peicha G, Lajtai G, et al. Conventional radiography, CT, and MR imaging in patients with hyperflexion injuries of the foot: diagnostic accuracy in the detection of bony and ligamentous changes. *Am J Roentgenol* 1999;173(6):1673–1677.

215. Pretorius ES, Fishman EK. Volume-rendered three-dimensional spiral CT. *Radiographics* 1999;19:1143–1160.

216. Pruitt DL, Gilula LA, Manske PR, et al. Computed tomography scanning with image reconstruction in evaluation of distal radius fractures. *J Hand Surg [Am]* 1994;19:720–727.

217. Puhakka KB, Jurik AG, Egund N, et al. Imaging of sacroiliitis in early seronegative spondylarthropathy. Assessment of abnormalities by MR in comparison with radiography and CT. *Acta Radiol* 2003;44(2):218–229.

218. Pulisetti D, Ebraheim NA. CT-guided sacroiliac joint injections. *J Spinal Disord* 1999;12(4):310–312.

219. Puri L, Wixson RL, Stern SH, et al. Use of helical computed tomography for the assessment of acetabular osteolysis after total hip arthroplasty. *J Bone Joint Surg [AM]* 2002;84-A(4):609–614.

220. Quint LE, Gross BH, Glazer GM, et al. CT evaluation of chondroblastoma. *J Comput Assist Tomogr* 1984;8(5):907–910.

221. Rafii M, Firooznia H, Golimbu C, et al. Computed tomography of tibial plateau fractures. *Am J Roentgenol* 1984;142(6):1181–1186.

222. Rafii M, Firooznia H, Golimbu C, et al. Hematogenous osteomyelitis with fat-fluid level shown by CT. *Radiology* 1984; 153(2):493–494.

223. Rafii M, Minkoff J. Advanced arthrography of the shoulder with CT and MR imaging. *Radiol Clin North Am* 1998;36(4):609–633.

224. Ram PC, Martinez S, Korobkin M, et al. CT detection of intraosseous gas: a new sign of osteomyelitis. *Am J Roentgenol* 1981;137(4):721–723.

225. Renard M, Simonet J, Bencteux P, et al. Intermittent dislocation of the flexor hallucis longus tendon. *Skeletal Radiol* 2003;32(2): 78–81.

226. Resnick D. Additional congenital or heritable anomalies and syndromes. In: Resnick D, ed. *Diagnosis of bone and joint disorders*, 3rd ed. Philadelphia: W.B. Saunders, 1995; 4301.

227. Resnick D, Newell JD, Guerra J Jr, et al. Proximal tibiofibular joint: anatomic-pathologic-radiographic correlation. *Am J Roentgenol* 1978;131(1):133–138.

228. Resnik CS, Ammann AM, Walsh JW. Chronic septic arthritis of the adult hip: computed tomographic features. *Skeletal Radiol* 1987;16(7) 513–516.

229. Riddlesberger MM Jr. Computed tomography of the musculoskeletal system. *Radiol Clin North Am* 1981;19(3):463–477.

230. Rider LG. Outcome assessment in the adult and juvenile idiopathic inflammatory myopathies. *Rheum Dis Clin North Am* 2002;28(4):935–977.

231. Robbin MR, Murphey MD. Benign chondroid neoplasms of bone. *Semin Musculoskelet Radiol* 2000;4(1):45–58.

232. Robbin MR, Murphey MD, Temple HT, et al. Imaging of musculoskeletal fibromatosis. *Radiographics* 2001;21(3):585–600.

233. Robertson DD, Yuan J, Wang G, et al. Total hip prosthesis metal-artifact suppression using iterative deblurring reconstruction. *J Comput Assist Tomogr* 1997;21(2):293–298.

234. Robinson P, White LM. Soft-tissue and osseous impingement syndromes of the ankle: role of imaging in diagnosis and management. *Radiographics* 2002;22(6):1457–1469.

235. Rosenberg ZS, Cheung Y, Jahss MH, et al. Rupture of posterior tibial tendon: CT and MR imaging with surgical correlation. *Radiology* 1988;169(1):229–235.

236. Rosenthal DI, Aronow S, Murray WT. Iron content of pigmented villonodular synovitis detected by computed tomography. *Radiology* 1979;133(2):409–411.

237. Rosenthal DI, Hornicek FJ, Torriani M, et al. Osteoid osteoma: percutaneous treatment with radiofrequency energy. *Radiology* 2003;229(1):171–175.

238. Rosenthal DI, Hornicek FJ, Wolfe MW, et al. Percutaneous radiofrequency coagulation of osteoid osteoma compared with operative treatment. *J Bone Joint Surg [AM]* 1998;80(6):815–821.

239. Rosenthal DI, Springfield DS, Gebhardt MC, et al. Osteoid osteoma: percutaneous radio-frequency ablation. *Radiology* 1995;197(2):451–454.

240. Rozental TD, Khoury LD, Donthineni-Rao R, et al. Atypical lipomatous masses of the extremities: outcome of surgical treatment. *Clin Orthop* 2002;398:203–211.

241. Rydeberg J, Buckwalter KA, Caldemyer KS, et al. Multisection CT: scanning techniques and clinical applications. *Radiographics* 2000;20:1787–1806.

242. Sanders RK, Crim JR. Osteochondral injuries. *Semin Ultrasound CT MR* 2001;22(4):352–370.

243. Sanders WE. Evaluation of the humpback scaphoid by computed tomography in the longitudinal axial plane of the scaphoid. *J Hand Surg [Am]* 1988;13(2):182–187.

244. Sans N, Galy-Fourcade D, Assoun J, et al. Osteoid osteoma: CT-guided percutaneous resection and follow-up in 38 patients. *Radiology* 1999;212(3):687–692.

245. Santiago Restrepo C, Gimenez CR, McCarthy K. Imaging of osteomyelitis and musculoskeletal soft tissue infections: current concepts. *Rheum Dis Clin North Am* 2003;29(1):89–109.

246. Sartoris DJ, Kursunoglu S, Pineda C, et al. Detection of intra-articular osteochondral bodies in the knee using computed arthrotomography. *Radiology* 1985;155(2):447–450.

247. Schaefer O, Lohrmann C, Herling M, et al. Combined radiofrequency thermal ablation and percutaneous cementoplasty treatment of a pathologic fracture. *J Vasc Intervent Radiol* 2002; 13(10):1047–1050.

248. Scheck RJ, Romagnolo A, Hierner R, et al. The carpal ligaments in MR arthrography of the wrist: correlation with standard MRI and wrist arthroscopy. *J Magn Reson Imaging* 1999;9(3):468–474.

249. Schmitt R, Heinze A, Fillner F, et al. Imaging and staging of avascular osteonecroses at the wrist and hand. *Eur J Radiol* 1997; 25(2):92–103.

250. Schreiman JS, Crass JR, Wick MR, et al. Osteosarcoma: role of CT in limb-sparing treatment. *Radiology* 1986;161(2):485–488.

251. Schweitzer ME, Gannon FH, Deely DM, et al. Percutaneous skeletal aspiration and core biopsy: complementary techniques. *Am J Roentgenol* 1996;166(2):415–418.

252. Sciulli RL, Boutin RD, Brown RR, et al. Evaluation of the postoperative meniscus of the knee: a study comparing conventional arthrography, conventional MR imaging, MR arthrography with iodinated contrast material, and MR arthrography with gadolinium-based contrast material. *Skeletal Radiol* 1999;28(9):508–514.

253. Seinsheimer F III. Fractures of the distal femur. *Clin Orthop* 1980;153:169–179.

254. Shagam JY. Bone densitometry: an update. *Radiol Technol* 2003;74(4):321–338.

255. Sheafor DH, Paulson EK, Kliewer MA, et al. Comparison of sonographic and CT guidance techniques: does CT fluoroscopy decrease procedure time. *Am J Roentgenol* 2000;174(4):939–942.

256. Siebert W, Mai S, Kober R, et al. Technique and first clinical results of robot-assisted total knee replacement. *Knee* 2002;9:73–80.

257. Silverman SG, Tuncali K, Adams DF, et al. CT fluoroscopy-guided abdominal interventions: techniques, results, and radiation exposure. *Radiology* 1999;212(3):673–681.

258. Simon MA. Biopsy of musculoskeletal tumors. *J Bone Joint Surg [AM]* 1982;64:1253–1257.

259. Singson RD, Feldman F, Rosenberg ZS. Elbow joint: assessment with double-contrast CT arthrography. *Radiology* 1986;160(1):167–173.

260. Sirkin M, Sanders RK. The treatment of pilon fractures. *Orthop Clin North Am* 2001;32(1):91–102.

261. Skrzynski MC, Biermann JS, Montag A, et al. Diagnostic accuracy and charge-savings of outpatient core needle biopsy compared with open biopsy of musculoskeletal tumors. *J Bone Joint Surg [AM]* 1996;78(5):644–649.

262. Snedden MH, Shea JP. Diastasis with low distal fibula fractures: an anatomic rationale. *Clin Orthop* 2001;382:197–205.

263. Spaeth HJ, Chandnani VP, Beltran J, et al. Magnetic resonance imaging detection of early experimental periostitis. Comparison of magnetic resonance imaging, computed tomography, and plain radiography with histopathologic correlation. *Investigative Radiology* 1991;26(4):304–308.

264. Spitz DJ, Newberg AH. Imaging of stress fractures in the athlete. *Radiol Clin North Am* 2002;40(2):313–331.

265. Stallmeyer MJ, Ortiz AO. Facet blocks and sacroiliac joint injections. *Techniques in Vascular & Interventional Radiology* 2002;5(4):201–206.

266. Steinbach LS, Schwartz M. Elbow arthrography. *Radiol Clin North Am* 1998;36(4):635–649.

267. Stevens K, Tao C, Lee SU, et al. Subchondral fractures in osteonecrosis of the femoral head: comparison of radiography, CT, and MR imaging. *Am J Roentgenol* 2003;180(2):363–368.

268. Stevens MA, El-Khoury GY, Kathol MH, et al. Imaging features of avulsion injuries. *Radiographics* 1999;19(3):655–672.

269. Stewart NR, Gilula LA. CT of the wrist: a tailored approach. *Radiology* 1992;183(1):13–20.

270. Stindel E, Briard JL, Merloz P, et al. Bone morphing: 3D morphological data for total knee arthroplasty. *Comput Aided Surg* 2002;7(3):156–168.

271. Struk DW, Munk PL, Lee MJ, et al. Imaging of soft tissue infections. *Radiol Clin North Am* 2001;39(2):277–303.

272. Sturzenbecher A, Braun J, Paris S, et al. MR imaging of septic sacroiliitis. *Skeletal Radiol* 2000;29(8):439–446.

273. Sugimoto H, Tamura K, Fujii T. The SAPHO syndrome: defining the radiologic spectrum of diseases comprising the syndrome. *Eur Radiol* 1998;8(5):800–806.

274. Sundaram M, McGuire MH, Herbold DR. Magnetic resonance imaging of soft tissue masses: an evaluation of fifty-three histologically proven tumors. *Magn Reson Imaging* 1988;6(3):237–248.

275. Tay VK, Fitridge R, Tie ML. Computed tomography fluoroscopy-guided chemical lumbar sympathectomy: simple, safe and effective. *Australas Radiol* 2002;46(2):163–166.

276. Teeuwisse WM, Geleijns J, Broerse JJ, et al. Patient and staff dose during CT guided biopsy, drainage and coagulation. *Br J Radiol* 2001;74(884):720–726.

277. Tehranzadeh J, Mnaymneh W, Ghavam C, et al. Comparison of CT and MR imaging in musculoskeletal neoplasms. *J Comput Assist Tomogr* 1989;13(3):466–472.

278. Theodorou DJ, Theodorou SJ, Kakitsubata Y, et al. Fractures of proximal portion of fifth metatarsal bone: anatomic and imaging evidence of a pathogenesis of avulsion of the plantar aponeurosis and the short peroneal muscle tendon. *Radiology* 2003;226(3):857–865.

279. Thermann H, Krettek C, Hufner T, et al. Management of calcaneal fracturin adults. Conservative versus operative treatment. *Clin Orthop* 1998;353:107–124.

280. Tornetta P III, Gorup J. Axial computed tomography of pilon fractures. *Clin Orthop* 1996;323:273–276.

281. Totty WG, Murphy WA, Lee JK. Soft-tissue tumors: MR imaging. *Radiology* 1986;160(1):135–141.

282. Tscherne H, Lobenhoffer P. Tibial plateau fractures. Management and expected results. *Clin Orthop* 1993;292:87–100.

283. Tuite MJ, Rubin D. CT and MR Arthrography of the glenoid labroligamentous complex. *Semin Musculoskelet Radiol* 1998;2(4):363–376.

284. Uetani M, Hashmi R, Ito M, et al. Subchondral insufficiency fracture of the femoral head: magnetic resonance imaging findings correlated with micro-computed tomography and histopathology. *J Comput Assist Tomogr* 2003;27(2):189–193.

285. Vande Berg BC, Lecouvet FE, Poilvache P, et al. Dual-detector spiral CT arthrography of the knee: accuracy for detection of meniscal abnormalities and unstable meniscal tears. *Radiology* 2000;216(3):851–857.

286. Vande Berg BC, Lecouvet FE, Poilvache P, et al. Anterior cruciate ligament tears and associated meniscal lesions: assessment at dual-detector spiral CT arthrography. *Radiology* 2002;223(2):403–409.

287. Vande Berg BC, Lecouvet FE, Poilvache P, et al. Assessment of knee cartilage in cadavers with dual-detector spiral CT arthrography and MR imaging. *Radiology* 2002;222(2):430–436.

288. Vande Berg BC, Lecouvet FE, Poilvache P, et al. Spiral CT arthrography of the knee: technique and value in the assessment of internal derangement of the knee. *Eur Radiol* 2002;12(7):1800–1810.

289. Vanderschueren GM, Taminiau AH, Obermann WR, et al. Osteoid osteoma: clinical results with thermocoagulation. *Radiology* 2002;224(1):82–86.

290. Vannier MW, Hildebolt CF, Gilula LA, et al. Calcaneal and pelvic fractures: diagnostic evaluation by three-dimensional computed tomography scans. *J Digit Imaging* 1991;4(3):143–152.

291. Venbrux AC, Montague BJ, Murphy KP, et al. Image-guided percutaneous radiofrequency ablation for osteoid osteomas. *J Vasc Intervent Radiol* 2003;14(3):375–380.

292. Wadia N, Desai S, Bhatt M. Disseminated cysticercosis. New observations, including CT scan findings and experience with treatment by praziquantel. *Brain* 1988;111(Pt 3):597–614.

293. Wagner AL, Murtagh FR. Selective nerve root blocks. *Techniques in Vascular and Interventional Radiology* 2002;5(4):194–200.

294. Wang G, Frei T, Vannier MW. Fast iterative algorithm for metal artifact reduction in x-ray CT. *Acad Radiol* 2000;7(8):607–614.

295. Ward WG Sr, Kilpatrick S. Fine needle aspiration biopsy of primary bone tumors. *Clin Orthop* 2000;373:80–87.

296. Watson JT, Moed BR, Karges DE, et al. Pilon fractures. Treatment protocol based on severity of soft tissue injury. *Clin Orthop* 2000;375:78–90.

297. Wechsler RJ, Schweitzer ME, Karasick D, et al. Helical CT of calcaneal fractures: technique and imaging features. *Skeletal Radiol* 1998;27(1):1–6.

298. Weekes RG, McLeod RA, Reiman HM, et al. CT of soft-tissue neoplasms. *Am J Roentgenol* 1985;144(2):355–360.

299. Wehrli FW, Hopkins JA, Hwang SN, et al. Cross-sectional study of osteopenia with quantitative MR imaging and bone densitometry. *Radiology* 2000;217(2):527–538.

300. Weishaupt D, Zanetti M, Nyffeler RW, et al. Posterior glenoid rim deficiency in recurrent (atraumatic) posterior shoulder instability. *Skeletal Radiol* 2000;29(4):204–210.

301. White LM, Buckwalter KA. Technical considerations: CT and MR imaging in the postoperative orthopedic patient. *Semin Musculoskelet Radiol* 2002;6(1):5–17.

302. White MS. Three-dimensional computed tomography in the assessment of fractures of the acetabulum. *Injury* 1991;22(1):13–19.

303. Wicky S, Blaser PF, Blanc CH, et al. Comparison between standard radiography and spiral CT with 3D reconstruction in the evaluation, classification and management of tibial plateau fractures. *Eur Radiol* 2000;10:1227–1232.

304. Wing VW, Jeffrey RB Jr, Federle MP, et al. Chronic osteomyelitis examined by CT. *Radiology* 1985;154(1):171–174.

305. Wittram C, Whitehouse GH, Williams JW, et al. A comparison of MR and CT in suspected sacroiliitis. *J Comput Assist Tomogr* 1996;20(1):68–72.

306. Woertler K, Vestring T, Boettner F, et al. Osteoid osteoma: CT-guided percutaneous radiofrequency ablation and follow-up in 47 patients. *J Vasc Intervent Radiol* 2001;12(6):717–722.

307. Wunderbaldinger P, Bremer C, Schellenberger E, et al. Imaging features of iliopsoas bursitis. *Eur Radiol* 2002;12(2):409–415.

308. Yacoubian SV, Nevins RT, Sallis JG, et al. Impact of MRI on treatment plan and fracture classification of tibial plateau fractures. *J Orthop Trauma* 2002;16:632–637.

309. Yamaguchi T, Dortman HD. Radiographic and histologic patterns of calcification in chondromyxoid fibroma. *Skeletal Radiol* 1998;27(10):559–564.

310. Yamamato T, Kurosaka M, Soejima T, et al. Contrast-enhanced three-dimensional helical CT for soft tissue tumors in the extremities. *Skeletal Radiol* 2001;30(7):384–387.

311. Yao L, Eckardt JJ, Seeger LL. Fibrous dysplasia associated with cortical bony destruction: CT and MR findings. *J Comput Assist Tomogr* 1994;18(1):91–94.

312. Yao L, Nelson SD, Seeger LL, et al. Primary musculoskeletal neoplasms: effectiveness of core-needle biopsy. *Radiology* 1999;212(3):682–686.

313. Young JW. Pelvic Injuries. *Semin Musculoskelet Radiol* 1998;2(1):83–104.

314. Ziran BH, Smith WR, Towers J, et al. Iliosacral screw fixation of the posterior pelvic ring using local anaesthesia and computerised tomography. *J Bone Joint Surg* 2003;85(3):411–418.

315. Zornoza J, Bernardino ME, Ordonez NG, et al. Percutaneous needle biopsy of soft tissue tumors guided by ultrasound and computed tomography. *Skeletal Radiol* 1982;9(1):33–36.

The Spine

23

Zoran Rumboldt   Mauricio Castillo   J. Keith Smith

Magnetic resonance imaging (MRI) has become the modality of choice for evaluating the spine in a majority of clinical settings; however, computed tomography (CT) and MRI frequently provide complementary information. CT is generally better for assessment of cortical bone and trabeculae, while MRI is superior for analyzing soft tissues and bone marrow. This chapter presents an overview of spinal anatomy and the common pathologic entities that affect it. Congenital abnormalities and disorders that occur primarily in the meninges, subarachnoid spaces, and spinal cord are beyond the scope of this chapter and will not be discussed.

NORMAL ANATOMY

Cervical Spine

The cervical spine is composed of seven vertebrae. The first two differ in embryologic origin from the rest of the cervical spine and are best considered as part of the craniovertebral (or craniocervical) junction (CVJ) (Fig. 23-1A).

The anterior arch of C1 (atlas) contains a small ventral tubercle to which the anterior longitudinal ligament (ALL) attaches. The atlas and occiput are connected by anterior and posterior atlanto-occipital membranes. The transverse ligament (TL) extends between the two tubercles on the inner aspect of the anterior arch of C1 (Fig. 23-1B). The anterior arch continues laterally and joins the superior facets and lateral masses. The bulky lateral masses form the articular surfaces, contain the transverse foramina, and give origin to the transverse processes. C1 is completed by a posterior arch.

The second cervical vertebra (axis) has the most complex development of all vertebrae. It is formed from five primary (two for neural arches, two for odontoid process, and one for body) and one secondary (apex of the odontoid process) ossification centers. The dens is connected to the clivus by the medial apical ligament and paired lateral alar ligaments (Figs. 23-1C and 23-1D). The dens is held in apposition to the posterior surface of the anterior arch of C1 by the TL (Figs. 23-1E and 23-1F). The TL, together with longitudinal fibers extending from the axis to the occiput is referred to as the cruciform ligament. The anterior atlantoaxial ligament is located posterior to the ALL. The atlantodental space should not exceed 4 to 5 mm in children and 2 mm in adults (74).

Laterally, the vertebral body joins the transverse processes, which form the anterior margins of the transverse foramina. The medial and posterior margins of the transverse foramina are formed by the pedicles and the laminae. The laminae join posteriorly at the base of the spinous process.

Cervical vertebrae C3–C7 are derived from somites 7 to 12, and all have similar anatomic features. These vertebral bodies contain the uncinate processes (which form the uncovertebral joints) in their posterolateral margins. The uncovertebral joints contain loose areolar tissue or a synovial lining. They form the ventromedial margins of the neural foramina. The size of the vertebral bodies increases progressively from C3 to C7 (Figs. 23-2A and 23-2B). In their mid and dorsal portions, the vertebral bodies contain the basivertebral vein canal. All pedicles are short structures formed from cortical bone, which connect the vertebral bodies to the articular pillars (Fig. 23-2C). The articular pillars are composed of the inferior articular facet of one vertebra and the superior facet of the underlying vertebra. On axial images, the anteriorly located facet is the superior facet of the lower vertebra, whereas the posterior one is the inferior facet of the upper vertebra (Fig. 23-2D). The inferior articular facets join the laminae, which in turn join the spinous process. The spinous process of C7 is the largest in the cervical spine.

All cervical neural foramina are oriented in a 45-degree plane with respect to the vertebral bodies (24) (Fig. 23-2D). Although the anteroposterior diameter of the cervical spinal canal decreases from C3 through C7, 12 mm is considered to be the lower limit of normal in the cervical region. It is important to remember that there are eight pairs of cervical nerve roots. Each pair exits cephalad to its respective vertebral body. The C8 nerve roots exit at the C7–T1 neural foramina.

Thoracic Spine

The thoracic spine is composed of 12 vertebrae (Figs. 23-3A and 23-3B). The posterior ribs articulate with the vertebral bodies posterolaterally. The pedicles arise from the superior posterior aspect of the vertebral bodies and form

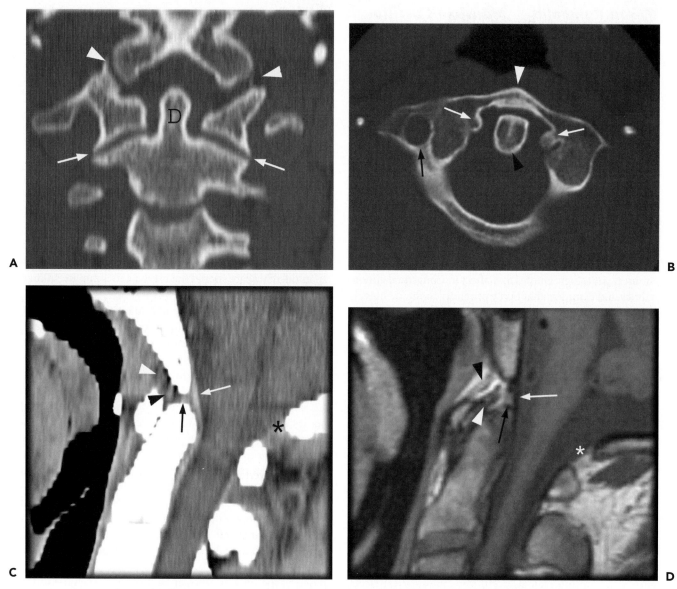

Figure 23-1 Normal craniovertebral junction (CVJ). **A:** Reformatted coronal CT image shows atlantoaxial (*arrowheads*) and atlanto-occipital (*arrows*) articulations. D, dens (odontoid process). **B:** Axial CT image at the level of C1 shows the anterior tubercle (*white arrowhead*) and very prominent tubercules on the inner aspect of the anterior arch (*white arrows*) representing the attachment of the transverse ligament. Right foramen transversarium (*black arrow*) for the vertebral artery and the dens (*black arrowhead*) are also seen. **C:** Reformatted midsagittal CT image demonstrates the main ligaments of the CVJ. The anterior atlanto-occipital membrane (*white arrowhead*), alar ligaments (*black arrowhead*), apical ligament (*black arrow*), and tectorial membrane (*white arrow*) are found anteriorly, while the posterior atlanto-occipital membrane (*) corresponds to the ligamenta flava between the vertebral bodies. **D:** Midsagittal T1-weighted image in a different patient shows the same structures: anterior atlanto-occipital membrane (*black arrowhead*), alar ligaments (*white arrowhead*), apical ligament (*black arrow*), tectorial membrane (*white arrow*), and posterior atlanto-occipital membrane (*).

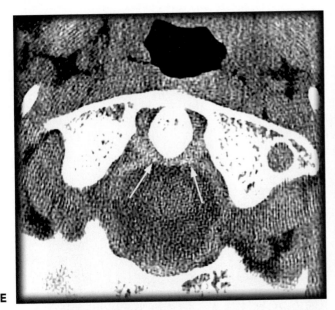
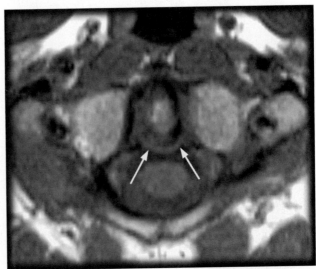

Figure 23-1 (*continued*) **E:** Axial CT image reveals the transverse ligament (*white arrows*) at the posterior aspect of the dens. **F:** The transverse ligament (*white arrows*) is well visualized on an axial T1-weighted image.

the superior and inferior margins of the neural foramina. The neural foramina are oriented laterally (Fig. 23-3C). The pedicles continue laterally with the transverse processes, which are located immediately posterior to the corresponding rib. The laminae originate from the dorsal aspects of the transverse processes and join posteriorly to form the spinous process. The superior articular facet is located at the junction between pedicle and lamina. The inferior facet arises from the lateral end of the lamina. The articular surfaces of both facets are flat. On axial images, the superior facet of the underlying vertebra is located anteriorly, and the inferior facet of the corresponding vertebra is located posteriorly. The spinal canal narrows slightly in the midthoracic region. The anteroposterior diameter of the thoracic spine is abnormal if less than 10 mm (36).

Lumbar Spine

The lumbar spine generally has five vertebrae; however, transitional vertebrae are common. Thus, the total number of vertebrae may vary between four and six. The lumbar vertebral bodies are massive and are larger in their transverse than in their anteroposterior dimension. The lumbar vertebral bodies are traversed by one or two venous channels in their mid portion. Thick pedicles are formed from dense cortical bone (Figs. 23-4A and 23-4B). As in the thoracic spine, the pedicles arise from the superior posterior vertebral body and form the superior and inferior margins of the neural foramina. The laminae are flat and join to

form the spinous process, and they do not overlap with each other (as they do in the thoracic spine). The transverse processes of L1 and L5 tend to be somewhat larger than those of other lumbar vertebrae. Again, on axial images, the superior articular facet of the vertebra below is seen anteriorly, whereas the inferior facet is located posteriorly. The neural foramina are oriented laterally (Figs. 23-4C and 23-4D). The L5 vertebral body may be identified on axial images by the lemon-like shape of its most caudal aspects (Fig. 23-4E). The anteroposterior diameter of the lumbar spinal canal increases caudally and should be considered abnormal if less than 12 mm. In the lumbar spine (as in the thoracic region), the nerve roots exit at their corresponding vertebrae. That is, the L3 nerve roots exit at the L3–L4 neural foramina.

Sacrum and Coccyx

The sacrum is formed by five fused vertebrae that contain residual disc spaces between them. The L5 vertebra may be fused to S1. The single median crest is flanked by the smaller intermediate crests. Located lateral to the intermediate crests are four paired neural foramina, which point anteriorly. The coccyx is generally formed by 3 to 5 articulating segments.

Special Imaging Features

On CT, all vertebral bodies are surrounded by well-demarcated cortical bone. The vertebral bodies contain fine

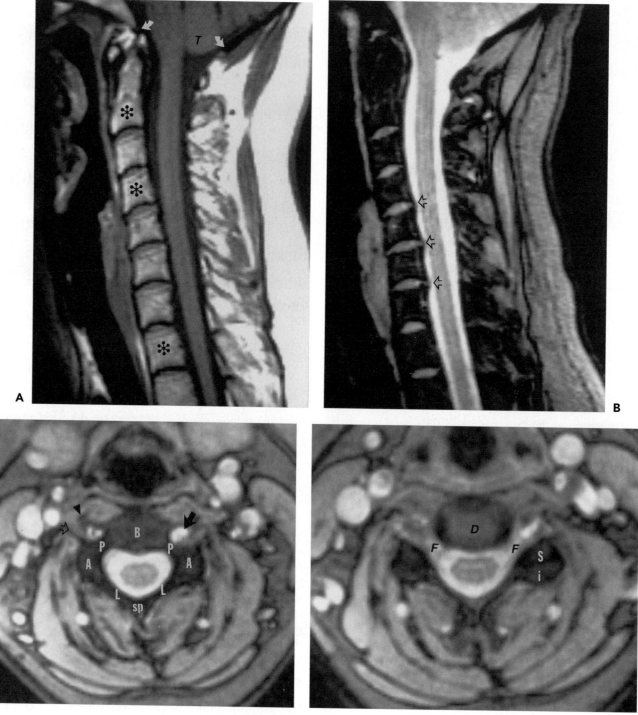

Figure 23-2 Normal cervical spine. **A:** Midsagittal T1-weighted image shows normal high signal intensity (*asterisks*) from vertebral bodies due to normal fatty bone marrow. The diameter of spinal cord decreases slightly and progressively from C3–C7. Cerebellar tonsils are above the foramen magnum (*arrows*). Signal intensity from discs is always less than that of the vertebral bodies. T, cerebellar tonsils. **B:** Midsagittal gradient echo T2*-weighted image shows the normal bone marrow to have low signal intensity. The discs are relatively bright. Spinal cord is normal in diameter and signal intensity. Minimal degenerative changes at C5–C7 (*arrows*) are seen. **C:** Axial gradient echo T2*-weighted image of a normal C5 vertebra. *Arrow,* flow-related enhancement in a vertebral artery coursing in the foramen transversarium; *arrowhead,* anterior tubercle of transverse process; *open arrow,* posterior tubercle of transverse process; B, vertebral body; P, pedicles; A, articular pillars; L, laminae; sp, spinous process. **D:** Axial gradient echo T2-weighted image at a normal C4–C5 disc space. Neural foramina are oriented in a 45-degree angle with respect to the vertebral body and thus are not clearly seen in the sagittal plane. The superior facet of C5 is located anteriorly, and the inferior facet of C4 is posterior. D, disc; F, neural foramina; S, superior articular facet; i, inferior articular facet.

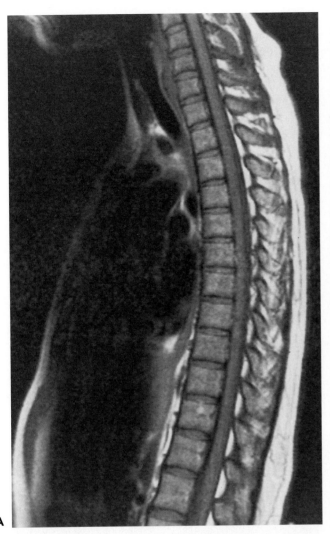

A

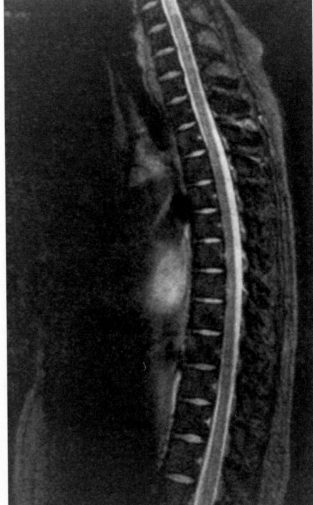

B

Figure 23-3 Normal thoracic spine. **A:** Midsagittal T1-weighted image obtained with the body coil, a high-resolution rectangular matrix (256 × 512) and a 50-cm FOV. This sequence allows for adequate visualization of the majority of the spinal cord. In cases of suspected cord compression, the cervical spine may be imaged with a dedicated surface coil. **B:** Midsagittal T2-weighted image shows normal bright discs, low signal intensity from bone marrow, and normal spinal cord. **C:** Axial T1-weighted image obtained through midthoracic vertebra. C, spinal cord; S, superior articular facet; i, inferior articular facet; L, lamina; sp, spinous process. The neural foramina (*curved arrows*) are oriented laterally. A spinal nerve root (*arrowhead*) is well seen. *Open arrow,* joint space.

C

bone trabeculae traversing the marrow space. These trabeculae are more prominent in the lumbar region. The pedicles and transverse processes are well corticated and contain little cancellous bone. The laminae and spinous processes in the cervical and thoracic spine contain cancellous bone; however, in the lumbar region they generally appear as single bony plates. The articular surfaces of the facets, which are dense and smooth, are generally biconvex in the cervical spine but flat in the thoracic and lumbar regions (Fig. 23-4C). The intervertebral discs are of homogeneous soft tissue density (50 to 100 HU) on CT, and the annulus fibrosus cannot be separated from the nucleus pulposus. The ligamentum flavum (LF), which is also of soft tissue density, joins the interlaminar spaces (see Figs. 23-4C and 23-4D). In the lumbar spine, the LF normally measures 3 to 5 mm and is considered thickened or buckled if larger than 5 mm. The posterior lon-

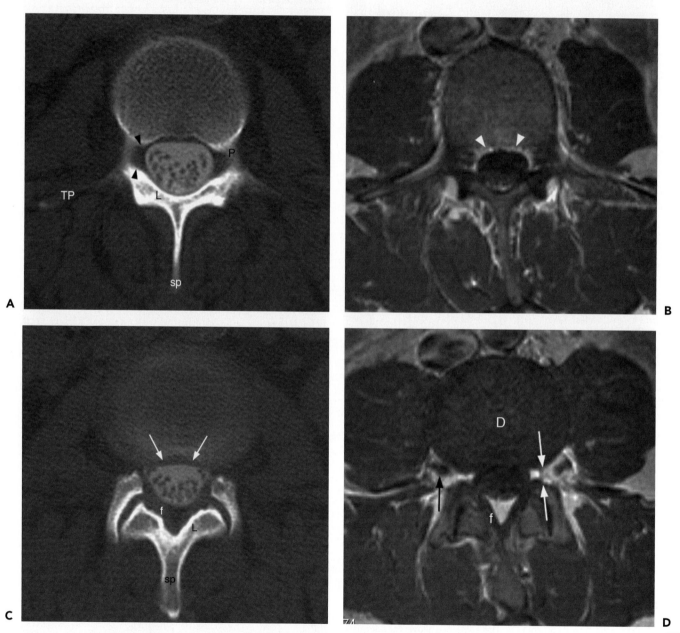

Figure 23-4   Normal lumbar spine. **A:** Postmyelogram axial computed tomography (CT) scan (bone windows) at L3. Nerve roots are seen as discrete round filling defects floating in opacified cerebrospinal fluid (CSF). Arrowheads, lateral recess; P, pedicle; T, transverse process; L, lamina; SP, spinous process. **B:** Axial T1-weighted image at L4 shows bright ventral epidural fat (*arrowheads*) creating a contrast between bone and CSF. **C:** Axial postmyelogram CT shows normal concavity of L3 to L4 disc (*arrows*) in its central portion. SP, spinous process; L, lamina; f, ligamentum flavum. **D:** Axial T1-weighted image at the L3 to L4 disc space. The neural foramina (*white arrows*) are oriented laterally and well imaged in sagittal sequences. The dorsal root ganglia (*black arrow*) are well seen and normally enhance after contrast administration. D, disc; f, ligamentum flavum.

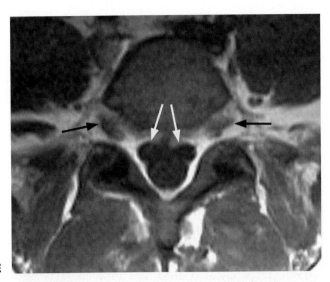

E

Figure 23-4 *(continued)* **E:** Axial T1-weighted image at L5. The vertebral body is characteristically lemon shaped. The L5 dorsal root ganglia (*black arrows*) and sleeves around the S1 nerve roots (*white arrows*) are well visualized.

gitudinal ligament (PLL) is contained in the ventral epidural space together with fat and blood vessels. The fat in the ventral epidural space extends into the lateral recesses, which carry the nerve roots into the neural foramina. In the lumbar region, the lateral recesses are bordered anteriorly by the vertebral bodies, laterally by the pedicles, and posteriorly by the superior articular facets (see Fig. 23-4A). The lateral recesses normally measure 3 to 5 mm and are considered narrowed if less than 3 mm.

On MRI, the vertebral cortex appears as an area of low signal intensity due to lack of mobile protons. Fatty marrow produces high signal intensity on T1-weighted spin echo and T2-weighted fast spin echo (FSE) images. However, patchy bone marrow may be seen at any age and by itself should not be considered pathologic (84). On T2-weighted spin echo or gradient echo images, the vertebral bodies are of low signal intensity (see Figs. 23-2B and 23-3B). However, they are of intermediate to high signal intensity with fast spin echo (FSE) sequences, which are most commonly performed due to their superior image quality along with decreased imaging time. Normal bone marrow enhances homogeneously after intravenous administration of gadolinium. The normal intervertebral discs are of similar or slightly lower signal intensity than marrow on T1-weighted images (18) (see Figs. 23-2A and 23-3A) and of higher signal intensity on T2-weighted images (see Fig. 23-3B). In the normal disc, the annulus fibrosus may be seen as a subtle and peripheral region of lower signal intensity on all T2-weighted sequences (76). The nucleus pulposus is of higher signal intensity and is traversed horizontally by a dark line that probably represents the normal internuclear cleft (2,76). The internuclear cleft is seen in more than 94% of patients 30 years of age or older (2). The ligaments are dark

on T2-weighted images and are usually inseparable from the cortical bone. The purpose of all T2-weighted sequences (in addition to detection of spinal cord lesions) is to provide a myelographic effect by making the cerebrospinal fluid (CSF) appear bright (see Figs. 23-2C and 23-2D). If FSE sequences are used, the bright CSF may be inseparable from adjacent fat-containing structures, and fat-suppression techniques may be needed to distinguish them.

IMAGING PROTOCOLS

Cervical Spine

Computed Tomography

For examination of degenerative disorders, on a multislice scanner we acquire 3-mm-thick contiguous sections C3 through T1. We reconstruct these at 2-mm-thick sections and do sagittal reformations at 1-mm-thick sections. In this type of scanner, pitch is not an issue as it is in single-slice spiral CT. If single-slice spiral CT is used, a pitch of 1 is recommended (acquire by 3-mm and reconstruct by 3-mm thicknesses). For trauma in the cervical spine, we cover the entire area (C1 to C7) and additionally perform coronal and sagittal 1-mm-thick reformations. For trauma in other regions, we scan the region of interest and obtain sagittal and coronal reformations too. All images are viewed using soft tissue and bone algorithm and window settings.

Magnetic Resonance Imaging

Sagittal T1-weighted spin echo images [500 to 600/15/2 (TR/TE/number of excitations)] are obtained initially with a field-of-view (FOV) of 270 to 280 mm and 3- to 4-mm sections with a 10% intersection gap, usually using a 256 × 256 matrix. This is followed by sagittal T2-weighted FSE images (3,000 to 4,000/80 to 120/1) with an echo train of 4 to 8 using the same FOV and section thickness, preferably with a 512 × 256 matrix. For the cervical spine, axial gradient echo T2*-weighted low-flip angle (25 degrees to 30 degrees) images (650 to 850/20/2) using FOV of 180 to 200 mm, and a 3- or 4-mm section thickness with a 0.4- to 0.6-mm intersection gap, are generally also obtained from C3 to T1. The gradient echo technique is preferred to fast spin echo sequences, which in the cervical and thoracic spine are commonly hampered by CSF flow artifacts. In patients with infection or tumor, precontrast axial T1-weighted images, as well as sagittal and axial T1-weighted postcontrast images, are performed. Administering gadolinium in the postoperative cervical spine is controversial because epidural scar formation does not occur. Gadolinium administration may be helpful to delineate questionable disc herniations.

Thoracic Spine

Computed Tomography

We use the same protocol described for the cervical spine. If only an area of interest will be imaged (and not the entire thoracic spine), then we scan one level above and below the lesion.

Magnetic Resonance Imaging

Sagittal T1-weighted images (600/15/2) are obtained first with an FOV of 250 to 300 mm and 4-mm section thickness with 0.4-mm intersection gap. This is followed by sagittal T2-weighted FSE images (3,500/90/1) with an echo train of 4 to 8, using the same FOV and section thickness, again preferably with a 512 × 256 matrix. Axial low flip angle (25 degrees to 30 degrees) images (650/20/2) are obtained with an FOV of 200 mm and 3- to 4-mm section thickness with 0.4- to 0.6-mm intersection gap. Axial T1-weighted images and sagittal and axial T1-weighted images after administration of gadolinium are obtained when indicated.

Lumbar Spine

Computed Tomography

Stacked (i.e., no angle) 2-mm sections are obtained from top of L3 through S1. Sagittal reformations are routinely performed at 1-mm thickness.

Magnetic Resonance Imaging

Sagittal T1-weighted images (600/15/2) are obtained first with an FOV of 250 mm and 4-mm section thickness with 0.4-mm intersection gap. These images are followed by sagittal T2-weighted FSE images (3,500/90/1) with an echo train of four, using the identical FOV and section thickness as described earlier. CSF flow artifacts are generally absent in the lumbar spine, so FSE is the preferred sequence for acquiring stacked axial images (3,000 to 4,000/90/1) from L3 through S1 with a FOV of 200, 512 × 256 matrix, and 4-mm section thickness with 0.4-mm intersection gap. Stacked axial T1-weighted images (650/15/2) are also obtained with a FOV of 200 mm and a 256 × 256 matrix. After intravenous administration of gadolinium, axial and sagittal T1-weighted images are obtained immediately after the injection. If the sacrum is to be studied, axial and coronal T1-weighted and T2-weighted sequences are useful.

If spinal cord compression is a consideration, the entire spine may be screened using a body coil or a multiple array coil. Sagittal T1-weighted images (560/18/4) are obtained with an FOV of 500 mm, 4-mm section thickness with 0.4-mm intersection gap, and a rectangular matrix of 256 × 512. These images can be obtained in approximately 9.5 minutes and include the base of the skull through L2. Low flip angle T2*-weighted gradient echo images (560/18/4/15), using the same FOV and section thickness as above, may be obtained in a similar amount of time. It is important to overlap the scans or to mark the skin of the patient (generally with a vitamin E capsule) to be able to count the vertebrae and localize a lesion. If bone lesions are suspected, such as in trauma, metastatic or primary bone tumors, fat-suppression techniques are added. These techniques include STIR (short tau inversion recov-

ery) as a T2-weighted sequence and frequency-selective fat saturation (commonly referred to as FatSat) for T1-weighted postcontrast images. Diffusion-weighted images (DWI) may be valuable in differentiating benign osteoporotic vertebral fractures from pathologic compression fractures (16).

For evaluation of extramedullary disease, intravenous gadolinium administration is recommended in patients with suspected infection, tumor, vascular malformations, and failed back surgery syndrome (epidural fibrosis versus recurrent herniated disc) (11,41,63,87,107). Gadolinium-enhanced MRI is also useful for highlighting nerve root abnormalities in unoperated lumbar spines (44). In general, all gadolinium compounds are administered at a standard dose of 0.1 mmol/kg. Increasing the dose of gadolinium to 0.3 mmol/kg may accentuate contrast enhancement of diseased areas and cause normal nerve roots to enhance (71).

ADVANTAGES AND DISADVANTAGES OF COMPUTED TOMOGRAPHY AND MAGNETIC RESONANCE IMAGING

All patients with frank and uncomplicated radiculopathy, whose symptoms are not relieved after 6 weeks of conservative treatment, may undergo either CT or MRI if surgery is being considered. If signs of intrinsic spinal cord lesions are present, MRI is preferred. In evaluating the postoperative spine, MRI (85% accuracy) is superior to CT (43% to 60% accuracy) for distinguishing scar tissue from disc (29). MRI is also the method of choice for evaluating infections and congenital anomalies, especially when a tethered cord is suspected. If a soft tissue tumor is suspected, MRI is preferred; if a bone tumor is suspected, CT is usually obtained.

Overall, CT and MRI are comparable in their ability to detect disc herniation. CT has greater than 90% accuracy (65). In one series, MRI detected 93% of all herniated discs (117).

Minor disadvantages of CT compared with MRI include nonvisualization of the spinal cord and other soft tissues (such as ligaments), the use of ionizing radiation, and occasionally, the need for iodinated contrast media. The inability of CT to scan in more than one plane is essentially not a disadvantage with multidetector scanners because high-quality reformations are easily obtained. On the other hand, MRI may not always be readily available, and the examination is generally more expensive and more time-consuming. Furthermore, patients with ferromagnetic intracranial aneurysm clips, cardiac pacemakers, cochlear implants, and nerve stimulators cannot undergo MRI. In addition, approximately 5% to 10% of patients are claustrophobic and are unable to tolerate MRI without sedation. Also, standard MRI in patients with spinal fusion hardware is frequently distorted, rendering the studies nondiagnostic. Single-shot FSE T2-weighted sequences, also known as HASTE, are less susceptible to metallic artifacts and in some cases provide images of diagnostic quality. Parallel MRI acquisition also decreases these artifacts. By using multidetector CT with very thin sections, most metal artifacts are minimized and thus the use of postmyelography CT is gradually increasing again.

It has recently been shown that a limited MRI protocol consisting of T1-weighted and STIR images in the sagittal plane may be the imaging modality of choice in patients with low back pain without radiculopathy that are unresponsive to conservative treatment. This limited protocol is sensitive to abnormalities (mostly fractures, pars defects, and tumors), its total acquisition time is approximately 6 minutes, and it has replaced radiographs at some institutions (61). Again, fast acquisition of routine studies in very short times using parallel imaging acquisition may negate the use of these abbreviated protocols.

SPINAL TRAUMA

Complementary roles of CT and MRI for the evaluation of spinal disorders are probably most evident in the assessment of trauma. Multidetector CT scanners provide axial images and high-quality reconstructions in any plane, allowing for precise delineation of fractures and visualization of bone fragments. Multiplanar reformatting of CT data has a crucial role in the assessment of injury, especially in the cervical spine. The fractures are better demonstrated by CT than by MRI, in particular when the posterior elements are affected (52).

MRI reveals injuries to the ligaments, intervertebral discs, and microfractures (also known as bone contusions or bruises). It also clearly shows spinal cord injury, intraspinal hematomas, and traumatic dissections of vertebral arteries (90). This is best accomplished with the STIR sequence, which should be included in all spinal trauma MRI protocols. This sequence is also used to determine whether an abnormal vertebral body is an acute injury or a long-standing one. Indications for MRI in trauma include neurologic deficit(s) or an injury with a potential to produce neurologic deficit. It has recently been reported that unsuspected vertebral body microfractures are found in over 40% of spinal injury patients (80).

The sensitivity and specificity of MRI in the detection of traumatic injuries to the ligaments and discs remain far from perfect. It has been shown that even high-resolution MRI of cervical spine specimens from trauma victims failed to reveal many lesions and that asymmetry of the alar ligaments, for instance, was found to be a frequent normal finding (77,102).

Upper Cervical Spine Fractures

The CVJ is well adapted to provide a remarkable range of motion, with approximately one half of neck rotation occurring at the C1–C2 articulation. This specialized structure also results in patterns of injuries that are specific to this region. Because of the relatively large spinal canal diameter at this level (approximately twice the spinal cord diameter), neurologic deficits may be mild or absent.

C1 (Atlas)

A burst fracture of C1 (Jefferson fracture) is the result of axial loading with bilateral outward displacement of the lateral masses of C1 (30). This injury can be diagnosed by recognizing the resultant fractures in both the anterior and posterior arches of C1 (Fig. 23-5).

An isolated fracture of the posterior arch of C1 may result from hyperextension with impaction of the posterior arch of C1 between the occiput and C2. This injury is distinguished from the C1 burst fracture by involvement of only the posterior arch.

An isolated fracture of the anterior arch of C1 is less common. It also results from hyperextension with avulsion of the attachment of the anterior spinal ligament. The small avulsed bone fragment is visible ventral to the anterior arch of C1.

C2 (Axis)

According to a scheme proposed by Anderson and D'Alonzo (4), fractures of the dens are commonly classified into types I, II, and III. Type II fractures are the most common, consisting of a fracture through the base of the dens at its junction with the body of C2 (Fig. 23-6). Such fractures have a high incidence of nonunion if not surgically fused (3). A fracture that extends through the upper body of C2 is classified as type III (37). Type III fractures usually heal completely with external immobilization. A type I fracture is an avulsion of the tip of the dens. This extremely rare injury should be differentiated from an os odontoideum (see Fig. 23-6).

Traumatic spondylolysis of C2 (hangman's fracture) is the most common fracture of C2. This injury is caused by hyperextension with resultant bilateral fractures of the pars interarticularis (the C2 vertebra is the only cervical vertebra with a true pars interarticularis) (Fig. 23-7). With more severe injuries, the body of C2 is displaced anteriorly with respect to C3, and spinal cord injury is more common.

Lower Cervical Spine Fractures

The majority of fractures in adults occur in the lower cervical spine, predominantly at the C6 and C7 levels. The classification of these fractures is based on the presumed mechanism of injury.

Hyperextension Injuries

Hyperextension injuries, caused by impact to the face or forehead, may result in either hyperextension dislocation or hyperextension teardrop fracture (40). Hyperextension dislocation is a disruption of the ligaments between adjacent vertebrae, including the ALL, annulus fibrosus, and facet capsular ligaments. As there may be no fracture, radiographs and CT may appear nearly normal, except for

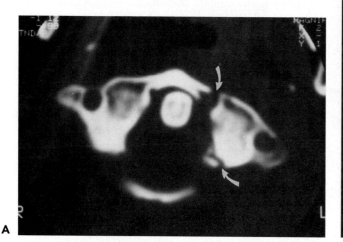

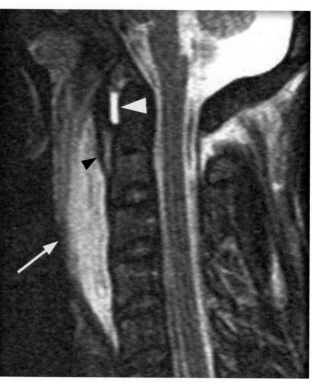

Figure 23-5   Jefferson-type fracture. **A:** Axial CT shows fractures of the anterior and posterior arches of C2 in this unilateral variation of a Jefferson fracture. **B:** Midsagittal STIR image in a different patient reveals high signal intensity in the atlantodental interval (*arrowhead*) and prevertebral swelling (*arrow*). There is no evidence of injury to the ligaments of the CVJ. The anterior atlantoaxial ligament (*black arrowhead*) is slightly displaced anteriorly.

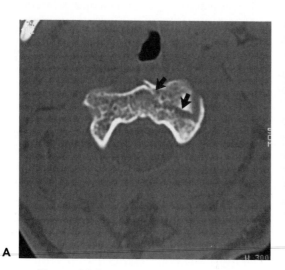

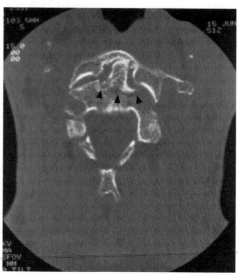

Figure 23-6   Dens fractures and os odontoideum. **A:** Axial CT shows fracture (*arrows*) involving the midportion and left lateral mass of C2. **B:** Oblique coronal CT in the same patient shows the low dens fracture (*arrowheads*). Hyperextension of the neck should not be done in these patients. Close to direct coronal images may occasionally be obtained (as in this case) solely by gantry angulation.

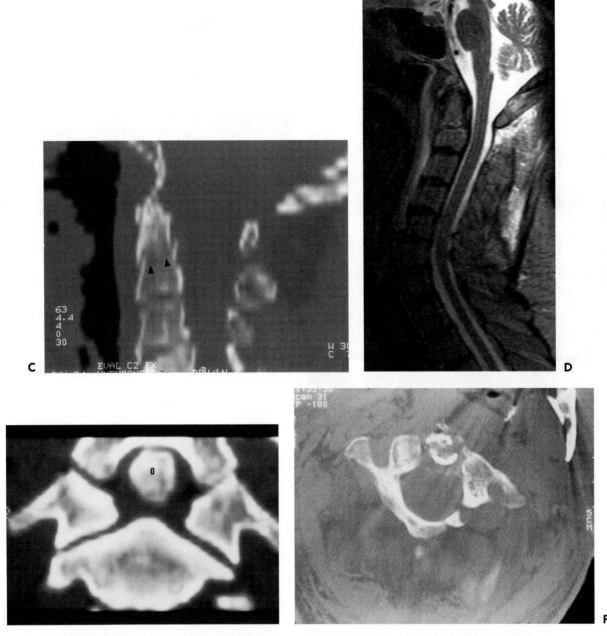

Figure 23-6 *(continued)* **C:** Sagittal CT reformation depicts the fracture (*arrowheads*). **D:** Midline sagittal T1-weighted image of the brain in a different patient shows a low dens fracture. **E:** In a different and asymptomatic patient, coronal CT reformation shows a well-corticated rounded os odontoideum (O). **F:** In a different patient, axial CT shows a rare vertically oriented fracture of the dens with extension into the body of C2. The left lamina is also fractured.

diffuse thickening of the prevertebral soft tissues (38). MRI identifies the prevertebral hematoma and discontinuity of ligaments (Fig. 23-8). This injury is frequently associated with severe spinal cord contusion, especially in patients with preexisting degenerative changes. In approximately two thirds of patients with hyperextension dislocation injury, the intact anterior annulus causes an avulsion fracture of the anteroinferior margin of the affected vertebral body (38). This fragment is larger in its transverse dimension than in its height, with an almost horizontally oriented fracture line.

Hyperextension teardrop fracture is an avulsion fracture of the anteroinferior margin of the vertebral body caused by excessive stress on the ALL (40). This injury occurs most commonly at C2, usually in older, osteoporotic individuals, although it may occur at lower levels in nonosteoporotic patients. The fracture fragment can be distinguished from the avulsion fracture of hyperextension dislocation by the obliquity of the fracture line (approximately 45 degrees from vertical) and the relatively greater height of the fragment.

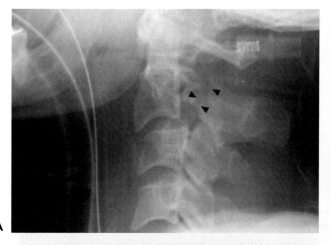

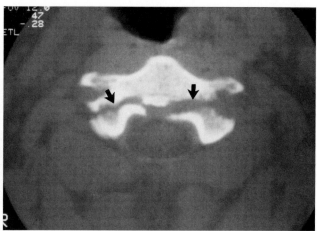

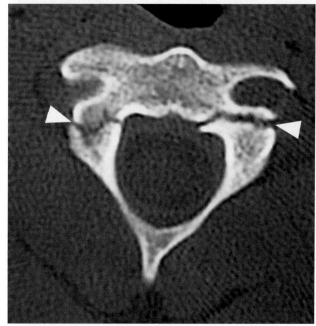

Figure 23-7 Hangman's fracture. **A:** Lateral radiograph shows fractures (*arrowheads*) through the pars interarticularis of C2. The vertebral body of C2 is slightly displaced anteriorly on C3. **B:** Axial CT in the same patient confirms the presence of bilateral pars interarticularis fractures (*arrows*). **C:** Axial CT in a different patient shows bilateral pars interarticularis fracture (*arrowheads*) with minimal displacement.

All hyperextension injuries may be associated with herniation of intervertebral discs, which may cause or worsen the associated spinal cord injury (see Fig. 23-8) (79). MRI provides excellent depiction of these herniated discs.

Hyperflexion Injuries

Hyperflexion injuries result from impact to the top or back of the head, with the neck in flexion (34,50). These injuries, which are especially common in divers, include hyperflexion sprain, wedge fracture, bilateral facet joint dislocation, and teardrop fracture.

Hyperflexion sprain refers to a disruption of the posterior ligamentous attachments between adjacent vertebrae (the nuchal ligament, interspinous ligaments, facet capsular ligaments, and PLL). On radiographs, this injury may be recognized by abnormal widening between adjacent posterior elements and by subtle, acute kyphotic angulation at the level of injury. On T2-weighted MRI, high signal intensity edema and blood products are seen in the posterior ligaments. Diagnosis of this injury is important because it may be associated with chronic neck pain and a high incidence of failed ligament healing in patients managed without surgery.

Wedge fractures consist of an impaction fracture of the superior endplate of the affected vertebral body in addition to posterior ligament disruption. The inferior endplate remains intact. There is greater loss of vertebral body height anteriorly, resulting in the typical wedge-shaped vertebral body seen on the lateral radiographs or sagittal CT reformations (Fig. 23-9).

Bilateral interfacet joint dislocations require greater forces than that associated with other hyperflexion injuries described above. In addition to disruption of the posterior ligamentous structures, this injury involves disruption of the ALL, the annular fibers of the intervertebral disc, and complete bilateral dislocation of the facet joints (101) (Fig. 23-10). The inferior articular processes of the upper vertebra become lodged in the neural foramina anterior to

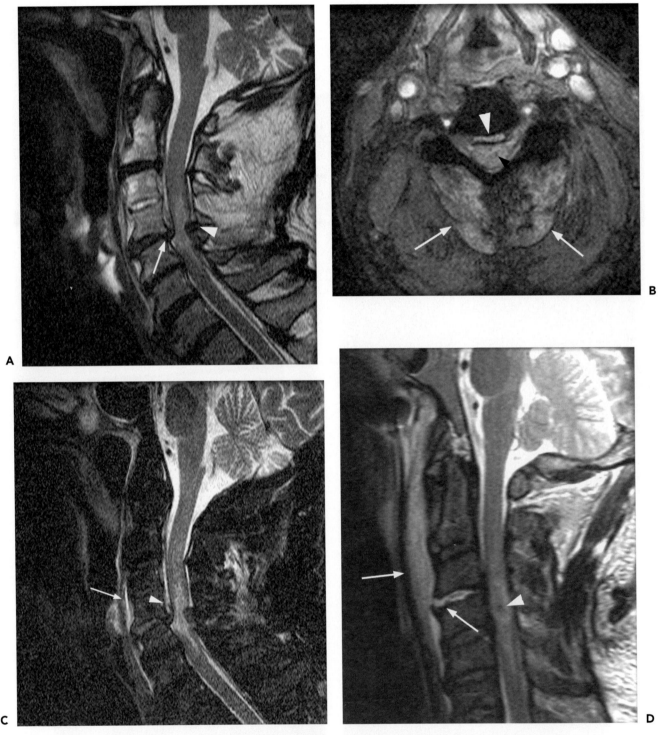

Figure 23-8 Hyperextension injury. **A:** Midline sagittal T2-weighted image shows slight posterior displacement of C4 on C5. There is increased signal in the C4–C5 vertebral disc that shows posterior herniation (*white arrow*). The spinal cord is impinged at that level, demonstrating edema. The narrowed spinal canal is partially due to thickening and buckling of ligamenta flava (*arrowhead*). The residual disc between the fused C3–C4 vertebrae is bright. **B:** A central disc herniation (*arrowhead*) is clearly seen on this axial gradient echo T2*- weighted image. A small hypointense lesion (*black arrowhead*) within the spinal cord represents deoxyhemoglobin in an acute hematoma (cord contusion). Increased signal intensity in the paraspinal muscles (*arrows*) is consistent with edema and hematoma. **C:** Increased signal within and adjacent to the anterior longitudinal ligament (*white arrow*) is better appreciated on this midsagittal STIR image. The disc herniation with displacement of the posterior longitudinal ligament (*white arrowhead*) is clearly seen. Spinal cord edema is more conspicuous, and muscle injury is also seen. The residual C3–C4 *disk* is no longer of high signal intensity. **D:** T2-weighted sagittal image in a different patient shows cord contusion (*arrowhead*), C3–C4 disc herniation with ALL rupture and prevertebral edema/hematoma (*arrows*).

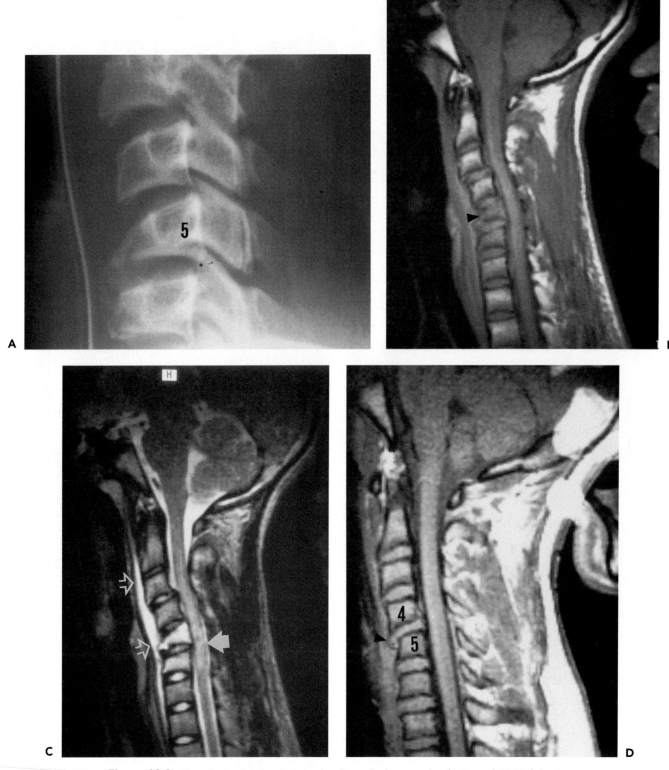

Figure 23-9   Hyperflexion injuries. **A:** Lateral radiograph shows wedge fracture of C5 (5) following diving accident. **B:** Sagittal T1-weighted image shows compression fracture of C5 (*arrowhead*). C5 is displaced posteriorly. C6 is also slightly wedged, and its superior endplate is disrupted. The C5–C6 vertebral bodies have low signal intensity, suggesting bone marrow edema. **C:** Corresponding T2-weighted image shows prevertebral swelling (*open arrows*) and spinal cord edema (*solid arrow*). Hyperintensity from C5 and C6 vertebral bodies compatible with bone marrow edema is present. **D:** Midline sagittal T1-weighted image in a different patient with a milder hyperflexion injury. There is slight anterior displacement of C4 (4) on C5 (5). Anterior disc herniation with disruption of the ALL (*arrowhead*) is present.

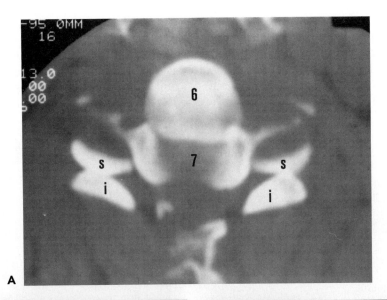

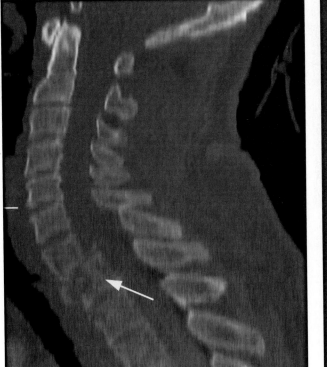

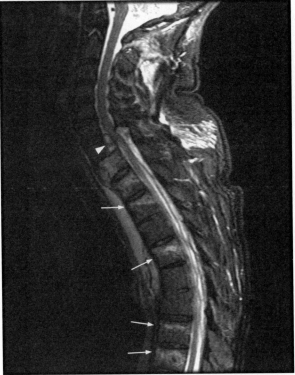

Figure 23-10 Bilateral facet dislocations. **A:** Axial CT shows that the superior facets (s) of C7 lie anterior to the inferior facets (i) of C6 (reverse of normal). The body of C6 (6) is severely anteriorly displaced on the body of C7 (7). The spinal canal is narrow. **B:** Reformatted midsagittal CT in a different patient shows severe anterior dislocation of C7 on T1 (*arrow*). The anterosuperior aspect of T1 is fractured and a bone fragment is displaced anteriorly. **C:** Sagittal STIR image shows disc herniation (*arrowhead*) with superior migration. The spinal cord is compressed without evidence of edema. In addition to the T1 compression fracture, the superior endplates of multiple vertebral bodies demonstrate high signal intensity consistent with microfractures (*arrows*).

the superior articular processes of the lower vertebra, preventing reduction. This injury is sometimes referred to as bilaterally locked facets, erroneously implying mechanical stability. On radiographs, this injury is diagnosed by anterior displacement of the upper vertebra by one half or more of the width of the lower vertebrae. The "naked" articular surfaces of the dislocated facets are usually visible on axial imaging. MRI not only reveals the previously mentioned features but also detects the presence of associated herniated discs, epidural hematoma, and cord and vertebral artery injuries. CT is helpful for detecting fractures of the articular masses that can interfere with attempts at reduction.

Hyperflexion teardrop fracture occurs with even greater magnitude forces. This injury shares the posterior ligamentous disruption of the other hyperflexion injuries, but it consists additionally of a large triangular fracture fragment arising from the anterior–inferior margin of the upper vertebral body (50,92) (Fig. 23-11). Associated severe narrowing of the spinal canal caused by retropulsed bone fragments almost universally produces severe spinal cord injury. This fracture can be distinguished from the similarly named hyperextension teardrop fracture by the larger size of the triangular fragment and distraction of the posterior elements, indicating the flexion mechanism.

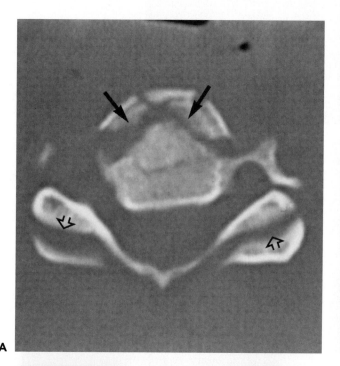

A

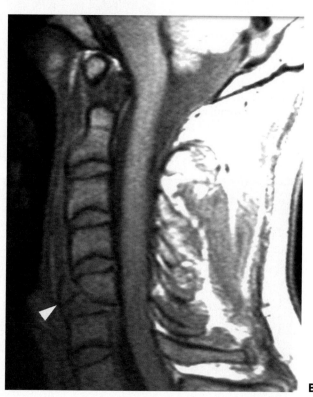

B

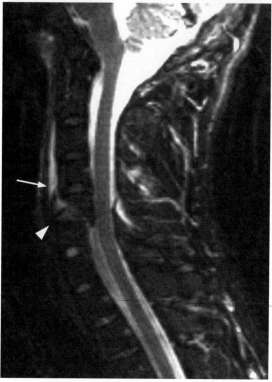

C

Figure 23-11   Hyperflexion teardrop fracture. **A:** Axial CT shows fracture (*arrows*) of the anteroinferior margin of C5. The facet joints are splayed (*open arrows*), indicating ruptured capsular ligaments. **B:** In a different patient, T1-weighted sagittal image shows a teardrop fracture of C5 with posterior displacement of the vertebral body (*arrowhead*). **C:** STIR sagittal image reveals ALL rupture (*arrow*). The fracture is of high signal intensity (*arrowhead*). The subarachnoid spaces are effaced without evidence of spinal cord lesions.

Vertical Compression Injuries

Vertical compression injuries result from impact to the top of the head with the spine straight (40). These injuries include the Jefferson fracture of C1 (discussed earlier) and burst fractures of the lower cervical spine.

Vertebral body burst fractures occur when vertical compressive forces are transmitted through the intervertebral disc with radial outward forces generated in the vertebral body (104). This type of injury causes a vertical fracture with lateral dispersion of the vertebral body fragments. On radiographs, the diagnosis is made by recognizing the widened uncovertebral joints or visualizing the vertical fracture line. CT may aid in identifying the vertical fracture line and the frequently associated fractures of the pedicles or laminae (Fig. 23-12). MRI is helpful in detecting herniated disc fragments, which also commonly accompany this injury.

Other Mechanisms

Less common mechanisms of injury also may lead to recognized fracture patterns. A combination of flexion and rotational forces can result in a unilateral facet dislocation (Fig. 23-13). This injury is distinguished from bilateral facet dislocations by the limited amount of anterolisthesis (approximately 25% versus 50% for bilateral). Lateral force vectors may lead to isolated fractures of the uncinate processes. Combined extension and rotation forces may result in pillar or pedicolaminar fractures.

Thoracic Spine

The normal thoracic spine is stabilized by the rib cage, thoracic musculature, and steeply oriented facet joints. Consequently, thoracic spine fractures are uncommon, except with severe trauma. The most common of these injuries are wedge-type fractures and flexion fracture dislocations (5). Radiographic evaluation of the thoracic spine may be difficult because of superimposition of the shoulder girdle and ribs. CT is valuable in all cases of suspected thoracic spine fracture (60).

Wedge fractures are considered simple if only the anterior vertebral body is involved. Severe wedge fractures involve the posterior vertebral body as well, with the potential for posterior displacement of bony fragments into the spinal canal (Fig. 23-14). CT and MRI can be used to assess spinal canal narrowing that results from hyperkyphotic angulation or retropulsed fragments.

Fracture dislocations occur with larger-magnitude forces, frequently resulting in severe spinal cord injury (Fig. 23-15). MRI provides valuable information regarding cord injury and the presence of associated epidural hematoma.

Thoracolumbar and Lumbar Spine

The thoracolumbar junction (T12 to L2) is the next most common site of spine fracture after the cervical spine (72). Most of the injuries to the lumbar spine and thoracolumbar junction are related to abnormal flexion or vertical

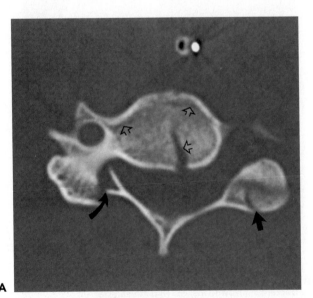
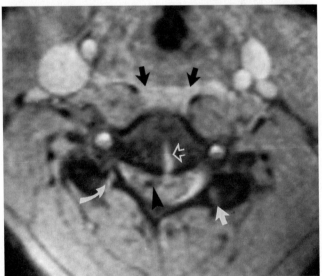

A   B

Figure 23-12 Vertical compression fracture. **A:** Axial CT shows multiple fractures (*open arrows*) in the C5 body. Also seen are fractures of the right lamina (*curved arrow*) and left articular pillar (*arrow*). **B:** Axial gradient echo image at the same level also shows fractures of vertebral body (*white open arrow*), right lamina (*white curved arrow*), and left articular pillar (*white solid arrow*). Low signal intensity (*black arrowhead*) in the spinal cord represents an acute hematoma. Prevertebral edema (*black solid arrows*) is also present.

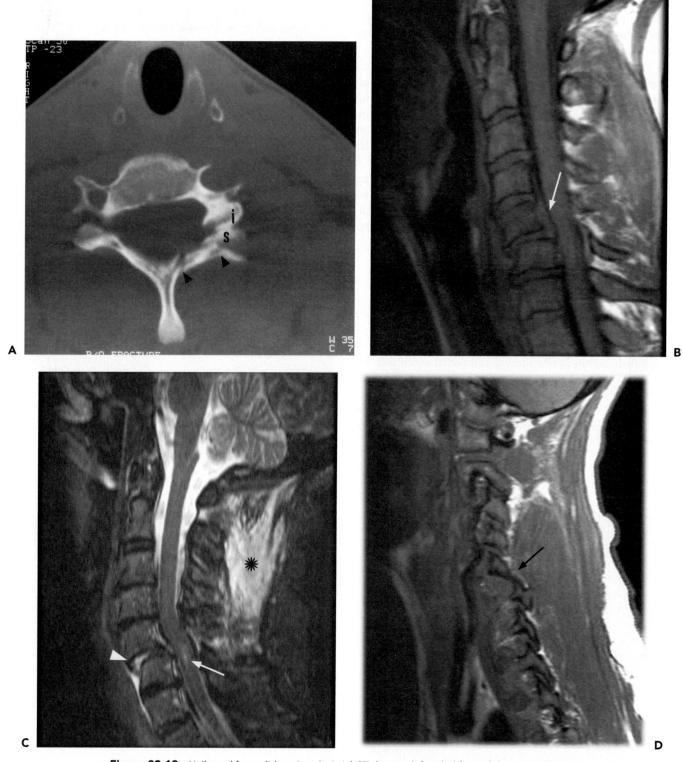

Figure 23-13 Unilateral facet dislocation. **A:** Axial CT shows a left-sided facet dislocation. The inferior facet (i) of C6 lies anterior to the superior facet (s) of C7 (reverse of normal). The C6 vertebral body is slightly rotated to the right. The left lamina is fractured (*arrowheads*). **B:** Midline sagittal T1-weighted image in a different patient shows mild anterior displacement of C5 on C6. The PLL is intact (*arrow*). **C:** Midsagittal STIR image reveals C5–C6 *disk* injury (*arrowhead*) and spinal cord edema (*arrow*). Note bright signal involving paraspinal muscles (*) consistent with edema/hemorrhage. **D:** Parasagittal T1-weighted image through left facet joints shows that the inferior facet of C7 is displaced anteriorly to the superior facet of C6 (*arrow*). Note the normal arrangement of facet joints in inferior levels.

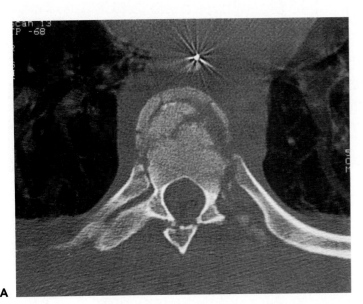

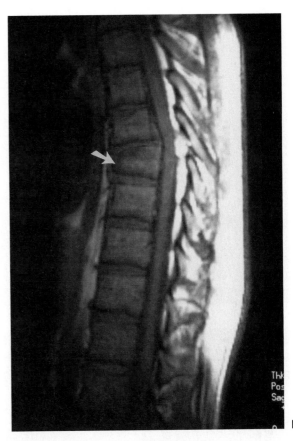

Figure 23-14 Thoracic spine compression fracture. **A:** Axial CT shows compression fracture involving mainly the anterior aspect of the T7 vertebral body. **B:** Midsagittal T1-weighted image (same patient) shows the wedged T7 vertebral body (*arrow*). The posterior margin is displaced into the spinal canal, producing spinal cord compression.

compression forces. Common types of injuries include wedge, burst, and Chance fractures.

Wedge (compression) fractures result when flexion forces lead to a fracture of the vertebral body only, without involvement of the posterior elements. Radiographs are diagnostic in most cases, and classification into simple or severe wedge fractures is similar to that of the thoracic spine. If there is a question of posterior element fractures or posterior displacement of fragments, CT and MRI provide clarification and assessment of the residual spinal canal diameter (Fig. 23-16).

Burst fractures in the lumbar spine consist of a vertically oriented fracture of the vertebral body with lateral dispersion of the fracture fragments (6). The posterior wall of the vertebral body is disrupted, which does not occur with wedge fractures. Usually, there are associated fractures in the posterior elements. This injury can be recognized on radiographs by identifying the vertical fracture line or by detecting a widened interpediculate distance. CT is useful for characterizing the associated posterior element fractures and for assessing spinal canal impingement (96). MRI provides assessment of the conus medullaris or spinal nerve roots in patients with neurologic deficits (Fig. 23-17).

The Chance fracture is defined as a horizontally oriented fracture that passes through the spinous process, laminae, and vertebral body (86). This fracture, which occurs nearly exclusively at the thoracolumbar junction, is thought to be the result of distractive forces generated when the spine is flexed about a fulcrum point, such as a car lap seat belt (99). This mechanism has prompted the term *seat-belt injury* to describe this and associated injuries. A horizontal disruption involves the intervertebral disc or posterior ligaments, rather than the vertebral body or posterior bony elements, and is considered a variation of the Chance fracture (Fig. 23-18). Usually, the fractures are visible on radiographs. MRI demonstrates the ligamentous components of the various forms of injury, along with any conus medullaris or nerve root injuries. The association of Chance fractures with significant intraperitoneal injuries in up to 50% of patients has prompted some authors to suggest routine CT of the abdomen in all patients with this type of injury (109).

Sacrum

Acute fractures of the sacrum are best considered within the category of pelvic fractures and will not be discussed here.

Insufficiency fractures of the sacrum occur when the elastic strength of the bone is not adequate to withstand

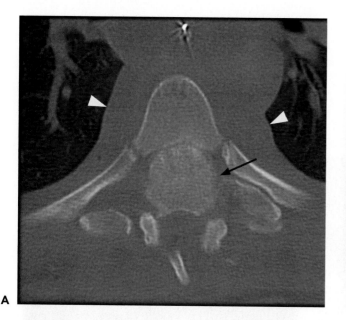

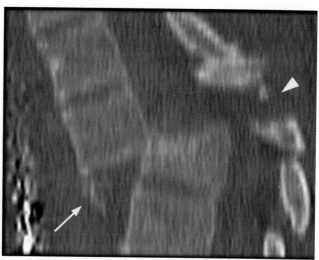

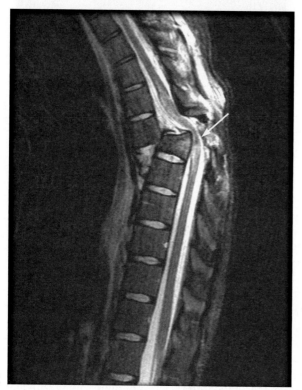

Figure 23-15 Thoracic spine fracture dislocation. **A:** Axial CT shows the T7 vertebral body (*arrow*) to be posterior to T6. There is associated prominent paravertebral swelling (*arrowheads*). **B:** Reformatted midsagittal CT demonstrates a fracture dislocation with a bone fragment arising from the inferior vertebral body (*arrow*). The fracture extends into the posterior elements (*arrowhead*). **C:** Midline sagittal T2-weighted image shows a fracture dislocation of T6 on T7 with severe compression of the spinal cord resulting in focal hematoma (*arrow*) and edema.

the stresses of normal activity (27). Such fractures occur in patients with metabolic bone disease or prior radiation therapy. Although insufficiency fractures of the sacrum are not uncommon, their radiographic diagnosis is frequently challenging. The typical radiographic finding is linear sclerosis running vertically within a sacral ala, parallel and adjacent to the sacroiliac joint (23). On radiographs and radionuclide bone scintigraphy, the fracture may be mistaken for a metastatic lesion. CT aids greatly in the diagnosis, demonstrating the fracture line traversing the sacrum

medial and parallel to the sacroiliac joint. A characteristic MRI finding is a wider area along the fracture line that is of low signal intensity on T1-weighted images and hyperintense on STIR images (Fig. 23-19).

Pathologic Fractures and Secondary Tumors

Metastases to the spine are most commonly the result of hematogenous spread. Approximately 20% to 35% of cancer patients develop symptomatic spine metastases (111).

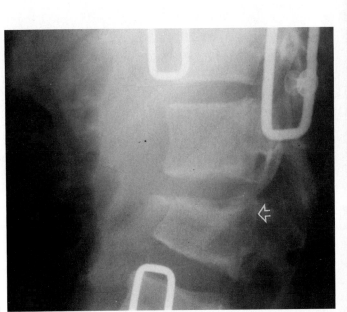

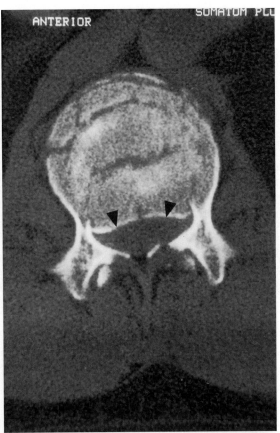

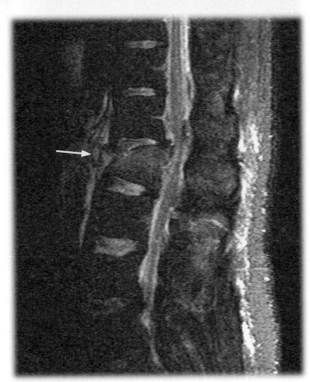

Figure 23-16 Lumbar vertebral body wedge fracture. **A:** Lateral radiograph shows typical wedge fracture of L1. Height loss in the anterior aspect of the vertebral body is greater than posteriorly. There is a questionable bone density (*arrow*) in the canal. Patient is in a brace. **B:** Axial CT shows fractures involving the vertebral body and confirms posterior displacement of dorsal cortex (*arrowheads*), which narrows the canal. **C:** Midsagittal STIR image in a different patient shows an L1 wedge compression fracture with a bright vertebral body and prevertebral swelling (*arrow*). Note spinal canal narrowing.

However, at autopsy, 70% of all cancer patients have spine metastases. The thoracic and lumbar regions are most commonly involved. Approximately 5% of patients develop symptoms of spinal cord compression due to collapse of one or more vertebrae, or epidural tumor spread. The most common primary tumors to produce spinal metastases are carcinomas of the breast, lung, prostate, and kidney, followed by lymphomas.

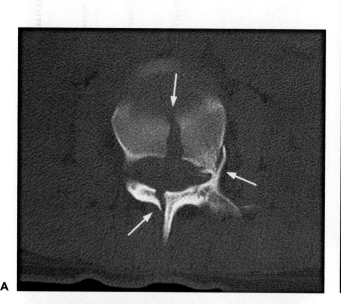

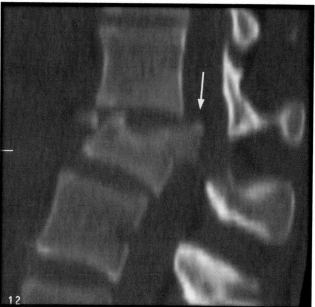

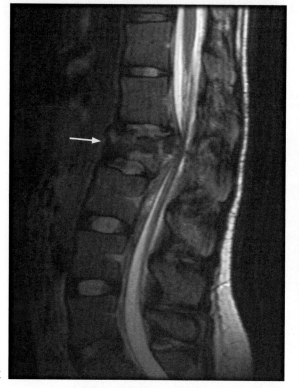

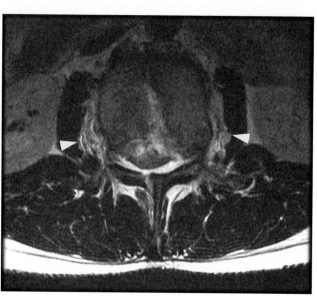

Figure 23-17 Lumbar burst fracture. **A:** Axial CT at L2 shows fractures involving the vertebral body, right lamina, and left pedicle (*arrows*). The spinal canal is narrowed. **B:** Reformatted sagittal CT confirms significant spinal canal narrowing caused by retropulsion of bone fragments (*arrow*). **C:** Midline sagittal T2-weighted image shows fracture of L2, posteriorly displaced bone fragment, and compression of the cauda equina. **D:** Axial T2-weighted image at L2 also demonstrates the fractures, which are less conspicuous in comparison with the CT study. The dural sac is compressed, and there is perivertebral soft tissue swelling (*arrowheads*).

CT is used mainly to confirm the presence of lesions suspected from a radionuclide bone scan. Depending on their origin, metastases may be lytic, sclerotic (prostate, carcinoid), or, more commonly, of mixed densities (Fig. 23-20).

MRI is more sensitive than CT and radionuclide bone scintigraphy for the detection of spinal metastases (31). On T1-weighted images, metastatic foci are usually of low signal intensity, whereas on T2-weighted images, the lesions

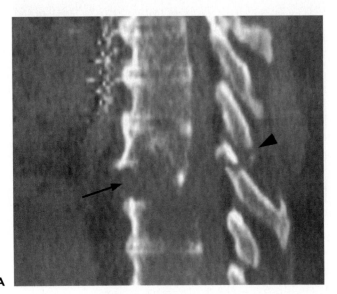
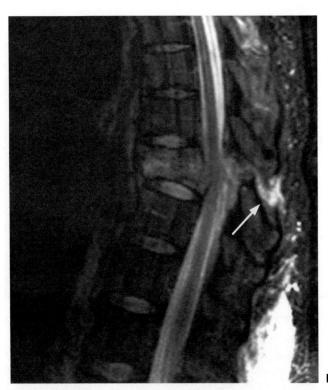

Figure 23-18 Chance fracture. **A:** Reformatted midline sagittal CT shows horizontal fracture involving L1 and L2 vertebral bodies (*arrow*). The fracture extends dorsally into the posterior elements of T12 and L1 (*arrowhead*). **B:** Midsagittal T2-weighted image in a different patient reveals disruption of the posterior ligament complex with widening of the interspinous space (*arrow*). The T11 vertebral body is slightly wedged and there is narrowing of the spinal canal with cord compression.

are bright and may be less conspicuous with FSE sequences (Fig. 23-21). After intravenous contrast medium administration, metastases enhance and their signal intensity may be such that they become isointense with surrounding bone marrow. Therefore, the precontrast sagittal T1-weighted images should always be obtained. Intravenous contrast enhancement aids in the evaluation of tumor extension into adjacent paraspinal and epidural compartments, and fat suppression is useful on postcontrast T1-weighted images. Extension of enhancing tissue beyond the margins of the affected vertebral body is commonly found in pathologic fractures (Fig. 23-22).

STIR images are very useful for detection of metastases to the spine, which are seen as bright lesions on a dark background (see Fig. 23-22). A recently reported useful sign is the high signal intensity of fluid commonly detected on sagittal STIR images within acute vertebral body compression fractures in patients with osteoporosis, but very rarely in metastatic fractures (9) (Fig. 23-23).

DWI has been found to be sensitive and specific in differentiating between benign osteoporotic spinal fractures and fractures resulting from metastatic deposits (10). On DWI, benign fractures remain hypointense, whereas tumor infiltration becomes bright (Figs. 23-23 and 23-24). More recent studies have shown that DWI may be less sensitive for metastatic spine involvement without fractures, especially

in patients with sclerotic metastases (17). Also, areas that are hyperintense on DWI are not necessarily malignant (16). The observed discrepancy in results is at least in part because of implementation of different techniques, and with further technologic advancements DWI may prove to be a reliable method for detection of spinal metastatic lesions (Fig. 23-25) (16).

Lymphoma and leukemia involving the spine generally show MRI findings identical to metastatic disease. However, lymphoma may present as a soft tissue mass that circumferentially compresses the spinal cord without bone involvement (31).

DEGENERATIVE SPINE DISEASE

Pain secondary to degenerative changes of the spine is one of the leading causes of disability among adults. Sixty percent to 80% of working-age adults at some point in their lives suffer from back pain (48). Most disorders of the spine result from degenerative changes that may arise in the bone, ligaments, or soft tissue components of the spine.

The intervertebral articulation consists of the intervertebral disc and two posterior facet joints. The major components of the intervertebral disc space consist of the hyaline cartilaginous endplates of the adjacent vertebral bodies,

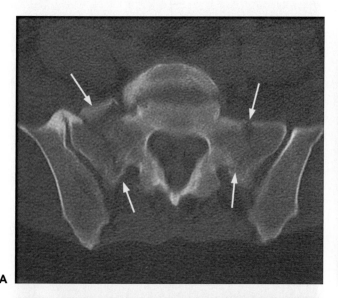

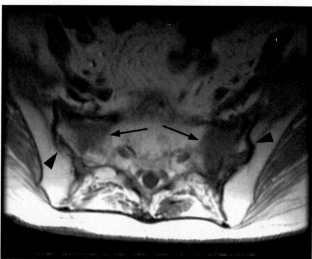

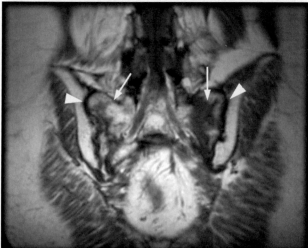

Figure 23-19 Sacral insufficiency fracture. **A:** Axial CT shows fractures running bilaterally through the sacral alae (*arrows*). The fractures are almost parallel to the sacroiliac joints. **B:** On an axial T1-weighted image the injuries are seen as decreased signal intensity (*arrows*), comprising a larger area. The sacroiliac joints (*arrowheads*) are adjacent to the fractures. **C:** Coronal T1-weighted image shows the fractures (*arrows*) running parallel to the sacroiliac joints (*arrowheads*).

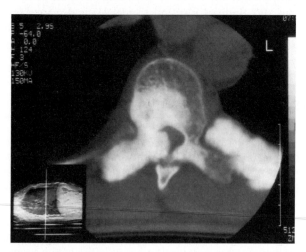

Figure 23-20 Sclerotic metastases. Axial CT, bone window setting, shows expansile, sclerotic metastases from bronchogenic carcinoid tumor. Note significant narrowing of the spinal canal by involved bone.

the gelatinous core of the intervertebral disc (nucleus pulposus), and its circumferential thick fibrous ring (annulus fibrosus). Degenerative alterations at any of these sites may alter the normal biomechanical forces and predispose the adjacent articulations to similar changes. Therefore, patients often present with manifestations of degenerative changes in multiple joints.

The degenerative process involving the disc begins as early as the late teens or early twenties. Initially, an increase in the water content of the nucleus pulposus predisposes it to generalized bulges or focal herniations through the cartilaginous endplates of the adjacent vertebra (Schmorl nodule) (51) (Fig. 23-26). With time, the nucleus pulposus undergoes progressive dehydration with resulting loss of height of the disc space. With further loss of water and proteoglycans, the disc becomes brittle and fibrotic and is unable to provide the necessary elasticity for proper support of the vertebral column, a process known as disc desiccation (115). Almost

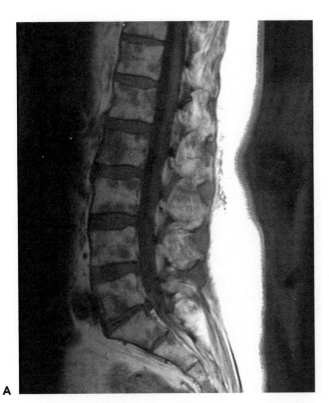
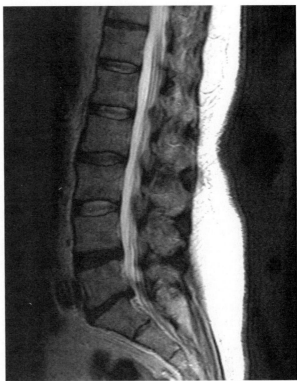

A

B

Figure 23-21 Metastases, T1- and T2-weighted imaging. **A:** Sagittal T1-weighted image shows numerous ill-defined areas of low signal intensity, predominantly oval in shape, throughout the bone marrow of the vertebral bodies. The finding is consistent with metastases. **B:** On the corresponding T2-weighted fast spin echo image, the lesions are inconspicuous. Note incidental degenerative changes of the L4–L5 and L5–S1 intervertebral discs.

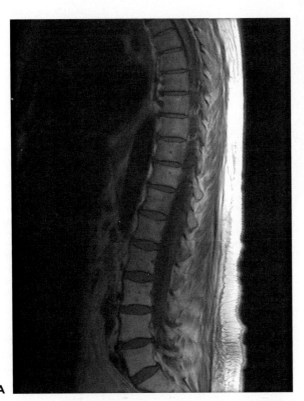
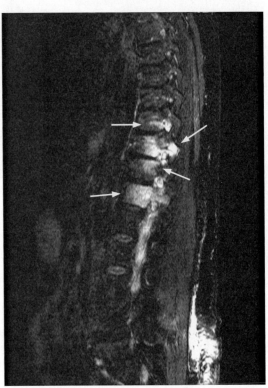

A

B

Figure 23-22 Lytic metastases, STIR and postcontrast images. **A:** Sagittal T1-weighted image in a patient with metastatic disease shows subtle areas of decreased signal intensity in the vertebral bodies of the lower thoracic and upper lumbar spine. **B:** Corresponding STIR image demonstrates bright signal of the involved vertebrae (*arrows*), both in the anterior and posterior elements, indicative of metastases. (*continued*)

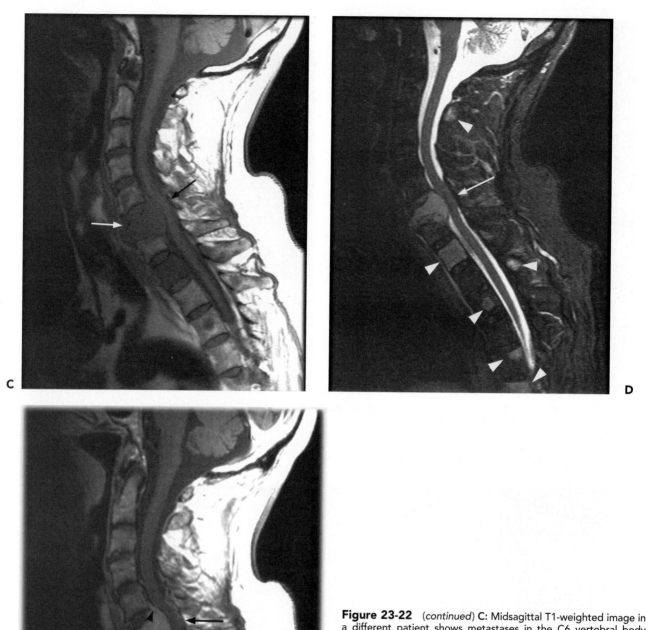

Figure 23-22 *(continued)* **C:** Midsagittal T1-weighted image in a different patient shows metastases in the C6 vertebral body *(white arrow)* producing spinal cord compression *(black arrow)*. Additional metastases are seen as hypointense areas. **D:** Corresponding STIR image confirms spinal cord compression *(arrow)* and widespread metastases *(arrowheads)*. Also identified are lesions in the posterior elements, which were not conspicuous on T1-weighted images. **E:** On a contrast-enhanced T1-weighted image there is enhancement of the C6 vertebral body *(white arrow)* and of the epidural extension of the tumor *(black arrowheads)*. Spinal cord compression *(black arrow)* is visualized to a better advantage compared to the precontrast image; however, many lesions have become inconspicuous *(white arrowhead)*.

all of the population over 60 years of age shows degenerative disc changes by MRI. The triad that characterizes disc degeneration includes bulging, loss of height, and loss of water, seen as decreased signal intensity on T2-weighted sequences. Occasionally, a diseased disc may be bright on precontrast T1-weighted images (Fig. 23-27). This probably implies the presence of intradiscal calcification (hydrated calcium) and/or hemorrhage. The mechanism by which a degenerated disc produces pain is unclear, but it is probably related to compression and repetitive firing of sensory nerve endings and the growth of nocioceptive pain fibers in adjacent granulation tissues. Causes of low back pain remain unknown in a majority of cases, and the diagnosis is based on concordance of symptoms, clinical findings, and imaging

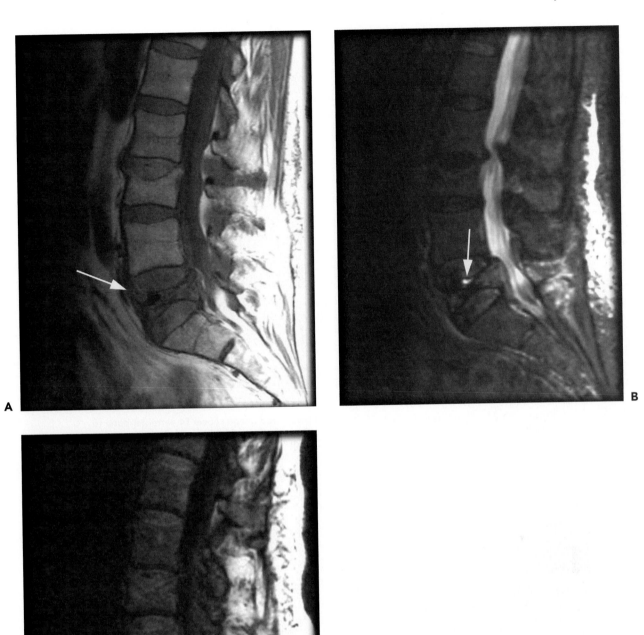

A

B

C

Figure 23-23 Acute benign compression fracture. **A:** Midsagittal T1-weighted image shows severe loss of height and signal intensity of L5 vertebral body (*arrow*). Note decreased height of L3 vertebral body with normal signal intensity indicative of a chronic osteoporotic fracture. **B:** STIR image reveals a small hyperintense area (*arrow*) within the diffusely bright L5 body, which is consistent with fluid and characteristic for a benign osteoporotic fracture. **C:** On steady-state free precession (SSFP) DWI (b = 165 s/mm²), the compressed verte-bra is hypointense (*arrow*), compatible with a benign fracture.

studies. Degenerative disc disease is common, but it is cer-tainly not the only cause of low back pain or radiculopathy, and it has been shown that a significant proportion of asymptomatic individuals harbor moderate and even severe lesions, with reported incidence of disc herniations between 27% to 67% and disc extrusions of 1% to 18% (43,114).

The imaging features of progressive degenerative disc dis-ease vary depending on the extent of the abnormality. CT is unable to detect early disc desiccation; however, it is useful for detecting late changes, such as disc space narrowing and sclerosis of the adjacent cartilaginous endplates. A reliable indicator of disc degeneration is the presence of intradiscal

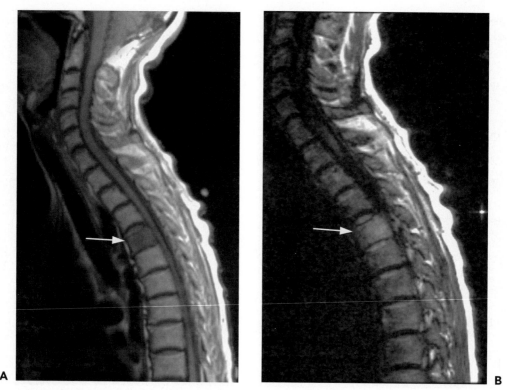

Figure 23-24 Metastases, DWI. **A:** Midsagittal T1-weighted image shows T4 vertebral body to have low signal intensity and preserved height (*arrow*). In a patient with history of malignant tumor, this finding raises concern of metastasis. **B:** SSFP DWI (b = 165 s/mm²) demonstrates relatively increased signal intensity of T4 (*arrow*), supporting the diagnosis is metastasis. Bone biopsy was performed and confirmed the presence tumor.

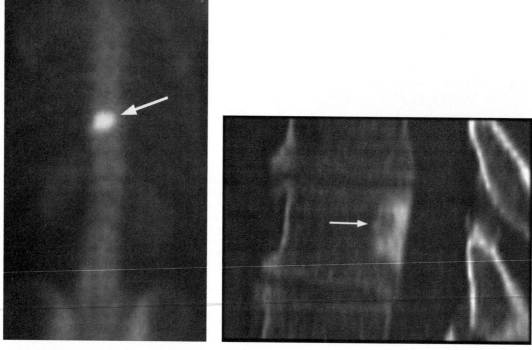

Figure 23-25 Solitary osteoblastic metastasis in a patient with prostate cancer. **A:** Radionuclide bone scan demonstrates increased tracer activity at T10 (*arrow*). **B:** Reformatted sagittal CT reveals a sclerotic lesion (*arrow*) in the posterior aspect of T10.

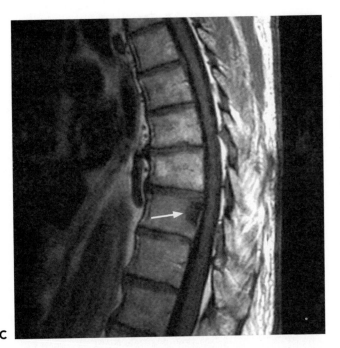

C

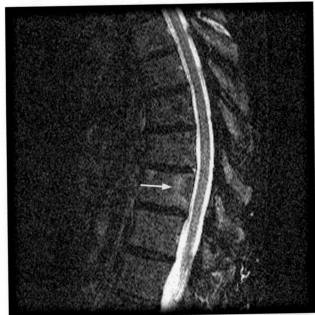

D

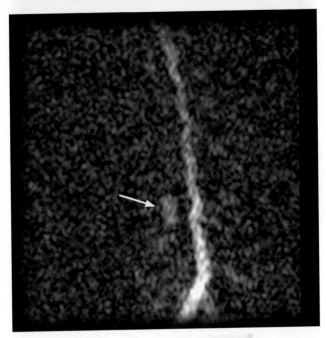

E

Figure 23-25 *(continued)* **C:** The lesion is hypointense on T1-weighted images *(arrow)* primarily corresponding to bone sclerosis. **D:** On STIR image there is no clear hyperintensity of the vertebral body lesion; a subtle increase in signal intensity is appreciated in its peripheral aspect *(arrow)*. **E:** Matching echo planar DWI (b = 1000 s/mm^2) has an overall low signal-to-noise ratio and shows that the posterior aspect of T10 is hyperintense *(arrow)*. Metastatic prostate cancer was confirmed by biopsy.

gas (Fig. 23-28A), which is referred to as vacuum phenomenon and may be visualized by radiographs or CT (83). The gas is predominantly nitrogen and is highly unusual in an infected disc space (65).

MRI may show signs of early degenerative changes that are not detected by CT, such as early disc desiccation reflected by loss of signal intensity on T2-weighted images (see Figs. 23-21B and 23-28B). MRI also detects marrow changes within endplates adjacent to degenerative discs. These changes are classified into three categories according to Modic (65). Type I changes show decreased signal on T1-weighted images and increased signal on T2-weighted

sequences (Fig. 23-29). Histologically, these changes correlate with vascularized fibrous tissue, with disruption, fissuring, and edema of the endplates. Type II changes, resulting from yellow (fatty) marrow replacement within the adjacent endplates, are characterized by increased signal on T1-weighted images, with decreased signal intensity on conventional spin echo T2-weighted images, but hyperintensity on FSE T2-weighted images (Fig. 23-30). Type III changes are advanced changes, characterized by decreased signal on both T1-weighted and T2-weighted images, correlating with extensive bone sclerosis of the involved endplates on radiographs and CT (Fig. 23-31). It is important to

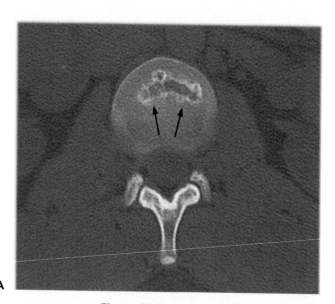

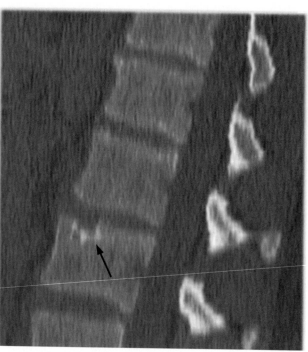

Figure 23-26 Schmorl nodules. **A:** Axial CT at the superior aspect of L2 shows areas of lower attenuation within the endplate surrounded by a sclerotic rim (*arrows*). This is the characteristic appearance of Schmorl nodules. **B:** Reformatted sagittal CT image confirms a typical Schmorl nodule (*arrow*).

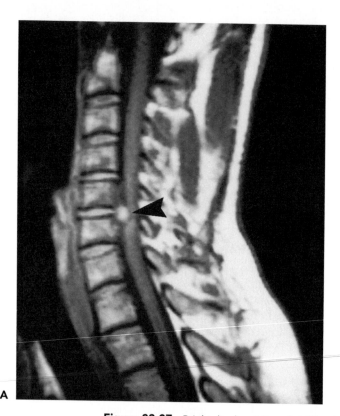

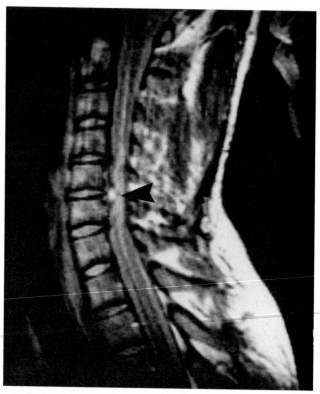

Figure 23-27 Bright disc herniation. **A:** Midsagittal T1-weighted image shows a bright disc herniation at the C5–C6 level (*arrowhead*). **B:** Midsagittal proton-density-weighted FSE image shows that the herniated disc fragment (*arrowhead*) remains hyperintense. Edema, hemorrhage, or hydrated calcium may account for the findings.

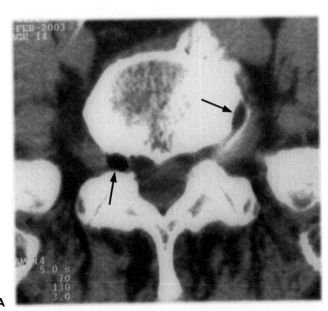

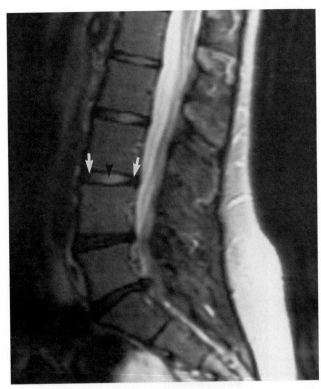

A

B

Figure 23-28 Degenerated lumbar disc. **A:** Axial CT at L5 demonstrates oval areas of low attenuation (*arrows*) adjacent to the vertebral body. These findings are consistent with a degenerated bulging disc. Note anterior osteophytes and bilateral facet disease. **B:** Midsagittal T2-weighted image shows low signal intensity and decreased height of the L4–L5 and L5–S1 discs. These findings are commonly referred to as degeneration and are probably related to loss of proteoglycans in the disc. The L4–L5 disc bulges posteriorly, and there is a probable herniation at the L5–S1 level. Note normal brightness of the L3–L4, L2–L3, and L1–L2 discs. In these normal discs the internuclear cleft (thin central linear hypointensity, *arrowhead*) and the annulus (peripheral zones of hypointensity, *white arrows*) are clearly identifiable.

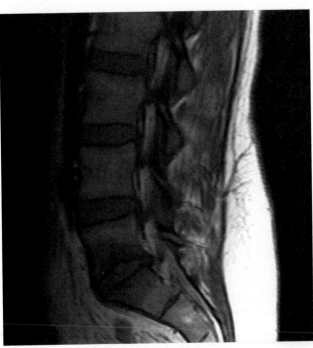

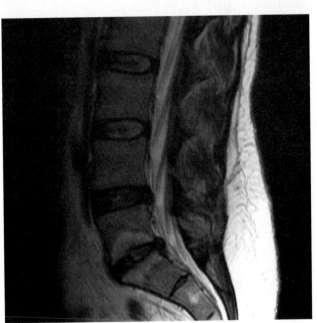

A

B

Figure 23-29 Type I, Modic changes. **A:** Midsagittal T1-weighted image shows low signal intensity from inferior endplate of L5 and superior endplate of S1. The corresponding disc space is narrowed. Findings are related to presence of vascularized fibrous tissue and edema. **B:** Matching FSE T2-weighted image shows the abnormalities to be hyperintense.

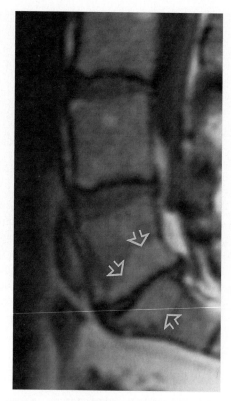

Figure 23-30 Type II, Modic changes. Midline sagittal T1-weighted image shows increased signal intensity from the inferior endplate of L4 and superior of L5 and narrowing of that disc space. These areas represent fatty infiltration.

recognize the above-described signal intensity changes as resulting from disc degeneration, so as not to confuse them with infection (discitis). There is, however, no correlation between these signal intensity changes and specific symptoms.

Disc Herniation

As the degenerative process progresses, small circumferential fissures develop in the annulus fibrosus, which later coalesce to form a radial tear. Distinction between focal extrusion of disc material and a circumferential enlargement is important, as the former is typically treated surgically, whereas the latter may be treated conservatively.

Disc *bulge* refers to a smooth circumferential (global) extension of the disc margin beyond the boundary of the adjacent vertebral end plates in greater than 50% of the disc circumference (Fig. 23-32). The annulus fibrosus is intact although weakened. There is usually loss of height of the involved disc space and desiccation of the nucleus pulposus. Patients rarely complain of nerve root compression unless there is coexisting spinal stenosis and facet joint disease (65).

Disc *herniation* refers to a focal, incomplete extension of the contents of the nucleus pulposus through an incomplete tear of the annulus fibrosus in less than 50% of the circumference of the disc. Disc herniation may be further subdivided into disc *protrusion* and disc *extrusion*.

A disc is protruded when the posterior extent of the involved disc material is limited by some intact outer fibers

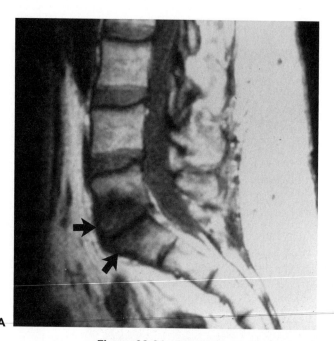

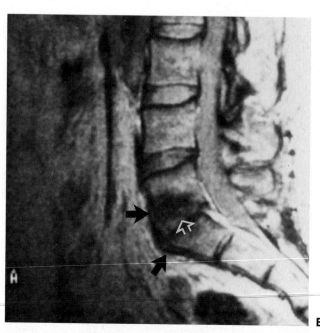

Figure 23-31 Type III, Modic changes. **A:** Midsagittal T1-weighted image shows low signal intensity from the inferior endplate of L5 and superior endplate of S1 (*arrows*). Corresponding disc space is narrow. **B:** Midsagittal conventional proton density-weighted image shows that the endplate abnormalities (*solid arrows*) remain hypointense (sclerosis was present on radiographs). The L5–S1 disc (*open arrow*) is also of low signal intensity.

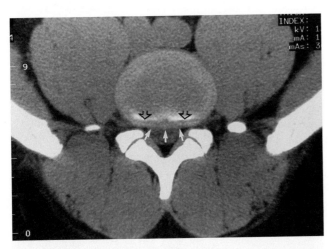

Figure 23-32 Disc bulge. Axial CT at L4–L5 level shows that the posterior margin of the disc (*solid arrows*) protrudes smoothly and in a generalized fashion from the edge of the vertebral body (*open arrows*). The disc has lost its normal posterior central concavity.

of the annulus fibrosus and an intact PLL. The term disc *protrusion* should be used when the greatest distance between the edges of the disc material beyond the disc space is less than the distance of the edges at the disc base in all planes (Fig. 23-33).

Disc *extrusion* is an extrusion of disc contents through complete tears of annulus fibrosus and the PLL resulting in an anterior epidural mass. In extrusion the distance between

the edges of the disc material beyond the disc space is greater than the distance between the edges of the base in at least one plane (Fig. 23-34). The extruded disc is often attached to the disc of origin. If the disc material is displaced in any direction away from the site of extrusion, it is called *migrated disc,* and if it has no continuity with the disc of origin it may be referred to as a *sequestered disc* or a *free fragment* (Fig. 23-35).

The proposed terminology used to describe the location of a herniated disc in the horizontal plane is central, left/right central ("paramedian"), subarticular ("lateral recess"), foraminal and extraforaminal ("far lateral") zone; in the craniocaudal plane the disc level may be infrapedicular, pedicular, and suprapedicular (32). Lumbar disc herniations most commonly occur posteriorly and are often paramedian because of the presence of the midline septum. Lumbar disc herniations generally produce symptoms involving the nerve root inferior to the level of the herniation. That is, an L3–L4 disc herniation will compress the L4 nerve root. An extraforaminal (far lateral) or foraminal disc herniation may produce symptoms involving the nerve root exiting at that same level (see Fig. 23-33D). Paramedian (the preferred term is left or right central) lumbar disc herniations occur most commonly at the L4-L5 and L5–S1 levels. In the cervical region, disc herniations most commonly involve the C5–C6 and C6–C7 spaces (Fig. 23-36). In the cervical spine, disc herniations tend to produce symptoms involving the nerve root at the same vertebral level (remember that there are eight paired cervical

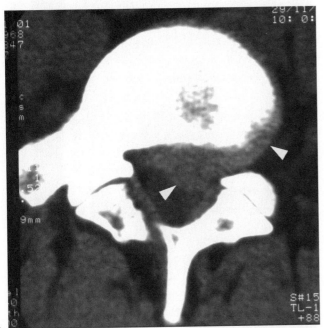

A

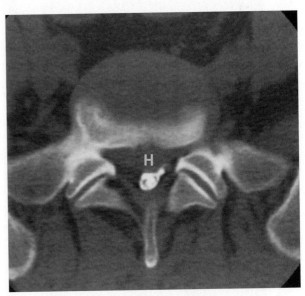

B

Figure 23-33 Disc protrusion. **A:** Transaxial CT image at L4–L5 shows left-sided disc herniation comprising less than 50% of the circumference (*arrowheads*). The base of the herniation is wider than the greatest distance between the edges of the disc material beyond the disc space. **B:** Axial post-myelogram CT in a different patient shows a right central herniated disc (H), located in the central and right paramedian ventral epidural compartment. The contrast-filled thecal sac is indented by the herniated disc. The right S1 nerve root is compressed and not seen. (*continued*)

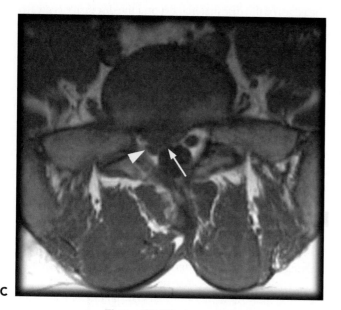

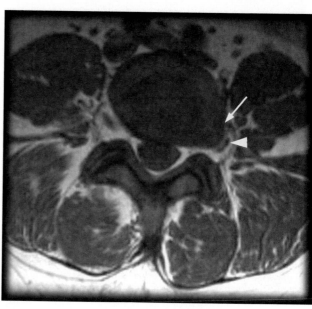

C

D

Figure 23-33 *(continued)* **C:** Axial T1-weighted image at L5–S1 level in a different patient demonstrates a right central *disk* protrusion *(arrowhead)* causing compression of the right S1 nerve root *(arrow)*. **D:** Axial T1-weighted image at L4–L5 (different patient) shows left extraforaminal disc protrusion *(arrow)* displacing the left L4 nerve root *(arrowhead)*.

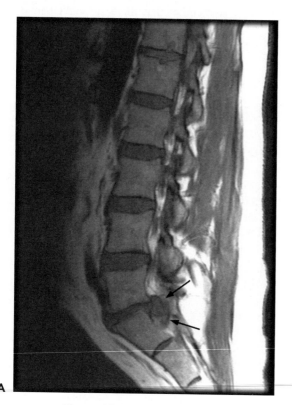

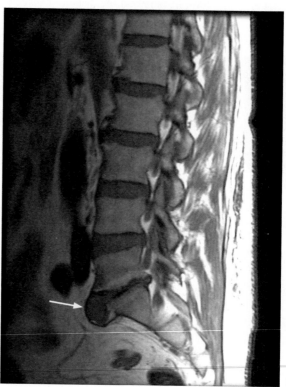

A

B

Figure 23-34 Disc extrusion. **A:** Sagittal T1-weighted image shows herniation of the L5–S1 intervertebral disc *(arrows)*. The distance between the edges of the herniated disc material is greater than the parent disc height, consistent with an extrusion. **B:** Sagittal T1-weighted image in a different patient reveals anterior disc extrusion *(arrow)*. Note decreased height of the L5–S1 interspace and Modic type 2 changes in the adjacent endplates.

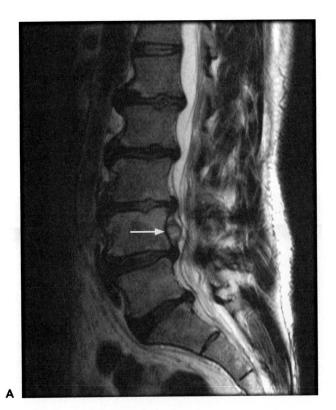

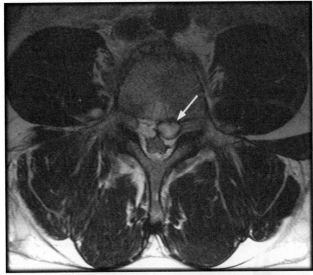

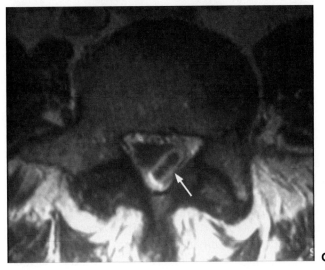

Figure 23-35 Sequestered disc fragment. **A:** Sagittal T2-weighted image shows an oval mass (*arrow*) behind L4. The mass has a central hyperintensity and no clear connection to either the L4–L5 or L5–S1 intervertebral disc. **B:** Axial T2-weighted shows a left central hyperintense epidural mass (*arrow*) corresponding to a free disc fragment. **C:** Axial T1-weighted image in another patient acquired immediately after gadolinium administration shows enhancing margins of a mass in the left posterior epidural space (*arrow*). At surgery, a sequestered disc surrounded by granulation tissues presumably arising from the L5–S1 interspace was found.

nerve roots). In the thoracic spine, the T11 and T12 discs herniate most commonly (Fig. 23-37).

The diagnosis of disc herniation can be made reliably with MRI, CT, or postmyelography CT. Although CT is more sensitive than MRI for the detection of intradiscal gas and calcification, MRI is used in most institutions for evaluating patients with radicular symptoms or symptoms referable to the conus medullaris, because of its multiplanar capabilities and superior tissue characterization. Although MRI and postmyelogram CT are similar in their ability to detect disc herniations, MRI is preferred to postmyelogram CT because it is less invasive and avoids the potential complications

associated with the intrathecal contrast administration. The benefits of intravenous gadolinium MRI for diagnosing lumbar disc herniation in the unoperated spine are somewhat unclear, and contrast enhancement may help in identifying subtle herniated discs (Fig. 23-38). Postcontrast MRI may show enhancing nerve roots. This finding corresponds to the level of clinical symptoms (Fig. 23-39) and probably reflects a breakdown of the nerve–blood barrier. In the absence of disc herniations, enhancement of a nerve merits no treatment. In some cases even large disc herniations may be successfully treated conservatively (118). The regression of the herniation may be, at least in part, due to resorption

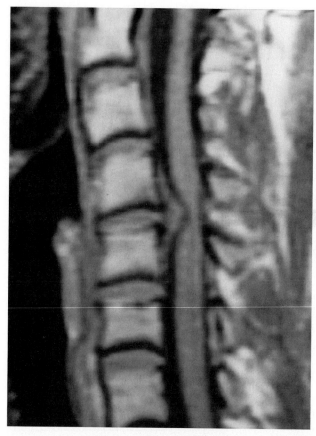

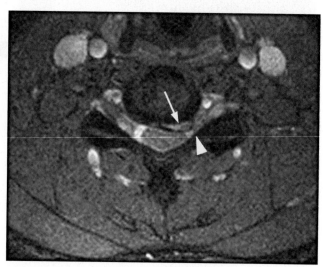

Figure 23-36 Cervical disc herniation. **A:** Midsagittal T1-weighted image shows a large herniated disc at C4–C5. Note significant indentation of ventral aspect of the spinal cord. The hypointense linear area posterior to the herniated disc is probably a combination of intact posterior longitudinal ligament and CSF. **B:** Axial T2*-weighted gradient echo image in a different patient shows left central/foraminal C5-C6 *disk* protrusion (*arrow*). The degenerated discs remain bright on T2*-weighted gradient echo sequences. The left anterior subarachnoid space is effaced and there is a significant foraminal stenosis (*arrowhead*).

of a hematoma, which accounts for a significant portion of the epidural mass, or it may be due to progressive disc dehydration. Contrast-enhanced MRI may also show faint radial areas of enhancement, which follow the configuration of the annulus fibrosus (Fig. 23-40). These may represent radial annular tears with ingrowth of granulation tissues, and they are typically hyperintense on T2-weighted images. Whether or not annular tears produce symptoms is debatable, and they are treated conservatively. In the cervical region, contrast-enhanced MRI results in increased signal intensity of the epidural space, highlighting disc herniations against the low signal intensity CSF on T1-weighted images. For MRI of the cervical spine, we use contrast enhancement only in cases in which the unenhanced images are equivocal, as the usefulness of routine contrast enhancement in the cervical spine has not been determined.

Spondylosis and Osteochondrosis

A common degenerative change of the spine is spondylosis deformans (also known as bridging osteophytes), which occurs in 60% to 80% of adults over the age of 50 years and is generally considered a consequence of aging. Spondylosis deformans essentially involves the annulus fibrosus and adjacent vertebral body apophyses, and it is characterized by anterior and lateral marginal osteophytes. The mucoid matrix of the disc is replaced by fibrous tissue, but the disc height is normal or only slightly decreased and the disc margins are regular (82).

Intervertebral osteochondrosis should be distinguished from spondylosis deformans, especially because the term "spondylosis" is often used as a synonym for degeneration, encompassing both entities. Osteochondrosis involves primarily the nucleus pulposus and the vertebral body endplates, with extensive fissuring of the annulus fibrosus. Osteochondrosis leads to significant disc space narrowing, vacuum phenomenon, reactive changes of the vertebral bodies, development of posterior osteophytes, and is an important factor in pathogenesis of spinal canal stenosis. In contrast to spondylosis deformans, intervertebral osteochondrosis is a clearly pathologic process, although not necessarily symptomatic (82).

Large posterior osteophytes and other bony overgrowths cause spinal stenosis with resultant compressive myelopathy, especially in the cervical region (Fig. 23-41). Patients with diffuse spondylitic ridging who are symptomatic may

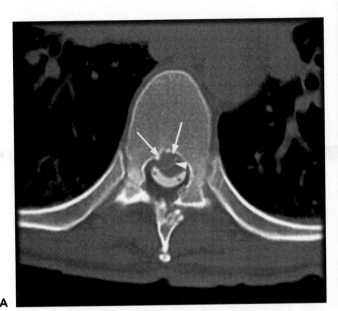
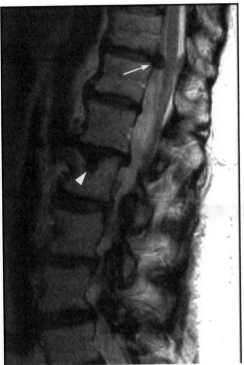

Figure 23-37 Thoracic disc herniation. **A:** Axial postmyelogram CT at T9 shows a ventral, epidural, soft tissue density (*arrows*) compressing the subarachnoid space and the spinal cord, which is displaced dorsally and to the left. A thin plane of contrast (*arrowhead*), corresponding to the anterior subarachnoid space, is seen between cord and mass. A migrated right central T8–T9 disc fragment was confirmed at surgery. **B:** A central T11–T12 disc herniation (*arrow*) is seen on this sagittal T2-weighted image. The cord is displaced posteriorly. There is also a dorsal disc herniation at L1–L2 and a Schmorl nodule (*arrowhead*) involving the superior L2 endplate.

require vertebral corpectomy with anterior cervical fusion for relief of their symptoms. Chronic spinal cord compression is sometimes associated with regions of increased T2 signal in the spinal cord, a finding suggestive of myelomalacia (see Figs. 23-41C and 23-41D). A zone of myelomalacia in the presence of multilevel osteophytosis may indicate the need for decompression at that level. Patients with myelomalacia generally respond less favorably to surgical decompression than those without spinal cord changes.

Facet Joint Disease

Degenerative changes of the facet joints may result from primary osteoarthritis or may be secondary to degenerative changes within the intervertebral disc. When facet joint and intervertebral changes are both present, it is impossible to ascertain the primary cause. The changes that occur with facet joint degeneration are similar to those seen in other osteoarthritides. Although the changes can be seen on MRI, they are better demonstrated on CT. The imaging findings consist of joint space narrowing with associated subchondral sclerosis of the articular surfaces, subchondral cyst formation, and hypertrophic new bone formation. In the cervical region, both the uncovertebral and facet joints may degenerate. The former tend to produce stenosis of the neural foramina, whereas the latter predominantly result in narrowing of the spinal canal diameter, and less frequently

foraminal stenosis (Fig. 23-42A). In the lumbar region, facet degeneration is usually accompanied by buckling (incorrectly called "hypertrophy") of the LF and degenerative disc disease, which when combined result in spinal canal stenosis. Inflammatory changes associated with hypertrophic facet degeneration enhance on postcontrast MRI and at times may mimic a neoplasm (Fig. 23-42B). A CT study usually confirms degenerative disease in such cases. Foraminal stenosis in the lumbar spine is generally best assessed on sagittal T1-weighted images (Fig. 23-42C).

An additional consequence of facet joint degeneration is the development of synovial cysts, which usually occur in the lower lumbar spine, most commonly at L4–5. These juxta-articular cysts are lined by synovium and communicate with the joint. They measure up to 10 mm in diameter, extend laterally or into the spinal canal, and may have a completely or partially calcified shell. The cysts may contain clear, mucinous, hemorrhagic fluid as well as gas. Their margins may show enhancement, which is probably related to the presence of granulation tissue (Fig. 23-43). Ganglion cysts occur in similar location, but they are not lined by synovium and do not communicate with the joint. Because synovial and ganglion cysts are usually not distinguished by imaging and management of both lesions is the same, the preferred term is juxta-articular (or degenerative intraspinal) cyst (95). On MRI the cysts are of high signal intensity on T2-weighted images (see Fig. 23-43C).

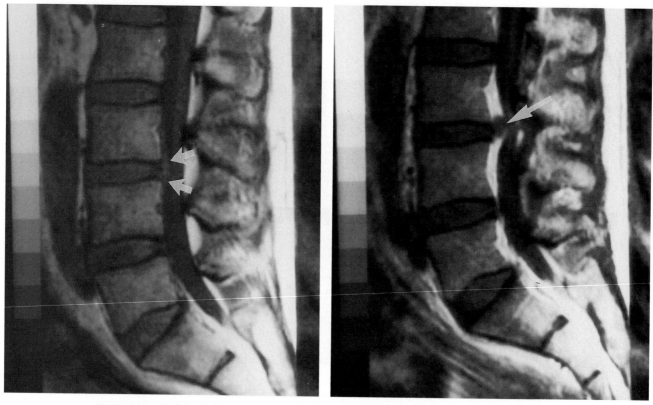

Figure 23-38 Disc herniation and gadolinium enhancement. **A:** Midsagittal T1-weighted image shows subtle prominence of the ventral epidural space (*arrows*) at L3–L4 but no definite disc herniation. **B:** After administration of contrast, T1-weighted midsagittal image shows a herniated disc (*arrow*) surrounded by enhancing epidural space, illustrating utility of contrast administration in the equivocal unoperated spine.

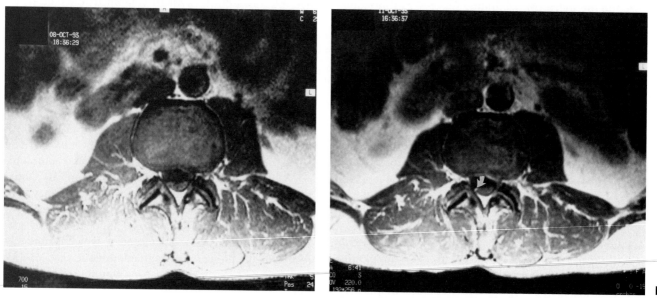

Figure 23-39 Enhancing nerve root, nonoperated back. **A:** Axial T1-weighted image at L4 in a patient with a right L5 radiculopathy and no history of surgery. The examination is normal. **B:** Image at the same level immediately after gadolinium administration shows enhancing right L5 nerve root (*arrow*) corresponding to clinical symptoms. The etiology of this enhancement is uncertain but confirms the location of the symptoms. Treatment is generally conservative.

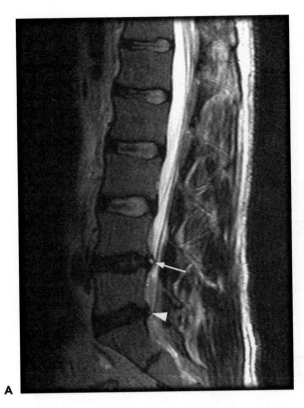

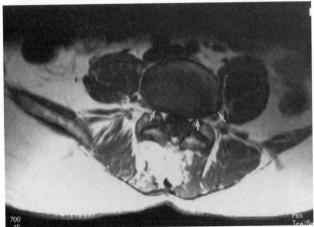

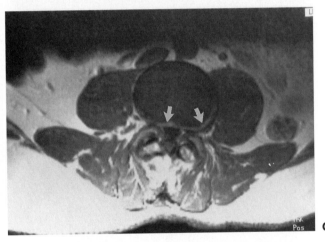

Figure 23-40 Radial annular tear. **A:** Sagittal T2-weighted image shows degenerative changes of L4–L5 and L5–S1 discs. The hyperintensity in the posterior aspect of the L4–L5 disc (*arrow*) corresponds to annulus fibrosus tear. A smaller bright spot at L5–S1 (*arrowhead*) may also represent a tear in the annulus fibrosus. **B:** Axial T1-weighted image at L4–L5 in a different patient shows minimal disc bulge (*arrows*). **C:** Comparable image after contrast administration shows linear zone of enhancement (*arrows*) in outer aspect of the annulus fibrosus representing granulation tissue in a radial tear.

They are commonly adjacent to a facet joint, which also shows abnormal high T2 signal intensity because of fluid in the intra-articular space. Hemorrhage into a cyst may cause acute exacerbation of chronic low-back pain.

Spinal Stenosis

Spinal stenosis refers to a reduction in the caliber of the spinal canal. Resultant symptoms depend on the level of involvement. If the cervical region is involved, the patient may present with a radiculopathy, myelopathy, or neck or shoulder pain. Stenosis of the lumbar region may cause neurogenic claudication, back pain, or paresthesia. In cases of superimposed acute lumbar disc herniation, patients may present with an acute cauda equina syndrome.

Spinal stenosis may be either primary or acquired. The most common cause of acquired stenosis is degenerative change. Degenerative spinal stenosis arises from changes occurring in three major locations: the disc space, the facet joints, and the LF. Narrowing of the disc space results in alterations in the mechanical forces exerted upon the facet joints and associated ligaments. As a result, the facet joints and LF often become thick. The canal may be narrowed anteriorly by a degenerative disc (bulging or herniated) and posterior osteophytes, posteriorly by hypertrophy of the LF and facet joints (see Figs. 23-41 to 23-43). Hypertrophic bone formation of the facet joints also contributes to lateral encroachment on the spinal canal with effacement of the lateral recesses. Other rare causes of acquired spinal canal stenosis include epidural lipomatosis and

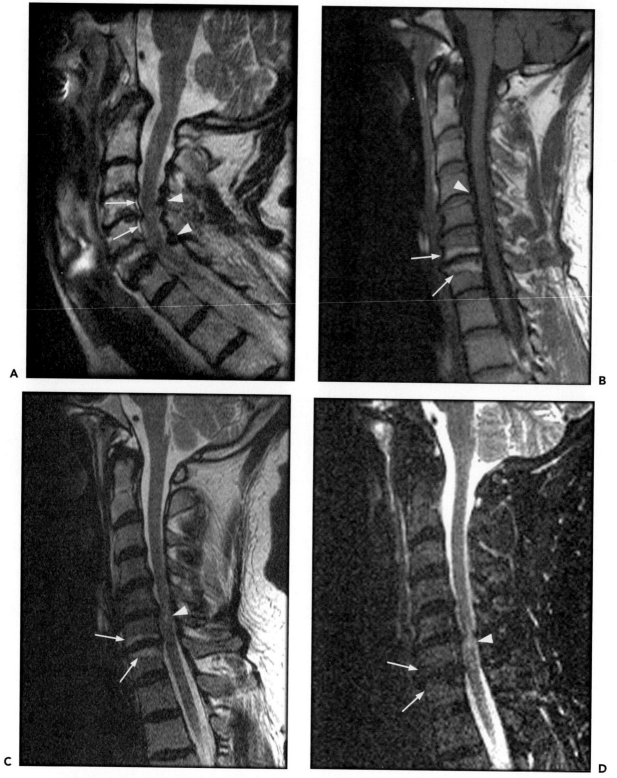

Figure 23-41 Osteochondrosis and cervical spinal canal stenosis. **A:** Midsagittal T2-weighted image shows extensive degenerative changes with loss of disc height, end plate degeneration, and anterolis-tesis of C6 on C7. The posterior disc-osteophyte complex has displaced the PLL (*arrows*). The spinal canal is further narrowed by thickened ligamenta flava (*arrowheads*). There is no abnormal signal in the spinal cord. **B:** Midline sagittal T1-weighted image in a different patient demonstrates cervical spinal canal stenosis, dorsal C4–C5 disc herniation (*arrowhead*), anterior and posterior osteophytes, and Modic type 2 changes (*arrows*). **C:** Midsagittal T2-weighted image reveals hyperintense spinal cord le-sion (*arrowhead*). Type 2 endplate degenerative changes caused by fat infiltration (*arrows*) are again seen. **D:** The spinal cord lesion (*arrowhead*) is more conspicuous on this STIR image. The high signal of the endplates has disappeared with nulling of the signal from fat, confirming type 2 changes (*arrows*).

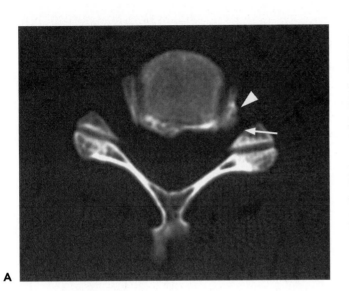

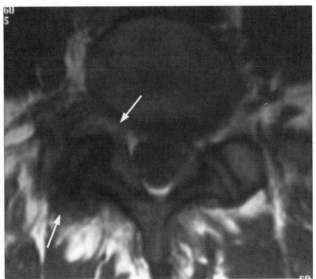

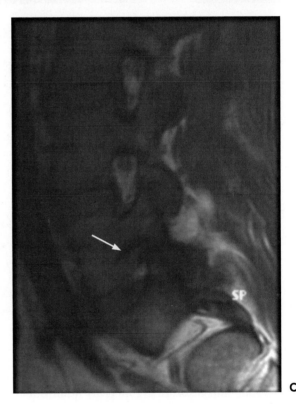

Figure 23-42   Neural foraminal stenosis. **A:** Axial CT at C4–C5 shows hypertrophic degenerative changes involving the left uncovertebral joint (*arrowhead*) causing significant narrowing of the left neural foramen (*arrow*). Note normal appearance of facet joints. **B:** Axial T1-weighted image in a different patient at L4–L5 shows prominent degenerative facet disease on the right (*arrows*). The joint space is replaced by sclerotic subchondral bone of low signal intensity, and the joint capsule is swollen due to acute inflammation. Such lesions also enhance with gadolinium and may mimic an infectious process. **C:** Sagittal T1-weighted image through the neural foramina clearly demonstrates narrowing of the L4–L5 neural foramen on the right (*arrow*) with loss of fat planes around the nerve root. Note normal appearance of the more superior neural foramina.

ossification of the PLL and/or the LF. Epidural lipomatosis may be seen in cases of endogenous or, more commonly, exogenous hypercortisolism. Epidural lipomatosis may also occur in the setting of morbid obesity. Most cases (70%) involve the thoracic spine and in some instances can produce a myelopathy and polyneuropathy (65). The lumbar region also may be involved.

Ossification of the posterior longitudinal ligament (OPLL) is endemic in Japan, where it is found in 3% of the population with neurologic findings referable to the cervical region (75). It is seen more often in the cervical region

(88%), but it also may involve the thoracic region (75). Its incidence is higher in patients with diffuse idiopathic skeletal hyperostosis. This type of ossification may be continuous or segmental. The ossified ligament is better seen with CT, but MRI may show a band of hypointensity posterior to the vertebral bodies (Fig. 23-44). The ossified ligament is not reliably detected by MRI unless it measures more than 3 mm in thickness. Patchy areas of increased T1 signal intensity, which occasionally are present in the hypertrophied ligament, probably represent areas of fatty or active bone marrow.

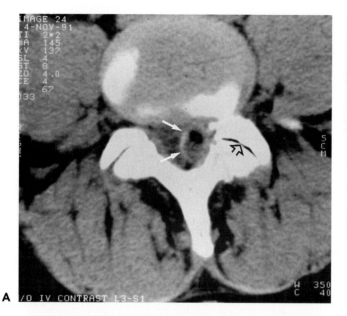

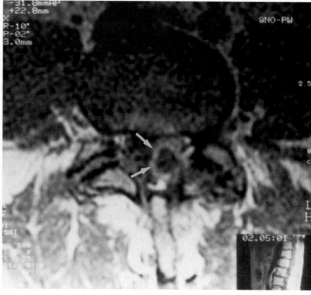

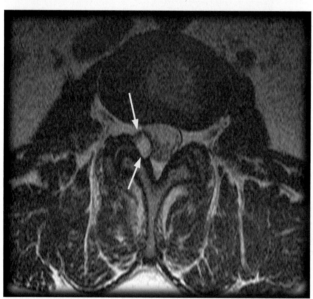

Figure 23-43 Synovial cyst. **A:** Axial CT shows a mass adjacent to a degenerated left facet joint at L4–L5 (*arrows*) that is compressing the thecal sac. Note gas (*open arrow*) in the facet joint, which extends into the synovial cyst. **B:** Postcontrast axial T1-weighted image shows the cyst (*arrows*) to have peripheral enhancement, presumably secondary to granulation tissue formation. **C:** Axial T2-weighted image in a different patient demonstrates a typical synovial cyst (*arrows*), hyperintense and adjacent to a facet joint. The thecal sac is compressed.

Ossification of the LF is generally seen in the setting of OPLL, but occasionally it occurs in an isolated form (Fig. 23-45). It is found most commonly in the cervical and thoracic regions (106). Another uncommon cause of acquired spinal stenosis is Paget disease (106). Congenital spinal stenosis is usually related to "short" pedicles, but it is seen also in children with achondroplasia and deposition disorders, such as mucopolysaccharidoses.

Although absolute measurements are not valuable in all cases, spinal canal stenosis should be considered if the anteroposterior diameter of the cervical and lumbar canals is less than 12 mm and in the thoracic region if its anteroposterior diameter is less than 10 mm. Kinematic MRI in flexion and extension may show cervical and lumbar spinal canal stenosis to a better advantage, because in many patients a

significant increase in spinal cord impingement is seen, especially in extension (68).

The dimensions of the spinal canal play an important role with regards to the development of symptoms in individuals with disc herniations. In symptomatic patients the cross-sectional area of the spinal canal has been found to be significantly smaller compared with asymptomatic individuals (28).

Spondylolisthesis and Spondylolysis

Spondylolisthesis refers to displacement of a vertebra in relation to an adjacent vertebra, resulting in a malalignment of the spinal column. The displacement can be either anterior (anterolisthesis) or posterior (retrolisthesis).

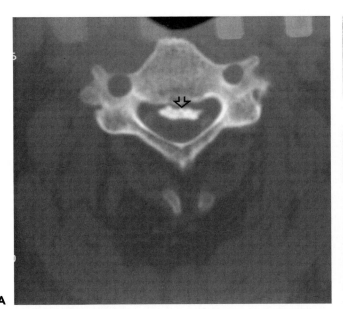

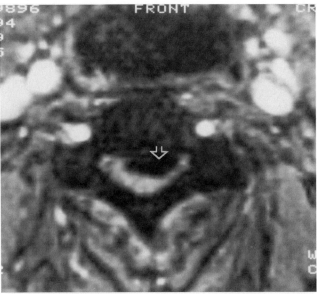

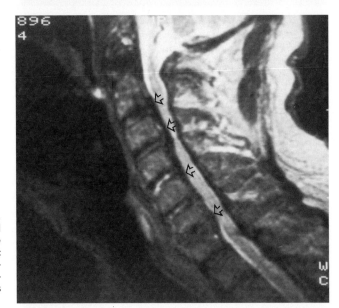

Figure 23-44 Ossified posterior longitudinal ligament (OPLL). **A:** Postmyelogram axial CT shows OPLL (*arrow*) causing spinal cord compression. **B:** Axial gradient echo image at same level shows the ligament (*arrow*) to be hypointense. Note that due to magnetic susceptibility artifact the abnormality appears larger on this sequence. **C:** Midsagittal T2-weighted image shows the ossified ligament (*arrows*) extending from C2–C7. There is spinal canal stenosis at the C3–C4 and C6–C7 levels.

The term *degenerative spondylolisthesis* is used to denote a malalignment that arose as a result of spinal instability due to degenerative changes involving the disc and facet joints. Spondylolisthesis may also result from acute trauma or from congenital or acquired fibrous defects in the pars interarticularis (spondylolysis).

Spondylolysis occurs in approximately 5% of the population, but a majority of these lesions occur without associated symptoms (65,103). It tends to be bilateral and most commonly involves the lower lumbar spine, but it may also be found in the cervical region. The most widely accepted explanation for spondylolysis is that repeated minor trauma leads to stress fractures of the pars interarticularis (65,103). Although both CT and MRI readily show the abnormality, CT is preferred when spondylolysis is suspected. Spondylolysis usually affects L5 (around 90% of cases),

with involvement of L4 (10%) and L3 (<1%) much less frequent (65,103). CT shows a lucent defect with irregular margins in one or both pars interarticulares (Fig. 23-46). The presence of "double facets" ("too many facets") in a CT examination should prompt the consideration of pars defects at the corresponding level. In cases of unilateral spondylolysis, the contralateral normal articular pillar supports all biomechanical stress at that level and may become sclerotic. If significant slippage of one vertebra over another has occurred, the "double canal" sign may be seen. Sagittal MRI shows the pars defects to be oriented perpendicular to the long axis of the adjacent facet joint. At times, the anterior portion of the defective pars interarticularis may show high signal intensity on T1-weighted images. On STIR images high signal intensity may be seen adjacent to the pars defects, and hyperintensity corresponding to stress

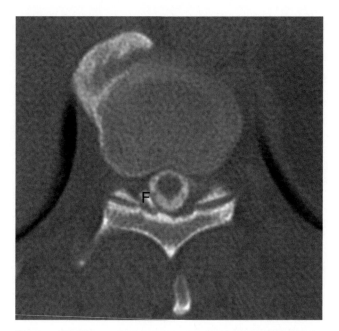

Figure 23-45 Ossified ligamentum flavum. Axial CT myelogram, bone window settings, shows heavily calcified ligamentum flavum (F).

fractures may be detected even before the fractures develop. The spondylolisthesis may impinge upon and stretch the nerve roots, producing a radiculopathy that tends to be bilateral.

POSTOPERATIVE SPINE

After lumbar spine surgery for disc disease, 10% to 40% of patients report recurrent pain, a condition referred to as "failed back surgery syndrome" (87). Causes for this pain include recurrent or residual disc herniations (or unrecognized far lateral disc herniation), epidural scar formation, arachnoiditis, postoperative infection, radiculitis, stenoses of the lateral recesses or neural foramina, failure of bone fusion, and failure to correctly identify the structural sources of pain. The dimensions of the neural foramina are best assessed on parasagittal images, and contrast-enhanced MRI is the method of choice for differentiating epidural scar from herniated disc. Herniated disc material is of intermediate signal intensity and blends with the intervertebral disc on T1-weighted images. Mass effect is seen in up to 69% of patients and may mimic the preoperative findings (87). The central substance of the herniated disc should not enhance. Peridiscal scar causes peripheral enhancement in the majority of recurrent/residual disc herniations (11,41) (Fig. 23-47). Postcontrast MRI should be obtained as quickly as possible after gadolinium administration, because homogeneous disc enhancement may be seen on images obtained more than 15 to 30 minutes after contrast administration. This delayed enhancement phenomenon is generally seen at least 3 to 6 weeks after surgery and reflects ingrowth of fibrosis into the disc with proliferation of capillaries that have "leaky" tight junctions (29).

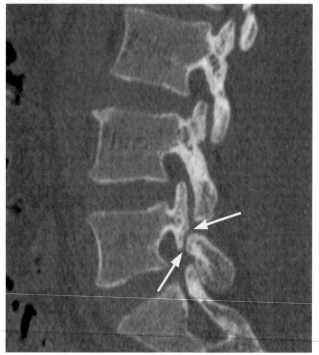
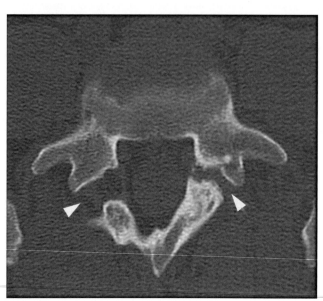

A   **B**

Figure 23-46 Spondylolysis. **A:** Sagittal reformatted CT shows a defect of L5 pars interarticularis (*arrows*). There is no evidence of spondylolisthesis. **B:** Axial CT at L5 shows bilateral lucent defects (*arrowheads*), right greater than left, involving the pars interarticulares. Cortical bone is seen adjacent to the defects indicating the chronic nature of the process.

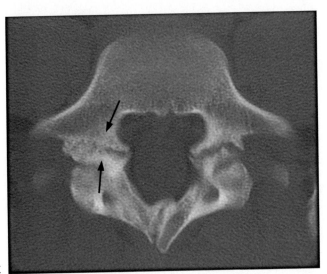

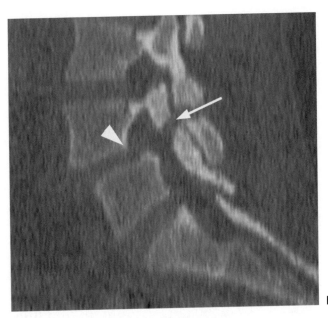

Figure 23-46 *(continued)* **C:** Axial CT at L5 in a different patient demonstrates a lucent defect of the left pars. The findings are subtler on the right *(arrows)*. Both of these lesions may be more acute in nature. **D:** Sagittal reformatted CT in a different patient reveals a wide L4 pars defect *(arrow)* and anterior spondylolistehesis of L4 *(arrowhead)*.

Epidural scar (fibrosis) is of intermediate signal intensity on T1-weighted images and of variable signal intensity on T2-weighted images. Although it is generally accepted that scar does not exert mass effect, occasionally it may produce significant compression of the thecal sac or neural structures (13). Scar, which normally contains abundant capillaries with "loose" tight junctions and wide extracellular spaces, enhances markedly, homogeneously, and immediately after MRI contrast medium administration (Fig. 23-48). It is usually better visualized in the transverse

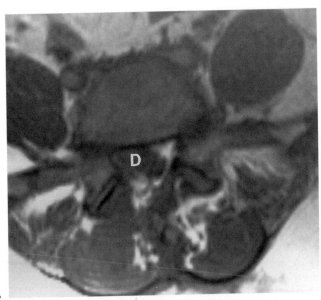

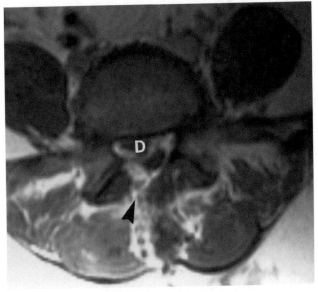

Figure 23-47 Recurrent disc herniation. **A:** T1-weighted image shows ventral and rightward epidural soft tissue (D) at the L5–S1 level in this patient with recurrent symptoms 2 months after surgery. **B:** Image at a comparable level immediately after contrast administration shows marginal enhancement of the lesion compatible with a disc fragment surrounded by granulation tissue. Laminectomy site *(arrowhead)* is clearly seen.

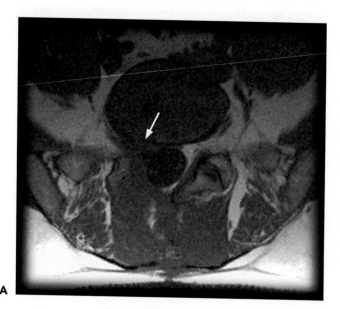
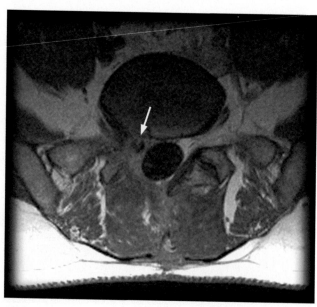

Figure 23-48 Epidural scar. **A:** Axial T1-weighted image at L5–S1 shows tissue isointense to the disc (*arrow*) that replaces the epidural fat on the right in this patient 1 year after a hemilaminectomy. **B:** Immediately after administration of gadolinium, the tissue demonstrates homogenous contrast enhancement compatible with fibrosis. The right S1 nerve root (*arrow*) is now visualized surrounded by the epidural scar.

plane, so axial images should be obtained first after gadolinium administration. At times, epidural scar may be separated from underlying disc fragments by a thin zone of low signal intensity on the postcontrast T1-weighted images. Scar located in the ventral epidural space may enhance for many years after the surgery, whereas enhancement of scar in the dorsal epidural space is temporary.

Linear enhancement of the end plates, the annulus fibrosus, and especially the disc space along the end plates may be a normal finding during the first 3 to 6 months after surgery (89,110). Infection should be strongly considered if the following MRI signs are present: complete enhancement of the residual intervertebral disc, enhancement of the vertebral endplates adjacent to the operated disc, and enhancing epidural and/or paravertebral tissue or fluid collections. Enhancement of the paravertebral soft tissues is a specific sign suggestive of septic spondylodiscitis, although it is not always present (110).

Arachnoiditis, an inflammatory process involving all three meningeal layers, is an important cause of the failed back surgery syndrome. Causes of arachnoiditis include surgery, infection, intrathecal administration of medications, trauma, subarachnoid hemorrhage, and prior myelography (88). Postmyelogram CT shows lack of nerve root sleeve filling, adhesion of nerve roots to the walls of the thecal sac (the "empty sac" sign), nerve root clumping, and soft tissue masses that may obliterate the canal (88) (Fig. 23-49A). MRI is less sensitive than postmyelogram CT in the detection of arachnoiditis. MRI reveals enhancement of thickened meninges in 50% of patients with

arachnoiditis shown on myelography (45). Nerve root clumping and enhancement are the most common signs of arachnoiditis by MRI (Figs. 23-49B and 23-49C).

Lumbar epidural anesthesia rarely induces a severe arachnoiditis that may lead to the formation of arachnoid cysts (98). These cysts can potentially compress the spinal cord and lead to development of syrinx. Such arachnoiditis may result from inadvertent introduction of medications into the subarachnoid space or may be related to the preservatives contained in anesthetic solutions. Other possible complications related to epidural anesthesia include infectious spondylodiscitis and spinal cord infarct (21).

Intrathecal droplets from prior myelography with Pantopaque (oil-based contrast medium) have a characteristic MRI appearance (14). These droplets, primarily localized in the dependent portions of the subarachnoid space, are very bright on T1-weighted images and of very low signal intensity on T2-weighted images (Fig. 23-50).

INFECTIONS OF THE SPINE

Infections that begin primarily in the intervertebral disc space are most frequently caused by staphylococci, enterobacteria, and, less commonly, *Pseudomonas*. Tuberculosis (TB) and *Brucella* usually involve the vertebral body first. Involvement of the epidural space is usually secondary to discitis or osteomyelitis. Predisposing risk factors include diabetes, intravenous drug use, renal failure, alcoholism, surgery, trauma, and immunosuppression (112). Routes of

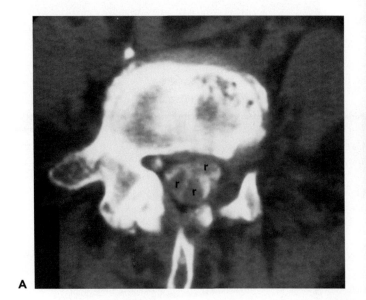

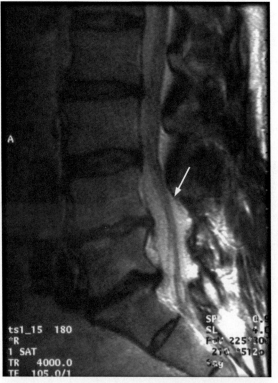

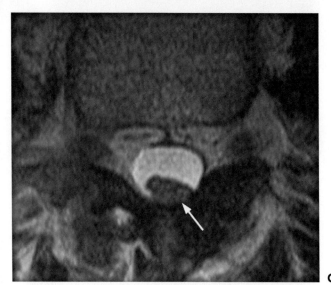

Figure 23-49 Arachnoiditis. **A:** Axial postmyelogram CT shows clumping of nerve roots (r) compatible with arachnoidal adhesions. **B:** On a midsagittal T2-weighted image (different patient) the nerve roots are thick and joined together (*arrow*). **C:** Axial T2-weighted image at L4 shows clumping of nerve roots (*arrow*) to a better advantage.

spread are hematogenous, ascending (via Batson plexus from pelvic infections), and direct implantation. The most common sites of infection are the lumbar and thoracic regions and less commonly the cervical spine (91). Usually, a period of 2 to 8 weeks elapses between the onset of clinical symptoms and the appearance of detectable morphologic changes on imaging studies. MRI is the method of choice for evaluation of suspected localized spinal infection. If symptoms are nonlocalizing, a radionuclide bone scan may be used as a screening test. CT is less sensitive and should be used as a confirmatory test

rather than as the initial imaging method. The earliest CT findings include narrowing of the disc space, erosion of the vertebral body endplates, and vertebral body osteopenia (22). Sagittal reformations are valuable when these findings are present. Later in the process, new bone formation giving rise to osteosclerosis may be seen (22). Extension to the paravertebral soft tissues occurs in approximately 20% of patients and is clearly demonstrated by CT (112), but spread into the epidural or subdural compartments is poorly visualized. Lumbar puncture for the introduction of contrast medium is contraindicated in this clinical setting,

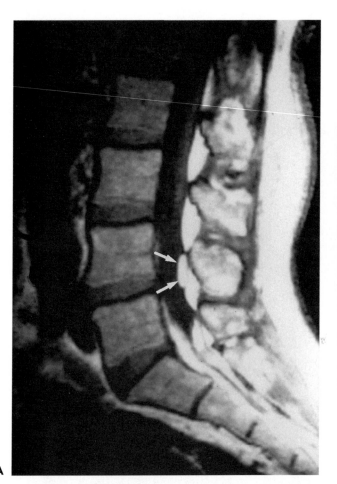
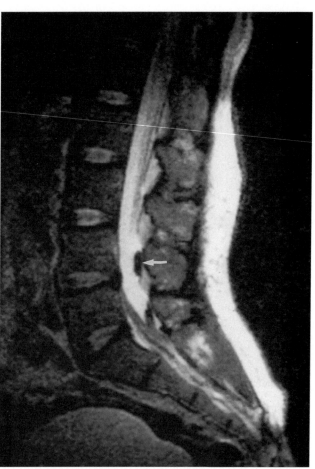

Figure 23-50 Intrathecal pantopaque. **A:** Midsagittal T1-weighted image shows pill-shaped hyperintense droplet (*arrows*) in the dependent aspect of the subarachnoid space at the L4–L5 level. **B:** Corresponding midsagittal T2-weighted image shows marked hypointensity from the Pantopaque (*arrow*).

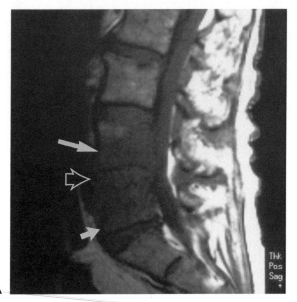
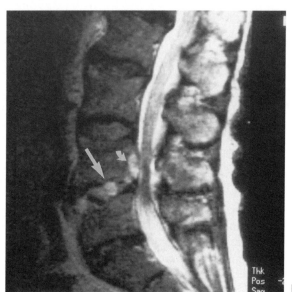

Figure 23-51 Bacterial discitis, osteomyelitis, and epidural abscess. **A:** Midsagittal T1-weighted image in a patient with L4–L5 discitis and osteomyelitis secondary to *Staphylococcus* species. There is low signal intensity from the L4 (*large solid arrow*) and L5 (*short solid arrow*) vertebrae. The inferior endplate of L4 and superior endplate of L5 are indistinct. The L4–L5 disc (*open arrow*) is hypointense. **B:** Midsagittal FSE T2-weighted image shows increased signal intensity (*large arrow*) from the infected L4–L5 disc. This sign is fairly specific for discitis. The epidural abscess (*small curved arrow*) is also hyperintense. Note that the normal internuclear cleft is not seen.

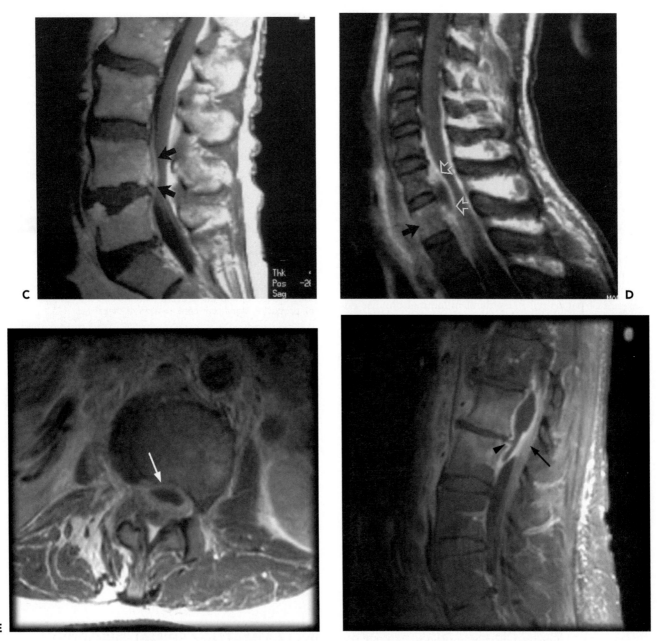

Figure 23-51 *(continued)* **C:** T1-weighted midsagittal image after contrast shows enhancement of L4 and L5 vertebral bodies. A small epidural abscess *(arrows)* narrows the thecal sac. **D:** In a different patient, midsagittal T1-weighted image after contrast administration shows epidural abscess *(open arrows)* at C7–T1. Note enhancement of T1 vertebral body *(solid arrow)* but intact disc space. The dorsal epidural space from C5–T2 also enhances and is thickened. Precervical inflammatory changes extend from the base of the skull to T3. **E:** Axial postcontrast T1-weighted image in a different patient with *Streptococcus* discitis–osteomyelitis shows an anterior epidural abscess *(arrow)* compressing the thecal sac. **F:** Sagittal postcontrast T1-weighted image with fat saturation reveals enhancement of L2 and L3 vertebral bodies and prevertebral space, as well as the anterior epidural abscess, which appears continuous with the superior L3 endplate *(arrowhead)*. The nerve roots within the thecal sac are compressed *(arrow)*.

as it may facilitate spread of infection into the subarachnoid space, resulting in meningitis.

MRI is 96% sensitive and 94% accurate in the detection of spinal infection (64). It is more sensitive than myelography and CT in the diagnosis of discitis, osteomyelitis, and epidural abscesses (78). T1-weighted MRI shows low signal intensity of the involved intervertebral disc and the adjacent vertebral bodies (Fig. 23-51). The cortical bone of the vertebral endplates is usually indistinct or clearly eroded on precontrast images. On T2-weighted sequences, the disc space and adjacent vertebrae are of increased signal intensity and the intranuclear cleft may be effaced. Extension into the paraspinal soft tissues is seen as focal or confluent areas of low signal intensity on T1-weighted and high signal intensity on T2-weighted images. Epidural infection, again bright on T2-weighted images and dark on T1-weighted images, may be isointense with CSF and blend with it imperceptibly. Therefore, intravenous gadolinium administration is imperative, because an epidural abscess may be separated from the thecal sac on postcontrast images (73,113) (Figs. 23-51D to 23-51F). Separating the enhancing epidural abscess from surrounding fat may be shown to a better advantage by the use of fat suppression techniques. Contrast enhancement of the disc and the adjacent vertebrae are also commonly seen after intravenous administration of contrast media (94). With successful treatment, contrast enhancement tends to become less pronounced. The most sensitive signs of spinal infection are presence of paraspinal or epidural inflammation, disc enhancement, and hyperintense disc on T2-weighted MRI, followed by erosion or destruction of vertebral endplate and effacement of the nuclear cleft. Paraspinal or epidural inflammation combined with any of the other four signs has a reported sensitivity of 100% (57).

In contradistinction to pyogenic discitis, TB is said to classically affect the vertebral bodies and the posterior elements. However, in a large series, TB was found to cause a variety of lesions, most of them indistinguishable from pyogenic infection (94). TB most commonly involves the thoracolumbar junction of older individuals in developed countries, while children are primarily affected in developing countries. The primary source of infection is identified in less than 10% of patients (22). Clinically, spinal TB is a more insidious process than its pyogenic counterpart. Multilevel disease results from a propensity to involve the anteroinferior aspect of the endplates, causing spread beneath the ALL (94,112). Chronic destruction of a vertebral body may lead to a sharply angulated kyphosis, known as a gibbus deformity. Although CT and MRI findings are usually nonspecific, on CT the presence of calcifications in the paraspinal muscles is characteristic of TB (Fig. 23-52). Other findings suggestive of TB include rim enhancement of vertebral body lesions and of paraspinal abscesses, spread underneath the longitudinal ligaments, relatively spared intervertebral discs, and skip lesions (64,67). Abscesses tend to be overall larger in TB than in pyogenic spondylitis. TB is also seen in patients with AIDS. The imaging finding of brucellosis and other granulomatous infections are identical to those of TB (112) (Fig. 23-53).

Almost all epidural abscesses are the sequelae of adjacent discitis/osteomyelitis. Isolated epidural abscesses are usually from hematogenous spread and seen in diabetics, intravenous drug users, and patients with a chronic illness or an underlying immunodeficiency (94). Dental abscesses and pneumonia also have been implicated. The most

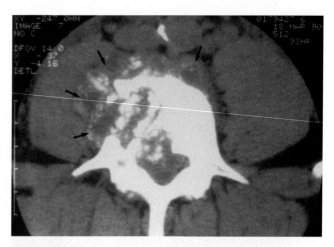

Figure 23-52   Tuberculosis. Axial CT in a patient with tuberculosis affecting L4. There is destruction of the right side of the vertebral body with extension of an abscess into right psoas muscle and prevertebral space (*arrows*). The posterior aspect of the vertebral body is eroded, and the process extends into the epidural space (e), producing significant compression of thecal sac.

common causative microorganism is *Staphylococcus aureus* (112). If treatment is delayed, paraplegia, quadriplegia, or death may ensue. Imaging is critical in these patients, as the correct diagnosis is made clinically in only 20% to 25% of patients. If a distinct sensory level is not present, the entire spine should be evaluated with contrast-enhanced MRI. The two most common MRI appearances include homogeneous or heterogeneous enhancement of the portion of the abscess and lack of enhancement of the liquefied portions of the abscess (113) (see Figs. 23-51 and 23-53). Abscess drainage may be performed under CT guidance and the obtained material sent for microbiological analysis. Follow-up contrast-enhanced MRI may be used to document a decrease in the abscess size with successful antibiotic treatment.

INFLAMMATORY SPINAL DISORDERS

Only the most common inflammatory disorders affecting the vertebral column, namely rheumatoid arthritis and ankylosing spondylitis, will be addressed in this section.

Rheumatoid Arthritis

The cervical spine, and the craniocervical junction in particular, are among the most common sites of rheumatoid arthritis (RA) in adults (involved in more than 80% of patients). The imaging findings include erosions, destruction of the dens, anterior atlantoaxial subluxation, and vertical subluxation. Erosion of the dens by inflammatory pannus (synovial hypertrophy) is common and is most frequently found in the retrodental space. If large, the pannus itself may compress the neural elements. Atlantoaxial dislocation

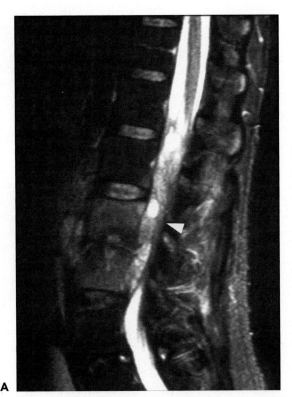 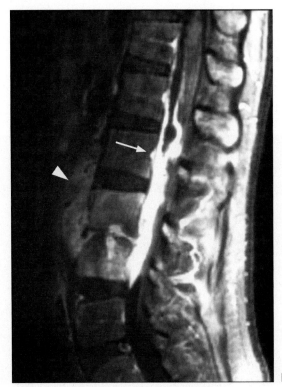

A   B

Figure 23-53 Brucellosis discitis-osteomyelitis. **A:** Midsagittal STIR image shows loss of the L2–L3 disc space and increased signal intensity involving entirely the L2–L3 vertebral bodies. The hyperintensity in the prevertebral space extends into the anterior epidural space (*arrowhead*) with posterior displacement of PLL. The conus medullaris is displaced posteriorly. **B:** On a corresponding postcontrast T1-weighted image with fat saturation there is enhancement of the affected vertebral bodies, disc space, prevertebral space, presumably under ALL (*arrowhead*), and an anterior epidural abscess (*arrow*) that extends cephalad beneath the PLL to the T12 level. Note that this appearance is similar to the one seen with pyogenic discitis-osteomyelitis in Figures 23-51E and F. The only possibly distinctive feature is the more prominent tracking underneath the longitudinal ligaments involving four vertebrae. Tuberculosis could present with the same appearance.

is secondary to ligamentous laxity, ligamentous disruption, or local synovitis and causes pain, instability, and cord compression leading to chronic myelopathy and progressive disability (47). Vertical subluxation, also known as cranial settling and basilar protrusion, causes upward vertical displacement of the cervical spine leading to brainstem compression, which occasionally results in death. Other, less common, types of cervical spine subluxations seen in patients with RA include posterior atlantoaxial, lateral, and subaxial. The subaxial type of subluxation is seen in 40% of patients with RA and leads to a "stepladder" appearance of the cervical spine. Occasionally, the subluxations are severe enough to produce compression of the vertebral arteries, which may lead to vascular insufficiency (47).

Only advanced stages of RA are detected on radiographs, and atlantoaxial subluxations may be demonstrated by obtaining flexion and extension views. In adults, a distance greater than 2 mm between the posterior arch of C1 and the anterior surface of the dens is diagnostic of subluxation. CT may be used to show bone erosions involving the dens, lateral C1–C2 articulations, facet and uncoverte-

bral joints (Fig. 23-54A). CT is also useful in assessing displacements and narrowing of the spinal canal. Pannus occasionally may be identified by CT, but it is better evaluated with MRI. MRI detects joint effusion and pannus tissue in a significant proportion of patients with negative radiographs. Also, it may discriminate between joint effusion and various forms of pannus, which all tend to be of low to intermediate signal intensity on precontrast T1-weighted sequences (Figs. 23-54B to 23-54D). Based on their appearances on T2-weighted and contrast-enhanced MRI, these lesions have been categorized into four groups: hypervascular pannus and joint effusion have high signal intensity on T2-weighted images, hypovascular pannus is relatively isointense, whereas fibrous pannus is of low signal intensity. Hypervascular pannus shows early homogenous enhancement in contrast to effusion, which enhances at the periphery, whereas hypovascular and fibrous pannus demonstrate negligible enhancement after gadolinium administration (105).

MRI readily shows compression of the dural sac, spinal cord, and brainstem. Dynamic MRI, using either gradient

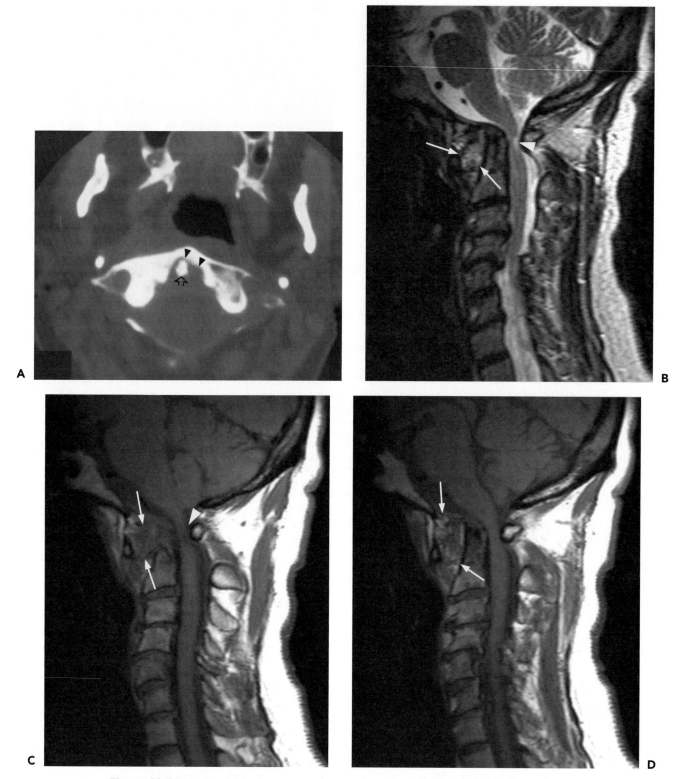

Figure 23-54 Rheumatoid arthritis. **A:** Axial CT, bone window setting, shows marked thinning of the dens (*open arrow*) secondary to surrounding pannus. The posterior margin of the anterior arch (*arrowheads*) of C1 is eroded. **B:** Midsagittal T2-weighted image in a different patient shows increased atlantodental space due to a predominantly hyperintense mass (*arrows*). The dens is displaced posteriorly, compressing the cervicomedullary spinal cord junction (*arrowhead*). Note also spinal canal stenosis at C4. **C:** The mass (*arrows*) is isointense with the cord on this T1-weighted image. The dural sac is compressed (*arrowhead*). Note malalignment of cervical spine and herniated discs. **D:** On post-contrast T1-weighted images the lesion shows some peripheral enhancement (*arrows*). These imaging findings are consistent with joint effusion surrounded by a rim of hypertrophied synovia.

echo or single-shot fast spin echo sequences, with the patient in varying degrees of neck flexion and extension, may be helpful in demonstrating atlantoaxial subluxations and, more important, compression of the brainstem with pannus or joint effusions.

Ankylosing Spondyloarthritis

Ankylosing spondylitis (AS) is one of the most common inflammatory diseases of the spine. It most commonly affects young men and is specifically associated with the histocompatibility antigen B27. It affects the sacroiliac joints, spine, and the bone insertions of ligaments. In the spine, it may give rise to ankylosis, subluxations, and fractures (which may produce epidural hematomas). Cauda equina syndrome is an unusual complication seen late in the course of AS. The etiology of involvement of the cauda equina is uncertain, but it may be secondary to inflammation of the neighboring ligaments, which in turn leads to radiculitis. Dural ectasia with scalloping of the posterior margins of the vertebral bodies and erosion of the posterior elements may sometimes occur (1) (Fig. 23-55A). The nerve roots may be adherent to the edges of the erosive dural ectasia. Atlantoaxial subluxation and destruction of endplates and adjacent discs are other rare complications.

Radiographs have been used to screen the sacroiliac joints for early involvement; however, it has been established that MRI reveals lesions at an even earlier stage of the disease (15). Radiographs also show the so-called bamboo spine in advanced stages. The presence of osteopenia, squaring of the vertebral body margins (due to erosions), symmetric sacroiliitis, marginal syndesmophytes, and fusion of facet joints establishes the diagnosis. Both CT and MRI demonstrate squaring and bridging of the vertebral bodies, as well as dural ectasia (Figs. 23-55B and 23-55C). Early MRI changes of the inflammatory process involving thoracolumbar spine have also been detected in the absence of radiographic abnormality. These lesions are hypointense on T1-weighted, and hyperintense on T2-weighted images, demonstrating homogeneous contrast enhancement. They involve several vertebral bodies, either confined to the corners or widely distributed, and the adjacent intervertebral discs and soft tissues are of normal appearance (55) (see Fig. 23-55C).

Patients with AS are prone to vertebral fractures, frequently leading to pseudoarthrosis which typically develops at the thoracolumbar junction. The fractures are identifiable on radiographs, but their detailed evaluation requires CT. Sterile discitis is best evaluated with MRI, which shows loss of the vertebral endplate cartilage and destruction of the disc. The cartilage is replaced by zones of heterogeneous signal intensity, and T2-weighted images show decreased signal intensity of the disc without a paraspinal soft tissue mass (49). These findings, presumably related to fibrous tissue replacement, serve to distinguish AS from infection.

PRIMARY BONE TUMORS OF THE SPINE

Numerous primary tumors may develop in and adjacent to the spine, and only the most frequent neoplasms arising from the bones of the spinal column will be discussed here.

Hemangioma

Vertebral body hemangiomas are found in more than 10% of autopsies and are frequently encountered on radiologic studies, especially on MRI (59). They are almost always asymptomatic, occur predominantly in women, and are most often located in the thoracic or lumbar regions. Hemangiomas are composed of low-pressure, thin-walled vessels with slow blood flow that are interspersed among thick bone trabeculae and fat. The CT and MRI appearance reflect this histology. On CT, hemangiomas are of low attenuation and contain coarse punctuate and striated areas of sclerosis, the so-called polka dot pattern on axial images (Fig. 23-56A). Cortical bone destruction is almost never present. Calcifications within soft tissue extension are detected occasionally. On MRI, the lesions are characteristically of high signal intensity on both T1-weighted and T2-weighted sequences (Figs. 23-56B to 23-56D). Enhancement after gadolinium administration reflects the extent of vascularization and is minimal or absent in typical indolent hemangiomas. The main differential diagnosis is that of focal fatty replacement of the vertebral bone marrow. In asymptomatic patients, distinction between these two entities is mostly academic.

Less than 1% of vertebral body hemangiomas behave aggressively and lead to compression fractures or soft tissue masses that may cause spinal cord compression. Such aggressive hemangiomas have been reported to involve the entire vertebral body (usually thoracic) and extend into the neural arch with a soft tissue mass and cortical expansion (56). On MRI, they are of low signal intensity on T1-weighted images, showing prominent enhancement with gadolinium, and they are thus generally indistinguishable from other malignancies (particularly metastases). In many cases they may be identified by their CT appearance of irregular honeycomb pattern and accompanying soft tissue masses.

Aneurysmal Bone Cyst

Aneurysmal bone cysts (ABC) account for only 1% to 2% of all primary bone tumors, and about 20% of all ABCs are found in the spine. Those located in the spine most often involve the neural arch, most commonly in the cervical and thoracic regions, but the sacrum may also be affected (111). Most ABCs are found in patients 20 years of age or younger. Histologically they are benign hamartomas, but biologically they show aggressive behavior. They may arise secondary to trauma or a tumor-induced anomalous vascular process, and a preexisting lesion can be clearly identified in approximately one third of cases. The most common predisposing lesions are giant cell tumor, followed by osteoblastoma, angioma, and chondroblastoma (53).

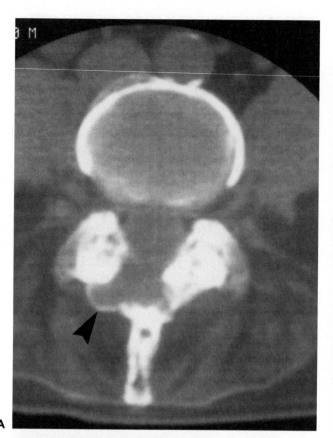

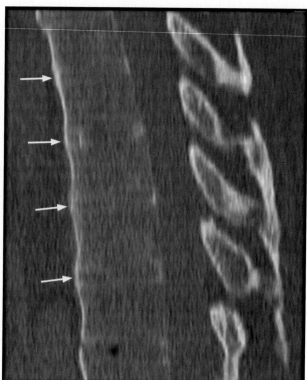

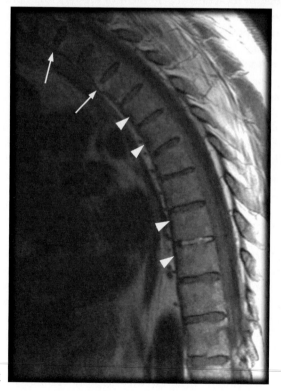

Figure 23-55 Ankylosing spondyloarthritis. **A:** Axial CT, bone window setting, shows marked dural ectasia that has eroded the right lamina (*arrow*). Also seen are multiple foci of hypodensity in the neural arch, particularly in the vicinity of the facet joints. The joint space is partially obliterated. A bridging syndesmophyte extends along the anterior and lateral borders of the vertebral body. **B:** Sagittal reformatted CT in a different patient demonstrates characteristic bridging syndesmophytes (*arrows*). There is squaring of vertebral bodies that are almost completely fused. **C:** Sagittal T1-weighted image in a different patient shows bridging osteophytes along the ALL (*arrows*) and PLL. A number of vertebral bodies contain hypointense areas (*arrowhead*), either diffusely or confined to their corners.

On CT, ABCs are typically eccentric, lytic, expansile, and surrounded by a thin shell of remodeled bone. Within the cyst, fluid-fluid levels are present (119) (Fig. 23-57). MRI shows similar features of "ballooned" bony contour of the host bone. The presence of paramagnetic blood-breakdown products gives rise to fluid levels of varying signal intensities ranging from very bright signal on T2-weighted images (representing extracellular methemoglobin) to very

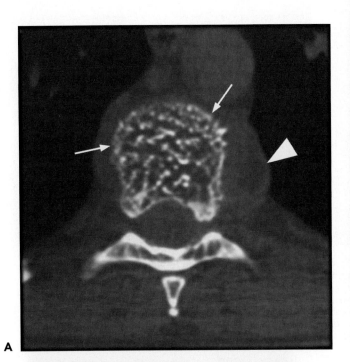

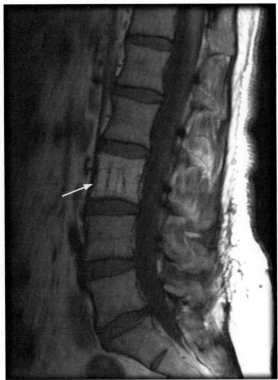

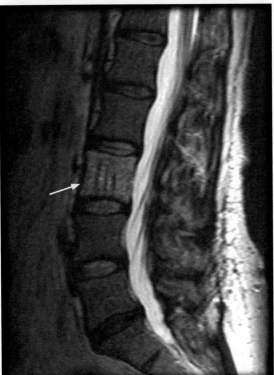

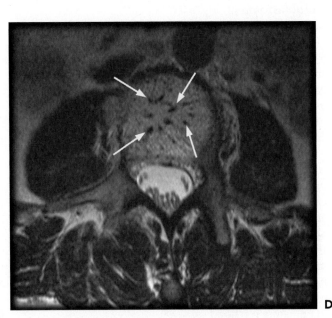

Figure 23-56 Vertebral body hemangioma. **A:** Axial CT shows characteristic "polka-dot" appearance of the involved thoracic vertebral body (*arrows*). An associated soft tissue mass (*arrowhead*) is seen, indicating a more aggressive hemangioma. **B:** Midsagittal T1-weighted image in a different patient shows a hyperintense L3 vertebral body (*arrow*) with internal linear hypointense structures representing hypertrophied trabeculae. **C:** The affected vertebral body remains of similar appearance and signal intensity (*arrow*) on the T2-weighted image. **D:** Axial T2-weighted image at L3 reveals that the hemangioma involves most of the vertebral body (compare its signal intensity with that of the pedicles and transverse processes). The internal hypointense areas (*arrow*) may correspond to hypertrophic secondary trabeculae or vascular flow-voids.

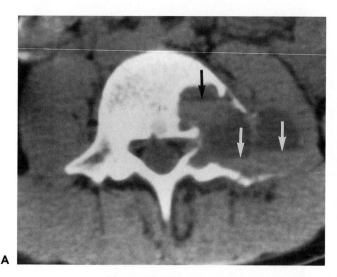

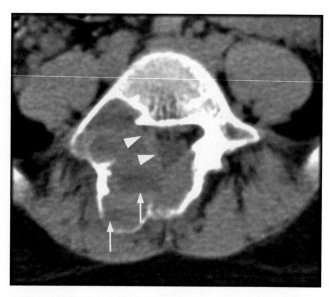

A   **B**

Figure 23-57   Aneurysmal bone cyst (ABC). **A:** Axial CT at L4 shows large ABC eroding the vertebral body, pedicle, transverse process, and lamina. The margins of the lesion are well defined, and the lesion contains multiple blood/fluid levels (*arrows*). There is extension into the left psoas muscle. **B:** Axial CT at L5 in a different patient shows a large mass involving both laminae, right pedicle, transverse process, and a portion of the vertebral body. Characteristic multiple blood/fluid levels are present (*arrows*). This ABC has completely destroyed the right pedicle and is extending into the epidural space and compressing the dural sac (*arrowheads*).

low signal (indicating the presence of deoxyhemoglobin or hemosiderin).

Osteoblastoma

Osteoblastoma (giant osteoid osteoma) is another tumor that preferentially involves the neural arch. Approximately 45% of all osteoblastomas occur in the spine, where they commonly cause scoliosis. Males in the second to fourth decades of life are primarily affected (54). The lesion may represent reactive changes rather than a true neoplasm. Osteoblastomas are generally larger than 2 cm in diameter when discovered.

CT shows a well-defined expansile and lytic lesion generally surrounded by a thin rim of calcium. Ossified matrix can be identified in up to 50% of cases, and extension into neighboring soft tissue structures also may be seen (54). Diffuse sclerosis of the vertebral body at that level may also occur (69). The MRI features are nonspecific, with lesion enhancement after intravenous administration of gadolinium (54,69). High signal intensity areas in the muscles and bone around the lesion are commonly found on T2-weighted images, presumably corresponding to an inflammatory reaction.

Osteoid Osteoma

Osteoid osteomas are histologically similar to osteoblastomas but smaller, generally measuring less than 1.5 to 2 cm in diameter. They are most common in males during the first two decades of life and represent approximately 6% of all benign bone tumors. Approximately 10% of osteoid osteomas are found in the spine, most often in the lumbar region, typically arising in the posterior elements, primarily in the neural arch (75%) (7). The nidus of an osteoid osteoma consists of vascular connective tissue with surrounding osteoid matrix. The classic symptoms include back pain (during the night and relieved by aspirin) and scoliosis and adjacent muscle spasm (particularly torticollis when the cervical spine is affected), and varying degrees of radiculopathy are occasionally encountered.

The initial localization of the lesion may be accomplished with radionuclide bone scintigraphy. CT shows a small rounded central area of low attenuation (nidus) with or without central calcification surrounded by variable zone of sclerosis. If the osteoid osteoma arises in cancellous bone, the surrounding sclerosis may not be present. CT is used primarily for precise localization of the lesion before excision. On MRI these lesions show a broad spectrum of appearances demonstrating variable signal intensities, while contrast enhancement is found within the tumor or in the adjacent reactive changes (26). The muscles surrounding the tumor are usually hyperintense on T2-weighted images and demonstrate contrast enhancement.

Giant Cell Tumor

Giant cell tumor (GCT) comprises fewer than 4% of all bone neoplasms. In the spine, they most often involve the sacrum. Women in their third decade of life are predominantly affected (25). Most GCTs are histologically benign, but up to 25% may show malignancy. CT and/or MRI are often needed for surgical planning. Total resection is the recommended treatment, as treatment with curettage alone results in a 50% recurrence rate (39).

As opposed to most other spinal tumors, these neoplasms primarily affect the vertebral body and not the posterior elements (69). When it involves the sacrum, it is generally located adjacent to the sacroiliac joint. On CT, a GCT is a well-demarcated, expansile, and lytic lesion, with shell-like calcifications and absence of mineralized matrix. Cortical disruption may be present. GCT enhances markedly on postcontrast images. In most patients, MRI shows the lesion to be of low-to-intermediate signal intensity on T1-weighted images and of heterogeneous intermediate signal intensity on T2-weighted images (39). Presence of hemosiderin and dense fibrous tissue leads to focal areas of low signal intensity on T2-weighted images. GCT may also show heterogenous enhancement following gadolinium administration.

Chordoma

Chordoma accounts for fewer than 4% of bone lesions (108,116). It arises from notochordal remnants in the vertebral body or within the disc space, which explains why these neoplasms characteristically occur in the midline. Histologically, chordomas are classified as either conventional (having a mucinous matrix) or chondroid. One half of all chordomas occur in the sacrum (mainly S4 and S5) followed by the clivus (35%) and the vertebrae (15%), particularly C2 (108). Men between the ages of 40 and 70 years are most commonly affected. Chordomas are slow-growing, locally aggressive tumors. Vertebral chordomas are more malignant than sacrococcygeal or clival ones. Metastases occur in about one fourth of patients.

On CT, chordomas are mainly lytic, but sclerotic chordomas are occasionally encountered (Fig. 23-58A). The low-density mass is surrounded by calcified rim and contains flecks of calcium within it. Low-density areas, representing necrosis or gelatinous myxoid material, also may be seen in the tumor. Paravertebral extension is not uncommon. On T1-weighted MRI, chordomas are of intermediate (75%) or low signal (25%) intensity (108), and the majority are heterogeneous. On T2-weighted images, conventional chordomas are of higher signal intensity than CSF, while chondroid chordomas also contain hypointense areas, due to abundant cartilage-like tissue. The tumor may contain large septa of low signal intensity radiating through the hyperintense areas and creating a multilobulated appearance (100). In some cases chordomas may mimic schwannomas, demonstrating no obvious bone involvement. After intravenous gadolinium administration, they show variable and mostly moderate enhancement (Fig. 23-58B).

Langerhans Cell Histiocytosis

Langerhans cell histiocytosis (LCH) and its solitary form, formerly referred to as eosinophilic granuloma, mostly occur in children in the first years of life. Vertebral involvement is found in 6% of patients (62). LCH is a rapidly growing lytic bone lesion that characteristically leads to a flattened and sclerotic vertebral body, known as *vertebra plana*. Partial restoration of vertebral body height may be spontaneous or follow treatment (46). LCH is the most common benign cause of the vertebra plana; however, it is seen in only about 15% of affected patients (46). The diagnosis is generally based on radiographs.

Active lesions are lytic (Fig. 23-59A), manifesting as nonspecific low signal intensity on T1-weighted sequences and high signal intensity on T2-weighted images. The adjacent intervertebral discs are normal. The inactive healing

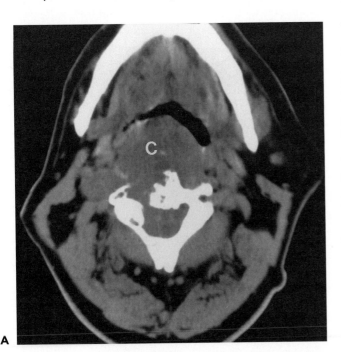
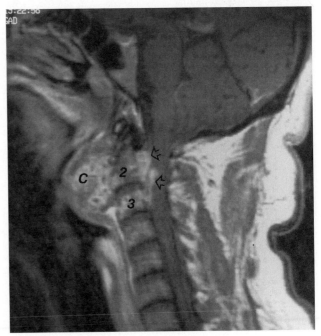

A   B

Figure 23-58 Chordoma. **A:** Axial CT at C2 shows a chordoma (C) arising in the vertebral body and extending into the prevertebral region. The vertebral body is partially destroyed. **B:** Postcontrast midsagittal T1-weighted image shows the chordoma (C) arising from the axis (2) and also involving C3 (3). There is extension into the epidural space (*arrows*) with compression of the upper cervical spinal cord.

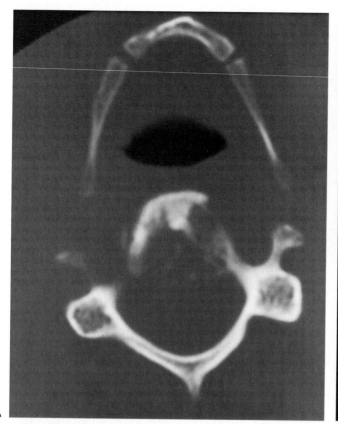

A

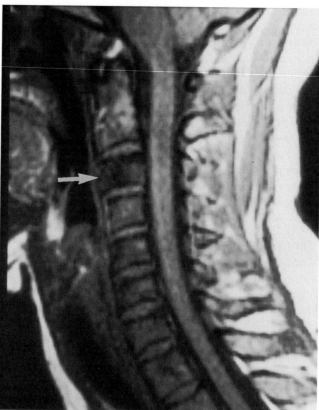

B

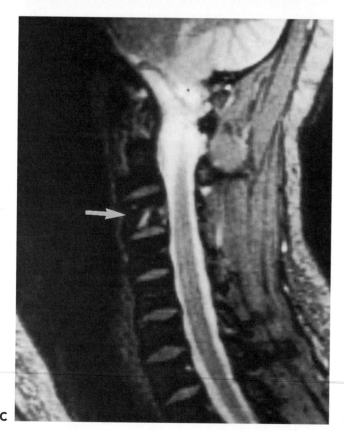

C

Figure 23-59 Eosinophilic granuloma. A: Axial CT, bone window setting, shows destructive lesion involving the body of C3. B: Midsagittal noncontrast T1-weighted image shows that the C3 vertebral body has predominantly low signal intensity (*arrow*). C: Midsagittal T2-weighted image shows inhomogeneous signal intensity from the C3 vertebral body (*arrow*).

lesions are usually of normal signal on T2-weighted images and hyperintense on T1-weighted images. This distinction may be important in guiding the biopsy in patients with multilevel involvement (46). The majority of affected vertebral bodies are of mixed signal intensities, corresponding to collapsed vertebral bodies and active lesions (Figs. 23-59B and 23-59C). CT and MRI are useful in outlining the extension of the lesion if surgery is considered. Propagation into the adjacent soft tissues is atypical and should prompt histologic confirmation of the lesion.

Multiple Myeloma and Plasmacytoma

Multiple myeloma is a disseminated disorder of bone marrow plasma cells (111), occurring mainly in middle- or advanced-age men. The vertebrae are affected in 66% of patients (111). The thoracic and lumbar regions are most commonly involved. During the course of the disease, nearly 50% of patients develop neurologic symptoms, most often secondary to compression of the spinal cord due to vertebral body compression fractures and/or epidural spread of disease. Plasmacytoma refers to a solitary plasma cell tumor of bone or soft tissue. Plasmacytomas occur in approximately 5% of patients and usually arise in the vertebral body. These lesions generally have an indolent course, but multiple myeloma eventually develops in most patients.

CT is very sensitive for detecting and confirming myeloma lesions. The typical CT appearance is predominantly that of "punched-out" lytic abnormalities that are devoid of surrounding sclerosis (Fig. 23-60A). However, the most common CT manifestation of myeloma is diffuse osteopenia. MRI is the most sensitive technique for detection of myeloma lesions (81,97). On MRI, the lesions are typically hypointense on T1-weighted images and hyperintense on T2-weighted images with respect to normal bone marrow (Figs. 23-60B and 23-60C). Thus, they cannot be distinguished from metastases. After radiation therapy, some lesions become hypointense on both T1-weighted and T2-weighted images, presumably due to fibrosis, but some lesions remain unchanged.

A pattern seen on axial MRI that is referred to as a "mini brain" has been reported as a characteristic of solitary vertebral plasmacytoma (58,93). This pattern is formed by curvilinear structures of low signal intensity on all pulse sequences that partially extend through the vertebral body. These structures, resembling sulci of the brain, are caused by hypertrophic residual trabecular bone, possibly due to the less aggressive nature of plasmacytoma.

SELECTED SPINAL VASCULAR DISORDERS

Vascular Malformations

Only radiculomeningeal vascular malformations will be addressed here. These rare lesions are usually acquired and consist of a fistula between the radicular (radiculomeningeal) arteries and veins. The shunt is located in the surface of the dura matter and drains via one or more dilated veins, which in turn drain to a large venous plexus located on the surface (most commonly dorsal) of the spinal cord. These malformations are known as spinal dural arterial-venous fistulae (SDAVF) and are most commonly found in the lower thoracic spine in men between 30 and 70 years of age (85). The patients typically present with slowly progressive sensory and motor deficits, corresponding to chronic progressive myelopathy, and the lesions are usually recognized late in the course of the disease. The cause of this syndrome is believed to be venous congestion, which leads to spinal cord ischemia.

Plain CT is not helpful, while postmyelogram CT (and myelography) may show rounded or serpentine filling defects, representing dilated veins, on the surface of the spinal cord. Spin echo MRI demonstrates long serpiginous areas of flow void, usually on the dorsal surface of the spinal cord. Although this sign is relatively specific, it is not always encountered. T2-weighted images in both axial and sagittal planes may serve to highlight the areas of signal void against the bright CSF (Fig. 23-61A). The most common MRI finding, seen in more than 80% of patients, is spinal cord swelling and increased signal intensity on T2-weighted images. This finding is nonspecific and is related to edema and, sometimes, infarcts caused by venous hypertension. A recently reported characteristic MRI finding is the presence of peripheral hypointensity of the involved portion of the cord (42). Postcontrast MRI may show enhancement of some of the vessels, particularly the veins with slow flow (Fig. 23-61B), and spinal cord enhancement is also frequently found. Magnetic resonance angiography, preferably contrast-enhanced, using 3D phase-contrast or time-resolved techniques, may demonstrate the vein(s) into which the fistula drains, thus allowing for noninvasive identification of the spinal level of the shunt (12). All patients with documented (or suspected) spinal arteriovenous malformation should undergo catheter angiography for precise localization of the malformation, followed by embolization and/or surgery.

Epidural Hematoma

The most common cause of an epidural hematoma is trauma, including spinal catheterization or spinal manipulation therapy. However, epidural hematomas are considered to be spontaneous in almost one half of patients, usually as a result of anticoagulation, vigorous exercise, hypertension, underlying vascular malformations, intervertebral disc surgery, or collagen vascular disorders (66). Clinically, an epidural hematoma is characterized by an acute onset of pain and motor and sensory deficits. Epidural hematomas are generally located in the dorsolateral aspect of the spinal canal and most commonly involve the upper thoracic region. Although the size of the hematoma decreases progressively with time, surgical decompression is

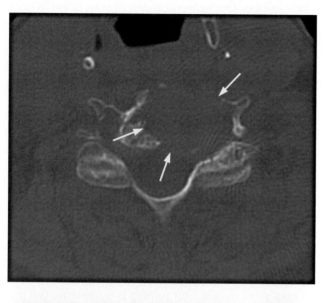

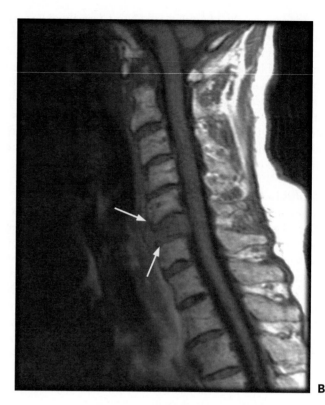

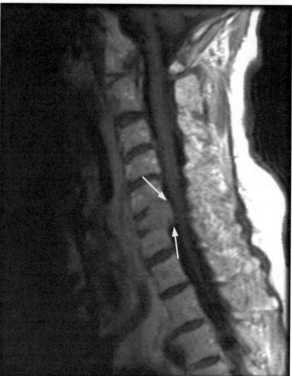

Figure 23-60 Plasmacytoma. **A:** Axial CT shows a lytic destructive lesion (*arrow*) replacing most of the C6 vertebral body. There is no evidence of sclerosis. **B:** Midsagittal T1-weighted image shows low signal intensity from the plasmacytoma (*arrows*). The vertebra is of normal height and indistinguishable from a solitary metastasis. **C:** After contrast administration, the lesion enhances and becomes isointense with the normal adjacent vertebrae. There is anterior epidural extension (*arrows*).

usually the treatment of choice. In a series of 18 patients with ventrally located epidural hematomas, two thirds were associated with herniated lumbar spine discs (35). It seems that the lumbar epidural hematomas are more common than previously believed and that their progressive resolution accounts for the improvement of symptoms in some of the conservatively treated patients with lumbar disc herniations.

Unenhanced CT shows a lentiform, high-density collection located adjacent to the neural arch (Fig. 23-62A). MRI is the modality of choice, as CT does not always reveal the

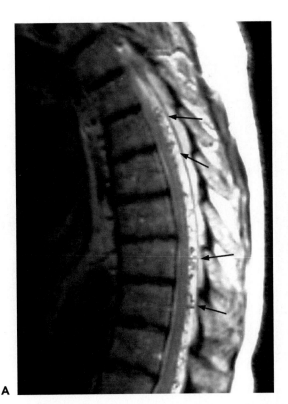
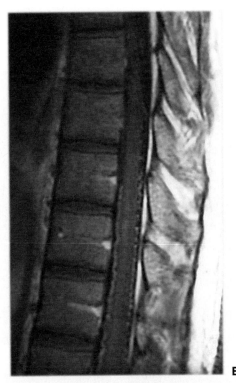

Figure 23-61 Spinal dural arteriovenous fistula. **A:** Midline sagittal T2-weighted image shows multiple flow voids in the dorsal subarachnoid space along most of the thoracic spinal cord. These represent enlarged draining veins from a radicular arteriovenous fistula. The signal intensity of cord is normal. **B:** Midline sagittal postcontrast T1-weighted image in a different patient demonstrates gadolinium accumulating in draining veins along the anterior and posterior cord surface.

epidural hematoma. Heterogeneous hyperintensity outside the cord with focal hypointensity on T2-weighted images should suggest the diagnosis of acute spinal epidural hematoma (33). A gradient echo T2*-weighted sequence should be added to the imaging protocol, as it is very sensitive to deoxyhemoglobin (present within the initial 24 to 48 hours) and makes the hematoma appear black in contrast to the bright CSF and relatively hyperintense fat. Deoxyhemoglobin is generally isointense to CSF, while methemoglobin is seen as areas of high signal, similar to fat, on T1-weighted images (Fig. 23-62B). The appearance on T1-weighted images does not always correlate with time elapsed before imaging (33). The most reliable way to distinguish an epidural from a subdural hematoma is the absence of a low-intensity plane (corresponding to dura) between the bright methemoglobin and bright fat on T1-weighted images (Fig. 23-62C). Fat-suppression MRI is helpful to distinguish normal epidural fat from methemoglobin. Contrast-enhanced MRI is not routinely indicated, and if performed it may show enhancement of the hematoma (20). Cases of chronic spinal epidural hematomas causing progressive myelopathy have also been described (70).

FUTURE TRENDS IN SPINE MRI

Considerable effort has been placed in developing DWI of the spine. At present the different ways to acquire DWI in spine include: a diffusion-sensitized steady-state free precession (SSFP) technique, navigator echo-corrected techniques (spin echo, fat-suppressed spin echo, stimulated echo), line scan diffusion imaging, and conventional DWI. SSFP is mostly used to image the bone marrow. Presumably, using low and high diffusion strengths, metastases and malignant compression fractures show higher signal intensity than noninvolved vertebrae. The problem with this sequence is that T2 effects contribute to the findings; thus, the signal intensity of the abnormality is a reflection of many factors and not only diffusion characteristics (16). Because of this, false- positive results are not uncommon (that is, a lesion that is T2 bright is also bright on SSFP without having restricted diffusion). Navigator echo techniques are time-consuming and will not be addressed here. Line diffusion scanning is also time-consuming but offers the possibility of using two b values and thus provides apparent diffusion coefficient values and adequate signal-to-noise ratio (SNR). Using this sequence, high ADC values are found in benign

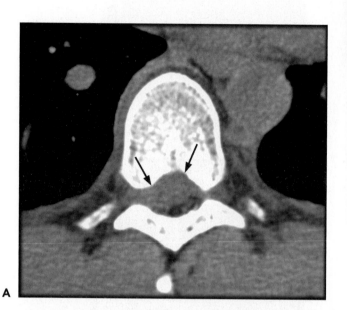

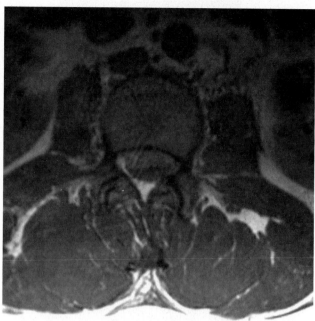

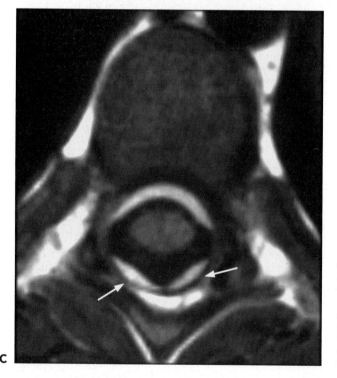

Figure 23-62 Epidural and subdural hematomas. **A:** Axial CT shows replacement of anterior and right lateral epidural fat in the thoracic spine with isodense mass (*arrows*), corresponding to epidural hematoma. **B:** Axial T1-weighted image in a different patient shows a crescentic shaped ventral epidural hematoma at the L1 level. **C:** Axial T1-weighted image in a child with a clotting disorder reveals hyperintense subdural hematomas anterior and posterior to the spinal cord. In contrast to epidural hematomas, a dark line (*arrow*), corresponding to dura, is visualized between the epidural fat and hematoma. This appearance is due to the presence of the meningospinal ligaments.

compression fractures, reflecting the presence of edema. Conventional DWI is difficult to obtain because of low SNR and significant susceptibility artifacts (16).

Parallel MRI (called by some manufacturers SENSE, SMASH, and so on) uses several receiver channels simultaneously attached to an array coil. The basic idea is that of combining reduced Fourier encoding with spatially distinct coil sensitivity patterns to produce the images. The benefits

of this technique are a reduced readout length (which reduces image distortions and indirectly increases the number of slices) and increased spatial resolution (by 30% to 50% pixel size reduction). In spine imaging this translates to decreasing the acquisition time by one half while maintaining good SNR (Fig. 23-63). It is possible to decrease the acquisition time more, but the images typically have lower SNR. Other disadvantages are larger raw data

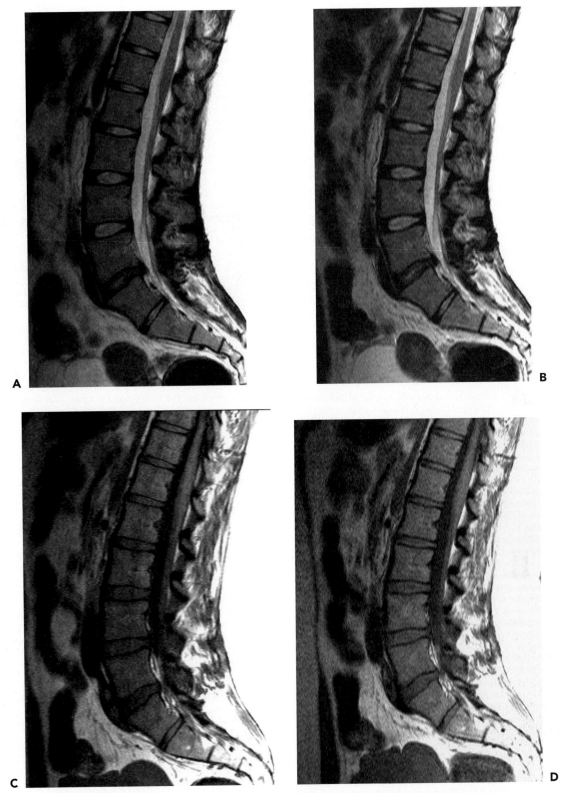

Figure 23-63 Conventional spine versus parallel MRI. **A:** Midline sagittal FSE T2-weighted image shows a small disc bulge at L5–S1. **B:** Parallel (multireceiver coil) image at same level is of good quality, although the noise is minimally increased. This image was obtained in one-half the time of the image A. **C:** Midline sagittal conventional T1-weighted image in the same patient. **D:** Corresponding T1-weighted image obtained using parallel imaging is slightly more grainy but otherwise is of comparable quality.

requirements and a more complicated image reconstruction operation, both of which translate into the need to use special hardware (array coil with high-speed data acquisition channels) and special software. It is also possible that parallel imaging may decrease artifacts caused by surgical hardware. Because time requirements are decreased by 50% at least, there should be no need for abbreviated "screening studies" of the spine when this technique is available.

Parallel imaging may also have an impact in the implementation of diffusion tensor imaging (DTI) in the spine (19). Using SENSE and DTI results in images of the cervical cord that provide information regarding the fractional direction of water motion with what appears to be little contamination from the surrounding CSF. DTI is also feasible in its standard acquisition fashion but suffers from the magnetic susceptibility artifacts associated with echo-planar imaging. It is also possible that parallel imaging may be helpful in functional MRI studies of the spinal cord (8). Visualization of segmental cord activation may be easier with parallel imaging because of lesser susceptibility artifacts when compared with standard echo-planar functional MRI.

REFERENCES

1. Abello R, Rovira M, Sanz MP, et al. MRI and CT of ankylosing spondylitis with vertebral scalloping. *Neuroradiology*. 1988; 30: 272–275.
2. Aguila LA, Piraino DW, Modic MT, et al. The internuclear cleft of the intervertebral disc: magnetic resonance imaging. *Radiology*. 1985;155: 155–158.
3. Amyes EW, Anderson FM. Fracture of the odontoid process: report of sixty-three cases. *Arch Surg*. 1956;72:377–393.
4. Anderson LD, D'Alonzo RT. Fractures of the odontoid process of the axis. *J Bone Joint Surg Am*. 1974;56:1663–1674.
5. Antuaco EJ, Binet EF. *Radiology* of thoracic and lumbar fractures. Clin Orthop. 1984;189:43–57.
6. Atlas SW, Regenbogen V, Rogers LF, et al. The radiographic characterization of burst fractures of the spine. *AJR Am J Roentgenol*. 1986;147:575–582.
7. Azouz EM, Kozlowski K, Marton D, et al. Osteoid osteoma and osteoblastoma of spine in children. Report of 22 cases with brief literature review. *Pediatr Radiol*. 1986;16:25–31.
8. Backes WH, Mess WH, Wilmink JT. Functional MR imaging of the cervical spinal cord by use of median nerve stimulation and fist clenching. *AJNR Am J Neuroradiol*. 2001;22:1854-1859
9. Baur A, Stabler A, Arbogast S, et al. Acute osteoporotic and neoplastic vertebral compression fractures: fluid sign at MR imaging. *Radiology*. 2002;225:730-735.
10. Baur A, Stabler A, Bruning R, et al. Diffusion-weighted MR imaging of bone marrow: differentiation of benign versus pathologic compression fractures. *Radiology*. 1998;207:349-356.
11. Boden SD, Davis DO, Dina TS, et al. Contrast-enhanced MR imaging performed after successful lumbar disc surgery: prospective study. *Radiology*. 1992;182:59–64.
12. Bowen BC, Pattany PM. MR angiography of the spine. *Magn Reson Imaging Clin N Am*. 1998;6:165-178.
13. Braun IF, Hoffman JC, Davis PC, Landman JA, Tindall GT. Contrast enhancement in CT differentiation between recurrent disc herniation and postoperative scar: prospective study. *AJNR Am J Neuroradiol*. 1985;6:607–612.
14. Braun IF, Malko JA, Davis PC, Hoffman JC, Jacobs LH. The behavior of Pantopaque on MR: in vivo and in vitro analyses. *AJNR Am J Neuroradiol*. 1986;7:997–1001.
15. Braun J, Golder W, Bollow M, et al. Imaging and scoring in ankylosing spondylitis. *Clin Exp Rheumatol*. 2002;20:S178-184.

16. Castillo M. Diffusion-weighted imaging of the spine: is it reliable? *AJNR Am J Neuroradiol*. 2003;24:1251-1253.
17. Castillo M, Arbelaez A, Smith JK, et al. Diffusion-weighted MR imaging offers no advantage over routine noncontrast MR imaging in the detection of vertebral metastases. *AJNR Am J Neuroradiol*. 2000;21:948-953.
18. Castillo M, Malko JA, Hoffman JC. The bright intervertebral disc: an indirect sign of abnormal spinal bone marrow on T1-weighted MR images. *AJNR Am J Neuroradiol*. 1990;11:23–26.
19. Cercignani M, Horsfiled MA, Agosta F, Filippi M. Sensitivity-encoded diffusion tensor MR imaging of the cervical cord. *AJNR Am J Neuroradiol*. 2003;24:1254-1256
20. Chang FC, Lirng JF, Chen SS, et al. Contrast enhancement patterns of acute spinal epidural hematomas: a report of two cases. *AJNR Am J Neuroradiol*. 2003;24:366-369.
21. Chiapparini L, Sghirlanzoni A, Pareyson D, et al. Imaging and outcome in severe complications of lumbar epidural anaesthesia: report of 16 cases. *Neuroradiology*. 2000;42:564-571.
22. Colombo N, Berry I, Norman D. Infections of the spine. In: Manelfe C, ed. *Imaging of the spine and spinal cord*. New York: Raven Press, 1992;489–512.
23. Cooper KL, Beabout JW, Swee RG. Insufficiency fractures of the sacrum. *Radiology*. 1985;156:15–20.
24. Czervionke LF, Daniels DL, Ho PSP, et al. Cervical neural foramina: correlative anatomic and MR imaging study. *Radiology*. 1988;169:753–759.
25. Dahlin DC, Cupps RE, Johnson EW. Giant-cell tumor: a study of 195 cases. *Cancer*. 1970;25:1061–1068.
26. Davies M, Cassar-Pullicino VN, Davies AM, et al. The diagnostic accuracy of MR imaging in osteoid osteoma. *Skeletal Radiol*. 2002;31:559-569.
27. Denis F, Denis S, Comfort T. Sacral fractures: an important problem. Retrospective analysis of 236 cases. *Clin Orthop*. 1988;277:67–81.
28. Dora C, Walchli B, Gal I, et al. The significance of spinal canal dimensions in discriminating symptomatic from asymptomatic disc herniations. *Eur Spine J*. 2002;11:575-581.
29. Duda JJ Jr, Ross JS. The postoperative lumbar spine: imaging considerations. *Semin Ultrasound CT MR*. 1993;14:425-436.
30. Effendi B, Roy D, Cornish B, et al. Fractures of the ring of the axis: a classification based on the analysis of 131 cases. *J Bone Joint Surg Br*. 1981;63:319–327.
31. Enzmann DR, DeLaPaz RL. Tumor. In: Enzman DR, DeLaPaz RL, Rubin JB, eds. Magnetic resonance imaging of the spine. St. Louis, MO: CV Mosby, 1990;365–372.
32. Fardon DF, Milette PC. Nomenclature and classification of lumbar disc pathology: recommendations of the combined task forces of the north american spine society, american society of spine radiology, and american society of neuroradiology. *Spine*. 2001;26:E93-E113.
33. Fukui MB, Swarnkar AS, Williams RL. Acute spontaneous spinal epidural hematomas. *AJNR Am J Neuroradiol*. 1999;20:1365-1372.
34. Green JD, Harle TS, Harris JH Jr. Anterior subluxation of the cervical spine: hyperflexion sprain. *AJNR Am J Neuroradiol*. 1981;2:243-250.
35. Gundry CR, Heithoff KB. Epidural hematoma of the lumbar spine: 18 surgically confirmed cases. *Radiology*. 1993;187:427–431.
36. Hackney DB. Magnetic resonance imaging of the spine. Normal anatomy. *Top Magn Reson Imaging*. 1992;4:1–6.
37. Harris JH, Burke KT, Ray RD, et al. Low type (III) odontoid fracture: a new radiographic sign. *Radiology*. 1984;153:353–356.
38. Harris JH, Yeakley JS. Radiographically subtle soft tissue injuries of the cervical spine. *Top Magn Reson Imaging*. 1989;25:167–190.
39. Herman SD, Mesgarzadeh M, Bonakdarpour A. The role of magnetic resonance imaging in giant cell tumor of bone. *Skeletal Radiol*. 1987;16:635–643.
40. Holdsworth F. Review article: dislocations and fracture–dislocations of the spine. *J Bone Joint Surg Am*. 1970;52:1534–1551.
41. Hueftle MG, Modic MT, Ross JS, et al. Lumbar spine: postoperative MR imaging with Gd-DTPA. *Radiology*. 1988;167:817–824.

42. Hurst RW, Grossman RI. Peripheral spinal cord hypointensity on T2-weighted MR images: a reliable imaging sign of venous hypertensive myelopathy. *AJNR Am J Neuroradiol.* 2000;21:781-786.

43. Jensen MC, Brant-Zawadzki MN, Obuchowski N, et al. Magnetic resonance imaging of the lumbar spine in people without back pain. *N Engl J Med.* 1994;331:69-73.

44. Jinkins JR. MR of enhancing nerve roots in the unoperated lumbosacral spine. *AJNR Am J Neuroradiol.* 1993;14:193–202.

45. Johnson CE, Sze G. Benign lumbar arachnoiditis: MR imaging with gadopentetate dimeglumine. *AJNR Am J Neuroradiol.* 1990;11:763–770.

46. Kaplan GR, Saifuddin A, Pringle JA, et al. Langerhans' cell histiocytosis of the spine: use of MRI in guiding biopsy. *Skeletal Radiol.* 1998;27:673-676.

47. Kawaida H, Sakou T, Morizono Y, Yoshikuni N. Magnetic resonance imaging of upper cervical disorders in rheumatoid arthritis. *Spine.* 1989;17:1144–1148.

48. Kelsey JL, White AA, Pastides H, et al. The impact of musculoskeletal disorders in the population of the United States. *J Bone Joint Surg Am.* 1979;61:959–964.

49. Kenny JB, Hughes PL, Whitehouse GH. Discovertebral destruction in ankylosing spondylitis: the role of computed tomography and magnetic resonance imaging. *Br J Radiol.* 1990;63:448–455.

50. Kim KS, Chen HH, Russell EJ, Roger LF. Flexion tear-drop fractures of the cervical spine: radiographic characteristics. *AJR Am J Roentgenol.* 1989;152:319–326.

51. Kirkwood JR. *Spine.* In: *Essentials of neuroimaging.* New York: Churchill Livingstone, 1990;365–452.

52. Klein GR, Vaccaro AR, Albert TJ, et al. Efficacy of magnetic resonance imaging in the evaluation of posterior cervical spine fractures. *Spine.* 1999;24:771-774.

53. Kransdorf MJ, Sweet DE. Aneurysmal bone cyst: concept, controversy, clinical presentation, and imaging. *AJR Am J Roentgenol.* 1995;164:573-580.

54. Kroon HM, Schurman J. Osteoblastoma: clinical and radiographic findings in 98 new cases. *Radiology.* 1990;175:783–790.

55. Kurugoglu S, Kanberoglu K, Kanberoglu A, et al. MRI appearances of inflammatory vertebral osteitis in early ankylosing spondylitis. *Pediatr Radiol.* 2002;32:191-194.

56. Laredo JD, Assouline E, Gelbert F, et al. Vertebral hemangiomas: fat content as signal of aggressiveness. *Radiology.* 1990;177:467–472.

57. Ledermann HP, Schweitzer ME, Morrison WB, et al. MR imaging findings in spinal infections: rules or myths? *Radiology.* 2003;228:506-514.

58. Major NM, Helms CA, Richardson WJ. The "mini brain": plasmacytoma in a vertebral body on MR imaging. *AJR Am J Roentgenol.* 2000;175:261-263.

59. Masaryk TJ. Neoplastic disease of the spine. *Radiol Clin North Am.* 1991;4:829–845.

60. McAfee PC, Yuan HA, Fredickson BE, et al. The value of computed tomography in thoracolumbar fractures. *J Bone Joint Surg Am.* 1983;65:461–472.

61. McNally EG, Wilson DJ, Ostlere SJ. Limited magnetic resonance imaging in low back pain instead of plain radiographs: experience with first 1000 cases. *Clin Radiol.* 2001;56:922-925.

62. Meyer JS, Harty MP, Mahboubi S, et al. Langerhans cell histiocytosis: Presentation and evolution of radiological findings with clinical correlation. *Radiographics.* 1995;15:1135-1146.

63. Minami S, Sagoh T, Nishimura K, et al. Spinal arteriovenous malformation: MR imaging. *Radiology.* 1988;169:109–115.

64. Modic MT, Feiglin DH, Piraino DW, et al. Vertebral osteomyelitis: assessment using MR. *Radiology.* 1985;157:157–166.

65. Modic MT, Masaryk TJ, Ross JS, Carter JR. Imaging of degenerative disc disease. *Radiology.* 1988;168:177–186.

66. Mohazab HR, Langer B, Spigos D. Spinal epidural hematoma in a patient with lupus coagulopathy: MR findings. *AJR Am J Roentgenol.* 1993;160:853–854.

67. Moorthy S, Prabhu NK. Spectrum of MR imaging findings in spinal tuberculosis. *AJR Am J Roentgenol.* 2002;179:979-983.

68. Muhle C, Metzner J, Weinert D, et al. Classification system based on kinematic MR imaging in cervical spondylitic myelopathy. *AJNR Am J Neuroradiol.* 1998;19:1763-1771.

69. Murphey MD, Andrews CL, Flemming DJ, et al. From the archives of the AFIP. Primary tumors of the spine. Radiologic pathologic correlation. *Radiographics.* 1996;16:1131-1158.

70. Muthukumar N. Chronic spontaneous spinal epidural hematoma - a rare cause of cervical myelopathy. *Eur Spine J.* 2003;12:100-103.

71. Nguyen CM, Haughton VM, Ho KC, An HS. MR contrast enhancement: an experimental study in postlaminectomy epidural fibrosis. *AJNR Am J Neuroradiol.* 1993;14:997–1002.

72. Nicoll EA. Fractures of the dorso-lumbar spine. *J Bone Joint Surg Br.* 1949;31:376–394.

73. Numaguchi Y, Rigamonti D, Rothman MI, et al. Spinal epidural abscess: evaluation with Gadolinium-enhanced MR imaging. *Radiographics.* 1993;13:545–559.

74. Olsen WL, Chakeres DW, Berry I, Richaud R. Spine and spinal cord trauma. In: Manelfe C, ed. *Imaging of the spine and spinal cord.* New York: Raven Press 1992;413–416.

75. Otake S, Marcuo N, Nishizawa S, et al. Ossification of the posterior longitudinal ligament in MR evaluation. *AJNR Am J Neuroradiol.* 1992;13:1059–1067.

76. Pech P, Haughton VM. Lumbar intervertebral disc: correlative MR and anatomic study. *Radiology.* 1985;156:699–701.

77. Pfirrmann CW, Binkert CA, Zanetti M, et al. MR morphology of alar ligaments and occipitoatlantoaxial joints: study in 50 asymptomatic subjects. *Radiology.* 2001;218:133-137.

78. Post MJD, Quencer RM, Montalvo BM, et al. Spinal infection: evaluation with MR imaging and intraoperative ultrasound. *Radiology.* 1988;169:765–771.

79. Pratt ES, Green DA, Sengler DM. Herniated intervertebral discs associated with unstable spine injuries. *Spine.* 1990;15:662–666.

80. Qaiyum M, Tyrrell PN, McCall IW, et al. MRI detection of unsuspected vertebral injury in acute spinal trauma: incidence and significance. *Skeletal Radiol.* 2001;30:299-304.

81. Rahmouni A, Divine K, Mathieu D, et al. Detection of multiple myeloma involving the spine: efficacy of fat-suppression and contrast-enhanced MR imaging. *AJR Am J Roentgenol.* 1993;160:1049–1052.

82. Resnick D, Niwayama G. Degenerative disease of the spine. In: Resnick D (ed): *Diagnosis of Bone and Joint Disorders,* ed 3. Philadelphia: WB Saunders, 1995;1372-1462.

83. Resnick D, Niwayama G, Guerra J, et al. Spinal vacuum phenomena: anatomical study and review. *Radiology.* 1981;139:341–348.

84. Ricci C, Cova M, Kang YS, et al. Normal age-related patterns of cellular and fatty bone marrow distribution in the axial skeleton: MR imaging study. *Radiology.* 1990;177:83–88.

85. Rodesch G, Berenstein A, Lasjaunias P. Vasculature and vascular lesions of the spine and spinal cord. In: Manelfe C, ed. *Imaging of the spine and spinal cord.* New York: Raven Press, 1992;565–598.

86. Rogers LF. The roentgenographic appearance of transverse or Chance fracture of the spine: the seat belt fracture. *AJR Am J Roentgenol.* 1971;111:844–849.

87. Ross JS, Masaryk TJ, Modic MT, et al. Lumbar spine: postoperative assessment with surface-coil MR imaging. *Radiology.* 1987;164:851–860.

88. Ross JS, Masaryk TJ, Modic MT, et al. MR imaging of lumbar arachnoiditis. *AJR Am J Roentgenol.* 1987;149:1025-1032.

89. Ross JS, Zepp R, Modic MT. The postoperative lumbar spine: enhanced MR evaluation of the intervertebral disk. *AJNR Am J Neuroradiol.* 1996;17:323-331.

90. Saifuddin A. MRI of acute spinal trauma. *Skeletal Radiol.* 2001;30:237-246.

91. Sapico FL, Montgomerie JZ. Vertebral osteomyelitis. *Infect Dis Clin North Am.* 1990;4:539–551.

92. Schneider RC, Kahn EA. Chronic neurologic sequelae of acute trauma to the spine and spinal cord. Part I: the significance of the acute flexion or "tear-drop" fracture-dislocation of the cervical spine. *J Bone Joint Surg Am.* 1956;38-A:985-97.

93. Shah BK, Saifuddin A, Price GJ. Magnetic resonance imaging of spinal plasmacytoma. *Clin Radiol.* 2000;55:439-445.

94. Sharif HS. Role of MR imaging in the management of spinal infections. *AJR Am J Roentgenol.* 1992;158:1333–1345.

95. Shima Y, Rothman SLG, Yasura K, et al. Degenerative intraspinal cyst of the cervical spine: case report and literature review. *Spine.* 2002;27:E18-E22.

96. Shuman WP, Rogers JB, Sickler ME, et al. Thoracolumbar burst fractures: CT dimensions of the spinal canal relative to post surgical improvement. *AJR Am J Roentgenol.* 1985;145:337–341.

97. Sigimura K, Yamasaki K, Kitagaki H, Tanaka Y, Kono M. Bone marrow diseases of the spine: differentiation with T1- and T2-relaxation time in MR imaging. *Radiology.* 1987;165:541–544.

98. Sklar EML, Quencer RM, Green BA, et al. Complications of epidural anesthesia: MR appearance of abnormalities. *Radiology.* 1991;181:549–554.

99. Smith WS, Kaufer H. Patterns and mechanisms of lumbar injuries associated with lap seat belts. *J Bone Joint Surg Am.* 1969;51:239–254.

100. Smolders D, Wang X, Drevelengas A, et al. Value of MRI in the diagnosis of non-clival, non-sacral chordoma. *Skeletal Radiol.* 2003;32:343-350.

101. Sonntag VKH. Management of bilateral locked facets of the cervical spine. *Neurosurgery.* 1981;8:150–152.

102. Stabler A, Eck J, Penning R, et al. Cervical spine: postmortem assessment of accident injuries-comparison of radiographic, MR imaging, anatomic, and pathologic findings. *Radiology.* 2001;221:340-346.

103. Standaert CJ, Herring SA. Spondylolysis: a critical review. *Br J Sports Med.* 2000;34:415-422.

104. Starr KH, Hanely EN. Junctional burst fractures. *Spine.* 1992;17:551–558.

105. Stiskal MA, Neuhold A, Szolar DH, et al. Rheumatoid arthritis of the craniocervical region by MR imaging: detection and characterization. *AJR Am J Roentgenol.* 1995;165:585-592.

106. Sugimura H, Kakitsubata Y, Suzuki Y, et al. MR of ossification of ligamentum flavum. *J Comput Assist Tomogr.* 1992;16:73–76.

107. Sze G, Bravo S, Krol G. Spinal lesions: quantitative and qualitative temporal evolution of gadopentetate dimeglumine enhancement in MR imaging. *Radiology.* 1989;170:849–856.

108. Sze G, Uichanco LS, Brant-Zawadzki M, Davis R, et al. Chordomas: MR imaging. *Radiology.* 1988;166:187–191.

109. Tyroch AH, McGuire EL, McLean SF, et al. The association between Chance fractures and intra-abdominal injuries revisited: a multicenter review. *Am Surg.* 2005;7:434-438.

110. Van Goethem JWM, Parizel PM, Jinkins JR. Review article: MRI of the postoperative lumbar spine. *Neuroradiology.* 2002;44:723-739.

111. Van Goethem JW, van den Hauwe L, Ozsarlak O, et al. Spinal tumors. *Eur J Radiol.* 2004;50:159-176.

112. Van Tassel P. MR imaging of spinal infections. *Top Magn Reson Imaging.* 1994;6:69–81.

113. Weaver P, Lifeso RM. The radiological diagnosis of tuberculosis of the adult spine. *Skeletal Radiol.* 1984;12:178–186.

114. Weishaupt D, Zanetti M, Hodler J, et al. MR imaging of the lumbar spine: prevalence of intervertebral disk extrusion and sequestration, nerve root compression, end plate abnormalities, and osteoarthritis of the facet joints in asymptomatic volunteers. *Radiology.* 1998;209:661-666.

115. Yu S, Haughton VM, Sether LA, Wagner M. Annulus fibrosus in bulging intervertebral discs. *Radiology.* 1988;169:761–763.

116. Yuh WTC, Flickinger FW, Barloon TJ, Montgomery WJ. MR imaging of unusual chordomas. *J Comput Assist Tomogr.* 1988;12:30–35.

117. Yussen PS, Swartz JD. The acute lumbar disc herniation: imaging diagnosis. *Semin Ultrasound CT MR.* 1993;14:389-398.

118. Zenter J, Schneider B, Schramm J. Efficacy of conservative treatment of lumbar disc herniation. *J Neurosurg Sci.* 1997;41:263–268.

119. Zimmer WD, Berquist TH, McLeod RA, et al. Bone tumors, magnetic resonance imaging versus computed tomography. *Radiology.* 1985;155:709–718.

Pediatric Applications

Marilyn J. Siegel

Both computed tomography (CT) and magnetic resonance imaging (MRI) are important imaging techniques in nearly every part of the pediatric body. CT is usually the study of choice to further evaluate abnormalities of the chest, abdomen, and pelvis detected on conventional radiographic studies or ultrasonography (US), and it is accepted as the primary imaging test to evaluate blunt abdominal trauma. MRI is the primary study to evaluate soft tissue and paraspinal masses as well as joint abnormalities, and it is employed as a secondary test to assess abnormalities observed on plain radiographs or CT scans. This chapter highlights the diagnostic applications of CT and MRI in a wide variety of disease processes of the chest, abdomen, pelvis, and musculoskeletal system in children. General guidelines to assist in appropriately selecting imaging examinations also are provided.

PATIENT PREPARATION/TECHNIQUE

Imaging pediatric patients has several inherent problems that are not present in adults, in particular, patient motion, small body size, and lack of perivisceral fat. These problems can be minimized or eliminated by appropriate use of sedation and intravenous contrast medium (247).

Sedation

Initial reports suggest that the use of multidetector CT has reduced the frequency of sedation in infants and children 5 years of age and younger (116,188). Early experience suggests that the sedation rate for young children undergoing multidetector CT is equal to or less than 5% (3). These studies have included small groups of patients, so further experience is required to determine the precise sedation rate in a young patient population. Sedation likely still will be required for some uncooperative children, but in general, children older than 5 years of age will cooperate after verbal reassurance and an explanation of the procedure.

Sedation for imaging examinations is nearly always conscious sedation (70). Conscious sedation is defined as a minimally depressed level of consciousness that retains the patient's abilities to maintain a patent airway, independently and continuously, and respond appropriately to physical stimulation and/or verbal command.

The drugs most frequently used for sedation are oral chloral hydrate and intravenous pentobarbital sodium. Oral chloral hydrate, 50 to 100 mg/kg, with a maximum dosage of 2,000 mg, is the drug of choice for children younger than 18 months. Intravenous pentobarbital sodium, 6 mg/kg with a maximum dose of 200 mg, is advocated in children older than 18 months. It is injected slowly in fractions of one fourth the total dose and is titrated against the patient's response. This is an effective form of sedation, with a failure rate of less than 5%. Regardless of the choice of drug, the use of parenteral sedation requires the facility and ability to resuscitate and maintain adequate cardiorespiratory support during and after the examination (4,43).

Patients who are to receive parenteral sedation should have no liquids by mouth for 3 hours and no solid foods for 6 hours prior to their examination. Patients who are not sedated but are to receive intravenous contrast medium should be NPO (nothing by mouth) for 3 hours to minimize the likelihood of nausea or vomiting with possible aspiration during a bolus injection of intravenous contrast medium.

After being sedated, the infant or child is placed on a blanket on the CT or MRI table. The arms routinely are extended above the head to avoid streak artifacts and to provide an easily accessible route for intravenous injection. The upper arms can be restrained with sandbags, adhesive tape, or Velcro straps.

Computed Tomography: Special Considerations

Intravenous Contrast Material

Scanning after intravenous administration of iodinated contrast material is helpful to confirm a lesion thought to be of vascular origin, or to establish its relationship to vascular structures, in addition to improving differentiation between normal and pathologic parenchyma, especially in the liver and kidneys. If intravenous contrast material is to be administered, it is helpful to have an intravenous line in place when the child arrives in the radiology department. This reduces patient agitation that otherwise would be associated with a venipuncture performed just prior to administration of contrast material. The largest gauge cannula that can be placed is recommended.

The contrast dose is 2 mL/kg (not to exceed 4 mL/kg or 125 mL). A nonionic contrast medium should be used. The advantages of nonionic agents over ionic agents are less discomfort at the injection site, fewer side effects such as nausea and vomiting, and decreased patient motion during contrast administration.

Contrast can be administered by mechanical or hand injection (18,240,247). The former type of administration should be performed if a 22-gauge or larger cannula can be placed into an antecubital vein. The contrast injection rate is determined by the caliber of the intravenous catheter. Contrast is infused at 1.5 to 2.0 mL per second for a 22-gauge catheter and 2.0 to 3.0 mL per second for a 20-gauge catheter. The site of injection is closely monitored during the initial injection of contrast to minimize the risk of contrast extravasation. A power injection also can be used to administer contrast media via a central venous catheter or 24-gauge catheter if the rate of injection is slow (1 mL per second). The contrast medium should be administered by a hand injection using a bolus technique if intravenous access is through a peripheral access line or a smaller caliber antecubital catheter. The complication rates for manual and power injections are similar (less than 0.4%), provided that the catheter is positioned properly and functions well (117).

An automated bolus tracking technique can be used to monitor contrast enhancement and initiate scanning. This technique allows on-line monitoring of contrast enhancement by acquiring very low mA scans and region of interest measurements at a predetermined level. Once an arbitrary threshold level of contrast enhancement has been reached, diagnostic scanning is initiated.

Bowel Opacification

Opacification of the small and large bowel is necessary for most examinations of the abdomen, as unopacified bowel loops can simulate a mass or abnormal fluid collection. The exceptions are patients with depressed mental status who are at risk of aspiration and those with acute blunt abdominal trauma for whom there may be insufficient time

TABLE 24-1

ORAL CONTRAST VERSUS PATIENT AGE

Patient age	Minimum amount given at least 45 min before scanning	Additional volume given 15 min prior to scanning
Less than 1 month	2–3 ounces (60–90 mL)	1–1.5 ounces (30–45 mL)
1 month to 1 year	4–8 ounces (120–240 mL)	2–4 ounces (60–120 mL)
1 to 5 years	8–16 ounces (240–480 mL)	4–8 ounces (120–180 mL)
6 to 12 years	16–36 ounces (480–1,000 mL)	8–18 ounces (180–540 mL)
13 years and older	36 ounces (1,000 mL)	18 ounces (500 mL)

to administer oral contrast material. A dilute water-soluble, iodine-based oral contrast agent is given by mouth, or through a nasogastric tube if necessary. The oral contrast agent can be mixed with Kool-Aid or fruit juice if needed to mask the unpleasant taste.

The gastrointestinal tract from the stomach to the terminal ileum usually can be well opacified if the contrast agent is given in two volumes, one 45 to 60 minutes before the examination and the other 15 minutes prior to scanning. The first volume should approximate that of an average feeding. The second volume should be approximately one half that of the first. Appropriate volumes of contrast medium with respect to patient age are shown in Table 24-1.

CT Technical Considerations

Scan Delay Times

The scan delay time is the time between the start of the contrast injection and the start of data acquisition. Routine chest examinations (i.e., screening for pathology, tumor staging, evaluation of a mediastinal mass or congenital lung anomaly) are acquired with a scan delay of 25 to 30 seconds. For CT angiography, a scan delay of 12 to 15 seconds is used in neonates and infants weighing less than 10 kg. In larger children, a bolus tracking method is used. A predetermined enhancement level in the aorta of 100 to 120 Hounsfield units (HU) is used to trigger the examination (240,242).

For routine abdominal and pelvic examinations (i.e., evaluation of abdominal tumor, trauma, or abscess), the scan delay time is 55 to 60 seconds. CT angiography is used in the evaluation of hepatic masses and for preoperative vascular mapping. The time delay for an arterial phase acquisition is 12 to 15 seconds in infants and small children weighing less than 10 kg. In larger children and ado-

TABLE 24-2
MILLIAMPERAGE SETTINGS

Weight (kg)	Chest CT mAs	Abdomen CT mAs
<10	40	50
10–15	50	60
16–25	60	70
26–35	70	90
36–45	80	100
>45	100 or >	120 or >

lescents, the time delay for arterial phase imaging is 20 seconds. The venous phase is initiated 55 to 60 seconds after the start of contrast administration.

Technical Parameters

Strategies that minimize radiation dose are mandatory for CT examinations in children (53,86,190,259). A variety of parameters can affect the amount of radiation from CT, including tube current, kilovoltage, table speed, and detector collimation. The current (in mA) for pediatric CT examinations needs to be the lowest possible that maintains image quality. General guidelines for tube current based on patient weight are shown in Table 24-2. Kilovoltage is another factor that affects scan quality and radiation dose. A kVp of 80 should be considered for patients weighing less than 50 kg. In larger patients, a higher kVp (100 to 120) should be used to compensate for the higher noise (224).

For optimal examination of children, CT examinations should be performed with scan times of 1 second or less. Detector collimation and pitch vary depending on the type of scanner used. For a four-row detector scanner, a 2.5-mm collimation with a pitch of 1.5 to 2.0 is adequate for routine scanning. For a 16-row detector, 1.25 to 1.5 mm collimation with a pitch of 1.0 to 1.5 suffices. For a 64-row detector, 0.6 to 1.25-mm collimation and a pitch of 1.0 to 1.5 suffices (see Protocols 1 to 5 at the end of this chapter).

CT examinations are performed with breath-holding at suspended inspiration in cooperative patients, usually children over 5 to 6 years of age. Scans are obtained during quiet respiration in children who are unable to cooperate with breath-holding instructions and in patients who are sedated.

Magnetic Resonance Imaging: Technical Considerations

Imaging Parameters

Lesion detectability is dependent on the signal-to-noise (S/N) ratio, spatial resolution, and contrast resolution. These parameters vary with the size of the receiver coil, slice thickness, field of view (FOV), matrix size, and number of acquisitions. For optimal S/N ratio and spatial resolution, MRI examinations should be performed with the smallest coil that fits tightly around the body part being studied (5,12,195). A head coil usually is adequate in infants and small children, whereas a whole-body or phased-array surface coil is needed for larger children and adolescents. Surface coils can be useful in the evaluation of superficial structures, such as the spine, but the drop-off in signal strength with increasing distance from the center of the coil limits the value of these coils in the evaluation of deeper abdominal structures.

Slice thickness varies with patient size and the area of interest. Thinner slices (3 to 4 mm) are used in the evaluation of small lesions and through areas of maximum interest, whereas thicker slices (6 to 8 mm) suffice for a general survey of the chest and abdomen and for larger lesions. The FOV can have a square or rectangular shape. A square shape is used when the body part being examined fills the FOV. An asymmetric rectangular FOV is ideal for body parts that are narrow in one direction, such as the abdomen in a thin patient. One or two signal acquisitions generally are used in pediatric MRI examinations to shorten imaging time.

Pulse Sequences
Spin-Echo Sequence

T1-weighted sequences [short repetition time (TR), short echo time (TE)] are obtained in virtually all patients because they provide excellent contrast between soft tissue structures and fat and thus help in tissue characterization (i.e., fluid, fat, or blood). Fat-suppressed T1-weighted images are useful to improve conspicuity of diseased tissues.

T2-weighted sequences (long TR, long TE) are used in most examinations of the chest (excluding heart and great vessels), abdomen, and musculoskeletal system. They provide excellent contrast between tumor and adjacent soft tissues and are useful for tissue characterization. The T2-weighted sequences can be acquired with conventional or echo-train (fast/turbo) techniques. Echo-train spin-echo sequences are useful when decreased imaging time is desired, although these images may lead to a decrease in contrast and can at times render liver lesions imperceptible. To increase lesion conspicuity, fat-suppression techniques can be used in conjunction with T2-weighted echo-train sequences.

Most lesions have low signal intensity on T1-weighted images and high signal intensity on T2-weighted images. The T1 signal can increase if the lesion contains fat, blood, proteinaceous fluid, or cartilage. Mineralization and gadolinium chelate enhancement also result in high T1 signal intensity. A low T2 signal intensity is seen with mineralization, hemosiderin and other blood products, iron oxide, and fibrosis.

Other Magnetic Resonance Imaging Techniques

Fat-suppressed sequences are useful to increase contrast between normal and pathologic tissues on T2-weighted images. Two basic methods of fat suppression are widely available: short tau inversion recovery (STIR) and radiofrequency presaturation of the lipid peak (fat saturation). Signal from fat is nulled on STIR and fat-saturated images, whereas most pathologic lesions, with increased free water and prolonged T1 and T2 values, are bright on the fat-suppressed sequences.

Gradient-echo (GRE) time of flight images are useful for detecting flowing blood. Flowing blood typically appears bright on GRE images (214). By comparison, flowing blood appears as a flow void or decreased signal within the vessel lumen on spin echo sequences. GRE imaging is most effective in cooperative children who can suspend respiration, but it can be used in children of any age. The evaluation of blood flow with the GRE sequence requires the use of technical parameters that are tailored for vascular imaging.

Chemical shift imaging is a method that is helpful to detect and characterize lesions suspected of containing microscopic fat. This technique uses GRE images obtained in phase and out of phase to exploit differences in precessional frequencies of fat and water. The presence of fat and water within a voxel results in phase cancellation and decreased signal intensity on out-of-phase images. The shortest possible TE should be used for out-of-phase imaging to reduce $T2^*$ effects.

Contrast-Enhanced Imaging

Gadolinium, a paramagnetic metal ion, is most frequently used in MRI for contrast enhancement (5,12,195). When used as an MR contrast agent, gadolinium is chelated with another substance, such as dimeglumine or diethylenetriamine penta-acetic acid. Gadolinium chelates are extracellular contrast agents that cause T1 shortening of tissues in which the agent is taken up. The usual dose is 0.1 mmol/kg. Gadolinium-enhanced T1-weighted imaging with fat suppression is used in the evaluation of tumors to improve contrast between normal and pathologic tissue and to help in lesion characterization. For gadolinium-enhanced MR angiography, a three-dimensional (3D) spoiled gradient-echo is used and the data are obtained in a volume, typically during suspended respiration (88,273).

Single-shot echo train imaging is the sequence used for MR cholangiopancreatography (170) and urography (25). The single-shot fast spin echo uses long echo train lengths and half Fourier imaging to provide fast images.

Optimizing Image Quality

As a result of the relatively long time required to perform abdominal MRI in children, gross voluntary motion or physiologic motion, such as respiration and blood flow, may produce artifacts that degrade the MR image. Voluntary motion can be minimized or eliminated with the use of sedation, whereas physiologic motion and its resultant artifacts—ghosting and blurring—can be suppressed by adjusting technical parameters (169). Newer techniques,

such as respiratory triggering using an abdominal belt or by monitoring diaphragmatic motion, can be used to reduce breathing artifact. GRE, fast spin-echo, and single-shot fast spin-echo sequences, and signal averaging, or increasing the number of excitations in the MR examination, are simple methods to reduce respiratory motion artifacts. Spatial presaturation, an additional technique for motion suppression, uses selective radiofrequency pulses to saturate spins that are outside of the area of interest being imaged. Thus, blood flowing into the imaged section has little signal and consequently produces little or no artifact. Presaturation also can eliminate abdominal wall motion artifact even it if is in the same cross-sectional image.

Electrocardiographic (ECG) gating reduces motion unsharpness and is used in MRI examinations of the thorax. This technique entails an increase in scan time, but it markedly improves the image quality. Imaging is triggered to the R-wave of the ECG, with data acquisition taking place during diastole.

CHEST

Mediastinum

Cross-sectional CT and MR images are particularly helpful in detecting or clarifying abnormalities in the mediastinum, chest wall, and peridiaphragmatic and subpleural regions of the lung. The information provided by these techniques can directly affect the treatment or aid in determining the prognosis of a patient.

Indications for CT and MRI of the mediastinum include (a) characterization of mediastinal widening or evaluation of a mass suspected or detected on chest radiography; (b) determination of the extent of a proved mediastinal tumor; (c) detection of mediastinal involvement in children who have an underlying disease that may be associated with a mediastinal mass but who have a normal chest radiograph; and (d) assessment of the response of a mediastinal mass to therapy.

Normal Anatomy
Thymus

In the pediatric population, the normal thymus is seen in virtually every patient. In individuals under age 20, there are wide variations in size and shape of the normal thymus. Recognition of the various appearances of the normal thymus is important if errors in diagnosis are to be avoided (217,228,237). In patients younger than 5 years, the thymus usually has a quadrilateral shape with convex or straight lateral margins (Fig. 24-1). Later in the first decade, the thymus is triangular or arrowhead-shaped with straight or concave margins, and by 15 years of age, it is triangular in nearly all individuals (Fig. 24-2). In general, in the first two decades of life, the thymus abuts the sternum, separating the two lungs. A distinct anterior junction line

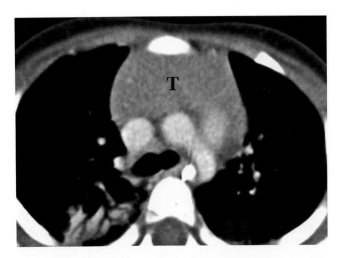

Figure 24-1 Normal computed tomography appearance of thymus, 6-month-old boy. The thymus (T) is quadrilateral in shape with slightly convex lateral borders and a wide retrosternal component. The density of the thymus is equal to that of chest wall musculature. A nasogastric tube is present in the esophagus. There is minimal right upper lobe atelectasis.

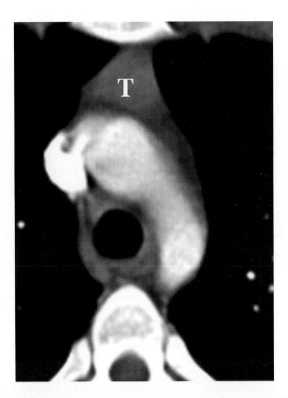

Figure 24-2 Normal computed tomography appearance of thymus, 10-year-old boy. The thymus (T) has assumed a triangular shape, but it still abuts the sternum and has a density equal to that of chest wall musculature.

between the lungs is usually not seen until the third decade of life.

The thymus in prepubertal children and most adolescents is homogeneous, with an attenuation value equal to that of chest wall musculature. In approximately 30% of adolescents, the thymus is heterogeneous, containing low-density areas of fat deposition. Thymic lobar width (largest dimension parallel to the long axis of the lobe) shows little change with age. Thymic lobar thickness (the largest dimension perpendicular to the long axis of the lobe) correlates inversely with advancing age, decreasing from 1.50 ± 0.46 (mean ± standard deviation) cm for the 0 to 10 year age group to 1.05 ± 0.36 cm for patients between 10 and 20 years of age. For infiltrative diseases of the thymus, increased thickness is a fairly sensitive indicator of an abnormality.

Signal intensity of the thymus on MR images also varies with patient age. The signal intensity of the prepubertal thymus is slightly greater than that of muscle on T1-weighted images, slightly less than or equal to that of fat on T2-weighted images, and greater than that of fat on fat-suppressed T2-weighted images (Fig. 24-3). After puberty, the signal intensity on T1-weighted images increases, reflecting fatty replacement (Fig. 24-4). Measurements of thymic thickness are slightly greater on MRI than on CT, probably reflecting the lower lung volumes on MR images (217). MR images are obtained during quiet respiration, whereas CT images generally are obtained in suspended or full inspiration. This difference produces some flattening of the thymus in the craniocaudal dimension on MRI, which increases thickness.

Occasionally, the thymus extends either cranially above the brachiocephalic vessels or into the posterior thorax.

The CT or MRI findings of the abnormally positioned thymus are: its direct continuity with the thymic tissue in the anterior mediastinum, an attenuation value or signal intensity similar to that of normal thymic tissue, and the lack of compression of adjacent mediastinal vessels or the tracheobronchial tree.

Lymph Nodes

Mediastinal lymph nodes generally are not seen on CT or MRI in children prior to puberty, and their presence should be considered abnormal (237). In adolescents, small normal nodes (not exceeding 1 cm in widest dimension) occasionally can be identified. Nodes are of soft tissue attenuation on CT and have signal intensity between those of muscle and fat on both T1- and T2-weighted images.

Azygoesophageal Recess

The configuration of the azygoesophageal recess varies with patient age. The contour of the recess is convex laterally in children under 6 years of age, straight in children between 5 and 12 years of age, and concave in adolescents and young adults (167) (Fig. 24-5). Recognition of the normal dextroconvex appearance in young children is important so that it is not mistaken for lymphadenopathy.

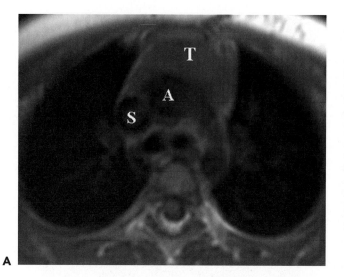

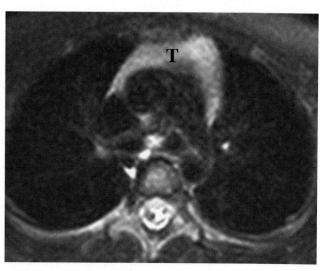

Figure 24-3   Normal magnetic resonance imaging (MRI) appearance of the thymus, 2-year-old boy. **A:** T1-weighted transaxial MR image shows a quadrilateral-shaped thymus (T) anterior to the superior vena cava (S) and aortic arch (A). The signal intensity is equal to that of the chest wall musculature but is less than that of subcutaneous fat. **B:** Fat-saturated T2-weighted transaxial MRI. The signal intensity of the thymus (T) is greater than that of subcutaneous fat.

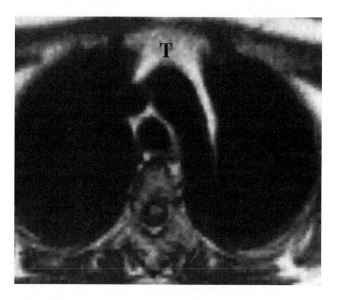

Figure 24-4   Normal magnetic resonance (MR) imaging appearance of the thymus, 15-year-old boy. T1-weighted axial MR image shows a high signal intensity thymus (T), indicating the presence of fatty replacement.

Mediastinal Pathology

A widened mediastinum in infants and children often is the result of a mass, usually a lymphoma, neurogenic tumor, teratoma, or cyst of foregut origin. Abundant mediastinal fat, aneurysms, or tortuosity of the mediastinal vessels are rare in children. CT and MRI have the capability of differentiating among lesions composed predominantly of fat, water, or soft tissues and, therefore, can provide a more definitive diagnosis than can conventional radiographic techniques (161,166,237).

Fat-containing masses in children usually are teratomas. Rarely, they represent thymolipomas or herniation of omental fat through the foramen of Morgagni. Lesions that can present with attenuation values near that of water include pericardial cysts, thymic cysts, lymphangiomas, and duplication cysts of foregut origin. Rarely, bronchogenic cysts or duplication cysts have a density equal to that of soft tissue, because they contain thick viscid contents, rather than simple serous fluid. Vascular causes of mediastinal widening, such as aortic aneurysm or a congenital anomaly of the thoracic vascular system, also can be identified with confidence on CT scans or on MRI.

CT can be valuable in determining the extent or origin of most soft tissue attenuation mediastinal masses, but a specific pathologic diagnosis generally is not possible. Determining the location of the mass in the mediastinum, however, can narrow the differential diagnosis.

Anterior Mediastinal Masses: Soft Tissue Attenuation

Lymphoma

Lymphoma is the most common cause of an anterior mediastinal mass of soft tissue attenuation in children, with Hodgkin disease occurring three to four times more frequently than non-Hodgkin lymphoma (102,213). Approximately 65% of pediatric patients with Hodgkin disease have intrathoracic involvement at clinical presentation, and 90% of the chest involvement is mediastinal. In contradistinction, about 40% of pediatric patients with non-Hodgkin lymphoma have chest disease at diagnosis, and only 50% of this disease involves the mediastinum. CT plays an important role in the identification and staging of disease, the planning of treatment, and the follow-up evaluation of patients with lymphoma (28,89,149).

Lymphomatous masses in Hodgkin disease are most common in the anterior mediastinum and reflect lym-

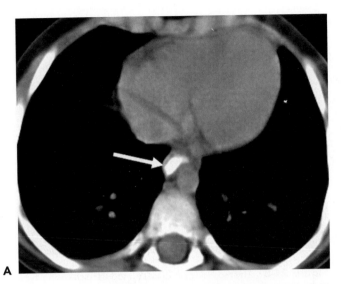
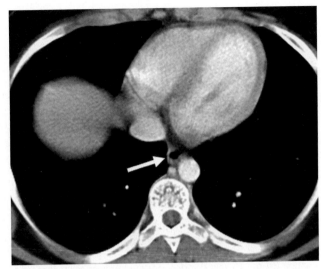

Figure 24-5 Azygoesophageal recess. **A:** In this 5-year-old boy, the recess (*arrow*) has a convex lateral shape, resulting from intrusion of the esophagus into the recess. **B:** A 15-year-old boy has a concave azygoesophageal recess (*arrow*).

phadenopathy or infiltration and enlargement of the thymus. The enlarged thymus has a quadrilateral shape with convex, lobular lateral borders (Fig. 24-6). On CT, the attenuation of the lymphomatous organ is equal to that of soft tissue (20,89,217,228). The MR signal intensity is slightly greater than that of muscle on T1-weighted pulse sequences and similar to or slightly greater than that of fat on T2-weighted pulse sequences (217) (Fig. 24-7). Calcifications or cystic areas resulting from ischemic necrosis consequent to rapid tumor growth can be seen within the tumor (137) (Fig. 24-8). Additional findings include mediastinal or hilar lymph node enlargement, airway narrowing, and compression of vascular structures.

Intrathoracic lymphadenopathy from lymphoma has varied appearances, ranging from mildly enlarged nodes in a single area to large conglomerate soft tissue masses in multiple regions. Typically, the enlarged nodes have well-defined margins and show little enhancement after intravenous administration of contrast medium (Fig. 24-9). Hodgkin disease usually causes enlargement of the thymus or anterior mediastinal nodes, whereas non-Hodgkin lymphoma predominantly affects middle mediastinal lymph nodes.

Successfully treated lymphomas usually decrease in size, but residual mediastinal masses may remain on serial CT examinations (28,149). Differential diagnostic considerations in these cases include fibrosis versus persistent or recurrent lymphoma. Serial CT examinations can usually distinguish between these two conditions. In general, masses resulting fibrosis remain stable or decrease in size, whereas tumor is likely to increase in size.

MR, gallium-67 scintigraphy, and positron emission tomography (PET) with 2-[F-18]-fluoro-2-deoxy-D-glucose (FDG) have been used to assess treatment response in the instances in which CT is not diagnostic (69,181,263). Fi-

brosis has low signal intensity (similar to that of muscle) on T1- and T2-weighed and fat-suppressed sequences, whereas active neoplasm has high signal intensity on T2-weighted sequences. However, increased signal intensity is not specific for tumor and it also may be associated with infection, hemorrhage, acute radiation pneumonitis, necrosis, and immature fibrotic tissue early in the post-treatment course. Gallium and FDG accumulate in viable tumor, but not in fibrotic tissue.

Thymic Hyperplasia

Thymic hyperplasia is another cause of diffuse thymic enlargement. In childhood, thymic hyperplasia is most often "rebound" hyperplasia associated with chemotherapy, particularly therapy with corticosteroids. Rebound hyperplasia may be observed during the course of chemotherapy or after the completion of therapy. The mechanism of hyperplasia in these cases is believed to be initial depletion of lymphocytes from the cortical portion of the gland because of high serum levels of glucocorticoids, followed by repopulation of the cortical lymphocytes when the cortisone levels return to normal. Rare causes of hyperplasia include myasthenia gravis, red cell aplasia, and hyperthyroidism.

On CT and MRI, hyperplasia appears as diffuse enlargement of the thymus with preservation of the normal triangular shape (20,228,237) (Fig. 24-10). The attenuation value and the signal intensity of the hyperplastic thymus on spin-echo sequences are similar to those of the normal organ and also tumor. The absence of other active disease and a gradual decrease in size of the thymus on serial CT scans or MRI supports the diagnosis of rebound hyperplasia as the cause of thymic enlargement. Limited experience suggests that chemical shift MRI also may be useful in the diagnosis of thymic hyperplasia and in its differentiation

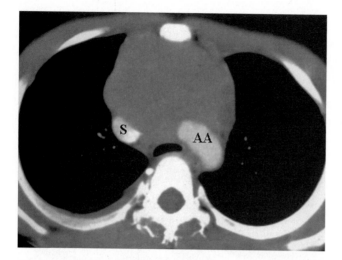

Figure 24-6 Thymic Hodgkin disease, nodular sclerosing type, 11-year-old girl. Contrast-enhanced computed tomography image shows a markedly enlarged thymus with a lobulated contour. The infiltrated thymus displaces the ascending aorta (AA) and superior vena cava (S) posteriorly. Note the compressive effects on the cava and trachea.

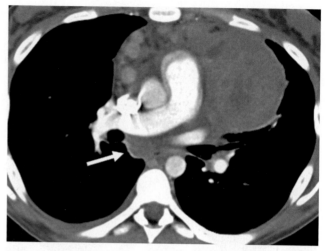

Figure 24-8 Thymic Hodgkin disease, nodular sclerosing type with cystic changes, 15-year-old girl. Contrast-enhanced computed tomography scan shows an enlarged thymus with cystic components, resulting from necrosis, in the left lobe. Multiple enlarged lymph nodes are noted in the anterior mediastinum and subcarinal (arrow) area. There is also a small right pleural effusion.

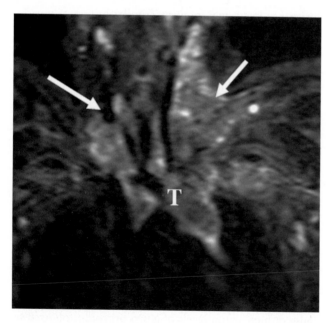

Figure 24-7 Thymic Hodgkin disease, nodular sclerosing type, 15-year-old girl. A: Coronal short tau inversion recovery magnetic resonance image shows thymic infiltration (T). The thymus is heterogeneous and has a signal intensity slightly greater than that of subcutaneous fat. Tumor is also present in both supraclavicular areas (arrows).

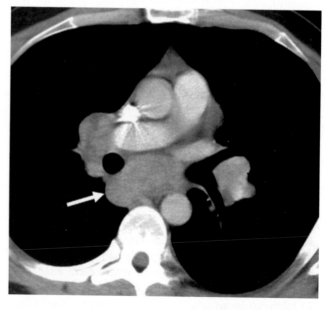

Figure 24-9 Lymphadenopathy, non-Hodgkin disease. Computed tomography scan shows enlarged nodes in the hilar and subcarinal (arrow) areas. The anterior mediastinum is normal.

from neoplastic processes. Normal and hyperplastic thymic tissues show lower intensity on opposed-phase GRE images than on in-phase imaging. The neoplastic thymus reveals no signal change between in-phase and opposed-phase chemical shift MR images (270).

Thymoma

Thymomas account for less than 5% of all mediastinal tumors in children. Nearly all thymomas are benign and occur sporadically, but they can be found in association

with myasthenia gravis, red cell aplasia, or hypogammaglobulinemia. Benign thymomas appear as well-defined, round or oval masses bulging the lateral thymic margin. On CT, they are of intermediate soft tissue density, but sometimes they contain calcifications or lower density areas of necrosis (228,237). On T1-weighted MR images, thymomas have signal intensity similar to that of muscle; the signal intensity increases on T2-weighted images, approaching that of fat (217). Approximately 10% to 15% of thymomas are invasive (i.e., malignant). The CT and MRI appearance of invasive thymoma is that of an anterior me-

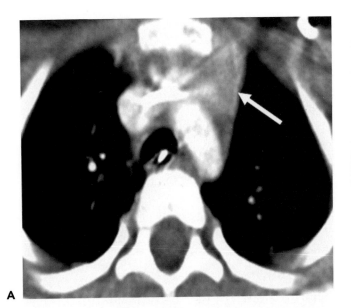

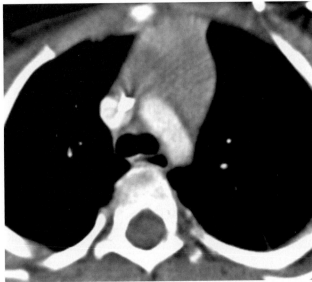

A

B

Figure 24-10 Rebound thymic hyperplasia, 4-year-old boy receiving chemotherapy for Wilms tumor. **A:** Computed tomography (CT) image of the chest at the time of diagnosis shows a normal thymus (*arrow*). **B:** CT image 3 month after the start of chemotherapy shows enlargement of both lobes of the thymus. The patient was clinically doing well. A follow-up CT study 6 months later showed spontaneous reduction in the size of the thymus.

diastinal mass associated with mediastinal or chest wall extension or metastatic implants along mediastinal, pleural, or pericardial surfaces, usually limited to one side of the thoracic cavity.

Miscellaneous Lesions

Other differential diagnostic considerations for diffuse thymic enlargement include leukemia, Langerhans cell histiocytosis, and histoplasmosis. Diagnosis requires tissue sampling.

Thyroid abnormalities are a rare cause of an anterior mediastinal mass in children. In childhood, an intrathoracic thyroid gland is more likely to represent true ectopic thyroid tissue rather than substernal extension of a cervical thyroid gland. The CT features of intrathoracic thyroid are a well-defined, intensely enhancing soft tissue mass anterior to the trachea.

Anterior Mediastinal Masses: Fat Attenuation
Germ Cell Tumors

Germ cell tumors are the second most common cause of an anterior mediastinal mass in children and the most common cause of a fat-containing lesion. They are derived from one or more of the three embryonic germ cell layers and usually arise in the thymus. Approximately 90% are benign and histologically are either dermoid cysts (containing only ectodermal elements) or teratomas (containing tissue from all three germinal layers). On CT, both lesions are well defined, thick-walled cystic masses containing a variable admixture of tissues: water, calcium, fat, and soft tissue (193,206) (Fig. 24-11). A fat–fluid level and amorphous bone or teeth occasionally can be seen

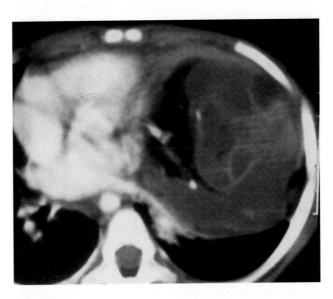

Figure 24-11 Benign teratoma. A large, well-circumscribed, heterogeneous mass containing low-density fluid, calcifications, and fat occupies most of the left hemithorax. The mass displaces but does not invade vascular structures. Pathologic examination showed a benign cystic teratoma, which contained sebaceous fluid, a small amount of fat, and embryonic teeth.

within these tumors. On MRI, germ cell tumors are heterogeneous masses with variable signal intensities depending on the relative amounts of fluid and fat (217). Fluid components usually have a signal intensity less than or equal to that of muscle on T1-weighted images. The signal intensity can be greater than that of muscle if the contents contain blood or proteinaceous material. The signal intensity of fluid usually is hyperintense to fat on T2-weighted images. Fat components have high signal intensity on both

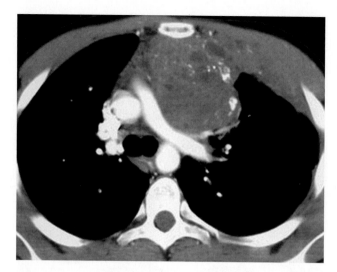

Figure 24-12 Teratocarcinoma. A large anterior mediastinal, soft tissue mass, containing calcifications and some low-density areas representing necrosis, displaces the main pulmonary to the right and posteriorly.

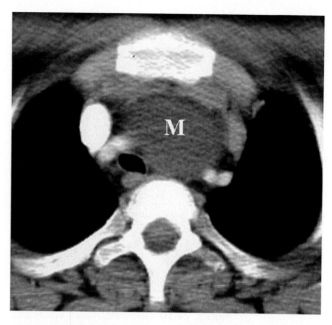

Figure 24-13 Thymic cyst. Contrast-enhanced computed tomography demonstrates replacement of the thymus by a homogeneous, water-attenuation mass (M).

T1- and T2-weighted images. Calcification and bone have low signal intensity on all imaging sequences.

A malignant teratoma generally appears on CT and MRI as a poorly defined, soft tissue mass, sometimes containing calcification and fat. Local infiltration into the adjacent mediastinum with encasement or invasion of mediastinal vessels or airways also is frequent. Other malignant germ cell tumors arising in the anterior mediastinum are seminoma, embryonal cell carcinoma, choriocarcinoma, and endodermal sinus tumor. These tumors typically are heterogeneous, soft tissue density masses containing some low-density areas of necrosis (Fig. 24-12). Rarely, they contain calcifications (206).

Thymolipoma

Thymolipoma is an infrequent cause of an intrathymic tumor. Pathologically, the tumor contains mature fat and strands of thymic tissue. Most cases in the pediatric population occur in the second decade and are discovered incidentally on plain radiographs. The tumor often is large, extending caudally to the diaphragm, and may mimic cardiomegaly or a cardiophrenic mass. On CT and MRI, it appears as a heterogeneous mass containing fat and some soft tissue elements. Thymolipoma does not compress or invade adjacent structures (204).

Anterior Mediastinal Masses: Fluid Attenuation
Thymic Cysts

Thymic cysts usually are congenital lesions resulting from persistence of the thymopharyngeal duct, but they can occur after thoracotomy. Typically, they are thin-walled, homogeneous masses of near water density on CT (Fig. 24-13), low signal intensity on T1-weighted MR images, and high signal intensity on T2-weighted sequences. The attenuation value or the signal intensity on T1-weighted images

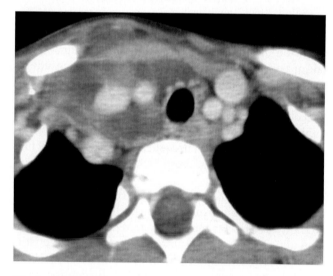

Figure 24-14 Cystic hygroma, 6-month-old girl. Computed tomography scan through the superior mediastinum shows a low-density mass infiltrating the superior mediastinum. The tumor encases the mediastinal vessels.

may be higher than that of simple cysts when the cyst's contents are proteinaceous or hemorrhagic rather than serous. Multiple thymic cysts have also been described in children with HIV infection and Langerhans cell histiocytosis (10,142).

Cystic Hygroma

Cystic hygromas (lymphangiomas) are developmental tumors of the lymphatic system that occur in the anterosuperior mediastinum and are almost always inferior extensions of cervical hygromas. On CT, they appear as nonenhancing, thin-walled, multiloculated masses with near-water attenuation value (Fig. 24-14). The presence of

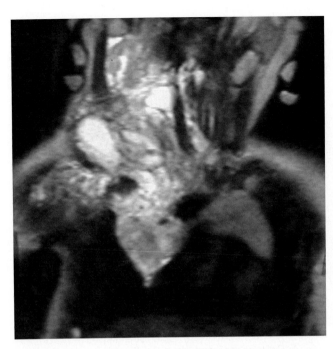

Figure 24-15 Cystic hygroma, newborn girl. T2-weighted coronal magnetic resonance image shows a heterogeneous high signal intensity mass infiltrating the superior mediastinum and right neck. The tumor extends into the right thymic lobe.

contrast enhancement of the wall or internal septations suggests superimposed infection or a hemangiomatous component. On MRI, cystic hygroma has signal intensity equal to or slightly less than that of muscle on T1-weighted images and greater than that of fat on T2-weighted images (216) (Fig. 24-15). The surrounding fascial planes are obliterated if the tumor infiltrates the adjacent soft tissues. Hemorrhage can cause a sudden increase in tumor size and can increase the CT attenuation value or the signal intensity on T1-weighted MR images (216). Occasionally, marked dilatation of adjacent veins is noted (113).

Middle Mediastinal Masses

The frequent causes of middle mediastinal masses are lymph node enlargement and congenital foregut cysts.

Lymphadenopathy

Lymph node enlargement, as a cause of a middle mediastinal mass, is usually caused by lymphoma or granulomatous disease. On CT, adenopathy can appear as discrete, round soft tissue masses, or as a single soft tissue mass with poorly defined margins. Calcification within lymph nodes suggests old granulomatous disease, such as histoplasmosis or tuberculosis. On T1-weighted MR images, lymph nodes involved by infection or tumor have a signal intensity similar to or slightly greater than that of muscle. On T2-weighted MR images, the signal intensity is high, similar to that of fat. Most lymph nodes are homogeneous on MRI, but they can appear heterogeneous if they contain calcification or necrosis. Neither CT nor MRI is able to pro-

vide a specific histologic diagnosis, but they can be useful for determining whether mediastinoscopy or thoracotomy would be better to yield a diagnosis.

Mediastinal nodes involved by granulomatous disease usually undergo spontaneous regression, frequently with resultant calcification. In some cases, healing occurs with extensive fibrosis, resulting in airway or vascular (e.g., superior vena caval) obstruction (Fig. 24-16). CT is superior to MRI for showing calcifications, which are important for establishing the diagnosis of inflammation. MRI, however, can provide complementary information about vascular patency, especially if there is a contraindication to the administration of iodinated contrast media. On MRI, calcifications and fibrotic tissue are of low intensity on both T1- and T2-weighted sequences (127).

Foregut Cysts

Foregut cysts in the middle mediastinum are classified as either bronchogenic or enteric, depending on their histology (87). Bronchogenic cysts are lined by respiratory epithelium, and most are located in the subcarinal or right paratracheal area. Enteric cysts are lined by gastrointestinal mucosa and are located in a paraspinal position in the middle to posterior mediastinum. In children, most foregut cysts are discovered because they produce symptoms of airway or esophageal compression; occasionally they are detected incidentally on a chest radiograph.

The CT appearance of a foregut cyst is usually that of a well-defined, round nonenhancing mass of near-water density, reflecting serous contents (Fig. 24-17). Air or an air–fluid level can be present when a communication between the cyst and the bronchial tree or gastrointestinal tract develops (152). On MRI, foregut cysts typically have a low signal intensity on T1-weighted images and a very high signal intensity on T2-weighted images. Some cysts have a soft tissue density on CT or a high signal intensity on T1-weighted images, because the fluid is proteinaceous or contains calcium carbonate or oxalate.

Posterior Mediastinal Masses

Posterior mediastinal masses are of neural origin in approximately 95% of cases and may arise from sympathetic ganglion cells (neuroblastoma, ganglioneuroblastoma, or ganglioneuroma) or from nerve sheaths (neurofibroma or schwannoma). Rarer causes of posterior mediastinal masses in children include paraspinal abscess, lymphoma, neurenteric cyst, lateral meningocele, and extramedullary hematopoiesis.

On CT, ganglion cell tumors appear as paraspinal masses, extending over the length of several vertebral bodies (237). They are fusiform in shape, of soft tissue density, and contain calcifications in up to 50% of cases (Fig. 24-18). Nerve root tumors tend to be smaller, spherical, and occur near the junction of a vertebral body with an adjacent rib. Both types of tumors may cause pressure erosion of a rib. On MRI, most neurogenic tumors have low signal intensity on T1-weighted images and relatively high signal

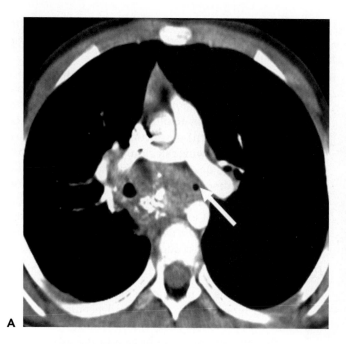

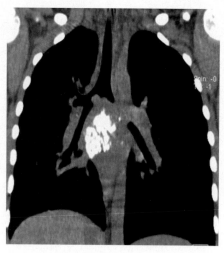

Figure 24-16 Fibrosing mediastinitis, 14-year-old girl. **A:** Contrast-enhanced computed tomography scan shows calcified subcarinal lymph nodes, with secondary narrowing of the left mainstem bronchus (*arrows*). **B:** Coronal multiplanar reformatted image shows the full extent of the subcarinal nodal mass and compression of right and left main bronchi.

intensity on T2-weighted images (Fig. 24-19). Some tumors have low attenuation on CT and intermediate to high signal intensity on T1-weighted images because of their myelin content. Because of their origin from neural tissue, neurogenic tumors have a tendency to invade the spinal canal (Fig. 24-19). Intraspinal extension is extradural in location, displacing and occasionally compressing the cord. Recognition of intraspinal invasion is critical because such

involvement usually requires radiation therapy or a laminectomy prior to tumor debulking.

Other causes of posterior mediastinal masses include neurenteric cyst, lateral meningocele, extralobar sequestration, and hemangioma. Neurenteric cysts and lateral meningoceles demonstrate water attenuation on CT, low signal intensity on T1-weighted images, and very high signal intensity on T2-weighted and fat-suppressed images. The former are associated with a midline defect in one or more vertebral bodies. Hemangioma typically is a unilateral highly vascular paraspinal mass (52). Sequestration sometimes appears as a paraspinal rather than intraparenchymal mass. Identification of an anomalous feeding artery or vein can confirm the diagnosis.

Vascular Masses

Abnormalities of the aorta and its branches and of the superior or inferior vena cava (IVC) can cause a mass or mediastinal widening on plain chest radiography. Either CT or MRI can be used to detect and characterize vascular anomalies (16,21,93,94,98,118,140,197,240). Both provide equivalent anatomic data.

Aortic Arch

The right arch with aberrant left subclavian artery and the double arch are common congenital anomalies of the aorta that produce an abnormal mediastinum on plain chest radiography (16) (Fig. 24-20). The double arch is characterized by two arches that surround the trachea and esophagus. The arches arise from a single ascending aorta and reunite to form a single descending aorta after giving

Figure 24-17 Duplication cyst, 15-year-old girl. Contrast-enhanced computed tomography shows a homogeneous, near-water-density cyst (C) in the middle mediastinum, posterior to the trachea.

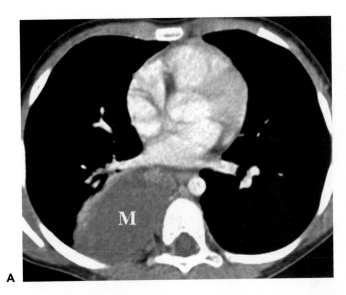
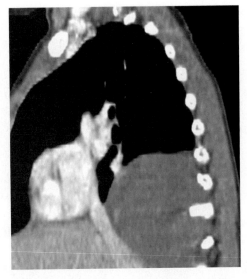

Figure 24-18 Neuroblastoma, 2-year-old girl. **A:** Contrast-enhanced computed tomography shows a large right paraspinal soft tissue mass (M). **B:** Sagittal multiplanar reformatted image shows the tumor extending over the length of several vertebral bodies. The craniocaudal extent of the mass is better defined on the coronal image.

rise to the subclavian and carotid arteries. The right arch component of a double arch anomaly usually is more cephalad and larger than the left arch component. Both aortic arches usually are patent, but occasionally the left arch is atretic. In the right arch with aberrant subclavian artery, the subclavian artery arises as the last branch from the aortic arch and traverses the mediastinum behind the

esophagus to reach the left arm. The vascular ring is completed by the ligamentum arteriosum. Airway compression may be a result of a tight ligamentum arteriosum, a Kommerell's diverticulum, or a midline descending aorta (54).

Aneurysm of the thoracic aorta is another cause of a vascular mediastinal mass. The most common cause of aneurysms in children is Marfan syndrome. Less commonly, bacterial infections or Ehlers-Danlos syndrome is the cause. Most aneurysms are fusiform in configuration. They may be focal or extend the entire length of the vessel.

Superior Vena Cava

Venous anomalies producing mediastinal widening include persistent left superior vena cava and interruption of the IVC (13,49). Persistent left superior vena cava, resulting from failure of regression of the left common and anterior cardinal veins, drains the left jugular and subclavian veins, and in some cases, the left superior intercostal vein. The persistent vena cava lies lateral to the left common carotid artery and anterior to the left subclavian artery, descends lateral to the main pulmonary artery, and drains into the coronary sinus posterior to the left ventricle.

Dilatation of the azygos or hemiazygos vein is a cause of a posterior mediastinal or right paratracheal mass. When the infrahepatic segment of the IVC above the renal veins fails to develop, blood from below the renal veins returns to the heart via the azygos or hemiazygos veins, with resultant dilatation of these structures. Typically, the hemiazygos vein crosses behind the aorta to join the dilated azygos vein, which in turn drains into the azygos arch (Fig. 24-21). The suprarenal portion of the IVC also is absent, and the hepatic veins drain directly into the right atrium.

Figure 24-19 Neurofibroma, 15-year-old boy. **A:** Axial T2-weighted magnetic resonance image shows a large, relatively high signal intensity, paraspinal mass invading the spinal canal (*arrow*), displacing the cord slightly to the right.

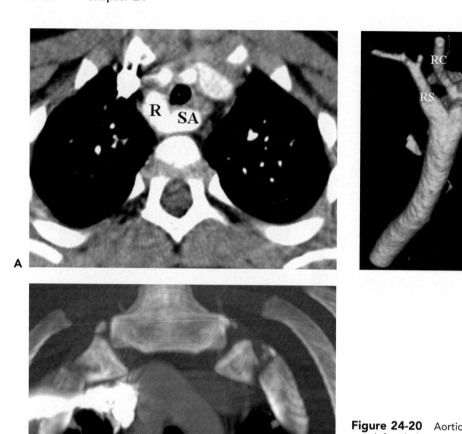

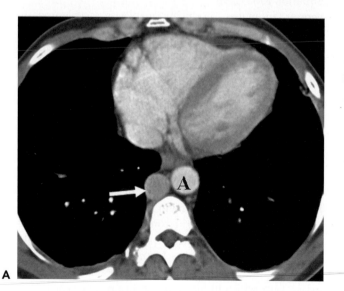

Figure 24-20   Aortic arch anomalies. **A:** Right arch with an aberrant left subclavian artery, 3-year-old girl. Contrast-enhanced computed tomography (CT) scan demonstrates a right aortic arch (R) giving rise to the left subclavian artery (SA), which passes behind the trachea and esophagus to reach the left arm. **B:** Three-dimensional reconstruction shows the left subclavian artery (*arrow*) arising as the last branch off the right-sided aorta. RS, right subclavian artery; RC, right carotid artery; LC, left carotid artery. **C:** Double arch in an 17-year-old girl. CT shows the two limbs of the double arch encircling the trachea and esophagus. R, right arch; L, left arch. (**C** reprinted from Siegel MJ. Multiplanar and three-dimensional row CT of thoracic vessels and airways in the pediatric population. *Radiology* 2003;229:641–650, with permission.)

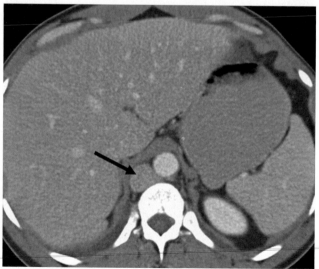

Figure 24-21   Azygos continuation of inferior vena cava. **A:** Computed tomography scan at the level of the distal aorta (A) shows a markedly dilated azygos vein (*arrow*). **B:** A dilated azygos vein (*arrow*) is noted at the level of the liver. The inferior vena cava is absent.

Comparative Imaging and Clinical Applications

CT and MRI are both sensitive for detection of mediastinal masses and provide comparable information on the presence and size of a lesion. CT usually suffices for assessing anterior and middle mediastinal masses, with the exception of cystic hygroma. In patients with cystic hygroma, MRI is superior to CT in defining the extent of the tumor, particularly soft tissue infiltration. MRI is the method of choice for evaluating patients with posterior mediastinal masses suspected of being of neurogenic origin, because of the high likelihood of intraspinal extension.

Lungs

Congenital Anomalies

Congenital lung anomalies include a variety of conditions involving the pulmonary parenchyma, the pulmonary vasculature, or a combination of both. Because many of these conditions are associated with either a parenchymal lesion or anomalous vessels, they are well suited for analysis by CT scanning. In selected cases, MRI can provide complementary information about the presence or absence of an anomalous vessel.

Anomalies With Normal Vasculature

Congenital lobar emphysema, cystic adenomatoid malformation, and bronchial atresia are anomalies resulting from abnormal bronchial development. Chest radiography often suffices for diagnosis. CT is performed to confirm the diagnosis and to determine its extent in patients in whom surgery is contemplated.

Congenital lobar emphysema is characterized by hyperinflation of a lobe (42). The exact etiology is unknown, but many cases are believed to be caused by bronchial obstruction. The affected patient usually presents in the first six months of life with respiratory distress. CT shows a hyperinflated lobe with attenuated vascularity, compression of ipsilateral adjacent lobes, and mediastinal shift to the opposite side (Fig. 24-22). The left upper lobe is involved in about 45% of cases, the right middle lobe in 30%, the right upper lobe in 20%, and two lobes in 5% of cases (42).

Cystic adenomatoid malformation is characterized by an overgrowth of distal bronchial tissue, with formation of a cystic mass. Symptoms of respiratory distress usually occur soon after birth. Histologically, there are three types of cystic adenomatoid malformation: type I (50% of cases) contains a single cyst or multiple large cysts (greater than 10 mm in diameter); type II (41%) contains multiple small cysts (1 to 10 mm in diameter); and type III (9%) is a solid lesion to visual inspection, but contains microscopic cysts (42,125). The anomaly occurs with equal frequency in both lungs, although there is slight upper lobe predominance. On CT, cystic adenomatoid malformation appears as a parenchymal mass that may be predominantly cystic or solid or contain an admixture of cystic and solid com-

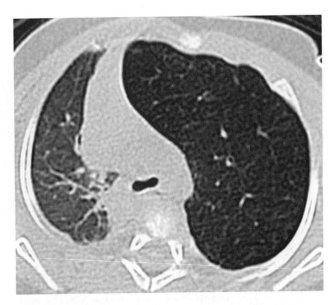

Figure 24-22 Congenital lobar emphysema, 6-month-old boy. Computed tomography through the upper thorax shows a hyperinflated left upper lobe with attenuated vascularity.

ponents (42,125,205) (Fig. 24-23). Air–fluid levels occasionally can be seen within the cysts.

Bronchial atresia results from abnormal development of a segmental or subsegmental bronchus. It rarely causes symptoms and is usually discovered on chest radiographs performed for other indications. The CT features of bronchial atresia include over-aerated lung distal to the atresia and a round, ovoid, or branching density near the hilum, representing mucoid impaction just beyond the atretic bronchus (3) (Fig. 24-24).

Anomalies With Abnormal Vasculature

Sequestration, hypogenetic lung syndrome, and arteriovenous malformation (AVM) are congenital anomalies with abnormal vasculature. Chronic or recurrent segmental or subsegmental pneumonitis in children, especially at a lung base, is a finding suggestive of sequestration. Pathologically, a sequestered portion of lung has no normal connection with the tracheobronchial tree and is supplied by an anomalous artery, usually arising from the aorta. When the sequestered lung is confined within the normal visceral pleura and has venous drainage to the pulmonary veins, it is termed "intralobar." The sequestered lung is termed "extralobar" when it has its own pleura and venous drainage to systemic veins.

Although plain chest radiography or conventional tomography occasionally may demonstrate an anomalous vessel, CT and MRI are more sensitive for identifying such a vessel (66,67,128). CT scanning after an injection of contrast material demonstrates opacification of the anomalous vessel immediately following enhancement of the descending thoracic aorta. The anomalous vessel often can be traced to the sequestered lung. The CT appearance of

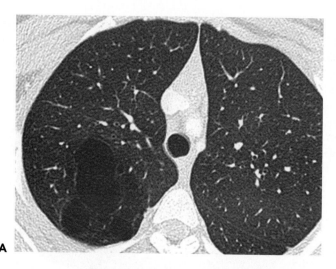
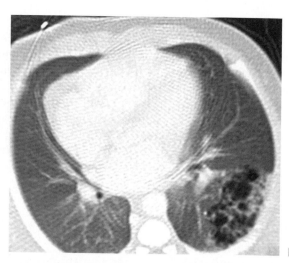

Figure 24-23 Cystic adenomatoid malformation. **A:** Type I lesion, 15-year-old girl, multilocular mass in the right upper lobe containing numerous large cysts. **B:** Type II malformation, infant girl, a complex mass in the left lower lobe containing multiple small cysts.

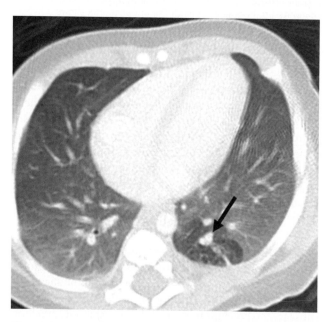

Figure 24-24 Bronchial atresia, infant girl. Computed tomography shows an ovoid soft tissue nodule (*arrow*) in the left lower lobe. The nodule is surrounded by over-aerated lung resulting from collateral air drift.

the pulmonary parenchyma depends on whether or not the sequestered lung is aerated. When the sequestration communicates with the remainder of the lung, usually after being infected, it appears cystic; a sequestration that does not communicate appears as a homogeneous density, usually in the posterior portion of the lower lobe (Figs. 24-25 and 24-26). On MRI, the feeding vessel appears as an area of signal void on T1-weighted spin-echo images and as a hyperintense area on GRE sequences. The parenchymal portion of the sequestration appears as an area of intermediate or high signal intensity.

An additional congenital lung abnormality with vascular anomalies that can be diagnosed by CT or MRI is the hypogenetic lung or scimitar syndrome (82,130,285). CT and MRI findings include a small right lung, ipsilateral mediastinal displacement, a corresponding small pulmonary artery, and occasionally partial anomalous pulmonary venous return from the right lung to the IVC (Fig. 24-27). Other associated anomalies include systemic arterial supply to the hypogenetic lung, accessory diaphragm, and horseshoe lung. Horseshoe lung is a rare anomaly in which the posterobasal segments of both lungs are fused behind the pericardial sac.

Pulmonary AVM is characterized by a direct communication between a pulmonary artery and vein without an intervening capillary bed. When the diagnosis is suspected on chest radiographs, CT and MRI are useful to establish the definitive diagnosis (82,96,138,196,207). However, if surgery or embolization is planned, arteriography may be needed to demonstrate the precise vascular anatomy of complex fistulae or the presence of multiple tiny AVMs that may not be visible on CT or MRI. On CT and MRI, AVMs appear as rounded or lobular masses with rapid enhancement and washout after intravenous contrast medium administration. Enhancement typically occurs after enhancement of the right ventricle and before enhancement of the left atrium and left ventricle.

Pulmonary Metastases

CT is a valuable technique for detection of pulmonary metastases in patients with known malignancies with a high propensity for lung dissemination, such as Wilms tumor, osteogenic sarcoma, and rhabdomyosarcoma. Demonstration of one or more pulmonary nodules in such patients, or documentation of additional nodules in a patient with an apparent solitary metastasis for whom surgery is planned, may be critical to treatment planning.

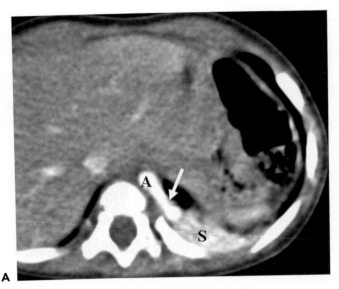

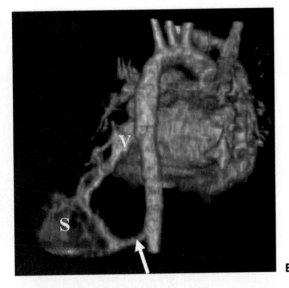

Figure 24-25 Intralobar sequestration, 6-month-old girl with recurrent left lower lobe pneumonia. **A:** Computed tomography demonstrates the anomalous arterial supply (*arrow*) to the sequestered lung (S) arising from the thoracic aorta (A). **B:** Posterior three-dimensional volume-rendered image shows the anomalous arterial supply (*arrow*) from the descending aorta to the sequestered lung (S) and the anomalous venous drainage (V) to the left atrium. (Reprinted from Siegel MJ. Multiplanar and three-dimensional row CT of thoracic vessels and airways in the pediatric population. *Radiology* 2003;229:641–650, with permission.)

In the first instance, such detection may lead to additional treatment (surgery, chemotherapy, or radiation), whereas in the latter setting, demonstration of several metastatic nodules may negate surgical plans. Confusion with benign granulomas does not appear to be as significant a clinical problem in children as it is in adults; in children, almost all noncalcified nodules depicted by CT are a result of metastases (Fig. 24-28) rather than granulomatous disease or a primary neoplasm.

MRI can detect large parenchymal nodules, but it is not as sensitive as CT in detecting nodules less than 1 cm in diameter because of its poorer spatial resolution. Hence, CT remains the imaging method of choice for detecting and characterizing pulmonary nodules.

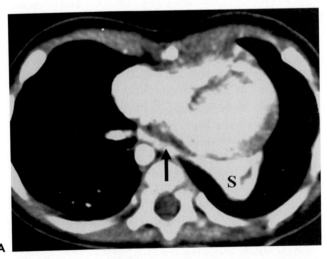

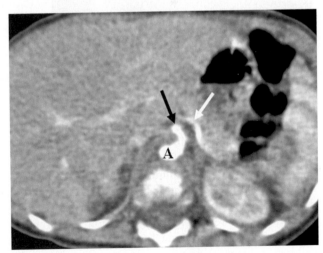

Figure 24-26 Extralobar pulmonary sequestration, 6-month-old boy with a left paraspinal mass on chest radiographs. **A:** Computed tomography (CT) scan shows the anomalous vein (*arrow*) arising from the sequestered lung (S) and crossing the midline to the right hemithorax. **B:** More caudal CT image demonstrates the anomalous arterial vessel (*white arrow*) arising from the celiac artery (*black arrow*). A, aorta. (Reprinted from Lee E, Siegel MJ, Foglia R. Evaluation of angioarchitecture of pulmonary sequestration in pediatric patients using 3D MDCT angiography. *AJR Am J Roentgenol* 2004;183:183–188, with permission.)

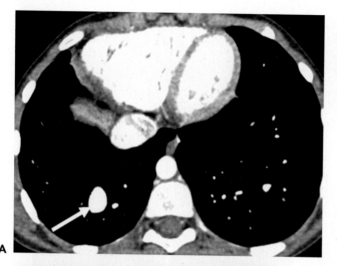

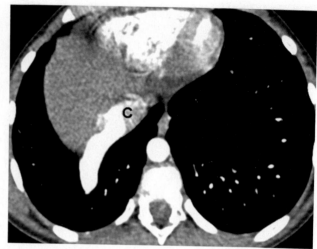

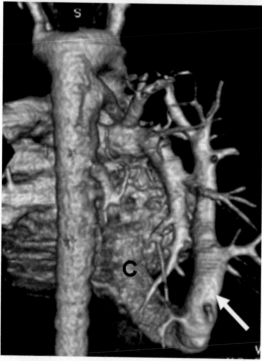

Figure 24-27 Scimitar syndrome with partial anomalous venous return, 10-year-old girl. **A:** Axial computed tomography scan at the level of the ventricles shows part of the anomalous pulmonary vein (*arrow*). **B:** Several centimeters lower, the anomalous vessel enters the intrahepatic inferior vena cava (C). Note that the right hemithorax is smaller than the left and that there is mediastinal shift to the right. **C:** Volume-rendered three-dimensional display depicts the entire course of the anomalous vessel on one image. C, inferior vena cava; arrow, anomalous vein.

Diffuse Parenchymal Disease

Chest radiography remains the imaging study of choice for evaluating diffuse parenchymal lung disease. CT, however, can be useful to better define and characterize an abnormality suspected on conventional chest radiography, especially when the CT examination is performed with high-resolution technique using narrow (1- to 2-mm) collimation and a high spatial frequency reconstruction algorithm. Indications for high-resolution CT of the lung parenchyma in children include: (a) detection of disease in children who are at increased risk for lung disease (e.g., immunocompromised patients) and who have respiratory symptoms but a normal chest radiograph; (b) determination of the extent, distribution, and character of lung diseases; (c) localization of abnormal lung for biopsy; and (d) assessment of the response to treatment (135,151,159,160,172,234).

Although many lung diseases in children have nonspecific findings, some have characteristic appearances. Cystic fibrosis is characterized by diffuse hyperinflation, bronchiectasis, and peribronchial soft tissue thickening (Fig. 24-29), whereas bronchopulmonary dysplasia is characterized by hyperinflation, cystic airspaces, and septal lines, without bronchiectasis (135,151,172,186,234) (Fig. 24-30). Bronchiolitis obliterans is manifested as patchy areas of overinflation with resultant attenuation of pulmonary vessels, sometimes in conjunction with bronchiectasis (35,136). In older children who are able to suspend respiration, dynamic CT with inspiratory and expiratory imaging may aid in confirming the diagnosis of focal air-trapping (Fig. 24-31) (215).

The common interstitial lung diseases in children include Langerhans cell histiocytosis and pulmonary fibro-

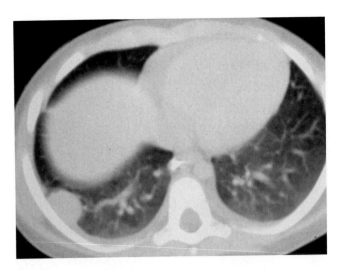

Figure 24-28 Metastatic Wilms tumor. A large, soft tissue nodule is seen in the right lower lobe.

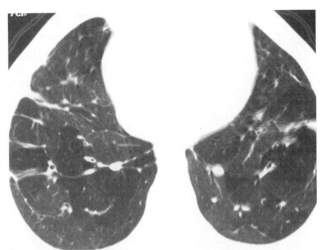

Figure 24-30 Bronchopulmonary dysplasia. High-resolution computed tomography shows diffuse septal lines without bronchiectasis.

sis. CT findings of Langerhans cell histiocytosis include small pulmonary nodules (less than 5 mm) in the early stages of the disease and thin-walled cysts and septal thickening in later stages of the disease (162) (Fig. 24-32). Pulmonary fibrosis is characterized by septal thickening, traction bronchiectasis, and subpleural honeycombing with architectural distortion. The most common airspace disease is pulmonary alveolar proteinosis, which is characterized by ground-glass opacity and alveolar consolidation (2) (Fig. 24-33).

Pulmonary Infections

Conventional chest radiography remains the imaging technique of choice to exclude or confirm a clinically suspected pulmonary infection, to evaluate for the presence of parapneumonic effusion, and to assess the response to

treatment. In patients who do not respond to appropriate therapy, CT is useful to assess suspected complications, including pneumatocele formation, abscess, lung necrosis (i.e., necrotizing pneumonia), and empyema (56,57).

On CT, pneumatoceles appear as single or multiple, thin-walled, cystic lesions, whereas abscesses have thick, irregular walls and may contain an air–fluid level if they develop a communication with the bronchus (Fig. 24-34). Necrotizing pneumonia manifests as cavitary lesions within an area of consolidation in conjunction with decreased parenchymal enhancement after administration of intravenous contrast medium (Fig. 24-35). Necrotizing pneumonia is important to recognize, because most children with this finding need to be hospitalized and require a longer course of antibiotic therapy than do children with uncomplicated pneumonia. Empyema is characterized by

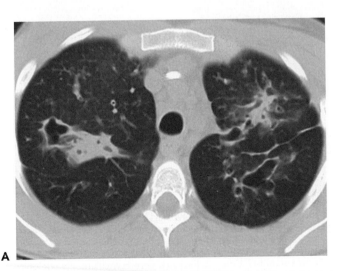

A

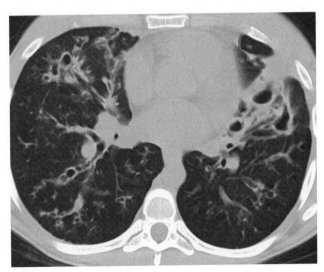

B

Figure 24-29 Cystic fibrosis. **A, B:** High-resolution computed tomography sections at two levels demonstrate diffuse cystic bronchiectasis and peribronchial thickening.

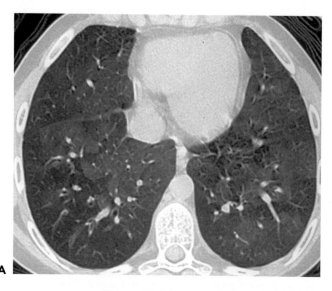

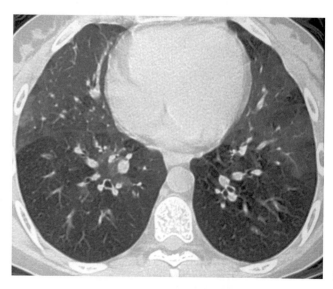

Figure 24-31 Bronchiolitis obliterans after bilateral lung transplantation, 14-year-old girl. **A:** Axial computed tomography section at inspiration shows mild mosaic attenuation. **B:** Image during expiration shows more prominent mosaic attenuation. The lower attenuation areas indicate air trapping in small airways.

pleural fluid and thickening of the adjacent visceral and parietal pleura. Frequently, there is edema/inflammation of the extrapleural tissues as well.

Parenchymal or Pleural Disease

In some patients, CT can be helpful in distinguishing between a parenchymal process and a pleural or extrapleural process. The features of parenchymal lesions are a rounded or oval shape, acute or abrupt angles at the interface with the chest wall, and poorly defined margins with the adjacent lung. The CT features of pleural disease are a lenticular or crescentic shape, obtuse or tapering angles at the interface with the chest wall, and well-defined margins with adjacent lung, bone, and soft tissues. Extrapleural lesions

are lenticular in shape with poorly defined margins and obtuse or tapering angles at the interface with the pleura. Two-dimensional (2D) and 3D reconstructions in coronal and sagittal planes may be helpful in characterizing a lesion as intraparenchymal or pleural based.

MRI currently has a limited role in evaluating pulmonary disease, including pleural processes. Although it is sensitive for detection of a variety of pleural and parenchymal disorders, it adds little clinically important information over that gained with CT.

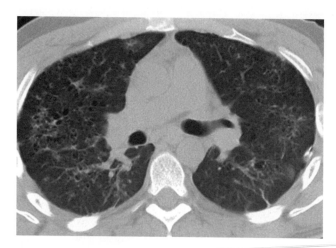

Figure 24-32 Langerhans cell histiocytosis. High-resolution computed tomography shows multiple small air-filled, thin-walled cysts.

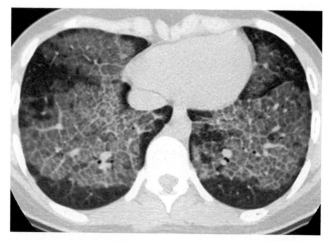

Figure 24-33 Pulmonary alveolar proteinosis, 15-year-old girl with shortness of breath. High-resolution computed tomography through the lung bases shows extensive ground-glass opacity and interstitial thickening, creating a "crazy paving" appearance. (From Siegel MJ, Coley B. Pediatric core curriculum. Philadelphia: Lippincott Williams & Wilkins, 2005, with permission.)

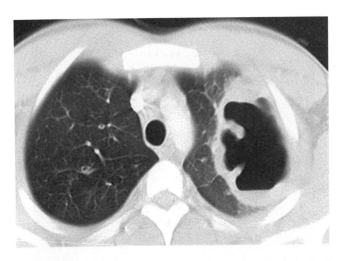

Figure 24-34 Lung abscess, 15-year-old boy. Contrast-enhanced computed tomography shows a thick-walled cavitary lesion adjacent to the pleural surface.

Airway Disease

The tracheobronchial tree, including the trachea, carina, and mainstem and lobar bronchi, are easily seen by CT. CT images of the airways are acquired in the axial plane and postprocessed with both multiplanar reformations in the coronal, oblique, and sagittal planes and 3D volume-rendering techniques (261). Axial images are mandatory for assessing extraluminal disease, including the lung parenchyma and mediastinal structures. Multiplanar and volume renderings are helpful in delineating mild stenoses and complex congenital airway abnormalities, such as abnormal origins of the bronchi or bronchoesophageal fistu-

las. They also can assist in showing the relationship of the airway to surrounding vessels.

The more frequent indications prompting CT of the airway are: (a) evaluation of congenital tracheobronchial anomalies (73,286), (b) assessment of tracheal narrowing (99,160,187), and (c) detection or confirmation of tracheomalacia (76). Tracheobronchial neoplasia is a rare indication for CT in children. The common congenital anomalies are the tracheal and cardiac bronchi. The tracheal or pig bronchus arises almost always on the right side of the trachea and usually within 2 cm of the carina (73,286) (Fig. 24-36). The accessory cardiac bronchus nearly always arises from the inferior medial wall of the right main or intermediate bronchus. Both types of bronchi may serve as reservoirs for infectious organisms leading to recurrent pneumonia. Tracheal strictures are usually the sequelae of intubation, tracheostomy placement, or surgical anastomoses.

Tracheomalacia refers to an abnormal weakness of the tracheal walls and supporting tissues, resulting in luminal collapse during expiration. When tracheomalacia is suspected, scans are acquired at both end-inspiration and end-expiration and then reformatted in the coronal and sagittal planes. This technique is limited to cooperative patients or to patients who are on assisted ventilation. The diagnosis of tracheomalacia can be made by CT when there is 50% or greater reduction in transluminal diameter during expiration.

A less frequent indication for airway CT is foreign body aspiration (132). The foreign body can be precisely localized by spiral CT prior to bronchoscopic retrieval. Dynamic CT with inspiratory and expiratory imaging can show the air trapping distal to the bronchial obstruction.

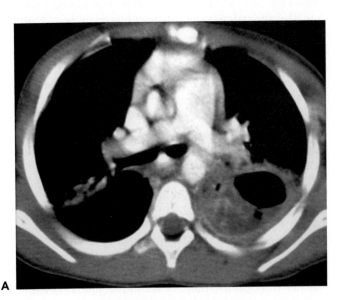
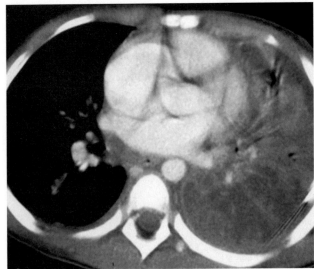

A   B

Figure 24-35 Necrotizing pneumonia. **A, B:** Two contrast-enhanced computed tomography images show left lung consolidation without contrast enhancement and cavitary changes indicating lung necrosis.

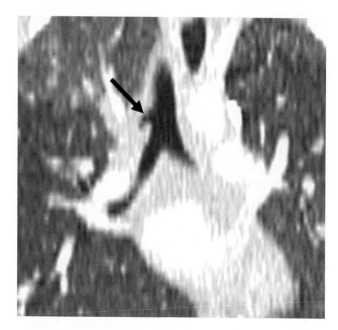

Figure 24-36 Tracheal bronchus. Coronal reconstruction computed tomography scan shows an ectopic right upper lobe bronchus (*arrow*) arising from the proximal trachea.

Pulmonary Arteries and Veins

Congenital anomalies of the pulmonary arteries and veins are also well suited to CT and MR angiography. The common anomalies of the pulmonary arteries are agenesis or hypoplasia and anomalous origin of the left pulmonary artery from the right pulmonary artery (pulmonary sling) (Fig. 24-37) (189).

The common anomaly of the pulmonary veins is anomalous return, which occurs when a pulmonary vein

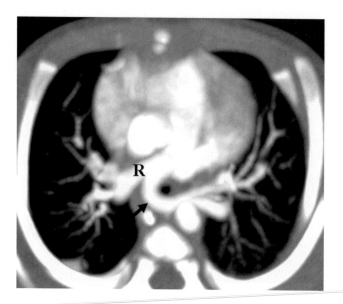

Figure 24-37 Pulmonary sling, 3-month-old girl. Contrast-enhanced axial computed tomography image shows anomalous left pulmonary artery (*arrow*) arising from right pulmonary artery (R) and compressing trachea. (Courtesy of Joseph Schoepf, MD.)

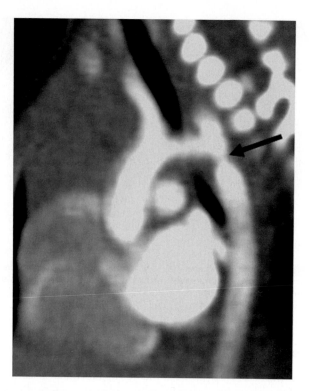

Figure 24-38 Aortic coarctation. Sagittal computed tomography reconstruction shows mild hypoplasia of the transverse aortic arch and an area of high-grade coarctation (*arrow*) just distal to the origin of the subclavian artery.

enters the right heart or a systemic vein. The anomalous connection commonly involves the left superior, right inferior, and right superior pulmonary veins (50,277). The anomalous left superior pulmonary vein drains into the left brachiocephalic vein, producing a vertical vein that courses lateral to the aortic arch and aortopulmonary window. The anomalous right inferior pulmonary vein drains cephalad into the azygous vein or caudal into the subdiaphragmatic IVC or portal vein. The right superior pulmonary vein drains into the superior vena cava and is often associated with a secundum atrial septal defect. Anomalous return to the right lung can occur in association with the hypogenetic lung syndrome (see Fig. 24-27).

Cardiac Disease

The presence of most congenital and acquired cardiac lesions can be determined with echocardiography in combination with Doppler sonography, but CT and MRI can be of use when echocardiography provides inadequate information (26,37,75,77,83,95,141). The major indications for CT and MRI in congenital cardiac anomalies include: (a) evaluation of the size and patency of the pulmonary arteries in patients with cyanotic heart disease, such as pulmonary atresia and tetrology of Fallot (283), (b) assessment of the extent and severity of aortic coarctation (41,129,141) (Fig. 24-38) and the degree of supravalvar aortic stenosis, (c) detection of anomalous origin of the coronary artery, (d) de-

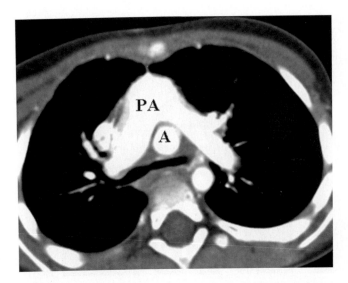

Figure 24-39 Jatene procedure. Contrast-enhanced computed tomography after an arterial switch procedure shows characteristic draping of the pulmonary arteries (PA) around the aorta (A).

termination of the extracardiac anatomy in patients with complex congenital heart disease (e.g., great vessel relationships, bronchial collateral vessels, abdominal situs) (38,55, 124), (e) evaluation of postoperative anatomy and surgically created systemic-to-pulmonary artery shunts and intracardiac baffles (201) (Figs. 24-39 and 24-40), and (f) detection of arrhythmogenic right ventricular cardiomyopathy (11). CT and MRI also can provide information about acquired lesions, including intracardiac or pericardial masses (225).

ABDOMEN

The appearance of the abdomen on CT and MR examinations is similar in adults and children, except for the limitations imposed by the small size of the structures being

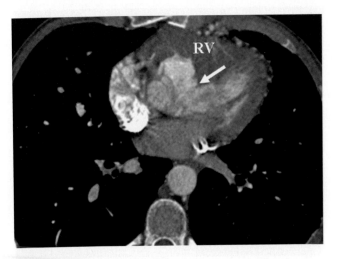

Figure 24-40 Tetralogy of Fallot. Patient had undergone palliative Blalock Taussig shunt in infancy. Axial image shows ventricular septal defect (*arrow*) and right ventricular hypertrophy (RV).

examined and the relative paucity of perivisceral fat. The major clinical questions usually prompting CT examination of the abdomen are: (a) determination of the site of origin, extent, and character of an abdominal mass; (b) determination of the extent of a proven lymphoma; (c) evaluation of the extent of injury from blunt abdominal trauma; and (d) determination of the presence or absence of a suspected abscess. Less often, CT is used to evaluate non-neoplastic, parenchymal disease of the kidney, liver, pancreas, and gastrointestinal tract or to assess abnormalities of the major abdominal vessels.

Abdominal masses in the pediatric population are predominantly retroperitoneal in location, with the kidney being the source in more than half of the cases. In neonates, most abdominal masses are benign; beyond the neonatal period, the percentage of malignant neoplasms increases. CT and MRI have an important role in older infants and children in determining the site of origin, characteristics, and extent of a mass, as well as the presence or absence of metastatic disease (165,227,238,239,249).

Renal Masses

Solid Renal Tumors
Wilms Tumor

Wilms tumor is the most common primary malignant renal tumor of childhood (71,78,148). Affected patients generally are under 4 years of age. They present most frequently with a palpable abdominal mass, and less often with abdominal pain, fever, and microscopic or gross hematuria. Approximately 10% of children have metastatic disease at presentation (78). Metastases are characteristically to the lungs and less frequently to the liver.

Wilms tumor appears as a large, spherical, at least partially intrarenal mass with a soft tissue density on CT and an MR signal intensity equal to or lower than that of normal renal cortex on T1-weighted images and equal to or higher than that of normal parenchyma on T2-weighted images (71,148,163,238,239,249) (Figs. 24-41 and 24-42). The tumor enhances after intravenous administration of contrast medium, but usually to a lesser extent than the adjacent parenchyma. Approximately 80% of tumors are heterogeneous, because they contain areas of necrosis or hemorrhage. Less than 15% of Wilms tumors contain calcifications or fat as a minor component. Poor or absent function of the involved kidney occurs in about 10% of patients, resulting from invasion or compression of hilar vessels or the renal pelvis, or from extensive infiltration of tumor throughout the kidney (180). Bilateral synchronous tumors occur in 5% to 10% of patients (Fig. 24-43).

Local spread of tumor may take the form of extension through the capsule into the perinephric space (20% of cases), retroperitoneal lymphadenopathy (20%), or renal vein or IVC thrombosis (5% to 10%) (78). Perinephric extension may be seen as a thickened renal capsule or as nodular or streaky densities in the perinephric fat. The

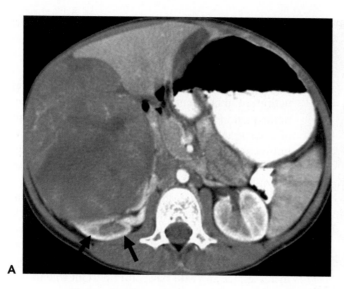
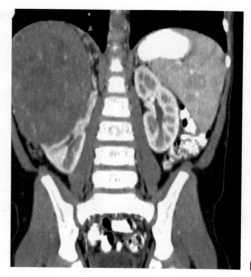

Figure 24-41 Wilms tumor in a 2-year-old boy. **A, B:** Contrast-enhanced axial computed tomography and coronal multiplanar reconstruction demonstrate a large, round, low-density mass that distorts and displaces the enhancing parenchyma (*arrows*) in the lower pole of the right kidney.

diagnosis of lymph node involvement is based on demonstration of perirenal, periaortic, paracaval, or retroperitoneal lymph nodes. Any identified retroperitoneal lymph node, regardless of size, should be regarded with suspicion. Although normal-size nodes are commonly demonstrated on abdominal CT and MRI in adults, such nodes are rarely, if ever, seen in infants and young children.

Neither CT nor MRI can detect tumor thrombus in the small intrarenal veins, but both imaging techniques are capable of identifying tumor in the main renal vein or IVC. The presence or absence of IVC invasion is an important determinant of the surgical approach. A thoracoabdomi-

nal approach is required for removal of tumor thrombus extending to or above the confluence of the hepatic veins, whereas an abdominal approach alone is satisfactory for intravascular thrombus below the hepatic veins. On CT, the thrombus is seen as a low-density intraluminal mass. On MRI, tumor thrombus is hyperintense to flowing blood on spin-echo sequences and is hypointense to flowing blood on GRE images.

After therapy, CT or MRI can be used to detect local recurrence and hepatic metastases. Patients with incomplete resection of tumor, lymph node involvement, and vascular invasion have the highest risk for postoperative recurrence. Features that suggest localized recurrence are a soft tissue

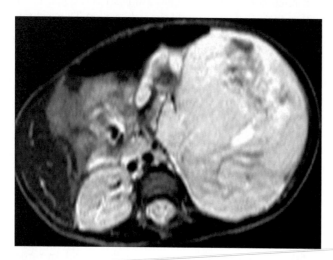

Figure 24-42 Wilms tumor in a 2-year-old girl. T2-weighted transaxial magnetic resonance image shows a large mass replacing most of the left kidney. The predominant signal intensity is similar to that of normal parenchyma. Several areas of low signal intensity, representing necrosis, are noted in the tumor.

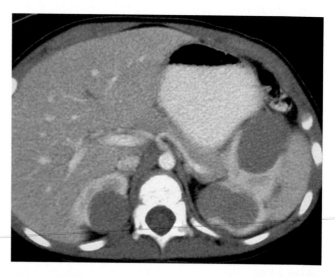

Figure 24-43 Bilateral Wilms tumors. Computed tomography scan shows two nonenhancing low-attenuation Wilms tumors in the left kidney and one in the right kidney.

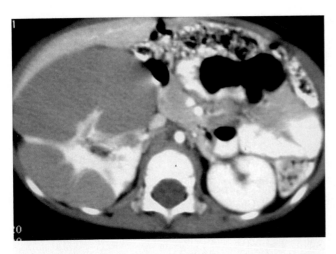

Figure 24-44 Nephroblastomatosis, 12-month-old girl. Computed tomography demonstrates an enlarged right kidney with a rind of soft tissue in the subcapsular space compressing the enhancing renal cortex.

mass in the empty renal fossa and ipsilateral psoas muscle enlargement.

Nephroblastomatosis

Nephroblastomatosis is an abnormality of nephrogenesis characterized by persistence of fetal renal blastema beyond 36 weeks of intrauterine gestation. Nephroblastomatosis itself is not a malignant condition, but it is a precursor to Wilms tumor. Renal involvement by nephroblastomatosis is often bilateral. The CT findings of nephroblastomatosis include (a) nephromegaly, (b) low-attenuation subcapsular masses or nodules, and (c) poor corticomedullary differentiation (84,145,174,202) (Fig. 24-44). On gadolinium-enhanced T1-weighted MR images, nephroblastomatosis is hypointense relative to normal renal tissue (84). On T2-weighted images, nephrogenic rests usually are

isointense or slightly hyperintense to renal cortex, but occasionally they can be hypointense.

Mesoblastic Nephroma

Mesoblastic nephroma, also termed fetal renal hamartoma, is a benign neoplasm usually presenting in the first year of life as an abdominal mass. The CT and MRI findings are those of a fairly uniform intrarenal mass that enhances after intravenous contrast medium injection, although not to the extent of normal renal parenchyma (30,199,249). Occasionally, areas of cystic degeneration and necrosis are seen as low-density foci within the tumor. Invasion of the vascular pedicle or extension into the renal pelvis is rare, although the tumor can penetrate the renal capsule and invade the perinephric space. Differentiation between Wilms tumor and mesoblastic nephroma usually is not possible without a biopsy.

Lymphoma

Renal involvement by lymphoma occurs infrequently during the course of disease, but it is not uncommon at autopsy. This complication is more often associated with the non-Hodgkin than with the Hodgkin form of disease, and it is often bilateral. The most common CT appearance of renal lymphoma in childhood is that of multiple bilateral nodules, occurring in approximately 70% of cases (Fig. 24-45A), followed in frequency by direct invasion from contiguous lymph node masses (20% of cases) and solitary nodules (10% of cases) (Fig. 24-45B) (36,103). Typically, the intrarenal tumors are hypodense relative to normal renal parenchyma and show minimal enhancement. The CT appearance of solitary renal lymphoma is indistinguishable from that of other solid intrarenal masses, but the diagnosis is possible when there is coexisting splenomegaly or widespread lymph node enlargement. On T1-weighted MR images, lymphomatous nodes have a signal

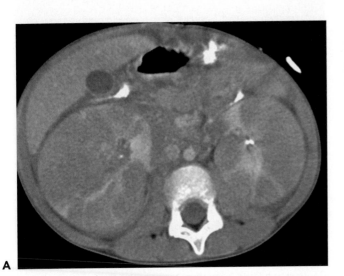

A

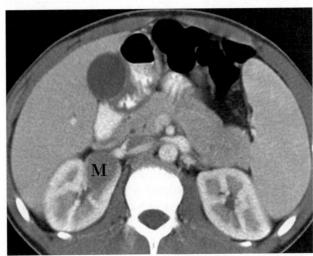

B

Figure 24-45 Renal lymphoma. **A:** Computed tomography (CT) scan in a 1-year-old boy shows bilateral nephromegaly and renal masses. **B:** CT in a 14-year-old boy shows a solitary mass (M) in the right kidney.

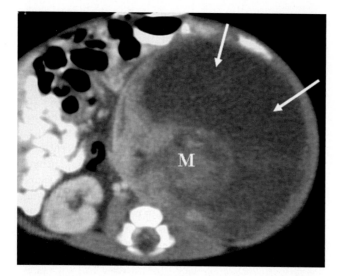

Figure 24-46 Rhabdoid tumor. Computed tomography scan through the upper abdomen demonstrates an irregular, poorly defined soft tissue mass (M) replacing the parenchyma of the left kidney. Also noted is perirenal fluid (*arrows*).

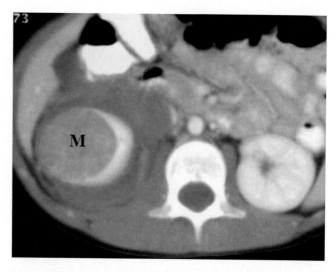

Figure 24-47 Renal cell carcinoma, 10-year-old boy. Contrast-enhanced computed tomography scan demonstrates a soft tissue mass (M) in the right kidney and a surrounding perirenal hematoma. The hemorrhage was secondary to trauma and tumor rupture.

intensity that is slightly higher than that of muscle and lower than that of fat. On T2-weighted images, the signal intensity of lymphomatous nodes is equal to or higher than that of retroperitoneal fat.

Rare Renal Tumors

Clear cell sarcoma and malignant rhabdoid tumor are rare pediatric renal masses (6,30,40,90,251). The former tends to affect children between 3 and 5 years of age, whereas the latter is more frequent in infants, with a median age of 13 months. Presenting signs are similar to those of Wilms tumor. On CT and MRI, these tumors appear as solid intrarenal masses, replacing or compressing the remaining normal kidney. The tumors may involve one or both kidneys. Additional findings include renal capsular thickening and subcapsular or perinephric fluid collection with tumor implants (6,40,90,251) (Fig. 24-46). Concomitant primary tumors of the posterior cranial fossa, soft tissues, and thymus occur in association with malignant rhabdoid tumor. Clear cell sarcoma commonly metastasizes to bone.

Renal cell carcinoma accounts for less than 1% of pediatric renal neoplasms. Mean age of presentation of children with renal cell carcinoma is approximately 9 years, in contrast to Wilms tumor with a mean patient age at presentation of 3 years. Presenting signs and symptoms are nonspecific and include mass, pain, and hematuria. On CT and MRI, renal cell carcinoma is indistinguishable from Wilms tumor and appears as a solid intrarenal mass with ill-defined margins (114) (Fig. 24-47). After the intravenous administration of contrast medium, the mass enhances, but less than that of the surrounding normal renal parenchyma. Calcification occurs in approximately 25% of tumors. Like Wilms tumor, renal cell carcinoma may

spread to retroperitoneal lymph nodes or may invade the renal vein and metastasize to lung and liver.

Renal medullary carcinoma is an unusual tumor associated with sickle cell trait (47). Most patients are diagnosed in the second or third decades of life. The tumor is extremely aggressive, arises centrally within the kidney, grows in an infiltrative pattern, and invades the renal sinus. Contrast enhancement is heterogeneous, reflecting tumor necrosis.

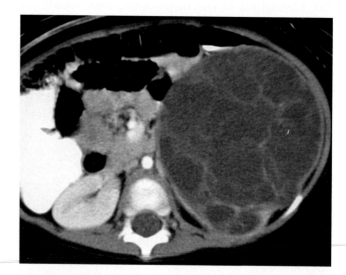

Figure 24-48 Multilocular cystic nephroma in a 4-year-old boy. Contrast-enhanced computed tomography scan shows a low-attenuation mass containing several enhancing septations in the upper pole of the left kidney.

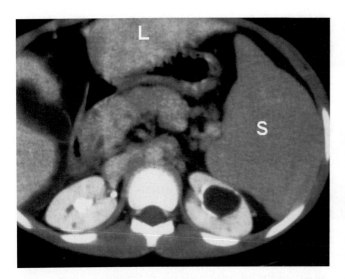

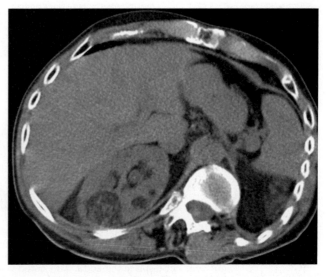

Figure 24-49 Autosomal recessive polycystic disease and hepatic fibrosis. Contrast-enhanced computed tomography scan shows multiple, small renal cysts. Splenomegaly (S) and hypertrophy of the left hepatic lobe (L) secondary to hepatic fibrosis are also noted.

Figure 24-50 Angiomyolipomas in an adolescent boy with tuberous sclerosis. Unenhanced computed tomography scan demonstrates small masses of low attenuation, approaching fat density, in the right kidney.

Cystic Renal Masses
Multilocular Cystic Nephroma
Multilocular cystic nephroma (also termed benign cystic nephroma, cystic hamartoma, cystic lymphangioma, and partial polycystic kidney) is a unilateral, nonhereditary cystic mass. The lesion has a biphasic age and sex distribution, affecting boys under 4 years of age and women over 40 years of age. Presenting signs are a nonpainful abdominal mass or hematuria. On CT and MRI, the lesion appears as a well-defined intrarenal mass with multiple, water-density cysts separated by soft tissue septa (7,97) (Fig. 24-48). The cystic spaces do not communicate with each other and do not enhance, but the septa are vascular and do enhance after intravenous administration of contrast medium. Curvilinear calcifications may be seen within the wall or the septa.

Cystic Disease
Renal cysts in children usually are bilateral and found in association with hereditary polycystic disease and tuberous sclerosis. Nonhereditary simple cortical cysts are distinctly uncommon in children. The clinical features of autosomal recessive polycystic disease are dependent on the age of presentation. Infants present with large kidneys, poor renal function, and minimal hepatic disease. In older children, portal hypertension and esophageal varices secondary to hepatic fibrosis predominate. CT or MRI is done to search for collateral vessels, abscess, or hemorrhage. The kidneys are enlarged with smooth margins. The cysts, which represent dilated tubules, usually are centrally located and exhibit near-water attenuation on CT (Fig. 24-49), low signal intensity on T1-weighted MR images, and high signal intensity on T2-weighted MR images (146). Some cysts are hyperdense on CT and hyperintense on T1-

weighted MR images, because the contents are mucoid or hemorrhagic. Dilated bile ducts resulting from hepatic fibrosis also can be seen on CT or MRI.

Autosomal dominant polycystic disease also has age-dependent clinical features. Affected neonates have palpable abdominal masses, whereas children and adolescents present with hypertension or hematuria. In the latter age groups, the kidneys may be of normal size or enlarged and have lobulated or smooth borders. The cysts are multiple, unequal in size, and cortical or medullary in location and have an attenuation value and signal intensity similar to those of cysts elsewhere in the body. Associated hepatic, splenic, and pancreatic cysts also can be identified by CT or MRI.

Fatty Renal Masses
Angiomyolipoma
Angiomyolipoma is a benign renal tumor composed of angiomatous, myomatous, and lipomatous tissue. It is rare as an isolated lesion in the general pediatric population, but is present in as many as 80% of children with tuberous sclerosis. The lesions usually are detected as an incidental finding, but some patients present with abdominal pain or anemia secondary to intratumoral or retroperitoneal hemorrhage, or with renal failure because of extensive parenchymal replacement by tumor. On CT, these tumors are small, multiple, bilateral, and of low attenuation, usually containing at least some areas of identifiable fat (Fig. 24-50). Occasionally, they coexist with cystic renal disease. Differentiation with CT usually is possible based on differences in the attenuation values of cystic and lipomatous tissue. On MRI, angiomyolipomas demonstrate high signal intensity on T1- and T2-weighted sequences and low signal intensity on fat-suppressed images.

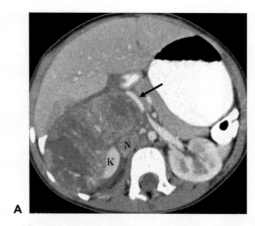
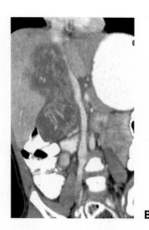

Figure 24-51 Neuroblastoma. **A:** Contrast-enhanced computed tomography (CT) in a 2-year-old girl shows a suprarenal low-density mass displacing the right kidney (K) inferiorly. The inferior vena cava (*arrow*) is compressed and displaced anteriorly. The tumor extends to the midline and abuts but does not displace the aorta. Also noted is a small retroperitoneal lymph node (N). **B:** Coronal multiplanar CT shows the craniocaudal extent of the tumor.

Adrenal Masses

Hemorrhage

Hemorrhage is the most common cause of an adrenal mass in the neonate, occurring as a result of birth trauma, septicemia, or hypoxia. Adrenal hemorrhage is less frequent in infants and children and is usually the result of trauma (184,254). The CT attenuation varies with the age of the hematoma. Acute hematoma has a high attenuation, whereas subacute and chronic hematomas are of low attenuation. The signal characteristics of the blood vary with the age of the hemorrhage. Acute blood has a low signal intensity on T1-weighted images and high signal intensity on T2-weighted images. Subacute hemorrhage has high signal intensity on T1- and T2-weighted sequences. As the blood clots and lyses, the intensity of the hemorrhage decreases over time. A chronic hematoma appears hypointense on T1-weighted images and hyperintense on T2-weighted images.

Neonatal neuroblastoma can be hemorrhagic and, thus, have an appearance similar to that of benign hemorrhage. Differentiating between these two conditions is possible when there are hepatic metastases or when serum vanillylmandelic acid (VMA) levels are elevated. Serial imaging also can help to differentiate between these lesions. A hematoma decreases in size over 1 to 2 weeks, whereas neuroblastoma either remains the same size or enlarges.

Neuroblastoma

Neuroblastoma is the most common malignant abdominal tumor in children, usually affecting children under the age of 4 years. More than half of all neuroblastomas originate in the abdomen, and two thirds of these arise in the adrenal gland (1,29,147). The extra-adrenal tumors originate in the sympathetic ganglion cells or para-aortic bodies and may be found anywhere from the cervical region to the pelvis. Neuroblastoma tends to metastasize early and more than half of all patients have bone marrow, skeletal, liver, or skin metastases when initially diagnosed. Lung metastases are rare.

On CT, neuroblastoma appears as a homogeneous or heterogeneous, pararenal or paraspinal, soft tissue mass with lobulated margins (1,147,227,284). The tumor enhances less than that of surrounding tissues after intravenous administration of contrast material (Fig. 24-51). Calcifications within the tumor, which may be coarse, mottled, solid, or ring-shaped, are observed in approximately 85% of neuroblastomas on CT.

On T1-weighted MR images, neuroblastoma appears either hypointense or isointense relative to the liver. On T2-weighted and gadolinium-enhanced sequences, it appears slightly to markedly hyperintense relative to liver (Fig. 24-52). The center of the tumor is often heterogeneous, reflecting the presence of hemorrhage, necrosis, or calcification. Hemorrhage may appear as a low or high signal intensity focus on T1-weighted pulse sequences, depending on the age of the blood; it usually has high signal intensity on T2-weighted images. Focal necrosis produces signal hypointensity on T1-weighted images and hyperintensity on T2-weighted sequences. Calcifications are hypointense on all sequences (1,24,147,238,239,284). Findings of local spread, such as prevertebral extension across the midline (Fig. 24-53), vascular encasement (Fig. 24-53), hepatic metastases, intraspinal extension (Fig. 24-54), and renal invasion or infarction, can be seen on both CT and MRI. CT and MRI can also show skeletal involvement (209,221,260). Knowledge of tumor extent is important for understanding the many appearances of neuroblastoma, for treatment planning, and for prognosis.

Following surgery or chemotherapy, CT or MRI may be used to monitor treatment response and detect recurrent disease. Serial CT examinations after therapy often suffice to determine the adequacy of treatment. In patients with residual masses, MRI and FDG-PET imaging may be able

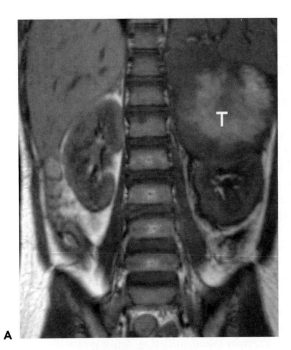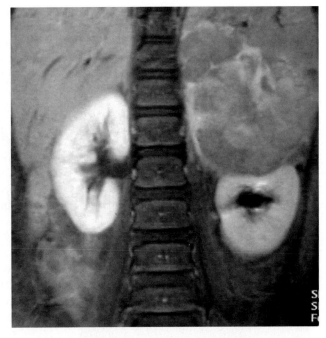

Figure 24-52 Neuroblastoma. **A:** T1-weighted coronal magnetic resonance (MR) image in a 3-year-old girl shows a large left suprarenal tumor (T). The area of relatively high signal intensity within the tumor represents hemorrhage. **B:** T1-weighted MR image after gadolinium chelate administration shows heterogeneous enhancement.

to separate fibrosis and tumor involvement. Demonstration of a residual mass with low signal intensity on both T1- and T2-weighted images favors the diagnosis of fibrosis, whereas high signal on the T2-weighted sequence suggests residual tumor.

Adrenocortical Neoplasms

Adrenal lesions, other than neuroblastomas, are rare in childhood, accounting for 5% or less of all adrenal tumors

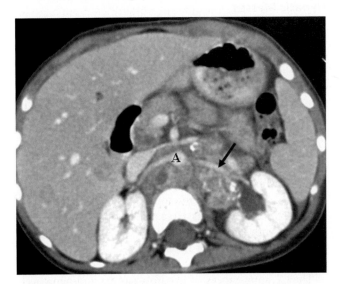

Figure 24-53 Neuroblastoma with midline extension. Contrast-enhanced computed tomography scan demonstrates extension of tumor, with calcifications anterior to the vertebral body and with encasement of the left renal artery (*arrow*) and aorta (A). There is mild left hydronephrosis.

(1,198). Of these, carcinoma is the most common, followed in frequency by adenoma. The mean ages at presentation of patients with carcinoma and adenoma are approximately 6 years and 3 years, respectively. Adrenal carcinomas are usually hormonally active, producing virilization, feminization, or Cushing syndrome. Adenomas can cause Cushing syndrome or primary aldosteronism, but they also may be detected incidentally.

Adrenal carcinomas are typically large masses at the time of presentation, often greater than 4 cm in diameter, with an attenuation value equal to that of soft tissue (Fig. 24-55). Many contain low-density areas from prior hemorrhage and necrosis; some contain calcifications. Cortisol-producing adenomas range between 2 and 5 cm in diameter, whereas aldosterone-secreting tumors are usually less than 2 cm in diameter. Both types of adenomas tend to be homogeneous and of low attenuation because of their high lipid content (227). Carcinomas exhibit a low signal intensity on T1-weighted MR images and high signal intensity on T2-weighted MR images. Adenomas may have a high signal intensity on both pulse sequences.

Pheochromocytoma

Pheochromocytomas are catecholamine-producing tumors that cause paroxysmal hypertension in children (1,284). Most pheochromocytomas in children are sporadic; however, they may be associated with multiple endocrine neoplastic (MEN) syndromes and the phakomatoses, including neurofibromatosis, tuberous sclerosis, von Hippel-Lindau disease, and Sturge-Weber disease. Approximately 75% of childhood pheochromocytomas arise

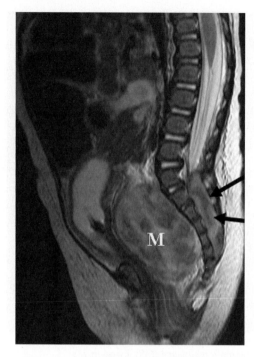

Figure 24-54   Neuroblastoma with intraspinal invasion. Sagittal turbo-spin-echo T2-weighted image shows a large intermediate signal intensity pelvic mass (M) invading the spinal canal (*arrows*).

in the adrenal medulla; the remainder are extra-adrenal, occurring in the sympathetic ganglia adjacent to the vena cava or aorta, near the organ of Zuckerkandl, or in the wall of the urinary bladder. Up to 70% of tumors are bilateral and about 5% to 10% are malignant. Most are at least 3 cm in diameter at the time of diagnosis. On CT, pheochromocytomas are of soft tissue density and frequently enhance

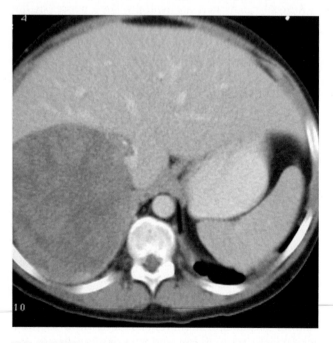

Figure 24-55   Adrenal carcinoma in a 9-year-old girl with virilization. A large soft tissue mass is present in the right adrenal gland.

after intravenous administration of contrast medium (Fig. 24-56A). On T1-weighted MR images, they have a signal intensity similar to that of muscle; on T2-weighted images, the signal intensity is equal to or greater than that of fat (Fig. 24-56B). Small pheochromocytomas often are homogeneous, whereas larger tumors appear heterogeneous with both cystic and solid components. Calcifications within the tumor are rare.

Retroperitoneal Soft Tissue Masses

Although rare, both benign and malignant primary tumors occur in the retroperitoneal soft tissues. Benign tumors include teratoma, lymphangioma, neurofibroma, and lipomatosis. Teratomas appear as well-defined, fluid-filled masses with a variable amount of fat or calcium (Fig. 24-57). Lymphangiomas are well-circumscribed, multiloculated fluid-filled masses. Neurofibromas are usually well-defined, cylindrical, soft tissue lesions with a characteristic location in the neurovascular bundle. Lipomatosis appears as a diffuse, infiltrative mass with an attenuation value or signal intensity equal to that of fat; it grows along fascial planes and may invade muscle.

Rhabdomyosarcoma is the most common malignant tumor of the retroperitoneum, followed by neurofibrosarcoma, fibrosarcoma, and extragonadal germ cell tumors. These tumors appear as bulky soft tissue masses with attenuation values slightly less than or equal to that of muscle. On T1-weighted MR images, they appear either hypo- or isointense to liver, kidney, and muscle. On T2-weighted images, rhabdomyosarcoma has a signal intensity equal to or greater than that of fat. Vessel displacement or encasement sometimes occurs and can be seen easily with GRE imaging (214).

Hepatic Masses
Primary Malignant Neoplasms

Primary hepatic tumor is the third most frequent solid abdominal mass in children, following Wilms tumor and neuroblastoma. Two thirds of hepatic tumors are malignant, with hepatoblastoma and hepatocellular carcinoma accounting for the majority (34,79). The former occurs in children under the age of 3 years, whereas the latter is more frequent in older children. The tumors are discovered as asymptomatic upper abdominal masses, occasionally associated with anorexia and weight loss.

At gross examination, hepatoblastoma contains small, primitive epithelial cells, resembling fetal liver. Hepatocellular carcinoma contains large, pleomorphic multinucleated cells with variable degrees of differentiation (34,79). Invasion of the portal or hepatic veins is frequent in both tumors.

The CT appearances of hepatoblastoma and hepatocellular carcinoma are similar. Both tumors usually are confined to a single lobe, with the right lobe affected twice as often as the left, but they may involve both lobes or they may be multicentric. They generally have a density equal

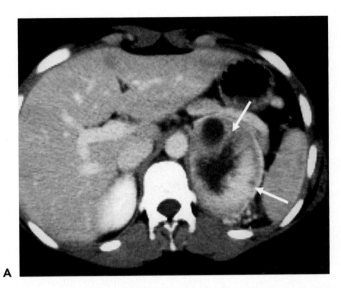
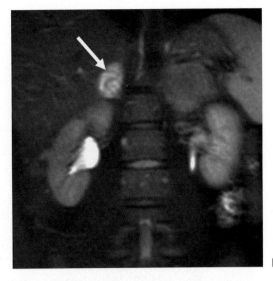

A

B

Figure 24-56 Adrenal pheochromocytomas. **A:** Contrast-enhanced computed tomography scan shows a left adrenal mass (*arrows*) with central necrosis. The soft tissue components show moderate enhancement. **B:** Fat-saturated T2-weighted magnetic resonance image in another patient shows high signal intensity mass (*arrow*) in the right adrenal gland.

to or lower than that of normal hepatic parenchyma on unenhanced scans (46,52,100,107,191,233). On arterial phase imaging, they enhance more than adjacent normal liver (Fig. 24-58). They become hypointense to liver on portal venous phase imaging. Both tumors often are heterogeneous because they contain hemorrhage, necrosis, or focal steatosis. Calcifications occur in approximately 50% of hepatoblastomas and in 25% of hepatocellular carcinomas. Tumor thrombus appears as a low-attenuation area within the portal or hepatic veins.

Malignant hepatic lesions are hypointense with respect to liver on T1-weighted MR images and hyperintense on T2-weighted sequences (52,191,192,223). On gadolinium-enhanced images, both hepatoblastoma and hepatocellular carcinoma demonstrate diffuse, heterogeneous enhancement (Fig. 24-59). Tumor thrombus is seen as a hyperintense focus within a normally signal-free vessel on spin-echo images or as a hypointense area on GRE imaging (Fig. 24-60). Hemorrhage can appear hypo- or hyperintense on T1-weighted pulse sequences, depending on the

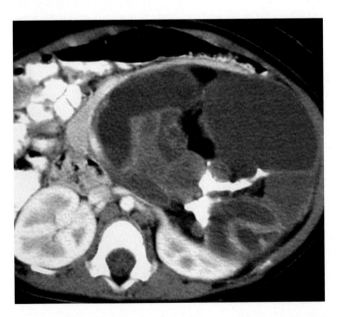

Figure 24-57 Retroperitoneal teratoma. Contrast-enhanced computed tomography scan demonstrates a large predominantly fluid-filled mass containing areas of fat and calcification.

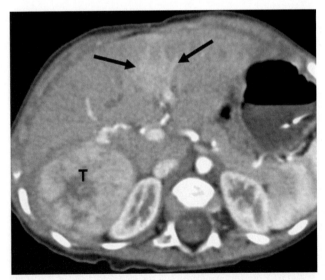

Figure 24-58 Hepatoblastoma in a 2-year-old girl with a right upper quadrant mass. Arterial phase computed tomography image obtained 12 seconds after the start of contrast administration shows a large, heterogeneously enhancing soft tissue tumor (T) occupying the posterior right lobe of the liver and a smaller homogeneous mass (*arrows*) in the medial segment of the left lobe.

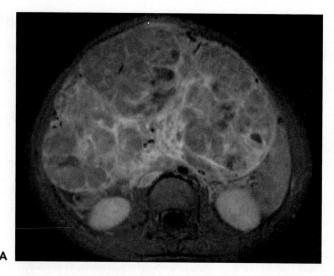

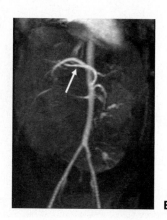

Figure 24-59 Hepatoblastoma, 7-year-old boy. **A:** Gadolinium-enhanced T1-weighted axial magnetic resonance (MR) image with fat saturation shows a large, heterogeneously enhancing tumor replacing most of the upper abdomen. **B:** MR angiogram shows a large hepatic artery (*arrow*) feeding the tumor. (Case courtesy of Fred Hoffer, MD, Memphis, TN.)

age of the blood; it usually is hyperintense on T2-weighted images. Focal steatosis produces signal hyperintensity on both T1- and T2-weighted pulse sequences and low signal intensity on fat-suppressed images. Calcifications are hypointense on all sequences.

Fibrolamellar hepatocellular carcinoma, which is a subtype of hepatocellular carcinoma, is a rare malignant tumor in children and adolescents. The prognosis for patients with unresectable tumor is better than that for patients with the usual variety of hepatocellular carcinoma (average survival, 32 and 6 months, respectively). On CT and MRI, fibrolamellar hepatocellular carcinoma is usu-

ally solitary and well delineated with variable contrast enhancement. Small central calcifications are seen in about 40% of tumors and a central scar in 30% (104,158,265). The imaging features of fibrolamellar carcinoma are similar to those of the other malignant hepatic tumors, and so biopsy is needed for definitive diagnosis.

Undifferentiated embryonal sarcoma, also known as mesenchymal sarcoma, embryonal sarcoma, and malignant mesenchymoma, is the third most common primary malignant tumor in children after hepatoblastoma and hepatocellular carcinoma. It primarily affects older children and adolescents. The usual presenting features are abdominal mass and pain. On CT, the tumor is a hypodense multilocular mass with multiple septations and a thick peripheral rim, which may enhance after injection of contrast medium (32,183) (Fig. 24-61). The MRI appearance is that

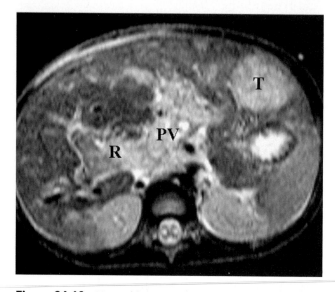

Figure 24-60 Hepatoblastoma in a 3-year-old boy. T2-weighted image shows a high signal intensity tumor (T) in the lateral segment of the left lobe of the liver and in the right (R) and main portal vein (PV).

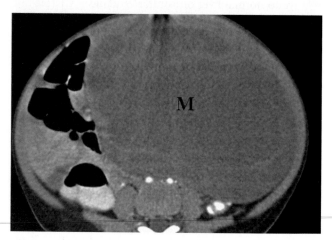

Figure 24-61 Undifferentiated embryonal sarcoma in a 9-year-old boy. Contrast-enhanced computed tomography shows a predominantly cystic mass (M) with several thin septations.

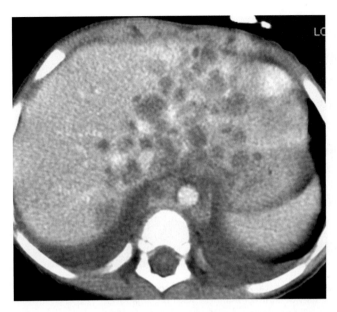

Figure 24-62 Hepatic metastases in a neonate with neuroblastoma. Contrast-enhanced computed tomography scan shows multiple low-density hepatic metastases and bilateral pleural effusions.

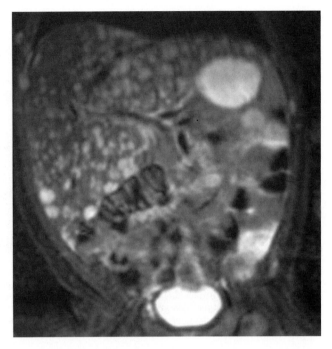

Figure 24-63 Multiple hemangioendotheliomas in a newborn girl. T2-weighted spin-echo image shows multiple lesions that are markedly hyperintense to normal liver parenchyma. (Courtesy of Sudha Appunirni, MD, Boston, MA.)

of a heterogeneous, septated mass with predominantly hypointense contents on T1-weighted images and hyperintense contents on T2-weighted images. The fibrous rim has low signal intensity on both imaging sequences. After gadolinium administration, the solid areas enhance, whereas the cystic spaces remain hypointense.

Hepatic Metastases

The malignant tumors of childhood that most frequently metastasize to the liver are Wilms tumor, neuroblastoma, and lymphoma. Clinically, patients with hepatic metastases present with hepatomegaly, jaundice, abdominal pain or mass, or abnormal hepatic function tests.

Hepatic metastases are typically multiple, hypodense relative to normal liver on contrast-enhanced CT (Fig. 24-62), hypointense on T1-weighted images, and hyperintense on T2-weighted images. Although the signal intensity is high on T2-weighted images, it is not as high as that seen with hemangiomas or cysts. Other findings include central necrosis and mass effect with displacement of vessels. Hepatic metastases in children may exhibit some degree of heterogeneous central enhancement on postcontrast images.

Benign Neoplasms

Benign tumors account for about one third of all hepatic tumors in children. The majority are of vascular origin and usually hemangioendotheliomas (34). Most patients with hemangioendotheliomas are under 6 months of age and present with hepatomegaly or congestive heart failure because of high-output overcirculation. Occasionally, affected patients present with bleeding diathesis secondary

to platelet sequestration (Kasabach-Merritt syndrome) or massive hemoperitoneum resulting from spontaneous tumor rupture. By comparison with adults, cavernous hemangioma is infrequently found in children, although it is sometimes encountered as an incidental finding.

On gross examination, hemangioendothelioma is a relatively bloodless tumor composed of multiple nodules ranging from 2 to 15 cm in diameter (34). Histologically, it is composed of vascular channels lined by plump endothelial cells that are supported by reticular fibers. The tumor is usually solitary and has a slight predilection for the posterior segment of the right lobe, but it may be multicentric and involve both lobes. Areas of fibrosis, calcification, hemorrhage, and cystic degeneration are frequent.

Hemangioendothelioma and cavernous hemangioma have similar appearances on CT and MRI. On non–contrast-enhanced CT, both lesions are hypoattenuating relative to the liver and both are hypointense on T1-weighted MR images (52,107,121,191,223,233). On T2-weighted images, the lesions are hyperintense (Fig. 24-63). A heterogeneous appearance may be noted because of areas of fibrosis, necrosis, or hemorrhage. Images after administration of iodinated contrast medium or gadolinium chelates demonstrate centripetal enhancement with variable degrees of delayed central enhancement (Fig. 24-64) (175,223,233). Small tumors may rapidly become hyperdense without showing peripheral enhancement. Larger lesions, particularly solitary lesions, may not completely enhance on delayed scans (51), reflecting areas of fibrosis or thrombosis.

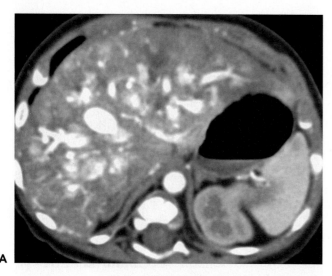
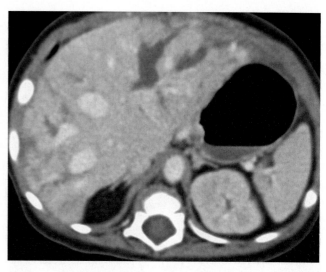

A   B

Figure 24-64   Diffuse hemangioendotheliomatosis in a neonate. **A:** Arterial phase computed tomography (CT) image obtained 12 seconds after the start of contrast administration demonstrates multiple high-attenuation lesions in the liver. **B:** Portal venous phase CT scan obtained 50 seconds after injection of contrast medium demonstrates nearly complete washout of the lesions.

After the vascular lesions, mesenchymal hamartoma is the next most common benign hepatic tumor of childhood. It is the benign counterpart to the undifferentiated embryonal sarcoma. This tumor usually is found as an asymptomatic mass in boys under 2 years of age. Rarely, the hamartoma has a large vascular component and produces arteriovenous shunting, leading to congestive heart failure. On CT, the lesion appears as a well-circumscribed multilocular mass containing multiple low-density areas separated by solid tissue (Fig. 24-65) (52,107,191,233).

After intravenous administration of contrast medium, the central contents do not enhance, but the thicker septa may increase in attenuation. T1-weighted MR images show a low-intensity mass; T2-weighted images demonstrate a hyperintense mass containing septations of low signal intensity (192,223). Differentiation between mesenchymal hamartoma and undifferentiated embryonal sarcoma by imaging findings is difficult. A younger age and absence of symptoms favors a benign hamartoma, but definitive diagnosis requires tissue sampling.

Biliary Masses

Choledochal cyst is the most common mass arising in the biliary ductal tree (212). Classically, patients present with jaundice, pain, and a palpable abdominal mass, although the complete triad is present in only about one third of patients. The diagnosis usually can be made by sonography. CT and MR cholangiography have proved to be useful, noninvasive alternatives to endoscopic retrograde pancreatography to delineate the anatomy of the biliary system when the results of other studies are indeterminate or additional information is needed for surgical planning (105,123,171) (Figs. 24-66 and 24-67). The intrahepatic dilatation is limited to the central portions of the left and right hepatic ducts. Generalized ductal dilatation, with gradual tapering to the periphery, characteristic of acquired obstruction, is absent.

Rhabdomyosarcoma of the biliary tract is rare, but it is the most common malignant neoplasm of the biliary tract in children. Most biliary tract rhabdomyosarcomas arise in the porta hepatis and involve the cystic duct. Imaging findings are intra- and extrahepatic ductal dilatation and a mass in the porta hepatis (200,211).

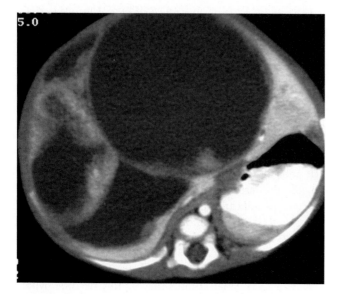

Figure 24-65   Mesenchymal hamartoma. Computed tomography image during the portal venous phase shows a well-circumscribed mass containing low-attenuation locules separated by soft tissue septations. (Courtesy of James Meyer, MD, Philadelphia, PA)

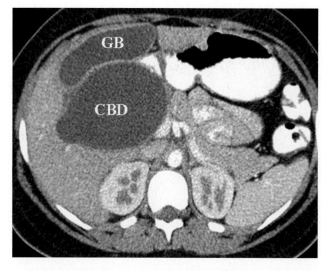

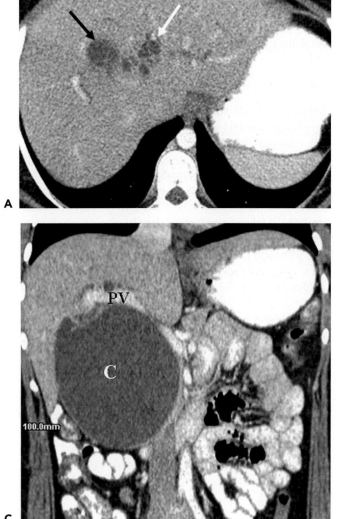

Figure 24-66 Choledochal cyst, 13-year-old girl with abdominal pain. **A:** Postcontrast computed tomography (CT) scan demonstrates mildly dilated right (*black arrow*) and left (*white arrow*) hepatic ducts. The peripheral branches are not dilated. **B:** CT image 4 cm caudal shows a dilated common bile duct (CBD), representing the choledochal cyst, separate from the gallbladder (GB). **C:** Coronal multiplanar reformatted image shows the relationship of the cyst (C) to the portal vein (PV).

Pancreatic Masses

Focal pancreatic lesions in children are usually exocrine neoplasms or cystic lesions. Pancreaticoblastoma is the most common exocrine pancreatic neoplasm in young children. It is an encapsulated, epithelial tumor composed of tissue resembling fetal pancreas, has a favorable prognosis, and usually arises in the pancreatic head. On contrast-enhanced CT, the tumor appears as a focal mass of homogeneous or heterogeneous soft tissue density (81,92,150) (Fig. 24-68). Secondary signs include hepatic and lymph node metastases and vascular encasement.

Solid and papillary epithelial neoplasm of the pancreas is the most common exocrine tumor in adolescents, usually affecting females more than males (31,92,278). The tumor has a low potential for malignancy, is well encapsulated, and usually occurs in the tail. On CT, this neoplasm appears as a large (mean 11.5 cm), well-defined, thick-walled cystic mass containing papillary projections and occasionally septa.

Cystic lesions are usually associated with inherited disorders including cystic fibrosis, von Hippel-Lindau disease, and autosomal dominant polycystic disease. The cysts in cystic fibrosis are believed to be the result of inspissated secretions leading to ductal dilatation.

Splenic Masses

Focal splenic lesions in children include abscesses, neoplasms (most commonly lymphoma and rarely hamartoma), vascular malformations (lymphangioma, hemangioma), and cysts (246). Abscesses, vascular malformations, and cysts have a low attenuation value on CT, a low signal intensity on T1-weighted MR images, and a signal intensity greater than that of fat on T2-weighted images (275,280). Solid tumors are of soft tissue density on

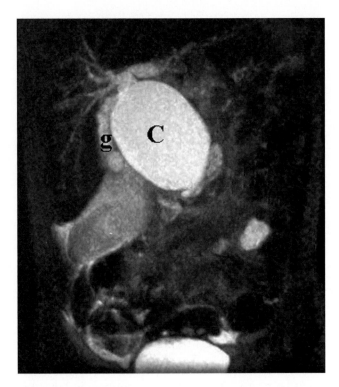

Figure 24-67 Choledochal cyst in a 2-year-old boy with jaundice. Coronal fat-suppressed turbo T2-weighted image demonstrates a high-signal intensity cyst (C) in the porta hepatis separate from the gallbladder (g). (Courtesy of Peter Strouse, MD, Ann Arbor, MI.)

CT and have intermediate signal intensity on T1-weighted images and high signal intensity on T2-weighted images (Fig. 24-69). On MRI, they show a signal intensity greater than that of muscle and less than that of fat on T1-weighted images, and a signal intensity nearly equal to that of fat on T2-weighted sequences. Vascular malformations enhance after intravenous contrast medium administration (62).

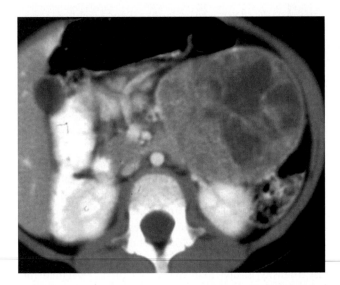

Figure 24-68 Pancreaticoblastoma in a 3-year-old girl with a left upper quadrant mass. A 7-cm, heterogeneous mass is present in the tail of the pancreas. Low-density areas represent necrosis.

In some children, the spleen is highly mobile because of the failure of fusion of the gastric mesentery with the dorsal peritoneum, and presents as a mass in the anterior abdomen. CT or MRI demonstrates absence of the spleen in the left upper quadrant and a lower abdominal or pelvic soft tissue mass. The mobile spleen enhances after administration of intravenous contrast medium unless it has undergone torsion with resultant vascular compromise (91).

Gastrointestinal and Mesenteric Masses

Lymphangiomatous malformations, also termed mesenteric cysts, and enteric duplications account for most benign gastrointestinal/mesenteric masses (208,246). On CT, a mesenteric cyst is a near-water density mass with a barely discernible wall (Fig. 24-70), whereas an enteric duplication appears as a cystic mass with a thick wall (155,208, 246,266). Both lesions have a signal intensity equal to or slightly less than that of muscle on T1-weighted MR images, although the signal intensity may be higher if the lesions contain blood or proteinaceous material. On T2-weighted images, the signal intensity is greater than that of fat.

Lymphoma is the most common malignant neoplasm of the bowel and mesentery. The CT features of bowel lymphoma include bowel wall–thickening greater than 1 cm in diameter, extraluminal soft tissue mass, and mesenteric invasion. The CT features of mesenteric involvement by lymphoma range from multiple small soft tissue masses to a large soft tissue mass displacing adjacent structures (Fig. 24-71). On MRI, lymphomatous masses have a signal intensity similar to that of muscle on T1-weighted images and similar to that of fat on T2-weighted sequences.

Lymphoma

Intra-abdominal lymphoma most often affects the retroperitoneal and mesenteric lymph nodes, bowel, and mesentery. Although CT and MRI occasionally demonstrate normal-size lymph nodes in the retroperitoneum and pelvis in the adult, these are rarely recognized in children. However, lymphoma and metastatic disease of any cause may produce sufficient lymph node enlargement to be demonstrable on CT and MRI. The CT appearance of such lymphadenopathy varies from individually enlarged lymph nodes of soft tissue density to a large mass obscuring normal structures (Fig. 24-71). On MRI, lymph nodes involved by lymphoma have a signal intensity greater than or equal to that of muscle on T1-weighted images and close to that of fat on T2-weighted sequences. As in the adult, these imaging studies cannot differentiate normal lymph nodes from nodes that are of normal size but replaced with tumor. In addition, it is impossible to distinguish between mild enlargement of lymph nodes resulting from inflammatory conditions, such as Crohn disease, giardiasis, tuberculosis, sarcoidosis, and acquired immune deficiency syndrome, and enlargement resulting from neoplastic involvement.

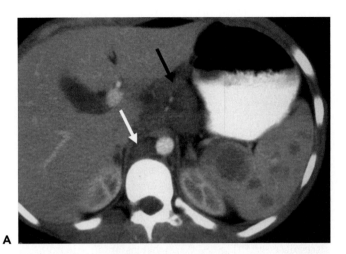
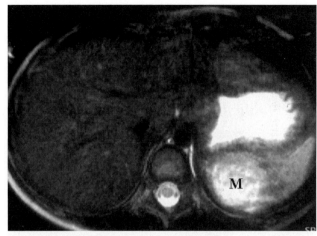

Figure 24-69 Splenic masses. **A:** Hodgkin lymphoma. Contrast-enhanced computed tomography shows multiple low-attenuation masses in the spleen. Also noted is mesenteric (*black arrow*) and retrocrural (*white arrow*) lymphadenopathy. **B:** Hamartoma. T2-weighted image shows high signal intensity mass (M) in the medial part of the spleen.

Rarely, rhabdomyosarcoma is a cause of intraperitoneal nodal masses. The CT and MR appearances are similar to those of lymphoma (39).

Abdominal Abscess

Most abdominal abscesses in children are caused by appendicitis, Crohn disease, and/or postoperative complications. The typical CT appearance of an abscess is that of a mass of relatively low density, with or without a rim that often is enhanced after intravenous administration of contrast material (Fig. 24-72). Gas is present in slightly more than one third of abscesses and may appear as multiple small bubbles or as a large collection with an air–fluid level. The size and shape are affected by location, because abscesses usu-ally are confined to fascial or intraperitoneal compartments, expanding the spaces and displacing contiguous structures. Abscesses commonly produce obliteration of adjacent fat planes and thickening of surrounding muscles, mesentery, or bowel wall.

Blunt Abdominal Trauma

Abdominal injuries in children are most often the result of blunt trauma caused by motor vehicle accidents and less frequently caused by bicycle, skateboard, and all-terrain vehicle accidents, falls, gunshot injuries, and child abuse (248,250). CT is employed as the initial imaging procedure for severely traumatized children whose vital signs are stable enough to permit the examination. CT provides

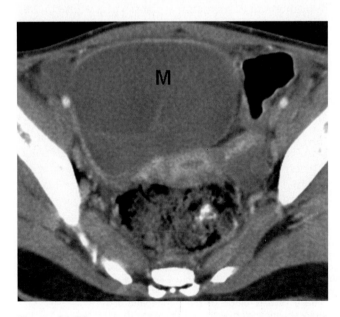

Figure 24-70 Mesenteric cyst, 15-year-old girl. A well-defined, low-density mass (M), containing several thin septations, is noted in the lower pelvis. The lesion involved the small bowel mesentery.

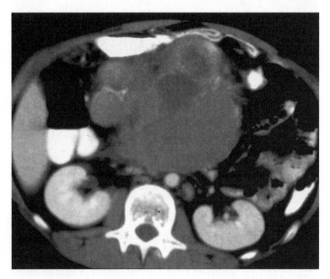

Figure 24-71 Mesenteric lymphoma, 12-year-old boy. A large conglomerate mesenteric mass of lymphomatous nodes, some with necrosis, extends from the anterior abdominal wall to the retroperitoneum.

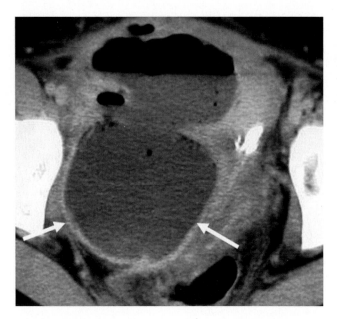

Figure 24-72 Appendiceal abscess. Contrast-enhanced computed tomography demonstrates a low-attenuation bilobed mass with small air bubbles and an air–fluid level in the lower pelvis. The mass is partially surrounded by an enhancing rim (*arrows*) and streaky soft tissue densities extending into the adjacent pelvic fat.

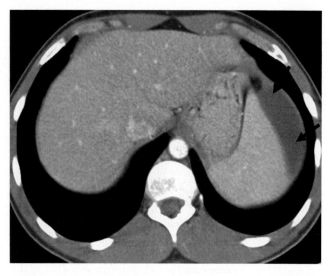

Figure 24-74 Subcapsular splenic hematoma. A low-attenuation lenticular-shaped subcapsular hematoma (*arrows*) flattens the lateral splenic contour. The patient had a small splenic laceration, seen on other levels.

a radiologic display of the entire abdomen following nonpenetrating injuries and can document injury to both solid and hollow organs, intraperitoneal or retroperitoneal hemorrhage, sites of active bleeding, and unsuspected thoracic or skeletal injuries (271,272). Unstable pediatric patients generally proceed directly to surgery without imaging examinations.

The CT appearance of intra-abdominal injuries depends on whether the injury is to a solid or hollow organ. The liver is the most commonly injured abdominal organ, followed by the spleen, kidney, adrenal gland, and pancreas. The spectrum of injuries in solid organs ranges from small intraparenchymal and subcapsular hematomas to large lacerations or fractures with capsular disruption (15,119, 231). Typically, intraparenchymal hematomas appear on CT as round or oval fluid collections. Fractures and lac-

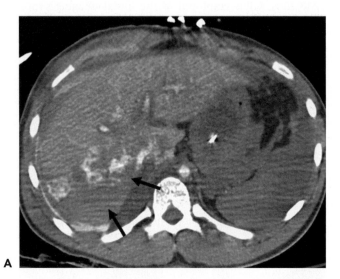

A

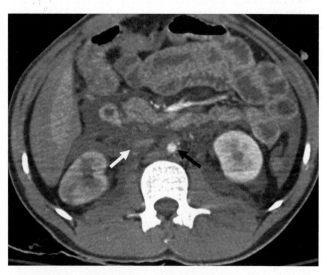

B

Figure 24-73 Liver fracture with hypovolemic shock. **A:** Computed tomography (CT) image through the upper abdomen shows a deep parenchymal laceration extending through the right hepatic lobe, resulting in an avulsed, nonperfused posterior segment (*arrows*). High-attenuation extravasated contrast material representing active hemorrhage is evident at the fracture site. The decreased splenic enhancement is related to the hypotension and should not be misinterpreted as representing splenic injury. **B:** A more caudal CT image reveals blood in the perihepatic and perisplenic spaces, dilated small bowel loops with intensely enhancing walls, a small aorta (*black arrow*) and inferior vena cava (*white arrow*), indicating hypovolemic shock.

erations appear as irregular, linear areas of low density within an organ (Fig. 24-73). Subcapsular hematomas are lenticular or oval in configuration and flatten or indent the underlying parenchyma (Fig. 24-74). Acute blood generally has a density lower than that of surrounding tissue on contrast-enhanced CT images. Other CT findings reported with hepatic injuries include subcapsular or intraparenchymal gas, resulting from acute tissue necrosis, and periportal areas of low attenuation. Periportal low-attenuation zones, presumably representing edema, have been noted in 65% of children with blunt abdominal trauma, and in 30% of patients they are the only CT abnormality (219).

Intra- or extraperitoneal fluid may be seen with fractures or lacerations extending to the surface of an organ (255). In fact, a localized fluid collection may be more readily appreciated than the underlying parenchymal injury, and thus may be a radiologic clue to the diagnosis (255). A large intraperitoneal fluid collection suggests a more severe injury. Fluid collections in the perirenal and pararenal spaces, interfascial spaces, and psoas space are indicative of injury to retroperitoneal organs (253).

In injuries to hollow organs, such as the intestine, CT findings include bowel wall or mucosal fold thickening, free intra- or retroperitoneal gas, peritoneal fluid, and small bowel obstruction resulting from an acute hematoma or a subsequent stricture (267). Lap-belt ecchymosis occurs in approximately 70% of children with bowel injuries and is a clinical clue to the diagnosis (257). Findings associated with rupture of the urinary bladder include thickening of the bladder wall and leakage of contrast-enhanced urine into the peritoneal or extraperitoneal spaces (252).

Hypoperfusion associated with hypovolemic shock has a characteristic CT appearance, evidenced by diffusely dilated, fluid-filled small bowel loops; intense contrast-enhancement of the kidneys, bowel wall, and mesentery; a flattened or collapsed IVC and a small aorta; and intraperitoneal fluid (256) (see Fig. 24-73). It is critical that the radiologist recognize the CT findings of hypoperfusion, as they are indicative of a severe injury and a poorer prognosis.

Diffuse Liver Diseases

Diagnoses of diffuse diseases of the liver can be made with either CT or MRI (179). Cirrhosis is the result of diffuse, irreversible hepatocyte damage and replacement by fibrosis, usually as a consequence of chronic hepatitis, bile stasis, metabolic disorders, congenital hepatic fibrosis, or toxins. Characteristic findings include a small right hepatic lobe and medial segment of the left lobe, enlargement of the caudate lobe and lateral segment of the left lobe, heterogeneous parenchyma, and nodular hepatic margins. The regenerating nodules of cirrhosis may be macronodular or micronodular. Regenerating nodules are often isodense to liver on CT and isointense on MRI. Some nodules may

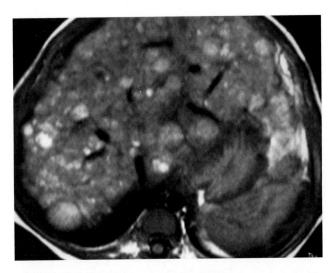

Figure 24-75 Cirrhosis in a 3-year-old girl with tyrosinemia. T1-weighted magnetic resonance image shows a heterogeneous liver with irregular margins and multiple high-signal-intensity lesions in both hepatic lobes, representing siderotic nodules.

show iron deposition. Siderotic nodules can show a high attenuation on CT, high signal intensity on T1-weighted MR images, and low signal intensity on T2-weighted images (Fig. 24-75). Extrahepatic findings, indicative of portal hypertension, include splenomegaly, ascites, and dilated collateral vessels in the porta hepatis and umbilical and splenic regions.

Attenuation values higher than normal can occur with hepatic iron overload, usually associated with repeated blood transfusions and occasionally with glycogen storage disease (72,176). As a result of the increased CT density, the hepatic vessels appear as low-density branching structures against the background of the hyperdense liver on unenhanced scans. Although CT can be used to evaluate iron overload, MRI is more sensitive for the diagnosis. On MRI, the paramagnetic effect of the ferric ions in the stored iron leads to a low signal intensity on both T1- and T2-weighted images.

Fatty change, often associated with fulminant liver diseases, severe malnutrition, cystic fibrosis, and chemotherapy, is clearly recognized on CT as diminished hepatic density (176) (Fig. 24-76A). The decrease in hepatic attenuation may be focal or diffuse and directly corresponds to the amount of fat deposited in the liver. With diffuse fatty change, the portal veins appear as high-density structures against the background of the lower density hepatic parenchyma. MR with in- and opposed-phase imaging can be used to corroborate CT findings (Fig. 24-76B).

Ultrasonography (US) is the procedure of choice to screen for diffuse infiltrative diseases of the liver. The role of CT and MRI is to clarify equivocal sonographic findings. CT and MRI also are recommended to provide additional information about vascular anatomy in patients who are scheduled to undergo liver transplantation. After liver

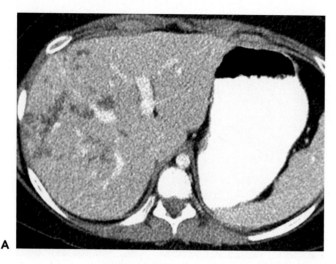
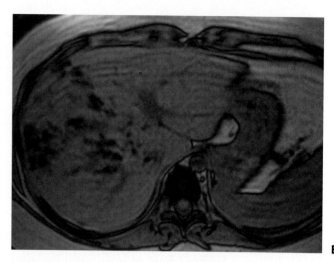

Figure 24-76 Focal fatty liver in an adolescent boy with Crohn disease. **A:** Computed tomography shows multiple low-attenuation areas in the liver. **B:** On the opposed-phase magnetic resonance image, these areas have low signal intensity, indicating the presence of fat.

transplantation, US, CT, or MRI can be used to evaluate biliary or vascular complications.

Biliary Tract Obstruction

Biliary tract obstruction in children usually is the result of ductal calculi or acute pancreatitis. A rare cause of ductal obstruction is rhabdomyosarcoma. The CT diagnosis is based on demonstration of dilated intra- or extrahepatic bile ducts of near-water attenuation. Associated findings include ductal calcifications, pancreatic enlargement, or a soft tissue mass in the porta hepatis (200,211).

In jaundiced patients, US is the preliminary imaging procedure to detect intrahepatic ductal dilatation associated with obstruction, as well as cystic diseases. Sonography can be supplemented with radionuclide studies using hepatobiliary imaging agents. Although the ability of CT to document the presence of dilated bile ducts is well known, CT should be reserved for cases in which the level or cause of obstruction cannot be determined by these other radiologic methods (80). MRI can also detect biliary dilatation, but it offers no additional information over that provided by US or CT.

Renal Parenchymal Disease

Most renal calcifications in children are associated with obstruction and infection, and less frequently are a result of metabolic disorders, cortical necrosis, glomerulonephritis, or adrenocorticotropic hormone (ACTH) therapy. CT may be of value in confirming lithiasis or nephrocalcinosis suspected on clinical evaluation or sonography (120).

Acute pyelonephritis can present as uniform enlargement of the kidney. Non–contrast-enhanced CT images usually are normal, whereas contrast-enhanced images may show single or multiple low-density areas, presumably related to inflammatory hypovascularity, vasoconstriction, or microabscesses (120,226,243) (Fig. 24-77). In

some cases, a striated pattern, characterized by bands of alternating increased and decreased density, can be observed. This is believed to represent capillary stasis or hyperdense urine within tubules plugged by inflammatory debris. Associated findings include caliceal distortion and perinephric inflammation, manifested by thickening of Gerota's fascia and strands of increased density in the perinephric fat. More severe infection can produce a renal abscess. The CT appearance of renal abscess is that of a spherical, low-density mass with thick, irregular walls. A CT diagnosis of chronic pyelonephritis is based on recognition of a small kidney with cortical scars overlying clubbed calyces. Unilateral renal hypoplasia or renal artery stenosis,

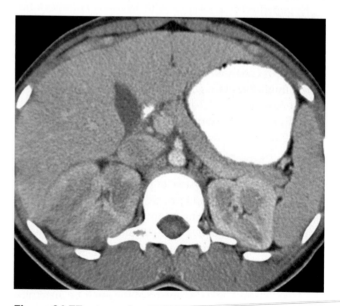

Figure 24-77 Acute bacterial pyelonephritis, 4-year-old girl. Contrast-enhanced computed tomography shows an enlarged right kidney with several poorly enhancing areas, representing more severe areas of bacterial nephritis. Urine cultures grew *Escherichia coli.*

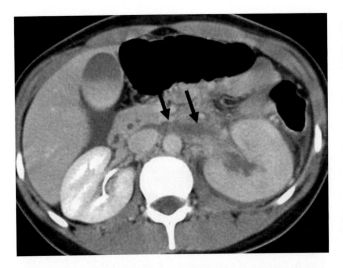

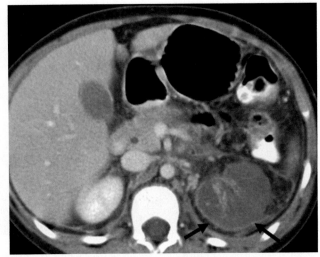

Figure 24-78 Renal vein thrombosis in a 4-year-old boy with left flank pain. Contrast-enhanced computed tomography during the excretory phase shows an enlarged left kidney with poor excretion. Thrombus is noted in the left renal vein (*arrows*).

Figure 24-79 Renal artery occlusion. Computed tomography shows an absent left nephrogram with an enhancing cortical rim (*arrows*).

in contradistinction, is associated with a small, smooth kidney. MRI does not offer additional information over that provided by CT.

A voiding cystourethrogram (VCUG) and a sonogram are the initial imaging examinations in a child with an initial urinary tract infection. The VCUG is used to investigate the possibility of reflux. CT may be a valuable ancillary examination in patients with acute pyelonephritis suspected of having perinephric extension or a complicating abscess, because it provides a better topographic display of the kidney and its adjacent structures than does sonography.

Renal Vascular Diseases

Sonography is considered the imaging test of choice for diagnosis of renovascular disease, but in equivocal cases CT or MRI can confirm the diagnosis. Renal vein thrombosis in children occurs as a result of trauma, neoplastic invasion of the renal vein, or dehydration. CT and MRI findings of acute thrombosis include unilateral renal enlargement, a prolonged corticomedullary phase of enhancement, diminished contrast excretion into the collecting system, thrombus in the renal vein or IVC, and thickening of Gerota's fascia (Fig. 24-78).

Acute renal infarction in children is most often a global event and a complication of traumatic or neoplastic occlusion of the renal artery. CT and MRI findings include a normal-size kidney and absent parenchymal enhancement. Peripheral rim enhancement may be seen as a result of perfusion by capsular vessels (185) (Fig. 24-79). The occlusion usually occurs within the proximal 2 cm of the renal artery. Segmental infarction is less common and may result from a vasculitis or embolus from an indwelling arterial line. Segmental infarction appears as a sharply demarcated, often wedge-shaped area that has a low density

on contrast-enhanced CT, low signal intensity on T1-weighted and gadolinium-enhanced images, and high signal intensity on T2-weighted images.

Pancreatic Disorders

Hereditary Diseases

Hereditary pancreatic diseases include cystic fibrosis (CF) and Shwachman-Diamond syndrome, which are autosomal recessive disorders, and von Hippel-Lindau disease and hereditary pancreatitis, which are autosomal dominant diseases (92,143). Involvement of the pancreas in CF takes the form of a fatty pancreas, parenchymal calcifications, or single or multiple large cysts, referred to as pancreatic cystosis (92,262) (Fig. 24-80). Shwachman-

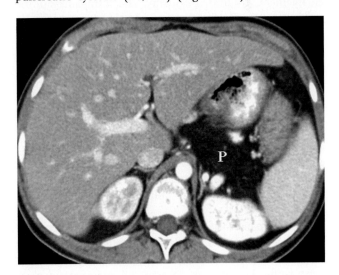

Figure 24-80 Cystic fibrosis, 15-year-old boy. The pancreas (P) is completely replaced by fatty tissue. The liver has diminished density, also secondary to fatty replacement.

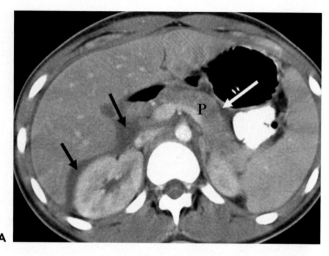
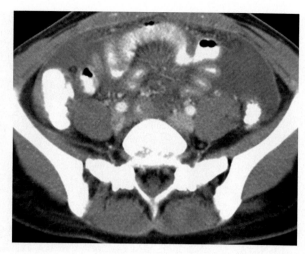

Figure 24-81 Acute pancreatitis in a 7-year-old boy. **A:** Computed tomography (CT) image at the level of the pancreatic body and tail shows fluid in the lesser sac (*white arrow*) and in the subhepatic space (*black arrows*). The pancreas (P) is minimally enlarged. **B:** CT image at a more caudal level demonstrates fluid in the paracolic gutters and edema in the small bowel mesentery.

Diamond syndrome (exocrine pancreatic insufficiency, neutropenia, metaphyseal dysostosis, and dwarfism) also is characterized by fatty replacement of the pancreas, causing a low attenuation value on CT and high signal intensity on MRI (92). In Von Hippel-Lindau disease, the pancreas contains multiple cysts. Findings in patients with hereditary pancreatitis include ductal dilatation, parenchymal and ductal calcifications, and pancreatic atrophy (92).

Pancreatitis

Acute pancreatitis in childhood is most often a result of blunt abdominal trauma, but other causes include operative trauma, chemotherapy, CF, mumps, and congenital anomalies, such as pancreas divisum and duplication cyst. The CT changes of pancreatitis include diffuse glandular enlargement, contour irregularity, and intrapancreatic or extrapancreatic fluid collections (126). Extrapancreatic fluid in children is seen most often in the anterior pararenal space, followed by the lesser sac, lesser omentum, and transverse mesocolon (126) (Fig. 24-81). The fluid collections in acute pancreatitis are of water density and variable in size and shape, distending an already existing space in the retroperitoneal or intraperitoneal compartment. They are not considered pseudocysts. Pseudocysts have a thick fibrous capsule, are usually found in close proximity to the pancreas, and contain homogeneous fluid of near-water attenuation value. They are more permanent in nature and unlikely to resolve spontaneously (218).

Chronic pancreatitis in childhood usually is a result of hereditary pancreatitis, and less frequently a result of malnutrition, hyperparathyroidism, CF, idiopathic fibrosing pancreatitis, or pancreas divisum. CT manifestations of chronic pancreatitis include calcifications, focal or diffuse pancreatic enlargement or atrophy, pancreatic or biliary ductal dilatation, increased density of the peripancreatic fat, and thickening of the peripancreatic fascia.

In patients with good clinical evidence supporting the diagnosis of uncomplicated acute pancreatitis, neither US or CT is necessary. Diagnostic evaluation is reserved for patients suspected of having complications. US is preferred as the screening examination because it does not require ionizing radiation. In cases in which US is suboptimal because of bowel gas, commonly present in patients with acute pancreatitis, CT may be used to provide the needed information. CT is considered the procedure of choice for displaying calcification in patients suspected of having hereditary pancreatitis. MRI does not contribute useful information in pancreatitis over that provided by CT.

Bowel Diseases

Several congenital and acquired anomalies can affect the bowel in childhood, but only the more common ones evaluated by CT or MRI are discussed here.

Congenital Anomalies

Anorectal malformations are characterized by varying degrees of atresia of the distal hindgut and the levator sling. Preoperative CT and MRI can provide information about the level of atresia and the thickness of the puborectalis muscle and external anal sphincter. Postoperatively, they can show the position of the neorectum in the levator ani sling (276) (Fig. 24-82). The neorectum needs to be positioned within both the puborectalis and external sphincter muscles if rectal continence is to be achieved. An additional congenital anomaly that can be diagnosed by CT or MRI is malrotation. CT and MRI findings include inversion of the superior mesenteric vessels, with the artery lying anterior or to the right of the vein; positioning of the jejunum on the right and the colon on the left; and a whirl-like appearance of the small bowel mesentery (Fig. 24-83) (288).

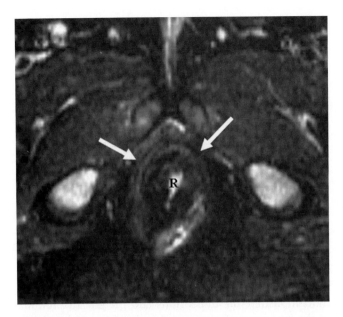

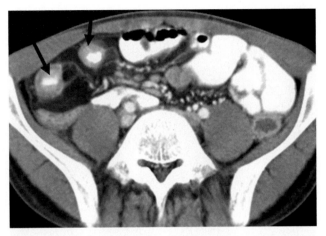

Figure 24-84 Crohn disease. A 14-year-old boy with a palpable right lower quadrant mass. Computed tomography shows circumferential thickening of the wall of the distal ileum (*arrows*) and an increased amount of mesenteric fat in the right lower quadrant.

Figure 24-82 Congenital anorectal anomaly. A 10-year-old boy with rectal incontinence after a pull-through operation for treatment of an imperforate anus. Transaxial T2-weighted magnetic resonance image shows the neorectum (R) lying within a hypoplastic puborectalis sling (*arrows*) located in the midline.

Inflammation

Crohn disease is the most frequent inflammatory condition affecting the small bowel in children. CT has been shown to be useful to diagnose extraluminal extension or abscess (106,229). CT findings in the early stage of Crohn disease include circumferential bowel wall thickening, inflammation of the adjacent mesenteric fat, and enlarged regional lymph nodes (106,229) (Fig. 24-84). Increased amounts of mesenteric fat, segmental narrowed areas of bowel, and fistulas, sinus tracts, or abscesses may be seen in advanced disease. Other inflammatory small bowel conditions that can be imaged by CT include Yersinia ileitis,

tuberculosis, and histoplasmosis. The CT appearances of these diseases are similar to those of Crohn disease.

Inflammatory diseases of the colon and appendix also can be easily diagnosed by CT. In patients with ulcerative colitis, there is concentric colonic wall thickening, which usually is heterogeneous. The CT findings in granulomatous colitis are similar to those seen in the small bowel, except that the colonic wall tends to be thicker (106,229).

Acute appendicitis is manifested as a dilated appendix, measuring between 8 and 12 mm in diameter, with a thick enhancing wall (Fig. 24-85) (68,115,178,258). By comparison, in children without appendicitis, appendiceal diameter ranges between 3 and 8 mm and the appendiceal wall is barely perceptible. Other findings of appendicitis include an appendicolith (see Fig. 24-85) and pericecal

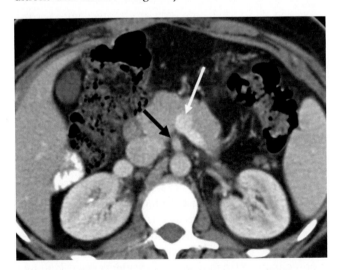

Figure 24-83 Malrotation. Contrast-enhanced computed tomography shows reversal of the normal orientation of the superior mesenteric vessels, with the artery (*black arrow*) lying to the right of the vein (*white arrow*).

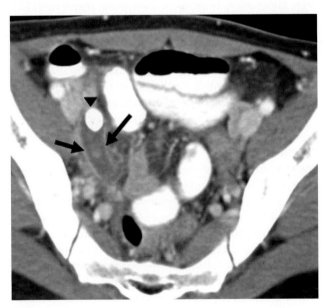

Figure 24-85 Acute appendicitis, 7-year-old girl. Computed tomography demonstrates a dilated, fluid-filled appendix (*arrows*) with an enhancing wall and an appendicolith (*arrowhead*).

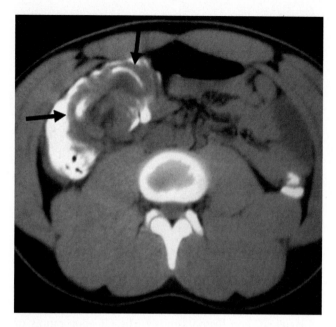

Figure 24-86 Intussusception. Computed tomography of a 9-year-old girl with abdominal pain. The bowel has a target-like appearance (*arrows*) with a central soft tissue density a surrounding layer of mesenteric fat, and an outer layer of contrast and soft tissue.

inflammation, appearing as streaky opacities in the adjacent fat. An abscess, as expected, appears as a walled-off fluid collection with an enhancing wall (see Fig. 24-72).

Noninflammatory bowel diseases, such as Henoch-Schönlein purpura and graft-versus-host disease (GVHD), are also easily recognized by CT. In patients with Henoch-Schönlein purpura, a nonthrombocytopenic vasculitis, there is small bowel wall thickening, which usually has a high attenuation because of intramural bleeding (112). The CT findings of GVHD, which is a complication of heterotopic bone marrow transplantation, are dilated fluid-filled loops of large and small bowel with thickened walls and enhancing mucosa (58,59). Extraintestinal findings include ring-like mucosal enhancement of the gallbladder and urinary bladder wall, inflammation of the mesenteric fat, increased mesenteric vascularity, and ascites.

Obstruction

The most frequent lesions producing obstruction are adhesions, hernias, and intussusception. In obstruction, bowel loops proximal to an obstructing lesion are dilated and filled with fluid or contrast, compared to loops distal to the site of obstruction. The CT diagnosis of hernia is based on the demonstration of bowel or a combination of bowel, mesenteric fat, and vessels within a hernia sac. The CT appearance of intussusception is that of a target sign, with a collapsed segment of proximal bowel (the intussusceptum) and its surrounding layer of fat-containing mesentery lying within a segment of distal bowel (the intussuscipiens) (45) (Fig. 24-86). Regardless of the cause,

the bowel loops distal to the site of obstruction are collapsed, whereas those more proximal are dilated and filled with fluid, gas, or contrast medium.

Vascular Lesions

Aneurysms are rare in children and occur most frequently in association with Marfan syndrome, collagen vascular diseases, sepsis, or trauma. Thrombosis also is uncommon and usually is the result of severe illness associated with intense dehydration, tumor extension, or trauma. In addition, various developmental anomalies of the venous system can occur, and their recognition is important lest they be misinterpreted as pathology. CT or MRI can be used to diagnose congenital anomalies or acquired lesions of the abdominal vascular structures (14,268).

US is the preferred examination for confirming a suspected aneurysm or venous thrombosis, because it can easily demonstrate the dimensions and the effective lumina of the aorta or vena cava and their branches in longitudinal and transverse sections. However, if the abdomen is obscured by bowel gas, CT or MRI can provide the necessary information.

PELVIS

The major indications for CT and MRI examination of the pediatric pelvis are the evaluation of a suspected or known pelvic mass and the determination of the presence or absence of a suspected abscess. In addition to facilitating evaluation of patients suspected of having masses or abscesses, CT and MRI can be useful in characterizing congenital uterine malformations, localizing nonpalpable testes, and evaluating the response of malignant tumors to therapy (23,236,244,264).

Pelvic Masses

Ovarian Masses

Nonneoplastic functional cysts, resulting from exaggerated development of follicular or corpus luteum cysts, are the most common ovarian masses in infant and adolescent girls. An ovarian cyst appears as a large (greater than 3 cm), unilocular, thin-walled mass that has near-water density contents. On MRI, the cyst has very low signal intensity on T1-weighted images and an extremely high signal intensity on T2-weighted images (23,236,244,264). Intracystic bleeding can increase the CT attenuation or the signal intensity on T1-weighted images. In some cases, layering of fluid and high signal intensity blood can be observed.

Mature teratomas or dermoid cysts are the most common pediatric ovarian neoplasms. Patients usually present between 6 and 11 years of age with a palpable mass or with pain resulting from torsion or hemorrhage. The CT diagnosis of teratoma is based on identification of a cystic

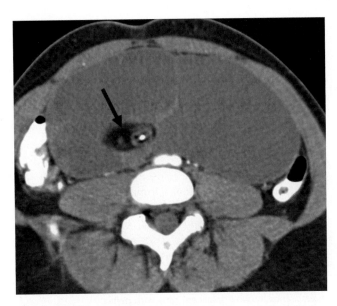

Figure 24-87 Benign ovarian teratoma, 13-year-old girl. Contrast-enhanced computed tomography shows a low-density teratoma, with an attenuation value close to that of water, lying anterior to the spine. The teratoma contains a mural nodule with calcification and fat (arrow).

mass containing fat or a combination of fatty tissue, calcification, ossification, or teeth (108,194,236,245) (Fig. 24-87). MRI findings vary depending on the tissue composition. On T1-weighted images, fat appears as an area of high signal intensity, whereas serous fluid and calcifications have low signal intensity. On T2-weighted images, fat and serous fluid show high signal intensity, whereas calcifications, bone, and hair demonstrate low signal intensity (287).

Malignant ovarian neoplasms are most commonly (60% to 90%) germ cell tumors (dysgerminoma, immature teratoma, endodermal sinus tumor, embryonal carcinoma, and choriocarcinoma) and less commonly stromal tumors (Sertoli-Leydig, granulosa theca) or epithelial carcinomas (33). On CT, malignant tumors are large (average diameter 15 cm), heterogeneous, soft tissue masses, containing low-attenuation areas of necrosis, calcifications, thick septations, or papillary projections (27,194,244) (Fig. 24-88). Cul-de-sac fluid, ascites, peritoneal implants, lymphadenopathy, and hepatic metastases also may be noted. On MRI, malignant ovarian neoplasms appear as heterogeneous masses with intermediate signal intensity on T1-weighted images and intermediate or high signal intensity on T2-weighted images (27,194,236).

Other causes of an adnexal mass include ovarian torsion and tubo-ovarian abscess. The features of ovarian torsion are an enlarged ovary of soft tissue density on CT (74,244). The ovary has a low signal intensity on T1-weighted MR images and very high signal intensity on T2-weighted MR images, reflecting vascular engorgement and edema (236). Abscesses have an appearance similar to that of abscesses in other parts of the body.

Vaginal/Uterine Masses

Hydrocolpos or hydrometrocolpos is the most common cause of vaginal or uterine enlargement. Hydrocolpos refers to dilatation of the vagina, usually by serous fluid or some-

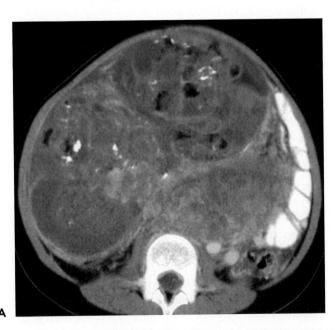

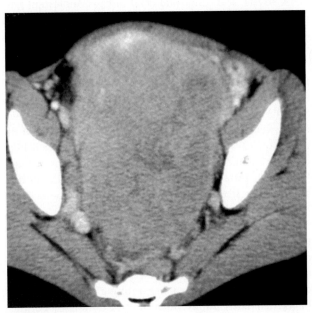

A   B

Figure 24-88 Malignant ovarian tumors. **A:** Malignant teratoma, 11-year-old girl. Computed tomography (CT) shows a large, predominantly soft tissue mass containing foci of calcification and fat that fills the lower abdomen. **B:** Dysgerminoma, 11-year-old girl. Contrast-enhanced CT shows a solid heterogeneously enhancing soft tissue tumor filling the pelvis and displacing bowel superiorly and to the left. The predominance of soft tissue elements in both tumors should suggest that these lesions are malignant rather than benign.

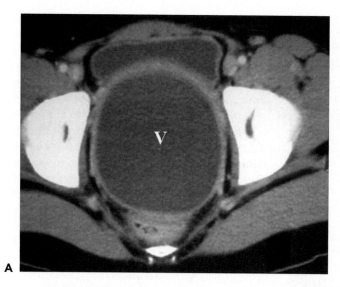
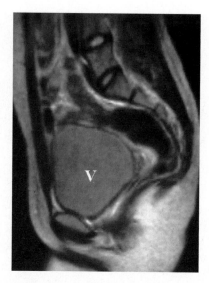

Figure 24-89 Hydrocolpos as a result of vaginal membranes in two adolescent girls with pelvic pain. **A:** Computed tomography scan shows a dilated, fluid-filled vagina (V). **B:** Sagittal T1-weighted magnetic resonance image shows an enlarged, intermediate signal intensity vagina (V). The fluid in both patients represented blood products.

times urine if there is a urogenital sinus; hydrometrocolpos refers to dilatation of both the uterus and the vagina. Both conditions are caused by vaginal obstruction, resulting from vaginal atresia or stenosis or an imperforate membrane. The clinical features vary with patient age. Affected neonates present with a pelvic or lower abdominal mass or associated anomalies, including imperforate anus, esophageal or duodenal atresia, and congenital heart disease. Adolescent girls present with a pelvic mass or pain. The dilated vagina in this age group often contains blood (i.e., hematocolpos) as a result of physiologic hormonal stimulation.

On CT, the dilated vagina and uterus appear as midline, near-water density masses. The walls may enhance after administration of intravenous contrast medium (Fig. 24-89A) (244,264). On MRI, they have low signal intensity on T1-weighted images (Fig. 24-89B) and high signal intensity on T2-weighted images. The signal intensity is high on T1-weighted images if the contents are hemorrhagic (236,245). Intra-abdominal extension and hydronephrosis resulting from ureteral compression can be seen in long-standing obstruction.

Rhabdomyosarcoma is the most common malignant uterine and vaginal tumor in childhood. On CT, rhabdomyosarcoma appears as a soft tissue mass with an attenuation value approximating that of muscle. Necrosis or calcification also can be present, along with variable enhancement after intravenous administration of contrast material. Metastases to pelvic lymph nodes can be seen if the involved nodes are enlarged. Rhabdomyosarcoma usually has low signal intensity on T1-weighted MR images and high signal intensity on T2-weighted MR images (8,64,220).

Bladder and Prostate Masses

Rhabdomyosarcoma accounts for most neoplasms of the bladder and prostate in children. It typically affects children under 10 years of age and usually metastasizes early, either by a lymphatic route to regional lymph nodes or by a hematogenous route to lung, bone, and liver. The CT and MRI features are similar to those of vaginal rhabdomyosarcoma (8,64,220) (Fig. 24-90).

Less common bladder neoplasms include hemangioma, neurofibroma, pheochromocytoma, leiomyoma, and transitional cell carcinoma. On CT and MRI, these appear as pedunculated or sessile soft tissue masses projecting into the bladder lumen. Based on CT or MRI findings alone, it is usually impossible to differentiate a benign lesion from a malignant one. However, when there is extension into the perivesical fat or adjacent structures, malignancy should be suspected.

Presacral Masses

Sacrococcygeal teratoma, neuroblastoma, anterior meningocele, and lymphoma are the most frequent presacral masses. Sacrococcygeal teratomas are congenital tumors containing derivatives of all three germinal layers. Most teratomas are benign in patients under 2 months of age, but in children beyond the neonatal period, they have a higher frequency of malignancy, nearing 90%. Affected children usually present with a large soft tissue mass in the sacrococcygeal or gluteal region and less often with constipation or pelvic pain. On CT, the diagnosis of sacrococcygeal teratoma can be confirmed by identification of a cystic mass containing fat, calcification, bone, or teeth. Usually there are no associated osseous anomalies

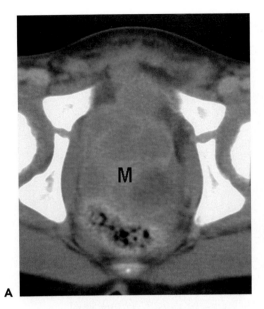 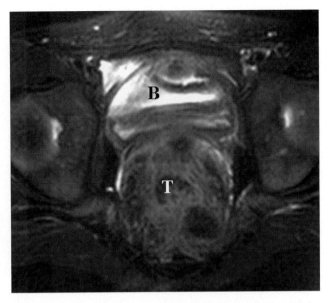

Figure 24-90 Prostatic rhabdomyosarcoma. **A:** Contrast-enhanced computed tomography at the level of the pubic symphysis in a 3-year-old boy with urinary retention shows a large, heterogeneous soft tissue mass (M) in the expected location of the prostate gland. **B:** Axial T2-weighted magnetic resonance image in a 2-year-old boy demonstrates a large heterogeneous soft tissue tumor (T) posterior to the bladder (B).

(122,220). In general, predominantly fluid-filled teratomas are benign (Fig. 24-91), whereas tumors containing predominantly solid components are more likely to be malignant (Fig. 24-92) (194). Fluid-filled, cystic sacrococcygeal teratomas have a low signal intensity on T1-weighted MR images and a high signal intensity on T2-weighted MR images. Fat appears as high signal intensity foci on T1-weighted images, and calcification, bone, or hair appears as foci of low signal intensity on both T1- and T2-weighted images (Fig. 24-93) (122,220).

Anterior meningoceles are herniations of spinal contents through a congenital defect in the vertebral body (an-

terior dysraphism) and are most common in the sacral region and at the lumbosacral junction. The mass is termed a myelomeningocele in cases in which the contents of the herniated sac contain neural elements in addition to meninges and cerebrospinal fluid, and is termed a lipomeningocele in cases in which fat and cerebrospinal fluid are present. Meningoceles or myelomeningoceles are recognized on CT by their relatively low attenuation values

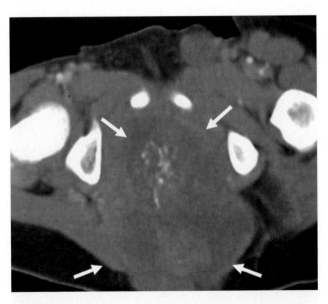

Figure 24-92 Malignant sacrococcygeal teratoma in an adolescent. Contrast-enhanced computed tomography scan shows a predominantly soft tissue mass (*arrows*) with a cluster of calcifications in the presacral area. The tumor extends into the right gluteal area.

Figure 24-91 Benign sacrococcygeal teratoma in a newborn with a palpable pelvic mass. Axial computed tomography shows a cystic mass (*arrows*) with several septations in the presacral area.

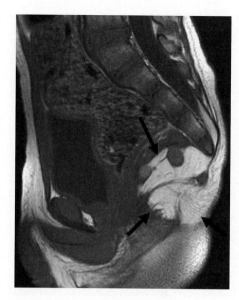

Figure 24-93   Benign sacrococcygeal teratoma in a newborn. Sagittal T1-weighted magnetic resonance image shows a presacral mass (*arrows*), with a predominant signal intensity equal to that of fat. The mass contains several lower signal intensity nodules, representing fluid components. The sacrum was normal.

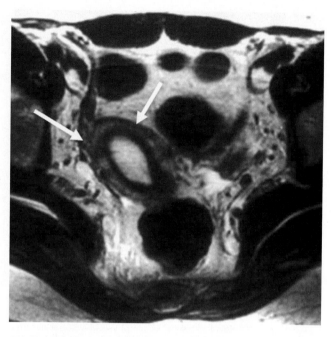

Figure 24-95   Unicornuate uterus with a noncommunicating rudimentary horn. Axial T1-weighted image shows a single fusiform uterine cavity (*arrows*), which is deviated to the right. The high signal intensity focus within the right endometrial cavity represents blood.

(cerebrospinal fluid or fat), their position anterior to the sacrum, and the associated sacral defects. The soft tissue contents of the herniated sac, especially the presence of a tethered cord, and the communication between the meningocele and the thecal sac can be demonstrated best with MRI. Neuroblastoma and lymphoma arise less frequently in the pelvis than in the abdomen or chest. On CT,

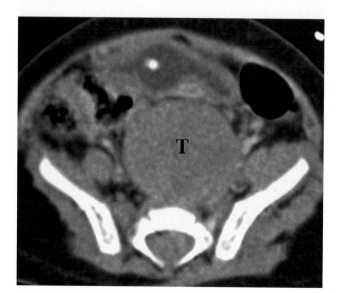

Figure 24-94   Presacral neuroblastoma in a 2-year-old. Contrast-enhanced computed tomography shows a soft tissue tumor (T) anterior to the sacrum.

both appear as presacral soft tissue masses. Neuroblastomas and lymphomas have a signal intensity slightly higher than that of striated muscle on T1-weighted MR images. On T2-weighted images, the signal intensity is close to that of urine or fat (Fig. 24-94).

Congenital Uterine Malformations

Congenital uterine malformations are easily recognized and characterized by MRI. CT also can detect and differentiate congenital anomalies, but it is not performed routinely because it uses ionizing radiation and has suboptimal soft tissue contrast compared with MRI (63,274).

Uterine Agenesis or Hypoplasia

Uterine malformations occur in 0.1% to 0.5% of all women. Uterine agenesis or hypoplasia is best displayed on T2-weighted sagittal images. In agenesis, there is no recognizable uterine tissue. In uterine hypoplasia, the uterus is small and exhibits poorly differentiated zonal anatomy and reduced endometrial and myometrial width (63,274).

Unicornuate Uterus

The classic appearance of a unicornuate uterus is the banana shaped uterus (single fusiform uterine cavity with lateral deviation). In some patients, a rudimentary contralateral horn, which may or may not communicate with the main uterine body, may be seen (Fig. 24-95). Renal anomalies occur in about 25% of cases (63,274).

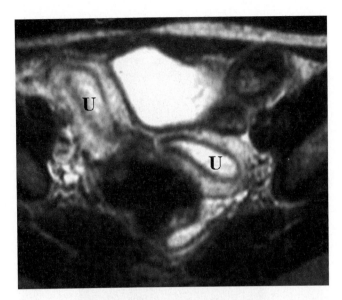

Figure 24-96 Uterus didelphys. Axial T2-weighted magnetic resonance image demonstrates duplicated uterine horns (U) with a widened intercornual distance. Two vaginas and cervices were seen on more caudal images. (Case courtesy of Shirley McCarthy, MD, New Haven, CT.)

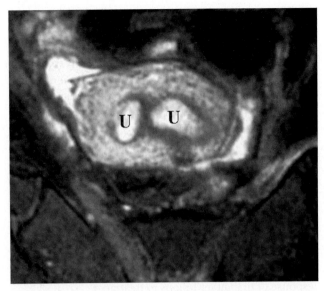

Figure 24-97 Uterus septate, 18-year-old girl. Angled coronal T2-weighted image shows two uterine horns (U) with normal zonal anatomy. A continuous band of myometrium surrounds the horns.

Uterine Duplication

The spectrum of duplication anomalies includes: uterus didelphys (two vaginas, two cervices, and two uterine corpora); uterus bicornuate, either bicollis uterus (single vagina, two cervices, and two uteri) or unicollis uterus (one vagina, one cervix, and two uteri); and uterus septus (single uterus, cervix, and vagina with a septum dividing the uterus into two compartments). MRI is particularly valuable in differentiating uterus didelphys from a bicornuate or septate uterus. Hydrocolpos or hydrometrocolpos associated with congenital vaginal obstruction also can be evaluated (63,274).

Uterus didelphys and uterus bicornuate have a bilobed shape with a concave fundal contour and myometrium separating the two endometrial cavities (Fig. 24-96). The appearance of septate uterus is that of a single uterine fundus with a convex, flat or minimally dimpled fundal contour and a central septum dividing the endometrium into two cavities (Fig. 24-97).

Impalpable Testes

Identification of an undescended testis or cryptorchidism is important because of the increased risk of infertility if the testis remains undescended and because of the increased incidence of malignancy, particularly with an intra-abdominal testis. Early surgery, either orchiopexy in younger patients or orchiectomy in patients past puberty, limit but do not eliminate these risks. Preoperative localization of a nonpalpable testis by CT or MRI is helpful in expediting surgical management and shortening the anesthesia time. The CT and MRI diagnosis of an undescended testis is based on detection of a soft-tissue mass, often oval in shape, in the expected course of testicular descent. The more normal the testis is in size and shape, the lower is its attenuation value or signal intensity on T1-weighted MR images. A very atrophic testis appears as a small focus of soft tissue with a density or signal intensity similar to that of abdominal wall musculature. The diagnosis of an undescended testis is easier if the testis is in the inguinal canal or lower pelvis, where structures usually are symmetrical. Differentiation of an undescended testis from adjacent structures, such as bowel loops, vessels, and lymph nodes, is more of a problem in the upper pelvis and lower abdomen.

US can detect an impalpable undescended testis when it is in a high scrotal or intracanalicular position, which occurs in about 90% of cases. Because it does not involve ionizing radiation, US is recommended as the initial imaging examination of choice for localizing impalpable testes. US, however, usually is not reliable for identifying undescended testes located higher in the pelvis or in the abdomen. Therefore, if sonographic findings are equivocal or negative and preoperative localization of the testis is desired, either CT or MRI can be performed, although MRI is preferred because it does not use ionizing radiation.

MUSCULOSKELETAL SYSTEM

Skeletal abnormalities are nearly always first identified by conventional radiography. Scintigraphy is helpful to confirm the presence of a skeletal lesion if the initial radiograph is nonconfirmatory and to determine the presence of metastatic disease. CT and MRI are used as complementary studies to conventional radiographs and scintigraphy when further definition of an abnormality is needed (173,241).

The frequent indications for CT of the skeleton in children include: (a) characterization of congenital abnormalities in areas of complex anatomy, (b) assessment of the extent of complex fractures and sequelae of skeletal trauma, and (c) determination of the origin and extent of nidus in osteoid osteoma.

Indications for MRI are more diverse than those for CT and include: (a) evaluation of the extent of skeletal and soft tissue neoplasms, (b) determination of the extent of infection, (c) evaluation of sequelae of skeletal trauma, (d) assessment of intra-articular derangement, (e) definition of anatomy in selected congenital anomalies, (f) assessment of possible bone infarction and osteonecrosis, (g) evaluation of unexplained pain in patients with normal conventional imaging studies, and (h) assessment of the response of malignant lesions to treatment.

Bone Marrow

The appearance of the normal bone marrow varies with the age of the patient (173,222,269,279,281). At birth, hematopoietic or red marrow predominates. Shortly thereafter, there is conversion of red to yellow marrow. In the shafts of the long bones, this conversion begins in the diaphysis and progresses proximally and distally to the physeal plate. By late adolescence, the appendicular skeleton contains predominantly yellow marrow. Epiphyseal conversion occurs within a few months of the appearance of the ossification center (111). Red marrow has low signal intensity on T1- weighted MR images and high signal intensity on T2-weighted images, whereas yellow marrow appears as high signal intensity on both T1- and T2- weighted sequences.

Infiltrative disorders, including tumor, infection, and edema alter marrow characteristics on MRI, producing low to intermediate signal intensity on T1-weighted images and high signal intensity on T2-weighted images (210,222, 232) (Fig. 24-98). Abnormalities are easier to identify in bones with predominantly yellow marrow. In bones with a predominance of red marrow, such as those in infants and young children and patients with red cell hyperplasia, differentiation between low signal tumor and red marrow can be difficult. In these individuals, the use of fat suppression techniques can enhance lesion conspicuity. Because the MRI appearance is not specific, a final diagnosis depends on correlation with the patient's history and other clinical information and possibly tissue sampling.

Osseous Neoplasms

Ninety percent of malignant skeletal tumors are osteosarcoma or Ewing sarcoma. Virtually all malignant bone tumors have a nonspecific MR appearance with lesions displaying a low signal intensity on T1-weighted MR images, high signal intensity greater than that of fat on T2-weighted

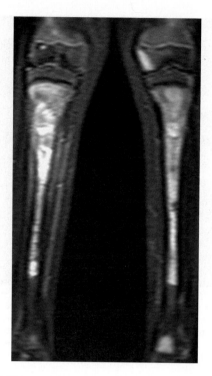

Figure 24-98 Metastatic neuroblastoma, 2-year-old boy. Coronal short tau inversion recovery image of the lower extremities shows diffusely high signal intensity marrow, indicating widespread metastases.

images (Fig. 24-99), and variable enhancement on gadolinium-enhanced T1-weighted images depending on the extent of necrosis (17,65,110,168,173). Low signal intensity on T2-weighted images suggests sclerosis, partially ossified matrix, tumor hypocellularity, or large amounts of collagen, whereas marked hyperintensity suggests highly cellular tumors with a high water content or hemorrhage. Fluid–fluid levels resulting from layering of new and old hemorrhage can be found in telangiectatic osteosarcomas, although they are not specific and also occur in aneurysmal bone cysts, fibrous dysplasia, and giant cell tumors.

Plain skeletal radiography remains the initial technique for the diagnosis of skeletal tumors. CT and MRI are helpful to further characterize a lesion if plain radiographs are equivocal and to determine the full extent of a lesion prior to treatment. The primary role of MRI in evaluating malignant tumors is establishing the extent of marrow involvement, soft tissue and intra-articular extension, and neurovascular encasement for staging. Neurovascular involvement is best assessed by sequences that are tailored to blood flow, such as GRE images. Slow or absent flow, encasement, and displacement are features suggesting tumor involvement of the neurovascular bundles. MRI and CT are comparable in detecting extensive cortical bone destruction, but CT is more sensitive for diagnosing subtle cortical erosion. MRI is also used to evaluate the response to chemotherapy and radiation treatment.

In the evaluation of benign osseous neoplasms of the skeleton, CT and MRI can be of value in determining the

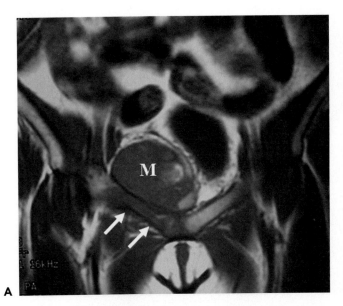

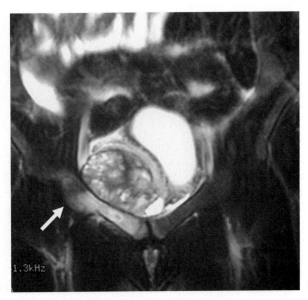

Figure 24-99   Ewing sarcoma, 16-year-old boy. **A:** Coronal T1-weighted magnetic resonance (MR) image shows low-intensity tumor in the right pubic ramus (*arrows*) with an associated soft tissue mass (M). **B:** Coronal fat-saturated T2-weighted MR image shows increased signal intensity in the intramedullary portion of the tumor and the extramedullary soft tissue component of the tumor. Tumor extension through the cortex inferiorly (*arrow*) is better seen on the T2-weighted image.

extent of a lesion or its spatial relationships for preoperative planning. Benign osseous lesions usually have well-defined margins on CT and MRI examinations (Fig. 24-100). The attenuation value and signal intensity of the matrix is generally nonspecific so that correlation with radiographs or tissue sampling is needed for a final diagnosis. Another indication for CT and MRI is determination of the precise location of the nidus in osteoid osteomas prior to surgical resection (9) (Fig. 24-101).

Soft Tissue Neoplasms

The common benign soft tissue masses in childhood are ganglion cyst, lipoma, neurofibroma, hematoma, abscess, and the vascular tumors (e.g., hemangioma, venous malformations, and cystic hygroma). The most frequent malignant mass is rhabdomyosarcoma. Sonography is the initial examination of choice for the study of most soft tissue masses to determine whether they are cystic or solid. MRI, however, has become the examination of choice for large lesions to define the extent of the mass and its local relationships (22,235). Small size, well-defined margins with a capsule,

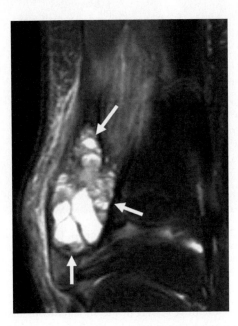

Figure 24-100   Aneurysmal bone cyst. T2-weighted coronal magnetic resonance image shows a sharply marginated lesion (*arrows*) containing multiple high signal intensity locular components expanding the distal right fibula.

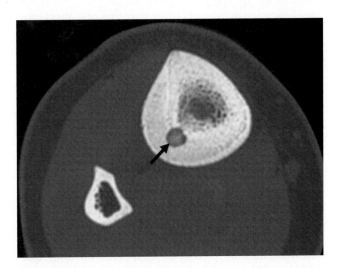

Figure 24-101   Osteoid osteoma in an 11-year-old boy. Axial image shows a lytic nidus (*arrow*) with faint calcification in the lateral cortex of the proximal right femur. The cortex around the nidus is thickened.

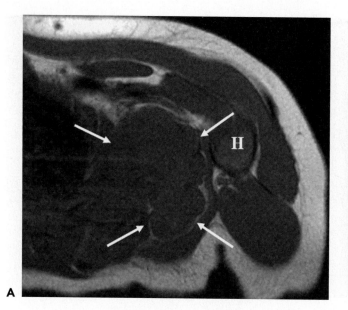
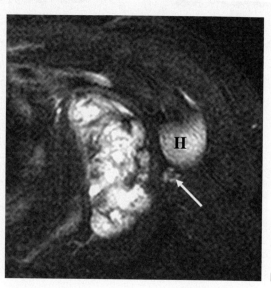

Figure 24-102 Rhabdomyosarcoma in a 2-year-old girl. **A:** T1-weighted magnetic resonance image shows an intermediate signal intensity mass (*arrows*) in the left axilla. **B:** On a fat-saturated T2-weighted image the mass has high signal intensity. The heterogeneity is typical of a malignant tumor. Also seen is an enlarged lymph node (*arrow*) adjacent to the humeral head (H).

homogenous matrix on T2-weighted MR images, and absence of edema suggest a benign lesion (22,154,177,235). Poorly defined margins and a heterogeneous matrix on T2-weighted images favor an aggressive process (Fig. 24-102). Bone erosion and infiltration of the neurovascular bundles are confirmatory evidence of malignancy. Unfortunately, some acute hematomas, abscesses, and benign neoplasms can have an aggressive appearance, whereas some malignant neoplasms can have a benign appearance.

Certain soft tissue lesions have specific MR characteristics (22,154,177,235). Lipomas appear as well-defined masses with a signal intensity equal to that of subcutaneous fat on T1- and T2-weighted images (134). Ganglion cysts have a signal intensity lower than that of skeletal muscle on T1-weighted images and greater than that of fat on T2-weighted and fat-suppressed images. Neurofibromas appear as well-circumscribed, round or ovoid masses with low to intermediate signal intensity on T1-weighted images and high signal intensity on T2-weighted and gadolinium-enhanced images. Most benign neural tumors exhibit a target sign, characterized by a low intensity center and a hyperintense rim on T2-weighted images and on contrast-enhanced T1-weighted images (19) (Fig. 24-103).

Hemangiomas are relatively common tumors of the appendicular skeleton (131,164). The blood-filled spaces of hemangiomas are isointense to muscle on T1-weighted images and hyperintense on T2-weighted images. They enhance diffusely after injection of gadolinium chelate. Focal heterogeneities are present in most cases, on both spin-echo and GRE images, related to hemosiderin deposits, fibrosis, fat, calcification, thrombosis, or stagnant blood (Fig. 24-104). Associated findings include the presence of

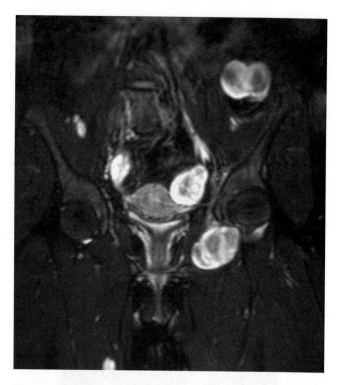

Figure 24-103 Plexiform neurofibromas. Coronal T2-weighted magnetic resonance image with fat saturation demonstrates the typical target appearance of benign neural tumors, with a central zone of low signal intensity and a peripheral zone of high signal intensity.

feeding or draining vessels in the subcutaneous tissues and muscle atrophy. Other vascular malformations include venous malformations (characterized by dilated venous spaces and a normal arterial component) (Fig. 24-105), arteriove-

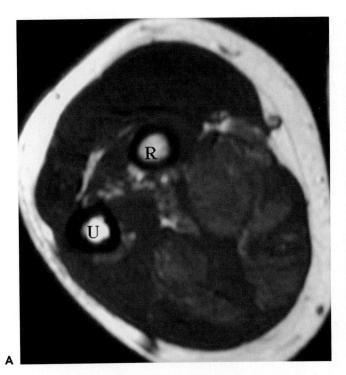

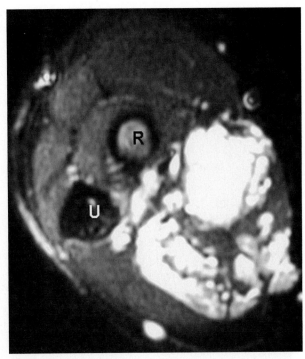

Figure 24-104 Hemangioma, right forearm. **A:** Axial T1-weighted image demonstrates a hetero-geneous mass of intermediate signal intensity replacing the posterior muscles. Low signal intensity foci represent fibrosis; foci of high signal intensity are related to fat. **B:** On axial T2-weighted image with fat saturation, the dilated vascular channels comprising the mass have high signal intensity. In-terspersed throughout the lesion is low signal intensity fibrous tissue. The involved muscle is atro-phied evidenced by the absence of mass effect given the large size of the hemangioma. Dilated ves-sels are also seen in the subcutaneous fat. U, ulna; R, radius.

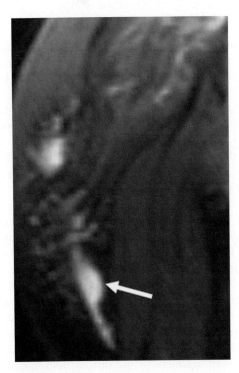

Figure 24-105 Venous malformation in a 5-month-old boy. Coronal three-dimensional gradient-echo image of the thigh after gadolinium chelate administration shows enlargement of the greater saphenous vein (*arrow*) and multiple small high signal intensity venous channels.

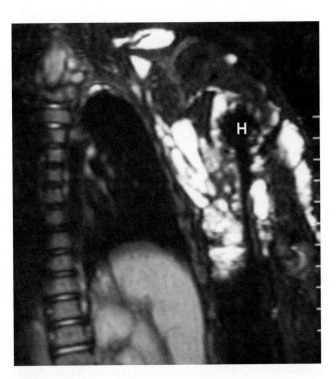

Figure 24-106 Cystic hygroma, 18-year-old girl. Axial T2-weighted image with fat saturation demonstrates multiple high signal intensity cysts of varying size in the subcutaneous tissues of the left upper extremity. H, humeral head.

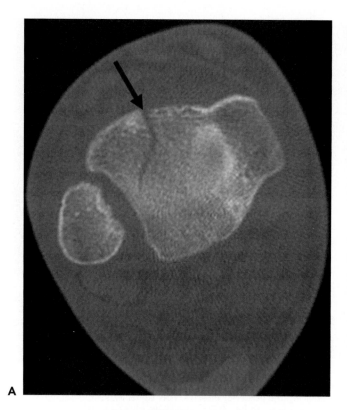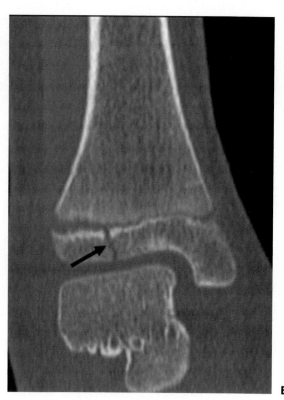

Figure 24-107 Epiphyseal fracture in an 11-year-old girl. **A:** Axial computed tomography image of the distal right tibial epiphysis shows a linear fracture (*arrow*). The relationship of the fracture line to the physis is difficult to appreciate on axial sections. **B:** Coronal multiplanar image shows extension of the fracture (*arrow*) to the physis and widening of the physis laterally.

nous malformations (characterized by enlarged feeding arteries and draining veins without an intervening capillary bed), and lymphatic malformations (characterized by fluid-filled spaces and fibrous septations) (Fig. 24-106).

Hematomas can be distinguished from hemangiomas on the basis of signal intensity characteristics (230). Very acute hematomas (1 to 24 hours of age) are generally hypo- or isointense to muscle on T1-weighted images and hyperintense to muscle on T2-weighted images. Acute hematomas (1 to 7 days of age) tend to be hypo- or isointense to muscle on T1-weighted images and hypointense on T2-weighted images. Subacute hematomas (one week to several months old) are hyperintense to fat on T1-weighted images. Chronic hematomas have MR characteristics similar to those of other fluid collections, which include a low signal intensity on T1-weighted images and a high signal intensity on T2-weighted and fat-suppressed images.

Infection

Cross-sectional imaging is useful in children in whom complications of osteomyelitis are suspected or drainage is considered. Both CT and MRI can be used to evaluate osteomyelitis, but MRI is especially well suited for the detection of marrow abnormality (e.g., Brodie abscess and sequestrum) and extension into the periosteum and soft tissues (85,133,156). Cortical destruction and sequestra are more reliably diagnosed with CT (153).

Bone and Joint Trauma

Traditional radiographs remain the initial examination of choice in the evaluation of acute trauma. When radiographs are not confirmatory, scintigraphy, CT, or MRI can be used to establish the presence and extent of a fracture (44) (Fig. 24-107), and in particular, growth plate injuries, which if unrecognized lead to growth disturbance. CT, with 2D or 3D imaging, is especially useful in the evaluation of the axial skeleton and pelvis, which are difficult to evaluate with plain radiographs because of superimposition of osseous parts (241).

After the injury has healed, CT or MR imaging can be used to define the size and location of a posttraumatic bony bridge and the severity of the associated growth deformity (61,144) (Fig. 24-108). CT is useful in the diagnosis of posttraumatic osteochondral loose bodies.

MRI is the examination of choice for detecting meniscal and ligamentous tears (109). Tears appear as alterations in morphology and signal intensity within the substance of the meniscus or ligament. MRI has also been shown to be an effective method for evaluating bone marrow edema associated with ligamentous and cartilaginous injuries.

Joint Disorders

The most common arthropathies in childhood are juvenile rheumatoid arthritis (JRA), hemophilia, and pigmented

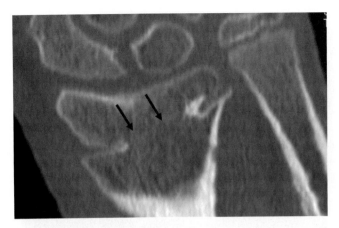

Figure 24-108 Posttraumatic epiphyseal closure, 14-year-old boy. Computed tomography image of the right wrist obtained 18 months after a Salter-Harris type IV fracture shows an osseous bridge crossing the central portion of the physeal plate (*arrows*).

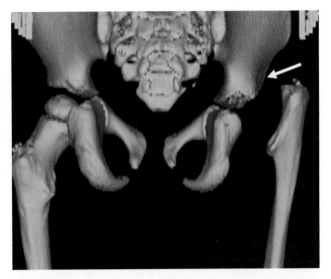

Figure 24-109 Developmental dysplasia of the hip. Computed tomography scan with three-dimensional reconstruction demonstrates lateral and superior dislocation of the proximal left femur. The femoral head is deformed, and there is a shallow pseudoacetabulum (*arrow*).

villonodular synovitis (PVNS). MRI is used to demonstrate the extent of cartilaginous and synovial involvement. MRI findings of early JRA and hemophilia include thickened synovium, which has a low signal on T1-weighted images and mixed intensity on T2-weighted images, reflecting the presence of inflammation and hemosiderin deposition. Late changes include cartilage loss and bone erosions. Gadolinium-enhanced MRI is superior to unenhanced MRI for showing cartilage loss, joint effusion, and synovial thickening. PVNS appears as an intra-articular mass containing areas of decreased signal intensity on all sequences, corresponding to hemosiderin deposition.

Congenital Anomalies

Developmental hip dysplasia and tarsal coalition are congenital anomalies that are well suited for CT. Plain radiographs can diagnose these conditions, but CT is useful to show the precise relationship between the bony acetabulum and the femoral head or neck (101). 3D reconstructions are particularly useful for assessing acetabular coverage and deformity of the femoral head (Fig. 24-109). In selected cases, MR imaging can be useful to provide information about coverage of the cartilaginous portion of the femoral head.

Tarsal coalition is a cause of rigid flatfoot and peroneal spasm in children. Nearly 70% of tarsal coalitions are talocalcaneal and 30% are calcaneonavicular. For talocalcaneal coalitions, scans should be obtained perpendicular to the foot, whereas for calcaneonavicular coalition, scans should parallel the long axis of the foot (60,182,282) (Fig. 24-110). Less frequent indications for CT include measurement of the amount of femoral anteversion or tibial torsion (241).

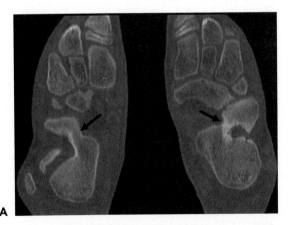

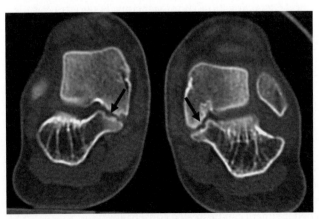

A   B

Figure 24-110 Tarsal coalition. **A:** Computed tomography (CT) in a 13-year-old boy through the long axis of the hind feet shows bilateral calcaneonavicular coalitions (*arrows*). **B:** Short-axis CT image in a 14-year-old boy shows narrowing and irregularity of the cortical surfaces of the talocalcaneal joints bilaterally (*arrows*), indicating fibrous coalition.

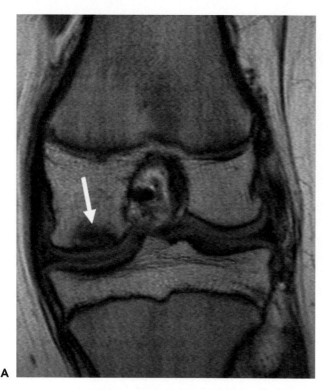
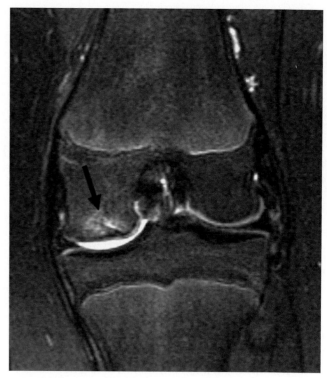

Figure 24-111 Osteochondritis desiccans. **A:** T1-weighted coronal magnetic resonance image shows a low signal intensity subarticular defect (*arrow*) in the medial femoral condyle of the left femur. **B:** Increased signal intensity is noted in the subchondral bone (*arrow*) on fat-saturated T2-weighted image. The absence of signal around the fragment implies lesion stability.

Bone Infarction

Bone infarction can involve the subarticular or the metadiaphyseal marrow of long bones. The more common causes in children include sickle cell disease, steroid therapy, and Legg-Calve-Perthes disease (109). MRI has become the primary imaging examination for diagnosis of infarction. Acute avascular necrosis of the femoral head usually exhibits a low signal intensity on T1-weighted images and high signal intensity on T2-weighted images. Varying patterns of devascularization (homogeneous, heterogeneous, and ring) have been described.

Osteochondritis dissecans is a subarticular osteonecrosis that often involves the femoral condyles, particularly the medial condyle. The necrotic fragment of bone may or may not have intact overlying cartilage. Fat-suppressed T2-weighted fast spin echo and STIR images are best for showing fluid within the subchondral fragment and adjacent medullary bone (Fig. 24-111). A high signal intensity interface on T2-weighted images between the bone fragment and native bone suggests a loose fragment. Knowledge of the stability of the osteochondral fragment is important because a loose fragment may need to be removed, whereas an attached fragment can be treated conservatively.

Acute medullary bone infarction is seen as a region of low signal intensity on T1-weighted images and high sig-

nal intensity on T2-weighted images. Chronic infarcts may appear as a central area of high signal intensity, representing fatty marrow, with a surrounding hypointense rim, corresponding to reactive bone (173,222).

REFERENCES

1. Abramson SJ. Adrenal neoplasms in children. *Radiol Clin North Am* 1997;35:1415–1453.
2. Albafouille V, Sayegh N, Coudenhove S, et al. CT scan patterns of pulmonary alveolar proteinosis in children. *Pediatr Radiol* 1999;29:147–152.
3. al-Nakshabandi N, Lingawi S, Muller NL. Congenital bronchial atresia. *Can Assoc Radiol J* 2000;51:47–48.
4. American Society of Anesthesiologists Task Force. Practice guidelines for sedation and analgesia by non-anesthesiologists: a report by the American Society of Anesthesiologists Task Force on sedation and analgesia by non-anesthesiologists. *Anesthesiology* 1996;84:459–471.
5. Anupindi S, Jaramillo D. Pediatric magnetic resonance imaging techniques. *Magn Reson Imaging Clin N Am* 2002;10:189–207.
6. Argons GA, Kingsman KD, Wagner BJ, et al. Rhabdoid tumor of the kidney in children: a comparison of 21 cases. *AJR Am J Roentgenol* 1997;168:447–451.
7. Argons GA, Wagner BJ, Davidson AJ, et al. Multilocular cystic renal tumor in children: radiologic-pathologic correlation. *Radiographics* 1995;15:654–669.
8. Argons GA, Wagner BJ, Lonergan GJ, et al. Genitourinary rhabdomyosarcoma in children: radiologic-pathologic correlation. *Radiographics* 1997;17:919–937.

9. Assoun J, Richardi G, Railhac JJ, et al. Osteoid osteoma: MR imaging versus CT. *Radiology* 1994;191:217–223.

10. Avila NA, Mueller BU, Carrasquillo JA, et al. Multilocular thymic cysts: imaging features in children with human immunodeficiency virus infection. *Radiology* 1996;201:130–134.

11. Aviram G, Fishman J, Young ML, et al. MR evaluation of arrhythmogenic right ventricular cardiomyopathy in pediatric patients. *AJR Am J Roentgenol* 2003;180:1135–1141.

12. Barnewolt CE, Chung T. Techniques, coils, pulse sequences, and contrast enhancement in pediatric musculoskeletal MR imaging. *Magn Reson Imaging Clin N Am* 1998;6:441–453.

13. Bass JE, Redqine MD, Kramer LA, et al. Spectrum of congenital anomalies of the inferior vena cava: cross-sectional imaging findings. *Radiographics* 2000;20:639–652.

14. Bass JE, Redwine MD, Kramer LA, et al. Spectrum of congenital anomalies of the inferior vena cava: cross-sectional imaging findings. *Radiographics* 2000;20:639–652.

15. Benya EC, Bulas DI, Eichelberger MR, et al. Splenic injury from blunt abdominal trauma in children: follow-up evaluation with CT. *Radiology* 1995;195:685–688.

16. Berdon WE. Rings, slings, and other things: vascular compression of the infant trachea updated from the mid-century to the millennium—the legacy of Robert E. Gross, MD, and Edward B. D. Neuhauser, MD. *Radiology* 2000;216:624–632.

17. Berger FH, Verstraete KL, Gooding CA, et al. MR imaging of musculoskeletal neoplasm. *Magn Reson Imaging Clin N Am* 2000;8:929–951.

18. Bhalla S, Siegel MJ. Multislice computed tomography in pediatrics. In: Silverman PM, ed. *Multislice computed tomography: a practical approach to clinical protocols.* Philadelphia: Lippincott Williams & Wilkins, 2002;231–282.

19. Bhargava R, Parham DM, Lasater OE, et al. MR imaging differentiation of benign and malignant peripheral nerve sheath tumors: use of the target sign. *Pediatr Radiol* 1997;27:124–129.

20. Bisset GS III. Hodgkin's disease. In: Siegel BA, Proto AV, eds. *Pediatric disease (fourth series) test and syllabus.* Reston, VA: American College of Radiology, 1995:130–164.

21. Bisset GS. Anomalies of the great vessels. In: Siegel BA, Proto AV, eds. *Pediatric disease (fourth series) test and syllabus.* Reston, VA: American College of Radiology, 1995:198–219.

22 Bisset GS. MR imaging of soft-tissue masses in children. *Magn Reson Imaging Clin N Am* 1996;4:697–719.

23 Boechat IN. MR imaging of the pediatric pelvis. *Magn Reson Imaging Clin N Am* 1996;4:679–697.

24. Borrello JA, Mirowitz SA, Siegel MJ. Neuroblastoma. In: Siegel BA, Proto AV, eds. *Pediatric disease (fourth series) test and syllabus.* Reston, VA: American College of Radiology, 1993:640–665.

25. Borthne A, Nordshus T, Reiseter T et al. MR urography: the future gold standard in paediatric urogenital imaging? *Pediatr Radiol* 1999;29:694–701.

26 Boxt LM. MR imaging of congenital heart disease. *Magn Reson Imaging Clin N Am* 1996;4:327–359.

27. Brammer HM, Buck JL, Hayes WS, et al. Malignant germ cell tumors of the ovary: radiologic-pathologic correlation. *Radiographics* 1990;10:715–724.

28. Brisse H, Pacquement H, Burdairon E, et al. Outcome of residual mediastinal masses of thoracic lymphomas in children: impact on management and radiological follow-up strategy. *Pediatr Radiol* 1998;28:444–450.

29. Brodeur GM, Maris JM. Neuroblastoma. In: Devita VT, Hellman S, Rosenberg SA, eds. *Cancer: principles and practice of oncology.* Philadelphia: Lippincott Williams & Wilkins, 2001:895–933.

30 Broecker B. Non-Wilms renal tumors in children. *Urol Clin North Am* 2000;27:463–469.

31. Buetow PC, Buck JL, Pantongrag-Brown L, et al. Solid and papillary epithelial neoplasm of the pancreas: imaging-pathologic correlation in 56 cases. *Radiology* 1996;199:707–711.

32. Buetow PC, Buck JL, Pantongrag-Brown L, et al. Undifferentiated (embryonal) sarcoma of the liver: pathologic basis of imaging findings in 28 cases. *Radiology* 1997;203:779–783.

33. Castleberry RP, Cushing B, Perlman E, et al. Germ cell tumors. In: Pizzo PA, Poplack DG, et al., eds. *Principles and practice of pediatric oncology.* Philadelphia: Lippincott–Raven Publishers, 1997:921–945.

34. Chandra RS, Stocker JT, Dehner LP. Liver, gallbladder, and biliary tract. In: Stocker JT, Dehner LP, eds. *Pediatric pathology.* Philadelphia: J.B. Lippincott Co., 1992:703–789.

35. Chang AB, Masel JP, Masters B. Post-infectious bronchiolitis obliterans: clinical, radiological and pulmonary function sequelae. *Pediatr Radiol* 1998;28:23–29.

36. Chepuri NB, Strouse PJ, Yanik GA. CT of renal lymphoma in children. *AJR Am J Roentgenol* 2003;180:419–431.

37. Choe YH, Kim YM, Han BK, et al. MR imaging in the morphologic diagnosis of congenital heart disease. *Radiographics* 1997;17:403–422.

38. Choi BW, Park YH, Choi JY, et al. Using electron beam CT to evaluate conotruncal anomalies in pediatric and adult patients. *AJR Am J Roentgenol* 2001;177:1045–1049.

39. Chung CJ, Fordham L, Little S, et al. Intraperitoneal rhabdomyosarcoma in children: incidence and imaging characteristics on CT. *AJR Am J Roentgenol* 1998;170:1385–1387.

40. Chung CJ, Lorenzo R, Rayder S, et al. Rhabdoid tumors of the kidney in children: CT findings. *AJR Am J Roentgenol* 1995;164:697–700.

41. Cinar A, Haliloglu M, Kragoz T, et al. Interrupted aortic arch in a neonate: multidetector CT diagnosis. *Pediatr Radiol* 2004;34:901–903.

42. Cleveland RH. Congenital lobar emphysema. In: Siegel BA, Proto AV, eds. *Pediatric disease (fourth series) test and syllabus.* Reston, VA: American College of Radiology, 1993:96–129.

43. Committee on Drugs, American Academy of Pediatrics. Guidelines for monitoring and management of pediatric patients during and after sedation for diagnostic and therapeutic procedures. *Pediatrics* 1992;89:1110–1115.

44. Connolly SA, Connolly LP, Jaramillo D. Imaging of sports injuries in children and adolescents. *Radiol Clin North Am* 2001;39:773–790.

45. Cox TD, Winters WD, Weinberger E. CT of intussusception in the pediatric patient: diagnosis and pitfalls. *Pediatr Radiol* 1996;26:26–32.

46. Davey MS, Cohen MD. Imaging of gastrointestinal malignancy in childhood. *Radiol Clin North Am* 1996;34:717–742.

47. Davidson AJ, Choyke PL, Hartman DS, et al. Renal medullary carcinoma associated with sickle cell trait: radiologic findings. *Radiology* 1995;195:83–85.

48. Demos TC, Posniak HV, Harmath C, et al. Cystic lesions of the pancreas. *AJR Am J Roentgenol* 2002;179:1375–1388.

49. Demos TC, Posniak HV, Pierce KL, et al. Venous anomalies of the thorax. *AJR Am J Roentgenol* 2004;182:1139–1150.

50. Dillon EH, Camputaro C. Partial anomalous pulmonary venous drainage of the left upper lobe vs duplication of the superior vena cava: distinction based on CT findings. *AJR Am J Roentgenol* 1993;160:375–379.

51. Donaldson JS. Hemangioendothelioma of the liver. In: Siegel BA, Proto AV, eds. *Pediatric disease (fourth series) test and syllabus.* Reston, VA: American College of Radiology, 1993:436–462.

52. Donnelly LF, Bisset GS III. Pediatric hepatic imaging. *Radiol Clin North Am* 1998;36:413–427.

53. Donnelly LF, Emery KH, Brody AS, et al. Minimizing radiation dose for pediatric body applications for single-detector helical CT: strategies at a large children's hospital. *AJR Am J Roentgenol* 2001;176:303–306.

54. Donnelly LF, Fleck RJ, Pacharn P, et al. Aberrant subclavian arteries: cross-sectional imaging findings in infants and children referred for evaluation of extrinsic airway compression. *AJR Am J Roentgenol* 2002;178:1269–1274.

55. Donnelly LF, Higgins CB. MR imaging of conotruncal abnormalities. *AJR Am J Roentgenol* 1996;166:925–928.

56. Donnelly LF, Klosterman LA. Pneumonia in children: decreased parenchymal contrast enhancement-CT sign of intense illness and impending cavitary necrosis. *Radiology* 1997;205:817–820.

57. Donnelly LF, Klosterman LA. The yield of CT of children who have complicated pneumonia and noncontributory chest radiography. *AJR Am J Roentgenol* 1998;170:1627–1631.

58. Donnelly LF, Morris CL. Acute graft-versus-host disease in children: abdominal CT findings. *Radiology* 1996;199:265–268.

59. Donnelly LF. Graft-versus-host disease. In: Siegel BA, Siegel MJ, eds. *Pediatric disease (fifth series) test and syllabus*. Reston, VA: American College of Radiology, 2002:87–97.

60. Donnelly LF. Tarsal coalition. In: Siegel BA, Siegel MJ, eds. *Pediatric disease (fifth series) test and syllabus*. Reston, VA: American College of Radiology, 2002;181–191.

61. Ecklund K, Jaramillo D. Imaging of growth disturbance in children. *Radiol Clin North Am* 2001;39:823–841.

62. Ferrozzi F, Bova D, Draghi F, et al. CT Findings in primary vascular tumors of the spleen. *AJR Am J Roentgenol* 1996; 166:1097–1101.

63. Fielding JR. MR imaging of müllerian anomalies: impact on therapy. *AJR Am J Roentgenol* 1996;167:1491–1495.

64. Fletcher BD, Kaste SC. Magnetic resonance imaging for diagnosis and follow-up of genitourinary, pelvic, and perineal rhabdomyosarcoma. *Urol Radiol* 1992;14:262–272.

65. Fletcher BD. Imaging pediatric bone sarcomas. *Radiol Clin North Am* 1997;35:1477–1494.

66. Franco J, Aliaga R, Domingo ML, et al. Diagnosis of pulmonary sequestration by spiral CT angiography. *Thorax* 1998;53: 1089–1092.

67. Frazier AA, Rosado de Christenson ML, Stocker JT et al. Intralobar sequestration: radiologic-pathologic correlation. *Radiographics* 1997;17:725–745.

68. Friedland J, Siegel MJ. CT appearance of acute appendicitis in childhood. *AJR Am J Roentgenol* 1997;168:439–442.

69. Front D, Ben-Haim S, Israel O, et al. Lymphoma: predictive value of Ga-67 scintigraphy after treatment. *Radiology* 1992; 182:359–363.

70. Frush DP, Bisset GS 3rd, Hall SC. Pediatric sedation in radiology: the practice of safe sleep. *AJR Am J Roentgenol* 1997;167: 1381–1387.

71. Geller E, Smergel E, Lowry P. Renal neoplasms of childhood. *Radiol Clin North Am* 1997;35:1391–1413.

72. Gerety BM. Hemochromatosis. In: Freeny PC, Stevenson GW, eds. *Alimentary tract radiology*. St. Louis: Mosby, 1994:1560–1665.

73. Ghaye B, Szapiro D, Fanchamps J-M, et al. Congenital bronchial abnormalities revisited. *Radiographics* 2001;21:105–119.

74. Ghossain MA, Buy NJ, Bazot M et al. CT in adnexal torsion with emphasis on tubal findings: correlation with US. *J Comput Assist Tomogr* 1994;18:619–625.

75. Gilkeson RC, Ciancibello L, Zahka K. Multidetector CT evaluation of congenital heart disease in pediatric and adult patients. *AJR Am J Roentgenol* 2003;180:973–980.

76. Gilkeson RC, Ciancibello LM, Hejal RB, et al. Tracheobronchomalacia dynamic airway evaluation with multidetector CT. *AJR Am J Roentgenol* 2001;176:205–210.

77. Goo HW, Park IS, Ko JK, et al. CT of congenital heart disease: normal anatomy and typical pathologic conditions. *Radiographics* 2003;23:S147–S165.

78. Green DM, Coppes MJ, Breslow NE, et al. Wilms tumor. In: Pizzo PA, Poplack DG, eds. *Principles and practice of pediatric oncology*. Philadelphia: Lippincott–Raven Publishers, 1997: 733–759.

79. Greenberg M, Filler RM. Hepatic tumors. In: Pizzo PA, Poplack DC, eds. *Principles and practice of pediatric oncology*. Philadelphia: Lippincott–Raven Publishers, 1997:717–732.

80. Gubernick JA, Rosenberg HK, Ilaslan H, et al. US approach to jaundice in infants and children. *Radiographics* 2000; 20:173–195.

81. Gupta AK, Mitra DK, Berry M, et al. Sonography and CT of pancreatoblastoma in children. *AJR Am J Roentgenol* 2000;174: 1639–1641.

82. Gupta H, Mayo-Smith WW, Mainiero MB, et al. Helical CT of pulmonary vascular abnormalities. *AJR Am J Roentgenol* 2002; 178:487–492.

83. Gutierrez FR, Siegel MJ, Fallah JH, et al. Magnetic resonance imaging of cyanotic and noncyanotic congenital heart disease. *Magn Reson Imaging Clin N Am* 2002;10:209–235.

84. Gylys-Morin V, Hoffer FA, Kozakewich H, et al. Wilms tumor and nephroblastomatosis: imaging characteristics at gadolinium-enhanced MR imaging. *Radiology* 1993;188:517–521.

85. Gylys-Morin VM. MR imaging of pediatric musculoskeletal inflammatory and infectious disorders. *Magn Reson Imaging Clin N Am* 1998;6:537–559.

86. Haaga JR. Commentary. Radiation dose management: weighing risk versus benefit. *AJR Am J Roentgenol* 2001;177:289–291.

87. Haddon MJ, Bowen A. Bronchopulmonary and neurenteric forms of foregut anomalies. Imaging for diagnosis and management. *Radiol Clin North Am* 1991;29: 241–254.

88. Haliloglu M, Hoffer FA, Gronemeyer SA, et al. Applications of 3D contrast-enhanced MR angiography in pediatric oncology. *Pediatr Radiol* 1999;29:863–868.

89. Hammrick-Turner JE, Saif MF, Powers CI, et al. Imaging of childhood non-Hodgkin lymphoma: assessment by histologic subtype. *Radiographics* 1994;14:11–28.

90. Han TI, Kim MJ, Yoon HK, et al. Rhabdoid tumour of the kidney: imaging findings. *Pediatr Radiol* 2001;31:233–237.

91. Herman TE, Siegel MJ. CT of acute spleen torsion in children with wandering spleen. *AJR Am J Roentgenol* 1991;156:151–153.

92. Herman TE, Siegel MJ. CT of the pancreas in children. *AJR Am J Roentgenol* 1991;157:375–379.

93. Hernandez RJ. Cardiovascular MR imaging of children. *Magn Reson Imaging Clin N Am* 1996;4:615–636.

94. Hernandez RJ. Magnetic resonance imaging of mediastinal vessels. *Magn Reson Imaging Clin N Am* 2002;10:237–251.

95. Higgins CB. Congenital heart disease. In: Higgins CB, Hricak H, Helms CA, eds. *Magnetic resonance imaging of the body*, 3rd ed. Philadelphia: Lippincott–Raven Publishers, 1997:461–518.

96. Hoffman LV, Kuszyk BS, Mitchell SE, et al. Angioarchitecture of pulmonary arteriovenous malformation: characterization using volume-rendered 3D CT angiography. *Cardiovasc Intervent Radiol* 2000;23:165–170.

97. Hopkins JK, Giles HW, Wyatt-Ashmead J, et al. Cystic nephroma. *Radiographics* 2004;24:589–593.

98. Hopkins KL, Patrick LE, Simoneaux SF, et al. Pediatric great vessel anomalies: initial clinical experience with spiral CT angiography. *Radiology* 1996;200:811–815.

99. Hoppe H, Walder B, Sonnenschein M, et al. Multidetector CT virtual bronchoscopy to grade tracheobronchial stenosis. *AJR Am J Roentgenol* 2002;178:1195–2000.

100. Horton KM, Bluemke DA, Hruban RH, et al. CT and MR imaging of benign hepatic and biliary tumors. *Radiographics* 1999; 19:431–451.

101 Hubbard AM. Imaging of pediatric hip disorders. *Radiol Clin North Am* 2001;39:721–732.

102. Hudson MM, Donaldson SS. Hodgkin's disease. In: Pizzo PA, Poplack DG, eds. *Principles and practice of pediatric oncology*, 3rd ed. Philadelphia: Lippincott–Raven Publishers, 1997:523–543.

103. Hugosson C, Mahr MA, Sabbah R. Primary unilateral renal lymphoblastic lymphoma. *Pediatr Radiol* 1997;27:23–25.

104. Ichikawa T, Federle MP, Grazioli L, et al. Fibrolamellar hepatocellular carcinoma: imaging and pathologic findings in 31 recent cases. *Radiology* 1999;213:352–361.

105. Irie H, Honda J, Jimi M, et al. Value of MR cholangiopancreatography in evaluating choledochal cysts. *AJR Am J Roentgenol* 1998;171:1381–1385.

106. Jabra AA, Fishman EK, Taylor GA. CT findings in inflammatory bowel disease in children. *AJR Am J Roentgenol* 1994;162: 975–979.

107. Jabra AA, Fishman EK, Taylor GA. Hepatic masses in infants and children: CT evaluation. *AJR Am J Roentgenol* 1992;158: 143–149.

108. Jabra AA, Fishman EK, Taylor GA. Primary ovarian tumors in the pediatric patient: CT evaluation. *Clin Imaging* 1993;17: 199–203.

109. Jaramillo D, Kasser JR, Villegas-Medina OL, et al. Cartilaginous abnormalities and growth disturbances in Legg-Calvé-Perthes disease: evaluation with MR imaging. *Radiology* 1995;197: 767–777.

110. Jaramillo D, Laor T, Gebhardt MC. Pediatric musculoskeletal neoplasms. *Magn Reson Imaging Clin N Am* 1996;4:749–770.

111. Jaramillo D, Laor T, Hoffer FA, et al. Epiphyseal marrow in infancy: MR imaging. *Radiology* 1991;180:809–812.

112. Jeong YK, Ha HK, Yoon CH, et al. Gastrointestinal involvement in Henoch-Schönlein syndrome: CT findings. *AJR Am J Roentgenol* 1997;168:965–968.

113. Joseph AE, Donaldson JS, Reynolds M. Neck and thorax venous aneurysm: association with cystic hygroma. *Radiology* 1989; 170:109–112.

114. Kabala JE, Shield J, Duncan A. Renal cell carcinoma in childhood. *Pediatr Radiol* 1992;22:203–205.

115. Kaiser S, Finnbogason T, Jorulf HK, et al. Suspected appendicitis in children: diagnosis with contrast-enhanced versus nonenhanced helical CT. *Radiology* 2004;23:427–433.

116. Kaste SC, Young CW, Holmes TP, et al. Effect of helical CT on the frequency of sedation in pediatric patients. *AJR Am J Roentgenol* 1997;168:1001–1003.

117. Kaste SC, Young CW. Safe use of power injectors with central and peripheral venous access devices for pediatric CT. *Pediatr Radiol* 1995;26:499–501.

118. Katz M, Konen E, Rozenman, et al. Spiral CT and 3D image reconstruction of vascular rings and associated tracheobronchial anomalies. *J Comput Assist Tomogr* 1995;19:564–568.

119. Kawashima A, Sandler CM, Corl FM, et al. Imaging of renal trauma: a comprehensive review. *Radiographics* 2001;21:557–584.

120. Kawashima A, Sandler CM, Goldman SM, et al. CT of renal inflammatory disease. *Radiographics* 1997;17:851–866.

121. Kesslar PJ, Buck JL, Selby DM. Infantile hemangioendothelioma of the liver revisited. *Radiographics* 1993;13:657–670.

122. Kesslar PJ, Buck JL, Suarez ES. Germ cell tumors of the sacrococcygeal region: radiologic-pathologic correlation. *Radiographics* 1994;14:607–620.

123. Kim OH, Chung HJ, Choi BG. Imaging of the choledochal cyst. *Radiographics* 1995;15:69–88.

124. Kim TH, Kim YM, Suh CH, et al. Helical CT angiography and three-dimensional reconstruction of total anomalous pulmonary venous connections in neonates and infants. *AJR Am J Roentgenol* 2000;175:1381–1386.

125. Kim WS, Lee KS, Kim IO, et al. Congenital cystic adenomatoid malformation of the lung: CT-pathologic correlation. *AJR Am J Roentgenol* 1997;168:47–53.

126. King L, Siegel MJ, Balfe DM. Acute pancreatitis in children: CT findings of intra-and extrapancreatic fluid collections. *Radiology* 1995;195:196–200.

127. Kirchner SG, Hernanz-Schulman M, Stein SM, et al. Imaging of pediatric mediastinal histoplasmosis. *Radiographics* 1991;11:365–381.

128. Ko SF, Ng SH, Lee TY, et al. Noninvasive imaging of bronchopulmonary sequestration. *AJR Am J Roentgenol* 2000;175:1005–1012.

129. Konen E, Merchant N, Provost Y, et al. Coarctation of the aorta before and after correction. The role of cardiovascular MRI. *AJR Am J Roentgenol* 2004;182:1333–1339.

130. Konen E, Raviv-Zilka L, Cohen RA, et al. Congenital pulmonary venolobar syndrome: spectrum of helical CT findings with emphasis on computerized reformatting. *Radiographics* 2003;23:1175–1184.

131. Konez O, Burrows PE. Magnetic resonance imaging of vascular anomalies. *Magn Reson Imaging Clin N Am* 2002;10:363–388.

132. Kosucu P, Ahmetoglu A, Koramaz I, et al. Low-dose MDCT and virtual bronchoscopy in pediatric patients with foreign body aspiration. *AJR Am J Roentgenol* 2004;183:1171–1777.

133. Kothari NA, Pelchovitz DJ, Meyer JS. Imaging of musculoskeletal infections. *Radiol Clin North Am* 2001;39:653–671.

134. Kransdorf MJ, Moser RP Jr, Meis JM, et al. Fat-containing soft-tissue masses of the extremities. *Radiographics* 1991;11:81–106.

135. Kuhn JP, Brody AS. High resolution CT of pediatric lung disease. *Radiol Clin North Am* 2002;40:89–110.

136. Lau DM, Siegel MJ, Hildebolt CF, et al. Bronchiolitis obliterans syndrome: thin-section CT diagnosis of obstructive changes in infants and young children after lung transplantation. *Radiology* 1998;208:783–788.

137. Lautin EM, Rosenblatt M, Friedman AC, et al. Calcification in non-Hodgkin lymphoma occurring before therapy: identification on plain films and CT. *AJR Am J Roentgenol* 1990;155: 739–740.

138. Lawler LP, Fishman EK. Arteriovenous malformations and systemic lung supply: evaluation by multidetector CT and three-dimensional volume rendering. *AJR Am J Roentgenol* 2002;178: 493–494.

139. Lee E, Siegel MJ, Foglia R. Evaluation of angioarchitecture of pulmonary sequestration in pediatric patients using 3D MDCT angiography. *AJR Am J Roentgenol* 2004;183:183–188.

140. Lee E, Siegel MJ, Guttierez F, et al. Multidetector CT evaluation of thoracic aortic anomalies in pediatric patients and young adults: comparison of thoracic axial, multiplanar, and 3D images. *AJR Am J Roentgenol* 2004;182:777–784.

141. Lee E, Siegel MJ, Guttierez F, et al. Multidetector CT evaluation of thoracic aortic anomalies in pediatric patients and young adults: comparison of thoracic axial, multiplanar, and 3D images. *AJR Am J Roentgenol* 2004;182:777–784.

142. Leonidas JC, Berdon WE, Valderrama E, et al. Human immunodeficiency virus infection and multilocular thymic cysts. *Radiology* 1996;198:377–379.

143. Lerner A, Branski D, Lebental E. Pancreatic diseases in children. *Pediatr Clin North Am* 1996;43:125–156.

144. Loder RT, Kuhns LR, Swinford AE. The use of helical computed tomographic scan to assess bony physeal bridges. *J Pediatr Orthop* 1997;17:356–359.

145. Lonergan GJ, Martinez-Leon MI, Agrons GA, et al. Nephrogenic rests, nephroblastomatosis, and associated lesions of the kidney. *Radiographics* 1998;18:947–968.

146. Lonergan GJ, Rice RR, Suarez ES. Autosomal recessive polycystic kidney disease: radiologic-pathologic correlation. *Radiographics* 2000;20:837–855.

147. Lonnergan GJ, Schwab CM, Suarez ES, et al. Neuroblastoma, ganglioneuroblastoma and ganglioneuroma: radiologic-pathologic correlation. *Radiographics* 2002;22:911–934.

148. Lowe LH, Isuani BH, Heller RM, et al. Pediatric renal masses: Wilms tumor and beyond. *Radiographics* 2000;20:1585–1603.

149. Luker GD, Siegel MJ. Mediastinal Hodgkin disease in children: response to therapy. *Radiology* 1993;189:737–740.

150. Lumkin B, Anderson MW, Ablin DS, et al. CT, MRI, and color Doppler ultrasound correlation of pancreatoblastoma: a case report. *Pediatr Radiol* 1993;23:61–62.

151. Koh DM, Hansell DM. Computed tomography of diffuse interstitial lung disease in children. *Clin Radiol* 2000;55:659–667.

152. Lyon RD, McAdams HP. Mediastinal bronchogenic cyst: demonstration of a fluid-fluid level at MR imaging. *Radiology* 1993; 186:427–428.

153. Ma LD, Frassica FJ, Bluemke DA, et al. CT and MRI evaluation of musculoskeletal infection. *Crit Rev Diagn Imaging* 1997;36: 535–568.

154. Ma LD, Frassica FJ, Scott WW Jr, et al. Differentiation of benign and malignant musculoskeletal tumors: potential pitfalls with MR imaging. *Radiographics* 1995;15:349–366.

155. Macpherson RI. Gastrointestinal tract duplications: clinical, pathologic, etiologic, and radiologic considerations. *Radiographics* 1993;13:1063–1080.

156. Mazur J, Ross G, Cummings RJ, et al. Usefulness of magnetic resonance imaging for the diagnosis of acute musculoskeletal infections in children. *J Pediatr Orthop* 1995;15:144–147.

157. McAdams HP, Rosado-de-Christenson ML, Moran CA. Mediastinal hemangioma: radiographic and CT features in 14 patients. *Radiology* 1994;193:399–402.

158. McLarney JK, Rucker PT, Bender GN, et al. Fibrolamellar carcinoma of the liver: radiologic-pathologic correlation. *Radiographics* 1999;19:453–471.

159. Medina LS, Siegel MJ, Glazer HS et al. Diagnosis of pulmonary complications associated with lung transplantation in children: value of CT vs histopathologic studies. *AJR Am J Roentgenol* 1994;162:969–974.

160. Medina LS, Siegel MJ. CT of complications in pediatric lung transplantation. *Radiographics* 1994;14:1341–1349.

161. Merten DF. Diagnostic imaging of mediastinal masses in children. *AJR Am J Roentgenol* 1992;158:825–832.

162. Meyer JS, Harry MP, Mahboubi S, et al. Langerhans cell histiocytosis: presentation and evolution of radiologic findings with clinical correlation. *Radiographics* 1995;15:1135–1146.

163. Meyer JS, Harty MP, Khademian Z. Imaging of neuroblastoma and Wilms tumor. *Magn Reson Imaging Clin N Am* 2002;10: 175–302.

164. Meyer JS, Hoffer FA, Barnes PD, et al. Biological classification of soft-tissue vascular anomalies: MR correlation. *AJR Am J Roentgenol* 1991;157:559–564.

165. Meyer JS. Retroperitoneal MR imaging in children. *Magn Reson Imaging Clin N Am* 1996;4:657–678.

166. Meza MP, Benson M, Slovis TL. Imaging of mediastinal masses in children. *Radiol Clin North Am* 1993;31:583–604.

167. Miller FH, Fitzgerald SW, Donaldson JS. CT of the azygoesophageal recess in infants and children. *Radiographics* 1993; 13:623–634.

168. Miller SL, Hoffer FA. Malignant and benign bone tumors. *Radiol Clin North Am* 2001;39:673–699.

169. Mirowitz SA. MR imaging artifacts. Challenges and solutions. *Magn Reson Imaging Clin N Am* 1999;7:717–32.

170. Miyazaki T, Yamashita Y, Tang Y, et al. Single-shot MR cholangiopancreatography of neonates, infants, and young children. *AJR Am J Roentgenol* 1998;170:33–37.

171. Miyazaki T, Yamashita Y, Tang Y, et al. Single-shot MR cholangiopancreatography of neonates, infants, and young children. *AJR Am J Roentgenol* 1998;170:33–37.

172. Moon WK, Kin WS, Kim IO, et al. Diffuse pulmonary disease in children: high-resolution CT findings. *AJR Am J Roentgenol* 1996;167:1405–1408.

173. Moore SG, Bisset GS, Siegel MJ, et al. Pediatric musculoskeletal MR imaging. *Radiology* 1991;179:345–360.

174. Morello FP, Donaldson JS. Nephroblastomatosis. In: Siegel BA, Proto AV, eds. *Pediatric disease (fourth series) test and syllabus.* Reston, VA: American College of Radiology, 1993:584–615.

175. Mortele K, Mergo PJ, Urrutia M, et al. Dynamic gadolinium-enhanced MR findings in infantile hepatic hemangioendothelioma. *J Comput Assist Tomogr* 1998;22:714–717.

176. Mortele KJ, Ros PR. Imaging of diffuse liver disease. *Semin Liver Dis* 2001;21:195–212.

177. Moulton JS, Blebea JS, Dunco DM, et al. MR imaging of soft-tissue masses: diagnostic efficacy and value of distinguishing between benign and malignant lesions. *AJR Am J Roentgenol* 1995;164:1191–1199.

178. Mullins ME, Kircher MF, Ryan DP, et al. Evaluation of suspected appendicitis in children using limited helical CT and colonic contrast material. *AJR Am J Roentgenol* 2001;176:37–41.

179. Murakami T, Mochizuki K, Nakamura H. Imaging evaluation of the cirrhotic liver. *Semin Liver Dis* 2001;21:213–224.

180. Navoy JE, Royal SA, Vaid YN, et al. Wilms tumor: unusual manifestations. *Pediatr Radiol* 1995;25:S76–S86.

181. Newman JS, Francis IR, Kaminski MS, et al. Imaging of lymphoma with PET with 2-[F-18]-fluoro-2-deoxy-D-glucose: correlation with CT. *Radiology* 1994;190:111–116.

182. Newman JS, Newberg AH. Congenital tarsal coalition: multimodality evaluation with emphasis on CT and MR imaging. *Radiographics* 2000;20:321–332.

183. Newman KD, Schisgall R, Rearman G, et al. Malignant mesenchymoma of the liver in children. *J Pediatr Surg* 1989;24:781–783.

184. Nimick K, Teeger S, Wallach MT, et al. Adrenal hemorrhage in abused children: imaging and postmortem findings. *AJR Am J Roentgenol* 1994;162:661–663.

185. Nunez D, Becerra JL, Fuentes D, et al. Traumatic occlusion of the renal artery: helical CT diagnosis. *AJR Am J Roentgenol* 1996;167:777–780.

186. Oppenheim C, Mamou-Mani T, Sayegh N, et al. Bronchopulmonary dysplasia: value of CT in identifying pulmonary sequelae. *AJR Am J Roentgenol* 1994;163:169–172.

187. Pacharn P, Poe SA, Donnelly LF. Low-tube current multidetector CT for children with suspected extrinsic airway compression. *AJR Am J Roentgenol* 2002;179:1523–1527.

188. Pappas JN, Donnelly LF, Frush DP. Reduced frequency of sedation of young children using new multi-slice helical CT. *Radiology* 2000;215:897–899.

189. Park HS, Im JG, Jung JW, et al. Anomalous left pulmonary artery with complete cartilaginous ring. *J Comput Assist Tomogr* 1997;21:478–480.

190. Patterson A, Frush DP, Donnelly L. Helical CT of the body: are settings adjusted for pediatric patients. *AJR Am J Roentgenol* 2001;176:297–301.

191. Pobeil RS, Bisset GS. Pictorial essay: imaging of liver tumors in the infant and child. *Pediatr Radiol* 1995;25:495–506.

192. Powers C, Ros PR, Stoupis C, et al. Primary liver neoplasms: MR imaging with pathologic correlation. *Radiographics* 1994;14:459–482.

193. Quillin SP, Siegel MJ. CT features of benign and malignant teratomas in children. *J Comput Assist Tomogr* 1992;16:723–726.

194. Quillin SP, Siegel MJ. CT features of benign and malignant teratomas in children. *J Comput Assist Tomogr* 1992;16:722–726.

195. Rawson JV, Siegel MJ. Techniques and strategies in pediatric body MR imaging. *Magn Reson Imaging Clin N Am* 1996;4:589–598.

196. Remy J, Remy-Jardin M, Giraud F, et al. Angioarchitecture of pulmonary arteriovenous malformations: clinical utility of three-dimensional helical CT. *Radiology* 1994;191:657–664.

197. Remy-Jardin M, Remy J, Mayo JR, et al. Thoracic aorta. In: *CT angiography of the chest.* Philadelphia: Lippincott Williams & Wilkins, 2001:29–50.

198. Riberio J, Ribeiro RC, Fletcher BD. Imaging findings in pediatric adrenocortical carcinoma. *Pediatr Radiol* 2000;30:45–51.

199. Rieumont MJ, Whitman GJ. Mesoblastic nephroma. *AJR Am J Roentgenol* 1994;162:76.

200. Roebuck DJ, Yang WT, Lam WWM, et al. Hepatobiliary rhabdomyosarcoma in children: diagnostic radiology. *Pediatr Radiol* 1998;28:101–108.

201. Roest AA, Helbing WA, van der Wall EE. Postoperative evaluation of congenital heart disease by magnetic resonance imaging. *J Magn Reson Imaging* 1999;10:656–666.

202. Rohrschneider WK, Weirich A, Rieden K, et al. US, CT and MR imaging characteristics of nephroblastomatosis. *Pediatr Radiol* 1998;28:435–443.

203. Rosado-de-Christenson ML, Frazier AA, Stocker JT, et al. Extralobar sequestration: radiologic-pathologic correlation. *Radiographics* 1993;13:425–441.

204. Rosado-de-Christenson ML, Pugatch RD, Moran CA, et al. Thymolipoma: analysis of 27 cases. *Radiology* 1994;193:121–126.

205. Rosado-de-Christenson ML, Stocker JT. Congenital cystic adenomatoid malformation. *Radiographics* 1991;11:865–886.

206. Rosado-de-Christenson ML, Templeton PA, Moran CA. Mediastinal germ cell tumors: radiologic and pathologic correlation. *Radiographics* 1992;12:1013–1030.

207. Rotondo A, Scialpi M, Scapati C. Pulmonary arteriovenous malformation: evaluation by MR angiography. *AJR Am J Roentgenol* 1997;168:847–849.

208. Ruess L, Frazier AA, Sivit C. CT of the mesentery, omentum, and peritoneum in children. *Radiographics* 1995;15:89–104.

209. Ruzal-Shapiro C, Berdon WE, Cohen MD, et al. MR imaging of diffuse bone marrow replacement in pediatric patients with cancer. *Radiology* 1991;181:587–589.

210. Ruzal-Shapiro C, Berdon WE, Cohen MD, et al. MR imaging of diffuse bone marrow replacement in pediatric patients with cancer. *Radiology* 1991;181:587–589.

211. Sanz N, de Mingo L, Florez F, et al. Rhabdomyosarcoma of the biliary tree. *Pediatr Surg Int* 1997;12:200–201.

212. Savader SJ, Benenati JF, Venbrux AC, et al. Choledochal cysts: classification and cholangiographic appearance. *AJR Am J Roentgenol* 1991;156:327–331.

213. Shad A, Magrath I. Malignant non-Hodgkin's lymphoma in children. In: Pizzo PA, Poplack DG, eds. *Principles and practice of pediatric oncology,* 3rd ed. Philadelphia: Lippincott–Raven Publishers, 1997:545–587.

214. Shady KL, Siegel MJ, Brown JJ. Preoperative evaluation of intraabdominal tumors in children: gradient-recalled echo vs spin-echo MR imaging. *AJR Am J Roentgenol* 1993;161:843–847.

215. Siegel MJ, Bhallah S, Gutierrez F, et al. Post-lung transplantation bronchiolitis obliterans: usefulness of expiratory thin-section CT for diagnosis. *Radiology* 2001;220:455–462.

216. Siegel MJ, Glazer HS, St. Amour TE, et al. Lymphangiomas in children: MR imaging. *Radiology* 1989;170:467–470.

217. Siegel MJ, Glazer HS, Wiener JI, et al. Normal and abnormal thymus in childhood: MR imaging. *Radiology* 1989;172:367–371.

218. Siegel MJ, Herman TE. Pancreatic pseudocyst. In: Siegel BA, Proto AV, eds. *Pediatric disease (fourth series) test and syllabus.* Reston, VA: American College of Radiology, 1993:532–555.

219. Siegel MJ, Herman TE. Periportal low attenuation at CT in childhood. *Radiology* 1992;183:685–688.

220. Siegel MJ, Hoffer FA. Magnetic resonance imaging of nongynecologic pelvic masses in children. *Magn Reson Imaging Clin N Am* 2002;10:325–344.

221. Siegel MJ, Ishwaran H, Fletcher B, et al. Staging of neuroblastoma with computed tomography and magnetic resonance imaging: report of the Radiology Diagnostic Oncology Group. *Radiology* 2002;223:168–175.

222. Siegel MJ, Luker GD. Bone marrow imaging in children. *Magn Reson Imaging Clin N Am* 1996;4:771–796.

223. Siegel MJ, Luker GD. MR imaging of the liver in children. *Magn Reson Imaging Clin N Am* 1996;4:637–656.

224. Siegel MJ, Suess C, Schmidt B, et al. Radiation dose and image quality in pediatric CT: effect of technical factors and phantom size and shape. *Radiology* 2004;233:515–522.

225. Siegel MJ, Weber CK. Cardiac and paracardiac masses. In: Guttierez FR, Brown JJ, Mirowitz SA, eds. *Cardiovascular magnetic resonance imaging*. St. Louis: Mosby–Year Book, 1992:112–123.

226. Siegel MJ. Acute pyelonephritis. In: Siegel BA, Siegel MJ, eds. *Pediatric disease (fifth series) test and syllabus*. Reston, VA: American College of Radiology, 2002:71–97.

227. Siegel MJ. Adrenal glands, pancreas and other retroperitoneal structures. In: Siegel MJ, ed. *Pediatric body CT*. Philadelphia: Lippincott Williams & Wilkins, 1999:253–286.

228. Siegel MJ. Diseases of the thymus in children and adolescents. *Postgrad Radiol* 1993;13:106–132.

229. Siegel MJ. Gastrointestinal tract. In: Siegel MJ, ed. *Pediatric body CT*. Philadelphia: Lippincott Williams & Wilkins, 1999:201–225.

230. Siegel MJ. Hematoma. In: Siegel BA, Siegel MJ, eds. *Magnetic resonance imaging (second series) test and syllabus*. Reston, VA: American College of Radiology, 2000:1–16.

231. Siegel MJ. Hepatic fracture with hypovolemic shock. In: Siegel BA, Proto AV, eds. *Pediatric disease (fourth series) test and syllabus*. Reston, VA: American College of Radiology, 1993:490–508.

232. Siegel MJ. Leukemia. In: Siegel BA, Choplin RH, Siegel MJ, et al., eds. *Body MRI test and syllabus*. Reston, VA: American College of Radiology, 2000:173–189.

233. Siegel MJ. Liver and biliary tract. In: Siegel MJ, ed. *Pediatric body CT*. Philadelphia: Lippincott Williams & Wilkins, 1999: 141–174.

234. Siegel MJ. Lung, pleural and chest wall. In: *Pediatric body CT*. Philadelphia: Lippincott Williams & Wilkins, 1999:101–140.

235. Siegel MJ. Magnetic resonance imaging of musculoskeletal soft tissue masses. *Radiol Clin North Am* 2001;39:701–720.

236. Siegel MJ. Magnetic resonance imaging of the adolescent female pelvis. *Magn Reson Imaging Clin N Am* 2002;10:303–324.

237. Siegel MJ. Mediastinum. In: Siegel MJ, ed. *Pediatric body CT*. Philadelphia: Lippincott Williams & Wilkins, 1999:65–100.

238. Siegel MJ. MR imaging of pediatric abdominal neoplasms. *Magn Reson Imaging Clin N Am* 2000;8:837–851.

239. Siegel MJ. MRI of the pediatric abdomen. *Magn Reson Imaging Clin N Am* 1995;3:161–182.

240. Siegel MJ. Multiplanar and three-dimensional row CT of thoracic vessels and airways in the pediatric population. *Radiology* 2003;229:641–650.

241. Siegel MJ. Musculoskeletal system and spine. In: Siegel MJ, ed. *Pediatric body CT*. Philadelphia: Lippincott Williams & Wilkins, 1999:312–345.

242. Siegel MJ. Pediatric chest applications. In: Fishman EK, Jeffrey B, eds. *Multislice helical CT*, 3rd ed. Philadelphia: Lippincott Williams & Wilkins, 2003:159–182.

243. Siegel MJ. Pediatric urinary tract infection. In: Pollack HM, McClennan BL, eds. *Clinical urography*. Philadelphia: WB Saunders, 2000:1103–1121.

244. Siegel MJ. Pelvic organs and soft tissues. In: Siegel MJ, ed. *Pediatric body CT*. Philadelphia: Lippincott Williams & Wilkins, 1999:287–311.

245. Siegel MJ. Pelvic tumors. *Radiol Clin North Am* 1997;35: 1455–1475.

246. Siegel MJ. Spleen, peritoneum and abdominal wall. In: Siegel MJ, ed. *Pediatric body CT*. Philadelphia, PA: Lippincott Williams & Wilkins, 1999:175–200.

247. Siegel MJ. Techniques. In: Siegel MJ, ed. *Pediatric body CT*. Philadelphia: Lippincott Williams & Wilkins, 1999:1–41.

248. Siegel MJ. The child with abdominal trauma. In: Hilton SVW, Edwards DK. *Practical pediatric radiology*, 3rd ed. Philadelphia: W.B. Saunders Co., 2005. In press.

249. Siegel MJ. The kidney. In: Siegel MJ, ed. *Pediatric body CT*. Philadelphia: Lippincott Williams & Wilkins, 1999:226–252.

250. Siegel MJ. Thoracoabdominal trauma. In: Siegel MJ, ed. *Pediatric body CT*. Philadelphia: Lippincott Williams & Wilkins, 1999: 346–371.

251. Sisler CL, Siegel, MJ. Malignant rhabdoid tumor of the kidney: radiologic features. *Radiology* 1989;172:211–212.

252. Sivit CJ, Cutting JP, Eichelberger MR. CT diagnosis and localization of rupture of the bladder in children with blunt abdominal trauma: significance of contrast material extravasation in the pelvis. *AJR Am J Roentgenol* 1995;164:1243–1246.

253. Sivit CJ, Eichelberger MR, Taylor GA, et al. Blunt pancreatic trauma in children: CT diagnosis. *AJR Am J Roentgenol* 1992;158: 1097–1100.

254. Sivit CJ, Ingram JD, Taylor GA, et al. Post-traumatic adrenal hemorrhage in children: CT findings in 34 patients. *AJR Am J Roentgenol* 1992;158:1299–1302.

255. Sivit CJ, Taylor GA, Bulas DI, et al. Blunt trauma in children: significance of peritoneal fluid. *Radiology* 1991;178:185–188.

256. Sivit CJ, Taylor GA, Bulas DI, et al. Posttraumatic shock in children: CT findings associated with hemodynamic instability. *Radiology* 1992;182:723–726.

257. Sivit CJ, Taylor GA, Newman KD. Safety-belt injuries in children with lap-belt ecchymosis: CT findings in 61 patients. *AJR Am J Roentgenol* 1991;157:111–114.

258. Sivit CJ. Siegel MJ, Applegate KE, et al. Special focus session. When appendicitis is suspected in children. *Radiographics* 2001;21:247–262.

259 Slovis TL. The ALARA concept in pediatric CT: myth or reality. *Radiology* 2002;223:5–6.

260. Sofka CM, Semelka RC, Kelekis NL, et al. Magnetic resonance imaging of neuroblastoma using current techniques. *Magn Reson Imaging* 1999;17: 193–198.

261. Sorantin E, Geiger B, Lindbichler F, et al. CT based virtual tracheobronchoscopy in children—comparison with axial CT and multiplanar reconstructions: preliminary results. *Pediatr Radiol* 2002;32:8–15.

262. Soyer P, Spelle L, Pelage JP, et al. Cystic fibrosis in adolescents and adults: fatty replacement of the pancreas—CT evaluation and functional correlation. *Radiology* 1999;210:611–615.

263. Spiers AS, Husband JES, MacVicar AD. Treated thymic lymphoma: comparison of MR imaging with CT. *Radiology* 1997;203: 369–376.

264. States LJ, Bellah RD. Imaging of the pediatric female pelvis. *Semin Roentgenol* 1996;31:312–329.

265. Stevens WR, Johnson CD, Stephens DH, et al. Fibrolamellar hepatocellular carcinomas: stage at presentation and results of aggressive surgical management. *AJR Am J Roentgenol* 1995;164: 1153–1158.

266. Stoupis C, Ros PR, Abbitt PL, et al. Bubbles in the belly: imaging of cystic mesenteric or omental masses. *Radiographics* 1994;14: 729–737.

267. Strouse PJ, Close BJ, Marshall KW, et al. CT of bowel and mesenteric trauma in children. *Radiographics* 1999;19: 1237–1250.

268 Strouse PJ. Magnetic resonance angiography of the pediatric abdomen and pelvis. *Magn Reson Imaging Clin N Am* 2002;10: 345–361.

269. Taccone A, Oddone M, Dell'Acqua A, et al. MRI "road-map" of normal age-related bone marrow. *Pediatr Radiol* 1995;25: 596–606.

270. Takahashi K, Inasoka T, Murakami N, et al. Characterization of the normal and hyperplastic thymus on chemical-shift MR imaging. *AJR Am J Roentgenol* 2003;180:1265–1269.

271. Taylor GA, Kaufman RA, Sivit CJ. Active hemorrhage in children after thoracoabdominal trauma: clinical and CT features. *AJR Am J Roentgenol* 1994;162:401–404.

272 Taylor GA. Imaging of pediatric blunt abdominal trauma: what have we learned in the past decade? *Radiology* 1995;195: 600–601.

273. Teo EL, Strouse PJ, Prince MR. Applications of magnetic resonance imaging and magnetic resonance angiography to evaluate the hepatic vasculature in the pediatric patient. *Pediatr Radiol* 1999;29:238–243.

274. Trojiano RN, McCarthy SM. Mullerian duct anomalies: imaging and clinical issues. *Radiology* 2004;233:19–34.

275. Urrutia M, Mergo PJ, Ros LH, et al. Cystic masses of the spleen: radiologic-pathologic correlation. *Radiographics* 1996;16:107–129.

276. Vade A, Reyes H, Wilbur A, et al. The anorectal sphincter after rectal pull-through surgery for anorectal anomalies: MRI evaluation. *Pediatr Radiol* 1989;19:179–183.

277. Van Praagh S, Carrera ME, Sanders S, et al. Partial or total direct pulmonary venous drainage to the right atrium due to malposition of septum primum. *Chest* 1995;107:1488–1498.

278. Vaughn DD, Jabra AA, Fishman EK. Pancreatic disease in children and young adults: evaluation with CT. *Radiographics* 1998;18:1171–1187.

279. Vogler JB III, Murphy WA. Bone marrow imaging. *Radiology* 1998;168:679–693.

280. Wadsworth DT, Newman B, Abramson SJ, et al. Splenic lymphangiomatosis in children. *Radiology* 1997;202:173–176.

281. Waitches G, Zawin JK, Poznanski AK. Sequence and rate of bone marrow conversion in the femora of children as seen on MR imaging: are accepted standards accurate? *AJR Am J Roentgenol* 1994;162:1399–1406.

282. Wechsler RJ, Schweitzer ME, Deely DM, et al. Tarsal coalition: depiction and characterization with CT and MR imaging. *Radiology* 1994;193:447–452.

283. Westra SJ, Hill JA, Alejos JC, et al. Three-dimensional helical CT of pulmonary arteries in infants and children with congenital heart disease. *AJR Am J Roentgenol* 1999;173:109–115.

284. Westra SJ, Zaninovic AC, Hall TR, et al. Imaging of the adrenal gland in children. *Radiographics* 1994;14:1323–1340.

285. Woodring JH, Howard TA, Kanga JF. Congenital pulmonary venolobar syndrome revisited. *Radiographics* 1994;14:349–369.

286. Wu JW, White CS, Meyer CA, et al. Variant bronchial anatomy: CT appearance and classification. *AJR Am J Roentgenol* 1999;172:741–744.

287. Yamashita Y, Hatanka Y, Torashima M et al. Mature cystic teratomas of the ovary without fat in the cystic cavity: MR features in 12 cases. AJR *Am J Roentgenol* 1994;163:613–616.

288. Zerin JM, DiPietro MA. Mesenteric vascular anatomy at CT: normal and abnormal appearances. *Radiology* 1991;179:739–742.

289. Zobel MS, Borrello J, Siegel MJ, et al. Pediatric knee MR imaging: pattern of injuries in the immature skeleton. 1994;190:397–401.

PROTOCOL 1

INDICATION:	**Standard Lung/Mediastinum** (oncologic staging, detection of metastases, characterization of mediastinal or pulmonary mass, evaluation of trauma)
Extent	Lung apices to caudal bases
Scanner settings	kVp: 80 for patients weighing <50 kg; higher kVp for larger patients mA: lowest possible based on patient weight
Detector collimation	4 row: 2.5 mm 16 row: 1.25–1.5 mm 64 row: 0.6–1.25 mm
Pitch	4 row: 1.5–2.0 16 row: 1.0–1.5 64 row: 1.0–1.5
Slice reconstruction thickness	3–5 mm for viewing
IV Contrast	Nonionic 280–320 mg iodine/mL
Contrast volume	2 mL/kg (maximum of 4 mL/kg or 125 mL, whichever is lower)

Contrast injection rate	Hand injection: rapid push bolus
	Power injector:
	  22 gauge: 1.5–2.0 mL/sec
	  20 gauge: 2.0–3.0 mL/sec

Scan delay	25 to 30 sec
Miscellaneous	1. Contrast medium used at discretion of radiologist in the evaluation of metastases. Routinely given for evaluation of mediastinal and pulmonary masses and trauma. 2. Use a standard reconstruction algorithm.

PROTOCOL 2

INDICATION:	**CT Angiography** (cardiovascular anomalies, postoperative shunts)
Extent	Lung apices to caudal bases
Scanner settings	kVp: 80 for patients weighing <50 kg; higher kVp for larger patients mA: lowest possible based on patient weight
Detector collimation	4 row: 2.5 mm 16 row: 1.25–1.5 mm 64 row: 0.6–1.25 mm
Pitch	4 row: 1.5–2.0 16 row: 1.0–1.5 64 row: 1.0–1.5
Slice reconstruction thickness	2–5 mm for viewing
IV Contrast	Nonionic 280–320 mg iodine/mL
Contrast volume	2 mL/kg (maximum of 4 mL/kg or 125 mL, whichever is lower)

Contrast injection rate	Hand injection: rapid push bolus
	Power injector:
	  22 gauge: 1.5–2.0 mL/sec
	  20 gauge: 2.0–3.0 mL/sec

Scan delay	Patient weight <10 kg: 12–15 sec Patient weight >10 kg: automated scan initiation
Miscellaneous	1. If sequestration is suspected, scanning should extend through the upper abdominal aorta. 2. Precontrast images are not needed for most examinations, but they are used in the evaluation of endovascular stents. 3. Use standard reconstruction algorithm.

PROTOCOL 3

INDICATION:	**Tracheobronchial Tree** (congenital anomalies, stricture, tumor, tracheomalacia)
Extent	Vocal cords to mainstem bronchi, just below carina
Scanner settings	kVp: 80 for patients weighing <50 kg; higher kVp for larger patients mA: lowest possible based on patient weight
Detector collimation	4 row: 2.5 mm 16 row: 1.25–1.5 mm 64 row: 0.6–1.25 mm
Pitch	4 row: 1.5–2.0 16 row: 1.0–1.5 64 row: 1.0–1.5
Slice reconstruction thickness	2–3 mm
Patient instructions	Suspended inspiration
Contrast type	None
Comments	1. Select pitch so that the area of interest can be scanned in a single breath-hold in cooperative patients. 2. Use high spatial resolution reconstruction (bone) algorithm. 3. Multiplanar and 3D reconstructions are useful to provide an overview of anatomy for surgical planning. 4. If tracheomalacia is suspected, obtain scans in inspiration and expiration.

PROTOCOL 4

INDICATION:	**Abdomen/Pelvis Survey** (tumor, trauma, appendicitis)
Extent	Diaphragm to pubic symphysis
Scanner settings	kVp: 80 for patients weighing <50 kg; higher kVp for larger patients mA: lowest possible based on patient weight
Detector collimation	4 row: 2.5 mm 16 row: 1.25–1.5 mm 64 row: 0.6–1.25 mm
Pitch	4 row: 1.5–2.0 16 row: 1.0–1.5 64 row: 1.0–1.5
Slice reconstruction thickness	3–5 mm for viewing
Oral contrast	Water-soluble contrast material given 45 to 60 minutes prior to scan. Additional volume given 15 minutes prior to scan. Oral contrast medium should be used with caution if patient has a depressed level of consciousness.
Intravenous contrast volume	2 mL/kg (maximum of 4 mL/kg or 125 mL, whichever is lower)
Contrast injection rate	Hand injection: rapid bolus administration Power injector: 　　22 gauge: 1.5–2.0 mL/sec 　　20 gauge: 2.0–3.0 mL/sec
Scan delay	55 to 60 seconds after onset of contrast injection (i.e., scan in portal venous phase of enhancement).
Miscellaneous	1. Multiplanar or 3D reconstructions can help define the full longitudinal extent of a tumor. 2. In setting of trauma, delayed images may be helpful if an abnormality of the bladder or renal collecting system is suspected. 3. Our preference for evaluation of appendicitis is a nonfocused technique performed with oral and intravenous contrast medium. We also will perform appendiceal imaging of the entire abdomen and pelvis with the use of only IV contrast material.

PROTOCOL 5

INDICATION:	**Liver: Dual-Phase Imaging** (hepatic tumor)
Extent	Arterial phase: dome to tip of liver Portal venous phase: Diaphragm to pubic symphysis
Scanner settings	kVp: 80 for patients weighing <50 kg; higher kVp for larger patients mA: lowest possible based on patient weight
Detector collimation	4 row: 2.5 mm 16 row: 1.25–1.5 mm 64 row: 0.6–1.25 mm
Pitch	4 row: 1.5–2.0 16 row: 1.0–1.5 64 row: 1.0–1.5
Slice reconstruction thickness	3–5 mm for viewing
Oral contrast	Water-soluble contrast material given 45 to 60 minutes prior to scan. Additional volume given 15 minutes prior to scan.
Intravenous contrast volume	2 mL/kg (maximum of 4 mL/kg or 125 mL, whichever is lower)

Contrast injection rate	Hand injection: rapid bolus administration
	Power injector:
	    22 gauge: 1.5–2.0 mL/sec
	    20 gauge: 2.0–3.0 mL/sec

Scan delay	Patient weight <10 kg: 12–15 sec delay Patient weight >10 kg: 20 sec delay 55- to 60-second delay time for portal venous phase
Miscellaneous	If the child is sedated or uncooperative, CT scans are obtained at quiet breathing.

Index